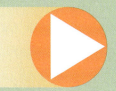

THERAPYED'S
PTA Examination Review & Study Guide

6th Edition

SUSAN B. O'SULLIVAN, PT, EdD
Professor Emerita
Department of Physical Therapy
College of Health Sciences
Lowell, Massachusetts

RAYMOND P. SIEGELMAN, PT, DPT, MS
President Emeritus
TherapyEd
Boston, Massachusetts

KAREN E. RYAN, PTA, BS
Editor and Director Physical Therapist Assistant Education
TherapyEd
Evanston, Illinois

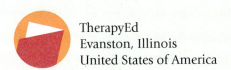

TherapyEd
Evanston, Illinois
United States of America

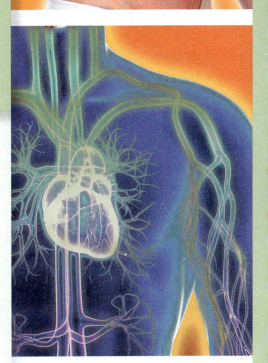
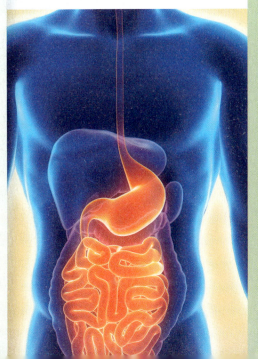

Copyright © 2003, 2008, 2010, 2013, 2018, 2019 TherapyEd

Library of Congress Control Number: 2003/012202

ISBN: 978-0-9904162-9-6

Printed in the United States of America. All rights reserved. No portion of this book or accompanying software may be reproduced, stored in a data base retrieval system or transmitted electronically or in any other way without written permission from the publisher.

The authors and contributors have made a faithful attempt to include relevant summaries of current physical therapy practice and other information at the time of publication. It is recognized that recommended practices, equipment, devices, governmental regulations, administrative procedures, and other protocols and factors may change or be open to other interpretations. Assistants should take responsibility for being aware of technological advances, new information or conclusions available through research, new governmental regulations, or ethical guidelines.

The publisher disclaims any liability or loss incurred as a result of direct or indirect use of this book. Use of this book does not guarantee successful passage of the National PTA Examination.

Copies of this book and software may be obtained from:
TherapyEd
500 Davis St., Suite 512
Evanston, IL 60201
Telephone (888) 369-0743
FAX (847) 328-5049
www.TherapyEd.com

Preface

One of the final hurdles to becoming a licensed physical therapist assistant in the United States is the successful completion of the National Physical Therapist Assistant Examination. This examination requires candidates to combine entry-level information with clinical experience in order to solve problems that occur in clinical situations. The results of the examination are the main resource the licensing boards use to determine whether a candidate for licensure has demonstrated minimal standards necessary to be a safe and effective clinician.

Founded in 1988, TherapyEd publishes Review and Study Guides and teaches exam preparation courses for tens of thousands of physical therapists, physical therapist assistants, occupational therapists, and occupational therapist assistants.

The PTA Examination Review and Study Guide includes a comprehensive content review, study and test-taking strategies, information about licensure, and three complete practice exams online. All the exam items are categorized according to the content outline and challenge students to prepare for the breadth, depth, and rigor of the PTA exam.

The content of this publication was developed exclusively for the physical therapist assistant licensure examination; areas not covered in this publication are not contributing elements for the examination. The purpose of this book is to assist the candidate in focusing their studies on the information necessary to pass the licensure examination and to streamline study time for the examination.

The authors and contributors hope that all examination candidates are successful on their examination and reap the rewards of practicing as a physical therapist assistant in the United States.

Table of Contents

Introduction I-1

Chapter 1: Therapeutic Exercise Foundations 1

Chapter 2: Musculoskeletal Physical Therapy 21

Chapter 3: Neuromuscular Physical Therapy 83

Chapter 4: Cardiac, Vascular, and Lymphatic Physical Therapy 139

Chapter 5: Pulmonary Physical Therapy 189

Chapter 6: Other Systems 219

Chapter 7: Integumentary Physical Therapy 273

Chapter 8: Geriatric Physical Therapy 297

Chapter 9: Pediatric Physical Therapy 333

Chapter 10: Therapeutic Modalities 365

Chapter 11: Functional Training, Equipment, and Devices 395

Chapter 12: Teaching and Learning 435

Chapter 13: Management, Safety, and Professional Roles 447

Chapter 14: Research and Evidence-Based Practice 483

Chapter 15: Chapter Review Questions and Answers 493

Chapter 16: Online Examinations 519

Examination A 520

Examination B 616

Examination C 707

References 801

Quick Facts Index 805

Index 809

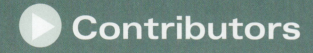
Contributors

Michele Avery, PTA, MS
PTA Program and Clinical Coordinator
Assistant Professor
Kansas City Kansas Community College
Kansas City, Kansas

Jane Baldwin, PT, DPT
Board Certified Clinical Specialist in Neurological
    Physical Therapy
Assistant Professor
MGH Institute of Health Professions
Advanced Clinician
Spaulding Rehabilitation Hospital Network
Boston, Massachusetts

Thomas Bianco, PT, MSPT
President
Sensible Ergonomic Solutions
Wilbraham, Massachusetts

Wendy Bircher, PT, EdD
Retired Program Director
San Juan College PTA Program
Farmington, New Mexico

Tiffany Bohm, PT, DPT
Dean of Health Professions
Co-Coordinator of Academic Assessment
Kansas City Kansas Community College
Kansas City, Kansas

Cindy Brandehoff, PTA, BS
PTA Program Faculty and Academic Coordinator of
    Clinical Education
Rhodes State College
Lima, Ohio

Bridget Brauns, RN, BSN, CWOCN
Regional Clinical Consultant
Celleration
Denver, Colorado

Michael Crowell, PT, DPT, DSc, OCS, SCS,
    FAAOMPT
Associate Professor
Baylor University-Keller Army Community Hospital
Division 1 Sports Physical Therapy Fellowship
West Point, New York

Jodi Cusack, MHS, PA-C
Gastrointestinal Medical Associates
Cranston, Rhode Island

Suzanne M. Giuffre, PT, EdD
Associate Professor and Program Director
Doctor of Physical Therapy Program
Cleveland State University
Cleveland, Ohio

Kari Inda, OTR, PhD
Professor
Occupational Therapy Department Chairperson
Mount Mary College
Milwaukee, Wisconsin

Steven G. Lesh, PhD, PT, SCS, ATC
Board-Certified Clinical Specialist in Sports Physical
    Therapy
Chair and Professor of Physical Therapy
Southwest Baptist University
Bolivar, Missouri

Kelly Macauley, PT, EdD, DPT, CCS, GCS
Interprofessional Faculty
School of Physical Therapy
Husson University
Bangor, Maine

Kelly Maxcy, PTA
Physical Therapist Assistant
Iowa Health Systems
Des Moines, Iowa

Becky S. McKnight, PT, MS
Educational Consultant
Reach Consulting
Forsyth, Missouri

Susan B. O'Sullivan, PT, EdD
Professor Emerita
Department of Physical Therapy
College of Health Sciences
Lowell, Massachusetts

Robert Rowe, PT, DPT, DMT, MHS, FAAOMPT
Director
Brooks Institute of Higher Learning
Brooks Rehabilitation
Jacksonville, Florida

Karen E. Ryan, PTA, BS
Editor and Director Physical Therapist Assistant
  Education
TherapyEd
Evanston, Illinois

Laura Sage, PT, DPT, MEd
Geriatric Clinical Specialist, Wound Care
  Certified
Director of Clinical Education PTA Program
Pima Medical Institute
Denver, Colorado

Todd Sander, PT, PhD, SCS, ATC
Associate Professor
Doctoral Program in Physical Therapy
Army-Baylor University
JBSA-Fort Sam Houston, Texas

Kelly Sass, PT, PhD
Clinical Assistant Professor
Academic Coordinator of Clinical Education
Department of Physical therapy & Rehabilitation Science
University of Iowa
Iowa City, Iowa

Raymond Siegelman, PT, DPT, MS
President Emeritus
TherapyEd
Boston, Massachusetts

Lori Slettehaugh, PT, MPT
Assistant Professor
Physical Therapist Assistant Program
Kansas City Kansas Community College
Kansas City, Kansas

Julie Ann Starr, PT, DPT, MS, CCS
Clinical Associate Professor
Physical Therapy Program
Department of Rehabilitation Sciences
Sargent College of Health and Rehabilitation Sciences
Boston University
Boston, Massachusetts

Thomas Sutlive, PT, PhD, OCS
Professor
Doctoral Program in Physical Therapy
Army-Baylor University
JBSA-Fort Sam Houston, Texas

Bradley Tragord, PT, DSc, OCS, FAAOMPT
Assistant Professor
Director of Clinical Education
Doctoral Program in Physical Therapy
Army-Baylor University
JBSA-Fort Sam Houston, Texas

Jason M. Wilken, PT, PhD
Associate Professor
Director, Collaborative Research and Development
Department of Physical therapy & Rehabilitation Science
University of Iowa
Iowa City, Iowa

Reviewers

Carol Fawcett, PTA, BS, MEd
Dean, Allied Health & Emergency Services
Prairie State College
Chicago Heights, Illinois

Julie Feeny, PT, MS
Program Director
Physical Therapist Assistant Program
Illinois Central College
East Peoria, Illinois

Angela M. Heaton, PT, MSEd
Assistant Dean Health Sciences/Allied Health
PTA Program Chair, Assistant Professor
Rhodes State College
Lima, Ohio

Ron Meade, PT, DPT
PTA Program Director
Somerset Community College
Somerset, Kentucky

Maggie Thomas, PT, MA
Program Director
Physical Therapist Assistant Program
Kirkwood Community College
Cedar Rapids, Iowa

Acknowledgments

This is my fourth revision of this Review and Study Guide, and I have to say that editing and authoring are truly a labor of love, not to mention a lot of long hours at the computer! Each time I complete a revision, I can't wait for the next one to start because I have so many great ideas about what to add and how to better help students pass their exam.

This edition has been such a pleasure to work on because I have had the consistent support and input from our core group of PTA Instructors: Jane Baldwin, PT, DPT; Tiffany Bohm, PT, DPT; Cindy Brandehoff, PTA, BS; Angie Heaton, PT, MSEd; Steven Lesh, PhD, PT, SCS, ATC; and Michele Avery, PTA, MS. Thank you from the bottom of my heart for all of the knowledge, ideas, and energy you bring to this project and to our on-site licensure preparation course. I am truly blessed to have such dedicated and talented individuals committed to making these products be the best they can be.

No book comes together without a lot of work from the copyeditors, creative staff, and project managers within the publishing company. Thank you to Christine Becker, Project Manager for her consistent follow up and gentle reminders of upcoming deadlines. I also thank those of you I don't know by name who have contributed time and talent to this project.

I will end on a personal note. I would like to acknowledge my parents for always telling me I could accomplish whatever I wanted to do—and believing it. I love you both and thank you for that. Thank you to my dear friends Kathy McGovern and Ben Lager for being great role models of serenity in the face of pressure. And last, but definitely not least, I want to thank my wonderful husband Mike. Thank you for all of your hard work turning "the Pod" into my office and for putting up with me missing all those hours building our home. I love you, Mike.

Karen E. Ryan, PTA, BS

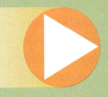

Introduction

RAYMOND P. SIEGELMAN
KAREN E. RYAN
KARI INDA

Review > Practice > Motivate > Analyze > Apply

 Purpose of This Book and Software

TherapyEd's PTA Exam Review & Study Guide, 6th Edition, is designed to help physical therapist assistant (PTA) candidates focus their preparation for the PTA Exam. Each chapter is presented in an easy-to-read outline format and emphasizes the major elements presented in the Federation of State Boards of Physical Therapy (FSBPT) Content Outline for the PTA Exam. Because a main emphasis of the licensure exam is PTA interventions, the first chapter is dedicated to therapeutic exercise. The next four chapters in the book focus on the body systems most heavily tested: musculoskeletal, neuromuscular and nervous, cardiovascular, and pulmonary. Successful candidates will be able to incorporate a solid understanding of disease states and conditions into treating the patient (applying interventions) and basing interventions on data collected regarding the patient/clients current state. Additionally, the candidate will be able to adapt, modify, or discontinue the intervention based upon assessment of the patient/client. In addition, specific emphasis is placed upon important areas of physical therapy practice (e.g., pediatric, geriatrics, and therapeutic exercise foundations). It is vital for the PTA candidate to be able to incorporate knowledge of normal anatomy, physiology, and kinesiology into the treatment and management of individuals of all ages. The PTA candidate must also be able to measure and make adaptions to an individual's response to intervention. This text will help candidates plan their review and prepare to take the licensure examination. The outlined contents will help organize and focus review and help each student prepare in an efficient and effective manner.

The three practice exams are designed to enable candidates to determine whether they understand a particular content area and are able to apply it to a clinical situation described in a question. The practice examination format mimics the actual PTA Exam format. The exam programming analyzes results and provides feedback to help identify areas for additional study. The answers and rationales to the practice exam questions are provided in the back of this text. The process of reading and interpreting these practice questions should help candidates prepare for the actual PTA Exam. The online exams also feature short mini-tests, drawn from the three full practice exams, to allow students to focus on specific content areas. Students can test their knowledge in specific domains, categories, or critical reasoning skills, or take a 150-question exam to test their physical and mental endurance.

How Is the Examination Developed?

The FSBPT is the organization that helps the various regulatory boards coordinate the practice of physical therapy. The FSBPT owns the National Physical Therapy Examinations for both PTAs and physical therapists. The American Physical Therapy Association does not develop, oversee, or administer the examination.

A large number of practitioners, educators, and others contribute questions to the FSBPT. These items are designed to test knowledge and problem solving that reflect entry-level competency and the current practice expectations for PTAs. The exam covers knowledge of both entry-level academic and clinical training.

Various committees and psychometricians of the Federation help develop the PTA Exam. From a large pool of items, a group selects those that will be used on each examination.

Currently, the Federation does not publish the number of forms that exist for the exam; however, they do identify that a test taker can take the exam three times and not get the same items or same exam. Each examination adheres to the content outline in order to comprehensively and fairly assess a candidate's competency to practice. There is a degree of stability, consistency, and continuity from examination to examination in terms of what is being assessed. Questions are not derived from one specific textbook or point of view. A list of texts commonly used in PTA programs can be found on the FSBPT website. Terminology is consistent with the *Guide to Physical Therapist Practice* and other commonly used texts. There is usually a retooling of the examination questions every year; however, the Content Outline changes only every five years.

Each candidate who sits for the PTA Exam must accept the NPTE Security Agreement. In part, this agreement states that it is illegal and unethical to recall (memorize) and share questions that are on the PTA Exam or to solicit questions that are on the PTA Exam from candidates who have taken the exam. The FSBPT has and will continue to actively prosecute individuals who violate the Security Agreement. This Security Agreement is necessary because questions may be reused on subsequent examinations.

What Areas Does the Examination Cover?

There is a great emphasis on the clinical application of knowledge to the management of patient/client clinical situations and problems in safely and effectively treating patients consistent with the principles of best practice and current best evidence. The exam also covers the implementation and adjustment for effective use of equipment, devices, technologies, and therapeutic modalities. To a lesser extent, knowledge of pharmacology and medical management of individuals may also be tested. The examination can deal with topics peripheral to direct patient care. These topics might include the PTA's role in safety, federal/state regulations, accrediting standards, knowledge of professional roles, documentation, patient/client rights, cultural and socioeconomic factors impacting patient/client management, patient/peer teaching and learning, and evidence-based practice.

The examination is comprehensive. Ensure your preparation reflects the composition of the current content outline. Naturally, not every item or subitem listed below will be covered on each examination. The examination consists of 200 questions. Of those, only 150 questions are graded and will count toward your score. The test is delivered in four blocks of 50 questions at a time. The additional 50 questions are used by the Federation to check for validity and reliability for future use. This content outline is based on the 150 questions that are scored.

Examination Content for the PTA

The current content outline is divided into three large groups of questions centered on the body systems. This accounts for approximately 81% of the examination. The focus of these questions places the PTA candidate in the position of making clinical decisions based on diseases and conditions that may affect treatment, performing data collection or assessing the meaning of data collected, in addition to performing/monitoring/assessing/adjusting interventions. Of these questions, the musculoskeletal, cardiovascular/pulmonary, and neuromuscular/nervous systems represent the greatest percentage of body systems—about 62%. About 19% of the examination includes questions on the lymphatic, integumentary, metabolic and endocrine, gastrointestinal, and genitourinary systems. The remaining 19% of the examination covers content that is non-body-system based. The non-body-system questions cover equipment and devices, therapeutic modalities, professional responsibilities, safety and protection, and research and evidence-based practice.

The following categories and division designations identify content areas covered in the PTA Exam. In addition, they are used to report scores on the practice exams included with this text. This will allow candidates to assess areas of strength and areas that require improvement as studies proceed.

Category A

Physical Therapy Data Collection

Items in this section will assess the test takers' knowledge and application of types of tests/measures, according to current best evidence, to appropriately and effectively assess the body systems and/or conditions. The candidate will need to understand the reaction of the body systems to the tests/measures as well as to intervention. The candidate will also need to have an understanding of the mechanics of movement as it relates to the various body systems. The test items will cover patient/client management as it relates to treatment, rehabilitation, and health promotion for patients/clients throughout the life span. This section is approximately 22% of the exam and candidates can expect approximately 33 questions from this content area on the exam. This category includes:

1. Clinical application of tests/measures, including outcome measures according to current best evidence.
2. Movement analysis as it relates to the body systems.
3. Anatomy and physiology of the body systems, as well as physiological response.
4. Kinesiology and kinematics application.
5. For number of questions by body system, see Table 1.

Table 1

Number of Questions by Body System

CONTENT AREA	EXAM PERCENTAGE	ITEM BREAKDOWN PER DOMAIN
Physical Therapy Data Collection	22%	Cardiovascular & Pulmonary = 6–8 Musculoskeletal = 12–14 Neuromuscular & Nervous = 8–10 Integumentary = 2–3
Diseases and Conditions Impacting Effective Intervention	27%	Cardiovascular & Pulmonary = 6–7 Musculoskeletal = 9–11 Neuromuscular & Nervous = 8–10 Integumentary = 1–3 Metabolic & Endocrine = 3–4 Gastrointestinal, Genitourinary = 0–2, each Lymphatic = 1–2 System Interactions = 5–7
Interventions	32%	Cardiovascular & Pulmonary = 9–11 Musculoskeletal = 15–16 Neuromuscular & Nervous = 12–14 Integumentary = 2–4 Metabolic & Endocrine = 2–3 Gastrointestinal, Genitourinary = 0–2, each Lymphatic = 1–2
Equipment, Devices, & Technologies **Therapeutic Modalities**	12%	Assistive and adaptive devices/technologies Application and adjustment of Indications/Contraindications/Precautions Between 16 and 20 questions
Safety & Professional Roles **Professional Responsibilities** **Research & Evidence-Based Practice**	7%	Factors influencing safety (patient handling, equipment handling, emergency preparedness, environment) Standards, laws, and regulations (state, federal, accrediting bodies) Professional Standards (patient/client rights, reporting) Terminology, methodology, levels of evidence, interpretation of Between 9 and 13 questions

Category B

Diseases and Conditions Impacting Intervention

Items in this section will assess the test taker's ability to link knowledge of diseases and conditions to an understanding of the involvement of the body systems in management (treatment, intervention), rehabilitation, and health promotion for patients/clients throughout the life span. This section is approximately 27% of the exam and candidates can expect approximately 40 questions. This category includes:

1. Anatomy and physiology of the body systems.
2. Pathologies/conditions of the body systems.
3. Diseases or conditions of the body systems.
4. Medical management of the body systems (e.g., imaging, laboratory test values).
5. Pharmacological management of the body systems, including polypharmacy.
6. For number of questions by body system, see Table 1.

Category C

Intervention

Items in this section will assess the candidate's ability to link knowledge of interventions (types, applications, responses and potential complications thereof, according to current best evidence) and their impact on the body system being treated as well as other body systems that may be affected. The test items will cover patient/client management as it relates to treatment, rehabilitation, and health promotion for patients/clients throughout the life span. This section is approximately 32% of the exam and candidates can expect approximately 48 questions. This category includes:

1. Application of interventions to the body systems, including secondary effects or complications from physical therapy and medical interventions on single, as well as multiple, body systems.
2. Appropriate types and application of interventions, according to current best evidence; it includes bowel/bladder programs, pelvic floor retraining, and positioning for reflux.
3. Physiologic response as it relates to interventions, daily activities, and environmental factors (e.g., heat, humidity, etc.).
4. Anatomy and physiology of body systems.
5. Motor control and motor learning related to neuromuscular/nervous systems and physical therapy intervention.
6. Wound management techniques.
7. Implement knowledge of teaching and learning strategies that are appropriate to specified audience.
8. For number of questions by body system, see Table 1.

Category D

Equipment, Devices, & Technologies, and Therapeutic Modalities

Items in this category assess the candidates' knowledge and adjustment of equipment/devices/technologies to support effective and appropriate patient/client management. Items related to therapeutic modalities will require the test taker to consider the use requirements and patient/client context for identified outcomes. Test takers will need to incorporate an understanding of context and other factors influencing the use and adjustment of equipment/devices/technologies/therapeutic modalities for effective patient/client management. Test items relate to treatment, rehabilitation, and health promotion for patients/clients throughout the life span. This section is approximately 12% of the exam and candidates can expect approximately 18 questions. This category includes:

Equipment and Devices

1. Assistive and adaptive devices (walkers, wheelchairs, adaptive equipment, mechanical lifts, etc.)
2. Prosthetic and orthotic devices (upper/lower extremity, microprocessor-controlled components)
3. Protective and supportive devices
4. Bariatric equipment and devices

Therapeutic Modalities

1. Thermal modalities (indications, contraindications, precautions, contextual considerations for setup and adjustment, e.g., waveform/pulse/cycle parameters, electrode placement, selection of modality appropriate to condition or limitation).
2. Mechanical modalities including pneumatic compression therapies, mechanical motion devices, and traction.
3. Electrotherapy modalities (electrical stimulation, iontophoresis, phonophoresis, biofeedback).

Category E

Safety, Protection, Professional Responsibilities, Research and Evidence-Based Practice

Items in this category test the candidate's understanding of and ability to apply principles of patient/client safety, demonstrate an understanding of roles and responsibilities of health care personnel as well as apply concepts of patient/client rights (ADA, HIPAA, etc.). This category also includes items to test knowledge of documentation standards and human resource legal issues (e.g., OSHA and sexual harassment). In addition, items relating to an understanding of basic research concepts are included in this section. This section is approximately 7% of the exam and candidates can expect approximately 11 questions. For number of questions per content area, see Table 1. This category includes:

Safety and Protection
1. Factors related to safety and injury prevention (e.g., falls, safe patient handling, environment safety, equipment maintenance).
2. Preparedness for emergency situations (e.g., CPR, first aid, disaster response).
3. Understanding and implementation of infection control measures (e.g., standard and universal precautions, isolation, sterile technique).
4. The functions, implications, and precautions related to intravenous lines, tubes, catheters, and monitoring devices.
5. Signs and symptoms of abuse and neglect (physical, sexual, psychological).
6. Risk management, quality assurance measures.

Professional Responsibilities
1. Professional standards (documentation, billing/coding/reimbursement, reporting obligations).
2. Patients'/clients' rights as related to the law (ADA, HIPAA, IDEA, etc.).
3. Human resource and legal issues (e.g., OSHA, state/federal laws/regulations, standards for accrediting/licensing agencies).
4. Cultural and socioeconomic factors impacting patient/client management.

Research and Evidence-Based Practice
1. Knowledge of research methodology/interpretation (measures, level of evidence).
2. Methodology for data collection, measurement, assessing evidence (peer-reviewed publication, clinical prediction rules).

How Is the PTA Exam Graded and the Scores Reported?

All jurisdictions now employ the criterion-referenced performance standard. Using this system, a test score is interpreted in terms of an individual's mastery of a specified content domain. A passing criterion or standard is established by the FSBPT. A candidate must reach or exceed the designated cut score of competency to pass the examination. The cut score represents the minimal acceptable level of exam performance consistent with the safe and effective practice expected of the PTA. A panel of content experts establishes the passing score after screening questions for performance characteristics and bias. The examinee's performance is not compared with the performance of others who took the same examination. There are different forms of the examination that are used when taking the exam. Each form of the PTA Exam has its own raw passing grade. Thus, when taking the examination, your test might differ from another individual's and have a different raw passing grade. Grading on the curve, use of a fixed percentage, and the number of questions answered correctly are methods no longer in use for determining passing scores.

Reporting the grades to candidates can be confusing. Because versions of the examination might differ as to level of difficulty, scaled scores rather than the absolute number of questions answered correctly (raw score) are reported to candidates. The scaled scoring range is from 200 to 800, with 600 always reflecting the passing score. Thus, if the passing raw score was determined to be 105 out of 150 questions for a particular version of the PTA Exam, the 105 would equal a scaled score of 600. If a candidate achieved a score of 600 or better, the state licensing board would notify the candidate of his or her success and issue a license providing that all other conditions were satisfied.

Some states still convert the scaled passing score to another system based on the number 70 or 75. Thus, your score could be reported as being above or below the number 70 or 75. This does not necessarily mean that you scored above or below 70% or 75% or correctly or incorrectly answered 70 or 75 questions. It is merely an arbitrary numbering system used to denote a pass/fail line.

What Is the Procedure for Obtaining and Retaining a License to Practice as a PTA?

Regulation (licensure, registration, certification) of health care practitioners by the states and other jurisdictions of the United States is a means by which the public is protected from incompetent or immoral practitioners. In the United States, all jurisdictions require PTAs to be regulated in some manner to practice. Regulation is a function of the state or territorial governments, not the federal government. The onus is on the candidate for regulation to demonstrate competency.

All jurisdictions that regulate PTAs require the candidate to successfully complete the National Physical Therapy Examination for Physical Therapist Assistants. What can be confusing is that each state may have different requirements to fulfill in order to become eligible to take the PTA Exam. These requirements may differ from state to state or within the same state depending upon whether or not the candidate graduated from a PTA program accredited by the Commission on Accreditation in Physical Therapy (CAPTE). Each state has sovereignty over PTA regulation.

Contact the individual regulatory board in the state or jurisdiction in which you are seeking licensure to obtain applications and information about requirements and procedures. Complete the application materials and submit them to the regulatory authority in which you seek licensure along with required payment. On receiving and approving your application, the regulatory authority will approve your application and then notify the FSBPT of your eligibility to sit for the PTA Exam. When the FSBPT receives notification of your eligibility to sit for the examination, you will be sent an authorization-to-test letter. Schedule your exam time and desired testing location as soon as possible. You may schedule your examination at a Prometric testing center by phone or online using the information provided in your authorization letter. You will be required to pay a computer usage fee upon scheduling your examination. On completion, the examination will be scored by the FSBPT and results reported to the regulatory authority in the jurisdiction in which you applied for licensure. The regulatory authority will notify you of the results. Results are reported in approximately 7 days.

Candidates with documented disabilities may receive special accommodation during the examination. Special seating, extra time, a reader or other considerations are possible. Any special accommodation must be requested through and preapproved by the regulatory board. Candidates are encouraged to contact the FSBPT as well as review the *PTA Exam Candidate Handbook* for further information.

Some additional factors candidates may encounter are as follows:

Jurisprudence Examination: Some states require candidates to pass an examination concerning the rules, regulations, and laws governing practice of physical therapy in that state. This written examination is in addition to the PTA Exam. PTAs who are already licensed and wish to obtain another license when moving to a different state may have to successfully complete a jurisprudence examination if required by that state.

Fees: All states require a fee to apply for and renew a license. There are separate fees to sit for the PTA Exam, which are paid to the FSBPT. Computer usage fees must also be paid to Prometric upon scheduling your examination. Fees vary widely and can change yearly.

Tests of English Language Proficiency: Various tests of spoken, written or comprehended English may be required if English is not a first language. Standards and requirements differ from state to state. Personal interviews may also be required.

AIDS Awareness Training: A requirement for licensure in some states.

Fingerprinting, FBI Check, Vaccination, Malpractice Insurance: One or more may be required by some jurisdictions.

Credentials Evaluation: May be required for PTAs who graduated from programs that are outside the United States or from programs not accredited by the CAPTE. This process may be required to establish eligibility to take the PTA Exam.

Temporary License: Some states grant a temporary license to a candidate eligible to take the PTA Exam. This allows the individual to practice under supervision prior to taking and passing the PTA Exam. If a candidate fails the PTA Exam, the temporary license may be revoked or it may be extended if the candidate immediately reapplies to take the exam. Again, this depends upon the state. If a state does not offer a temporary license, a PTA may NOT practice in that state until all requirements for licensure have been satisfied. With the implementation of computer-based examinations, temporary licenses are being phased out in many jurisdictions.

Transfer of Scores to Other Jurisdictions: All jurisdictions use the criterion-referenced grading method that standardizes exam scoring and allows transfer of passing scores. The FSBPT is responsible for score transfer. Contact the Score Transfer Service at http://www.fsbpt.net/pt. You may transfer your scores online or download the Score Transfer Request Form and mail the completed form to the Federation. There is a fee for this service. If you maintain licensure, you should not have to retake the PTA Exam if you move to a different state. However, if you are not licensed or regulated, let your license lapse, or never took the examination, you will probably have to take it when seeking a license in jurisdictions that require PTA regulation.

Retaking the PTA Exam: Some states limit the number of times one may take the PTA Exam. If you fail, the state may impose a stipulation that you show evidence of some form of remedial work or study before retaking the PTA Exam. The state has an obligation to protect the public from practitioners who do not demonstrate competency.

License/Regulation Renewal: After one, two, or three years, licensure must be renewed to continue practicing. The state or jurisdiction typically sends out a renewal notice. Sometimes renewal is an easy procedure. One just pays the fee and returns the form. In some states, verification of continuing education units may be required to renew. If there is a failure to notify the state of a change of address, the applicant may not receive a renewal notice; if there is a failure to respond to a renewal notice in a timely fashion, or if other requirements are not met, the license may lapse. It is illegal to practice without a valid license. The state may require a number of conditions be met in order to reinstate lapsed regulation. One condition might include retaking the PTA Exam even if you had previously passed. Inform the regulatory board of any change of address. Do not let your license lapse!

Continuing Education: Many states require the PTA to acquire a specific number of continuing education units (CEUs) in order to renew licensure. Documentation, approval, and reporting of CEUs vary from state to state. The state may also require evidence of continuing active practice in order to renew. Continuing education requirements change from time to time; the license holder is responsible to know and meet any current requirements. Be sure to track the regulatory body's requirements on a regular basis. Currently, the American Physical Therapy Association and the Federation of State Boards are exploring alternative means for continued competency measurement or monitoring.

Endorsement: With valid regulation in one jurisdiction, a PTA may apply to another state for a "license by endorsement." All criteria established by the new state must be met. This can include taking a jurisprudence exam for that state, interviews, letters of recommendation, AIDS awareness, CEUs, and so on. Contact the regulatory board in the state where license by endorsement is sought to get information and applications. Start the process early—it can take months!

What Happens If You Have to Retake the PTA Exam?

Remember, most candidates are successful the first time! If you receive bad news about your PTA Exam results, life goes on but gets a bit more complicated. You might lose your temporary license if the state or jurisdiction has granted you one. If you are working as a PTA, you may not be able to keep your job or you may be moved to another position. If you have accepted a future position and fail to get a license, your employer might opt not to save the position for you.

Undoubtedly, you will experience various emotions that could include anger, frustration, depression, low self-esteem, and embarrassment.

What can be done? You can go online and download the Performance Feedback Request Form from the FSBPT. This report compares your test performance, in various categories, with that of other candidates who sat for the same examination. It gives the number of questions in a category, your percentage score and the average percentage score of others in that category. The current cost is $90 plus a small processing fee for this service. No personal checks are accepted. For examination security reasons, no one has access to or can revisit his or her actual examination. You may contact http://www.fsbpt.org or call 703-739-9420.

Our advice is not to dwell on past failures. Carefully evaluate your performance. Think about areas on the previous examination(s) with which you had some difficulty. Were there any gaps in your academic or clinical knowledge? Did you find it difficult to answer questions requiring judgment or application of knowledge?

Focus on the next examination. Reinstitute a program of disciplined self-study. Consider taking a preparation course if you had not previously attended one. Do not retake the PTA Exam too quickly. We have found that candidates who retake the examination without adjusting their behaviors or correcting deficiencies wind up with the same disappointing results. There is no magic potion that helps you pass the examination. The onus is on you to demonstrate competency to practice. Take a positive and determined outlook. Approach the next examination with self-confidence and a minimum of anxiety.

Useful Web Links and E-Mail Addresses

1. http://www.fsbpt.org
   The Federation of State Boards of Physical Therapy
   Information on licensure, addresses and links to state physical therapy boards, information about the PTA Exam and the role of the Federation.
2. http://www.2test.com
   Locations of Prometric Testing and Assessment Centers
3. http://www.apta.org
   The American Physical Therapy Association
   Information about the profession, policies regarding the role of the physical therapist assistant, resources in selected areas of practice, etc.
4. http://www.TherapyEd.com
   TherapyEd
   Information about examination preparatory courses and materials for physical and occupational therapists, PTAs and occupational therapy assistants.

Testing Success

You are likely now in the process of completing, or have just completed, your college education to become a physical therapist assistant. Good for you! Your next big step is taking (and passing!) the National PTA Exam. While you were in school, you successfully figured out how to answer questions from your instructors—based on set course objectives.

This examination is somewhat different; it is based on the Content Outline developed by the FSBPT (Federation) rather than your instructors' content outline (objectives). The PTA Exam does, however, cover your entire two years of education and is given based on the premise that you are a graduate of an accredited PTA program.

The National Physical Therapist Assistant Exam (PTA)

Purpose of the Licensure Examination

Protection of the Public
1. The "agreement" the Federation of State Boards of Physical Therapy has with individual jurisdictions (states) is that when physical therapist assistants pass this examination, they are "SAFE" and competent to work with patients/clients in that state.
2. A "SAFE" clinician is a clinician who:
   a. Recognizes and makes decisions that are within their scope of practice and refers out when not.
   b. Performs interventions that follow standard protocols and that meet the patient's/client's condition, stage of healing, diagnosis, etc.; recognizes when the patient/client is not tolerating the intervention or is demonstrating signs/symptoms inconsistent with what would be expected.
   c. Comprehends anatomy and physiology, pathology, indications and contraindications, red flags, and treatment progress—to make appropriate decisions.
3. A competent clinician is a clinician who:
   a. Adapts intervention to patient/client needs considering current medical or health condition—for patients/clients across their life span.
   b. Provides intervention and data collection appropriately/correctly.
   c. Applies knowledge of anatomy/physiology and pathology to patients/clients with differing pathology and/or conditions that are most representative of current physical therapy practice.
4. Test takers should always keep SAFETY in mind when answering exam items on the PTA Exam!

This Exam Is Not a "Jurisprudence" Examination
1. The PTA Exam DOES NOT ask questions about the test taker's knowledge of state (jurisdiction) rules and regulations or the practice act in the individual jurisdiction in which the test taker is seeking a license.

2. A "jurisprudence" examination:
   a. Is an exam covering the specific rules and regulations and state statute governing the practice of physical therapy in the jurisdiction requiring it.
   b. Is determined by the jurisdiction in which the test taker is seeking a license ("license" will be used to encompass licensure, certification, registration, regulation of the PTA).
   c. Will also be taken at a Prometric testing center.
   d. Can be taken prior to or following the PTA Exam; the test taker will not receive a license until this AND the PTA Exam have been successfully taken.
3. Be sure to check with the jurisdiction in which you are seeking a license to identify if a jurisprudence exam is required in that state.
   a. Several states do require this exam as well as the PTA Exam.
   b. Specific state information can be found on the Federation website, https://www.fsbpt.org/LicensingAuthorities/index.asp.

PTA Exam Format

The PTA Exam Is 200 Questions
1. Only 150 are counted toward the test taker's score.
2. The additional 50 test items are "trial run" questions being tested for validity and reliability for use on future exams. These items will have the same look and feel of all items on the exam; test takers will not know which questions are scored and which are "trial run" questions.

Breaks and Timing During the Exam
1. Total time allotted for the exam itself will be 4 hours. There is additional time for the candidate to participate in the tutorial and take the allowed 15-minute break.
   a. Candidates will be required to arrive a minimum of 30 minutes prior to scheduled start time for processing and identification verification.
   b. Candidates are allowed 4 hours to complete the exam. A clock will count backward from the 4 allotted hours and will be visible to the candidate on the screen throughout the examination.
   c. Time will be allotted at the beginning of the exam for the candidate to participate in the tutorial to the testing program if desired.
      - This time does not count against the 4-hour allotted exam time, and TherapyEd suggests that candidates participate in the tutorial.
   d. One 15-minute break is scheduled after item number 100 in the second block of questions is submitted; the exam clock stops counting during this time.
      - Candidates may choose to take a longer or shorter break during this exam. A shorter break will restart the clock as the candidate begins the exam again; a longer break will result in the clock initiating prior to the candidate being reseated.
   e. Two unscheduled breaks may also be taken during the exam; the clock does not stop during these breaks.
2. There are 200 questions on the exam. The questions are delivered in blocks of 50 questions at a time, over a time frame of 4 hours.
   a. This means the candidate will have access to 50 questions at a time. Upon completion of questions in each block, the candidate must submit the block and the next block of questions then becomes available.
      - There is no time limit within the blocks, just the 4-hour maximum time.
      - Each block will contain questions from various parts of the content outline as well as trial run questions.
      - On the screen with each question, candidates may choose to "mark" the question, thus flagging it for review at the end of the block.
      - At the end of the block, candidates will be given the opportunity to choose to "review marked items," "review all items," or "submit" the block of questions.
   b. Candidates can go back and forth through questions in each block as many times as they choose during the review process.
   c. Upon submitting the block of questions, that block becomes unavailable for further review.

Question (Item) Format
1. Each item is a multiple-choice item.
   a. Items do not relate to prior or upcoming items on the exam. Consider each separately on its own merits and information provided.
2. Each item will have four specific choices for the best answer.
   a. Individual choices do not link to each other (e.g., "both a. and b. are correct").
   b. There is only one correct/best answer provided for each item.
      - Bear in mind that there may be multiple correct ways to accomplish what the question is asking; however, only one of those ways will be listed as an answer choice.
3. Candidates are not "penalized" for incorrect responses.
   a. Do not leave answers blank; always select a response and mark the question for review if uncertain of the response.
   b. Even an "educated guess" gives the candidate a 25% chance of choosing the best response; a blank answer is always 100% incorrect!

Successfully Managing Examination Items/Questions

Test Item Difficulty

The greatest percentage of questions require problem solving at the middle to upper levels of cognitive functioning. Those types of questions are termed "application," "analysis," and "evaluation" level questions on *Bloom's Taxonomy* of thought processing. It is not important that candidates can identify or define these levels; however, it is important to understand the level of thought processing that is required to correctly determine the best response to exam items. Candidates may also find items on the exam written at less challenging cognitive levels, "remembering" or "understanding"; however, there likely will be very few of those.

See the Taxonomy Diagram below, which identifies five types of exam questions.

Review Table 2 on page I-11 to explore the levels of questions and how they might be used on the exam.

Item Strategies

Items on the PTA Exam are written to ascertain how a candidate will deal with a variety of different clinical situations in order to determine how the candidate is likely to function in the clinical setting. The exam is developed such that the candidate who passes the examination should be "minimally competent" to practice as an entry-level PTA. A "minimally competent" candidate makes clinical decisions that are SAFE and competent.

Most successful test takers use specific "strategies" to navigate exam items and answer correctly. This not only includes carefully reading the exam items to determine the best/correct response, it requires candidates to identify specific types of test items and use a strategy to narrow the potential responses.

Best Strategies for Answering Multiple-Choice Questions

Key Words

1. Look for key words/phrases/clues in the stem (question/item) that will set the scene for the answer. Some key terms will appear in all caps or bold within the exam (e.g., GREATEST BENEFIT, FIRST, ALWAYS). These words help to set priorities for the response, for example, "which would a PTA perform FIRST in this scenario," or "what is the MOST important symptom." Additional key words/phrases/clues to help guide thought processing include:

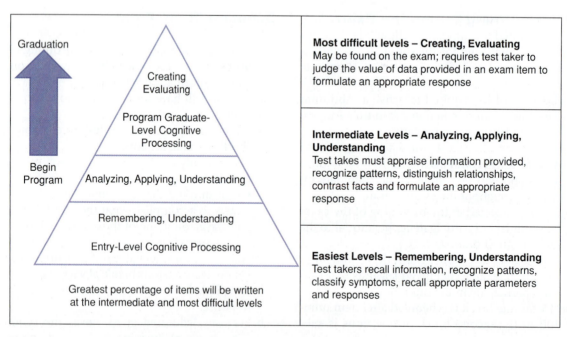

Taxonomy of Exam Item Difficulty (based on the work of Benjamin Bloom, Bloom's Taxonomy)

Table 2

Levels of Exam Questions

QUESTION LEVEL AND DESCRIPTION	RELEVANCE	EXAM PREPARATION STRATEGY
Remembering Recall of basic information and facts. For example, spinal cord levels, muscle attachments, diagnoses, wheelchair measurements.	A solid knowledge foundation of entry-level information is required to answer clinical scenario questions that will be posed on the NPTE. It is very unlikely that you will find a question written at this level on the exam.	A strong commitment to studying specific facts and information acquired during your PTA education is needed. This text provides extensive information in an outline format to ease your review. Memorization of specific facts and information you will need to apply to solving clinical problem posed in the questions is highly suggested.
Understanding Understanding of information to determine significance, consequences, or implications. For example, the impact of spasticity on function.	The exam is not a "matching" type of test. You will not be able to simply recall information to be successful in answering a question. You must be able to apply facts and knowledge to multiple clinical scenarios. You can expect to find many questions written at this level on the examination.	When studying the text to review basic content and foundational knowledge, ask yourself how and why this fundamental information is important, how you will use the information to administer and modify interventions to persons across the lifespan. Studying with a peer or a group can provide you with additional insights about the relevance, significance, consequences, and implications of the information.
Applying and Analyzing Use of information and application of rules, procedures, or theories to new situations. For example, the modification of a treatment for a patient who has a recent hip replacement in addition to an acute CVA.	The exam requires you to use your knowledge and comprehension as described above, along with the competencies you developed during your clinical experiences, in a manner that best fits the specific scenario identified in the exam item. You can expect to find many questions written at this level on the examination.	Continue to actively apply information that you review in the textbook to new and novel clinical situations. Consider how the information you are processing can be used for patients with different diagnoses, of different ages, and with differing levels of health and wellness. The exam items included on the CD in this text are constructed such that you must use these comprehension and application skills to correctly answer the items. Review the analysis of your performance after you have completed the exam to help identify how well you are applying your knowledge.
Evaluating Recognition of interrelationships between principles and interpretation or evaluation of data presented. For example, the most appropriate focus for discharge planning for a patient with a traumatic brain injury.	It is unlikely the exam for the physical therapist assistant will contain items that are written at the evaluating level.	Critically review the rationales provided in the text of the correct and incorrect responses to the exam questions. Review the content area(s) you did not get correct. Reflection with a peer or study group can be beneficial in helping to determine your gaps in analysis of exam items.

2. Those words indicating timing or criticality—first, most important.
3. A diagnosis and/or indication of stage of recovery.
4. An indication of care environment in which the scenario is taking place.

Clues

Identify clues in the stem that may be helpful in focusing thoughts. For example, the examiners present a recently discharged patient who can transfer independently but cannot ambulate independently for greater than 20 feet. The candidate's judgment should lead one to conclude that the patient is probably homebound. Therefore, if asked to choose among exercises or activities, the one best suited for home use might be most appropriate.

Similar Choices

Identify choices that are so similar to each other that it is difficult to distinguish between them. Perhaps the choices are saying the same thing but using slightly different terminology. Items that are difficult to discriminate between are likely the incorrect response as there is only one best/correct response. For example, if one answer choice is the *primary muscle of inspiration,* and the other choice is *the diaphragm,* they both are really identifying the same thing and should both be eliminated. The choice that is different, but not far-fetched, merits greater consideration in this type of question.

Opposites

Look for opposites in the four choices. Candidates may find two answer choices—one stating "positive" and the other stating "negative," or "inversion" versus "eversion," or "hypoglycemia" and "hyperglycemia." Examine these opposites first. If both cannot be eliminated, it is likely that one of the pair of opposites is the best response. If both can be easily eliminated, focus on the remaining two choices, thus elevating one's chances to 50%. This is certainly better than the 25% chance before eliminating anything!

Overlapping Facts

1. Look for overlapping facts in the choices. If one can ascertain that a fact or statement in a choice is incorrect and that same fact is included in another choice, both can be eliminated.
2. For example, given a patient problem, two options in the choices are
   a. Pallor and diaphoresis.
   b. Tachycardia and diaphoresis.
3. If one has determined that "diaphoresis" is incorrect, both choices can be eliminated without further consideration.

Crucial for Survival

1. Identify options that are crucial for patient/client survival, or relate to the safety of the patient/client. These choices should receive your highest priority, consider these choices carefully.

Overanalyze

Do not overanalyze the question or the choices. Each item is written so that it includes the information the test taker needs to answer the item correctly. Test takers will need to recall diseases, interventions, progression, signs and symptoms, and so forth, to answer the question correctly; however, if you find yourself developing a "story line" to go along with the question to determine the best response, it is likely that something was missed in the first review of the item. Go back and re-read the entire question and reassess key words, and so on, to determine the best response.

Negative Words or Phrases

There are few examples in the exam of "negative" questions, for example, *Which of the following would the PTA NOT perform?* If candidates find this type of question, it is helpful to label the answer choices TRUE or FALSE as relative to the scenario presented. The result should then be three TRUE responses and one FALSE; the FALSE response is likely then the best choice.

Avoid These Strategies

Patterns

Do not look for patterns or answer choices so that you alter your selection for best choice. For example, if you have chosen 2 as the best response, don't change that selection because you realize that you have answered 2 for the five immediately preceding responses. Questions, and the order of their choices, are randomly placed on the exam. Do not look for or think about the patterns for answers.

Change Answer

It is typically best to NOT CHANGE the answer originally chosen. The only time test takers should consider changing a response is when, upon re-reading a question, the test taker realizes that he or she read the question incorrectly the first time, or if upon re-reading the question new information is recalled (e.g., remembering a certain diagnosis or red flag, etc.). Often when an answer is changed based on the test taker's "feeling" or a "hunch" that he or she has chosen a wrong response, the test taker may ultimately end up getting it wrong.

The Role of Critical Reasoning in Licensure Exam Performance

Critical reasoning is the process of drawing conclusions—a process everyone goes through many times every day. Individuals use knowledge, skills, experiences, and logic to make conclusions about everyday situations. In order to successfully draw conclusions, one must make a concerted effort to embark on this decision-making process with purpose, clarity, accuracy, and thoroughness. Understanding what type(s) of critical reasoning you struggle with will provide significant insight into what strategies should be used during the exam and review process. How does this relate to the PTA Exam, and why should test takers spend time focusing attention on this process?

This text has already identified that the exam tests candidates' ability to solve clinical situations versus simply recalling facts that are readily found in textbooks. Although factual knowledge is an important foundation for the exam, the questions on the PTA Exam are designed to compel candidates to test their ability to reason out clinical scenarios, to make prudent decisions about the situation described in each question.

There are five types of critical reasoning. The circumstances surrounding a proposed situation in each exam item determine the critical reasoning strategy individuals need to employ to select the best response. Candidates will find that they excel at some types of critical reasoning and struggle in others; that is perfectly normal. The five subtypes of critical reasoning are inductive reasoning, deductive reasoning, analysis, inference and evaluation. These principles of critical reasoning are based on expert consensus of critical-thinking experts and reported by Peter and Noreen Facione (1990a, 1990b, 2006).

Five Subtypes of Critical Reasoning

Inductive Reasoning

1. Inductive reasoning requires clinical judgment and ongoing expansion of our knowledge base. It begins with observations and reasoning in specific situations

and progresses to the ability to draw conclusions from more generalized situations with a larger set of circumstances. It is important as it provides insight into understanding populations and not just individuals.
2. PTAs use critical reasoning skills for effective treatment planning in order to meet the goals set in the plan of care established by the PT. The PTA weighs all viable treatment options, rather than just one, and selects the most appropriate choice given the entire set of circumstances.
3. *Example*: When working with a patient with back pain, transcutaneous electrical nerve stimulation (TENS) was able to decrease pain for this specific patient when nothing else would work. One may initially assume that all back pain, therefore, will respond positively to TENS. While this thinking is flawed, it may lead us to further explore the use of TENS for pain management of areas other than low back pain, or may encourage us to consider the use of other modalities for addressing back pain in different individuals.

Deductive Reasoning
1. Deductive reasoning is the opposite of inductive reasoning; one begins with a larger set of circumstances and theories that we then apply to the specific situation being addressed. This type of reasoning involves drawing conclusions based on facts, laws, rules or accepted principles.
2. PTAs make decisions about patient care and situations using deductive reasoning. This type of reasoning helps provide a starting point as well as a structured process from which to work in the clinical decision-making process. The clinician must have good background knowledge of the information prior to making decisions in this fashion, as utilizing incorrect procedures or flawed knowledge will result in unsound conclusions.
3. *Example*: There is a standard protocol for using TENS for pain control based on data gathered over the course of its use on multiple individuals; therefore, we are able to utilize this protocol on a variety of individuals with various types of pain, rather than starting from the beginning each time.

Analysis
1. Analysis is the process of "making sense out of pieces"; interpreting the meaning of information, determining relationships within the information presented and then making assumptions or judgments about that information.

2. This type of reasoning is important to the PTA as it allows the individual to draw conclusions based on observations, a frequent occurrence in the implementation of the treatment plan. The PTA must continually determine what is relevant and irrelevant information in order to effectively analyze the situation.
3. *Example*: The PTA examines range of motion readings taken over the past week and makes a determination whether the patient is progressing as expected based on the diagnosis and outlined plan of care.

Inference
1. Inference involves making logical judgments based on concepts, beliefs, assumptions and evidence rather than direct observation. This process often relies on the PTA's prior clinical experiences in making predictions about future occurrences.
2. A PTA uses this skill to make assumptions as to what he or she can expect from a certain clinical situation. It is often employed to answer patients' questions about their future (e.g., length of stay, possible recovery, or ongoing disabilities to expect).
3. *Example*: The PTA reviews a patient chart prior to seeing the patient for the first time and finds a diagnosis of right anterior cerebral artery cerebral vascular accident. Immediately, the PTA begins to make predictions about what to expect when meeting the patient for the first time. The PTA should expect possible personality changes, greater LE involvement than UE, and urinary incontinence.

Evaluation
1. Evaluation involves relying on guiding principles to determine a course of action as well as validating the decision made. It involves the "gut instinct" utilized in decision making, often forcing us to rely on ethical principles to find solutions where there are no easy answers. It can be difficult for concrete thinkers to use evaluative reasoning as there is often not a black or white answer.
2. PTAs should not be scared off by the name of this type of critical reasoning—PTAs utilize evaluative thinking skills. A PTA will use evaluative reasoning when determining if a referral back to the PT for further evaluation is indicated.
3. *Example*: A patient who has had a recent myocardial infarction is completing shoulder rehabilitation exercises. During exercise the patient begins to sweat profusely and complain of nausea and light-headedness. The PTA must weigh what is happening and determine whether or not the symptoms being observed are related to the shoulder exercises or are symptomatic of a new heart problem.

Improving Your Critical Reasoning Skills

Critical reasoning is not learned or improved in a quick lesson or by simply reading basic definitions. It requires practice with items that test these skill areas and provide feedback on your performance. The good news is that you already have this information contained in this study guide! Each practice question answer in the book has an accompanying rationale for the correct and incorrect choices. Additionally, each question has an explanation about the subskill of critical reasoning and the knowledge or skill required to arrive at a correct conclusion. Paying attention to these areas will help you to build your knowledge and experiences with critical reasoning skills and prepare you for the NPTE and all its challenges.

After you receive the results of your online practice test, refer back to your incorrect responses. This may help you uncover a pattern in the types of questions you are answering incorrectly, as related to a subskill of critical reasoning. Do you notice that you have difficulty with certain types of questions, such as those that encourage evaluative or inferential reasoning? This will help you to identify a potential area for improvement and an area to help base study strategies. Once you have identified a weakness in critical reasoning, take some time to reflect on why this is so. See Table 3 for examples of strategies based on type of reasoning.

Table 3

Critical Reasoning Self-Assessment Questions

OBSERVED EXAM DIFFICULTY	REASONING CHALLENGE	EXAM PREPARATION STRATEGY
Do you: - Have difficulty with taking specific information and applying it to larger populations? - Select incorrect answers because you don't know how to generalize your knowledge?	Inductive	When studying a specific content area, think about how to apply the information you are reviewing to a diversity of situations. Use a reflective "what if" stance to think about how this information may be generalized to a broader context. This can be a fun and effective study group activity.
Do you: - Prefer to follow your instincts rather than the guidelines that a protocol may provide? - Select incorrect answers because you are unfamiliar with established practice standards or major theoretical approaches?	Deductive	When studying, be sure to master all major concepts, laws, rules, and accepted principles that guide PT practice. Carefully review all frames of reference, practice guidelines, and intervention protocols and procedures. Review the APTA Code of Ethics and Guidelines for Professional Conduct.
Do you: - Tend to misinterpret information provided and make poor judgments and apply inadequately conceived assumptions about it? - Select incorrect answers because you misjudged the effects of a clinical condition on functional performance?	Analytical	Obtain knowledge of all major clinical conditions, their symptoms, diagnostic testing and criteria, anticipated sequelae, and expected outcomes. This information is extensively reviewed in this text to help you make accurate judgments and correct assumptions about the potential impact of a clinical condition on functional performance. Review potential adverse effects (red flags in this text) and common errors associated with training.
Do you: - Have difficulty with thinking about how clinical conditions and practice situations may evolve over time? - Assume information is valid when it is not true? - Select incorrect answers because you have difficulty deciding the best course of action in a practice scenario?	Inferential	When studying clinical conditions, think about how the presentation of these conditions may sometimes vary from textbook descriptions. Use the knowledge and experience you acquired during your clinical education experiences to assess the trustworthiness of your assumptions. Study guidelines and models developed from evidence-based practice to develop a solid foundation on how to decide the best course of action.
Do you: - Feel anxious when you have questions that are ambiguous and you cannot find answers to them in a textbook? - Rely on protocols and guidelines more than gut instinct? - Select incorrect answers because you become overwhelmed by questions that present ethical dilemmas?	Evaluative	When reviewing specific content, think about the practice ambiguities and ethical dilemmas you observed during your clinical education experiences related to these areas. Review the APTA Code of Ethics and Guidelines for Professional Conduct and practice applying this information to determine a correct course of action using practice examples and case studies.

This table was adapted with permission from Dr. Kari Inda, from a table published in Fleming-Castaldy, R: National Occupational Therapy Certification Exam: Review & Study Guide, 6th ed. TherapyEd, 2012, p. 22.

Other Courses of Action. This study guide was designed to help you to identify potential weak areas and prepare you to succeed on the NPTE. More detailed information about critical reasoning is beyond the scope and focus of this book. However, if you would like additional information about critical reasoning and practice with questions that test critical thinking and reasoning skills, the following resources may help you practice honing these skill areas:

- **Insight Assessment, Inc.** www.insightassessment.com. Offers periodic free mini-tests with rationales for correct and incorrect answers. Also offers resources that discuss the various types of reasoning.
- Nosich, G. M. (2001). *Learning to Think Things Through: A Guide to Critical Thinking in the Curriculum*, 2nd ed. Prentice Hall. A handy guide to help students engage in critical thinking.

Reasoning References

Facione P (2006). *Critical Thinking: What It Is and Why It Counts.* Millbrae, CA: The California Academic Press.

Facione P (1990a). *Critical Thinking: A Statement of Expert Consensus for Purposes of Educational Assessment and Instruction: Research Findings and Recommendations.* Newark, DE: The American Psychological Association. ERIC Document Reproduction Service. No. ED 315423.

Facione P (1990b). *Critical Thinking: A Statement of Expert Consensus for Purposes of Educational Assessment and Instruction* ("Executive Summary: The Delphi Report"). Millbrae, CA: The California Academic Press.

Facione NC & Facione PA (2006). *The Health Sciences Reasoning Test HSRT: Test Manual 2006 Edition.* Millbrae, CA: The California Academic Press.

Organizing the Examination Review

Time and Structure of Study Sessions

Total Study Time Is 4 to 6 Weeks

1. Candidates should allow approximately 4 to 6 weeks of "full-time" studying prior to the scheduled exam date. See Table 4.
    a. Candidates for whom English is a second language may want to include additional time.
2. "Full-time" studying implies 4 to 6 days a week of 2 to 4 hours per day of structured content review and study.
3. Establish a regular schedule and follow it.

Structuring Each Individual Study Session

1. Individual study sessions should be focused on 1 to 3 areas of weakness, not entire chapters of texts.
2. Use time wisely by developing and sticking to objectives for each study session. Develop objectives for study sessions based on content that is most problematic, areas tested poorly on in didactic program, areas struggled with in clinical setting, areas identified from practice exam.
    a. Use the Content Outline to guide individual study objectives.
3. Integrate resources for studying.
    a. TherapyEd has developed this PTA Examination Review & Study Guide as well as the accompanying Course Manual (only available to students taking our PTA Examination Preparatory Course) as a comprehensive solution for candidates.

Table 4

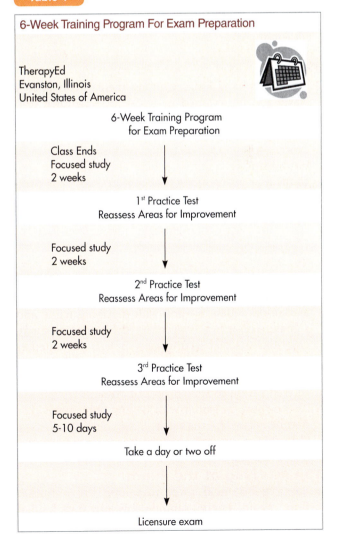

6-Week Training Program For Exam Preparation

TherapyEd
Evanston, Illinois
United States of America

b. If the candidate is not planning to take the PTA Examination Preparatory Course simply use appropriate textbooks from the PTA program attended in addition to this Review & Study Guide.

Take the Practice Exam(s) the Week Before the Exam
1. The week before the exam the candidate should take, or have taken, all three practice exams provided in this review and study guide. Candidates should spend time brushing up on the material that was most difficult or particularly troubling.

Planning for Success

Preplanning for the Day of the Examination

Scheduling
1. The PTA exam is offered four times per year, typically in January, April, July, and October. Specific dates are posted each year on the FSBPT website at www.fsbpt.org.
2. Choose an exam block (morning, mid-day, or early evening—contact selected exam site for specific times) during the time of day you are most alert and able to focus.

Travel
1. Make travel and lodging arrangements in advance if travel will be required to get to the scheduled testing site. Directions are available at the Prometric website, www.prometric.com. Take a trial drive to the test center during expected traffic conditions for exam to ensure timing is accurate. Plan ahead for congested traffic flow, bring along money if necessary for parking fees, and so forth.
2. Plan to **arrive a minimum of 30 minutes early** as it is required for documentation, identify verification, photographs, and fingerprinting.

Bring Required Identification
1. A government-issued, current and valid picture ID and a secondary identification with matching name and signature on it (e.g., student ID, debit or credit card). Note that a social security card IS NOT permitted as a secondary form of ID. Test takers will also need to present the "authorization to test" (ATT) letter from the Federation of State Boards of Physical Therapy.
2. Also be sure to gather with ID any other items that may be needed for the exam: glasses or contact lenses, maps/directions, and so forth.

The Morning of the Exam
1. **Eat** a good meal prior to taking the examination; avoid energy-sapping carbohydrate-loaded foods. Avoid excessive stimulants such as caffeine or energy drinks—they tend to create an immediate energy boost followed by a crash an hour or so following consumption! Avoid use of new medications such as antihistamines or muscle relaxants, alcohol, or other substances that may affect level of alertness.
2. **Dress** comfortably in moderate-weight clothing. Some test centers do not allow candidates to dress in layers (e.g., wearing a sweater or jacket), as these have been implicated in past cheating attempts.

During the Examination

Length of Time
1. Expect the entire examination procedure to last up to 4.5 hours or so. This includes processing prior to the exam, time to take the tutorial, and time for the allotted break. Time in the examination room is limited to allow for the next group to take their examination.

Personal Items
1. Test takers are not allowed to bring personal items, drinks, digital cell phones, watches, other digital devices, and so forth, into the examination room. Prometric test centers do provide lockers in which candidates can lock personal items during the exam.

Will be Provided
1. Test center personnel will orient test takers to specific procedures required prior to and throughout the examination process.
2. Test takers can request headphones or earplugs to dampen any noise in the room during the examination process.
3. Each candidate will be provided with one to two "white boards" for use during the examination.
   a. These boards may or may not be dry erase. If the boards are not dry erase, or you are not allowed to erase, you will be allowed to exchange the filled

board for another provided by the Prometric testing center.
  b. Use it to help with problem solving test items, recording important thoughts or creating diagrams/graphs/lists to help identify the best response for test items.

Tutorial
1. Take the tutorial prior to beginning the examination. This is a good time to focus thoughts and energy for success on the examination.

Attitude
1. Keeping a positive attitude is beneficial throughout the examination. You alone are in charge of your approach to the test taking process. It is best to come to the exam with a confident and prepared attitude toward the exam environment and process.

Time Management
1. Develop a strategy for each question; on average, exam items should take approximately 1 minute each. Stick to your time management strategy throughout the examination; do not be dissuaded or distracted by other test takers coming and going prior to your completing the examination.

Skipping Questions
1. Do not skip questions, even if the correct answer is unknown. An unanswered question submitted in a block is automatically wrong. Candidates are not penalized for "guessing."

Break
1. Take the 15-minute allowed break and take the opportunity to get up and move around, get a drink, use the restroom, and take some cleansing breaths. You may be allowed short breaks between submitting each block of questions; however, the 4-hour time clock only stops during the "scheduled break" after the second block of questions is submitted.

Communication
1. Once the examination has commenced, communicate only with Prometric personnel. An innocent remark to a nearby test taker or glancing at another computer screen may be mistaken for an attempt to cheat. Candidates attempting to cheat, by whatever means, can face serious consequences. Trying to obtain a license to practice as a PTA by fraudulent means is a crime, and the FSBPT will take allowable action to sanction your examination score.

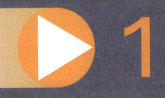

1

Therapeutic Exercise Foundations

THOMAS BIANCO and SUSAN B. O'SULLIVAN

Chapter Outline

- Training Programs, 2
  - Strength Training, 2
  - Types of Resistance Exercise, 4
  - Endurance Training, 6
  - Specific Weather Considerations, 9
  - Mobility and Flexibility Training, 9
  - Postural Stability Training, 12
  - Coordination and Balance Training, 14
  - Relaxation Training, 16
  - Aquatic Exercise, 17
  - Progression, 18
- Review Questions, 19

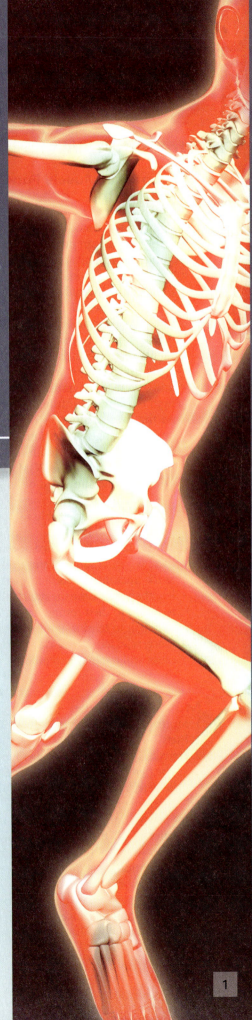

Training Programs

Strength Training

Concepts of Muscle Function and Strength

1. Strength is the force output of a contracting muscle and is directly related to the amount of tension a contracting muscle can produce.
2. Contractile elements of muscle.
   a. Muscles are composed of fibers, which are made up of myofibrils. Myofibrils are composed of sarcomeres that are connected in series. The overlapping cross bridges of actin and myosin make up a sarcomere.
   b. When a muscle contracts, the actin-myosin filaments slide together and the muscle shortens. The cross bridges slide apart when the muscle relaxes and returns to its resting length.
3. Length tension relationship.
   a. As the muscle shortens or lengthens through the available range of motion (ROM), the tension it produces varies. Maximum tension is generated at some midpoint in the ROM; less tension is developed in either shortened or lengthened ROM.
   b. The weight lifted or lowered cannot exceed that which the muscle is able to control at its weakest point in the ROM.
   c. When a muscle is stretched beyond the resting length, there is a mechanical disruption of the cross bridges as the microfilaments slide apart and the sarcomeres lengthen. Releasing the stretch allows the sarcomeres to return to their resting length. This change in ratio of length to tension is called elasticity.
   d. Once released, a muscle stretched into the elastic range will contract and produce a force or tension as the muscle returns to its original length.

Motor Fiber Type

1. Motor fibers are divided into 3 types. See Quick Facts 1-1.
2. Hereditary influences and fiber type distribution.
   a. The percentage of either FT or ST fibers in the body is determined by genetics. This ratio cannot be changed via normal exercise.
   b. Specific training can modify metabolic characteristics of all fiber types; e.g., high-intensity, anaerobic strength training will stimulate optimal FT adaptation.
3. Order of fiber type recruitment.
   a. Recruitment order depends upon type of activity, force required, movement pattern, and position of the body.

> **QUICK FACTS 1-1 ▶ MUSCLE FIBER TYPES**
>
> | Fiber Type | Qualities |
> |---|---|
> | Slow-twitch (ST) fibers Type I | • Slow contraction speed
• Low force (tension) production
• Highly resistant to fatigue
• Type I muscles: postural muscles (e.g., multifidi) |
> | Fast-twitch (FT) fibers Type IIa | • Fast contractions speed
• Fatigue resistant
• Characteristics can be influenced by type of training
• Type IIa muscles: strength and movement (e.g., gastrocnemius) |
> | Fast-twitch (FT) fibers Type IIb | • Fast contraction speed
• High force production
• Susceptible to quick fatigue
• Type IIb muscles: quick movement, eye muscles |

   b. ST motor units have the lowest functional thresholds and are recruited during lighter, slower efforts such as low-intensity, long-duration endurance activities.
   c. Higher forces with greater velocity cause the activation of more powerful, higher threshold FT motor units.
   d. Order of recruitment is ST, followed by FT IIa, and finally followed by FT IIb motor units.

Muscular Adaptations of Strength Training

1. Hypertrophy is an increase in muscle size as a result of resistance training and can be observed after at least 6–8 weeks of training.
2. Remodeling: individual muscle fibers are enlarged, contain more actin and myosin, and have more, larger myofibrils; sarcomeres are increased.
3. An increase in motor unit recruitment and synchronization of firing facilitates contraction and maximizes force production. This largely accounts for strength gains in the first 6 weeks of training.
4. The average person has a ratio of 50% fast- to slow-twitch motor units. Performing workloads of low intensity will challenge half of the body's muscle mass. High-intensity exercises for shorter durations (less than 20 repetitions) are needed to train the highly adaptable fast-twitch IIa fibers.

5. Disuse atrophy occurs when a muscle loses both size and strength from lack of use or when a limb is immobilized.
6. Cross-section area of a muscle highly correlates with strength gains. The larger the muscle, the greater the strength of that muscle.

Positive Changes in Response to Strengthening

1. Improvement in:
   a. Strength.
   b. Bone mass.
   c. Body composition: fat to lean body composition.
   d. Weight control and weight maintenance; decreased risk of adult-onset diabetes.
   e. Reaction time.
   f. Metabolism, calorie burning during and after exercise.
   g. Cardiovascular status: reduction in resting blood pressure.
   h. Immunological function.
2. Improved function and quality of life through improved:
   a. Balance and coordination.
   b. Gait and functional mobility.
   c. Activities of daily living.
   d. Job/recreational/athletic performance.
   e. Sense of well-being, posture, and self-image.

Guidelines to Develop Strength

1. Overload principle: to increase strength, the muscle must be loaded or challenged beyond its current force capability. Higher levels of tension will cause hypertrophy and recruitment of muscle fibers. This level will change with each adaptation.
2. Specificity of training: adaptations in the metabolic and physiological systems of the body depending on the type of overload imposed. Specific modes of exercise elicit specific adaptations, creating specific training effects.
3. Reversibility: benefits of training are not sustained unless muscles are continuously challenged. Detraining effects include decreased muscle recruitment and muscle fiber atrophy.
4. Metabolic effects of strength training.
   a. Muscle contraction to about 60% of its force-generating capacity causes a blockage of blood flow to the working muscle due to increased intramuscular pressure. The energy source for this level of muscle contraction is mainly anaerobic and does not improve with aerobic conditioning.
   b. Strength training of specific muscles has a brief activation period and uses a relatively small muscle mass, producing less cardiovascular metabolic demands than vigorous exercise, e.g., walking, running, swimming.
   c. Rhythmic activities increase blood flow to exercising muscles via a contraction and relaxation "milking action." The primary energy source is aerobic.
   d. Circuit training (cross-training) with high repetitions and low weights incorporates all modes of training and provides more general conditioning to improve body composition, muscular strength, and some cardiovascular fitness.
5. Common errors associated with resistance or strength training:
   a. Valsalva's maneuver: forcible exhalation with the glottis, nose, and mouth closed while contraction is being held. Valsalva's maneuver increases intrathoracic pressure, slows heart rate (HR), decreases return of blood to the heart, and increases venous pressure and cardiac work.
   b. Inadequate rest after vigorous exercise. Three to 4 minutes are needed to return the muscle to 90%–95% of preexercise capacity. Most rapid recovery occurs in the first minute.
   c. Increasing exercise progression too quickly (intensity, duration, frequency) can overwork muscles and cause injuries.
   d. Substitute motions occur from too much resistance, incorrect stabilization, and when muscles are weak from fatigue, paralysis, or pain.

Exercises to Improve Strength and Range

1. Manual resistance: a type of active exercise in which another person provides resistance.
   a. Advantages.
      - Useful in the early stages of an exercise program when the muscle is weak. The therapist can judge the capability of muscle to safely meet demands of exercise.
      - Can be modified for a painful arc in the joint range of motion.
      - Safe resistance exercise when the joint movement needs to be carefully controlled and the resistance is mild to moderate.
      - Can be easily changed to include diagonal or functional patterns of movement (e.g., proprioceptive neuromuscular facilitation [PNF]) or appropriate facilitation techniques (e.g., quick stretch).
   b. Disadvantages.
      - The amount of resistance cannot be measured quantitatively.
      - It may be difficult to maintain the same resistance during the full joint ROM and to consistently repeat the same resistance.
      - The amount of resistance is limited by the strength of the therapist or caregiver.

2. Mechanical resistance: a type of active exercise in which resistance is applied through the use of equipment or mechanical apparatus.
   a. Advantages.
      - The amount of resistance can be measured quantitatively and increased over time.
      - Can be used when amounts of resistance are greater than the therapist can apply manually.
   b. Disadvantages.
      - Not easily modified to exercise in diagonal or functional patterns.
      - May not be safe if resistance needs to be carefully controlled or maintained at low levels.
3. Goals and indications for resistance exercise.
   a. Increase strength in a muscle group that lifts, lowers, or controls heavy loads for relatively low number of repetitions.
   b. Increase muscular endurance by performing low-intensity repetitive exercise over a prolonged period.
   c. Improve muscular performance related to strength and speed of movement.
4. Precautions.
   a. Local muscle fatigue is a normal response of the muscle from repeated dynamic or static contractions over a period of time. Fatigue is due to depleted energy stores, insufficient oxygen, and build-up of lactic acid. It is characterized by a decline in peak torque and increased muscle pain with occasional spasm and decreased active ROM (AROM).
   b. General muscular fatigue affects the whole body after prolonged activities such as walking or jogging; usually due to low blood sugar, decreased glycogen stores in muscle and liver, depletion of potassium.
   c. Fatigue may be associated with specific clinical diseases; e.g., multiple sclerosis, cardiac disease, peripheral vascular dysfunction, and pulmonary diseases. These patients fatigue more rapidly and require longer rest periods.
   d. Overwork or overtraining causes temporary or permanent loss of strength as a result of exercise. In normal individuals, fatigue causes discomfort, so overtraining and muscle weakness does not usually occur. Patients with lower motor neuron disease who participate in vigorous resistance exercise programs can have a deterioration of strength; e.g., postpolio syndrome. Overwork can be avoided with slow progression of the exercise intensity, duration, and progression.
   e. Osteoporosis makes the bone unable to withstand normal stresses and highly susceptible to pathological fracture. May develop as a result of prolonged immobilization, bed rest, inability to bear weight on an extremity, and nutritional or hormonal factors.
   f. Acute muscle soreness develops during or directly after strenuous anaerobic exercise performed to the point of fatigue. Decreased blood flow and reduced oxygen (ischemia) creates a temporary build-up of lactic acid and potassium. A cool-down period of low-intensity exercise can facilitate the return of oxygen to the muscle and reduce soreness.
   g. Delayed-onset muscle soreness (DOMS) can begin 12–24 hours after vigorous exercise or muscular overexertion. Peaks at 24–48 hours after exercise. Muscle tenderness and stiffness can last up to 5–7 days. Usually greater after muscle lengthening or eccentric exercise. Severity of soreness can be lessened by gradually increasing the intensity and duration of exercises.
5. **CONTRAINDICATIONS.**
   a. Inflammation: resistance exercises can increase swelling and cause damage to muscles or joints.
   b. Pain: severe joint or muscle pain during exercise or for more than 24 hours after exercise requires elimination or reduction of the exercise.

Types of Resistance Exercise

Isometric Exercise
1. Is a static exercise that occurs when a muscle contracts without a length change (Table 1-1).
2. Resistance is variable and accommodating to patient ability. Contractions are held for at least 6 seconds to obtain adaptive changes in the muscle.
   a. Strengthening of muscles is developed at a point in the ROM, not over the entire length of the muscle.
   b. This type of resistance exercise can increase blood pressure and should be used cautiously with the patient with a cardiac condition.
   c. Monitor for potential Valsalva's maneuver.

Isotonic Exercise
1. Is dynamic and can have a constant (free weights) or variable (machine) load as the muscle lengthens or shortens through the available ROM. Speed can be variable for this type of exercise.
   a. Weight-lifting machines have an oval shaped cam or wheel that mimics the length-tension curve of the muscle; e.g., Nautilus or Cybex. These machines vary resistance as the muscle goes through the ROM, providing resistance that the muscle can safely complete at various points of the ROM.
   b. Free weights do not vary the resistance through the ROM of a muscle. The weakest point along the length-tension curve of each muscle limits the amount of weight lifted.

60°–120° = painful arc for Rotator Cuff Tendonitis

Table 1-1

Types of Resistance Exercises

TYPE	DESCRIPTION	TECHNIQUE	BENEFITS	PRECAUTIONS/CONTRAINDICATIONS
Isometric	Static muscle contraction No change in muscle length	Patient holds contraction for at least 6 seconds.	Strengthens muscle at a specific point in the ROM	Can cause an increase in blood pressure Monitor for Valsalva's maneuver
Isotonic	Dynamic muscle contraction Constant or variable resistance Concentric and eccentric contractions	Patient moves a resistance through a range of motion. Uses weight lifting machines, free-weights, manual resistance, theraband, etc.	Constant resistance primarily strengthens muscle at the weakest point in the range. Variable resistance strengthens muscle throughout the range of motion utilized.	Incorrect use of machines or free weights can lead to injury.
Isokinetic	Dynamic muscle contraction Speed controlled Resistance is variable and accommodating	Use of isokinetic equipment	Provides maximum resistance at all points of the range of motion	No additional precautions other than those for all resistive exercises
Eccentric	Dynamic lengthening contraction Constant or variable resistance	For weakened muscles, the clinician places the muscle in a shorted position and has the patient lower the extremity with gravity. For stronger muscles, can use hand weights through same procedure or isokinetic equipment	Eccentric contractions require less energy than concentric contraction. Useful for muscles that are unable to perform a concentric contraction Useful to prepare muscles for functional activities such as stand to sit	More apt to cause DOMS when working max contractions

c. Weight-lifting machines are safer than free weights; used early in a resistance exercise or rehabilitation program.

Isokinetic Exercise

1. Is dynamic and has a speed control for muscle shortening and lengthening. Resistance is accommodating and variable.
   a. Peak torque, the maximum force generated through the ROM, is inversely related to angular velocity (speed) as the body segment moves through ROM; e.g., increasing angular velocity decreases peak torque production.
   b. Concentric or eccentric resistance exercise can be performed on isokinetic equipment.
   c. Isokinetic exercise provides maximum resistance at all points in the ROM as the muscle contracts.
   d. During isokinetic testing, the weight of a body segment creates a torque output around the joint; e.g., the lower leg around the knee joint in sitting knee flexion. This gravity-produced torque adds to the force generated by the muscle when it contracts and gives a higher torque output than is actually created by the muscle. The higher value can affect the testing values of the muscle group and which muscle group needs to be strengthened. Software can correct for the effects of gravity.

Eccentric versus Concentric Exercise

1. Eccentric exercise—muscle is working as it lengthens.
2. Concentric exercise—muscle is working as it shortens.
   a. Maximum eccentric contraction produces more force than maximal concentric contraction.
   b. Resistance training performed concentrically improves concentric muscle strength, and eccentric training improves eccentric muscle strength (specificity of training).
   c. Eccentric contractions occur in a wide variety of functional activities, such as lowering the body against gravity; e.g., sitting down or descending stairs.
   d. Eccentric contractions provide a source of shock absorption during closed-chain functional activities.
   e. Eccentric contractions consume less oxygen and fewer energy stores than concentric contractions against similar loads.

Other Exercise Considerations

1. Range of motion.
   a. Short-arc exercise: resistance exercise performed through a limited ROM; e.g., initial exercise post–knee surgery (anterior cruciate repair), painful full-range movement.

b. Full-arc exercise: resistance exercise performed through full ROM.
2. Open-versus closed-chain exercises.
   a. Open-chain exercise occurs when the distal segment (hand or foot) moves freely in space; e.g., when an arm lifts or lowers a hand-held weight.
   b. Resistance exercises usually are open chain, which may be the only option if weight bearing is contraindicated.
   c. Open-chain exercise does not adequately prepare a patient for functional weight-bearing activities.
   d. Closed-chain exercise occurs when the body moves over a fixed distal segment; e.g., stair climbing or squatting activities.
   e. Closed-chain exercise loads muscles, bones, joints, and noncontractile soft tissues such as ligaments, tendons, and joint capsules.
   f. Mechanoreceptors are stimulated by closed-chain exercises, adding to joint stability, balance, coordination, and agility in functional weight-bearing postures.

Specific Exercise Regimens

1. Progressive resistive exercise (PRE): uses the repetition maximum (RM), or the greatest amount of weight a muscle can move through the ROM a specific number of times (e.g., DeLorme used 10 RM as baseline). Three sets of 10 repetitions are completed with brief rests (1–2 minutes) between sets. Progression (DeLorme): exercise begins with 10 repetitions at 50% RM, followed by 10 repetitions at 75% RM, and finally 10 repetitions at 100% RM (Table 1-2).
2. Circuit weight training: a sequence of exercises for total-body conditioning. A rest period of usually 30 seconds to 1 minute is taken between each exercise. Exercises can be done with free weights or weight-training machines.
3. Plyometric training, or stretch-shortening activity: an isotonic exercise that combines speed, strength, and functional activities. Used in later stages of rehabilitation to achieve high level of performance; e.g., jumping off of a platform, then up onto the platform at a rapid pace to improve vertical jumping abilities.
4. Brief, repetitive isometric exercise: occurs with up to 20 maximum contractions held for 5–6 seconds and performed daily. A 20-second rest after each contraction is recommended to prevent increases in blood pressure. Strength gains occur in 6 weeks.

Endurance Training

Muscular Endurance Strategies

1. Muscular endurance: the ability of an isolated muscle group to perform repeated contractions over time.
2. Muscular endurance is improved by performing low-load resistance exercise for many repetitions. Exercise programs that increase strength also increase muscular endurance.
3. Muscular endurance programs are indicated after injuries to joints and soft tissues. Dynamic exercises at a high number of repetitions against light resistance are more comfortable and create less joint irritation than heavy resistance exercises.
4. Early in a strength-training program, high repetitions and low-load exercises cause less muscle soreness and reduce the risk of muscle injury.

Cardiovascular Endurance Strategies

1. Cardiovascular endurance: the ability to perform large-muscle, dynamic exercise, such as walking, swimming, and/or biking, for long periods of time.
2. Overload principle: used to enhance physiological improvement and bring about a training change. Specific exercise overload must be applied.
   a. Training adaptation occurs by exercising at a level above normal.
   b. The appropriate overload for each person can be achieved by manipulating combinations of training frequency, intensity, and duration.
3. Specificity principle: adaptations in the metabolic and physiological systems, depending on the type of overload imposed.
   a. Specific exercise elicits specific adaptations, creating specific training effects; e.g., swim training will increase cardiovascular conditioning only when tested in swimming. There is not crossover for conditioning from swimming to running.

Table 1-2

Resistance Training Specificity Chart

RELATIVE LOADING	OUTCOME	% 1 RM	REPETITION RANGE	# OF SETS	REST BETWEEN SETS
Light	Muscular endurance	<70	12–20	1–3	20–30 seconds
Moderate	Hypertrophy and strength	70–80	8–12	1–6	30–120 seconds
Heavy	Maximum strength	80–100	1–8	1–5+	2–5 minutes

Training Programs

4. Individual differences principle: training benefits are optimized when programs are planned to meet the individual needs and capacities of the participants.
5. Reversibility principle: detraining occurs rapidly, after only 2 weeks, when a person stops exercising. Beneficial effects of exercise training are transient and reversible.
6. FITT equation: includes factors that affect training; frequency, intensity, time, and type. Intensity is interrelated with both duration (time) and frequency. See Quick Facts 1-2.

Pulmonary Endurance Strategies

1. Pulmonary endurance is related to the ventilation of the lungs and oxygen consumption.
2. Ventilation is the process of air exchange in the lungs. The volume of air breathed each minute, or minute ventilation ($\dot{V}_E$), is 6 liters. $\dot{V}_E$ = breathing rate × tidal volume. In maximum exercise, increases in breathing rate and depth may produce ventilation as high as 200 liters per minute.
3. Energy is produced aerobically as oxygen is supplied to exercising muscles. Oxygen consumption

QUICK FACTS 1-2 ▶ FITT EQUATION

Parameter	Considerations	Variables
Frequency	The number of exercise sessions per week Training at lower intensities should be performed with greater frequency	• If intensity is constant, the benefit from two versus four or three versus five times/week is the same • For weight loss, 5–7 days/week increases the caloric expenditure more than 2 days/week • Exercise <2 days/week fails to produce adequate changes in aerobic capacity or body composition
Intensity (overload)	Primary method to improve cardiovascular endurance	• Relative intensity for an individual is calculated as a percentage of maximum function (e.g., maximum oxygen consumption [VO_2 max] or maximum heart rate [HR_{max}]) • The VO_2 max or HR_{max} can be measured directly or indirectly based on different methods (e.g., 3-minute step, 12-minute run, or 1-mile walk test) • HR_{max} can be estimated using 220 minus the age of the individual. Training level or target (THR) can be established at 70% of maximum to increase aerobic capacity. • Karvonen's formula is used to predict heart rate reserve (HRR) or HR_{max} minus the resting heart rate (RHR) and correlates directly to VO_2 max. THR = (HR_{max} – RHR) × % of desired training intensity + RHR. • Rating of perceived exertion (RPE) can be used to evaluate training at submaximal levels. A cardiorespiratory training effect can be achieved at a rating of "somewhat hard" or "hard" (13–16 on original Borg scale of 6–19). An appropriate level of training should result in conversational exercise or "tale test"; moderate exercise that is not too strenuous and can improve endurance.
Duration (time)	Can be used when fitness level is limited	• If initial fitness level is limited, increase duration to achieve effect. Improvements in aerobic capacity, therefore, depend on increasing exercise duration and frequency (e.g., 3–5 minutes per day produces training effects in poorly conditioned individuals, whereas 23–30 minutes, three to five times per week is optimal for conditioned people). • Multiple sessions of short durations are also indicated when intensity is limited by environmental conditions, such as heat and humidity or by medical conditions, such as intermittent claudication or congestive heart failure. • Obese individuals should exercise at longer durations and lower intensities. At this exercise level, the person can speak without gasping and does not have muscle ache or burn from lactic acid accumulation. • Obesity increases the mechanical work of the heart and can lead to cardiac and left ventricular dysfunction.
Type	Multiple types may be used	• To increase cardiovascular endurance select exercise to involve large muscle groups activated in rhythmic aerobic nature. • Specificity of training should be considered. • Additional information can be found in Chapter 4 for application to patients with cardiovascular conditions.

rises rapidly during the first minutes of exercise, and then levels off as the aerobic metabolism supplies the energy required by the working muscles (steady state).
4. The more fit a person is, the more capable their respiratory system is of delivering oxygen to sustain aerobic energy production at increasingly higher levels of intensity.
   a. Obesity can impair pulmonary function because of the added effort to move the chest wall.
5. In severe pulmonary disease, the cost of breathing can reach 40% of the total exercise oxygen consumption. This decreases the oxygen available to the exercising nonrespiratory muscles and limits exercise capabilities. Obesity can significantly increase the level of impairments.
6. Exercise-induced asthma (EIA) can occur when the normal initial bronchodilatation is followed by bronchoconstriction. The reduction in air-flow from airway obstruction affects the ability of the lungs to provide oxygen to exercising muscles.
   a. EIA is an acute, reversible airway obstruction that develops 5–15 minutes after strenuous exercise when a person does not breathe through the nose, which warms and humidifies the air.
   b. When a person mouth-breathes, the air is cold and dry, contributing to the bronchoconstriction.
   c. Lowering the intensity level and allowing the person to breathe through the nose can allow prolonged aerobic exercise to continue.
   d. The problem is rare in activities that require only short bursts of activity such as baseball, and is more likely to occur in endurance activities such as soccer.
   e. When exercising in humid versus dry environments, the exercise-induced asthmatic response is considerably reduced. See Chapter 5 for application with patients with pulmonary conditions.

Aerobic Training
1. Aerobic training (cardiorespiratory endurance training) can result in higher fitness levels for healthy individuals, slow the decrease in functional capacity in the elderly, and recondition those with illness or chronic disease.
2. Positive effects of aerobic training on the cardiovascular and respiratory systems.
   a. Improve breathing volumes and increased VO_2 max.
   b. Increase heart weight and volume; cardiac hypertrophy is normal with long-term aerobic training.
   c. Increase total hemoglobin and oxygen delivery capacity.
   d. Decrease resting and submaximal exercise heart rates. Can be utilized to measure improvements from aerobic training.
   e. Increase cardiac output and stroke volume.
   f. Improve distribution of blood to working muscles and enhanced capacity of trained muscles to extract and use oxygen.
   g. Reduce resting blood pressure.
3. Continuous training at a submaximal energy requirement can be prolonged for 20–60 minutes without exhausting the oxygen transport system.
   a. Work rate is increased progressively as training improvements are achieved; overload can be accomplished by increasing the exercise duration.
   b. In healthy individuals, continuous training is the most effective way to improve endurance.
4. Circuit training uses a series of exercise activities that are repeated several times.
   a. Several exercise modes can be utilized, involving large and small muscle groups both statically and dynamically.
   b. Circuit training improves endurance and strength by stressing the aerobic and anaerobic energy systems.
5. Interval training includes an exercise period followed by a prescribed rest interval. It is perceived to be less demanding than continuous training, and tends to improve strength and power more than endurance.
   a. The relief interval can be passive or active; its duration ranges from a few seconds to several minutes. Active or work recovery involves doing the exercise at a reduced level. During the relief period, a portion of the adenosine triphosphate (ATP) and oxygen used by the muscles during the work period is replenished by the aerobic system.
   b. The longer the work interval, the more the aerobic system is stressed.
   c. With appropriate spacing of work-relief intervals, a significant amount of high-intensity work can be achieved. The total amount of work completed with interval training is greater than the amount of work accomplished with continuous training.
6. Warm-up and cool-down periods: each exercise session includes a 5- to 15-minute warm-up and a 5- to 15-minute cool-down period.
   a. The warm-up period prevents the heart and circulatory system from being suddenly taxed. It includes low-intensity cardiorespiratory activities and flexibility exercises.
   b. The cool-down period also consists of exercising at a lower intensity. It reduces abrupt physiological alterations that can occur with sudden cessation of strenuous exercise; e.g., venous pooling in the lower extremities, which causes decreased venous return to the heart.
   c. Longer warm-up and cool-down periods may be needed for deconditioned or older individuals.

Common Training Errors to Avoid

1. Lack of exercise tolerance testing (ETT) before the exercise prescription is determined could result in a training program set too high or too low for that individual.
2. Starting out at too high a level can overly stress the cardiorespiratory and muscular systems and potentially cause injuries.
3. Increasing intensity too fast can create a problem for an individual during endurance training.
4. Exercising at too intense a level can use the anaerobic energy system, not the aerobic system; this increases strength and power, not endurance.
5. Insufficient warm-up or cool-down results in inadequate cardiorespiratory and muscular adaptation; there is inadequate time to prepare for or recover from higher intense activity.
6. Inconsistent training frequency, duration, or intensity does not properly stress or overload the aerobic system to create training effects.

Specific Weather Considerations

Exercising at High Altitudes

1. At altitudes of 6,000 feet (1,829 meters [m]) or higher, there can be a noticeable drop in performance of aerobic activities.
2. The partial pressure of oxygen is reduced, resulting in poor oxygenation of hemoglobin.
3. This hypoxia at altitude can result in immediate compensatory hyperventilation (stimulation of the baroreceptors) and increased heart rate.
4. Reduction in CO_2 from hyperventilation results in more alkaline body fluids.
5. Adjustments or acclimatization to higher altitude.
   a. Takes 2 weeks at 2,300 m and an additional week for every additional 600 m in altitude.
   b. There is a decrease in plasma volume (concentrating red blood cells) and an increase in total red blood cells and hemoglobin improving oxygenation.
   c. Changes in local circulation may facilitate oxygen transport.
   d. Adjustments do not fully compensate for altitude. VO_2 max is decreased 2% for every 300 m above 1,500 m. Thus, there is a drop in performance for endurance activities.
   e. Training at altitude does not provide any improvement in sea-level performance.
6. The air in mountainous regions tends to be cool and dry. Body fluids can be rapidly lost through evaporation and result in dehydration.
   a. Ensure adequate hydration for those exercising or engaged in sports at altitude.

Exercising in Hot Weather Conditions

1. When exercising in the heat, muscles require oxygen to produce energy.
2. To decrease metabolic heat, blood is shunted to the periphery; thus, working muscles are deprived of needed oxygen.

RED FLAG: Core temperature increases and sweating increases. Fluids must be continually replaced or core temperatures can rise to dangerous levels.

3. Hot, humid environments diminish the evaporative cooling component, even with profuse sweating. Excess fluid loss can compromise cardiovascular function.
4. Fluid replacement.
   a. Maintain plasma volume.
   b. Colder fluids are emptied from the stomach more rapidly than room-temperature fluids.
   c. Concentrated carbohydrate drinks impair gastric emptying and slow fluid replacement.
   d. Glucose-polymer drinks do not impair physiological functioning. They may also resupply lost electrolytes.
5. Repeated heat stress results in acclimatization in about 10 days of exposure.
   a. Exercise capacity is increased.
   b. Cardiac output is better regulated.
   c. Sweating is more efficient.
   d. Acclimatization to heat stress does not seriously deteriorate with age.
6. Men and women can adapt equally well to heat, even though the mechanisms of thermoregulation differ slightly. The menstrual cycle is not a factor.
7. Obesity is a major consideration when exercising in the heat.
8. Exercise recommendations for individuals with obesity (see Chapter 6).

Mobility and Flexibility Training

Flexibility

1. Flexibility refers to the ability to move a joint through an unrestricted, pain-free ROM; the musculotendinous unit elongates as the body segment moves through the ROM.
2. Dynamic flexibility refers to the active ROM of a joint, and is dependent upon the amount of tissue resistance met during active movement.
3. Passive flexibility is the degree to which a joint can be passively moved through the available ROM, and is dependent upon the extensibility of the muscle and connective tissue around the joint.

Stretching

1. Stretching involves any therapeutic technique that lengthens shortened soft-tissue structures and increases ROM.
2. Effective stretching must include positioning the joint such that the origin and insertion is near or at the end of its available range of motion.
   a. Stretching multi-joint muscles requires considering the range of motion of the muscle across both joints.
3. Type of stretching is determined by the type of force applied, the intensity of stretch, and duration of stretch to contractile and noncontractile tissues.
   a. Manual static, passive stretching takes the structures beyond the free ROM to elongate tissues beyond their resting length.
      - To be effective with lasting results, the stretch force should be applied for 30 seconds to 2 minutes and be repeated several times during a treatment session. It should be noted that research identifying optimal stretch "hold" times is highly variable.
      - Manual stretching is considered a short-duration stretch, and is maintained statically for less time than mechanical stretching.
      - Intensity and duration depend on patient tolerance and therapist strength and endurance.
      - Low-intensity manual stretch, applied as long as possible, is better tolerated and results in optimal improvement in tissue length with minimal risk of injury to any weakened tissue.

   > **RED FLAG:** Static stretching does diminish the torque producing ability of the muscle and is NOT INDICATED prior to sport or activity in non-injured tissue.

   b. Dynamic stretching is an active or passive stretch performed actively by moving joints, either in a body weighted or eliminated position, through available range of motion. Gradually increasing range and speed of movement as the musculature warms up.
      - Motion is controlled and is performed at moderate speed within available range of motion.
      - It DOES NOT diminish peak torque producing ability of muscles and IS MORE appropriately used prior to sport or activity than static stretching.
   c. Ballistic stretching is a high-frequency, short-duration "bouncing" stretch performed beyond the available range of motion. The stretch is performed by contracting the opposite muscle group, and/or using body weight and momentum.

   > **RED FLAG:** Ballistic stretching is considered unsafe to perform initially following surgery, with weakened or injured tissues, and in instances of poor neuromotor control. A potential of rupturing weakened tissues does exist with this technique.

   - Ballistic stretch facilitates the stretch reflex, causing an increase in tension in the muscle that is being stretched. Ballistic stretching may, in fact, be indicated prior to sport performance of a sport requiring ballistic movements.
   - It is contraindicated in spastic muscles.
   - Do not perform ballistic stretching on tissues that have not been warmed up.
   - Frequencies for the ballistic movements are highly variable.

   d. Prolonged mechanical stretching is a low-intensity, external force (5–15 lb to 10% of body weight) applied over a prolonged period by positioning a patient with weighted pulley and traction systems. Dynamic splints or serial casts may also be used.
      - Prolonged stretch may be maintained for 20–30 minutes or as long as several hours.
      - Dynamic splints are applied for 8–10 hours to increase ROM.
      - Low-intensity, prolonged mechanical stretching has been shown to be more effective than manual, passive stretching with long-standing flexion contractures.
   e. Active stretching occurs when voluntary, unassisted movement by the patient provides the stretch force to a joint. It requires strength and muscular contraction of the prime mover to actively stretch the antagonist muscle group.
      - The force is controlled by the patient and is considered low-intensity (to tolerance). The risk of tissue injury is low.
      - Duration is equal to passive, manual stretching, or about 15–30 seconds, and is limited by prime mover muscular endurance.
   f. Facilitated stretching (active inhibition) refers to techniques in which the patient reflexively relaxes the muscle to be elongated prior to or during the stretching technique; e.g., PNF.
      - Hold-relax (HR): a relaxation technique usually performed at the point of limited ROM in the agonist pattern; an isometric contraction of the range-limiting antagonist is performed against slowly increasing resistance, followed by voluntary relaxation, and passive movement by the therapist into the newly gained range of the agonist pattern. The muscle relaxes as a result of autogenic inhibition, possibly from the Golgi

tendon organ (GTO) firing and decreasing muscular tension.
- Hold-relax-active contraction (HRAC): following hold-relax technique, active contraction into the newly gained range of the agonist pattern is performed. The muscle is further relaxed through the inhibitory effects of reciprocal inhibition.
- Contract-relax-active contraction (CRAC): a relaxation technique usually performed at a point of limited ROM in the agonist pattern; isotonic movement in rotation is performed followed by an isometric hold of the range-limiting muscles in the antagonist pattern against slowly increasing resistance, voluntary relaxation, and active movement into the new range of the agonist pattern.
- Indications for active inhibition techniques include limitations in ROM caused by muscle tightness or muscle spasm. CR techniques may be more painful, especially if muscle cocontraction is present.

4. Contractile tissue.
   a. A muscle that is lengthened over a prolonged period will have an increase in the number of sarcomeres in series. The muscle will adjust its length over time.
   b. A muscle immobilized in a shortened position will have a decrease in the number of sarcomeres and an increase in connective tissue.
   c. The sarcomere adaptation is transient. A muscle allowed to resume its normal length will produce or absorb sarcomeres (lengthen or shorten).

5. Neurophysiological properties of contractile tissue.
   a. The muscle spindle monitors the velocity and length changes in muscle.
   b. A quick stretch to a muscle stimulates the alpha motoneurons and facilitates muscle contraction via the monosynaptic stretch reflex. This can increase tension in a muscle to be lengthened.
   c. The GTO inhibits contraction of the muscle. When excessive tension develops, the GTO fires, inhibiting alpha motoneuron activity and decreasing tension in the muscle.
   d. Slow stretching, especially applied at end range, causes the GTO to fire and inhibit the muscle (autogenic inhibition), allowing the muscle to lengthen (stretch-protection reflex).

6. Noncontractile connective tissue, including ligaments, tendons, joint capsules, fasciae and skin, can affect joint flexibility and requires remodeling to increase length.
   a. Low-magnitude loads over long periods increase the deformation of noncontractile tissue, allowing a gradual rearrangement of collagen bonds (remodeling). This type of stretch is better tolerated by the patient.
   b. 15–20 minutes of low-intensity sustained stretch, repeated on five consecutive days, can cause a change in the length of muscles and connective tissue.
   c. Intensive stretching is usually not done every day in order to allow time for healing. Without healing time, a breakdown of tissue will occur, as in overuse syndromes and stress fractures.
   d. With aging, collagen loses its elasticity and tissue blood supply is decreased, reducing healing capability. Stretching in older adults should be performed cautiously.

7. Overstretch is a stretch well beyond the normal joint ROM, resulting in hypermobility. If the supporting structures of a joint are insufficient and weak, they cannot hold a joint in a stable, functional position during functional activities. This is known as stretch weakness.

8. Contracture is the adaptive shortening of muscle or other soft tissues that cross a joint; contracture results in decreased ROM.
   a. Myostatic contracture (pertaining to muscle) involves a musculotendinous unit that has adaptively shortened with loss of ROM. Usually occurs without specific tissue pathology and in two-joint muscles such as the hamstrings, rectus femoris, or gastrocnemius. Can typically be resolved in a short time with gentle stretching exercises and active inhibition techniques.
   b. Adhesions can occur if tissue is immobilized in a shortened position for extended periods of time, resulting in a loss of mobility.
   c. Scar tissue adhesions develop due to injury and the inflammatory response. Initially, new fibers develop in a disorganized pattern and will restrict motion unless remodeled along lines of stress; e.g., the patient with burns.
   d. Irreversible contracture: a permanent loss of soft tissue extensibility that cannot be released by nonsurgical treatment. Occurs when normal soft tissue is replaced by an excessive amount of nonextensible tissue, such as bone or fibrotic tissue.

Relaxation of Muscles

1. Local relaxation techniques can assist in the lengthening of contractile and noncontractile tissue.
2. Heat increases the extensibility of the shortened tissues. Warm muscles relax and lengthen more easily, reducing the discomfort of stretching. Connective tissue stretches with less force and shorter duration.
   a. GTO sensitivity is increased, making it more likely to fire and inhibit muscle tension.
   b. Low-intensity active exercise performed prior to stretching will increase circulation to soft tissue and warm the tissues to be stretched.

c. Heat without stretching has little or no effect on long-term improvement in muscle flexibility. The combination of heat and stretching produces greater long-term gains in tissue length than stretching alone.
3. Massage increases local circulation to the muscle and reduces muscle spasm and stiffness.
4. Biofeedback helps the patient reduce the amount of tension in a muscle and improves flexibility while decreasing pain. Increased level of feedback signals (auditory, visual) assists the patient in recognizing tense muscles.

Common Errors in Mobility and Flexibility Training

1. Passively forcing a joint beyond its normal ROM.
2. Aggressively stretching a patient with a newly united fracture or osteoporosis may result in fracture.
3. Using high-intensity, short-duration (ballistic) stretching procedures on muscles and connective tissues that have been immobilized over a long time or recovering from injury or surgery.
4. Stretching muscles around joints without using strengthening exercises to develop an appropriate balance between flexibility and strength.
5. Overstretching of weak muscles, especially postural muscles that support the body against gravity.
6. Failure to properly stabilize the affected and adjacent joints while applying the stretch can result in an ineffective stretch, or stretch to the incorrect segment, e.g., standing hip flexor stretch performed with the lumbar spine hyperextended or the gastric stretch performed with the knee in the flexed position.

Postural Stability Training

Stability (Static Postural Control)

1. Refers to the synergistic coordination of the neuromuscular system that enables an individual to maintain a stable position in an antigravity, weight-bearing position.
2. Postural stability control involves prolonged holding of core muscles.

Dynamic Stabilization, Controlled Mobility

1. Proximal segments and trunk provide a stable base for functional movements.
   a. An individual maintains postural stability of the trunk while weight shifting.
   b. Distal segments are fixed, while proximal segments are moving.
   c. Movement normally occurs through increments of range (small range to large range).
2. Patients with hyperkinetic movement disorders (e.g., ataxia) should be progressed from large range to small range movements, and finally to holding steady (stability control).

Dynamic Stabilization, Static-Dynamic Control

1. An individual maintains postural stability of the trunk during dynamic extremity movements (e.g., reaching, kicking a ball).
2. Strength, endurance, flexibility, and coordination are needed for static and dynamic stabilization.

Guidelines to Develop Postural Stability

1. Core musculature: Consider exercise protocols that effectively challenge core muscle groups and create adequate stability to perform functional activities. Stability requires the recruitment of tonic, slow-twitch muscle fibers for sustained periods of time.
2. Initiation of training: Start training by teaching safe spinal ROM in a variety of basic postures. Teach chin tucking with axial extension of the cervical spine and pelvic tilting with ROM of the lumbar spine.
3. Kinesthetic awareness: Incorporate procedures to retrain kinesthetic awareness of postural position. Teach the neutral pelvis position first to ensure a stable base.
   a. Emphasis is placed on strength and endurance of back multifidi and oblique abdominals rather than erector spinae.
   b. Focus patient's awareness on normal alignment of the spine and pelvis, and on muscles required to maintain that position.
   c. Visual, verbal, and proprioceptive cues, e.g., resistance of elastic bands or light manual resistance, can be used to improve postural awareness.
4. To safely develop strength and endurance in the stabilizing muscles, practice maintained holding in a variety of postures. The higher the center of mass (COM) and smaller the base of support (BOS), the greater the degree of postural challenge; e.g., sitting versus standing.
5. Movements of the extremities challenge trunk and neck stabilization; functional position must be maintained as movements are carried out.
6. Resistance can be applied to the trunk or the moving extremities; functional position must be maintained as resistance is increased.
7. Alternating isometric contractions between antagonists can enhance stabilizing contractions and develop postural control.
   a. Stabilizing reversals: isometric holding is facilitated first on one side of the joint, followed by alternate holding of the antagonist muscle groups. May be applied in a variety of directions; e.g., anterior-posterior, medial-lateral, diagonal.

b. Rhythmic stabilization (RS): simultaneous isometric contractions of both agonist and antagonist patterns performed without relaxation, using careful grading of resistance; results in cocontraction of opposing muscle groups; RS emphasizes rotational stability control.
8. During early training, emphasize muscles needed for trunk support in the upright posture, for performing basic body mechanics, and for upper extremity lifting.
9. Teach control of functional positions while moving from one position to another. This is called transitional stabilization and requires graded contractions and adjustments between the trunk flexors and extensors. Consider moving out of a posture (eccentric control) before moving into a posture (concentric control).
10. Introduce simple patterns of motion that develop safe body mechanics and movement.
11. Closed-chain tasks are good choices to enhance postural stabilization (e.g., partial squats and controlled lunges); add arm motions and weights as tolerated.
12. More complex patterns of movement (e.g., rotation and diagonal motions) can be added (e.g., PNF trunk patterns of chop/reverse chop, or lift/reverse lift). Postures can be progressed to add difficulty (e.g., supine to sitting to standing).
13. Incorporate stretching into the postural exercise program. Adequate flexibility is necessary for postural muscles to hold body parts in proper alignment.

Common Errors in Postural Stability Training

1. Inadequate stretching of tight muscles (e.g., tight hip flexors that hold the pelvis in an anterior pelvic tilt or tight hamstrings that hold the pelvis in a posterior tilt); both prevent a stable postural base (neutral pelvis and spine position).
2. Inadequate control of core muscles could place excessive stress on proximal structures during functional activities; e.g., the vertebrae and discs of the spine during sitting.
3. Progressing too quickly or starting at too high a functional level for the patient to maintain postural stability.
4. Exercising past the point of fatigue, which is determined by the inability of the trunk or neck muscles to stabilize the spine in its functional position.
5. Attempting to force a patient into a general neutral position instead of finding the proper and safe position for each individual.

Stability Ball Training

1. Stability balls are commonly known as a Swiss ball, physio ball, or therapy ball.
2. Benefits and uses for.
   a. Promotes balance; provides an unstable base of support, requiring continuous adjustments in balance. Moving the feet and/or the ball changes the base of support and challenges balance. Allows safe practice of falling.
   b. Works muscles in functional, synergistic patterns.
      - Recruits and retrains core muscles (deep spinal and abdominal muscles).
      - Promotes postural relearning; e.g., neutral position in sitting, cervical, or trunk rotation.
      - Enhances coordination, movement combinations; e.g., arm and leg bilateral symmetrical, bilateral asymmetrical movements, four-limb Mexican hat dance.
   c. Heightens proprioception and sensory perception, awareness of the body moving in space.
   d. Improves range of motion, allows safe stretching; e.g., total body extension or flexion, upper or lower extremity stretches.
   e. Allows relaxation training; e.g., gentle bouncing combined with deep breathing. Gentle rocking can be used to decrease tone in hypertonic patient.
   f. Allows a safe, dynamic cardiovascular workout; e.g., dynamic bouncing with extremity movements.
   g. Increases strength. Can be combined with resistance training (e.g., lifting the ball with arms or legs), using hand weights or resistive bands while on the ball, or closed chain exercises (e.g., partial squats using the ball).
   h. Has been used to replace chairs in schools; improves posture and concentration, calms hyperactive children.
3. Advantages: light, portable, durable, and inexpensive.
4. Determining appropriate ball size.
   a. Sitting on ball with feet flat, the ball height should place the hips and knees at 90° angles.
   b. Supine with ball under knees, the ball height should equal the distance between the greater trochanter and the knee.
   c. Quadruped, the ball height should equal the distance between the shoulder and the wrist.
5. Firmness/inflation.
   a. Ball should be comfortable and have some bounce.
   b. A firm ball moves more quickly.
   c. A soft ball moves more slowly, may make patient feel safer, more secure.
   d. Surface affects movement of the ball: quicker on hard surface, slower on mat or soft surface.

6. Precautions.
   a. Obese individuals, exceeding ball weight limits.
   b. Avoid sharp belt buckles, zippers when over the ball; check surface for sharp objects.
   c. Lack of foot traction, feet slipping: use bare feet, rubber-soled shoes, or yoga sticky mat.
   d. Requires adequate space around exercising individual.
   e. Watch for sensory overload: sympathetic signs (e.g., children, adults with traumatic brain injury).
   f. Increased pain with mobility exercises and degenerative joint disease.
   g. Muscle fatigue.
7. Contraindications.
   a. Dizziness or nausea associated with vestibular pathology.
   b. Extreme anxiety or fear of being on the ball.

Coordination and Balance Training

Goals and Outcomes

1. Motor function (motor control and learning) is improved.
2. Postural control, biomechanical alignment, and symmetrical weight distribution are improved.
3. Strength, power, and endurance necessary for movement control and balance are improved.
4. Sensory control and integration of sensory systems (somatosensory, visual, and vestibular) necessary for movement control and balance are improved.
5. Performance, independence, and safety are improved in transfers, gait, and locomotion.
6. Performance, independence, and safety are improved in basic activities of daily living (BADL) and instrumental activities of daily living (IADL).
7. Aerobic capacity and endurance are improved.
8. Self-management of symptoms is improved.

Training Strategies for Coordination and Balance

1. Motor learning strategies are important to assist the central nervous system (CNS) in adaptation for movement control.
   a. Learning requires repetition. Practice schedules should be carefully organized. Initial practice may feel threatening to patient; e.g., patient may feel in danger of losing control or balance. Progression should be gradual; the therapist should ensure patient confidence and safety, continuing motivation.
   b. Sensory cues are used to enhance motor performance.
   c. Feedback should stress knowledge of results (KR). Attention is drawn to the success of the outcome. It is important to establish a reference of correctness during early, cognitive learning.
   d. Feedback should address knowledge of performance (KP). Attention is drawn to missing elements, how to recruit, correct responses, and sequence responses.
   e. Feedback schedules: feedback given frequently (after every trial) improves initial performance. Feedback given less frequently (summed after a given number of trials or fading with decreasing frequency) improves retention of skills.
   f. A variety of activities and environments should be used to promote adaptability and generalizability of skills. Practice is from a closed environment (fixed) to open variable environments.
   g. Patient decision-making skills are promoted.
2. Remedial strategies focus on use of involved body segments (e.g., affected extremities in the patient with stroke).
   a. Control is first developed in isolated movements and progressed to more complex movements. Developmental postures/functional activities can be used to isolate body segments and focus on specific body skills (e.g., weight shifts to improve hip control are practiced first in kneeling before standing).
   b. Control is first achieved in holding (stability) before moving in a posture (stability-dynamic control) and skill level function (e.g., gait).
   c. Specific techniques can be used to remediate impairments (weakness, incoordination, and adaptive shortening, abnormal tone); e.g., tapping to improve responses of a weak quadriceps in standing position.
   d. As quality of movement improves, speed of movement and control are increased.
   e. Active responses and active learning should be promoted; progression is to unassisted or unfacilitated movements as soon as possible.
3. Compensatory strategies are utilized as appropriate to promote safety and early resumption of functional skills; e.g., the patient with delayed or absent recovery, multiple comorbidities. Compensatory training may lead to learned nonuse of impaired extremities and delay recovery in those patients with recovery potential; e.g., the patient with stroke.
   a. Safety is improved by substitution: intact segments (sound limbs) for impaired segments; cognitive control for impaired motor control; e.g., the patient with ataxia.
   b. Safety is improved by altering postural strategies; e.g., widening the BOS and lowering the COM.
   c. Safety is improved by use of appropriate assistive devices and shoes; e.g., weighted walker, athletic shoe.
   d. Safety is improved through environmental adaptations; e.g., handrails, adequate lighting, contrast tape on stairs, and removal of throw rugs.

Interventions to Improve Coordination

1. Functional training.
   a. Initial focus is on postural stability activities: holding.
      - A number of different weight-bearing postures can be used; e.g., prone-on-elbows, sitting, quadruped, kneeling, plantigrade, and standing. Progression is to gradually decrease BOS while raising height of COM.
      - Specific exercise techniques to enhance stability include stabilizing reversals and rhythmic stabilization.
      - Use dynamic reversals by decreasing ROM with ataxic movements.
   b. Progress to controlled mobility activities: weight shifting through decrements (decreasing) ROM progressing to stability (steady holding); moving in and out of postures (movement transitions).
      - Specific exercise techniques include dynamic reversals by increasing ROM.
      - PNF patterns can be utilized to enhance synergistic control and reciprocal action of muscles; can be used to modulate timing and force output.
   c. Aquatic exercises: water increases proprioceptive loading, slows down ataxic movements, provides buoyancy and light resistance.
   d. Stabilization devices (e.g., air splints, soft neck collars, stabilize body segments and eliminate unwanted movement).
   e. Environment: patients with ataxia do better in a low-stimulus environment; allows better utilization of cognitive strategies.
2. Sensory training.
   a. Patients with proprioceptive losses.
      - Visual compensation strategies (e.g., exercises in which position is varied from supine to sitting to standing); movements are guided visually.
      - Light weights: wrist cuffs, ankle cuffs, weighted walkers, elastic resistance bands to increase proprioceptive loading.
   b. Patients with visual losses benefit from a combination of cognitive training strategies along with environmental adaptations and assistive devices.

Interventions to Improve Balance

1. Exercises to improve ROM, strength, and synergistic responses in order to withstand challenges to balance.
   a. "Kitchen sink exercises": heel-cord stretches, heel rises, toe-offs, partial wall squats, single-leg activities (side kicks, back kicks), marching in place, look-arounds (head and trunk rotation), hip circles. Progression from bilateral upper extremity (UE) touch-down support to unilateral UE support to no UE support.
   b. Postural awareness training: focus on control of body position, centering the COM within the limits of stability (LOS).
   c. Weight shifts (postural sway): training of ankle strategies, hip strategies. Can include postural sway biofeedback (e.g., Balance Master).
   d. Training of change-of-support strategies: stepping strategies (forward, backward, sideward, crossed-step); UE reaching and protective extension.
2. Functional training activities.
   a. Sit-to-stand (STS) and sit-down (SIT) activities. Practice moving body mass forward over BOS, extending lower extremities (LEs), and raising body mass over feet and reverse. Focus on balance control while pivoting body mass over feet.
   b. Floor-to-standing rises. Practice rising from floor to standing in the event of a fall; e.g., side-sit to quadruped to kneeling to half-kneeling to standing transitions.
   c. Gait activities: practice walking forward, backward, sideward; slow to fast; normal BOS to narrowed BOS; wide turns to the right and left; 360° turns; head turns right and left; crossed-step walking and braiding; over and around obstacles.
   d. Elevation activities: practice step-ups, lateral step-ups, stair climbing, and ramps.
   e. Dual-task training. In standing or walking, practice simultaneous UE activities (e.g., bouncing a ball, catching or throwing a ball); in standing, practice LE activities (e.g., kicking a ball, tracing letters with one foot).
   f. Community activities. Practice walking in open (variable) environments; e.g., pushing or pulling doors, car transfers, grocery shopping.
   g. Practice anticipatory timing activities; e.g., getting on/off elevator, escalator.
3. Disturbed balance activities, including manual perturbations, moveable BOS devices (stability ball, wobble board, split foam roller, dense foam).
   a. Carefully grade force of perturbations, range, and speed of movements.
   b. Stability ball training. Practice sitting, active weight shifts (e.g., pelvic clock), UE movements (e.g., arm circles, reaching), LE movements (e.g., stepping, marching), trunk movements (e.g., head and trunk turns).
   c. Wobble board/equilibrium boards. Practice both self-initiated and therapist-initiated shifts in sitting or standing. Gradually increase range and speed of shifts.
4. Sensory training.
   a. Visual changes. Practice standing and walking, eyes open (EO) to eyes closed (EC); full lighting to reduced lighting.
   b. Somatosensory changes. Practice standing and walking on tile floor to carpet (low pile to high), dense foam, outside terrain.

c. Vestibular changes. Practice standing, walking, and moving head side-to-side, up-and-down; on a moving surface (e.g., escalator, elevator, bus).
d. Introduce sensory conflict situations (e.g., standing on foam cushion with eyes closed).
5. Safety education/fall prevention.
a. Assist patient in identification of fall risk factors; e.g., effect of medications, postural hypotension.
b. Lifestyle counseling: assist patient in recognizing unsafe activities, harmful effects of a sedentary lifestyle (see Chapter 8).

Interventions to Improve Aerobic Capacity and Muscular Endurance

1. Treadmill walking: Focus on velocity control; progression is from slow to fast. Safety harness can be worn to provide partial body weight support (BWS) if patient is unstable.
2. Ergometers. Pace pedaling on a cycle ergometer; progression is from slow to fast. Resistance and distance can also be modified. Can include both LE and UE training.
3. Strength training.
a. Active/active assistive exercise.
b. Manual resistance; PNF patterns can be used to promote synergistic control, improve timing.
c. Weights, pulleys, hydraulics, elastic resistance bands, mechanical or electromechanical devices.
4. Stretching exercises.
5. Teach activity pacing and energy conservation strategies as appropriate.
a. The patient with ataxia has increased energy expenditure and can experience debilitating fatigue.

Relaxation Training

Relaxation

1. Relaxation refers to a conscious effort to relieve excess tension in muscles.
a. Excess muscle tension can cause pain leading to muscle spasm, which in turn produces more pain. To break the pain/spasm cycle, patients must learn to relax tense muscles.
b. Excess tension in tissues can result from maintaining a constant posture or sustaining muscle contractions for a period of time. Abnormal shortening or lengthening of muscles and ligaments is termed postural stress syndrome (PSS).
c. Habituation of compensatory movement patterns that contribute to the persistence of pain is termed movement adaptation syndrome (MAS).
2. Awareness of prolonged muscle tension is accompanied by techniques designed to promote relaxation, improve circulation, and maintain flexibility.

Training Strategies to Promote Relaxation

1. Start with the patient in a comfortable resting position, with all body parts well supported.
2. Jacobson's progressive relaxation technique includes a systematic distal to proximal progression of conscious contraction and relaxation of musculature.
a. A period of reflex relaxation follows active contraction of muscle. The stronger the contraction, the greater the relaxation.
b. Breathing control: deep breathing coupled with the progressive relaxation to further promote relaxation. In diaphragmatic breathing, the patient breathes in slowly and deeply through the nose, allowing the abdomen to expand and then relax. This allows air to be expired through the relaxed, open mouth.
3. Cognitive strategies/guided imagery: the patient is instructed to focus on relaxing the body, visualizing calmness and relaxation.
a. Patient focuses on letting go of all muscular effort, letting tension melt away.
b. Patient focuses on a relaxing environment or pleasant images to promote relaxation; e.g., lying on a tropical beach in the warm sunshine.
4. Active range of motion: AROM can be used to reduce tension by moving body segments slowly.
5. Rhythmic rotation (RRo) involves slow, passive, rotational movements of the limbs or trunk, and can be very effective in relieving muscular tension and spasticity; e.g., hooklying with both feet flat or with the LEs placed on a stability ball, gently rocking the knees from side-to-side.
6. Slow vestibular stimulation: applied with gentle rocking techniques; can also be used to enhance relaxation, e.g., gentle rocking of the infant with colic.
7. Biofeedback training can be an effective modality to promote relaxation; e.g., training to reduce the level of tension in the frontalis muscle.
8. Stress management/lifestyle adaptation techniques.
a. Careful identification and evaluation of life stressors is critical in developing an appropriate plan of care to reduce chronic stress.
b. Assessment scales used: Life Events Scale, Holmes-Rahe Social Readjustment Scale, Hassles Scale.
c. Lifestyle modification reduces frequency of high-stress situations and events. It is important to ensure adequate rest, activity, and nutrition.
d. Enhance coping skills: ensure that the patient maintains some level of control and decision making.
e. Maximize effective use of social support systems.

Common Errors in Relaxation Training

1. Lack of awareness of the effects of the environment on an individual. Failure to have the patient in a low-stress environment and comfortably positioned.

2. Lack of awareness of stress factors affecting the patient. Failure to evaluate stressors carefully and incorporate stress-management techniques.
3. When using progressive relaxation techniques, progressing too fast from one body segment to another; e.g., distal to proximal body parts. Failure to combine slow deep breaths with each contraction and relaxation.
4. Lack of effective training of kinesthetic awareness. Patients do not recognize when their muscles are tense. They perceive the tense muscle as normal, not needing any relaxation intervention.

Aquatic Exercise

Goals and Outcomes
1. Improvements in body function and structure:
    a. Motor function and learning.
    b. ROM and flexibility.
    c. Postural control, biomechanical alignment, and symmetrical weight distribution.
    d. Strength, power, and endurance.
    e. Sensory control and integration of sensory systems (somatosensory, visual, and vestibular).
2. Improvements in activities and participation:
    a. Performance, independence, and safety in balance, gait, and locomotion.
3. Improvements in relaxation and reduction of pain and decreased muscle spasm.

Strategies
1. Immersion in pools or tanks is used to facilitate exercise. Water buoyancy, buoyant devices, and various depths of immersion decrease body weight and enhance movement; similar movements on land may be more difficult or impossible to perform.
2. Allows greater freedom and range of movement than is permitted in whirlpools or Hubbard tanks.
3. Pools or tanks with a walking track, with or without a treadmill, are used to enhance gait and endurance.

Physics Related to Aquatic Exercise
1. Buoyancy: the upward force of water on an immersed or partially immersed body or body part. Equal to the weight of the water that it displaces (Archimedes' principle). This creates an apparent decrease in the weight and joint unloading of an immersed body part, allowing easier movement in water.
2. Cohesion: the tendency of water molecules to adhere to each other. The resistance encountered while moving through water is due to cohesion; some force is needed to separate water molecules.
3. Density: the mass per unit volume of a substance. The density of water is proportional to its depth; deeper water must support the water above it.
4. Hydrostatic pressure: the circumferential water pressure exerted on an immersed body part. A pressure gradient is established between the surface water and deeper water, due to the increase in water density at deeper levels.
    a. Pascal's law states that the pressure exerted on an immersed body part is equal on all surfaces.
    b. Increased pressure counteracts effusion and edema, and enhances peripheral blood flow.
5. Turbulence: movement of a body part through water creates circular motion of the water (eddy current) near the surface of the part, producing frictional drag.
    a. As speed of movement increases, greater resistance is encountered.
    b. Moving through turbulent water creates greater resistance as compared to calm water.
    c. Use of equipment (e.g., paddle or boot) increases resistance and drag as the patient moves through water.

Thermodynamics
1. Water temperature affects body temperature and performance.
2. Water temperature is determined by specific needs of patient and intervention goals.
    a. Cooler temperatures are used for higher intensity exercise.
    b. Warmer temperatures are used to enhance mobility, flexibility, and relaxation; e.g., patients with arthritis.
    c. Ambient air temperature should be close to water temperature (e.g., ±3°C or ±4°F).
3. There is decreased heat dissipation through sweating with immersion.
4. At temperatures >37°C (98.6°F), patients have increased cardiovascular demands at rest and during exercise.
5. At temperatures <25°C (77°F), patients have difficulty maintaining core temperature.

Special Equipment
1. Buoyancy assistance devices: inflatable cervical collar, flotation rings, buoyancy belt or vest, kickboard.
2. Buoyant dumbbells (swimmers): used for upright or horizontal support.
3. Webbed gloves and hand paddles: used to increase resistance to upper extremity movement.
4. Fins and boots: used to increase resistance to lower extremity movement.

Exercise Applications
1. Movement horizontal to or upward toward the water surface (active assistive exercise) is made easier due to the buoyancy of water. A flotation device may be needed to support very weak patients.

2. Movement downward into the water is more difficult because of the buoyancy of water.
   a. A flotation device or hand-held paddle can be used to increase resistance.
   b. A paddle turned to slice through the water decreases resistance.
3. Resistance exercise can be controlled by the speed of the movement.
   a. Resistance increases with increased velocity of movement due to the cohesion and turbulence of the water.
   b. Slower movements meet less resistance.
   c. Ataxic movements are slower and more controlled against the resistance of water.
4. Stretching exercises can be assisted by the buoyancy of water.
5. The amount of weight bearing on the lower extremities is determined by the height of the water/level of immersion (buoyancy) relative to the upright patient.
   a. The greater the water depth, the less the weight/loading on extremities.
   b. Can be used for partial weight-bearing (PWB) gait training.
6. Lower extremity reciprocal movements are enhanced by use of a kickboard and using kicking movements.
7. Aerobic conditioning is enhanced with deep-water walking or running, high-step marching. Progresses to reduced water levels and then to land walking/running.
   a. Immersed equipment (e.g., cycle ergometer, treadmill, or upper body ergometer) can be used to enhance conditioning.
   b. Swimming is an excellent aerobic training activity.
   c. Regular monitoring of exercise responses (e.g., heart rate, ratings of perceived exertion) is required.
8. Treatment time varies with the type of activity, patient tolerance, and level of skill.

CONTRAINDICATIONS
1. Bowel or bladder incontinence.
2. Severe kidney disease.
3. Severe epilepsy.
4. Severe cardiac or respiratory dysfunction; e.g., cardiac failure, unstable angina, severely reduced vital capacity, unstable blood pressure.
5. Severe peripheral vascular disease.
6. Large open wounds, skin infections, colostomy.
7. Bleeding or hemorrhage.
8. Water and airborne infections; e.g., influenza, gastrointestinal infections.

Precautions
1. Fear of water, inability to swim.
2. Patients with heat intolerance; e.g., patients with multiple sclerosis.
3. Use waterproof dressing on small open wounds and intravenous lines.

Progression

Follow These General Principles for Progression
1. Therapeutic exercises are progressed based upon:
   a. The Plan of Care; specific consideration is placed upon the identified goals.
   b. The patient's response to the intervention.
2. Parameters for progression are chased based upon each specific goal.
3. Table 1-3 outlines the general rules for progression of therapeutic exercise.

Table 1-3

General Principles of Progression Table

PRINCIPLES OF PROGRESSION		
Small range of motion	→	Large range of motion
Lower center of gravity	→	Higher center of gravity
Lower resistance	→	Higher resistance
Slow movements	→	Fast movements
Stable surface	→	Unstable/movable surface
Large base of support	→	Small base of support
Closed environment	→	Open environment
All sensory input available	→	Limited sensory input (e.g., eyes closed)
Lots of feedback	→	No feedback
Eccentric exercises	→	Concentric exercises

Review Questions

Therapeutic Exercise Foundations

1. Describe these three specific principles as they relate to developing muscle strength:
   Overload
   Specificity
   Reversibility

2. Identify the benefits and precautions/contraindications of the following types of resistance exercise: isometric, isotonic, isokinetic and eccentric.

3. Differentiate between dynamic, static and ballistic stretching techniques. Include how to perform the technique and what it is best used for. Identify any precautions or contraindications to each.

4. Discuss conditions or situations when precaution must be exercised when implementing a strengthening program that includes mechanical resistance. Describe a technique to reduce post-exercise muscle soreness.

5. Describe the body's response to exercise in hot weather. Identify appropriate precautions a physical therapy clinician should implement.

6. Outline the progression of developing controlled mobility for an individual with ataxia.

2
Musculoskeletal Physical Therapy

MICHAEL S. CROWELL, ROBERT ROWE, KAREN E. RYAN, and BRADLEY S. TRAGORD

Chapter Outline

- **Anatomy and Physiology of the Musculoskeletal System, 23**
  - Tissue Structure and Function, 23
  - Response to Stress, 24
  - Effects of Aging on Structure and Function, 27
  - Effects of Immobilization, 28
- **Principles of Kinesiology and Biomechanics, 28**
  - General Principles of Biomechanics, 28
- **Intervention Strategies for Patients with Musculoskeletal System Dysfunction, 31**
  - Connective Tissue Mobilization for Tissue Tension, 31
  - Connective Tissue Mobilization for Lengthening, 31
  - Joint Mobilization, 32
- **Physical Therapy Examination and Data Collection, 34**
  - Physical Therapist Assistant's Role and Responsibilities, 34
  - Medical Diagnostic Exams and Imaging, 36
  - Laboratory Tests, 41
  - Electrodiagnostic Testing, 41

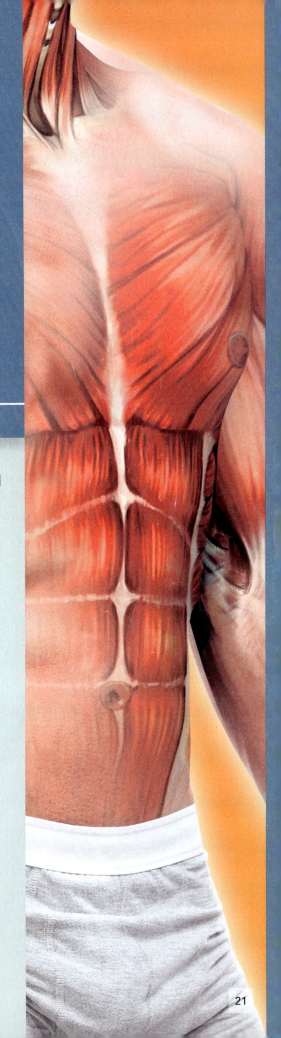

- Conditions/Pathology/Diseases with Intervention, 42
  - Arthritic Conditions, 42
  - Rheumatoid Conditions, 42
  - Skeletal Conditions, 44
  - Soft Tissue Conditions, 45
  - Upper Extremity Conditions—Shoulder, 48
  - Upper Extremity Conditions—Elbow, 51
  - Upper Extremity Conditions—Wrist & Hand, 54
  - Lower Extremity Conditions—Hip, 56
  - Lower Extremity Conditions—Knee, 58
  - Other Conditions of the Lower Leg, 60
  - Lower Extremity Conditions—Foot and Ankle, 61
  - Spinal Conditions, 64
  - Orthopedic Surgical Repairs—Upper Extremity, 68
  - Orthopedic Surgical Repairs—Lower Extremity, 70
- Interventions for Patients/Clients with Musculoskeletal Conditions, 73
  - Interventions for Patients/Clients with Acute Conditions, 73
  - Interventions for Patients/Clients with a Chronic Condition, 74
  - Specific Interventions, 74
  - Manual Therapy Approaches in Rehabilitation, 77
  - Modalities and Electrotherapeutic Agents, 77
  - Relevant Pharmacology, 77
  - Psychosocial Considerations, 80
- Review Questions, 81

Anatomy and Physiology of the Musculoskeletal System

Tissue Structure and Function

Collagen Types I and II
1. Type I: Tightly woven fibers collected into bundles; thick, rugged, and stiff.
   a. Demonstrate very little extensibility when placed under stress.
   b. Found in ligaments.
   c. Found in tendons.
   d. Found in joint capsule.
2. Type II: More loosely woven fibers collected into a network; more flexible than type I.
   a. Fiber network helps maintain shape and provide internal strength in tissues.
   b. Found in hyaline cartilage.

Elastin Fibers
1. Formed into an interwoven network within tissues.
2. Resist tensile (stretching) forces.
3. Elastin in tissues allows fibers to withstand a stretch and return readily to previous shape.
   a. Found in cartilage.
   b. Found in spinal ligaments.

Dense, Irregular Connective Tissue
1. Contains a high density of collagen type I fibers.
2. Has a high degree of tensile strength and low degree of extensibility.
3. Has multidirectional fiber orientation, contributing to its ability to withstand multidirectional forces.
4. Found in:
   a. Joint capsule
   b. Periosteum
   c. Aponeurosis
   d. Dermis
5. Contributes to joint stability.
6. Low vascularity and low water content contribute to slower healing time frame.
   a. The tension placed on these tissues during joint motion retrains undesirable motion.

Dense, Regular Connective Tissue
1. Contains a high density of collagen fibers that contribute to high tensile strength.
2. Has the most tensile strength and is the least extensible (stretchy) of connective tissue types.
3. Fiber orientation is unidirectional (parallel), contributing to its ability to withstand unidirectional forces.
4. Found in:
   a. Ligaments
   b. Tendons
5. Low vascularity and low water content contribute to slower healing time frame.

Loose, Irregular Connective Tissue
1. Contains lower density collagen fibers that exhibit multidirectional fiber organization.
2. Tissues are more pliable and extensible than dense regular or dense irregular connective tissues.
3. Found in:
   a. Superficial fascial sheaths.
   b. Muscle and nerve sheaths.
4. Relatively higher vasculature and water content contribute to faster healing times.
   a. Tissue is easiest tissue to mobilize following trauma or period of immobilization.

Articular Cartilage
1. Found on joint surfaces.
   a. Matrix at bottom layers firmly anchors it to the ends of bones.
   b. Fibers arranged in a scaffold-type arrangement; contributes to its significant strength.
   c. Responds well to compressive forces by dispersing stresses.
   d. Reduces friction between joint surfaces.
2. Is a type of hyaline cartilage; however, it is unable to nourish itself.
   a. Receives its nourishment from synovial fluid through the "milking" action that occurs when cartilage is deformed during joint loading.
3. Is avascular and aneural.

Fibrocartilage
1. Shares properties of dense, irregular connective tissue and articular cartilage.
2. Demonstrates significant ability to absorb and disperse multidirectional loads.
3. Found in:
   a. Intervertebral disc
   b. Labrum
   c. Meniscus
4. Nourishment obtained through "milking" action occurring through joint loading forces.
   a. In synovial joint, nutrients are diffused through synovial fluid.
   b. In joints such as the intervertebral disc and pubis symphysis, nutrients are diffused across fluid contained in surrounding trabecular bone.

5. Healing.
   a. Some tissue repair may occur where vascularized structures attach near it (e.g., ligaments of the spine, joint capsule in the knee).
   b. Portions that do not attach near a blood supply demonstrate poor healing ability (e.g., innermost portions of the meniscus).

Bone
1. Provides rigid support system for body.
2. Joints allow for a system of levers contributing to movement.
3. Composed of two basic layers:
   a. A strong, dense outer layer (compact bone) contributes to its strength.
      - Contains the haversian system that contributes to maintenance and repair of bone.
   b. A softer, mesh inner layer (cancellous bone) serves to store marrow.
4. Covered with periosteum, a fibrous connective tissue, which serves to provide blood supply to the bone as well as an attachment site for tendons and ligaments.
5. Is continuously remodeling and reshaping.
   a. Relies on compressive forces to maintain its health (e.g., those achieved by weight bearing and muscle contraction and relaxation).
   b. A balance between osteoblast (bond formation) and osteoclast (bone remodeling or absorbing) activity maintains this homeostatic state.

Muscle
1. Consists of light and dark bands of contractile fibers that respond to a stimulus to contract.
   a. Actin and myosin filaments interlink and become closer together during muscle contraction and slide farther apart during muscle relaxation.
2. Demonstrates elasticity.
3. Strength of muscle.
   a. Dependent on its cross-sectional area; greater cross-sectional area, greater strength and vice versa.
   b. Is weakest at the end ranges of complete relaxation and complete contraction.
   c. Is strongest at the mid ranges of its available range of motion (ROM).

Response to Stress

Soft Tissue
1. Connective tissues are designed to respond to stresses placed upon them at rest and at work (during activity).
2. Ability of the tissue to withstand stress, without tissue failure, is dependent upon:
   a. The health of the tissue prior to the load.
   b. The force applied to the tissue.
   c. The rate at which the force is applied.
   d. The viscoelastic qualities of the tissue.
   e. This action is depicted through the stress-strain curve (Figure 2-1).
3. Elasticity: When an external force is applied correctly, within the limits of the connective tissue's ability to withstand the force, an elastic change occurs.
   a. Maintenance of ROM of the tissue.
4. Plasticity: When an external force is applied correctly to the limits of the connective tissue's ability to withstand the force, a plastic change occurs.
   a. Increased ROM of the tissue.

Table 2-1

Tissue Healing Times

TISSUE	TISSUE TYPE CONSIDERATIONS	TIME FRAME	PHASE OF HEALING	INDICATED ACTIVITY LEVEL
Ligament	Primarily type 1 collagen—very strong in scars Generally hypovascular Contain mechanoreceptors—contribute to proprioception Contain free nerve endings—contribute to pain perception Varying intrinsic differences within ligaments lead to varying approaches to rehabilitation: extra-articular ligaments heal in an organized and predictable manner; intra-articular ligaments do not heal spontaneously	1 year postinjury—tensile strength approaching 50%–70% of normal		
		Day 3–14	Inflammation	RICE (rest, ice, compression, elevation) are indicated Pain modulation—TENS, oral anti-inflammatory and/or analgesics Protect ligament (soft or rigid dressing for short-term use) CPM within protected range of motion

Anatomy and Physiology of the Musculoskeletal System 25

Table 2-1

Tissue Healing Times (Continued)

TISSUE	TISSUE TYPE CONSIDERATIONS	TIME FRAME	PHASE OF HEALING	INDICATED ACTIVITY LEVEL
		Week 2 to Week 6	Proliferative	AROM and light resistance Avoid activities that cause pain Focus exercise on endurance rather than strength Supportive taping as appropriate
		Week 6 up to 1 year	Remodeling	AROM, resistive and plyometric activities WB activities Supportive taping with some functional activities and sport activities Reintegrate into function, sport, work activities
Muscle	Primarily made up of loose, irregular connective tissue, which makes the tissue more pliable and extensible High vascularization and water content lead to faster healing times Easiest tissue to mobilize following trauma or period of immobilization			
		Day 1 to Day 5	Inflammatory	RICE (rest, ice, compression, elevation) are indicated Pain modulation—TENS, oral anti-inflammatory and/or analgesics Isometrics PROM—pain free AROM
		Day 5 to Week 6	Proliferative	AROM—light resistance Continues use of pain relieving modalities AROM, resistive and plyometric activities WB activities
		Week 6 to Month 6	Remodeling	AROM, resistive and plyometric activities WB activities
Bone	Composed of two basic layers: Strong, dense outer layer—contributes to its strength Softer, mesh inner layer—stores marrow Covered with periosteum—provides blood to the bone Constantly remodeling—Wolf's Law			
		Day 1 to Day 14	Inflammatory	NWB to limited WB Stabilization/Protection PROM to AROM—no resistance RICE (rest, ice, compression, elevation) are indicated
		Week 2 to Week 12	Proliferative	Limited weight bearing to WBAT AROM to sub-max resistance exercises
		Week 12—can last years	Remodeling	FWB Max-resistance exercises

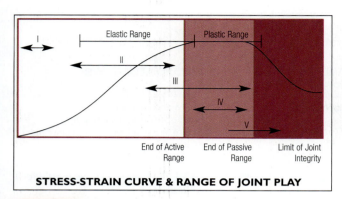

Figure 2-1 Grades of movement.

(Adapted from Grieve GP. *Mobilization of the Spine. A Primary Handbook of Clinical Method.* 5th ed. Churchill Livingstone, New York, 1991.)

5. When the force applied exceeds the tissue's ability to withstand the force, a tear (strain or sprain) occurs (e.g., "twisting" an ankle, hyperextending a shoulder).
    a. The extent of the injury to a muscle or tendon is identified as the "degree" of strain or sprain (Table 2-2).

Healing/Scar Tissue Formation in Soft Tissues

1. Occurs in three overlapping phases (Table 2-1).
2. Each phase responds differently to mobilization forces. Activity levels should match phase of healing to avoid further tissue damage.
3. Phases of scar tissue formation. See Quick Facts 2-1.
4. Response to tissue mobilization techniques.
    a. Cross-linking is diminished and new collagen is laid down in a more orderly fashion.

Table 2-2

Degree of Muscle Strain, Tendon Injury, and Ligament Sprain

	1° STRAIN	2° STRAIN	3° STRAIN	1° SPRAIN	2° SPRAIN	3° SPRAIN	TENDINITIS
Definition	A few fibers of muscle torn	Approximately ½ muscle fibers torn	All muscle fibers torn (rupture)	A few fibers of ligament torn	Approximately ½ ligament fibers torn	All ligament fibers torn	Inflammation of tendon, tendon degeneration
Mechanism of injury	Excessive load or stretch	Excessive load or stretch, crush injury	Excessive load or stretch	Excessive load or stretch	Excessive load or stretch	Excessive load or stretch	Overuse, excessive load or stretch; also aging
Weakness	Minor	Moderate, potentially >due to pain	Moderate to significant	Minor	Minor to significant	Minor to significant	Minor to significant
Muscle spasm	Minor	Moderate to significant	Moderate	Minor	Minor	Minor	Minor
Swelling	Minor	Moderate to significant	Moderate to significant	Minor	Moderate	Moderate to significant	Minor to significant, potential thickening
Disability, loss of function	Minor	Moderate to significant	Significant, reflex inhibition and pain	Minor	Moderate to significant	Moderate to significant, joint instability	Minor to significant
Pain with isometric contraction	Minor	Moderate to significant	Minor to no pain	No	No	No	Minor to significant
Pain with stretch	Yes	Yes	No, unless other tissues also damaged	Yes	Yes	No, unless other tissues also damaged	Yes
ROM	Decreased	Decreased	May increase or decrease, dependent on swelling	Decreased	Decreased	Decreased	May increase or decrease, dependent on swelling; dislocation of subluxation possible
Joint play	Normal	Normal	Normal	Normal	Normal	Normal to excessive	Normal

QUICK FACTS 2-1 ▶ SCAR TISSUE FORMATION – PHASES OF

Phase	Time Frame	Signs and Symptoms
Phase 1: Inflammatory/ proliferative phase	• Occurs immediately • Lasts from 24–36 hours • Essential to initiate healing process • Predominated by migration of fluids and macrophages to damaged site	Edema Erythema Heat Pain
Phase 2: Granulation/ fibroblastic phase	• Lasts 48 hours to 6 weeks (timing dependent on specific tissues; generally more vascular tissues heal more quickly; muscle and epithelial tissue heals faster; tendon and ligament heal more slowly) • Relative increase in vascularity	Granulation tissue forming

Phase 3: Remodeling or maturation phase	• 3 weeks to 6 months depending upon tissue vascularity
	• Characterized by increasing fibroblasts and collagen production (collagen is laid down in an unorganized fashion and begins binding to damaged areas)
	• Complications of healing:
	  ○ Chronic inflammation; ongoing inflammatory response
	  ○ Adhesions: scar tissue adheres to or connects with structures it does not normally connect to
	  ○ Fibrosis: scar tissue that develops in a space that is usually open or hollow
	  ○ Dehiscence: a wound that is closed and opens up before it is fully healed
		Scar tissue at this time can be easily remodeled with appropriate stresses

  b. Tissues become rehydrated and demonstrate improved viscosity.
  c. Adhesions are partially ruptured facilitating tissue elongation.

Bone Tissue
1. Bone tissue is designed to withstand stress.
2. Wolf's law.
  a. The process describing continuous bone remodeling and reshaping in response to stresses placed upon it.
  b. Muscle contraction and relaxation, such as that occurring during resisted exercise, places sufficient stress on bone to stimulate this remodeling and reshaping process.
  c. Weight-bearing activities are particularly effective in stimulating remodeling and reshaping of bone.
3. Excessive stress placed on bone results in fracture.
4. Fracture types:
  a. Complete: Bone is fractured all the way through, may be nondisplaced or displaced.
    • Will require immobilization.
    • Displaced will require relocation of the bone ends; may occur with local pain killers or under anesthesia.
    • May require open reduction internal fixation (ORIF); through surgical intervention the fracture is reduced and pins, screws, and/or plates are used to secure bone ends.
  b. Incomplete: Bone demonstrates a disruption in its integrity; the disruption does not completely separate and fragments are still somewhat connected.
    • Will require immobilization. Type used dependent upon location of fracture and whether it is a weight-bearing area or not.
  c. Stress fracture: Fine, hairline fracture occurring with little to no soft tissue damage.
    • Can be difficult to diagnose; often best seen on x-ray 3–4 weeks following incident.
  d. Open fracture: One in which the bone protrudes out of the skin.
    • Will require open reduction (surgical) and potentially internal fixation (placement of pins, screws, plates to secure bone segments).
  e. Greenstick: The bone is partially bent and partially broken (resembling what occurs when a green stick is bent); occurs in children (as their bones are more flexible than a teen's or adult's).

Effects of Aging on Structure and Function

Mechanical Properties
1. The ability to withstand forces diminishes with age.
2. Amount of deterioration is highly variable between individuals.
3. Accumulated microtrauma through normal "wear and tear" can contribute to structural failure.

QUICK FACTS 2-2 ▶ TISSUE IMMOBILIZATION – EFFECTS OF

Topic	Results
Histology and mechanics	• Immobilization alters the immediate and ultimate strength of tissues. • Decrease in strength can begin within days of immobilization. • Bone, cartilage, and muscle will lose mass, volume strength.
Fibrosis and adhesions	• Collagen being laid down to repair tissue is laid down in a "haphazard, disorganized" fashion (commonly called cross-linking) that further limits tissue mobility. • Water content of tissues decreases and contributes to cross-linking of collagen fibers.
Long term	• Studies demonstrate that ligaments that have been subjected to immobilization and subsequent rehabilitation do not regain the same tensile strength they had to begin with.

4. Tissues diminish in their ability to rehydrate, thus decreasing the ability to withstand forces placed upon them.
   a. Contributes to decreasing ability of tissue to distribute forces between bony surfaces.
5. With stress, bundles of fibers in connective tissues lose their ability to align themselves.
   a. Results in decreased ability to withstand more rapidly applied forces.

Effects of Aging Can Be Somewhat Modified
1. Good nutrition contributes to improved overall function as well as tissue function.
2. Proper hydration is important for all body systems to function normally.
3. Appropriate strengthening and aerobic activities can contribute to overall function and good health.

Effects of Immobilization

Tissue Immobilization
1. Tissue immobilization affects tissue histology, organization and mechanics. Long term effects can become problematic. See Quick Facts 2-2.

Principles of Kinesiology and Biomechanics

General Principles of Biomechanics

Levers: Rotations of a Rigid Surface About an Axis
1. First-class lever occurs when two forces are applied on either side of an axis.
   a. The effort is the force that attempts to cause movement.
   b. The resistance is the force that opposes movement.
   c. Example in human body is the contraction of triceps at elbow joint.
2. Second-class lever occurs when two forces are applied on one side of an axis.
   a. Resistance lies between the effort force and the axis of rotation.
   b. Few examples in human body (toe raises).
3. Third-class lever occurs when two forces are applied on one side of an axis.
   a. The effort force lies closer to the axis than the resistance force.
   b. Most muscles in the human body are third-class levers (elbow flexion).

Selected Kinematics
1. Arthrokinematics is defined as the movement between joint surfaces.
2. Three motions describe the movement of one joint surface on another.
   a. Roll consists of one joint surface rolling on another, such as a tire rolling on the road (e.g., movement between the femoral and tibial articular surfaces of knee).
   b. Glide consists of a pure translatory motion of one surface gliding on another, as when a braked wheel skids (e.g., movement of the joint surface of the

proximal phalanx at the head of the metacarpal bone of the hand).
c. Spin consists of a rotation of the movable component of the joint (e.g., movement between joint surfaces of radial head with humerus).
d. Combinations of all three motions can occur at joints (e.g., between joint surfaces of humerus and scapula of shoulder).
3. Osteokinematics: movement between two bones.
4. Convex-concave rule describes relationship between arthrokinematics and osteokinematics.
   a. When a convex surface is moving on a fixed concave surface, the convex surface moves opposite to the direction of the shaft of the bony lever.
   b. When a concave surface moves on a fixed convex surface, the concave articulating surface moves in the same direction as the bony lever (see Table 2-3).
   c. In the spine, the convex rule applies at the atlanto-occipital joint. Below the second vertebra, the concave rule applies.

Capsular Positions
1. Resting or loose-packed position (see Table 2-4).
   a. Joint position where capsule and other soft tissues are in most relaxed position.
   b. Minimal joint surface contact.
   c. May perform joint play and mobilization techniques in this joint position.
2. Close-packed position (see Table 2-4).
   a. Joint position where capsule and other soft tissues are maximally tensed.
   b. Maximal contact between joint surfaces.
   c. Joint play and mobilization cannot be properly performed in this position.
3. Selected capsular patterns (see Table 2-5).
4. End-feels.
   a. Normal physiological end-feel.
      - Soft: occurs with soft tissue approximation.
      - Firm: capsular and ligamentous stretching.
      - Hard: when bone and/or cartilage meet.
   b. Pathological end-feel.
      - Boggy: edema, joint swelling.
      - Firm with decreased elasticity: fibrosis of soft tissues.
      - Rubbery: muscle spasm.
      - Empty: loose, then very hard; associated with muscle guarding or patient avoiding painful part of range.
      - Hypermobility: end-feel at a later time than on opposite side.

Table 2-3

Concave-Convex Rule Application

ARTICULATION	FUNCTION	MOVING COMPONENT OF ARTICULATION	RELATIONSHIP OF CONVEX/CONCAVE RULE
Fingers	Flexion/extension	Distal phalanx	Concave moving on Convex
Metacarpal-phalangeal	Abduction/adduction	Proximal phalanx	Concave moving on Convex
Wrist	Flexion/extension	Capitate, scaphoid, lunate, triquetrum	Convex moving on Concave
		Trapezoid	Concave moving on Convex
Radioulnar			
Distal	Pronation/supination	Radius	Concave moving on Convex
Proximal	Pronation/supination	Radius	Convex moving on Concave
Humeroradial	Flexion/extension	Radius	Concave moving on Convex
Humeroulnar	Flexion/extension	Ulna	Concave moving on Convex
Glenohumeral	All movements	Humerus	Convex moving on Concave
Sternoclavicular	Elevation/depression	Clavicle	Convex moving on Concave
	Protraction/retraction	Clavicle	Concave moving on Convex
Acromioclavicular	All movements	Scapula	Concave moving on Convex
Toes	Flexion/extension	Distal phalanx	Concave moving on Convex
Metatarsal-phalangeal	Abduction/adduction	Proximal phalanx	Concave moving on Convex
Ankle/Foot			
Subtalar	All movements	Navicular, cuneiform	Concave moving on Convex
	Inversion/eversion	Cuboid, calcaneus	Convex moving on Concave
Talocrural	Dorsal/plantar flexion	Talus	Convex moving on Concave
Tibiofibular	All movements	Fibular head	Concave moving on Convex
Knee	All movements	Tibia	Concave moving on Convex
Hip	All movements	Femur	Convex moving on Concave
Temporomandibular	All movements	Mandible	Convex moving on Concave

Adapted from Kaltenborn F: Manual Mobilization of the Joints, Vol. 1: The Extremities, 8th ed. 2014.

Table 2-4

Joint Positions

ARTICULATIONS	RESTING POSITION	CLOSE-PACKED POSITION
Vertebral	Midway between flexion and extension	Maximal extension
Temporomandibular	Jaw slightly open (freeway space)	Maximal retrusion (mouth closed with teeth clenched) or maximal anterior position/mouth maximally opened/
Sternoclavicular	Arm resting by side	Arm maximally elevated
Acromioclavicular	Arm resting by side	Arm abducted 90°
Glenohumeral	40° to 55° abduction; 30° horizontal adduction (scapular plane)	Maximum abduction and ER
Elbow		
Humeroulnar	70° flexion and 10° supination	Full extension and supination
Humeroradial	Full extension and supination	90° flexion and 5° supination
Forearm		
Proximal radioulnar	70° flexion and 35° supination	5° supination
Distal radioulnar	10° supination	5° supination
Radio/ulnocarpal	Neutral with slight ulnar deviation	Full extension with radial deviation
Hand		
Midcarpal	Neutral or slight flexion with ulnar deviation	Extension with ulnar deviation
Carpometacarpal (2–5)	Midway between abduction-adduction and flexion-extension (thumb); midway between flexion and extension (fingers)	Full opposition (thumb); full flexion (fingers)
Metacarpophalangeal (MCP)	Slight flexion	Full opposition (thumb); full flexion (fingers)
Interphalangeal (IP)	Slight flexion	Full extension
Hip	30° flexion, 30° abduction, and slight lateral rotation	Full extension, abduction, internal rotation
Knee	25° flexion	Bony: 90° flexion, slight abduction, and slight ER Full extension and ER
Ankle/Foot		
Talocrural	Mid inversion/eversion and 10° plantar flexion	Full dorsiflexion
Subtalar	Midway between extremes of range of motion	Full inversion
Midtarsal	Midway between extremes of range of motion	Full supination
Tarsometatarsal	Midway between supination and pronation	Full supination
Toes		
Metatarsophalangeal	Neutral (extension 10°)	Full extension
Interphalangeal	Slight flexion	Full extension

Adapted from Magee DJ: Orthopedic Physical Assessment, 6th ed. 2014.

Table 2-5

Capsular Patterns

ARTICULATIONS	RELATIVE LIMITATIONS OF MOVEMENT
Temporomandibular	Limited mouth opening
Glenohumeral	Greater limitation of ER, followed by abduction and internal rotation
Sternoclavicular	Full elevation limited; pain at extreme range of motion
Acromioclavicular	Full elevation limited; pain at extreme range of motion
Humeroulnar	Loss of flexion more so than extension
Humeroradial	Loss of flexion more so than extension
Proximal radioulnar	Limitation: pronation = supination
Distal radioulnar	Limitation: pronation = supination
Wrist	Limitation: flexion = extension
Midcarpal	Limitation: equal all directions
Hip	Limited flexion/internal rotation; some limitation of abduction; no or little limitation of adduction and ER
Knee	Flexion grossly limited; slight limitation of extension
Talocrural	Loss of plantarflexion greater than dorsiflexion
Talocalcaneal (subtalar)	Increasing limitations of varus; joint fixed in valgus (inversion > eversion)
Midtarsal	Supination > pronation (limited dorsiflexion, plantar flexion, adduction, and medial rotation)

Adapted from Magee DJ: Orthopedic Physical Assessment, 6th ed. 2014.

5. Grading of accessory joint movement.
   a. Accessory joint movement or joint play is graded to assess arthrokinematic motion of the joint and/or when it is impractical or impossible to measure joint motion with a goniometer.
      - Movement is assessed in comparison to the uninvolved extremity or adjacent vertebral joints.
      - Graded normal, hypomobile, or hypermobile.
   b. Although interrater reliability is poor, intrarater reliability is acceptable.
   c. Data gleaned provide clinician with more specific data on source of patient's problem.

Muscle Substitutions

1. Occur when muscles have become shortened/lengthened, weakened, lost endurance, developed impaired coordination, or paralyzed.
2. Stronger muscles compensate for loss of motion.
3. Common muscle substitutions:
   a. Use of scapular stabilizers to initiate shoulder motion when shoulder abductors are weakened (reverse scapulothoracic rhythm).
   b. Use of lateral trunk muscles or tensor fascia latae (TFL) when hip abductors are weak.
   c. Use of passive finger flexion by contraction of wrist extensors when finger flexors are weak (tenodesis).
   d. Use of long head of biceps, coracobrachialis, and anterior deltoid when pectoralis major is weak.
   e. Use of lower back extensors, adductor magnus, and quadratus lumborum when hip extensors are weak.
   f. Use of lower abdominal, lower obliques, hip adductors, and latissimus dorsi when hip flexors are weak.

Intervention Strategies for Patients with Musculoskeletal System Dysfunction

Connective Tissue Mobilization for Tissue Tension

Transverse Friction Techniques

1. Press fingertip(s) perpendicular to tendon.
2. Press down through superficial tissues; move superficial tissues on tendon.
   a. Deeper tissues can most easily be accessed by placing the muscle on slack.
   b. Slight tension on a tendon allows effective transverse friction.
3. Use pressure in one direction on the tendon (e.g., always pull toward you and push away from you during each treatment session).
4. Apply for 5–6 minutes per tendon or tendon area.
5. Follow cross friction techniques with manual or active stretching of associated muscle.

Muscle Techniques

1. Apply a longitudinal stroke, using fingertips or thumbs, along the muscle fibers.
   a. This technique is designed to facilitate separating muscle bundles from each other.
2. Muscle tissue is best reached with the muscle on slack.

Transverse Muscle Techniques

1. Apply a transverse force to a muscle bundle along any portion of the muscle that demonstrates decreased mobility.
2. This technique helps mobilize the muscle fiber from its sheath.
3. This technique can improve ROM and active strength of the muscle.

Fascia Techniques

1. Use longitudinal strokes along fascial areas near bony surfaces that demonstrate limited mobility.
   a. For example, anterior-lateral border along the tibia in shin splints, iliotibial band (ITB) anterior to the lateral knee, junction between ITB and biceps femoris.

Connective Tissue Mobilization for Lengthening

Tissues Must Be Stretched Beyond Their Elastic Limit and Into Their Plastic Range

Speed

1. The stretching force must be applied slowly enough to avoid tissue damage, as well as to avoid stimulating contractile tissue in muscle (see Figure 2-1).
2. Gradually release the stretch.

Duration

1. The stretching force must be applied long enough to allow for remodeling (rearranging of collagen fiber

bonds) of collagen fibers and redistribution of water to surrounding tissues.
2. Long-duration stretches are typically recommended.
3. Terms typically used to describe long-duration stretching techniques include
   a. Static
   b. Sustained
   c. Prolonged
4. Terms typically used to describe short-duration stretching techniques include
   a. Cyclic
   b. Intermittent
   c. Ballistic
5. Evidence
   a. It is generally accepted that stretches applied for 30–60 seconds (whether it be one to two 30-second stretches or six 10-second stretches) are effective to gain ROM.
   b. Low-load and long-duration stretches yield the most significant elastic deformation and long-term plastic tissue responses.

Intensity
1. Stretching force should be a low-magnitude force that is applied over time.
2. Low-intensity stretching has been shown to elongate dense connective tissues more effectively, with less tissue damage and post-exercise soreness, than high-intensity stretch.

Frequency
1. There is little evidence to support a specified frequency of stretching.
2. Consider:
   a. Acuity or chronicity of condition.
   b. Cause of/for the condition.
   c. Stage of tissue healing.
   d. Severity of loss of ROM.

Mode of Stretch
1. See Chapter 10 for details.

Joint Mobilization

Indications and Contraindications
1. See Table 2-6 for indications and contraindications to the use of joint mobilization.

Systems of "Dosing"
1. Maitland (oscillatory techniques).
   a. Consists of four grades of movement designed to improve joint nutrition and increase joint range of motion. See Quick Facts 2-3.

Table 2-6

Indications and Contraindications to Joint Mobilization	
INDICATIONS	**CONTRAINDICATIONS/ PRECAUTIONS**
Pain Muscle spasm and guarding Joint hypomobility Functional limitation in joint ROM	Joint hypermobility Joint effusion Inflammation Precautions Malignancy Unhealed fracture Bone disease Hypermobility in adjacent joints Systemic connective tissue diseases (rheumatoid arthritis) Individual is on blood-thinning medications

QUICK FACTS 2-3 ▶ MOBILIZATION TECHNIQUES

Mobilization Grade	Maitland	Kaltenborn	Uses
Grade I	Small-amplitude oscillation at beginning of the range	Small-amplitude translation with no tension applied to the joint capsule	Distraction, increase joint nutrition Pain relief
Grade II	Large-amplitude oscillation that pushes into tissue resistance	Translation that stops just short of applying tension to the joint capsule	Joint nutrition Pain relief Stop translation just prior to applying tension
Grade III	Large-amplitude oscillation that pushes into tissue resistance	Translation that stretches/places tension on the joint capsule	Stretching of joint capsule
Grade IV	Small-amplitude, high-velocity manipulation past the end of passive range	N/A	

2. Uses of Maitland "doses."
   a. Grades I and II: primarily used to limit pain.
      - Joint oscillations stimulate mechanoreceptors that block nociceptive pathways at the brain or spinal cord level and inhibit the perception of pain.
   b. Grades III and IV: primarily used for stretch maneuvers.
   c. Either physiological or joint play motions are used in mobilization techniques.
3. Kaltenborn (sustained translation). See Figure 2-2.
   a. Consists of three grades of movement designed to improve joint nutrition and increase joint range of motion. See Quick Facts 2-3.
4. Uses of Kaltenborn "doses."
   a. Grade I: a distraction force used with all gliding motions; also used for pain relief.
   b. Grade II: distraction applied to assess joint reaction; this reaction indicated either increased or decreased distraction.
      - Gentle grade II distraction is used intermittently to inhibit pain; used to maintain joint play when ROM is not allowed.
   c. Grade III: Distractions and glides are used to stretch the joint structures to increase joint play.

> **Clinical Application:**
>
> Physical therapist assistant candidates should be prepared to answer questions about joint kinematics and kinesiology as they relate to the clinical application of physical therapy concepts and interventions to patients/clients on the licensure examination. This may include the application of, effects of, and responses to joint mobility techniques.

Assessment of Pain
1. Pain before limit in tissue ROM: indicates injury is still in the inflammatory or early granulation phase of tissue healing.
   a. Only small-amplitude rhythmic oscillation and/or distraction techniques are indicated.

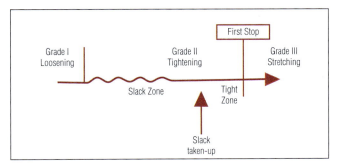

Figure 2-2 Manual mobilization of the joints.
(From Kaltenborn F. *Manual Mobilization of the Joints.* Vol II *The Spine.* 4th ed. Minneapolis, OPTP, 2003, with permission.)

2. Pain occurs concurrently with reaching the tissue limitation: indicates the tissues are in the granulation phase and are still healing.
   a. Small-amplitude and large-amplitude rhythmic oscillation techniques "within" the tissue ROM are indicated; helps maintain joint nutrition and begins to assist with remodeling disorganized (haphazardly organized) scar tissues.
3. Pain occurs after tissue limitation is met: indicates tissues are likely in the remodeling or maturation phase and can tolerate more aggressive stretching techniques.
   a. Small-and large-amplitude rhythmic oscillations into tissue resistance are indicated to stretch tissues.

Application Considerations
1. Position the joint so it is freely available and the muscles are relaxed.
   a. Position the joint capsule in the open packed position.
   b. May need to reposition the joint so that it is in the least painful position.
2. Examine joint play.
3. Initiate mobilization techniques.
   a. Begin with grades I and II.
   b. Progress to higher grades as indicated per outcome goals.

Force and Direction of Movements
1. Treatment force is applied close to the opposing joint surface.
   a. Position hand, fingers, thumb, and mobilization belt so the greatest surface area is in contact with the patient's tissues for increased comfort.
2. The entire bone is moved to accomplish the motion; do not use the bone as a lever so that the joint surface rolls.
3. The plane of the concave bone is used to determine direction of the force applied.
4. The treatment plane is perpendicular to a line running from the axis of rotation to the middle of the concave articular surface.
5. Distraction techniques are applied perpendicular to the treatment plane.
6. Gliding techniques are applied parallel to the treatment plane.
   a. Apply the concave-convex rule.
      - If the moving surface is convex, the treatment glide should be opposite the direction in which the moving bone swings.
      - If the moving surface is concave, the treatment glide should be in the same direction the bone swings.
7. Joint mobilization techniques should be used as part of a comprehensive treatment program to improve joint mobility and joint range of motion.

Physical Therapy Examination and Data Collection

Physical Therapist Assistant's Role and Responsibilities

Prior to and Throughout Patient Care
1. Tests and measures to determine if the patient is safe to participate in the planned intervention(s).
2. Tests and measures to monitor patient response(s) to intervention(s).
3. Document patient's status and progress or lack thereof.
4. Use the information in the physical therapist's plan of care to progress patient interventions appropriately.
5. Interpret patient response:
   a. Differentiate between appropriate and adverse changes.
   b. Determine what needs to be reported to the physical therapist.

Patient History and Medical Record Review
1. Current medical and therapy diagnoses.
2. Co-morbidities that might impact the physical therapy intervention.
3. Psychosocial history, living situation, and social support.
4. Diagnostic procedures completed.
   a. Review results that may affect physical therapy intervention.
   b. Examples include: imaging, laboratory results, electrodiagnostic testing.

Physical Therapist Special Tests
1. Musculoskeletal special tests:
   a. Utilized by the physical therapist.
   b. Primarily are diagnostic in nature providing information the PT uses in determining the patient's musculoskeletal condition or disorder (Table 2-7 for UE tests, Table 2-8 for LE tests).
   c. Are not typically performed by the PTA due to the diagnostic nature of the tests.
2. PTA's role regarding special tests:
   a. PTA needs to know what tissues are involved to be able to make appropriate decisions related to provision of interventions as outlined in the plan of care.
   b. Some special tests can be repeated to demonstrate progress. PTAs would perform the tests in these instances.
      - Example: Thomas' test.

Anthropometric Characteristics
1. Typically only performed by PT during the initial evaluation.
2. Height/weight/body mass index (BMI).
3. Girth: edema related to surgical limb.

Pain
1. Pain assessment performed:
   a. By PT at the initial evaluation.
   b. By PT and PTA during all interventions to monitor response to intervention and progression.
2. Numeric pain scale (NPS):
   a. 0 = no pain.
   b. 10 = worst possible pain.
3. Visual analog scale (VAS):
   a. 10 cm line.
4. McGill pain questionnaire.

Posture
1. Performed at initial evaluation by PT, ongoing by PT and PTA to determine progress.
2. Primarily done through observation.
   a. Anterior/posterior and both left and right views are observed.
3. Plumb bob, posture graph as reference point.
4. Pictures with grid film.
   a. Clinician notes deviations away from normal postural alignment.
5. Curvature may be measured with:
   a. Debrunner's kyphometer.
   b. Flexicure.

Range of Motion/Flexibility
1. Performed at initial evaluation by PT, ongoing by PT and PTA to determine progress.
2. Goniometric measurements.
3. Observation of ability to perform functional tasks.
4. Muscle length—two joint muscles.

Motor Function
1. Performed at initial evaluation by PT, ongoing by PT and PTA to determine progress.
2. Muscle performance.
   a. Strength, power, endurance.
3. Manual muscle testing.
4. Handheld dynamometry.
5. Isokinetic dynamometry.

Table 2-7

Special Tests used for the Upper Extremity

JOINT	TESTS FOR	TEST NAME & DESCRIPTION
Glenohumeral	Anterior instability	Apprehension test: Assessment of apprehension (anticipated pain) when subject is asked to maintain 90° abduction and ER of shoulder.
	Posterior and inferior instability	Jerk test: A sudden jerk or clunk occurs when subject is axial load is applied to shoulder positioned in 90° flexion and IR (humeral head subluxes off the back of the glenoid). Sulcus sign: An indentation (sulcus) occurs inferior to the acromion as distal distraction force is applied to humerus, also reproduces symptoms.
	Subacromial impingement	Hawkins-Kennedy test: Passive flexion (to 90°) and IR reproduce pain. Neer's test (see Figure 2-3): Passive IR and full abduction reproduce pain. Empty Can test (see Figure 2-4): Shoulder placed at 90° abduction and pain reproduced with resistance, or shoulder placed in "empty can" position (90° abduction and 30° horizontal adduction) and pain reproduced with resistance or weakness noted.
	Rotator cuff pathology	Drop arm test: Subject unable to slowly lower arm passively abducted to 120°. Lag signs (internal, external): Shoulder placed in full IR or ER and subject asked to hold position—positive when enable.
	Acromioclavicular joint	Horizontal adduction test: Shoulder flexed to 90°, then actively or passively fully adducted across body and results in localized pain at AC joint.
	SLAP lesion (superior labrum anterior to posterior)	Active compression (O'Brien) test: Painful pop or click occurs with shoulder in 90° flexion, 10–15° adduction and full IR when and a downward force is applied. Biceps load II test: Apprehension and/or pain occurs when subject asked to flex biceps against resistance with shoulder placed in 120° abduction. Yergason test: Provocative test for pathology of long head of biceps and SLAP lesion (tear of superior glenoid labrum in an anterior-to-posterior direction).
	Thoracic outlet syndrome	Adson's test (see Figure 2-5): Radial pulse diminishes or disappears and/or neurological symptoms occur when testing arm is extended and externally rotated, subject head rotated toward arm being tested. Roos elevated arm test: Radial pulse diminishes or disappears and/or neurological symptoms occur when testing arm is placed in 90° abduction, slight horizontal adduction and elbow flexed to 90°, subject then opens/closes hand for 3 minutes.
Elbow	Ligamentous instability	Varus/valgus stress tests: Laxity noted as clinician places varus and valgus stress on elbow placed in 20–0° flexion. Biceps rupture "Popeye" sign: Rupture of proximal long head of biceps when distal bunching of muscle is noted with complete loss of function.
	Neurological dysfunction	Elbow flexion test: Pain at the medial aspect of elbow and numbness and tingling in ulnar nerve distribution reproduce when subject holds position of full shoulder ER, maximal elbow flexion, and wrist extension for 1 minute; indicates cubital tunnel syndrome.
Wrist and hand	De Quervain's tenosynovitis (tendonitis of the abductor pollicis longus and/or extensor pollicis brevis)	Eichoff's test (see Figure 2-6): Pain reproduced when thumb is flexed across palm within confines of flexed fingers and examiner passive moves wrist into ulnar deviation. Note: must compare to uninvolved side as can produce pain with no pathology present. Finkelstein's test: Pain reproduced when examiner pulls wrist and thumb into ulnar deviation with distraction force.
	Neurological dysfunction	Phalen's (wrist flexion) test (see Figure 2-7): Tingling and paresthesia reproduced when subject maximally flexes wrists and holds against each other for 1 minute; indicative of carpal tunnel compression of median nerve. Tinel's sign: Tingling and paresthesia reproduced when tapping over area of carpal tunnel where median nerve passes; indicative of carpal tunnel compression of median nerve. Two-point discrimination test: Two-point discriminator tool or paperclip used over palmar aspect of fingers to assess ability to distinguish between 2 points of testing device. Examiner records smallest difference subject is able to discriminate; normal amount is generally less than 6 mm. Limited sensory ability correlates to decreased functional ability.

Table 2-8

Special Tests Used for the Lower Extremity

JOINT	TESTS FOR	TEST NAME & DESCRIPTION
Hip	Degenerative joint disease	Hip scour test (see Figure 2-8): Reproduction of hip pain (may also refer to knee and elsewhere) when a compressive force is applied to femur with hip in 90° flexion and knee fully flexed.
	Dysfunction, mobility restriction	Patrick (FABER) test (see Figure 2-9): Involved leg is unable to assume a relaxed posture and/or painful symptoms reproduced when subject positioned in hip flexion, abduction, and external rotation with foot placed proximal to knee on opposite limb (performed in supine position).
	Muscle length/strength involvement	Thomas test (see Figure 2-10): Straight limb flexes, or subject unable to remain flat on table, when opposite limb is fully flexed indicates muscle tightness of iliacus or psoas major. Test position: subject supine, one hip and knee maximally flexed to chest, opposing limb should remain straight on table. Limitation: does not differentiate which muscle is tight. Ober's test (see Figures 2-11 and 2-12): Indicates tightness of tensor fascia lata and/or iliotibial band when uppermost (involved) limb (positioned in passive hip extension and slowly lowered from abducted position) remains above horizontal position. Ely's test (see Figure 2-13): Indicates tightness of rectus femoris when hip of tested limb lifts off testing surface with knee flexion (tested in prone). Trendelenburg sign (see Figure 2-14): Observe pelvis of stance leg; positive if ipsilateral hip drops when limb support is removed. Indicative of weakness of gluteus medius or unstable hip.
Knee	1-Plane anterior instability	Lachman test (see Figure 2-15): Positive test is excessive anterior translation of the tibia compared to the uninvolved limb and lack of a firm end-feel. Anterior drawer test: positive test is excessive anterior translation of the tibia compared to the uninvolved limb.
	1-Plane posterior instability	Posterior drawer test: Positive test is excessive posterior translation of the tibia compared to the uninvolved limb. Posterior sag sign: Tibia "sags" posteriorly (normally extends 1 cm anteriorly beyond femoral condyle) when positioned supine, hip flexed to 45°, and knee flexed to 90°.
	1-Plane medial-lateral instability	Varus stress tests: Positive test is excessive lateral movement and/or pain at the knee. Valgus stress test: Positive test is excessive medial movement and/or pain at the knee (both tests performed at 0° and 30° flexion, positive test at 0° flexion indicates major disruption of the knee and one or more rotary tests also positive).
	Meniscus tear	McMurray test (see Figure 2-16): Positive test is reproduction of click and/or pain in knee joint with rotary force applied.

Functional Mobility and Use of Devices

1. Performed at initial evaluation by PT, ongoing by PT and PTA to determine progress.
2. Gait and locomotion (see Chapter 11).
3. Environmental, home, and work (job/school/play) barriers.
   a. Analysis of barriers.
   b. Analysis of activities the patient needs to perform.
4. Assistive/adaptive devices/orthotic, prosthetic, and supportive devices.
   a. Observe ability to:
      - Don/doff.
      - Monitor skin.
      - Maintain the device.
5. Self-care and home management (including activities of daily living).

Integumentary Integrity

1. Observation of surgical wound.
2. Skin integrity in association with use of devices and/or equipment.

Medical Diagnostic Exams and Imaging

Plain Film Radiograph (X-Ray)

1. Used to demonstrate integrity of bony tissues. X-ray beams pass through the tissues resulting in varying shades of gray on the film depending on the density of the tissue they pass through. The more dense the structure (bone), the more white the structure will appear.
2. A negative to this exam is that it exposes the patient to radiation.

Computed Tomography (CT Scan)

1. Uses plain film x-ray slices that are enhanced by a computer to improve resolution. It is multiplanar so it can be viewed from multiple directions.
2. Typically used to assess complex fractures as well as facet dysfunction, disc disease, or stenosis of the spinal canal, or intervertebral foramen.

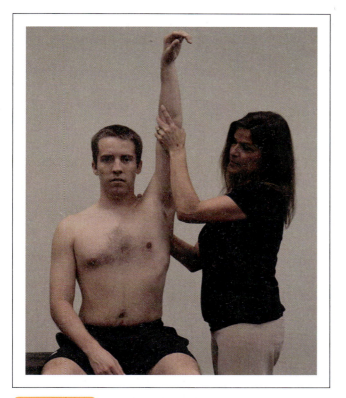

Figure 2-3 Neer's test.

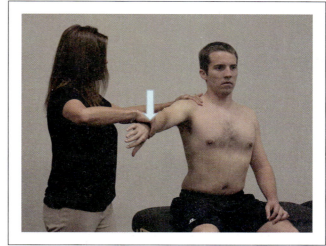

Figure 2-4 Supraspinatus (empty can) test.

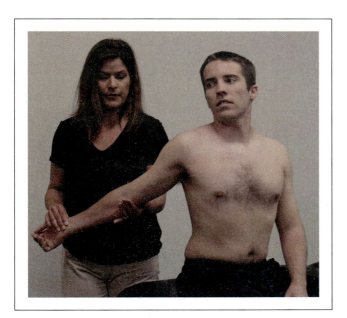

Figure 2-5 Adson's test.

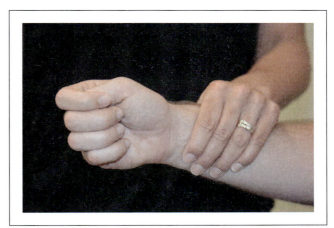

Figure 2-6a Eichhoff's test; start position.

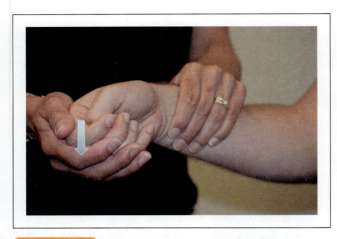

Figure 2-6b Eichhoff's test; passive movement into ulnar deviation.

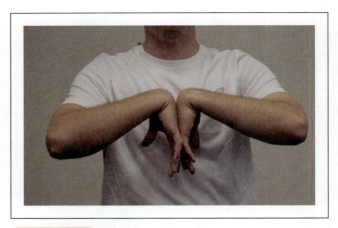

Figure 2-7 Phalen's test.

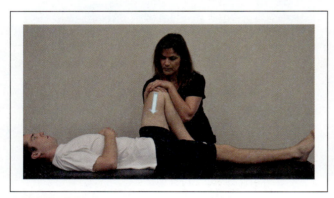

Figure 2-8 Grind (Scouring) test.

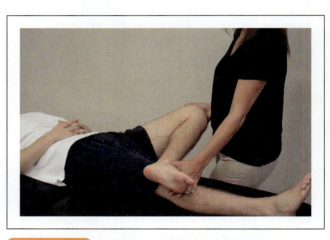

Figure 2-9 Patrick's (FABER) test.

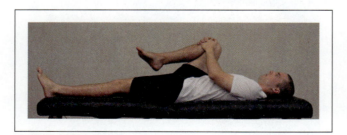

Figure 2-10a Thomas test; negative.

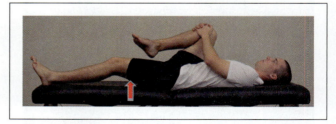

Figure 2-10b Thomas test; positive.

Physical Therapy Examination and Data Collection 39

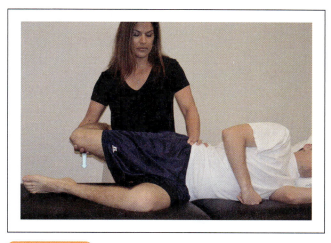

Figure 2-11   Ober test.

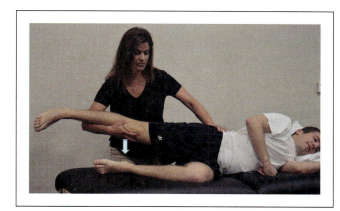

Figure 2-12   Modified Ober test.

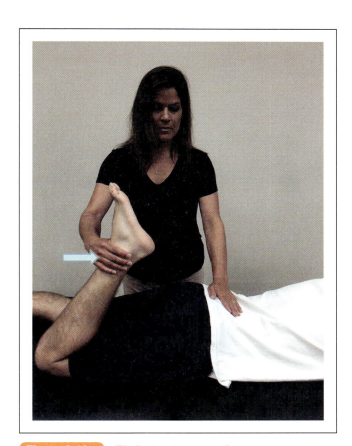

Figure 2-13a   Ely's test; negative.

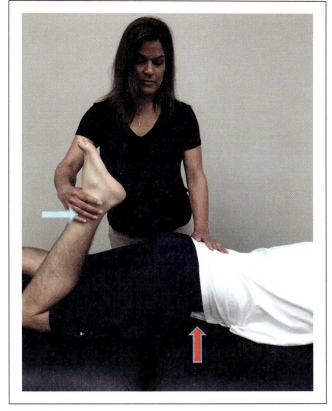

Figure 2-13b   Ely's test; positive.

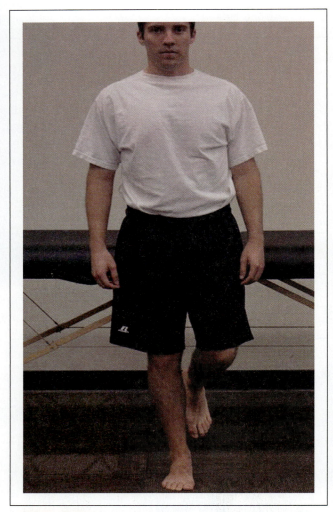

Figure 2-14a Trendelenburg sign; negative test.

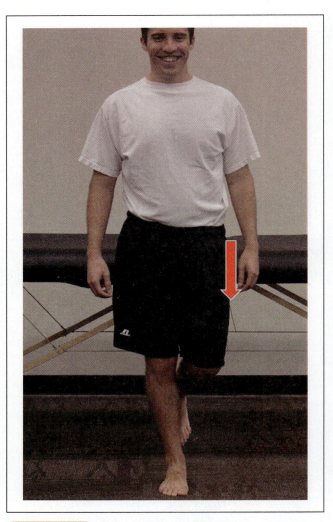

Figure 2-14b Trendelenburg sign; positive test; dropped pelvis.

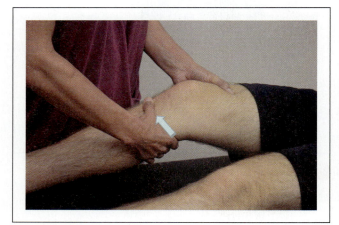

Figure 2-15 Lachman stress test.

3. CT does have the ability to demonstrate soft tissues, although not as well as magnetic resonance imaging (MRI).

Discography
1. Radiopaque dye is injected into the disc to identify abnormalities within the disc (annulus or nucleus). The needle is inserted into the disc with the assistance of radiography (fluoroscopy).

MRI
1. Uses magnetic fields rather than radiation.
2. Offers excellent visualization of tissue anatomy. Utilizes two types of imaging known as T1 and T2. T1 demonstrates fat within the tissues and is typically used to assess bony anatomy; T2 suppresses

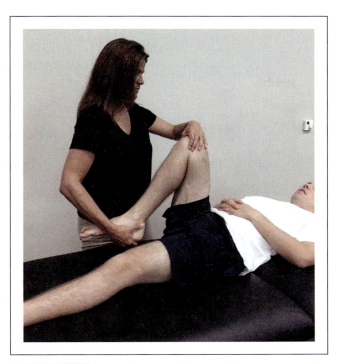

Figure 2-16a McMurray's test; knee flexion.

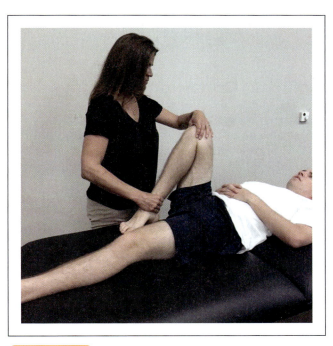

Figure 2-16b McMurray's test; tibial internal rotation.

fat and demonstrates tissues with high water content. T2 is used to assess soft tissue structures.

Arthrography
1. Invasive technique injects water-soluble dye into area and is observed with a radiograph. Dye is observed as it surrounds tissues, demonstrating the process whereby fluid moves within the joint.
2. Typically used to identify abnormalities with joints such as tendon ruptures.

Bone Scan (Osteoscintigraphy)
1. Chemicals laced with radioactive tracers are injected.
2. Isotope settles in areas where there is a high metabolic activity of bone.
3. Radiograph is taken; demonstrates any "hot spots" of increased metabolic activity.
4. Patients with dysfunctions, such as rheumatoid arthritis, possible stress fracture, bone cancer, infection within the bone, will often receive a bone scan because these dysfunctions are known to have an increase in metabolic activity of bone in affected area.

Diagnostic Ultrasound
1. Utilizes transmission of high-frequency sound waves, similar to therapeutic ultrasound.
2. Provides real-time dynamic images and able to assess soft tissue dysfunctions.
3. No harmful effects are known at this time.

Myelography
1. Invasive technique using water-soluble dye. Dye is visualized as it passes through vertebral canal to observe anatomy within region.
2. Seldom used because of many side effects.

Laboratory Tests

Rationale for
1. Laboratory tests can help diagnostic decision making.
2. Potential tests.
   a. Blood tests
   b. Serum chemistries
   c. Immunological tests
   d. Pulmonary function tests
   e. Arterial blood gases
   f. Fluid analysis

Electrodiagnostic Testing

Electroneuromyography (ENMG)
1. Evaluates the health and/or innervation of a muscle.

Nerve Conduction Velocity (NCV)
1. Evaluates nerve function that may be affected by a musculoskeletal disorder (i.e., carpal tunnel syndrome).

Conditions/Pathology/Diseases with Intervention

Arthritic Conditions

Degenerative Joint Disease (DJD)
1. May also be referred to as degenerative osteoarthritis (OA) or osteoarthrosis. It is a degenerative process of varied etiology which includes mechanical changes, diseases, and/or joint trauma. See Table 2-9.
2. Most common form or arthritis, affecting men more than women before age 50 and then more women after age 50. Differentiated in two ways: primary (idiopathic) and secondary disease (i.e., due to trauma).
3. Slowly progressive condition with pain initially episodic and triggered with activity. Eventually, pain and stiffness become chronic. DJD/OA is a progressive and chronic condition. Knee OA is considered the leading cause of disability in the elderly.
4. Many different medications are used to control pain, including corticosteroids and nonsteroidal anti-inflammatory drugs (NSAIDs). Glucocorticoids injected into joints that are inflamed and not responsive to NSAIDs. Viscosupplementation (e.g., Synvisc) or intra-articular injections of the knee with a form of hyaluronic acid (HA) can be used.
5. Diagnostic tests utilized: plain film imaging demonstrates characteristic findings of OA (diminished joint space, decreased height of articular cartilage, presence of osteophytes), and lab tests help to rule out other disorders such as rheumatoid arthritis (RA).
6. Clinical examination will assist in confirming diagnosis.
7. Physical therapy goals, outcomes, and interventions:
   a. Joint protection strategies to maintain joint and soft tissue mobility.
   b. Flexibility and general strengthening to maintain/improve joint mechanics and connective tissue functions.
   c. Implementation of aerobic capacity/endurance conditioning or reconditioning, such as aquatic programs.

Rheumatoid Conditions

Ankylosing Spondylitis (Marie-Strümpell, Bechterew's, Rheumatoid Spondylitis)
1. Progressive inflammatory disorder of unknown etiology that initially affects axial skeleton. Table 2-10 identifies how ankylosing spondylitis can be differeniated from spinal stenosis by the PT.
2. Initial onset (usually mid- and low-back pain for 3 months or more) before fourth decade of life.
3. First symptoms include mid- and low-back pain, morning stiffness, and sacroiliitis.
4. Results in kyphotic deformity of the cervical and thoracic spine and a decrease in lumbar lordosis.
5. Degeneration of peripheral and costovertebral joints may be observed in advanced stages.

Table 2-9

Summary of Symptoms Observed in Common and Uncommon Dysfunctions

DYSFUNCTION	SYMPTOMS OBSERVED
Degenerative joint disease/ Osteoarthritis	Pain and stiffness upon rising Pain eases through the morning (4–5 hours) Pain increases with repetitive bending activities Constant awareness of discomfort with episodes of exacerbation Describes pain as more soreness and nagging
Facet joint dysfunction	Stiff upon rising. Pain eases within an hour Loss of motion accompanied by pain Patient will describe pain as sharp with certain movements Movement in pain-free range usually reduces symptoms Stationary positions increase symptoms
Discal with nerve root compromise	No pain in reclined or semireclined position Pain increases with increasing weight-bearing activities Describes pain as shooting, burning, or stabbing Patient may describe altered strength or ability to perform activities of daily living
Spinal stenosis	Pain is related to position Flexed positions decrease pain, and extended positions increase pain Describes symptoms as a numbness, tightness or cramping Walking for any distance brings on symptoms Pain may persist for hours after assuming a resting position
Vascular claudication	Pain is consistent in all spinal positions Pain is brought on by physical exertion Pain is relieved promptly with rest (1–5 minutes) Pain is described as a numbness Patient usually has decreased or absent pulses
Neoplastic disease	Patient will describe pain as gnawing, intense or penetrating Pain is not resolved by changes in position, time of day, or activity level Pain will wake the patient

Table 2-10

Differentiating Ankylosing Spondylitis and Spinal Stenosis

	ANKYLOSING SPONDYLITIS	SPINAL STENOSIS
History	Morning stiffness Male predominance Sharp pain → ache Bilateral sacroiliac pain may refer to posterior thigh	Intermittent aching pain Pain may refer to both legs with walking (neurogenic intermittent claudication)
Active movements	Restricted	May be normal
Passive movements	Restricted	May be normal
Resisted isometric movements	Normal (in beginning of disorder)	Normal
Posture	Flexed posture of entire spine	Flexed posture of lumbar spine
Special tests	None	Bicycle test of van Gelderen may be positive; Stoop test may be positive
Reflexes	Normal (in beginning of disorder)	May be affected in long-standing cases
Sensory deficit	None (in beginning of disorder)	Usually temporary
Diagnostic imaging	Plain films are diagnostic	Computed tomography scans are diagnostic

Adapted from Magee D: Orthopedic Physical Assessment, 6th ed. 2014.

6. Affects men three times more often than women.
7. Medications: NSAIDs such as aspirin are used to reduce inflammation and pain associated with condition. Corticosteroid therapy or medications to suppress immune system may be used to control various symptoms. Cytotoxic drugs (drugs that block cell growth) may be used in people who do not respond well to corticosteroids or who are dependent on high doses of corticosteroids. Tumor necrosis factor (TNF) inhibitors have been shown to improve some symptoms of ankylosing spondylitis.
8. Diagnostic tests utilized: HLA-B27 antigen may be helpful, but not diagnostic by itself.
9. Clinical examination will assist in confirming diagnosis.
10. Physical therapy goals, outcomes, and interventions:
    a. Implementation of flexibility exercises for trunk to maintain/improve normal joint motion and length of muscles in all directions, especially extension.
    b. Implementation of aerobic capacity/endurance conditioning or reconditioning, such as aquatic programs.
    c. Implementation of relaxation activities to maintain/improve respiratory function.
       - Breathing strategies to maintain/improve vital capacity.

Gout

1. Genetic disorder of purine metabolism characterized by elevated serum uric acid (hyperuricemia). Uric acid changes into crystals and deposits into peripheral joints and other tissues (e.g., kidneys).
2. Most frequently observed at knee and great toe of foot.
3. Medications: NSAIDS (specifically indomethacin), COX-2 inhibitors (cardiac side effects may limit use), colchicine, corticosteroids, adrenocorticotropic hormone (ACTH), allopurinol, probenecid, and sulfinpyrazone.
4. Diagnostic tests utilized: lab tests identify monosodium urate crystals in synovial fluid and/or connective tissue samples.
5. Clinical examination will assist in confirming diagnosis.
6. Physical therapy goals, outcomes, and interventions:
    a. Patient/client education for injury prevention and reduction of involved joint(s).
    b. Early identification of condition with fast implementation of intervention is very important.

Psoriatic Arthritis

1. Chronic, erosive inflammatory disorder of unknown etiology associated with psoriasis.
2. Erosive degeneration usually occurs in joints of digits as well as axial skeleton.
3. Both sexes are affected equally.
4. Medications: acetaminophen for pain, NSAIDs, corticosteroids, disease-modifying antirheumatic drugs (DMARDs) can slow the progression of psoriatic arthritis, and biological response modifiers (BRMs) such as Enbrel (etanercept) are a newly developed class of medicines.
5. Diagnostic tests utilized: lab tests are not useful except to rule out rheumatoid arthritis.
6. Clinical examination will assist in confirming diagnosis.
7. Physical therapy goals, outcomes, and interventions:
    a. Joint protection strategies.
    b. Maintain/improve joint mechanics and connective tissue functions.
    c. Implementation of aerobic capacity/endurance conditioning or reconditioning such as aquatic programs.

Rheumatoid Arthritis (RA) (also See Chapter 8)

1. Chronic systemic autoimmune disorder of unknown etiology thought to have a genetic basis.
2. Individuals with RA produce antibodies to their own immunoglobulins, such as rheumatoid factor (RF) and anti-citrullinated protein antibody (ACPA). The disease is commonly characterized by periods of exacerbation and remission.
   a. Women have two to four times greater incidence than men, with an onset between 40–60 years of age.
   b. Systemic features of RA include weight loss, fever, and extreme fatigue.
   c. Juvenile rheumatoid arthritis (JRA) onset prior to age 16 with complete remission in 75% of children.
   d. Pharmacological management varies with disease progression and may include gold compounds and antirheumatic drugs (DMARDs) (e.g., hydroxychloroquine and methotrexate) early. NSAIDs (e.g., ibuprofen), immunosuppressive agents (e.g., cyclosporine, azathioprine, and mycophenolate) or corticosteroids are commonly prescribed for long-term management.
   e. Diagnostic tests utilized: plain film imaging demonstrating symmetrical involvement within joints as well as laboratory testing. Positive test findings include an increased white blood cell count and erythrocyte sedimentation rate. Hemoglobin and hematocrit tests will show anemia, and rheumatoid factor will be elevated.
   f. Clinical examination will assist in confirming diagnosis.
   g. Physical therapy goals, outcomes, and interventions:
      - Joint protection strategies.
      - Maintain/improve joint mechanics and connective tissue functions.
      - Implementation of aerobic capacity/endurance conditioning or reconditioning such as aquatic programs.

Skeletal Conditions

Osteomalacia
1. Characterized by decalcification of bones as result of a vitamin D deficiency.
2. Symptoms include: severe pain, fractures, weakness and deformities.
3. Medications: calcium, vitamin D, and vitamin D injection in the form of calciferol (vitamin D2).
4. Diagnostic tests utilized: Plain films, lab tests (urinalysis and blood work), bone scan, and potentially a bone biopsy.
5. PT clinical examination will assist in confirming diagnosis.

Physical Therapy Goals, Outcomes, and Interventions
1. Joint/bone protection strategies.
2. Maintain/improve joint mechanics and connective tissue functions.
3. Implementation of aerobic capacity/endurance conditioning or reconditioning such as aquatic programs.

Osteomyelitis
1. An inflammatory response within bone caused by an infection.
2. Usually caused by *Staphylococcus aureus* but could be another organism.
3. More common in children and immunosuppressed adults than healthy adults and more common in males than females.
4. Medical treatment consists of antibiotics. Proper nutrition is important as well. Surgery may be indicated if infection spreads to joints.
5. Diagnostic tests utilized: lab tests for infection and possibly a bone biopsy.
6. Clinical examination will assist in confirming diagnosis.
7. Physical therapy goals, outcomes, and interventions:
   a. Joint/bone protection strategies as well as cast care.
   b. Maintain/improve joint mechanics and connective tissue functions.

Osteochondritis Dissecans
1. A separation of articular cartilage from underlying bone (osteochondral fracture), usually involving medial femoral condyle near intercondylar notch and observed less frequently at femoral head and talar dome. Also affects the humeral capitellum.
2. Surgical intervention is indicated if fracture is displaced.
3. Diagnostic tests utilized: plain film or CT scan imaging to identify defect.
4. Clinical examination will assist in confirming diagnosis.
5. Physical therapy goals, outcomes, and interventions:
   a. Joint/bone protection strategies.
   b. Implementation of flexibility exercises to maintain/improve normal joint motion and length of muscles.
   c. Implementation of aerobic capacity/endurance conditioning or reconditioning such as aquatic programs.
   d. Implementation of strength, power, and endurance exercises.

Other Conditions
1. Osteoporosis. For a full description, see Chapter 8.
2. Arthrogryposis multiplex congenita. For a full description, see Chapter 9.
3. Osteogenesis imperfecta. For a full description, see Chapter 9.

Soft Tissue Conditions

Myofascial Pain Syndrome
1. Characterized by clinical entity known as a "trigger point," which is a focal point of irritability found within a muscle. Trigger points can be identified as a taut palpable band within the muscle.
2. Trigger points may be active or latent. Active trigger points are tender to palpation and have a characteristic referral pattern of pain when provoked. Latent trigger points are palpable taut bands that are not tender to palpation but can be converted into active trigger points.
3. Onset is hypothesized to sudden overload, overstretching, and/or repetitive/sustained muscle activities.
4. Medical intervention may include dry needling and/or injection of analgesic, possibly combined with a corticosteroid.
5. Diagnosis is made by clinical assessment with no diagnostic tests available.
6. Clinical examination will assist in confirming diagnosis.
7. Physical therapy goals, outcomes, and interventions:
   a. Implementation of flexibility exercises to maintain/improve normal joint motion and length of muscles.
   b. Implementation of manual therapy for maintenance of normal joint mechanics.
      - Soft tissue/massage techniques and joint oscillations to reduce pain and/or muscle guarding.
      - Biomechanical faults caused by joint restrictions should be corrected with joint mobilization to the specific restrictions identified during the examination.
      - Use of "spray and stretch" technique.
      - Cryotherapy, thermotherapy, hydrotherapy, sound agents, and transcutaneous electrical nerve stimulation (TENS) for symptomatic relief of pain.
      - Desensitization of trigger point with manual pressure.
   c. Implementation of strength, power, and endurance exercises.
      - Active assistive, active, and resistive exercises.
      - Task-specific performance training.

Tendinitis
1. An inflammation of tendon as result of microtrauma from overuse, direct blows, and/or excessive tensile forces. See Quick Facts 2-4.
2. Medications: acetaminophen, NSAIDs and/or steroid injection.
3. Diagnostic tests utilized: possibly MRI.
4. Clinical examination will assist in confirming diagnosis. Specific special tests are available to assist with making diagnosis within each region/joint.
5. Physical therapy goals, outcomes, and interventions:
   a. Implementation of flexibility exercises to maintain/improve normal joint motion and length of muscles.
   b. Implementation of manual therapy for maintenance of normal joint mechanics.
      - Soft tissue/massage techniques and joint oscillations to reduce pain and/or muscle guarding.
      - Biomechanical faults caused by joint restrictions should be corrected with joint mobilization to the specific restrictions identified during the examination.
   c. Implementation of aerobic capacity/endurance conditioning or reconditioning.
   d. Application of thermal agents for pain reduction, edema reduction, and muscle performance.
      - Cryotherapy, thermotherapy, hydrotherapy, and sound agents.
   e. Patient/client education and training/retraining for instrumental activities of daily living (IADLs).
      - Household chores, yard work, shopping, caring for dependents, and home maintenance.

QUICK FACTS 2-4 ▶ TENDINITIS VS. TENDINOSIS

Tendinitis	Tendinosis
Acute inflammation of a tendon caused by microtears when the musculotendinous unit is overloaded with a tensile force that is too heavy and/or too sudden.	**Degeneration** of a tendon's collagen as a response to chronic overuse and continued overuse without allowing rest and healing time. This is a repetitive strain injury, which can occur with even small movements.
Intervention focus:	Intervention focus:
• Rest	• Stretch tendon, soft tissue work
• Short-term use of anti-inflammatories	• Strengthen surrounding muscles
• Bracing, protection	• Medical intervention may include injection (platelet-rich plasma [PRP])
*Key point: typical recovery is several weeks	*Key Point: may take months to treat, heal

Tendonosis

1. Common chronic tendon dysfunction whose cause and pathogenesis are poorly understood. Often referred to as chronic tendinitis; however, there is no inflammatory response noted.
2. Common in many tendons throughout body (supraspinatus, common extensor tendon of elbow, patella, Achilles').
3. Medications: acetaminophen, NSAIDs and/or steroid injection.
4. Diagnostic tests utilized: possibly MRI.
5. Clinical examination will assist in confirming diagnosis. Specific special tests are available to assist with making diagnosis within each region/joint.
6. Physical therapy goals, outcomes, and interventions:
   a. Implementation of flexibility exercises to maintain/improve normal joint motion and length of muscles.
   b. Implementation of manual therapy for maintenance of normal joint mechanics.
      - Soft tissue/massage techniques and joint oscillations to reduce pain and/or muscle guarding.
      - Biomechanical faults caused by joint restrictions should be corrected with joint mobilization to the specific restrictions identified during the examination.
   c. Implementation of aerobic capacity/endurance conditioning or reconditioning.
   d. Application of thermal agents for pain reduction, edema reduction, and muscle performance.
      - Cryotherapy, thermotherapy, hydrotherapy, and sound agents.
   e. Patient/client education and training/retraining for IADLs.
      - Household chores, yard work, shopping, caring for dependents, and home maintenance.

Bursitis

1. Bursitis is an inflammation of bursa secondary to overuse, trauma, gout, or infection.
2. Signs and symptoms of bursitis.
   a. Pain with rest.
   b. Passive ROM (PROM) and active ROM (AROM) are limited due to pain but not in a capsular pattern.
3. Medications: acetaminophen, NSAIDs, and/or steroid injection.
4. Clinical examination will assist in confirming diagnosis.
5. Physical therapy goals, outcomes, and interventions:
   a. Implementation of flexibility exercises to maintain/improve normal joint motion and length of muscles.
   b. Implementation of manual therapy for maintenance of normal joint mechanics.
      - Soft tissue/massage techniques and joint oscillations to reduce pain and/or muscle guarding.
      - Biomechanical faults caused by joint restrictions should be corrected with joint mobilization to the specific restrictions identified during the examination.
   c. Implementation of aerobic capacity/endurance conditioning or reconditioning.
   d. Application of thermal agents for pain reduction, edema reduction, and muscle performance.
      - Cryotherapy, thermotherapy, hydrotherapy, and sound agents.
   e. Patient/client education and training/retraining for IADLs.
      - Household chores, yard work, shopping, caring for dependents, and home maintenance.

Muscle Strains

1. Characterized by an inflammatory response within a muscle following a traumatic event that caused microtearing of the musculotendinous fibers.
2. Pain and tenderness within that muscle.
3. Seen within muscles throughout the body.
4. Medications: acetaminophen and/or NSAIDs.
5. Diagnostic tests utilized: MRI if necessary.
6. Clinical examination will assist in confirming diagnosis.
7. Physical therapy goals, outcomes, and interventions:
   a. Implementation of flexibility exercises to maintain/improve normal joint motion and length of muscles.
   b. Implementation of manual therapy for maintenance of normal joint mechanics.
      - Soft tissue/massage techniques and joint oscillations to reduce pain and/or muscle guarding.
      - Biomechanical faults caused by joint restrictions should be corrected with joint mobilization to the specific restrictions identified during the examination.
   c. Implementation of aerobic capacity/endurance conditioning or reconditioning.
   d. Application of thermal agents for pain reduction, edema reduction, and muscle performance.
      - Cryotherapy, thermotherapy, hydrotherapy, and sound agents.
   e. Patient/client education and training/retraining for IADL.
      - Household chores, yard work, shopping, caring for dependents, and home maintenance.

Myositis Ossificans

1. Painful condition of abnormal calcification within a muscle belly.
2. Usually precipitated by direct trauma that results in hematoma and calcification of the muscle.

3. Can also be induced by early mobilization and stretching with aggressive physical therapy following trauma to muscle.
4. Most frequent locations are quadriceps, brachialis, and biceps brachii muscles.
5. Medications: acetaminophen and/or NSAIDs.
6. Surgical care is warranted only in patients with non-hereditary myositis ossificans and only after maturation of the lesion (6–24 months). Surgery is indicated when lesions mechanically interfere with joint movement or impinge on nerves.
7. Diagnostic tests utilized: imaging (plain films, CT scan, and/or MRI).
8. Clinical examination will assist in confirming diagnosis.
9. Physical therapy goals, outcomes, and interventions:
   a. Implementation of flexibility exercises to maintain/improve normal joint motion and length of muscles. Must avoid being overly aggressive with muscle flexibility exercises, which may worsen condition.
   b. Implementation of manual therapy for maintenance of normal joint mechanics.
      - Soft tissue/massage techniques and joint oscillations to reduce pain and/or muscle guarding. Avoid aggressive soft tissue/massage techniques, which may worsen condition.
      - Biomechanical faults caused by joint restrictions should be corrected with joint mobilization to the specific restrictions identified during the examination.
   c. Implementation of aerobic capacity/endurance conditioning or reconditioning, such as aquatic programs.

Complex Regional Pain Syndrome (CRPS)
1. See Chapter 3 for full description.

Paget's Disease (Osteitis Deformans)
1. See Chapter 8 for full description.

Idiopathic Scoliosis
1. Two types: structural and nonstructural, both of unknown etiology.
2. Structural scoliosis is an irreversible lateral curvature of spine with a rotational component.
3. Nonstructural scoliosis is a reversible lateral curvature of spine without a rotational component and straightening as individual flexes spine.
4. Intervention for structural scoliosis includes bracing and possible surgery with placement of Harrington rod instrumentation. Rule of thumb is <25 degrees, do conservative physical therapy (see below); between 25 and 45 degrees use spinal orthoses. Surgery is generally performed for curves >45 degrees.
5. Diagnostic tests utilized: plain film imaging using full-length Cobb's method. CT scan and/or MRI may be used to rule out associated conditions.
6. Clinical examination will assist in confirming diagnosis.
7. Physical therapy goals, outcomes and interventions:
   a. Implementation of flexibility exercises to maintain/improve normal joint motion and length of muscles throughout trunk and pelvis.
   b. Implementation of strength, power, and endurance exercises.
   c. Electrical stimulation to improve muscle performance.
   d. Application and patient education regarding spinal orthoses.

Torticollis
1. Spasm and/or tightness of sternocleidomastoid (SCM) muscle with varied etiology.
2. Dysfunction observed is side-bending toward and rotation away from the affected SCM.
3. Medications: acetaminophen, muscle relaxants, and/or NSAIDs.
4. Diagnostic tests utilized: none.
5. Physical therapy goals, outcomes and interventions:
   a. Implementation of flexibility exercises to maintain/improve normal joint motion and length of muscles.
   b. Implementation of manual therapy for maintenance of normal joint mechanics.
      - Soft tissue/massage techniques and joint oscillations to reduce pain and/or muscle guarding.
      - Biomechanical faults caused by joint restrictions should be corrected with joint mobilization to the specific restrictions identified during the examination.

TMJ Conditions
1. Common signs and symptoms include joint noise (i.e., clicking, popping, and/or crepitation), joint locking, limited flexibility of jaw, lateral deviation of mandible during depression or elevation of mandible, decreased strength/endurance of muscles of mastication, tinnitus, headaches, forward head posture, and pain with movement of mandible.
2. Cervical spine must be thoroughly examined because of close biomechanical and functional relationships between TMJ and cervical region. Many patients with a TMJ condition have a component of cervical dysfunction.
3. Dysfunctions fall into three diagnostic categories:
   a. DJD such as osteoarthritis (OA) or rheumatoid arthritis (RA) in the TMJ (refer to OA and RA for causes, characteristic findings, diagnostic methods, medical and physical therapy intervention).
   b. Myofascial pain is the most common form of temporomandibular dysfunction (TMD), which

is discomfort or pain in muscles that control jaw function, as well as neck and shoulder muscles. (Refer to myofascial pain syndrome for causes, characteristic findings, diagnostic methods, medical and physical therapy intervention.)
  c. Internal derangement of joint, meaning a dislocated jaw, displaced articular disc, or injury to condyle.
     - Loss of functional mobility may result from increased activity in muscles of mastication as result of stress and anxiety.
     - Causes:
       ○ Trauma, leading to joint edema, capsulitis, hypomobility/hypermobility or abnormal function of ligaments, capsule and/or muscles.
       ○ Congenital anatomical anomalies: change in shape of palate.
       ○ Abnormal function such as repeatedly chewing ice or hard candy, paranormal breathing (mouth breather), forward head posture.
4. Diagnostic tests utilized:
   a. Plain film imaging and/or MRI if necessary.
   b. Clinical examination helps to identify this condition.
5. Medications:
   a. Acetaminophen for pain.
   b. NSAIDs for pain and/or inflammation.
   c. Muscle relaxants.
   d. Trigger point injections.
   e. Corticosteroid injection or by mouth.
6. Physical therapy goals, outcomes, and interventions:
   a. Postural reeducation regarding regaining the normal anterior-posterior curves and left-right symmetry of the spine.
   b. Modalities for reduction of pain and inflammation.
   c. Biofeedback to minimize effects of stress and/or anxiety.
   d. Joint mobilization if restriction in TMJ is present. Primary glide is inferior, which gaps joint, stretches the capsule, and allows relocation of anteriorly displaced disc.
   e. Flexibility and muscle-strengthening exercises (e.g., Rocobado's jaw opening while maintaining the tongue in contact with the palate and isometric mandibular exercises).
   f. Patient education (e.g., foods to avoid and maintaining proper postural alignment).
   g. Night splints may be prescribed by the dentist to maintain resting jaw position.
   h. Educate patient regarding resting position of tongue on hard palate.
   i. It is critical to normalize the cervical spine posture prior to the patient receiving any permanent dental procedures and/or appliances.

Upper Extremity Conditions—Shoulder

Glenohumeral Subluxation and Dislocation

1. Most dislocations (95%) occur in anterior-inferior direction.
2. Anterior-inferior dislocation occurs when abducted upper extremity is forcefully externally rotated causing tearing of inferior glenohumeral ligament, anterior capsule, and occasionally glenoid labrum.
3. Posterior dislocations are rare and occur with multi-directional laxity of glenohumeral joint.
4. Posterior dislocation occurs with horizontal adduction and internal rotation of glenohumeral joint.
5. Complications may include compression fracture of posterior humeral head (Hill-Sachs lesion), tearing of superior glenoid labrum from posterior to anterior (SLAP lesion), an avulsion of anteroinferior capsule and ligaments associated with glenoid rim (Bankart's lesion), and bruising of axillary nerve.
6. Following surgical repair for dislocation/chronic subluxation, patients should avoid apprehension position (flexion to 90 degrees or greater, horizontal abduction to 90 degrees or greater, and external rotation to 80 degrees).
7. Diagnostic tests utilized: Plain film imaging, CT scan, and/or MRI.
8. PT clinical examination. Apprehension tests will be positive.
9. Medications:
   a. Acetaminophen for pain.
   b. NSAIDs for pain and/or inflammation.
10. Physical therapy goals, outcomes, and interventions:
    a. Physical therapy intervention is varied dependent upon the specific patient problems and whether surgery is performed.
    b. Biomechanical faults caused by joint restrictions should be corrected with joint mobilization to the specific restrictions identified during the examination.
    c. Restoration of normal shoulder mechanics via strengthening/endurance/coordination exercises that focus on regaining dynamic scapulothoracic and glenohumeral stabilization and muscular reeducation.

Instability

1. Divided into two categories: traumatic (common in young throwing athletes) and atraumatic (individuals with congenitally loose connective tissue around the shoulder).
2. Characterized by popping/clicking and repeated dislocation/subluxation of the glenohumeral joint.

3. Unstable injuries will require surgery to reattach the labrum to the glenoid. Bankart's lesions will require surgery.
4. Diagnosis made by clinical examination by comparing results of patient history with the AROM, PROM, resistive tests, and palpation. MRI arthrograms are very effective in identifying labral tears.
5. Medications:
   a. Acetaminophen for pain.
   b. NSAIDS for pain and/or inflammation.
6. Physical therapy goals, outcomes, and interventions:
   a. Physical therapy intervention emphasizes return of function without pain.
   b. Functional training and restoration of muscle imbalances using exercise to normalize strength, endurance, coordination, and flexibility.
   c. Biomechanical faults caused by joint restrictions should be corrected with joint mobilization to the specific restrictions identified during the examination.
   d. For patients requiring surgery, the shoulder will usually be kept in a sling for 3 or 4 weeks. After 6 weeks, more sport-specific training can be done, although full fitness may take 3 or 4 months.

Labral Tears

1. Glenoid labrum injuries are classified as either superior (toward the top of the glenoid socket) or inferior toward the bottom of the glenoid socket.
   a. A superior injury is known as a SLAP lesion (superior labrum, anterior [front] to posterior [back]) and is a tear of the rim above the middle of the socket which may also involve the biceps tendon.
   b. A tear of the rim below the middle of the glenoid socket is called a Bankart lesion and also involves the inferior glenohumeral ligament.
   c. Tears of the glenoid labrum may often occur with other shoulder injuries, such as a dislocated shoulder.
2. Characterized by the following signs and symptoms:
   a. Shoulder pain that cannot be localized to a specific point.
   b. Pain is made worse by overhead activities or when the arm is held behind the back.
   c. Weakness.
   d. Instability in the shoulder.
   e. Pain on resisted flexion of the biceps (bending the elbow against resistance).
   f. Tenderness over the front of the shoulder.
3. Unstable injuries will require surgery to reattach the labrum to the glenoid. Bankart's lesions will require surgery.
4. Diagnosis made by clinical examination by comparing results of AROM, PROM, resistive tests, and palpation. MRI arthrograms are very effective in identifying labral tears. The "gold" standard for identifying a labral tear is through arthroscopic surgery of the shoulder.
5. Medications:
   a. Acetaminophen for pain.
   b. NSAIDs for pain and/or inflammation.
6. Physical therapy goals, outcomes, and interventions:
   a. Physical therapy intervention emphasizes return of function without pain.
   b. Functional training and restoration of muscle imbalances using exercise to normalize strength, endurance, coordination, and flexibility.
   c. Any underlying causes that contributed to the injury such as shoulder instability should be addressed.
   d. Biomechanical faults caused by joint restrictions should be corrected with joint mobilization to the specific restrictions identified during the examination.
   e. Following surgery, the shoulder will usually be kept in a sling for 3 or 4 weeks. After 6 weeks, more sport-specific training can be done, although full fitness may take 3 or 4 months.

Thoracic Outlet Syndrome (TOS)

1. Compression of neurovascular bundle (brachial plexus, subclavian artery and vein, vagus and phrenic nerves, and the sympathetic trunk) in thoracic outlet between bony and soft tissue structures.
2. Compression occurs when size or shape of thoracic outlet is altered.
3. Common areas of compression are:
   a. Superior thoracic outlet.
   b. Scalene triangle.
   c. Between clavicle and first rib.
   d. Between pectoralis minor and thoracic wall.
4. Surgery may be performed to remove a cervical rib or a release of anterior and/or middle scalene muscle.
5. Diagnostic tests utilized: plain film imaging to identify abnormal bony anatomy and MRI to identify abnormal soft tissue anatomy. Electrodiagnostic test to assess nerve dysfunction.
6. PT clinical examination may include special tests (e.g., Adson's or Roos' test).
7. Medications:
   a. Acetaminophen for pain.
   b. NSAIDs for pain and/or inflammation.
8. Physical therapy goals, outcomes, and interventions:
   a. Physical therapy intervention will vary depending on the exact cause.
   b. Includes postural reeducation.
   c. Functional training and restoration of muscle imbalances using exercise to normalize strength, endurance, coordination, and flexibility.
   d. Biomechanical faults caused by joint restrictions should be corrected with joint mobilization to

the specific restrictions identified during the examination.
  e. Manipulations (typically first rib articulation) to diminish pain and soft tissue guarding.

Acromioclavicular and Sternoclavicular Joint Disorders
1. Mechanism of injury is a fall onto shoulder with upper extremity adducted or a collision with another individual during a sporting event.
2. Traditionally, degree of injury is graded from first to third degree.
3. Upper extremity is positioned in neutral with use of sling in acute phase. Avoid shoulder elevation during the acute phase of healing.
4. Diagnostic tests utilized: plain film imaging.
5. PT clinical examination may include the shear test.
6. Surgical repair is rare due to tendency of acromioclavicular joint degeneration following the repair.
7. Medications:
  a. Acetaminophen for pain.
  b. NSAIDs for pain and/or inflammation.
8. Physical therapy goals, outcomes, and interventions:
  a. Emphasize return of function without pain.
  b. Functional training and restoration of muscle imbalances using exercise to normalize strength, endurance, coordination, and flexibility.
  c. Manual therapy techniques to AC and SC joints and surrounding connective tissues such as soft tissue/massage, joint oscillations and mobilizations to normalize soft tissue and joint biomechanics.

Subacromial/Subdeltoid Bursitis
1. Subacromial and subdeltoid bursae (which may be continuous) have a close relationship to rotator cuff tendons, which makes them susceptible to overuse.
2. They can also become impinged beneath the acromial arch.
3. Diagnosis made by PT clinical examination. Differentiate from contractile condition by comparing results of AROM, PROM, and resistive tests.
4. Medications:
  a. Acetaminophen for pain.
  b. NSAIDs for pain and/or inflammation.
5. Physical therapy goals, outcomes, and interventions:
  a. Refer to intervention for general bursitis/tendinitis/tendonosis. (See Interventions listed pages 53–60.)

Rotator Cuff Tendinitis
1. Tendons of rotator cuff are susceptible to tendinitis due to relatively poor blood supply near insertion of muscles.
2. Results from mechanical impingement of the distal attachment of the rotator cuff on the anterior acromion and/or coracoacromial ligament with repetitive overhead activities.
3. Diagnostic tests utilized: MRI may be used, but sometimes not sensitive enough for accurate assessment.
4. PT clinical examination including the following special tests will be useful to make diagnosis.
  a. Supraspinatus test.
  b. Neer's impingement test.
5. Medications:
  a. Acetaminophen for pain.
  b. NSAIDs for pain and/or inflammation.
6. Physical therapy goals, outcomes, and interventions:
  a. Refer to intervention for general bursitis/tendinitis/tendonosis. (See Interventions listed pages 53–60.)

Impingement Syndrome
1. Characterized by soft tissue inflammation of the shoulder from impingement against the acromion with repetitive overhead AROM.
2. Diagnostic tests utilized: arthrogram or MRI may be used.
3. PT clinical examination including the following special tests will be useful to make diagnosis.
  a. Neer's impingement test.
  b. Supraspinatus test.
  c. Drop arm test.
4. Surgical repair of shoulder impingement.
  a. The patient should avoid shoulder elevation >90 degrees.
5. Medications:
  a. Acetaminophen for pain.
  b. NSAIDs for pain and/or inflammation.
6. Physical therapy goals, outcomes, and interventions:
  a. Restoration of posture.
  b. Correction of muscle imbalances and biomechanical faults using strengthening, endurance, coordination, and flexibility exercises to gain restoration of normal function.
  c. Biomechanical faults caused by joint restrictions should be corrected with joint mobilization to the specific restrictions identified during the examination.

Internal (Posterior) Impingement
1. Characterized by an irritation between the rotator cuff and greater tuberosity or posterior glenoid and labrum.
2. Often seen in athletes performing overhead activities. Pain commonly noted in posterior shoulder.
3. Diagnostic tests utilized: none.
4. PT clinical examination including posterior internal impingement test helps to identify this condition.
5. Medications:
  a. Acetaminophen for pain.
  b. NSAIDs for pain and/or inflammation.

6. Physical therapy goals, outcomes, and interventions:
   a. Correction of muscle imbalances and biomechanical faults using strengthening, endurance, coordination, and flexibility exercises to gain restoration of normal function.
   b. Biomechanical faults caused by joint restrictions should be corrected with joint mobilization to the specific restrictions identified during the examination.

Bicipital Tendinitis
1. Most commonly an inflammation of the long head of the biceps.
2. Results from mechanical impingement of the proximal tendon between the anterior acromion and the bicipital groove of the humerus.
3. Diagnostic tests utilized: MRI may be used, but sometimes not sensitive enough for accurate assessment.
4. PT clinical examination including the following special test will be useful to make diagnosis.
   a. Speed's test.
5. Medications:
   a. Acetaminophen for pain.
   b. NSAIDs for pain and/or inflammation.
6. Physical therapy goals, outcomes and interventions:
   a. Refer to intervention for general bursitis/tendinitis/tendonosis. (See Interventions listed pages 53–60.)

Proximal Humeral Fractures
1. Humeral neck fractures frequently occur with a fall onto an outstretched upper extremity among older osteoporotic women. Generally do not require immobilization or surgical repair because they are fairly stable fractures.
2. Greater tuberosity fractures are more common in middle-aged and elder adults. They are also usually related to a fall onto the shoulder and do not require immobilization for healing.
3. Diagnostic tests utilized: plain film imaging.
4. Medications:
   a. Acetaminophen for pain.
   b. NSAIDs for pain and/or inflammation.
5. Physical therapy goals, outcomes, and interventions:
   a. Physical therapy intervention emphasizes return of function without pain.
   b. Functional training and restoration of muscle imbalances using exercise to normalize strength, endurance, coordination, and flexibility.
   c. Biomechanical faults caused by joint restrictions should be corrected with joint mobilization to the specific restrictions identified during the examination.
   d. Early PROM is important in preventing capsular adhesions.

Adhesive Capsulitis (Frozen Shoulder)
1. Characterized by a restriction in shoulder motion as a result of inflammation and fibrosis of the shoulder capsule, usually due to disuse following injury or repetitive microtrauma.
2. Restriction follows a capsular pattern of limitation:
   a. Greatest limitation in external rotation, followed by abduction and flexion, and least restricted in internal rotation.
3. Commonly seen in association with diabetes mellitus.
4. Diagnosis made by clinical examination by comparing results of AROM, PROM, resistive tests, and palpation.
5. Medications:
   a. Acetaminophen for pain.
   b. NSAIDs for pain and/or inflammation.
6. Physical therapy goals, outcomes, and interventions:
   a. Physical therapy intervention emphasizes return of function without pain.
   b. Functional training and restoration of muscle imbalances using exercise to normalize strength, endurance, coordination, and flexibility.
   c. Biomechanical faults caused by joint restrictions should be corrected with joint mobilization to the specific restrictions identified during the examination.

Upper Extremity Conditions—Elbow

Elbow Contractures
1. Loss of motion in capsular pattern (loss of flexion greater than extension).
2. Loss of motion in noncapsular pattern as the result of a loose body in the joint, ligamentous sprain, and/or complex regional pain syndrome.
3. Diagnosis made by clinical examination by comparing results of AROM, PROM, resistive tests, and palpation.
4. Medications:
   a. Acetaminophen for pain.
   b. NSAIDs for pain and/or inflammation.
5. Physical therapy goals, outcomes, and interventions:
   a. Biomechanical faults caused by joint restrictions should be corrected with joint mobilization to the specific restrictions identified during the examination.
   b. Soft tissue/massage techniques, modalities, flexibility exercises, and functional exercises including strengthening, endurance, and coordination.
   c. Splinting may be an effective adjunct to physical therapy management in regaining loss of motion for capsular restrictions.

Lateral Epicondylitis ("Tennis Elbow")
1. Most often a chronic inflammation of the extensor carpi radialis brevis (ECRB) tendon at its proximal attachment to the lateral epicondyle of the humerus.
2. Onset is gradual, usually the result of sports activities or occupations that require repetitive wrist extension or strong grip with the wrist extended, resulting in overloading the ECRB.
3. PT clinical examination includes:
   a. Tests to rule out involvement or relationship to cervical spine condition.
   b. Lateral epicondylitis tests to clearly identify condition.
4. Medications:
   a. Acetaminophen for pain.
   b. NSAIDs for pain and/or inflammation.
5. Physical therapy goals, outcomes, and interventions:
   a. Correction of muscle imbalances and biomechanical faults using strengthening, endurance, coordination, and flexibility exercises to gain restoration of normal function.
   b. Biomechanical faults caused by joint restrictions should be corrected with joint mobilization to the specific restrictions identified during the examination.
   c. Education regarding prevention.
   d. Cryotherapy, thermotherapy, hydrotherapy, sound agents, and TENS for symptomatic relief of pain.
   e. Counterforce bracing is frequently used to reduce forces along the ECRB.

Medial Epicondylitis ("Golfer's Elbow")
1. Usually an inflammation of the pronator teres and flexor carpi radialis tendons at their attachment to the medial epicondyle of the humerus.
2. Occurs as the result of chronic overuse in sports such as baseball pitching, driving golf swings, swimming, or occupations that require a strong hand grip and excessive pronation of the forearm.
3. Diagnostic tests utilized: none.
4. PT clinical examination including medial epicondylitis test helps to identify this condition.
5. Physical therapy goals, outcomes, and interventions: Intervention is similar to lateral epicondylitis.

Distal Humeral Fracture
1. Complications can include loss of motion, myositis ossificans, malalignment, neurovascular compromise, ligamentous injury, and CRPS.
2. Supracondylar fractures must be examined quickly for neurovascular status due to high number of neurological (typically radial nerve involvement) and vascular structures that pass through this region (may lead to Volkmann's ischemia). In youth, it is important to assess growth plate as well. These fractures have high incidence of malunion.
3. Lateral epicondyle fractures are fairly common in young people and typically require an open reduction internal fixation (ORIF) to ensure absolute alignment.
4. Diagnostic tests utilized: plain film imaging.
5. Medications:
   a. Acetaminophen for pain.
   b. NSAIDs for pain and/or inflammation.
6. Physical therapy goals, outcomes, and interventions:
   a. Physical therapy intervention includes pain reduction and limiting the inflammatory response following trauma and/or surgery.
   b. Improving flexibility of shortened structures, strengthening, and training to restore functional use of upper extremity (UE).

Osteochondrosis of Humeral Capitellum
1. Osteochondritis dissecans affects central and/or lateral aspect of capitellum or radial head. An osteochondral bone fragment becomes detached from articular surface, forming a loose body in joint. Caused by repetitive compressive forces between radial head and humeral capitellum. Occurs in adolescents between 12 and 15 years of age.
2. Panner's disease is a localized avascular necrosis of capitellum leading to loss of subchondral bone with fissuring and softening of articular surfaces of radiocapitellar joint. Etiology is unknown but occurs in children age 10 or younger.
3. Diagnostic tests utilized: plain film imaging.
4. Medications:
   a. Acetaminophen for pain.
   b. NSAIDs for pain and/or inflammation.
5. Physical therapy goals, outcomes, and interventions:
   a. Physical therapy intervention includes rest with avoidance of any throwing or UE loading activities (e.g., gymnastics).
   b. When patient is pain free, initiate flexibility and strengthening/endurance/coordination exercises.
   c. During late phases of rehabilitation, a program to slowly increase load on joint is initiated. If symptoms persist, surgical intervention is necessary.
   d. After surgery, initial focus of rehabilitation is to minimize pain and swelling using modalities. Flexibility exercises are begun immediately following surgery.
   e. Thereafter, a progressive strengthening program is initiated.
   f. Biomechanical faults caused by joint restrictions should be corrected with joint mobilization to the specific restrictions identified during the examination.

Ulnar Collateral Ligament Injuries
1. Occur as result of repetitive valgus stresses to medial elbow with overhead throwing.
2. Clinical signs include pain along medial elbow at distal insertion of ligament. In some cases, paresthesias are reported in ulnar nerve distribution with positive Tinel's sign.
3. Diagnostic tests utilized: MRI.
4. PT clinical examination including medial ligament instability test helps to identify this condition.
5. Medications:
   a. Acetaminophen for pain.
   b. NSAIDs for pain and/or inflammation.
6. Physical therapy goals, outcomes, and interventions:
   a. Initial intervention includes rest and pain management.
   b. After resolution of pain and inflammation, strengthening exercises that focus on elbow flexors are initiated. Taping can also be used for protection during return to activities.

Nerve Entrapments
1. Ulnar nerve entrapment.
   a. Various causes that include direct trauma at the cubital tunnel, traction due to laxity at medial aspect of elbow, compression due to a thickened retinaculum or hypertrophy of flexor carpi ulnaris muscle, recurrent subluxation or dislocation, and DJD that affects the cubital tunnel.
   b. Clinical findings include medial elbow pain and paresthesias in ulnar distribution, and a positive Tinel's sign.
2. Median nerve entrapment.
   a. Occurs within pronator teres muscle and under superficial head of flexor digitorum superficialis with repetitive gripping activities required in occupations (e.g., electricians) and with leisure time activities (e.g., tennis).
   b. Clinical signs include an aching pain with weakness of forearm muscles and positive Tinel's sign with paresthesias in median nerve distribution.
3. Radial nerve entrapment.
   a. Entrapment of distal branches (posterior interosseous nerve) occurs within radial tunnel (radial tunnel syndrome) as result of overhead activities and throwing.
   b. Clinical signs include lateral elbow pain that can be confused with lateral epicondylitis, pain over supinator muscle, and paresthesias in a radial nerve distribution. Tinel's sign may be positive.
4. Diagnosis.
   a. Electrodiagnostic tests are used.
   b. Clinical examination can help to identify this condition as well.
5. Medications:
   a. Acetaminophen for pain.
   b. NSAIDs for pain and/or inflammation.
   c. Neurontin for neuropathic pain.
6. Physical therapy goals, outcomes, and interventions:
   a. Early intervention includes rest, avoiding exacerbating activities, use of NSAIDs, modalities, and soft tissue/massage techniques to reduce inflammation and pain.
   b. Protective padding and night splints to maintain slackened position of involved nerves.
   c. Nerve gliding to improve neurodynamics.
   d. With reduction in pain and paresthesias, rehabilitation program should focus on strengthening/endurance/coordination exercise of involved muscles to achieve muscle balance between agonists and antagonists, normal flexibility of shortened structures, and normalization of strength/endurance/coordination.
   e. Intervention should also include functional training, patient education, and self-management techniques.

Elbow Dislocations
1. Posterior dislocations account for most dislocations occurring at elbow.
   a. Posterior dislocations are defined by position of olecranon relative to the humerus.
   b. Posterolateral dislocations are most common and occur as the result of elbow hyperextension from a fall on the outstretched upper extremity.
   c. Posterior dislocations frequently cause avulsion fractures of medial epicondyle secondary to traction pull of medial collateral ligament.
2. Anterior and radial head dislocations account for only 1%–2% of all elbow dislocations.
3. With a complete dislocation, ulnar collateral ligament will rupture with possible rupture of anterior capsule, lateral collateral ligament, brachialis muscle, and/or wrist flexor and extensor muscles.
4. Clinical signs include rapid swelling, severe pain at the elbow, and a deformity with olecranon pushed posteriorly.
5. Diagnostic tests utilized: plain film imaging.
6. Medications:
   a. Acetaminophen for pain.
   b. NSAIDs for pain and/or inflammation.
7. Physical therapy goals, outcomes, and interventions:
   a. Initial intervention includes reduction of the dislocation.
   b. If elbow is stable, there is an initial phase of immobilization followed by rehabilitation focusing on regaining flexibility within limits of stability and strengthening.
   c. If elbow is not stable, surgery is indicated.

Upper Extremity Conditions— Wrist & Hand

Carpal Tunnel Syndrome (Repetitive Stress Syndrome)
1. Compression of the median nerve at the carpal tunnel of the wrist as the result of inflammation of the flexor tendons and/or median nerve.
2. Commonly occurs as result of repetitive wrist motions or gripping, with pregnancy, diabetes, and rheumatoid arthritis.
3. Must rule out potential of cervical spine dysfunction, thoracic outlet syndrome, or peripheral nerve entrapment that is mimicking this condition.
4. Diagnostic tests utilized: electrodiagnostic testing.
5. Common clinical findings include exacerbation of burning, tingling, pins and needles and numbness into median nerve distribution at night, and a positive Tinel's sign and/or Phalen's test. Long-term compression causes atrophy and weakness of thenar muscles and lateral two lumbricals.
6. Medications:
   a. Acetaminophen for pain.
   b. NSAIDs for pain and/or inflammation.
7. Physical therapy goals, outcomes, and interventions:
   a. Biomechanical faults caused by joint restrictions should be corrected with joint mobilization to the specific restrictions identified during the examination.
   b. Soft tissue/massage techniques, modalities, flexibility exercises, and functional exercises including strengthening, endurance and coordination.

DeQuervain's Tenosynovitis
1. Inflammation of extensor pollicis brevis and abductor pollicis longus tendons at first dorsal compartment.
2. Results from repetitive microtrauma or as a complication of swelling during pregnancy.
3. Diagnostic tests utilized: MRI, but usually not necessary to make diagnosis.
4. Clinical signs include: pain at anatomical snuffbox, swelling, decreased grip and pinch strength, positive Finkelstein's test (which places tendons on a stretch).
5. Medications:
   a. Acetaminophen for pain.
   b. NSAIDs for pain and/or inflammation.
6. Physical therapy goals, outcomes, and interventions:
   a. Biomechanical faults caused by joint restrictions should be corrected with joint mobilization to the specific restrictions identified during the examination.
   b. Soft tissue/massage techniques, modalities, flexibility exercises, and functional exercises including strengthening, endurance and coordination.

Colles' Fracture
1. Most common wrist fracture resulting from a fall onto an outstretched UE. These fractures are immobilized between 5 and 8 weeks. Complication of median nerve compression can occur with excessive edema.
2. Characteristic "dinner fork" deformity of wrist and hand results from dorsal or posterior displacement of distal fragment of radius with a radial shift of wrist and hand.
3. Diagnostic tests utilized: plain film imaging.
4. Complications may include loss of motion, decreased grip strength, CRPS, and carpal tunnel syndrome.
5. Medications:
   a. Acetaminophen for pain.
   b. NSAIDs for pain and/or inflammation.
6. Physical therapy goals, outcomes, and interventions:
   a. Early physical therapy intervention that focuses on normalizing flexibility is paramount to functional recovery of wrist and hand.
   b. Biomechanical faults caused by joint restrictions should be corrected with joint mobilization to the specific restrictions identified during the examination.
   c. Soft tissue/massage techniques, modalities, flexibility exercises, and functional exercises including strengthening, endurance, and coordination.

Smith's Fracture
1. Similar to Colles' fracture except distal fragment of radius dislocates in a volar direction causing a characteristic "garden spade deformity."
2. Diagnostic tests utilized: plain film imaging.
3. Medications:
   a. Acetaminophen for pain.
   b. NSAIDs for pain and/or inflammation.
4. Physical therapy goals, outcomes, and interventions:
   a. Intervention is similar to Colles' fracture.

Scaphoid Fracture
1. Results from a fall onto outstretched UE in a younger person. Most commonly fractured carpal.
2. Diagnostic tests utilized: plain film imaging.
3. Complications include a high incidence of avascular necrosis of the proximal fragment of the scaphoid secondary to poor vascular supply. Carpals are immobilized between 4 and 8 weeks.
4. Medications:
   a. Acetaminophen for pain.
   b. NSAIDs for pain and/or inflammation.
5. Physical therapy goals, outcomes, and interventions:
   a. Early intervention includes maintenance of flexibility of distal and proximal joints while UE is casted. Later intervention emphasizes strengthening, stretching, and joint and soft tissue mobilizations to regain full functional use of wrist and hand.

Dupuytren's Contracture
1. Observed as banding on palm and digit flexion contractures resulting from contracture of palmar fascia which adheres to skin. See Figure 2-17.
2. Affects men more often than women.
3. Contracture usually affects the metacarpophalangeal (MCP) and proximal interphalangeal (PIP) joints of fourth and fifth digits in nondiabetic individuals and affects third and fourth digits most often in individuals with diabetes.
4. Medications:
   a. Acetaminophen for pain.
   b. NSAIDs for pain and/or inflammation.
5. Physical therapy goals, outcomes, and interventions:
   a. Physical therapy intervention includes flexibility exercise to prevent further contracture and splint fabrication/application.
   b. Once contracture is under control, promote restoration of normal hand function through functional exercises.
   c. Physical therapy intervention following surgery includes wound management, edema control, and progression of functional exercise.

Boutonnière Deformity
1. Results from rupture of central tendinous slip of extensor hood. See Figure 2-18.
2. Observed deformity is extension of MCP and distal interphalangeal (DIP) with flexion of PIP.
3. Commonly occurs following trauma or in rheumatoid arthritis with degeneration of the central extensor tendon.
4. Medications:
   a. Acetaminophen for pain.
   b. NSAIDs for pain and/or inflammation.
5. Physical therapy goals, outcomes, and interventions:
   a. Physical therapy intervention includes edema management, flexibility exercises of involved and uninvolved joints, splinting or taping, and functional strengthening/endurance/coordination exercises.

Swan Neck Deformity
1. Results from contracture of intrinsic muscles with dorsal subluxation of lateral extensor tendons. See Figure 2-19.
2. Observed deformity is flexion of MCP and DIP with extension of PIP.
3. Commonly occurs following trauma or with rheumatoid arthritis following degeneration of lateral extensor tendons.
4. Diagnostic tests utilized: plain film imaging, but may not be necessary.
5. Medications:
   a. Acetaminophen for pain.
   b. NSAIDs for pain and/or inflammation.

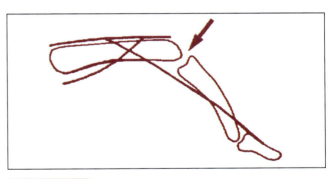

Figure 2-18 Boutonnière deformity.
(From Magee DJ. *Orthopedic Physical Assessment*. 2nd ed. Philadelphia, Saunders, 1992.)

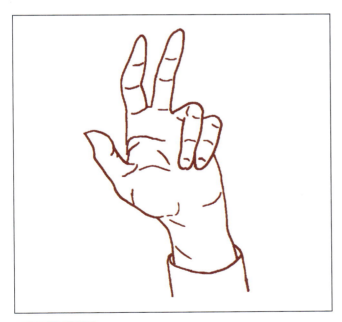

Figure 2-17 Dupuytren's contracture.
(Adapted from Magee DJ. *Orthopedic Physical Assessment*. 2nd ed. Philadelphia, Saunders, 1992.)

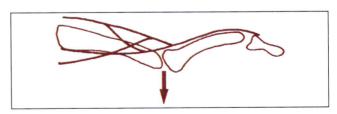

Figure 2-19 Swan neck deformity.
(From Magee DJ. *Orthopedic Physical Assessment*. 2nd ed. Philadelphia, Saunders, 1992.)

6. Physical therapy goals, outcomes, and interventions:
   a. Physical therapy intervention includes edema management, flexibility exercises of involved and uninvolved joints, splinting or taping, and functional strengthening/endurance/coordination exercises.

Ape Hand Deformity
1. Observed as thenar muscle wasting with first digit moving dorsally until it is in line with second digit. See Figure 2-20.
2. Results from median nerve dysfunction.
3. Diagnostic tests utilized: electrodiagnostic testing.
4. Medications:
   a. Acetaminophen for pain.
   b. NSAIDs for pain and/or inflammation.
5. Physical therapy goals, outcomes, and interventions:
   a. Physical therapy intervention includes edema management, flexibility exercises of involved and uninvolved joints, splinting or taping, and functional strengthening/endurance/coordination exercises.

Mallet Finger
1. Rupture or avulsion of extensor tendon at its insertion into distal phalanx of digit. See Figure 2-21.
2. Observed deformity is flexion of DIP joint.
3. Usually occurs from trauma forcing distal phalanx into a flexed position.
4. Diagnostic tests utilized: possibly MRI.
5. Medications:
   a. Acetaminophen for pain.
   b. NSAIDs for pain and/or inflammation.

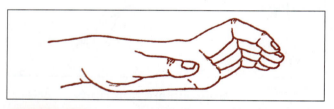

Figure 2-20 Ape hand deformity.
(From Magee DJ. *Orthopedic Physical Assessment*. 2nd ed. Philadelphia, Saunders, 1992.)

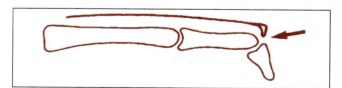

Figure 2-21 Mallet finger.
(From Magee DJ. *Orthopedic Physical Assessment*. 2nd ed. Philadelphia, Saunders, 1992.)

6. Physical therapy goals, outcomes, and interventions:
   a. Physical therapy intervention includes edema management, flexibility exercises of involved and uninvolved joints, splinting or taping, and functional strengthening/endurance/coordination exercises.

Gamekeeper's Thumb
1. A sprain/rupture of ulnar collateral ligament of MCP joint of first digit.
2. Results in medial instability of thumb.
3. Frequently occurs during a fall while skiing when increasing forces are placed on thumb through ski pole. Immobilized for 6 weeks.
4. Diagnostic tests utilized: possibly MRI.
5. Medications:
   a. Acetaminophen for pain.
   b. NSAIDs for pain and/or inflammation.
6. Physical therapy goals, outcomes, and interventions:
   a. Physical therapy intervention includes edema management, flexibility exercises of involved and uninvolved joints, splinting or taping, and functional strengthening/endurance/coordination exercises.

Boxer's Fracture
1. Fracture of neck of fifth metacarpal.
2. Frequently sustained during a fight or from punching a wall in anger or frustration.
3. Casted for 2–4 weeks.
4. Diagnostic tests utilized: plain film imaging.
5. Medications:
   a. Acetaminophen for pain.
   b. NSAIDs for pain and/or inflammation.
6. Physical therapy goals, outcomes, and interventions:
   a. Physical therapy intervention includes edema management, flexibility exercise initially at uninvolved joints followed by involved joints after sufficient healing has occurred.
   b. Initiation of functional strengthening/endurance/coordination occurs when flexibility is restored.

Lower Extremity Conditions—Hip

Avascular Necrosis—Hip (AVN, Osteonecrosis)
1. Multiple etiologies resulting in an impaired blood supply to the femoral head.
2. Hip ROM is decreased in flexion, internal rotation, and abduction.
3. Diagnostic tests utilized: Plain film imaging, bone scans, CT, and/or MRI.
4. Symptoms include pain in the groin and/or thigh and tenderness with palpation at the hip joint.
5. Coxalgic gait.

6. Medications:
   a. Acetaminophen for pain.
   b. NSAIDs for pain and/or inflammation.
   c. Corticosteroids contraindicated because they may be causative factor. Patient taking steroids for some other condition should have dose decreased.
7. Physical therapy goals, outcomes, and interventions:
   a. Joint/bone protection strategies.
   b. Maintain/improve joint mechanics and connective tissue functions.
   c. Implementation of aerobic capacity, endurance conditioning, or reconditioning such as aquatic programs.
   d. Postsurgical intervention includes regaining functional flexibility, improving strength/endurance/coordination, and gait training.

Femoral Anteversion and Antetorsion
1. Excessive femoral anteversion or antetorsion (30 degrees or greater) leads to squinting patellae and toeing in.
2. With an angle less than 0 degree (retroversion), femoral neck is rotated backward in relation to femoral condyles.
3. Diagnostic tests utilized: plain film imaging.
4. Clinical examination including Craig's test helps to identify this condition.
5. Physical therapy goals, outcomes, and interventions:
   a. Maintain/improve joint mechanics and connective tissue functions.

Coxa Vara and Coxa Valga
1. Angle of femoral neck with shaft of femur is <120 degrees; coxa vara results.
2. Angle of femoral neck with shaft of femur is >135 degrees; coxa valga results.
3. Coxa vara usually results from a defect in ossification of head of femur. Coxa vara and coxa valga may result from necrosis of femoral head occurring with septic arthritis.
4. Diagnostic tests utilized: plain film imaging.
5. Physical therapy goals, outcomes, and interventions:
   a. Maintain/improve joint mechanics and connective tissue functions.

Trochanteric Bursitis
1. An inflammation of deep trochanteric bursa from a direct blow, irritation by iliotibial band (ITB), and biomechanical/gait abnormalities causing repetitive microtrauma.
2. This condition is common in patients with rheumatoid arthritis.
3. Diagnostic tests utilized: none.
4. Diagnosis made by clinical examination.
   a. Differentiate from contractile condition by comparing results of AROM, PROM, and resistive tests.
5. Medications
   a. Acetaminophen for pain.
   b. NSAIDs for pain and/or inflammation.
6. Physical therapy goals, outcomes, and interventions:
   a. Refer to intervention for general bursitis/tendinitis/tendonosis. (See Interventions listed pages 53–60.)

ITB Tightness/Friction Disorder
1. Etiology: Tight ITB, abnormal gait patterns.
2. Results in inflammation of trochanteric bursa.
3. Noble compression test is positive when friction is introduced over the lateral femoral condyle during knee extension. Ober's test will also demonstrate tightness in ITB.
4. Medications:
   a. Acetaminophen for pain.
   b. NSAIDs for pain and/or inflammation.
5. Physical therapy goals, outcomes, and interventions:
   a. Reduction of pain and inflammation utilizing modalities, soft tissue techniques, and manual therapy techniques such as soft tissue/massage and joint oscillations.
   b. Correction of muscle imbalances and biomechanical faults using strengthening, endurance, coordination, and flexibility (ITB, hamstrings, quadriceps, and hip flexors) exercises to gain restoration of normal function.
   c. Biomechanical faults caused by joint restrictions should be corrected with joint mobilization to the specific restrictions identified during the examination.
   d. Gait training and patient education regarding the selection of running shoes and running surfaces. Orthoses may be fabricated.

Piriformis Syndrome
1. Piriformis muscle is an external rotator of hip and can become overworked with excessive pronation of foot, which causes abnormal femoral internal rotation. Considered a tonic muscle which is active with motion of sacroiliac joint, particularly sacrum.
2. Tightness or spasm of piriformis muscle can result in compression of sciatic nerve and/or sacroiliac dysfunction.
3. Diagnostic tests utilized: possibly electrodiagnostic tests for sciatic nerve.
4. Signs and symptoms include:
   a. Restriction in internal rotation.
   b. Pain with palpation of piriformis muscle.
   c. Referral of pain to posterior thigh.
   d. Weakness in external rotation, positive piriformis test.
   e. Uneven sacral base.
5. Perform lower extremity biomechanical examination to determine if abnormal biomechanics are the cause. Must rule out involvement of lumbar spine and/or sacroiliac joint.

6. Medications:
   a. Acetaminophen for pain.
   b. NSAIDs for pain and/or inflammation.
   c. Neurontin for neuropathic pain.
7. Physical therapy goals, outcomes, and interventions:
   a. Reduction of pain utilizing modalities and manual therapy techniques such as soft tissue/massage to piriformis muscle.
   b. Joint oscillations to hip or pelvis to inhibit pain.
   c. Correction of muscle imbalances and biomechanical faults using strengthening, endurance, coordination, and flexibility exercises to gain restoration of normal function.
   d. Restore muscle balance and patient education regarding protection of the sacroiliac joint (e.g., instruction not to step off a curb onto the dysfunctional lower extremity).
   e. Correction of biomechanical faults may include orthoses or orthotic devices for feet.

Other Hip Conditions
1. Legg-Calvé-Perthe's disease (osteochondrosis). See Chapter 9 for full explanation.
2. Slipped capital femoral epiphysis. See Chapter 9 for full explanation.

Lower Extremity Conditions—Knee

Ligament Sprains
1. Four major ligaments may be involved with knee sprains (anterior cruciate, posterior cruciate, medial collateral, and lateral collateral).
2. Injury to the ligaments may result in a single plane or rotary instability.
   a. Anterior cruciate ligament (ACL) laxity may result in single plane anterior instability.
   b. Posterior cruciate ligament (PCL) laxity may result in single plane posterior instability.
   c. ACL and medial collateral ligament (MCL) laxity may result in anteromedial rotary instability.
   d. ACL and lateral collateral ligament (LCL) laxity may result in anterolateral rotary instability.
   e. PCL and MCL laxity may result in posteromedial rotary instability.
   f. PCL and LCL laxity may result in posterolateral rotary instability.
3. Classification of injury:
   a. First degree, resulting in little or no instability.
   b. Second degree, resulting in minimal to moderate instability.
   c. Third degree, resulting in extreme instability.
4. "Unhappy triad" includes injury to the MCL, ACL, and the medial meniscus resulting from a combination of valgum, flexion, and external rotation forces applied to knee when the foot is planted.
5. Diagnostic tests utilized: MRI. Difficult to visualize complete ACL on MRI, so often read incorrectly as partially torn even if normal.
6. Refer to knee special tests that help to identify ligamentous instabilities of knee joint.
7. Reconstruction frequently involves a combination of intra-articular and extra-articular procedures.
8. Medications:
   a. Acetaminophen for pain.
   b. NSAIDs for pain and/or inflammation.
9. Physical therapy goals, outcomes, and interventions:
   a. Physical therapy intervention is varied depending on whether the patient undergoes a surgical procedure as well as type of surgery that is performed.
   b. Reduction of pain and inflammation utilizing modalities, soft tissue techniques, and manual therapy techniques such as oscillations.
   c. Postoperatively, continuous passive motion (CPM) devices may be used to maintain/promote flexibility of the joint.
   d. Correction of muscle imbalances and biomechanical faults using strengthening, endurance, coordination, and flexibility exercises to gain restoration of normal function.
   e. Biomechanical faults caused by joint restrictions should be corrected with joint mobilization to the specific restrictions identified during the examination.
   f. Progression to functional training based on patient's occupation and/or recreational goals.

Meniscal Injuries
1. Result from a combination of forces to include tibiofemoral joint flexion, compression, and rotation which places abnormal shear stresses on the meniscus.
2. Symptoms include lateral and/or medial joint pain, effusion, joint popping, knee giving way during walking, limitation in flexibility of knee joint, and joint locking.
3. Diagnostic tests utilized: MRI typically done, but not always sensitive enough to confirm tear.
4. PT clinical examination including the following special tests will be useful to make diagnosis.
   a. McMurray's test.
   b. Apley's test.
5. Medications:
   a. Acetaminophen for pain.
   b. NSAIDs for pain and/or inflammation.
6. Physical therapy goals, outcomes, and interventions:
   a. Reduction of pain and inflammation utilizing modalities, soft tissue/massage techniques to surrounding muscles, and manual therapy techniques such as joint oscillations to inhibit pain.
   b. Correction of muscle imbalances and biomechanical faults using strengthening, endurance,

coordination, and flexibility exercises to gain restoration of normal function.
   c. Biomechanical faults caused by joint restrictions should be corrected with joint mobilization to the specific restrictions identified during the examination.
   d. Progression to functional training based on patient's occupation and/or recreational goals.

Patellofemoral Conditions
1. Abnormal patella positions:
   a. Patella alta:
      - Malalignment in which patella tracks superiorly in femoral intercondylar notch.
      - May result in chronic patellar subluxation.
      - Positive camelback sign (two bumps over anterior knee region instead of typical one. Two bumps, because patella is riding high within femoral condyles so there is a superior bump; tibial tuberosity forms second bump inferiorly).
   b. Patella baja:
      - Malalignment in which patella tracks inferiorly in femoral intercondylar notch.
      - Results in restricted knee extension with abnormal cartilaginous wearing resulting in DJD.
   c. Lateral patellar tracking.
      - Could result if there is an increase in "Q angle" with a tendency for lateral subluxation or dislocation.
   d. Diagnostic tests utilized: plain film imaging including "sunrise" view.
   e. Physical therapy goals, outcomes, and interventions:
      - Regaining functional strength of structures surrounding knee, particularly vastus medialis oblique (VMO) muscle; regaining normal flexibility of ITB and hamstrings orthoses (if appropriate) and patellar bracing/taping.
2. Patellofemoral pain syndrome (PFPS).
   a. Common dysfunction that may occur on its own or in conjunction with other entities. May have been caused by trauma or by congenital/developmental dysfunction.
   b. May be interrelated with chondromalacia patellae and/or patella tendinitis.
   c. Common result is an abnormal patellofemoral tracking that leads to abnormal patellofemoral stress.
   d. Occasionally surgery is indicated.
   e. Diagnostic tests utilized: possibly MRI to rule out other dysfunctions.
   f. Medications:
      - Acetaminophen for pain.
      - NSAIDs for pain and/or inflammation.
   g. Physical therapy goals, outcomes, and interventions:
      - Patellofemoral (McConnell) taping is helpful to inhibit pain during rehabilitation.
      - Patella mobilization indicated with restrictions of patella glides (e.g., if patella is in a lateral glide position and has decreased medial glide, perform a medial glide joint mobilization to the patella).
      - Correction of muscle imbalances and biomechanical faults using strengthening, endurance, coordination, and flexibility exercises to gain restoration of normal function.
3. Patellar tendinitis.
   a. May be related to overload and/or jumping-related activities/sports.
   b. May also be interrelated to patellofemoral dysfunction.
   c. Diagnosis made by clinical examination.
   d. Medications:
      - Acetaminophen for pain.
      - NSAIDs for pain and/or inflammation.
      - Corticosteroid injection or by mouth.
   e. Physical therapy goals, outcomes, and interventions:
      - Refer to intervention for general bursitis/tendinitis/tendonosis. (See Interventions listed pages 53–60.)

Pes Anserine Bursitis
1. Typically caused by overuse or a contusion.
2. Must be differentiated from tendinitis.
3. Diagnosis made by PT clinical examination. Differentiate from contractile condition by comparing results of AROM, PROM, and resistive tests.
4. Medications:
   a. Acetaminophen for pain.
   b. NSAIDs for pain and/or inflammation.
   c. Corticosteroid injection or by mouth.
5. Physical therapy goals, outcomes, and interventions:
   a. Refer to intervention for general bursitis/tendinitis/tendonosis. (See Interventions listed pages 53–60.)

Osgood-Schlatter (Jumper's Knee)
1. Mechanical dysfunction resulting in traction apophysitis of the tibial tubercle at the patellar tendon insertion.
2. Diagnostic tests utilized: plain film findings demonstrate irregularities of the epiphyseal line.
3. Occasionally surgery is indicated.
4. Diagnosis made by clinical examination.
5. Medications:
   a. Acetaminophen for pain.
   b. NSAIDs for pain and/or inflammation.
6. Physical therapy goals, outcomes, and interventions.
   a. Modify activities to prevent excessive stress to irritated site.

Genu Varum and Valgum
1. Normal tibiofemoral shaft angle is 6 degrees of valgum.
2. Genu varum is an excessive medial tibial torsion commonly referred to as "bowlegs."

3. Genu varum results in excessive medial patellar positioning and the pigeon, toed orientation of the feet.
4. Genu valgum is an excessive lateral tibial torsion commonly referred to as "knock-knees."
5. Genu valgum results in excessive lateral patellar positioning.
6. Diagnostic tests utilized: plain film imaging.
7. Diagnosis made by clinical examination.
8. Physical therapy goals, outcomes, and interventions:
   a. Intervention includes decreased loading of knee while maintaining strength and endurance.

Fractures Involving the Knee Joint
1. Femoral condyle.
   a. Medial femoral most often involved due to its anatomical design.
   b. Numerous etiological factors include trauma, shearing, impacting, and avulsion forces.
   c. Common mechanism of injury is a fall with knee subjected to a shearing force.
2. Tibial plateau.
   a. Common mechanism of injury is a combination of valgum and compression forces to knee when knee is in a flexed position.
   b. Often occurs in conjunction with a medial collateral ligamentous injury.
3. Epiphyseal plate.
   a. Mechanism of injury is frequently a weight-bearing torsional stress.
   b. Presents more frequently in adolescents where an ACL injury would occur in an adult.
4. Patella.
   a. Most common mechanism of injury is a direct blow to patella as result of a fall.
5. Diagnostic tests utilized: plain film imaging most likely, unless complex fracture, which would benefit from CT.
6. Medications:
   a. Acetaminophen for pain.
   b. NSAIDs for pain and/or inflammation.
7. Physical therapy goals, outcomes, and interventions:
   a. Physical therapy intervention emphasizes return of function without pain.
   b. Early flexibility is important in preventing capsular adhesions.

Other Conditions of the Lower Leg

Anterior Compartment Syndrome (ACS)
1. Increased compartmental pressure resulting in a local ischemic condition.
2. Multiple etiologies; direct trauma, fracture, overuse, and/or muscle hypertrophy.
3. Symptoms of chronic or exertional compartment syndrome are produced by exercise or exertion and described as a deep cramping feeling.
4. Symptoms of acute ACS are produced by sudden trauma causing swelling within the compartment.
   a. Swelling.
   b. Parasthesia.
   c. Severe pain.
5. Diagnosis made by PT clinical examination.

> **RED FLAG:** Acute ACS is considered a medical emergency and requires immediate surgical intervention with fasciotomy to prevent tissue death and permanent disability.

Anterior Tibial Periostitis (Shin Splints)
1. Musculotendinous overuse condition.
2. Three common etiologies include:
   a. Abnormal biomechanical alignment.
   b. Poor conditioning.
   c. Improper training methods.
3. Muscles involved include anterior tibialis and extensor hallucis longus.
4. Pain elicited with palpation of lateral tibia and anterior compartment.
5. Diagnosis made by PT clinical examination.
6. Medications:
   a. Acetaminophen for pain.
   b. NSAIDs for pain and/or inflammation.
7. Physical therapy goals, outcomes, and interventions:
   a. Correction of muscle imbalances and biomechanical faults using strengthening, endurance, and coordination exercises.
   b. Flexibility exercises for anterior compartment muscles as well as the triceps surae to gain restoration of normal function.

Medial Tibial Stress Syndrome
1. Overuse injury of the posterior tibialis and/or the medial soleus resulting in periosteal inflammation at the muscular attachments.
2. Etiology is thought to be excessive pronation.
3. Pain elicited with palpation of the distal posteromedial border of the tibia.
4. Diagnosis made by PT clinical examination.
5. Medications:
   a. Acetaminophen for pain.
   b. NSAIDs for pain and/or inflammation.
6. Physical therapy goals, outcomes, and interventions:
   a. Correction of muscle imbalances and biomechanical faults using strengthening, endurance, and coordination exercises.
   b. Flexibility exercises for anterior compartment muscles as well as the triceps surae to gain restoration of normal function.

Stress Fractures
1. Overuse injury resulting most often in microfracture of the tibia or fibula.
2. 49% of all stress fractures involve the tibia, and 10% involve the fibula.
3. Three common etiologies: abnormal biomechanical alignment, poor conditioning, and improper training methods.
4. Diagnostic tests utilized: plain film imaging and bone scan.
5. Medications:
   a. Acetaminophen for pain.
   b. NSAIDs for pain and/or inflammation.
6. Physical therapy goals, outcomes, and interventions:
   a. Correction of muscle imbalances and biomechanical faults using strengthening, endurance, and coordination exercises.
   b. Flexibility exercises for anterior compartment muscles as well as the triceps surae to gain restoration of normal function.

Lower Extremity Conditions— Foot and Ankle

Ligament Sprains
1. 95% of all ankle sprains involve lateral ligaments.
2. With lateral sprains, foot is plantar flexed and inverted at time of injury.
3. The most common grading system is as follows:
   a. Grade I: No loss of function with minimal tearing of the anterior talofibular ligament.
   b. Grade II: Some loss of function with partial disruption of the anterior talofibular and calcaneofibular ligaments.
   c. Grade III: Complete loss of function with complete tearing of the anterior talofibular and calcaneofibular ligaments with partial tear of the posterior talofibular ligament.
4. Diagnostic tests utilized: MRI if necessary.
5. Instability is evaluated using anterior drawer and talar tilt special tests.
6. Medications:
   a. Acetaminophen for pain.
   b. NSAIDs for pain and/or inflammation.
7. Physical therapy goals, outcomes, and interventions:
   a. Physical therapy intervention is varied depending on whether the patient undergoes a surgical procedure as well as type of surgery performed.
   b. Reduction of pain and inflammation utilizing modalities, soft tissue techniques, and manual therapy techniques such as oscillations.
   c. Correction of muscle imbalances and biomechanical faults using strengthening, endurance, coordination, and flexibility exercises to gain restoration of normal function.
   d. Biomechanical faults caused by joint restrictions should be corrected with joint mobilization to the specific restrictions identified during the examination.
   e. Progression to functional training based on patient's occupation and/or recreational goals.

Achilles' Tendinitis/Tendonosis
1. Differentiate whether an inflammatory tendinitis or a chronic tendonosis.
2. PT clinical examination including Thompson's test helps to identify this condition.
3. Medications:
   a. Acetaminophen for pain.
   b. NSAIDs for pain and/or inflammation.
   c. Corticosteroid injection or by mouth.
4. Physical therapy goals, outcomes, and interventions:
   a. Refer to intervention for general bursitis/tendinitis/tendonosis. (See Interventions listed pages 53–60.)

Fractures of Foot and Ankle
1. Unimalleolar involves the medial or lateral malleolus.
2. Bimalleolar involves the medial and lateral malleoli.
3. Trimalleolar involves the medial and lateral malleoli and the posterior tubercle of the distal tibia.
4. Diagnostic tests utilized: plain film imaging.
5. Medications:
   a. Acetaminophen for pain.
   b. NSAIDs for pain and/or inflammation.
6. Physical therapy goals, outcomes, and interventions:
   a. Physical therapy intervention emphasizes return of function without pain.
   b. Functional training and restoration of muscle imbalances using exercise to normalize strength, endurance, coordination, and flexibility.
   c. Early PROM is important in preventing capsular adhesions.

Tarsal Tunnel Syndrome
1. Entrapment of the posterior tibial nerve or one of its branches within the tarsal tunnel.
2. Overpronation/excessive pronation, overuse problems resulting in tendinitis of the long flexor, and posterior tibialis tendon and trauma may compromise space in the tarsal tunnel.
3. Symptoms include pain, numbness, and paresthesias along the medial ankle to the plantar surface of the foot.
4. Diagnostic tests utilized: electrodiagnostic tests.
5. Positive Tinel's sign at the tarsal tunnel.
6. Medications:
   a. Acetaminophen for pain.
   b. NSAIDs for pain and/or inflammation.
   c. Neurontin for neuropathic pain.
7. Physical therapy goals, outcomes, and interventions:
   a. Intervention includes the use of orthoses to maintain neutral alignment of the foot.

Flexor Hallucis Tendonopathy
1. Identified as a tendinitis in the acute stage or can present as a chronic tendonosis. Commonly seen in ballet performers.
2. Medications:
   a. Acetaminophen for pain.
   b. NSAIDs for pain and/or inflammation.
   c. Corticosteroid injection or by mouth.
3. Physical therapy goals, outcomes, and interventions:
   a. Refer to intervention for general bursitis/tendinitis/tendonosis. (See Interventions listed pages 53–60.)

Pes Cavus (Hollow Foot)
1. Numerous etiologies to include genetic predisposition, neurological disorders resulting in muscle imbalances, and contracture of soft tissues.
2. Deformity observed includes an increased height of longitudinal arches, dropping of anterior arch, metatarsal heads lower than hindfoot, plantar flexion, and splaying of forefoot and claw toes.
3. Function is limited owing to altered arthrokinematics resulting in limited ability to absorb forces through foot.
4. Diagnosis made by clinical examination including thorough biomechanical lower quarter exam.
5. Physical therapy goals, outcomes, and interventions:
   a. Intervention includes patient education emphasizing limitation of high-impact sports (i.e., long-distance running and ballet), use of proper footwear, and fitting for orthoses.

Pes Planus (Flat Foot)
1. Etiologies include genetic predisposition, muscle weakness, ligamentous laxity, paralysis, excessive pronation, trauma, or disease (e.g., rheumatoid arthritis).
2. Normal in infant and toddler feet.
3. Deformity observed may include a reduction in height of medial longitudinal arch.
4. Decreased ability of foot to provide a rigid lever for push off during gait as result of altered arthrokinematics.
5. Diagnosis made by clinical examination including thorough biomechanical lower quarter exam.
6. Physical therapy goals, outcomes, and interventions:
   a. Intervention emphasizes patient education, use of proper footwear, and orthotic fitting.

Talipes Equinovarus (Clubfoot)
1. Two types: postural and talipes equinovarus.
2. Etiology.
   a. Postural, which results from intrauterine malposition.
   b. Talipes equinovarus, which is an abnormal development of the head and neck of the talus as the result of heredity or neuromuscular disorders (e.g., myelomeningocele).
3. Deformity observed:
   a. Plantar flexed, adducted, and inverted foot (postural).
   b. Talipes equinovarus has three components: plantar flexion at talocrural joint, inversion at subtalar, talocalcaneal, talonavicular, and calcaneocuboid joints. Supination is observed at midtarsal joints.
4. Diagnosis made by PT clinical examination including thorough biomechanical lower quarter exam.
5. Physical therapy goals, outcomes, and interventions:
   a. Manipulation followed by casting or splinting for postural condition.
   b. Talipes equinovarus requires surgical intervention to correct deformity followed by casting or splinting.

Equinus
1. Etiology can include congenital bone deformity, neurological disorders such as cerebral palsy, contracture of gastrocnemius and/or soleus muscles, trauma, or inflammatory disease.
2. Deformity observed: plantar flexed foot.
3. Compensation secondary to limited dorsiflexion includes subtalar or midtarsal pronation.
4. Diagnosis made by PT clinical examination including thorough biomechanical lower quarter exam.
5. Physical therapy goals, outcomes, and interventions:
   a. Physical therapy intervention includes flexibility exercises of shortened structures within foot, joint mobilization to joint restrictions identified in examination, strengthening to intrinsic and extrinsic foot muscles, and orthotic management.

Hallux Valgus
1. Etiology is varied to include biomechanical malalignment (excessive pronation), ligamentous laxity, heredity, weak muscles, and footwear that is too tight.
2. Deformity observed: a medial deviation of head of first metatarsal from midline of body; metatarsal and base of proximal first phalanx move medially, distal phalanx then moves laterally.
3. Normal metatarsophalangeal angle is 8–20 degrees.
4. Diagnosis made by clinical examination including thorough biomechanical lower quarter exam.
5. Physical therapy goals, outcomes, and interventions:
   a. Early orthotic fitting and patient education.
   b. Later management requires surgery followed by flexibility exercises to restore normal function, strengthening exercises, and possible joint mobilization to identified restrictions.

Metatarsalgia
1. Etiologies.
   a. Mechanical: tight triceps surae group and/or Achilles' tendon, collapse of transverse arch, short first ray, pronation of forefoot.

b. Structural changes in transverse arch possibly leading to vascular and/or neural compromise in tissues of forefoot.
c. Changes in footwear.
2. Complaint frequently heard is pain at first and second metatarsal heads after long periods of weight bearing.
3. Diagnosis made by PT clinical examination including thorough biomechanical lower quarter exam.
4. Medications:
   a. Acetaminophen for pain.
   b. NSAIDs for pain and/or inflammation.
   c. Neurontin for neuropathic pain.
5. Physical therapy goals, outcomes, and interventions:
   a. Intervention includes correction of biomechanical abnormality (improving flexibility of triceps surae), modalities to decrease pain.
   b. Prescription and/or creation of orthoses.
   c. Patient education regarding selection of footwear.

Metatarsus Adductus
1. Etiology: Congenital, muscle imbalance, or neuromuscular diseases such as polio.
2. Two types: rigid and flexible.
3. Deformity observed.
   a. Rigid deformity: results in a medial subluxation of tarsometatarsal joints. Hindfoot is slightly in valgus with navicular lateral to head of talus.
   b. Flexible deformity: is observed as adduction of all five metatarsals at the tarsometatarsal joints.
4. Diagnosis made by PT clinical examination including thorough biomechanical lower quarter exam.
5. Physical therapy goals, outcomes, and interventions:
   a. Intervention includes strengthening and regaining proper alignment of foot (i.e., through use of orthoses).

Charcot-Marie-Tooth Disease
1. Peroneal muscular atrophy that affects motor and sensory nerves.
2. May begin in childhood or adulthood.
3. Initially affects muscles in lower leg and foot, but eventually progresses to muscles of hands and forearm.
4. Slowly progressive disorder that has varying degrees of involvement depending on degree of genetic dominance.
5. Diagnostic tests utilized: electrodiagnostic tests.
6. Diagnosis made by PT clinical examination including thorough biomechanical lower quarter exam.
7. Medications:
   a. Acetaminophen for pain.
   b. NSAIDs for pain and/or inflammation.
   c. Neurontin for neuropathic pain.

8. Physical therapy goals, outcomes, and interventions:
   a. No specific treatment to prevent because it is an inherited disorder.
   b. Physical therapy intervention centers on preventing contractures/skin breakdown and maximizing patient's functional capacity to perform activities.
   c. Patient education and training regarding braces and ambulatory assistive devices.

Plantar Fasciitis
1. Etiology usually mechanical.
   a. Chronic irritation of plantar fascia from excessive pronation.
   b. Limited ROM of first metatarsophalangeal (MTP) and talocrural joint.
   c. Tight triceps surae.
   d. Acute injury from excessive loading of foot.
   e. Rigid cavus foot.
2. Results in microtears at attachment of plantar fascia.
3. Diagnostic tests utilized: none.
4. Diagnosis made by PT clinical examination including thorough biomechanical lower quarter exam. Differentiated from tarsal tunnel syndrome by a negative Tinel's sign.
5. Medications:
   a. Acetaminophen for pain.
   b. NSAIDs for pain and/or inflammation.
   c. Corticosteroid injection or by mouth.
6. Physical therapy goals, outcomes, and interventions:
   a. Physical therapy intervention includes regaining proper mechanical alignment.
   b. Modalities to reduce pain and inflammation.
   c. Flexibility of the plantar fascia for the pes cavus foot.
   d. Careful flexibility exercises for triceps surae.
   e. Joint mobilization to identified restrictions.
   f. Night splints.
   g. Strengthening of invertors of foot.
   h. Patient education regarding selection of footwear and orthotic fitting.

Forefoot/Rearfoot Deformities
1. Rearfoot varus (subtalar varus, calcaneal varus).
   a. Etiology: Abnormal mechanical alignment of tibia, shortened rearfoot soft tissues, or malunion of calcaneus.
   b. Deformity observed: rigid inversion of calcaneus when subtalar joint is in neutral position.
   c. Diagnosis made by PT clinical examination including thorough biomechanical lower quarter exam.
   d. Physical therapy goals, outcomes, and interventions:
   - Regaining proper mechanical alignment.
   - Improving flexibility of shortened soft tissues.
   - Orthotic fitting and patient education regarding selection of footwear.

2. Rearfoot valgus.
   a. Etiology: Abnormal mechanical alignment of the knee (genu valgum) or tibial valgus.
   b. Deformity observed: eversion of calcaneus with a neutral subtalar joint.
   c. Owing to increased mobility of hindfoot, fewer musculoskeletal problems develop from this deformity than occur with rearfoot varus.
   d. Diagnosis made by PT clinical examination including thorough biomechanical lower quarter exam.
   e. Physical therapy goals, outcomes, and interventions:
      - Regaining proper mechanical alignment.
      - Improving flexibility of shortened soft tissues.
      - Orthotic fitting and patient education regarding selection of footwear.
3. Forefoot varus.
   a. Etiology: congenital abnormal deviation of head and neck of talus.
   b. Deformity observed: inversion of forefoot when subtalar joint is in neutral.
   c. Diagnosis made by PT clinical examination including thorough biomechanical lower quarter exam.
   d. Physical therapy goals, outcomes, and interventions:
      - Regaining proper mechanical alignment.
      - Improving flexibility of shortened soft tissues.
      - Orthotic fitting and patient education regarding selection of footwear.
4. Forefoot valgus.
   a. Etiology: congenital abnormal development of head and neck of talus.
   b. Deformity observed: eversion of forefoot when the subtalar joint is in neutral.
   c. Diagnosis made by PT clinical examination including thorough biomechanical lower quarter exam.
   d. Physical therapy goals, outcomes, and interventions:
      - Regaining proper mechanical alignment.
      - Improving flexibility of shortened soft tissues.
      - Orthotic fitting and patient education regarding selection of footwear.

Spinal Conditions

Muscle Strain
1. May be related to sudden trauma, chronic or sustained overload, or abnormal muscle biomechanics secondary to faulty function (abnormal joint or muscle biomechanics).
2. Commonly will resolve without intervention, but if trauma is too great or if related to chronic etiology, will benefit from intervention.
3. Diagnosis made by PT clinical examination by comparing results of flexibility (AROM/PROM), resistive tests, and palpation.
4. Medications:
   a. Acetaminophen for pain.
   b. NSAIDs for pain and/or inflammation.
   c. Corticosteroid injection or by mouth.
   d. Muscle relaxants (e.g., Flexeril [cyclobenzaprine] or Valium [diazepam]).
   e. Trigger point injections.
5. Physical therapy goals, outcomes, and interventions:
   a. Biomechanical faults caused by joint restrictions should be corrected with joint mobilization.
   b. Patient education regarding the elimination of harmful positions and postural reeducation.
   c. Spinal manipulation for pain inhibition is generally indicated for this condition.

Spondylolysis/Spondylolisthesis
1. Etiology: thought to be congenitally defective pars interarticularis.
2. Spondylolysis is a fracture of the pars interarticularis with positive "Scotty dog" sign on oblique radiographic view of spine.
3. Spondylolisthesis is the actual anterior or posterior slippage of one vertebra on another following bilateral fracture of pars interarticularis.
4. Spondylolisthesis can be graded according to amount of slippage from 1 (25% slippage) to 4 (100% slippage).
5. Diagnostic tests utilized: plain film (oblique to see fracture and lateral views to see slippage).
6. PT clinical examination including stork test helps to identify this condition.
7. Medications:
   a. Acetaminophen for pain.
   b. NSAIDs for pain and/or inflammation.
   c. Corticosteroid injection or by mouth.
   d. Muscle relaxants.
   e. Trigger point injections.
8. Physical therapy goals, outcomes, and interventions:
   a. Biomechanical faults caused by joint restrictions should be corrected with joint mobilization to the specific restrictions identified during the examination.
   b. Exercise should focus on dynamic stabilization of trunk with particular emphasis on abdominals and trunk extension with multifidus muscle working from a fully flexed position of trunk up to neutral, but not into trunk extension.
   c. Avoid extension and/or other positions that add stress to defect (i.e., extension, ipsilateral side-bending, and contralateral rotation).
   d. Patient should be educated regarding the elimination of positions of extension and should be reeducated on posture.
   e. Braces such as Boston brace and TLSO (thoracolumbosacral orthosis) have traditionally been used, but frequency is decreasing.
   f. Spinal manipulation may be contraindicated for this condition, particularly at the level of defect.

Spinal or Intervertebral Stenosis

1. Etiology: congenital narrow spinal canal or intervertebral foramen coupled with hypertrophy of the spinal lamina and ligamentum flavum or facets as the result of age-related degenerative processes or disease.
2. Results in vascular and/or neural compromise.
3. Signs and symptoms (see Table 2-8).
   a. Bilateral pain and paresthesia in back, buttocks, thighs, calves, and feet.
   b. Pain is decreased in spinal flexion, increased in extension.
   c. Pain increases with walking.
   d. Pain relieved with prolonged rest.
4. Diagnostic tests utilized: imaging including plain films, MRI, and/or CT scan. Occasionally, myelography is helpful.
5. PT clinical examination including bicycle (van Gelderen's) test helps to identify this condition and differentiate it from intermittent claudication.
6. Medications:
   a. Acetaminophen for pain.
   b. NSAIDs for pain and/or inflammation.
   c. Corticosteroid injection or by mouth.
   d. Muscle relaxants.
   e. Trigger point injections.
7. Physical therapy goals, outcomes, and interventions:
   a. Biomechanical faults caused by joint restrictions should be corrected with joint mobilization to the specific restrictions identified during the examination.
   b. Perform flexion biased exercise and exercise that promotes dynamic stability throughout the trunk and pelvis.
   c. Avoid extension and/or other positions that narrow the spinal canal or intervertebral foramen (i.e., extension, ipsilateral side bending, and ipsilateral rotation).
   d. Manual and/or mechanical traction.
      - Traction:
        ○ Cervical spine positioning is at 15 degrees of flexion to provide the optimum intervertebral foraminal opening.
        ○ Contraindications include joint hypermobility, pregnancy, rheumatoid arthritis, Down syndrome, or any other systemic disease that affects ligamentous integrity.

Spinal Disc Conditions

1. Internal disc disruption.
   a. Internal structure of disc annulus is disrupted; however, external structures remain normal. Most common in lumbar region.
   b. Symptoms include constant deep achy pain, increased pain with movement, no objective neurological findings, although patient may have referred pain into lower extremity.
   c. Regular CT or myelogram will not demonstrate any abnormal findings. Can be diagnosed by CT discogram or an MRI.
   d. Clinical examination helps to identify this condition.
   e. Medications:
      - Acetaminophen for pain.
      - NSAIDs for pain and/or inflammation.
      - Muscle relaxants.
      - Trigger point injections.
      - Corticosteroid injection or by mouth.
   f. Physical therapy goals, outcomes, and interventions:
      - Biomechanical faults caused by joint restrictions should be corrected with joint mobilization to the specific restrictions identified during the examination.
      - Spinal manipulation may be contraindicated for this condition.
      - Patient education regarding proper body mechanics, positions to avoid, limiting repetitive bending and twisting movements, limiting upper extremity overhead and sitting activities, and carrying heavy loads.
2. Posterolateral bulge/herniation.
   a. Most commonly observed disc disorder of lumbar spine due to three structural deficiencies:
      - Posterior disc is narrower in height than anterior disc.
      - Posterior longitudinal ligament is not as strong and only centrally located in lumbar spine.
      - Posterior lamellae of annulus are thinner.
   b. Etiology: Overstretching and/or tearing of annular rings, vertebral endplate, and/or ligamentous structures from high compressive forces or repetitive microtrauma.
   c. Results in loss of strength, radicular pain, paresthesia, and inability to perform activities of daily living.
   d. Diagnostic tests utilized: MRI.
   e. PT clinical examination helps to identify this condition.
   f. Medications:
      - Acetaminophen for pain.
      - NSAIDs for pain and/or inflammation.
      - Muscle relaxants.
      - Trigger point injections.
      - Corticosteroid injection or by mouth.
   g. Physical therapy goals, outcomes, and interventions:
      - Exercise program to promote dynamic stability throughout trunk and pelvis as well as to provide optimal stimulus for regeneration of disc.
      - Positional gapping for 10 minutes to increase space within region of space occupying lesion (e.g., if left posterolateral lumbar herniation present).
        ○ Have patient lying on right side with pillow under right trunk (accentuating trunk side bending right).

- Flex both hips and knees.
- Rotate trunk to left (or pelvis to right).
- Patient can be taught to perform this at home.
• Spinal manipulation may be contraindicated for this condition, particularly at the level of the herniation.
• Patient education regarding proper body mechanics, positions to avoid, limiting repetitive bending and twisting movements, limiting upper extremity overhead and sitting activities, and carrying heavy loads.
• Manual and/or mechanical traction.
  - Traction: cervical spine positioning is at 15 degrees of flexion to provide the optimum intervertebral foraminal opening.
  - Contraindications include joint hypermobility, pregnancy, rheumatoid arthritis, Down syndrome, or any other systemic disease that affects ligamentous integrity.
  - Efficacy of traction for intervention of disc conditions is currently under scrutiny.

Central Posterior Bulge/Herniation

1. More commonly observed in the cervical spine but can be seen in the lumbar spine.
2. Etiology: Overstretching and/or tearing of annular rings, vertebral endplate, and/or ligamentous structures (posterior longitudinal ligament) from high compressive forces and/or long-term postural malalignment.
3. Results in loss of strength, radicular pain, paresthesia, inability to perform activities of daily living, and possible compression of the spinal cord with central nervous system symptoms (e.g., hyperreflexia and a positive Babinski's reflex) (Table 2-8).
4. Diagnostic tests utilized: MRI.
5. Clinical examination helps to identify this condition.
6. Medications:
   a. Acetaminophen for pain.
   b. NSAIDs for pain and/or inflammation.
   c. Muscle relaxants.
   d. Trigger point injections.
   e. Corticosteroid injection or by mouth.
7. Physical therapy goals, outcomes, and interventions:
   a. Refer to posterolateral intervention (section 2.g).
8. Anterior bulge/herniation is rare due to structural integrity of anterior intervertebral disc.

Facet Joint Conditions

1. DJD.
   a. Etiology: DJD is part of normal aging process because of weight-bearing properties of facets and intervertebral joints.
   b. Results in bone hypertrophy, capsular fibrosis, hypermobility or hypomobility of joint, and proliferation of synovium.
   c. Symptoms include reduction in mobility of the spine, pain and possible impingement of associated nerve root resulting in loss of strength and paresthesias (see Table 2-8).
   d. Diagnostic tests utilized: plain film imaging.
   e. Clinical examination including lumbar quadrant test helps to identify this condition.
   f. Medications:
      • Acetaminophen for pain.
      • NSAIDs for pain and/or inflammation.
      • Muscle relaxants.
      • Trigger point injections.
      • Corticosteroid injection or by mouth.
   g. Physical therapy goals, outcomes, and interventions:
      • Exercise program to promote dynamic stability throughout trunk and pelvis as well as to provide optimal stimulus for regeneration of facet cartilage and/or capsule.
      • Biomechanical faults caused by joint restrictions should be corrected with joint mobilization to the specific restrictions identified during the examination.
      • Spinal manipulation may be useful for this condition.
2. Facet extrapment (acute locked back).
   a. Caused by abnormal movement of fibroadipose meniscoid in facet during extension (from flexion). Meniscoid does not properly reenter joint cavity and bunches up, becoming a space-occupying lesion, which distends capsule, causing pain.
   b. Flexion is most comfortable for patient and extension increases pain.
   c. Medications:
      • Acetaminophen for pain.
      • NSAIDs for pain and/or inflammation.
      • Muscle relaxants.
      • Trigger point injections.
      • Corticosteroid injection or by mouth.
   d. Physical therapy goals, outcomes, and interventions:
      • Positional facet joint gapping and/or manipulation are appropriate treatments.

Acceleration/Deceleration Injuries of the Cervical Spine

1. Formerly known as "whiplash."
2. Occurs when excess shear and tensile forces are exerted on cervical structures.
3. Structures injured may include facets/articular processes, facet joint capsules, ligaments, disc, anterior/posterior muscles, fracture to odontoid process and spinous processes, temporomandibular joint (TMJ), sympathetic chain ganglia, spinal, and cranial nerves.
4. Signs and symptoms:
   a. Early include headaches, neck pain, limited flexibility, reversal of lower cervical lordosis and decrease

in upper cervical kyphosis, vertigo, change in vision and hearing, irritability to noise and light, dysesthesias of face and bilateral upper extremities, nausea, difficulty swallowing, and emotional lability.
   b. Late include chronic head and neck pain, limitation in flexibility, TMJ dysfunction, limited tolerance to ADL and IADL, disequilibrium, anxiety, and depression.
5. Common clinical findings include postural changes, excessive muscle guarding with soft tissue fibrosis, segmental hypermobility, and gradual development of restricted segmental motion cranial and caudal to the injury (segmental hypomobility).
6. Diagnostic tests utilized: plain film imaging, CT and/or MRI.
7. Medications:
   a. Acetaminophen for pain.
   b. NSAIDs for pain and/or inflammation.
   c. Muscle relaxants.
   d. Trigger point injections.
   e. Corticosteroid injection or by mouth.
8. Physical therapy goals, outcomes, and interventions:
   a. Spinal manipulation is generally indicated for this condition.
   b. Correction of muscle imbalances and biomechanical faults using strengthening, endurance, coordination, and flexibility exercises to gain restoration of normal function.
   c. Biomechanical faults caused by joint restrictions should be corrected with joint mobilization to the specific restrictions identified during the examination.
   d. Progression to functional training based on patient's occupation and/or recreational goals.
   e. Patient education regarding the elimination of harmful positions and postural reeducation.
   f. Manual and/or mechanical traction.
      - Traction.
        ○ Cervical spine positioning is at 15° of flexion to provide the optimum intervertebral foraminal opening.
        ○ Contraindications include joint hypermobility, pregnancy, rheumatoid arthritis, Down syndrome, or any other systemic disease that affects ligamentous integrity.

Hypermobile Spinal Segments
1. An abnormal increase in ROM at a joint due to insufficient soft tissue control (i.e., ligamentous, discal, muscle, or a combination of all three).
2. Diagnostic tests utilized: Plain film imaging, particularly dynamic flexion/extension views.
3. Medications:
   a. Acetaminophen for pain.
   b. NSAIDs for pain and/or inflammation.
   c. Muscle relaxants.
   d. Trigger point injections.
   e. Sclerosing injections.
   f. Corticosteroid injection or by mouth.
4. Physical therapy goals, outcomes, and interventions:
   a. Pain reduction modalities to reduce irritability of structures.
   b. Passive ROM within a normal range of movement.
   c. Passive stabilization with corsets, splints, casts, tape, and collars.
   d. Increase strength/endurance/coordination especially in the multifidus, abdominals, extensors, and gluteals, which control posture.
   e. Regain muscle balance.
   f. Patient education regarding postural reeducation, limiting excessive overloading, limiting sustained activities, and limiting end-range postures.

Sacroiliac Joint (SIJ) Conditions
1. Cause and specific pathology are unknown. Because this is a joint, it is assumed that it can become inflamed, develop degenerative changes or abnormal movement patterns.
2. Anatomically and functionally SIJ is closely related to lumbar spine, so a thorough examination of both regions is indicated if a patient presents with pain in either.
3. Diagnostic tests utilized: plain film imaging and possibly MRI. Occasionally double-blind injections may be used to assist in making the diagnosis (first injection is provocative in nature and second injection is analgesic. If increased "same" pain with first injection and decreased pain following second injection, joint is determined to be pathological.
4. Clinical examination including the following special tests will be useful to make diagnosis:
   a. Gillet's test.
   b. Ipsilateral anterior rotation test.
   c. Gaenslen's test.
   d. Long-sitting (supine to sit) test.
   e. Goldthwait's test.
5. Medications:
   a. Acetaminophen for pain.
   b. NSAIDs for pain and/or inflammation.
   c. Muscle relaxants.
   d. Trigger point injections.
   e. Corticosteroid injection or by mouth.
6. Physical therapy goals, outcomes, and interventions.
   a. Spinal manipulation such as SIJ gapping is generally indicated for this condition to inhibit pain, reduce muscle guarding, and restore normal joint motion.
   b. Correction of muscle imbalances throughout pelvis using strengthening, endurance, coordination, and flexibility exercises to gain restoration of normal function.

c. Biomechanical faults caused by joint restrictions should be corrected with joint mobilization to the specific restrictions identified during the examination.
d. Patient should be educated regarding the elimination of harmful positions and reeducated on posture.
e. Sacroiliac belts may be useful in some patients.

Repetitive/Cumulative Trauma to the Back

1. Disorders of the nerves, soft tissues, and bones precipitated or aggravated by repeated exertions or movements of the back, occurring most often in the workplace.
2. Repetitive trauma disorders account for 48% of all reported occupational diseases.
3. Diagnosis is difficult with up to 85% of back pain non-diagnosed.
4. Typically causes one of the conditions previously listed above: muscle, disc, and/or joint impairment.
5. Vocational factors that contribute to back pain include physically heavy static work postures, lifting, frequent bending and twisting, and repetitive work and vibration.
6. Chronic disability may be reduced by enrollment in a work-conditioning program that includes patient education, aerobic exercises, general strengthening, and functional stability exercises that promote endurance for work-related activities.
7. Intervention should be focused on prevention, consisting of education. If this phenomenon leads to a condition listed above, follow the specific intervention associated with that condition.

Other Conditions Affecting the Spine

1. Bone tumors.
   a. May be primary or metastatic.
      - Primary tumors include multiple myeloma (which is most common primary tumor of bone), Ewing's sarcoma, malignant lymphoma, chondrosarcoma, osteosarcoma, and chondromas.
      - Metastatic bone cancer has primary sites in lung, prostate, breast, kidney, and thyroid.
      - Patient history should always include questions about a prior episode of cancer.
      - Signs and symptoms include pain that is unvarying and progressive, is not relieved with rest or analgesics, and is more pronounced at night.
      - Diagnostic tests utilized: plain film imaging, CT and/or MRI, as well as laboratory tests.
2. Visceral tumors (Figure 2-22).
   a. Esophageal cancer symptomatology may include pain radiating to the back, pain with swallowing, dysphagia, and weight loss.
   b. Pancreatic cancer symptomatology includes a deep gnawing pain that may radiate from the chest to the back.
   c. Diagnostic tests utilized: plain film imaging, CT and/or MRI, as well as laboratory tests.
3. Gastrointestinal conditions:
   a. Acute pancreatitis may manifest itself as midepigastric pain that radiates through to back.
   b. Cholecystitis may present with abrupt severe abdominal pain and right upper quadrant tenderness, nausea, vomiting, and fever.
   c. Diagnostic tests utilized: plain film imaging, CT and/or MRI, as well as laboratory tests.
4. Cardiovascular and pulmonary conditions.
   a. Heart and lung disorders can refer pain to chest, back, neck, jaw, and upper extremity.
   b. Abdominal aortic aneurysm (AAA) usually appears as nonspecific lumbar pain.
   c. Diagnostic tests utilized: plain film imaging, CT and/or MRI, as well as laboratory tests.
   d. Will be identified as pain during examination of abdominal region.
5. Urological and gynecological conditions:
   a. Kidney, bladder, ovarian and uterine disorders can refer pain to the trunk, pelvis, and thighs.
   b. Diagnostic tests utilized: Plain film imaging, CT and/or MRI, as well as laboratory tests.

Orthopedic Surgical Repairs— Upper Extremity

Rotator Cuff Tears

1. Usually degenerative and occur over time with impingement of supraspinatus tendon between greater tuberosity and acromion.
2. Signs and symptoms include:
   - Significant reduction of AROM into abduction.
   - No reduction of PROM.
   - Drop arm test is positive.
   - Poor scapulothoracic and glenohumeral rhythm.
   a. Diagnostic tests utilized: arthrogram traditionally had been the "gold standard" test. MRI may be done but may not be as sensitive.
   b. Physical therapy goals, outcomes, and interventions:
      - Rehabilitation is initiated following a period of immobilization with surgical intervention.
      - Physical therapy intervention emphasizes return of normal strength/endurance/coordination of muscles, joint mechanics, flexibility (AROM/PROM), and scapulothoracic and glenohumeral rhythm with overhead function.

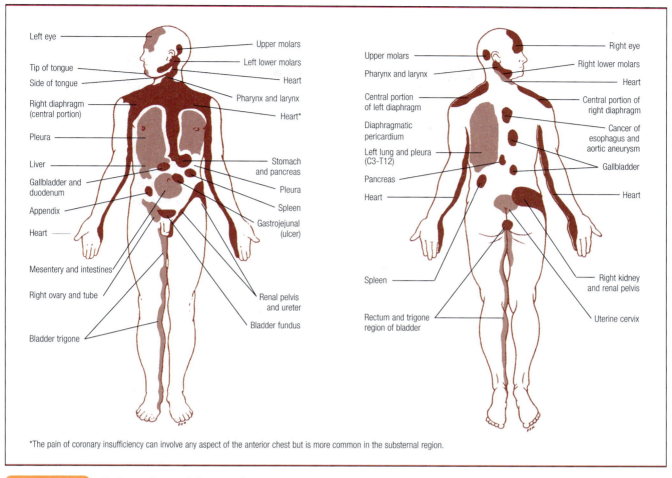

Figure 2-22 Pain referred from viscera.
(From Rothstein, J, Roy, S and Wolf, S: *Rehabilitation Specialist's Handbook*, 4th ed., Philadelphia, F A Davis, pg 412-413, with permission.)

*The pain of coronary insufficiency can involve any aspect of the anterior chest but is more common in the substernal region.

Tendon Injuries and Repairs of the Hand

1. Flexor tendon repairs.
   a. First 3–4 weeks, distal extremity is immobilized with a protective splint with wrist and digits flexed. Rubber band traction is applied to maintain interphalangeal joints in 30–50 degrees of passive flexion.
   b. Physical therapy goals, outcomes, and interventions:
      - Patient can perform resisted extension and passive flexion within constraints of splint. AROM to tolerance is initiated at 4 weeks.
      - Goal is to manage all soft tissues through wound-healing phases by providing collagen remodeling, which preserves free tendon gliding.
      - Early intervention consists of wound management, edema control, and passive exercises.
      - Active extension exercises are initiated first followed by flexion.
      - Resistive and functional exercises are introduced when full AROM is achieved.
   c. Extensor tendon repairs.
      - Distal repairs are immobilized such that the distal interphalangeal joints are in neutral for 6–8 weeks.
      - Physical therapy goals, outcomes, and interventions:
        ○ AROM is initiated at 6 weeks with proximal interphalangeal joints in neutral.
        ○ Goal is to manage all soft tissues through wound-healing phases by providing collagen remodeling, which preserves free tendon gliding.
        ○ Early intervention consists of wound management, edema control, and passive exercises.
        ○ Active extension exercises are initiated first, followed by flexion.
        ○ Resistive and functional exercises are introduced when full AROM is achieved.

- Proximal repairs are immobilized with the wrist and digital joints in extension for 4 weeks.
- Physical therapy goals, outcomes, and interventions:
  - Early AROM/PROM in flexion with metacarpophalangeal joint in extension. At 6 weeks, full AROM is initiated into flexion and extension.

Orthopedic Surgical Repairs—Lower Extremity

Total Hip Replacement (THR)/Arthroplasty

1. This information may vary depending on surgical procedure and/or MD preference/protocol. Must be familiar with postoperative protocol for each patient relative to procedure and/or MD.
2. Cemented versus noncemented.
   a. Cemented hips can tolerate full weight-bearing immediately following surgery.
   b. Cement may crack with aging causing a loosening of prosthesis. Noncemented technique is more stressful on bones during the surgical procedure.
   c. Noncemented procedures are typically used with younger and/or more active individuals. Cemented technique may be better for individuals with fragile bones or for those who will benefit from immediate ability to weight bear (e.g., those with dementia or significant debilitation).
3. Bed positioning with a wedge to prevent adduction.
4. Patient should avoid the position of hip flexion >90 degrees with adduction and internal rotation. Partial weight-bearing to tolerance is initiated on the second postsurgery day using crutches or a walker with typical surgical procedures. See Table 2-11.

> **RED FLAG:** Patients should avoid the positions of hip flexion >90°, adduction past midline, and internal rotation for the first 6 weeks after surgery. These positions place the hip at risk for dislocation and other complications.

5. Physical therapy goals, outcomes, and interventions:
   a. Physical therapy intervention focuses on bed mobility, transitional movements, ambulation, and return to premorbid ADL.

Table 2-11

Total Hip Replacement Guidelines/Precautions

ACTIVITY	CEMENTED	CEMENTLESS	
Internal rotation of hip joint	Do not perform for 3–6 months.	Do not perform for 3–6 months.	
Adduction of hip joint	Do not perform for 3–6 months.	Do not perform for 3–6 months.	
Flexion of hip joint beyond 90°	Do not perform for 3–6 months.	Do not perform for 3–6 months.	
Ambulation	Partial weight bearing (PWB) for approximately 3 weeks. Begin ambulation with cane at week 4 postop. Begin transition to full weight bearing at week 5.	Varies from weight bearing as tolerated (WBAT) to touch-down weight bearing (TDWB), based on the surgeon's philosophy and the surgical approach.	
		WBAT (WB as Tolerated)	**TDWB (Touch Down)**
		Partial weight bearing (PWB) for approximately 3 weeks. Begin ambulation with cane at week 4 postop. Begin transition to full weight bearing at week 6.	Progress to ⅓ weight bearing at week 6. Progress to ⅔ weight bearing at week 8. Progress to full weight bearing at week 10 with walker. Begin transition to cane at week 12. Progress to no assistive device when safe and no Trendelenberg gait.
Isometric exercise	Immediately postop as tolerated by the patient.	Immediately postop as tolerated by the patient.	
Active exercise	Initiation is variable between weeks 1 through 4, depending on the surgeon's guidelines.	Initiation is variable between weeks 1 through 4, depending on surgeon's guidelines.	

Open Reduction Internal Fixation (ORIF) After Femoral Fracture

1. Patient will typically be non-weight-bearing for 1–2 weeks using crutches or a walker. Thereafter, the patient will be partial weight-bearing as tolerated.
2. Physical therapy goals, outcomes, and interventions:
   a. Physical therapy intervention focuses on bed mobility, transitional movements, ambulation, and return to premorbid ADL.

Total Knee Replacement (TKR)/Arthroplasty

1. TKR surgery is typically performed as a result of severe DJD of the knee joint which has led to pain and impaired function.
2. Physical therapy goals, outcomes, and interventions:
   a. Goals of early rehabilitation (1–3 weeks) include muscle reeducation, soft tissue mobilization, lymphedema reduction, initiation of PROM (e.g., a continuous passive motion [CPM] machine is used in the hospital following surgery), AROM, and reduction of postsurgical swelling. See Table 2-12 for TKR guidelines and precautions.
   b. Goals of the second phase of rehabilitation include regaining endurance, coordination, and strength of the muscles surrounding the knee. Also functional activities to include progressive ambulation, stair climbing, and transitional training based on healing and the type of prosthesis used.
   c. Goals and outcomes of the last phase of rehabilitation include returning the patient to premorbid ADL. Functional and endurance training and proprioceptive exercises are introduced during this phase.
   d. The weight-bearing status of patients with a cemented prosthesis is at the level of the patient's tolerance. Patients with cementless prostheses are progressed according to the time frame for fracture healing. Weight bearing 1–7 weeks is 25%, 50% by week 8, 75% by week 10, and 100% weight-bearing without an assistive device by week 12.
   e. Treatment consideration: Avoid forceful mobilization and PROM into flexion because of the mechanical restraints of the prosthesis.
   f. Treatment consideration: Do not use continuous passive motion machines for postoperative management of patients following uncomplicated total knee replacement (White N, et al. Phys Ther. 2015).
   g. Biomechanical faults caused by joint restrictions should be corrected with joint mobilization to the specific restrictions identified during the examination.

Ligamentous Repairs of Knee

1. Six phases of rehabilitation are followed with ACL and PCL reconstructive surgery.
2. ACL reconstruction (Table 2-13).
   a. Immediately following surgery, a continuous passive motion (CPM) unit is utilized with PROM from 0–70 degrees of flexion.
   b. Motion is increased to 0–120 degrees by the sixth week.
   c. Reconstruction is usually protected with a hinged brace set at 20–70 degrees of flexion initially.
   d. Patient is non-weight-bearing for approximately 1 week.

Table 2-12

Total Knee Replacement Guidelines/Precautions

ACTIVITY	CEMENTED	CEMENTLESS	
Range of motion	0°–90° within 2 weeks 0°–120° within 3–4 weeks	0°–90° within 2 weeks 0°–120° within 3–4 weeks	
Ambulation	Weight bearing as tolerated with walker immediately postop. Ambulation with cane at week 3. Transition to full weight bearing at week 4.	Varies from weight bearing as tolerated (WBAT) to touch-down weight bearing (TDWB) based on surgeon's philosophy and surgical approach.	
		WBAT	**TDWB**
		Weight bearing as tolerated with walker immediately postop. Ambulation with cane at week 5–6. Transition to full weight bearing at week 6.	Touch down weight bearing with walker immediately postop. Weight bearing as tolerated with walker at week 6. Ambulation with cane at week 8–10. Transition to full weight bearing at week 10.
Isometric and active exercise	Immediately postop	Immediately postop	
Resisted exercise	Begin at week 2–3	Begin at week 2–3	

Table 2-13

Hamstring Versus Patella Tendon Graft For ACL Reconstruction

PROS/CONS	HAMSTRING GRAFTS	PATELLA TENDON GRAFTS
Pros	1. Typically fewer symptoms postoperatively 2. Greater return to pre-injury level of activity 3. Typically allows earlier rehabilitation	1. Better at maintaining graft tension postoperatively 2. Typically less expensive 3. Faster healing time
Cons	1. Typically more expensive 2. Believed to be more technically difficult procedure 3. Rehabilitation can be more difficult (i.e., slower).	1. Increased potential for anterior knee pain and later patellofemoral osteoarthrosis 2. Increased potential for knee extension deficit 3. Potential delay in rehabilitation secondary to more atrophy of quadriceps

e. Weight-bearing progresses as tolerated to full weight-bearing.
f. Patient is weaned from brace between the second and fourth weeks.
3. Posterior cruciate ligament reconstruction.
   a. Generally similar to ACL repair except patient is often initially in hinged brace at 0 degree during ambulation.
4. Physical therapy goals, outcomes, and interventions following ACL and PCL surgical repairs:
   a. Six phases of rehabilitation are as follows: preoperative, maximum protection, controlled motion, moderate protection, minimum protection, and return to activity.
   b. Specific interventions:
      - Soft tissue/massage techniques to quadriceps and hamstring muscles to reduce muscle guarding.
      - Joint oscillations to inhibit joint pain and muscle guarding.
      - Correction of muscle imbalances and biomechanical faults using strengthening, endurance, coordination, and flexibility exercises to gain restoration of normal function.
      - Biomechanical faults caused by joint restrictions should be corrected with joint mobilization to the specific restrictions identified during the examination.
      - Progression to functional training based on patient's occupation and/or recreational goals.

Lateral Retinacular Release
1. Typically performed as a result of patellofemoral pain syndrome (PFPS). Purpose of procedure is to restore normal tracking of the patella during contraction of the quadriceps muscle.
2. Physical therapy goals, outcomes, and interventions:
   a. Intervention should emphasize closed kinetic chain exercises to strengthen quadriceps muscles and regain dynamic balance of all structures (contractile and noncontractile) surrounding knee.
   b. Normalizing the flexibility of the hamstrings, triceps surae, and ITB will help restore mechanical alignment.
   c. Mobilization of patella is important to maintain nutrition and decrease the likelihood of adhesions.

Meniscal Arthroscopy
1. Partial meniscectomy.
   a. Partial weight-bearing as tolerated when full knee extension is obtained.
   b. Physical therapy goals, outcomes, and interventions:
      - Initial goals focus on edema/effusion control.
      - AROM is urged postsurgical day 1.
      - Isotonic and isokinetic strengthening by day 3.
      - Jogging on the ball of the foot or toes is recommended to decrease the loading of the knee joint.
   c. Repairs.
      - Patient will be non-weight-bearing for 3–6 weeks.
      - Rehabilitation of the joint begins within 7–10 days of procedure.
      - Physical therapy goals, outcomes, and interventions:
        ○ Soft tissue/massage techniques to quadriceps and hamstring muscles to reduce muscle guarding.
        ○ Joint oscillations to inhibit joint pain and muscle guarding.
        ○ Correction of muscle imbalances and biomechanical faults using strengthening, endurance, coordination, and flexibility exercises to gain restoration of normal function.
        ○ Biomechanical faults caused by joint restrictions should be corrected with joint mobilization to the specific restrictions identified during the examination.
        ○ Progression to functional training based on patient's occupation and/or recreational goals.

Surgical Repairs of Spine
1. Rehabilitation varies according to the type of surgery performed.
2. A back protection program and early mobilization exercises should be initiated prior to surgery.

3. Patients should avoid prolonged sitting, heavy lifting, and long car trips for approximately 3 months.
4. Repetitive bending with twisting should always be avoided.
5. With microdiscectomies, rehabilitation time is decreased because the fibers of the annulus fibrosus are not damaged.
6. With laminectomy/discectomy, early movement and activation of paraspinal musculature (especially multifidus) is necessary.

Multilevel Vertebral Fusion
1. Typically requires 6 weeks of trunk immobility with bracing.
2. Once brace is removed and movement is allowed, important to regain as much normal/functional movement as possible while restoring functional activation of muscles.
3. With combined anterior/posterior surgical approach, bracing is seldom used.
4. With Harrington rod placement for idiopathic scoliosis, rehabilitation goals focus on early mobilization in bed and effective coughing.
   a. The patient can begin ambulation between the fourth and seventh postoperative days.
   b. The patient should avoid heavy lifting and excessive twisting and bending.

Physical Therapy Goals, Outcomes, and Interventions Following Surgery
1. Soft tissue/massage techniques to paraspinal muscles to reduce muscle guarding.
2. Joint oscillations to inhibit joint pain and muscle guarding.
3. Correction of muscle imbalances using strengthening, endurance, coordination, and flexibility exercises to gain restoration of normal function. Make sure that multifidus function is restored.
4. Must develop dynamic stabilization for muscles of trunk and pelvis during all functional activities.
5. Biomechanical faults caused by joint restrictions should be corrected with joint mobilization to the specific restrictions identified during the examination.
6. Progression to functional training based on patient's occupation and/or recreational goals.

Interventions for Patients/Clients with Musculoskeletal Conditions

Interventions for Patients/Clients with Acute Conditions

Acute (Inflammatory) Phase/Maximal Protection
1. Patients in this phase often have pain at rest due to inflammation.
2. Limited mobilization:
   a. Limited bed rest in only some cases.
   b. Avoid activities that stress the injured tissues.
   c. Use braces, slings, corsets, cervical collars, assistive devices, and taping.
3. Control inflammatory response: follow PRICE: P = protect, R = rest, I = ice, C = compression, E = elevation.
   a. Physical agents: nonthermal modalities.
      - Ice
      - Electric stimulation
      - Ultrasound below 2 w/cm² has been shown to be effective in assisting with tendon healing.
   b. Compression and elevation to reduce and prevent effusion and swelling.
      - Edema should be controlled because excessive edema can lead to reduced circulation, increased pain and increased fibrosis, which restricts movement.
   c. NSAIDs.
   d. Rest/relaxation to reduce pain.
   e. Soft tissue/massage techniques.
      - Can help with circulation and prevent adhesions.
4. Assisted movement of injured tissues.
5. Joint oscillations (grades I and II) for pain relief.
6. Therapeutic exercise:
   a. Dose of 40%–60% of one repetition maximum (i.e., high repetition with low resistance) to stimulate regeneration of tissue and revascularization.
   b. Exercise should be nontraumatic, meaning no pain and/or increased edema as a result of the exercise.
   c. Pain-free AROM or gentle isometrics in a mid-range position can help with circulation and prevent the negative effects of immobilization.
7. Educate patient/client on joint protection strategies.
8. Lasts 24–48 hours or more if needed.
9. Stretching the involved tissue is contraindicated due to the weakness of the newly formed tissue.

Subacute Phase/Moderate Protection
1. Patients in this phase should only have pain with activities that overstress the healing tissues.
2. Avoidance of continued irritation and repetitive trauma.

3. Active movement and light resistance may be initiated—avoid activities that cause pain or delayed-onset muscle soreness.
4. Modify activities at home/work/recreation.
   a. Modify use of equipment or type of equipment at home/work/recreation.
5. Correct biomechanical faults such as leg length discrepancy, abnormal foot biomechanics, abnormal throwing motion.
6. Continued use of pain-relieving modalities, and/or supportive taping.
7. Joint mobilization.
8. Continued therapeutic exercise including flexibility/endurance/coordination exercise.
   a. Focus on endurance rather than strength.
   b. Stretching to regain flexibility is most effective during this phase of treatment.
   c. Progressive strengthening should be carefully monitored to prevent damage to the healing tissues.
9. Postural reeducation.
10. Biomechanical education.
11. Lasts 2–3 days up to 8–10 weeks depending upon:
    a. Type of tissue damage.
    b. Surgical procedure.

Functional Restoration/Minimal Protection Phase

1. Patients should have no pain by this phase and should gradually return to previous activities.
2. Continue increasing endurance and strength building, add active, resistive, and plyometric activities.
3. Incorporate weight-bearing proprioceptive activities.
4. Supportive taping may be necessary to tolerate increased functional activities such as participation in sports.
5. Modalities are unlikely at this phase.
6. Maintain or return to optimum level of patient function.
7. Normalize flexibility of joints and related soft tissues.
8. Restore loading capacity of connective tissues to normal strength.
9. Functional strengthening exercises.
10. Functional stabilization of the involved joint/region.

Interventions for Patients/Clients with a Chronic Condition

Determine Possible Causative Factors

1. Abnormal remodeling of injured tissues.
2. Chronic low-grade inflammation due to repetitive stresses of tissues.

Reduce Stresses to Tissues

1. Identify/eliminate the magnitude of loading.
2. Identify/eliminate direction of forces.
3. Identify and eliminate any biomechanical barriers that are preventing healing (e.g., a leg length discrepancy).
4. Educate patient regarding protection of joints and associated soft tissues.

Regain Structural Integrity

1. Improve flexibility.
2. Postural reeducation.
3. Increasing tissue's capacity to tolerate loading.
4. Functional strengthening/endurance/coordination exercises.

Resume Optimal Patient Function and Prevention of Reoccurrence

1. Patient education regarding causative factors in dysfunction.
2. Work conditioning.

Specific Interventions

Soft Tissue/Myofascial Techniques

1. These techniques aid in reduction of metabolites from muscle, reactivating a muscle that has not been functioning secondary to guarding and ischemia, revascularization of muscle, and decrease guarding in a muscle.
2. Autonomic: stimulation of skin and superficial fascia to facilitate a decrease in muscle tension.
3. Mechanical: movement of skin, fascia, and muscle causes histological and mechanical changes to occur in soft tissues to produce improved mobility and function. Examples include acupressure and osteopathic mechanical stretching techniques.
4. Goals: decrease pain, edema and muscle spasm, increase metabolism and cutaneous temperature, stretch tight muscles and other soft tissues, improve circulation, strengthen weak muscles, and mobilize joint restrictions.
5. Indications: patients with soft tissue and joint restriction that results in pain and limits ADL.
6. Contraindications:
   a. Absolute: soft tissue breakdown, infection, cellulitis, inflammation, and/or neoplasm.
   b. Relative: hypermobility and sensitivity.
7. Traditional massage techniques such as effleurage and petrissage.
8. Functional massage:
   a. Three techniques used to assist in reactivation of a debilitated muscle and/or to increase vascularity to a muscle.
      - Soft tissue without motion.
        ○ Traditional technique; however, hands do not slide over skin. Instead they stay in contact with skin while hands and skin move together over the muscle.

- Direction of force is parallel to muscle fibers and total stroke time should be 5–7 seconds.
- Soft tissue with passive pumping.
  - Place muscle in shortened position and with one hand place tension on muscle parallel to muscle fibers.
- Other hand passively lengthens muscle and simultaneously gradually releases tension of hand in contact with muscle.
- Soft tissue with active pumping.
  - Place muscle in lengthened position and with one hand place tension on muscle perpendicular to muscle fibers.
  - Other hand guides limb as patient actively shortens muscle. Simultaneously as muscle shortens, gradually release tension of hand in contact with muscle.
9. Transverse friction massage.
   a. Used to initiate an acute inflammatory response for tissue that is in metabolic stasis such as a tendonosis.
   b. Involved tendon is briskly massaged in a transverse fashion (perpendicular to the direction of the fibers).
   c. Performed for 5–10 minutes and tends to be very uncomfortable for the patient.
10. Movement approaches require the patient to actively participate in treatment. Examples include:
    a. Feldenkrais:
       - Facilitates development of normal movement patterns.
       - The practitioner uses skillful, supportive, gentle hands to create a sense of safety, maintain supportive contact, while introducing new movement possibilities in small, easily available increments.
    b. Muscle energy techniques.
       - Include voluntary contraction in a precisely controlled direction, at varying levels of intensity, against an applied counterforce from the clinician.
       - Purpose is to gain motion that is limited by restrictions of the neuromuscular system.
       - Modification of proprioceptive neuromuscular facilitation (PNF) technique.
    c. PNF hold-relax-contract technique.
       - Antagonist of the shortened muscle is contracted to achieve reciprocal inhibition and increased range.
       - Refer to Chapter 3.

Articulatory Techniques

1. Joint oscillation.
   a. Inhibits pain and/or muscle guarding.
   b. Lubricates joint surfaces.
   c. Provides nutrition to the joint structures.
   d. It is suggested by Maitland that grades III and IV oscillations are beneficial to stretch tight connective tissues.
   e. Grades of movement as described by Maitland (see Figure 2-1).
      - Five grades of joint play in neutral:
        - Grade I oscillations are small amplitude at the beginning of the range of joint play.
        - Grade II oscillations are large amplitude at the midrange of joint play.
      - Grade III oscillations are large amplitude at the end range of joint play.
      - Grade IV oscillations are small amplitude at the end range of joint play.
      - Grade V is a manipulation of high velocity and low amplitude to the anatomical endpoint of a joint. Technically this is not an oscillation because it is a single movement rather than a repetitive movement.
   f. Indications for use of oscillation grades per Maitland:
      - Grades I and II used to improve joint lubrication/nutrition as well as decrease pain and muscle guarding.
      - Grades III and IV used to stretch tight muscles, capsules and ligaments.
      - Grade V used to regain normal joint mechanics as well as decrease pain and muscle guarding.
   g. Contraindications:
      - Absolute: Joint ankylosis, malignancy involving bone, diseases that affect the integrity of ligaments (RA and Down syndrome), arterial insufficiency, and active inflammatory and/or infective process.
      - Relative: Arthrosis (DJD), metabolic bone disease (osteoporosis, Paget's disease and tuberculosis), hypermobility, total joint replacement, pregnancy, spondylolisthesis, use of steroids, and radicular symptoms.
2. Joint mobilization.
   a. To stretch/lengthen/deform collagen to normalize arthrokinematic glide of joint structures.
   b. Grades of translatoric glide as described by Kaltenborn (see Figure 2-2).
      - Grade I:
        - "Loosening" translatoric glide.
        - Movement is a very small amplitude traction force.
        - Used to relieve pain and/or decompress a joint during joint glides performed within examination or intervention.
      - Grade II:
        - "Tightening" translatoric glide.
        - Movement takes up slack in tissues surrounding joint.
        - Used to alleviate pain, assess joint play, and/or reduce muscle guarding.
      - Grade III:
        - "Stretching" translatoric glide.

- Movement stretches the tissues crossing joint.
- Used to assess end-feel or to increase movement (stretch tissue).
  c. Traction: Manual, mechanical, and self- or autotraction.
  - Vertebral bodies separating.
  - Distraction and gliding of facet joints.
  - Tensing of the ligamentous structures of the spinal segment.
  - Intervertebral foramen widening.
  - Spinal muscles stretching.

> **RED FLAG:** Contraindications for mobilization.
> - Absolute contraindications for joint mobilization/manipulation/traction include joint ankyloses, malignancy, disease that affect the integrity of ligaments (RA, Down syndrome), arterial insufficiency, and active inflammatory and/or infectious process.
> - Relative contraindications include arthorisis, metabolic bone disease (osteoporosis, Paget's disease, tuberculosis), hypermobility, total joint replacement, pregnancy, spondylolisthesis, use of steroids, and radicular symptoms.

3. Manipulation:
   a. Inhibit pain and/or muscle guarding.
   b. Improve translatory glide in cases of joint dysfunction due to restriction.
   c. Health care practitioners who commonly perform manipulative thrusts include physical therapists, osteopaths, chiropractors, and medical doctors.
   d. Types of manipulations:
      - Generalized:
        - Fairly forceful long-lever techniques that are intended to include as many vertebral segments as possible.
        - More commonly performed by chiropractic practitioners.
      - Specific:
        - Aimed at having an effect on either a specific segment or only a few vertebral segments.
        - Uses minimal force with short-lever arms.
        - Often includes "locking" techniques based on biomechanics to ensure that a specific vertebral segment receives the manipulative thrust.
        - More commonly performed by physical therapists.
      - Midrange:
        - Very gentle, short-lever arm techniques.
        - Barrier is created in midrange by specific positioning of patient as well as creating tautness in surrounding soft tissues.
        - More commonly performed by osteopathic practitioners.
   e. Contraindications:
      - Absolute: joint ankylosis, malignancy involving bone, diseases that affect the integrity of ligaments (RA and Down syndrome), arterial insufficiency, and active inflammatory and/or infective process.
      - Relative: arthrosis (DJD), metabolic bone disease (osteoporosis, Paget's disease and tuberculosis), hypermobility, total joint replacement, pregnancy, spondylolisthesis, use of steroids, and radicular symptoms.

Neural Tissue Mobilization
1. Movement of neural structures to regain normal mobility.
2. Tension tests for upper and lower extremities (i.e., dural stretch test).
   a. Movement of soft tissues that may be restricting neural structures (e.g., cross-friction massage for adhesions of the radial nerve to the humerus at a fracture site).
   b. Indications: used for patients who have some type of restriction in neural mobility anywhere along the course of the nerve.
   c. Postural reeducation: to open up the intervertebral foramen and decrease tension to tissues.
   d. Contraindications: extreme pain and/or increase in abnormal neurological signs.

Neurodynamic Exercises
1. Nerve entrapment by edema, scar tissue, or other tissue constrictions limits the nervous system's ability to dissipate tensile forces during movement.
2. Excessive tensile force (traction) on the nervous system can lead to pain, paresthesia, and muscle weakness.
3. Neurodynamic exercises are designed to maintain or regain lost nervous system mobility.
   a. Tension in a peripheral nerve is related to specific positions of the limbs and spine, much like tension in a muscle during a stretching exercise.
   b. A "nerve glide" exercise involves alternating tension between the distal and proximal portions of the nerve to achieve a gliding movement of the nerve.

Therapeutic Exercise for Musculoskeletal Conditions
1. Therapeutic exercise is indicated for the following reasons.
   a. Decrease muscle guarding.
   b. Decrease pain.
   c. Increase vascularity of tissue.
   d. Promote regeneration and/or speed up recovery of connective tissues such as cartilage, tendons, ligaments, capsules, intervertebral discs.
   e. Mobilize restricted tissue to increase flexibility.
   f. Increase endurance of muscle.

g. Increase coordination of muscle.
h. Increase strength of muscle.
i. Sensitize muscles to minimize joints going into excessive range in cases of hypermobility.
j. Develop dynamic stability and functional movement patterns allowing for optimal function within the environment.
2. Home exercise program for patients/clients with musculoskeletal conditions.
    a. Patient's home program will consist of exercises to reinforce clinical program.
    b. Necessary to perform enough repetitions to have the desired physiological effect on appropriate tissues as well as develop coordination and endurance to promote dynamic stability within functional patterns.
3. Refer to Chapter 10 for more details.

Manual Therapy Approaches in Rehabilitation

All Approaches Provide
1. A philosophical basis, subjective evaluation.
2. Objective examination.
3. A diagnosis.
4. A plan of care.

Approaches Can Be Divided Into Two Categories
1. Physician-generated.
    a. Mennell, who believed the joint is the dysfunctional unit.
    b. Osteopaths suggest any component of the somatic system is responsible for dysfunction.
    c. Cyriax, who contends that dysfunction is due to interplay between contractile and noncontractile tissues.
2. Clinician generated.
    a. McKenzie, who feels that postural factors precipitate discal dysfunction. Treatment emphasizes the use of extension exercises.
    b. Maitland, who proposes that the subjective evaluation should be integrated with objective measures in determining the dysfunctional area.
    c. Kaltenborn, who believes that abnormal joint mobility and soft tissue changes account for dysfunction.
3. Chiropractic generated.
    a. Focus is to restore normal joint function through soft tissue and joint manipulation. Chiropractors believe that restoration of normal biomechanical function affects other systems of the body as well, thus improving the patient's state of health in many ways.

Modalities and Electrotherapeutic Agents

Physical Agents
1. Modalities and electrotherapeutic agents are used to manage pain and inflammation throughout healing and rehabilitation.
2. Thermal agents (Table 2-14).
    a. Ice used to control edema.
        - Acute.
        - Sub-acute after introducing new activities.
    b. Heat.
        - Tissue extensibility.
3. Electrotherapeutic agents.
    a. Pain modulation.
    b. Edema management.
    c. Muscle stimulation.

Relevant Pharmacology

Nonsteroidal Anti-Inflammatory Drugs (NSAIDs)
1. Most commonly prescribed medication for pain relief for musculoskeletal dysfunction (Table 2-15).
2. Examples include ibuprofen (Motrin), naproxen sodium (Aleve), salsalate (Discalced), and indomethacin (Indocin).

Table 2-14

Pharmacokinetics and Therapeutic Modalities to Treat Soft Tissue and Skeletal Conditions

MODALITY	INDICATIONS	CONSIDERATION	EXAMPLE
Heat	Pain Tissue extensibility	Absorption: heat increases rate and extent of medication absorption	Hot packs, ultrasound, warm hydrotherapy
Electrotherapy	Pain Muscle guarding Muscle activation/weakness	Transdermal medication patches: potential for interaction between electromodality and any metallic backings on the patch; it may introduce a risk of increased heat and/or burns	Electromagnetic radiation (e.g., ultraviolet radiation, lasers, diathermy). Electrical current (e.g., TENS, NMES, etc.)
Cryotherapy	Pain Edema	Ice packs, cryo-units	

Table 2-15

Commonly Prescribed Medications and Associated Precautions—Musculoskeletal Conditions

MEDICATION	PRESCRIBED FOR	SIDE EFFECTS	INTERACTIONS	PHYSICAL THERAPY CONSIDERATIONS
Medications used to treat pain and/or inflammation				
Nonsteroidal antiinflammatory drugs (NSAIDS). Aspirin, ibuprofen (Motrin, Advil), meloxicam (Mobic), indomethacin (Indocin), naproxen (Aleve, Naprosyn), piroxicam (Feldene)	Inflammatory conditions and acute or chronic pain. Rheumatoid arthritis. Osteoarthritis	Stomach and gastrointestinal irritation, stomach ulcers, bleeding disorders. Can cause symptoms of dizziness, fatigue, dyspnea, tinnitus, headache. Processed in the liver and kidneys, can cause serious liver problems, alcohol increases risk	All have the potential to interact with warfarin and Coumadin (enhance effects) and are contraindicated. Should be avoided in individuals with congestive heart failure, kidney disease, stomach ulcers, kidney disorders, alcoholism.	Aspirin should be avoided in children <4 years of age.
COX-2 inhibitors				
Celecoxib (off the market: Vioxx)	Acute or chronic pain, inflammation	Produce less stomach and gastrointestinal irritation than NSAIDs; however, increased risk for potential heart problems. Liver dysfunction contributes to declining kidney function. Fluid accumulation mimicking congestive heart failure	When taken with anticoagulants, aspirin, corticosteroids, or SSRIs may cause increased risk of stomach bleeding. Effectiveness of ACE inhibitors or diuretics may be decreased by this medication. Should be avoided by persons allergic to sulfonamide antibiotics	
Narcotic analgesics and combination products. Acetaminophen + codeine phosphate (Tylenol #3), hydrocodone + acetaminophen (Lortab, Vicodin), oxycodone + acetaminophen (OxyContin), hydromorphone (Dilaudid), tramadol (Ultram)	Acute or chronic pain—mild to severe	Nausea, vomiting, constipation, lightheadedness, dizziness. Can create withdrawal reaction (restlessness, nausea, sweating, muscle aches, watering eyes) if it has been used regularly for extended period of time. Can cause serious liver problems if combined with alcohol	MAO inhibitors. Opioids are habit forming. Should be avoided/used under close supervision by persons with abnormal heart rhythm, abnormally low blood pressure, chronic and decreased lung function problems, inflammatory bowel disease, or liver failure.	Be cautious if patient/client experiences dizziness and lightheadedness; assume upright/standing positions slowly. Patient/client may tolerate better if taken an hour or so prior to PT.
Corticosteroids/glucocorticoids. Dexamethasone (Decadron, Hexadrol), cortisone, hydrocortisone (Cortef), prednisone (Deltasone)	Reduce or suppress the inflammatory process	Significant weakening of tendon, muscle, and bone can occur—especially with intraarticular injection. May weaken the immune system. Increased risk for high blood glucose, high blood pressure, abnormal fat distribution pattern, impaired wound healing	Can interact with and either increase or decrease effects of anticoagulant medications.	Clinician should pay careful attention to posture, monitor for changes that may reflect weakening of the spine or other support structures. Limit strenuous activity, high resistance and aggressive stretching in areas of injection

Table 2-15
Commonly Prescribed Medications and Associated Precautions—Musculoskeletal Conditions (Continued)

MEDICATION	PRESCRIBED FOR	SIDE EFFECTS	INTERACTIONS	PHYSICAL THERAPY CONSIDERATIONS
Medications used to treat bone resorption				
Bisphosphonates. Alendronate (Fosamax), ibandronate (Boniva), calcitonin (Miacalcin, Calcimar), raloxifene (Evista), zoledronic acid-IV (Reclast, Zometa), risedronate (Actonel)	Bone demineralization and disorders such as osteoporosis, Paget's disease	Constipation, indigestion, diarrhea, abdominal pain, deterioration (osteonecrosis) of the jaw, muscle cramps, headaches. Calcitonin: nasal spray can cause irritation in nose (e.g., sores, dryness, itching, bleeding). Injectable can cause: stomach pain, diarrhea, nausea or vomiting, flushing (face, ears, hands, feet), loss of appetite.	Can cause increases in abdominal distress if combined with use of aspirin. Calcium or antacids taken with medication can interfere with uptake of medication. Calcium intake should be monitored by doctor. Calcitonin: may interfere with other meds taken for Paget's disease. Calcium intake should be monitored by doctor. Raloxifene: may affect blood clotting (an increased risk of blood clots with this medication); individuals on warfarin (Coumadin). Calcium intake should be monitored by doctor as levels could become too high.	Alendronate: patient should take the medication on an empty stomach, should not lie down within 30 minutes of taking the medication; increased chance of irritation of esophagus. Raloxifene: monitor carefully for bruising. Ensure the patient is getting blood test for clotting times (prothrombin time, international ratio).
Medications used following surgical procedures				
Anticoagulants. Warfarin (Coumadin)	Prevent blood clot formation following surgery	Serious (possibly fatal) bleeding—particularly in new users. Nausea. Loss of appetite. Stomach/abdominal pain. Unusual or easy bruising. Prolonged bleeding from simple cuts/scrapes	Interacts with many prescription and non-prescription medications, vitamins and herbal products. Aspirin and NSAIDS are contraindicated. Many food interactions exist including, but not limited to: leafy green vegetables, soy, green tea, V-8 vegetable juice, cranberry.	Check with patient/client regarding most recent INR (blood clotting speed) test results. Be cautious when performing joint mobilization and soft tissue techniques
Antibiotics (a partial list, most can be administered orally or by injection). Penicillins—amoxicillin (Amoxil), tetracyclines (Sumycin, Achromycin), cephalosporins—cephalexin (Keflex) cefaclor (Ceclor)	Treat infection	Nausea, vomiting, diarrhea, loss of appetite, dizziness, headache. Can have increased effect in persons who are elderly. Oral or vaginal fungal infection	May be problematic for individuals with kidney or liver disease, esophagus problems (hiatal hernia, reflux disease—GERD). Some antibiotics can interact with calcium or magnesium supplements. Decreased effectiveness of oral contraceptives. Increased sensitivity to sunlight	Some antibiotics are best taken while sitting up and require ten or more minutes before the patient/client is allowed to lie down.

3. Provide analgesic, anti-inflammatory, and antipyretic capabilities.
4. Adverse side effects could include gastrointestinal irritation, fluid retention, renal or liver problems, and prolonged bleeding.
5. COX-2 inhibitors have decreased gastrointestinal irritation, but rofecoxib (Vioxx) was withdrawn from the market secondary to its relationship with heart-related conditions. Other COX-2 inhibitors such as colecoxib (Celebrex) and valdecoxib (Bextra) are being evaluated for their safety and possible association with heart-related conditions.

Muscle Relaxants
1. Commonly prescribed for skeletal muscle spasm.
2. Examples include cyclobenzaprine HCl (Flexeril), methocarbamol (Robaxin), and carisoprodol (Soma).
3. Act on the central nervous system to reduce skeletal muscle tone by depressing the internuncial neurons of the brain stem and spinal cord.
4. Adverse side effects could include drowsiness, lethargy, ataxia, and decreased alertness.

Nonnarcotic Analgesics
1. Prescribed when NSAIDs are contraindicated.
2. Examples include acetaminophen (Tylenol).
3. Act on the central nervous system to alter response to pain and have antipyretic capabilities.
4. Adverse side effects are negligible when taken in recommended doses. Excessive amounts of acetaminophen may lead to liver disease or acute liver shutdown.

Narcotic Analgesics
1. Prescribed for acute or moderate to severe pain.
2. Examples include codeine, fentanyl, hydrocodone, hydromorphone, and oxycodone.
3. Prevents pain input by binding to CNS opioid receptors.
4. Adverse side effects could include sedation, confusion, vertigo, orthostatic hypotension, constipation, incoordination, physical dependence, and tolerance.

> **RED FLAG:** Patients with a wide variety of musculoskeletal disorders may be prescribed narcotics (opioids). There is an increasing number of individuals who suffer from opioid dependency. Clinicians should recognize the signs and symptoms of the "opioid overdose triad": pinpoint pupils, respiratory depression, and unconsciousness. Clinicians should initiate emergency response procedures if a patient exhibits any signs or symptoms consistent with an opioid crisis (see APTA white paper on the opioid epidemic dated June 1, 2018).

Psychosocial Considerations

Malingering (Symptom Magnification Syndrome)
1. Defined as a behavioral response where displays of symptoms control the life of the patient, leading to functional disability.
2. There may be psychological advantages to illness:
   a. The patient may feel protected from the threatening world.
   b. Uncertainty or fear about the future.
   c. Social gain.
   d. Reduces stressors.
3. Therapist needs to recognize symptoms and respond to the patient.
   a. Tests to evaluate malingering back pain may include the Hoover's and Burn's tests and Waddell's signs.
      - Hoover's test involves the therapist's evaluation of the amount of pressure the patient's heels place on the therapist's hands when the patient is asked to raise one lower extremity while in a supine position.
      - Burn's test requires the patient to kneel and bend over a chair to touch the floor.
      - Waddell's signs evaluate tenderness, simulation tests, distraction tests, regional disturbances, and overreaction. Waddell's scores can be predictive of functional outcome.
   b. Functional capacity evaluations are used to evaluate psychosocial as well as physical components of disability.
   c. Emphasize regaining functional outcomes, not pain reduction.

Secondary Gain
1. Usually some type of financial gain for staying ill.
   a. Worker's compensation.
   b. Larger settlement for injury claims.
2. Frequently seen in clinics that manage industrial injuries.
3. May not want to return to work for various reasons associated with the work environment (e.g., stress, dislike of coworkers).

Review Questions

Musculoskeletal Physical Therapy

1. What joint accessory motion is used when performing mobilization techniques to increase joint range of motion? Identify and describe it.

2. In what circumstance might a physician order a plain film radiograph (x-ray) versus a CT scan?

3. Compare and contrast the symptoms a patient or client might describe for facet joint dysfunction versus spinal stenosis.

4. Compare and contrast physical therapy treatment strategies and goals for patients and clients with arthritic, soft tissue, and bony tissue conditions.

5. Describe the rehabilitation process for an individual rehabilitating from surgical repair of an anterior-inferior dislocation of the shoulder.

3

Neuromuscular Physical Therapy

TIFFANY BOHM and SUSAN B. O'SULLIVAN

Chapter Outline

- Anatomy and Physiology of the Neuromuscular System, 85
  - Organization of the Nervous System, 85
  - Structural Components, 85
  - Physiology, 86
  - Brain, 87
  - Spinal Cord, 90
- Physical Therapy Examination and Data Collection, 91
  - Physical Therapist Assistant's Role and Responsibilities, 91
  - Patient History and Medical Record Review, 91
  - Arousal, Mentation, and Cognition, 93
  - Aerobic Capacity and Endurance, 93
  - Sensory Testing, 94
  - Perceptual Dysfunction, 96
  - Motor Function, 97
  - Gait and Locomotion, 100
  - Balance, 100
  - Environment and Equipment Considerations, 104

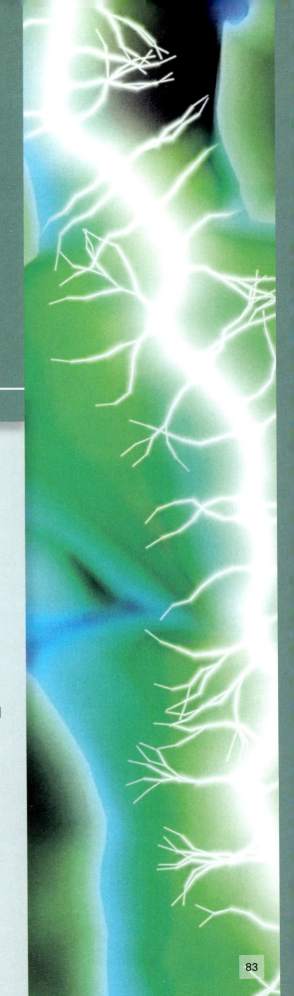

- Intervention Strategies for Patients with Neurological Dysfunction, 105
  - Physical Therapist Assistant's Role and Responsibilities, 105
  - Intervention Approaches, 106
  - Motor Control/Motor Learning, 109
  - Task-Specific Training Strategies, 113
  - Promote Ambulation Independence, 114
- Conditions/Pathology/Diseases with Intervention, 116
  - Infectious Disorders, 116
  - CNS Neoplasms, 116
  - Degenerative Diseases of the CNS, 117
  - Cerebral Vascular Accident (CVA, Stroke), 119
  - Medical Management, 121
  - Traumatic Brain Injury (TBI), 122
  - Medical Management, 123
  - Concussion, 125
  - Spinal Cord Injury (SCI), 126
  - Medical Management, 130
  - Epilepsy, 131
  - Medical Management, 133
  - Peripheral Nervous System (PNS) Disorders, 133
  - Medical Management, 136
- Painful Neurological Conditions, 136
  - Complex Regional Pain Syndrome (CRPS), 136
  - Medical Management, 137
- Review Questions, 138

Anatomy and Physiology of the Neuromuscular System

Organization of the Nervous System

Central Nervous System (CNS)
1. Brain (Figure 3-1).
2. Spinal cord.

Peripheral Nervous System (PNS)
1. Afferent system: conveys information from sensory receptors to the CNS.
2. Efferent system: conveys information from the CNS to muscles and glands.
   a. Somatic nervous system: conveys information to skeletal muscles.
   b. Autonomic nervous system (ANS): conveys information to smooth muscle, cardiac muscle, and glands.

Sympathetic Division
1. Stress responses (Figure 3-2).
2. Prepares body for "fight or flight" and emergency responses.
   a. Raises heart rate and blood pressure.
   b. Constricts peripheral blood vessels and redistributes blood to organs.
   c. Inhibits peristalsis.

Parasympathetic Division
1. Relaxation responses (Figure 3-3).
2. Conserves and restores homeostasis.
   a. Slows heart rate and reduces blood pressure.
   b. Increases peristalsis and glandular activity.

Structural Components

Neuron
1. Individual nerve cell that is responsible for conduction of impulses.
2. Parts.
   a. Soma (cell body).
   b. Dendrites: provide large surface area to receive information.
   c. Axons: conduct impulses away from the cell body, sometimes long distances.

Figure 3-1 Overview of the nervous system.

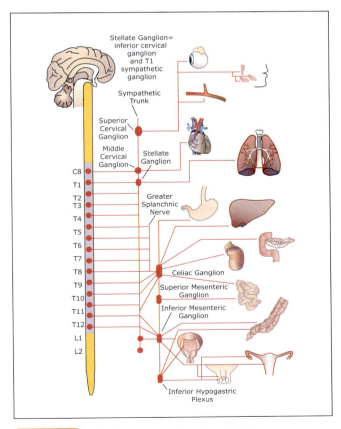

Figure 3-2 ANS-sympathetic division.

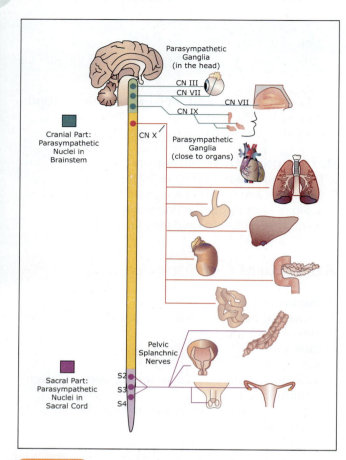

Figure 3-3 ANS-parasympathetic division.

Neuroglia
1. Support and protect neurons but do not transmit signals.
2. Includes astrocytes, oligodendrocytes, Schwann's cells, microglia.

Grouping of Neural Tissue
1. Nerve: grouping of neurons outside the CNS.
2. Tract: grouping of neurons inside the CNS.
3. Ganglia: grouping of neuron cell bodies outside the CNS.
4. White matter: myelinated axons from many neurons.
5. Gray matter: cell bodies and dendrites and/or unmyelinated axons.
6. Upper motor neuron: brain and spinal cord.
7. Lower motor neuron: peripheral nerve.

Physiology

Terminology
1. Resting potential: difference in electrical potential across the cell membrane when information is not being transmitted.
   a. Positive ion charge outside the membrane and negative ion charge inside the membrane that is maintained by sodium-potassium pumps.
2. Depolarization: potential becomes less negative than the resting potential via potassium rushing into the cell.
   a. Generates an action potential or nerve impulse that travels along the neuron.
3. Saltatory conduction.
   a. Nerve impulse jumps between spaces in the myelin sheath known as nodes of Ranvier.
   b. Increases speed of impulse conduction.
4. Synapse.
   a. Location of signal transmission between the presynaptic cell axon and postsynaptic cell dendrite or effector organ.
   b. Determines which chemical or electrical signals are released and transferred.
5. Neurotransmitters.
   a. Chemical messengers released by the presynaptic membrane.
   b. Bind to receptors on the postsynaptic membrane to cause excitation or inhibition of the postsynaptic membrane.
6. Neuromodulators.
   a. Alter neural function by activating membrane channels or genes within the cell.
   b. Effect occurs within seconds and can last from minutes to days.
7. All-or-none principle.
   a. If a stimulus is strong enough, it generates an action potential.
   b. If it is not, an action potential will not occur.
   c. No matter how strong the stimulus, the action potential is always the same as long as it is at the threshold level.
8. Refractory periods.
   a. Absolute refractory period: when the membrane is depolarized and it is not possible to create another action potential.
   b. Relative refractory period: hyperpolarization period when a stronger than normal stimulus would be required to produce another action potential.
9. Repolarization.
   a. Restoration of the membrane to resting potential when potassium is pushed out of the cell.

Types of Sensory Axons
1. Ia and Ib.
   a. Large and myelinated for fast conduction speed.
   b. Carry proprioceptive information (muscle, tendon or ligament stretch).
2. II and A-beta.
   a. Medium size and myelinated for medium speed of conduction.
   b. Carry fine touch information.

3. A-delta and C.
   a. Small with little or no myelination; therefore, they transmit slowly.
   b. Free nerve endings carrying temperature, coarse touch, and nociception.

Brain

The brain is a complex structure and plays a role in regulating most body functions (Figure 3-4). A good neurological clinician is able to recognize the patient's deficits and adapt their approach to and treatment with the patient based on anticipated and observed deficits. See the "Predictable Dysfunction" Clinical Application boxes in this section.

Brainstem

1. Midbrain.
   a. Connects pons to diencephalon.
   b. Contains ascending and descending tracts.
   c. Contains oculomotor and trochlear cranial nerve nuclei.
   d. Contains relay stations for visual and auditory reflexes.
   e. Substantia nigra.
      - Large motor nucleus connecting with the basal ganglia and cortex.
      - Important in motor control and muscle tone.
      - Substantia nigra and subthalamic nuclei function closely with basal ganglia and are often considered part of the basal ganglia.
2. Pons.
   a. Connects the medulla oblongata to the midbrain.
   b. Allows passage of ascending and descending tracts.
   c. Contains nuclei for trigeminal, abducens, facial and vestibulocochlear cranial nerves, and nuclei for regulation of respiration.
3. Medulla oblongata.
   a. Connects spinal cord with the pons.
   b. Contains all ascending and descending tracks.
   c. Contains glossopharyngeal, vagus, spinal accessory, and hypoglossal cranial nerve nuclei.
   d. Contains important centers for vital sign functioning: cardiac, respiratory, vasomotor centers, and reticular formation (maintenance of consciousness and arousal).

Diencephalon

1. Thalamus.
   a. Group of nuclei deep within the cerebrum.
   b. Receives all sensory stimuli except olfactory.
   c. Interprets crude sensory information.
2. Hypothalamus.
   a. Primary role is homeostasis.
   b. Regulates body temperature, sugar and fat metabolism, and water balance.
   c. Primitive drives for eating, sexual behavior, rage, aggression, emotion, thirst, hunger, and sleep/wake cycles.

Cerebrum

1. Constitutes the bulk of the brain and contains gray and white matter.
2. Convolutions of gray matter:
   a. Composed of unmyelinated axons with gyri and sulci.
   b. Separates lobes.
      - Lateral central fissure: separates temporal lobe from frontal and parietal lobes.
      - Longitudinal cerebral fissure: separates the two hemispheres.
      - Central sulcus: separates frontal lobe from the parietal lobe.
3. White matter: myelinated axons.
   a. Fibers connect the hemispheres and regions of the brain, allow for communication between the structures.
4. Deeper structures.
   a. Basal ganglia: caudate, putamen, and globus pallidus.
   b. Portions of limbic system.
      - Housed within cerebrum and diencephalon.
      - Associated with feeding, aggression, emotions, and endocrine aspects of sexual response.
5. Lobes (Table 3-1).
   a. Primary cortices: receive incoming messages.
   b. Association areas: link various parts of the cortex and integrate and interpret information.

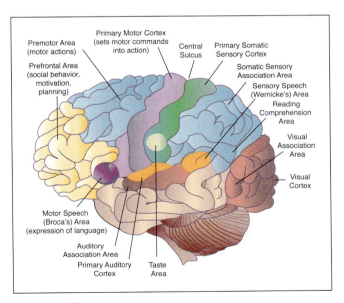

Figure 3-4 Functional areas of the brain.

Clinical Application: Predictable Dysfunction Patterns of the Brain Based on Area of Damage

Although no two insults are identical, each area of the brain has a specific function. Therefore, a patient with damage to a given area will likely follow predicted patterns of dysfunction and ensuing functional return based on the damaged area.

Frontal lobe
- Contralateral weakness
- Personality changes/antisocial behavior
- Ataxia
- Broca's aphasia
- Delayed or poor initiation

Parietal lobe
- Constructional apraxia and anosognosia (non-dominant)
- Wernicke's aphasia
- Homonymous visual deficits
- Impaired language comprehension

Occipital lobe
- Variety of visual deficit, including homonymous hemianopsia, visual agnosia, and cortical blindness
- Impaired extra-ocular muscle movement

Temporal lobe
- Hearing impairments (dominant)
- Memory and learning deficits
- Wernicke's aphasia
- Antisocial behaviors

Cerebellum
- Ataxia
- Lack of trunk and extremity coordination
- Intention tremors
- Balance deficits
- Dysdiadochokinesia
- Dysmetria

Basal ganglia
- Bradykinesia and akinesia
- Resting tremors
- Rigidity
- Athetosis
- Chorea

Thalamus
- Thalamic pain syndrome
- Altered relay of sensory information

Hypothalamus
- Altered basic life functions (body temp, thirst, hunger, sleep/wake cycles)
- Poor autonomic nervous system functioning
- Altered functioning of anterior pituitary gland (ADH secretion and reproduction)

Brainstem
- Altered consciousness
- Contralateral hemiparesis or hemiplegia
- Cranial nerve palsy
- Altered respiratory patterns
- Attention deficits

Anatomy and Physiology of the Neuromuscular System 89

Clinical Application: Predictable Presentation Related to Hemisphere Dominance

Although no two insults are identical, each hemisphere of the brain has a specific combination of functions. Therefore, a patient with damage to a given hemisphere will likely follow predicted patterns of overall presentation and dysfunction. Upon chart review a physical therapist assistant (PTA) can make certain predictions about how the patient may present to them upon ensuing treatment.

Left Hemisphere Injury	Right Hemisphere Injury
Right-sided sensory and motor deficits	Left-sided sensory and motor deficits
Difficulty understanding and producing language, both written and spoken	Unable to understand nonverbal communication
Difficulty sequencing movements	Difficulty sustaining movements
Poor logical and rational thought	Poor hand-eye coordination and kinesthetic awareness
Slow, cautious, anxious	Quick and impulsive
Self-deprecating	Overestimation of abilities

Table 3-1

Lobes of Cerebrum

LOBE	PRIMARY FUNCTIONS
Frontal	• Primary motor cortex (precentral gyrus): responsible for voluntary movements on contralateral side of the body • Broca's area: motor components of speech • Cognition, judgment, attention, abstract thinking, and emotional control
Parietal	• Primary sensory cortex (postcentral gyrus): integrates sensation from contralateral side of body • Short-term memory • Perception of touch, proprioception, pain, and temperature sensations
Temporal	• Primary auditory cortex: receives auditory information • Associative auditory cortex: processing of auditory information • Wernicke's area: comprehension of spoken word • Long-term memory • Visual perception • Primary visual cortex: receives visual information
Occipital	• Visual association cortex: processes visual information and applies meaning

Cerebellum
1. Located behind the pons and medulla in the posterior fossa.
2. Functions.
   a. Equilibrium.
   b. Regulation of muscle tone.
   c. Maintenance of posture and voluntary movement control.
   d. Coordinates smooth voluntary movements.
   e. Motor learning.
   f. Sequencing of movements.

Cranial Nerves
1. Cranial nerves identifies the 12 cranial nerves, names, and function (Table 3-2).

Blood Supply
1. Anterior system.
   a. Supplies the frontal, parietal, and parts of temporal lobe.
   b. Aortic arch: common carotid artery bifurcates to form internal and external carotid arteries; internal carotid enters cranium, bifurcates to form anterior and middle cerebral arteries.
2. Posterior system.
   a. Supplies brainstem, cerebellum, medial temporal lobe, and occipital lobes.
   b. Subclavian artery: vertebral arteries unite to form basilar artery, bifurcates to form posterior cerebral arteries.
3. Circle of Willis: anterior and posterior systems connect at the base of the brain to ensure adequate circulation to the brain.

Support Structures
1. Skull: rigid, bony chamber with an opening (foramen magnum) at its base.
2. Meninges: three membranes surrounding the brain.
   a. Dura mater: dense and fibrous outermost layer.
   b. Arachnoid layer: delicate, vascular middle layer.
   c. Pia mater: thin, vascular inner membrane covering the brain surface.
3. Cerebrospinal fluid.
   a. Protects the brain and aids in the exchange of nutrients and waste products.
   b. Produced in the choroid plexuses in the ventricles.
   c. Circulates within the subarachnoid space, ventricles, and central canal of the spinal cord.
4. Blood-brain barrier: protective structure that selects what can and cannot enter the CNS.

Table 3-2

Cranial Nerves

NUMBER	NAME	SENSORY/MOTOR	FUNCTION
I	Olfactory	Sensory	Smell
II	Optic	Sensory	Visual acuity
III	Oculomotor	Motor	Turns eye up, down, and in
IV	Trochlear	Motor	Turns adducted eye down
V	Trigeminal	Sensory	Facial sensation
		Motor	Muscles of mastication (temporalis and masseter)
VI	Abducens	Motor	Turns eye out
VII	Facial	Sensory	Taste on anterior two/thirds of tongue
		Motor	Facial expressions
VIII	Vestibulocochlear	Sensory	Vestibular: vestibular ocular reflex (VOR); balance
			Cochlear: hearing acuity
IX	Glossopharyngeal	Sensory	Taste on posterior one-third of tongue
		Motor	Gag reflex; pharynx control: soft palate rising with "ah" sound
X	Vagus	Sensory	Autonomic nervous system functions
		Motor	Gag reflex; pharynx control: soft palate rising with "ah" sound
XI	Spinal Accessory	Motor	Trapezius muscle: elevation of shoulders. Sternocleidomastoid muscle: turning head to side
XII	Hypoglossal	Motor	Tongue movements

Clinical Application: Function of Key Structures in the Brain

- Medulla oblongata: contains centers for vital sign functioning of the cardiac, respiratory, and vasomotor centers. It is responsible for the maintenance of consciousness and arousal.
- Hypothalamus: critical for maintaining homeostasis. Controls primitive drives including those related to rage, aggression, emotion, thirst and hunger, as well as the sleep/wake cycle. Damage can also cause problems with temperature, water, and behavioral regulation.
- Basal ganglia: regulates posture and muscle tone.
- Cerebellum regulates maintenance of posture and voluntary movement control.
- Brainstem: contains cranial nerve nuclei; damage can lead to a variety of cranial nerve dysfunctions.

Spinal Cord

Purpose and Structure
1. Purpose is to convey information to/from the brain and periphery.
2. Protection and coverings:
   a. Vertebral canal: bony structure formed by the vertebral foramina that houses the spinal cord and cauda equina.
   b. Meninges: continuous with the meninges of the brain.

Spinal Cord Cross-Section
1. Gray matter and white matter (Figure 3-5).
2. Divided into regions:
   a. Anterior/ventral regions carry motor information.
   b. Posterior/dorsal regions carry sensory information.

Spinal Nerves
1. Divided into 30 segments:
   a. Eight cervical, 12 thoracic, 5 lumbar, 5 sacral, and a few coccygeal segments.
   b. Cauda equina: nerves arising from the distal tip of the spinal cord.
   c. Dermatome distribution (Figure 3-6).
2. Dorsal and ventral roots branch off spinal cord and combine to form spinal nerve.
   a. Dorsal roots carry sensory information.
   b. Ventral roots carry motor information.

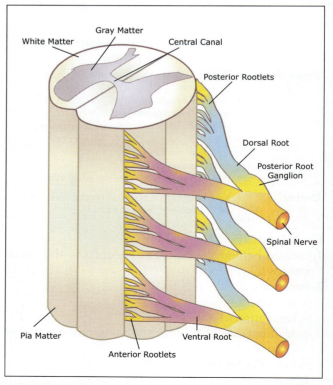

Figure 3-5 Spinal Cord: anterior cross section.

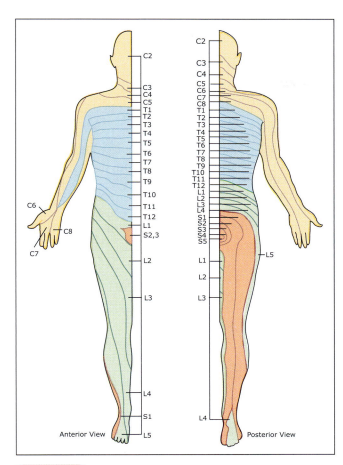

Figure 3-6 Dermatome distribution.

3. Spinal nerve splits into dorsal (posterior) and ventral (anterior) rami.
   a. Dorsal rami innervate the deep muscles and skin of the back.
   b. Ventral rami innervate the superficial back, lateral and anterior trunk and extremity muscles.
4. Plexuses.
   a. Network of adjoining nerves formed by ventral rami in the cervical and lumbosacral region.
   b. Brachial plexus (C5–T1) innervates the upper extremity and some cervical muscles.
   c. Lumbosacral plexus (T12–S2) innervates the lower extremity muscles.

Spinal Reflexes
1. Involuntary responses to stimuli.
2. Monosynaptic or stretch reflex.
   a. Stimulus: muscle stretch.
   b. Reflex arc: afferent Ia from muscle spindle to alpha motoneuron and back to muscle of origin.
   c. Aids with maintenance of muscle tone.
      - Autogenic facilitation: contraction of the agonist.
      - Reciprocal inhibition: inhibition of antagonist muscle.
3. Polysynaptic or inverse stretch reflex.
   a. Stimulus: muscle contraction.
   b. Reflex arc: afferent Ib from Golgi's tendon organ via inhibitory interneuron to muscle of origin.
   c. Functions for agonist inhibition and stretch-protection reflex.

Physical Therapy Examination and Data Collection

Physical Therapist Assistant's Role and Responsibilities

Data Collection
1. Demonstrate competence in performing specific data collection techniques as delegated by the supervising PT.

Prior to Treatments
1. Perform a thorough review of the patient's medical record.
2. Failure to review the medical chart for daily updates to identify subtle changes in the patient's status can lead to potential treatment when it is contraindicated.

Progress Interventions
1. Use information from data collection process to progress patient interventions within the plan of care established by the PT.

Monitor Changes
1. Differentiate appropriate and adverse changes that need to be reported to the physical therapist and other members of the health care team.

Patient History and Medical Record Review

Responsibilities
1. The physical therapist is responsible to perform the initial evaluation and develop the physical therapy plan of care.
2. The physical therapist assistant is responsible for reviewing and using the plan of care as well as medical documentation to implement the plan of care as directed by the physical therapist.

Review

1. Present symptoms.
2. Past medical history.
3. Psychosocial history.
   a. Current living situation.
   b. Family/social support.
4. The PT will review any diagnostic procedures ordered by the physician and review the results. Examples of potential diagnostic procedures follow
   a. Cerebral angiography: shows areas of increased and decreased vascularity.
   b. Computed tomography (CT): shows presence of abnormal changes in tissue density.
   c. Magnetic resonance imaging (MRI): identifies tumors, demyelination, and vascular abnormalities.
   d. Electroencephalography (EEG): records ongoing electrical activity of the brain, commonly used when assessing seizures.

Resting Posture

1. Performed at initial evaluation by PT, ongoing by PT and PTA to determine progress.
2. Observe in all functional positions.
3. Observe for typical patterns of spasticity following CNS insult (Table 3-3).

Level of Consciousness

1. Performed at initial evaluation by PT, ongoing by PT and PTA to determine progress
2. Orientation to person, place, and time (oriented × 3)
3. Response to stimuli
   a. Purposeful, nonpurposeful, no response.
   b. Verbal, tactile, painful stimuli, simple commands.

Table 3-3

Typical Patterns of Spasticity in Upper Motor Neuron Syndrome

UPPER LIMBS	ACTIONS	MUSCLES AFFECTED
Scapula	Retraction, downward rotation	Rhomboids
Shoulder	Adduction and internal rotation, depression	Pectoralis major, latissimus dorsi, teres major, subscapularis
Elbow	Flexion	Biceps, brachialis, brachioradialis
Forearm	Pronation	Pronator teres, pronator quadratus
Wrist	Flexion, adduction	F. carpi radialis
Hand	Finger flexion, clenched fist Thumb adducted in palm	F. dig. profundus/sublimis, add. pollicis brevis, F. pollicis brevis

LOWER LIMBS	ACTIONS	MUSCLES AFFECTED
Pelvis	Retraction (hip hiking)	Quadratus lumborum
Hip	Adduction (scissoring) Internal rotation Extension	Add. longus/brevis Add. magnus, gracilis Gluteus maximus
Knee	Extension	Quadriceps
Foot & ankle	Plantar flexion Inversion Equinovarus Toes claw (MP ext., PIP flex, DIP ext.) Toes curl (PIP, DIP flex)	Gastrocsoleus Tibialis posterior Long toe flexors Ext. hallucis longus Peroneus longus
Hip & knee (prolonged sitting posture)	Flexion Sacral sitting	Iliopsoas Rectus femoris, pectineus Hamstrings
Trunk	Lateral flexion with concavity rotation	Rotators Internal/external obliques
COG forward (prolonged sitting posture)	Excessive forward flexion Forward head	Rectus abdominis, external obliques Psoas minor

The form and intensity of spasticity may vary greatly, depending upon the CNS lesion site and extent of damage. The degree of spasticity can fluctuate within each individual (i.e., due to body position, level of excitation, sensory stimulation, and voluntary effort). Spasticity predominates in antigravity muscles (i.e., the flexors of the upper extremity and the extensors of the lower extremity). If left untreated, spasticity can result in movement deficiencies, subsequent contractures, degenerative joint changes, and deformity.

Adapted from Mayer NH, Esquenazi A, Childers MK. *Common patterns of clinical motor dysfunction.* Muscle and Nerve 6:S21, 1997.

Table 3-4

Glasgow Coma Scale

	MOTOR		VERBAL		EYE OPENING
6	Follows motor commands				
5	Localizes pain	5	Oriented		
4	Withdraws to pain	4	Confused conversation	4	Spontaneous
3	Decorticate posturing	3	Inappropriate words used	3	To verbal command
2	Decerebrate posturing	2	Incomprehensible sounds	2	To pain
1	No response	1	No response	1	No response

4. Level of arousal
   a. Alert: responds fully and appropriately to stimuli and examiner.
   b. Lethargic: appears drowsy; can respond to questions but falls asleep easily.
   c. Obtunded: responds slowly and is confused; decreased interest in environment.
   d. Stupor: only aroused from sleep with painful stimuli; minimal awareness of self and environment.
   e. Coma: cannot be aroused and no response to external stimuli or environment.

Glasgow Coma Scale
1. Consciousness is related to degree of eye opening, motor response, and verbal response (Table 3-4).
2. Score ranges from 3 to 15.
   a. Mild brain injury = score of 13 to 15.
   b. Moderate brain injury = score of 9 to 12.
   c. Severe brain injury (coma) = score ≤8.
   d. The typical scoring mechanism for verbal responses is modified for children ≤5 years of age.

Arousal, Mentation, and Cognition

Gather Information
1. Information used by PTA to correctly modify educational approach used during intervention

Attention
1. Length of attention span.
2. Sustained attention: ability to attend to task without redirection.
3. Divided attention: ability to shift attention from one task to another.
4. Focused attention: ability to stay on task in the presence of detractors.
5. Ability to follow single and multistep commands.

Memory
1. Immediate recall: recall of items after a brief interval (5 minutes).
2. Short-term recall: recall of recent events. (What did you have for breakfast?)
3. Long-term recall: remote recall of past events. (Where were you born?)

Emotional Responses/Behaviors
1. Safety, judgment: impulsivity, and lack of inhibition.
2. Affect, mood: irritability, agitation, depression, and withdrawal.
3. Egocentricity.
4. Insight into disability.
5. Ability to follow rules of social conduct.

> **RED FLAG:** A patient with impulsivity, lack of behavioral inhibition, and/or poor insight into his/her disability can be a safety concern to those around him/her as well as him/herself.

Higher-Level Cognitive Abilities
1. Judgment, problem solving.
2. Abstract reasoning.
3. Ability to learn new information and generalize learning to new situations.
4. Ability to order components of cognitive or functional task.

Mini-Mental Status Examination (MMSE)
1. Brief screening test for cognitive dysfunction.
2. Maximum score of 30.
   a. Mild cognitive impairment: 21–24.
   b. Moderate cognitive impairment: 16–20.
   c. Severe mental impairment: ≤15.

Aerobic Capacity and Endurance

Assessment Completed
1. Completed by PT and PTA prior to, during, and immediately following intervention.
2. Vital signs at rest, during, and after activity: heart rate, respiratory rate, blood pressure.

> **RED FLAG:** Failure to assess vital signs for an accurate baseline can lead to an emergency situation with patients demonstrating unstable cardiopulmonary functioning.

Autonomic Nervous System Responses Indicating Stress
1. Wide pupillary reactions.
2. Hyper alertness.
3. Increases in heart rate, pulse rate, and/or respiratory rate.
4. Nausea.
5. Diaphoresis.
6. Perceived exertion, dyspnea or angina. See Chapter 4 Cardiac, Vascular and Lymphatic Physical Therapy for measurement scales.

Observe for Signs of Postural Hypotension/Orthostatic Hypotension
1. Blood pressure drops with change from supine to sitting position.
2. Decrease of systolic blood pressure >20 mm Hg or diastolic blood pressure >10 mm Hg.
3. Lightheadedness, syncope, mental confusion, weakness.

> **RED FLAG:** Orthostatic hypotension must be identified immediately and the patient carefully monitored as he/she is at an increased risk of syncope and falls.

Sensory Testing

Assessment Completed
1. Sensory testing performed at initial evaluation by PT and on an ongoing basis by the PT and PTA to determine progress.
   a. Table 3-5 reviews sensory testing commonly performed.
   b. Table 3-6 reviews neural screens commonly performed.

Table 3-5

Sensory Testing

Exteroceptive (superficial) sensations

TEST	TEST	NORMAL RESPONSE
Sharp/dull discrimination	• Alternate between sharp and dull points applied on the tested location	• Identify touch as either sharp or dull
Temperature	• Patient is given test tubes with either hot or cold water.	• Correctly identify the test tube as having hot or cold water
Light touch	• Lightly touch the patient in the tested location with a cotton ball.	• Verbalize when the touch is felt

Proprioceptive (deep) sensations

TEST	TEST	NORMAL RESPONSE
Kinesthesia	• Therapist moves the patient's limb in various directions.	• Identifies the direction of motion (up/down, bent/straight, etc)
Proprioception	• Therapist places the joint/limb in a position.	• Able to mimic or verbalize the position of the joint
Vibration	• A tuning fork is applied to a bony prominence, vibrating or not.	• Identifies whether the tuning fork is vibrating or not

Combined (cortical) sensations

TEST	TEST	NORMAL RESPONSE
Stereognosis	• Object is placed in the patient's hand.	• Able to identify the object by touch only
Two-point discrimination	• Using calipers, test whether patient feels one or two points.	• Given normal ranges, accurately identifies 1 or 2 points
Texture recognition	• Patient is given objects with similar shape/size but of different textures.	• Able to identify the various textures (soft, hard, rough, etc)
Tactile localization	• Touch the patient in the tested location with a cotton ball or finger.	• Identifies when and where the touch occurs
Graphesthesia	• Draw a letter in palm of patient's hand.	• Able to identify the letter
Barognosis	• Place similar objects with varying weights in the patient's hand.	• Able to identify differences in weight

Table 3-6

Common Cranial Nerve Screens Performed by the PTA

NUMBER	NAME	SENSORY/MOTOR FUNCTION	SCREEN POTENTIAL ABNORMAL FINDINGS	POTENTIAL ASSOCIATED PATHOLOGIES
III IV VI	Oculomotor Trochlear Abducens	Motor Motor function: eye movements—smooth pursuits, saccades, convergence/divergence CN III: turns eye up, down, in, elevates eyelid CN IV: turns abducted eye down CN VI: turns eye out	Screen: observe position of eye; test pursuit eye movements Findings: impaired eye movements, eye deviation from normal position, ptosis (drooping) eyelid, pupillary dilation	Cerebrovascular accident Myasthenia gravis
V	Trigeminal	Both Motor function: temporal and masseter muscles Sensory function: face, cornea	Screen: • test pain: light touch sensations forehead, cheeks, jaw (eyes closed) • test corneal reflex: touch lightly with wisp of cotton • palpate muscles: have patient clench teeth, hold against resistance Findings: loss of facial sensation, numbness, loss of corneal reflex ipsilaterally; weakness, wasting of muscles of mastication	Trigeminal neuralgia Multiple sclerosis
VII	Facial	Both Motor function: facial expression Sensory function: taste	Screen: test motor function—raise eyebrows, frown, show teeth, smile, close eyes, puff out cheeks Findings: paralysis, ipsilateral facial muscles, inability to close eye, droop in corner of mouth, difficulty with speech articulation	Bell's palsy CNS facial paralysis stroke
VIII	Vestibulocochlear	Sensory Sensory function: vestibular ocular reflex (VOR), cochlear function	Screen vestibular function: test balance, eye-head coordination (VOR gaze stability) Screen cochlear function: test auditory acuity, use tuning fork top of head, on mastoid bone Findings vestibular: vertigo, disequilibrium, nystagmus (constant, involuntary cyclical movement of eyeball) Findings cochlear: deafness, impaired hearing, tinnitus (sensation of roaring or ringing in ears)	Balance deficits
X	Vagus	Both Sensory function: relays information about state of organs in body to brain (hunger, heartbeat, swallow) Motor function: throat, thorax and abdominal muscles	Screen: examine for difficulty swallowing, observe motion of soft palate (elevation, remains midline) and when patient says "ah" Findings: paralysis—palate fails to elevate, asymmetrical elevation, unilateral paralysis	Brainstem or hypothalamus dysfunction
XI	Spinal Accessory	Motor Motor function: trapezius, sternocleidomastoid muscle function	Screen: examine bulk of muscle, examine strength of muscle—shoulder shrug against resistance, turn head to each side against resistance Findings: atrophy, fasciculation, weakness (PNI); inability to shrug ipsilateral; (ell) shoulder; shoulder droops Inability to turn head to opposite side	Spinal cord injury Guillain-Barré syndrome

Testing Considerations
1. Ensure patient comprehends instructions and can communicate responses.
2. Occlude vision.
3. Apply stimulus in random, unpredictable order to avoid summation.
4. Always pose a choice. (Hot or cold?)
5. Check for objective manifestations: withdrawal, blinking, or wincing.
6. Document location of deficits by utilizing dermatome chart.

Exteroceptive (Superficial) Sensations
1. Sharp/dull discrimination.
2. Temperature.
3. Light touch.

Proprioceptive (Deep) Sensations
1. Movement sense (kinesthesia).
2. Joint position sense.
3. Vibration sense.

Combined (Cortical) Sensations
1. Stereognosis: ability to distinguish identity of small objects placed in the hand.
2. Two-point discrimination: ability to discern that two different points (typically sharp) that are touching the skin are distinctly two points and not one.
3. Texture recognition: ability to discern different textures touching the skin, e.g., cotton, burlap, sand paper.
4. Tactile localization: ability to identify exact point on the body where a tactile stimulus is applied—without looking.
5. Graphesthesia: while vision is occluded, the ability to recognize a number or letter drawn on the skin—typically hand.
6. Barognosis: the ability to assess the weight of, or differentiate objects of different weight placed in hands or by lifting them.

Perceptual Dysfunction

Use as Guide
1. Knowledge of perceptual dysfunction is used by the PT and PTA to correctly modify educational approach used during intervention.
2. The clinician should suspect perceptual dysfunction if patient has difficulty with functional mobility skills or activities of daily living for reasons that cannot be accounted for by specific sensory, motor, or comprehension deficits.
3. Language impairments, hearing loss, or visual disturbance can be masked as perceptual dysfunction.

Homonymous Hemianopsia
1. Loss of contralateral half of the visual field in each eye.
2. Results from a lesion in the optic tract.

> **RED FLAG:** The presence of homonymous hemianopsia is a safety concern for ambulatory patients because they are unable to fully visualize the environment and avoid potential dangers.

Body Scheme/Body Image Disorders
1. Body scheme disorder (somatognosia): inability to identify body parts or their relationship to each other.
2. Visual spatial neglect (unilateral neglect): ignores one side of the body and stimuli coming from that side.
3. Right/left discrimination disorder: unable to identify right and left sides of the body.
4. Anosognosia: severe denial, neglect, or lack of awareness of dysfunction.

> **RED FLAG:** Anosognosia presents a safety risk for the patient and those around him/her as he/she may not recognize the dangers and engage in activities unsafe for his/her functioning level.

Spatial Relations Disorders
1. Figure-ground discrimination disorder: inability to pick out an object from the background on which it rests.
2. Form constancy disorder: inability to pick out an object from an array of similarly shaped objects.
3. Spatial relations deficit: inability to properly place objects in relationship to one another.
4. Position in space deficit: inability to determine up/down, in/out, under/over.
5. Topographical disorientation: inability to navigate a familiar route on own.
6. Depth/distance perception disorder: unable to accurately judge depth or distance.
7. Vertical disorientation: unable to accurately determine what is upright.

> **RED FLAG:** The presence of spatial relations disorders makes independent ambulation a safety concern without extensive practice and development of compensatory strategies.

Agnosia
1. Inability to recognize familiar objects with one sensory modality.
2. Retains the ability to recognize the same object with other sensory modalities.

Apraxia
1. Inability to perform purposeful movements when there is no loss of sensation, strength, coordination, or comprehension.

2. Breakdown in ability to conceptualize and/or perform motor components of a task.
3. Ideomotor apraxia: cannot perform the task on command but can do the task when left on own.
4. Ideational apraxia: cannot perform the task at all either on command or on own.

Motor Function

Assessment
1. Performed at initial evaluation by PT, ongoing by PT and PTA to determine progress

Muscle Tone
1. Normal tone is necessary for skilled, coordinated, selective movement.
2. Types of tone abnormalities commonly found are identified in Table 3-7.
3. Quantification of tone.
   a. Modified Ashworth's scale for spasticity can be used to grade spasticity (Table 3-8).
      - No change in resistance with normal tone.
      - Faster movements will increase resistance if spasticity is present.
   b. Assess reflex integrity.
      - Deep tendon reflexes (DTRs).
      - Superficial cutaneous.
4. Signs of hypertonia.
   a. Increased resistance to passive range of motion.
      - Limb feels stiff, resistive to movement.
      - Increases further with increased velocity of quick stretch.
   b. Clonus.
      - Maintained stretch stimulus or quick stimulus produces a cyclical, spasmodic contraction.
      - Common in plantarflexors, wrist flexors, and jaw.
   c. Hyperactive reflexes.
5. Signs of hypotonia.
   a. Decreased or no resistance to passive range of motion.
   b. Hypoactive reflexes.
6. Influences on tone.
   a. Increased patient effort.
   b. Stress and anxiety.
   c. Position of patient and influence of tonic reflexes.
   d. Fever/infection increases tone.

Reflex Integrity
1. PT most likely to assess, PTA may or may not perform; however, should understand impact on intervention.
2. Deep tendon reflexes (DTR) (Table 3-9).
   a. Also called stretch reflex or monosynaptic stretch reflex.

Table 3-7

Muscle Tone Abnormalities

	HYPERTONIA
Spasticity	• Always an upper motor neuron (UMN) lesion
Decorticate rigidity	• Always an UMN lesion • Sustained flexor posturing in the upper extremities • Sustained extensor posturing in the lower extremities • Diencephalon lesion • Sign of severe impairment
Decerebrate rigidity	• Always an UMN lesion • Sustained extensor posturing in the upper and lower extremities • Brainstem lesion • Sign of severe impairment
Rigidity	• Always an UMN lesion • Resistance to passive stretch in agonist and antagonist • Basal ganglia lesion
Cogwheel rigidity	• Ratchet-like response to quick passive movement; catches/releases/catches
Leadpipe rigidity	• Constant rigidity
	HYPOTONIA
Flaccidity	• LMN lesion • Cerebellar lesion • Following spinal or cerebral shock—resolves or changes to spasticity

Table 3-8

Modified Ashworth Scale

GRADE	DESCRIPTION
0	• No increased tone
1 or 1+	• Slight increase in tone
2	• Moderate increase in tone
3	• PROM is difficult
4	• Affected joints are non-moveable (ankylosed)

Table 3-9

Deep Tendon Reflexes Commonly Tested

SITE	NERVE ROOT LEVEL
Biceps	C5-C6
Triceps	C7-C8
Brachioradialis	C5-C6
Hamstrings	L5-S3
Quadriceps	L2-L4
Achilles	S1-S2

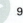

Table 3-10

Grading Scale for Muscle Stretch Reflexes

GRADE	DESCRIPTION
0	Absent
1+	Hyporeflexia
2+	Normal
3+	Hyperreflexia
4+ and 5+	Increasingly abnormal hyperreflexia

   b. Testing.
   - Position muscle in mid-range.
   - Tap tendon with reflex hammer or tips of fingers.
   - Jendrassik's maneuver: patient hooks fingers together and isometrically attempts to pull them apart to increase sensitivity of DTR in lower extremities.

   c. Grading (Table 3-10).
3. Babinski.
   a. Superficial cutaneous reflex.
   b. Test: quick stroke to lateral border of the sole of the foot.
   c. Normal response: flexion of 1st toe.
   d. Abnormal response: extension of 1st toe.

RED FLAG: Presence of a Babinski's reflex after 2 years of age is a sign of upper motor neuron dysfunction.

4. Developmental reflexes and reactions: refer to Chapter 9, Pediatric Physical Therapy.

RED FLAG: Persistent, absent, or asymmetric reflexes usually indicate early brain damage and affect normal development and rehabilitation at any age (refer to Table 9-1, Normal Responses and Reflexes).

Muscle Performance

1. Strength, power and endurance.
2. Upper motor neuron lesion (Table 3-11).
   a. Results from damage to the brain or spinal cord.
   b. Weakness.
   - May be present but masked by hypertonicity.
   - May be due to opposition from a spastic antagonist.
   - Resulting from disuse atrophy.
3. Lower motor neuron lesion (Table 3-11).
   a. Weakness and decreased muscle tone will be present in the involved muscles.
   b. May develop disuse atrophy in the involved and uninvolved muscles.

Table 3-11

Differential Diagnosis: Comparison of Upper Motor Neuron (UMN) and Lower Motor Neuron (LMN) Syndromes

	UMN LESION	LMN LESION
Location of lesion	Central nervous system	Peripheral nervous system
Structures involved	Cortex, brainstem, corticospinal tracts, spinal cord	SC: anterior horn cell, spinal roots, peripheral nerves CN: cranial nerves
Disorders	Stroke, traumatic brain injury, spinal cord injury	Polio, Guillain-Barré, PNI, peripheral neuropathy, radiculopathy
Tone	Increased: hypertonia Velocity-dependent	Decreased or absent: hypotonia, flaccidity Not velocity dependent
Reflexes	Increased: hyperreflexia, clonus Exaggerated cutaneous and autonomic reflexes: + Babinski response	Decreased or absent: hyporeflexia Cutaneous reflexes decreased or absent
Involuntary movements	Muscle spasms: flexor or extensor	With denervation: fasciculations
Strength	Stroke: weakness or paralysis on one side of the body Corticospinal lesions: contralateral if above decussation in medulla, ipsilateral if below Spinal cord lesions: bilateral loss below level of lesion	Limited distribution: segmental or focal pattern Root-innervated pattern
Muscle bulk	Variable, disuse atrophy	Neurogenic atrophy; rapid, focal, severe wasting
Voluntary movements	Impaired or absent: dyssynergic patterns, obligatory synergies	Weak or absent if nerve interrupted

Key: CN = cranial nerve; PNI = peripheral nerve injury; SC = spinal cord

Table 3-12

Abnormal Synergies

Synergy Patterns

	FLEXION SYNERGY	EXTENSION SYNERGY
Upper Extremity		
Scapula	Retraction & elevation	Protraction (pec minor)
Shoulder	Abduction & ER	Adduction & IR (subscapularis)
Elbow	Flexion	Extension
Forearm	Supination	Pronation
Wrist & finger	Flexion	Flexion
Lower Extremity		
Hip	Flexion, abduction, & ER	Extension and adduction
Knee	Flexion	Extension
Ankle	DF & inversion	PF & inversion
Toe	DF	PF

4. Testing protocols.
   a. Manual muscle testing.
      - Utilize traditional manual muscle testing when possible.
      - Make notations regarding alterations in test position/patient response.
   b. Handheld dynamometry.
   c. Isokinetic dynamometry.
   d. Timed tests for power and endurance.

Voluntary Movement Patterns

1. Coordinated movement requirements: control of speed, distance, direction, rhythm, varying levels of muscle tension, and trunk/proximal joint stability.
2. Common considerations associated with coordination impairments.
   a. Abnormal synergy patterns (Table 3-12).
   b. Associated reactions.
      - Ramiste's phenomenon: resisted hip abduction/adduction of uninvolved extremity causes the same reaction in the involved extremity.
      - Homolateral limb synkinesis: flexing involved UE causes flexion of involved LE.
   c. Substitution patterns due to pain or muscle weakness.
   d. Assess for signs of cerebellar dysfunction (Table 3-13).
   e. Assess for signs of basal ganglia dysfunction (Table 3-14).

RED FLAG: Presence of basal ganglia or cerebellar lesions can lead to decreased patient safety with balance activities and ambulation.

Table 3-13

Cerebellar Dysfunction Signs and Tests

TERM	DESCRIPTION	COMMON TEST
Ataxia	• General term used to describe uncoordinated movement, includes dysmetria, intention tremor	
Dysmetria	• Inability to accurately judge the distance to reach a goal or target • Hypermetria or hypometria	• Pointing, past pointing • Heel on shin
Hypotonia	• Low tone	• Passive movement • Deep tendon reflex testing
Dysdiadochokinesia	• Difficulty performing rapid alternating movements (RAM)	• Pronation/supination • Finger to nose • Knee flexion/extension
Movement decomposition	• Movements are performed in distinct segments instead of fluid motions	• AROM
Intention tremor	• Involuntary, oscillatory movement • Appears with voluntary movement, decreases/absent at rest	• Observation with movement
Postural tremor	• Appears while attempting to hold limb still or while holding trunk still during sitting or standing	• Observation with movement
Dysarthria	• Slurring of speech due to impaired motor control of speech structure	• Examined by the speech therapist

Table 3-14

Basal Ganglia Dysfunction Signs

TERM	DESCRIPTION	COMMON TEST
Bradykinesia	• Poverty of movement	• Observation of functional tasks
Akinesia	• Without movement • Unable to initiate movement	• Observation of attempts at functional tasks
Rigidity	• Cogwheel • Leadpipe • Present at rest	• Passive movement
Resting tremor	• Disappears with voluntary movement	• Observation at rest
Chorea	• Involuntary, relatively quick twitches or "dancing" movements	• Observation at rest
Athetosis	• Involuntary, slow irregular, twisting, sinuous movements • Occur more in upper extremities	• Observation at rest

3. Specific testing guidelines.
   a. Describe head, trunk and limb movement.
   b. Movement control.
      - Are movements precise?
      - Can the patient make continuous and appropriate motor adjustments if speed and direction of movement are changed?
      - Does occluding vision alter performance?
   c. Speed/rate control: does increasing the speed of performance affect quality of motor performance?
   d. Steadiness: can a position be maintained without swaying, tremors, or extra movements?
   e. Fatigue: does the patient fatigue rapidly, and does the quality of movement change with onset of fatigue?
   f. Reaction time: does movement occur in a reasonable amount of time?

> **RED FLAG:** Decreased reaction time should be identified and compensatory strategies outlined to prevent potential safety concerns.

4. Specific tests.
   a. Active ROM testing for examining abnormal synergy patterns.
   b. Nonequilibrium tests of coordination (Table 3-15).
   c. Equilibrium tests of coordination (Table 3-16).
   d. Scoring.
      - 0 (unable).
      - 1 (severe impairment).
      - 2 (moderate impairment).
      - 3 (minimal impairment).
      - 4 (normal performance).

Gait and Locomotion

Assessment of
1. Gait and locomotion assessment is initially performed by the PT. It is then completed on an ongoing basis by the PT and PTA to determine progress. See Quick Facts 3-1.
2. Observation for normal/abnormal patterns, timing, speed of ambulation, and wheelchair mobility.
   a. Indoor/outdoor surfaces.
   b. Level/uneven terrain.
   c. During functional activities such as opening/closing doors and on/off elevators.

> **RED FLAG:** Failure to assess and practice ambulation on a variety of surfaces and in all of the environments the patient will encounter does not adequately prepare the patient for safe ambulation upon discharge.

Balance

Assessment of
1. Balance assessment is initially performed by the PT. It is then completed on an ongoing basis by the PT and PTA to determine progress.
2. Performed at initial evaluation by PT, ongoing by PT and PTA to determine progress.

QUICK FACTS 3-1 ▶ GAIT DEVIATIONS – FOLLOWING CNS INSULT

Cerebellar Impairment	Basal Ganglia Impairment
• Wide base of support. • Arms at high guard (raised and away from body). • Slow initiation of swing with forceful termination.	• Narrow base of support, decreased step length, shuffling gait. • Decreased arm swing and trunk rotation. • Festination: increased velocity propulsion. • Akinesia or dyskinesia: difficulty starting and stopping gait.

Table 3-15

Nonequilibrium Coordination Tests

1.	Finger to nose	The shoulder is abducted to 90 degrees with the elbow extended. The patient is asked to bring the tip of the index finger to the tip of the nose. Alterations may be made in the initial starting position to assess performance from different planes of motion.
2.	Finger to assistant's finger	The patient and PTA sit opposite each other. The PTA's index finger is held in front of the patient. The patient is asked to touch the tip of their index finger to the PTA's index finger. The position of the PTA's finger may be altered during testing to assess ability to change distance, direction and force of movement.
3.	Finger to finger	Both shoulders are abducted to 90 degrees with the elbows extended. The patient is asked to bring both hands toward the midline and approximate the index fingers from opposing hands.
4.	Alternate nose to finger	The patient alternately touches the tip of the nose and the tip of the PTA's finger with the index finger. The position of the PTA's finger may be altered during testing to assess ability to change distance, direction and force of movement.
5.	Finger opposition	The patient touches the tip of the thumb to the tip of each finger in sequence.
6.	Mass grasp	An alternation is made between opening and closing fist (from finger flexion to full extension). Speed may be gradually increased.
7.	Pronation/ supination	With elbows flexed to 90 degrees and held close to body, the patient alternately turns the palms up and down. This test also may be performed with shoulders flexed to 90 degrees and elbows extended. The ability to reverse movements between opposing muscle groups can be assessed at many joints. Examples include active alternation between flexion and extension of the knee, ankle, elbow, fingers, and so forth.
8.	Rebound test	The patient is positioned with the elbow flexed. The examiner applies sufficient manual resistance to produce an isometric contraction of the biceps. Resistance is suddenly released. Normally, the opposing muscle group (triceps) will contract and "check" movement of the limb. Many other muscle groups can be tested for this phenomenon, such as the shoulder adductors or flexors and the elbow extensors.
9.	Tapping (hand)	With the elbow flexed and the forearm pronated, the patient is asked to "tap" his or her hand on the knee.
10.	Tapping (foot)	The patient is asked to "tap" the ball of one foot on the floor without raising the knee; heel maintains contact with floor.
11.	Pointing and past pointing	The patient and PTA are opposite each other, either sitting or standing. Both patient and PTA bring shoulders to a horizontal position of 90 degrees of flexion with elbows extended. Index fingers are touching or the patient's finger may rest lightly on the PTA's. The patient is asked to fully flex the shoulder (fingers will be pointing toward ceiling) and then return to the horizontal position such that index fingers will again approximate. Both arms should be tested, either separately or simultaneously. A normal response consists of an accurate return to the starting position. An abnormal response there is typically a "past pointing," or movement beyond the target. Several variations to this test include movements in other directions such as toward 90 degrees of shoulder abduction or toward 90 degrees of shoulder flexion (finger will point toward floor). Following each movement, the patient is asked to return to the initial horizontal starting position.
12.	Alternate heel to knee; heel to toe	From a supine position, the patient is asked to touch the knee and big toe alternately with the heel of the opposite extremity.
13.	Toe to examiner's finger	From a supine position, the patient is instructed to touch the great toe to the examiner's finger. The position of finger may be altered during testing to assess ability to change distance, direction, and force of movement.
14.	Heel on shin	From a supine position, the heel of one foot is slid up and down the shin of the opposite lower extremity.
15.	Drawing a circle	The patient draws an imaginary circle in the air with either upper or lower extremity (a table or the floor also may be used). This also may be done using a figure-eight pattern. This test may be performed in the supine position for lower extremity assessment.
16.	Fixation or position holding	Upper extremity: The patient holds arms horizontally in front (sitting or standing). Lower extremity: The patient is asked to hold the knee in an extended position (sitting).

Tests should be performed first with eyes open and then with eyes closed. Abnormal responses include a gradual deviation from the "holding" position and/or a diminished quality of response with vision occluded. Unless otherwise indicated, tests are performed with the patient in a sitting position. Vary speed from slow to fast, observe control.

From O'Sullivan S, Schmidtz T, Fulk G: Physical Rehabilitation, 6th ed, F. A. Davis, 2014, pg 218–219, with permission.

Balance Control

1. The control of relative position of body parts by skeletal muscles with respect to gravity and each other.
   a. Center of mass (COM): in anatomical position, it is located just anterior to S2.
   b. Base of support (BOS): body surface area in contact with the environmental surface.
   c. Limits of stability (LOS): perimeter of the base of support.

Systems Contributing to Balance

1. Visual system: visual acuity, depth perception, and visual field deficits.

Table 3-16

Equilibrium Coordination Tests and Interventions to Improve

POSTURE	TESTING POSITION	INTERVENTION TO IMPROVE
Standing, static	Maintain comfortable posture. Narrow base of support (feet close, then touching). Tandem stance (one foot directly in front of the other with distance in between, progress to toe-heel touching). Single limb stance.	Introduce arm movements bilaterally and symmetrical, progress to unilaterally and asymmetrical. Eyes open (EO) to eyes closed (EC) Romberg sign: ability to maintain an upright posture without visual input is referred to as a positive Romberg sign. Sharpened Romberg: standing in tandem with EO, progress to EC.
Standing, dynamic	Displace balance unexpectedly (clinician closely guarding patient). Actively flex/extend trunk, laterally flex to one side then the other. March in place.	Begin with smaller displacement and movements and progress to greater displacement and trunk movements through greater range of motion. Foot-placing activities; from stance, place foot on marked spots on floor; increase distance for greater COG displacement.
Walking	Walking. Walk following straight line drawn/taped to the floor. Tandem walking. Walk sideways, backward, or cross-stepping. Walk on heels or toes.	Alter speed of walking: faster-to-slower-to-faster, add starts and stops during walking. Walk placing feet on floor markers placed on floor, causing patient to step outside COG. Walk including horizontal and vertical head turns. Walk changing direction: pivot 90/180/360 degrees, in a circle-alternate direction.
Stepping	Step over or around obstacles. Stairclimbing beginning with handrails, one step at a time.	Progress to greater height or distances. Progress: without handrails, step-over-step.
Agility activities	Jumping jacks. Alternate UE or LE activities sitting on a balance ball.	Hopping forward-back, side-to-side. Sitting on balance ball: asymmetrical UE or LE activities, cross pattern (right UE and left LE, same side UE and LE, etc.).

Documentation should include: time, quality, distance, ability/inability to move outside center of gravity (COG), functional impact on ADLs/IADLs.

---

2. Somatosensory: proprioception and cutaneous sensation (touch, pressure) of lower extremities and trunk, especially feet and ankles.
3. Vestibular: motor responses to positional and movement changes.
4. Musculoskeletal: strength and range of motion of lower extremities and trunk. Since vision is a major component of balance, training of other systems must be incorporated in rehabilitation to assist patients with adapting to the visual changes that typically occur with age or are present with a number of neurological dysfunctions.

Assessing Balance and LOS

1. Observe maximum sway in any direction.
2. Check static balance.
   a. Sitting tests: holding a steady position, with and without upper extremity support.
   b. Standing tests: double limb and single limb support.
   c. Romberg's test.
      - Stand with feet together.
      - First with eyes open, then with eyes closed for 30 seconds each.
   d. Sharpened or tandem Romberg.
      - Stand in tandem heel to toe position.
      - First with eyes open, then with eyes closed for 30 seconds each.

> **RED FLAG:** Many clinicians fail to examine and rehabilitate static balance, tending more toward the dynamic balance tasks associated with ambulation. Both are equally important and, given the importance of static balance in daily function as well as a preparatory activity for dynamic balance, assessment of one should not be neglected.

3. Dynamic/functional balance.
   a. Standing up, walking, turning, and stopping.
   b. With ambulation, navigate an obstacle course or complete multiple tasks simultaneously (i.e., walking while talking).
   c. BOS challenges: sitting or standing on a moveable surface (Dynadisk, balance board, dense foam).

Testing

1. Functional balance tests (Table 3-17).
2. Functional balance grades (Table 3-18).

Table 3-17

Functional Balance Tests

TEST	DESCRIPTION	REFERENCE VALUES	BEST USED FOR
Performance-Oriented Mobility Assessment (POMA, Tinetti)	Examines balance (balance subset, nine items including sitting, sit-to-stand, standing, standing feet together, turn 360 degrees, sternal nudge, stand on one leg, tandem stand, reaching up, bending over, stand-to-sit, timed rising) and walking (gait subset, eight items including gait initiation, path, turning timed walk, step over obstacles)	Maximum score is 28; patients who score <19 are at high risk for falls; patients who score 19–24 are at moderate risk for falls.	Balance and mobility in the elderly population, residential care; demonstrates 68% sensitivity and 78% specificity
Berg Balance Scale	Examines functional balance (14 items) including sitting unsupported, sit-to-stand, stand-to-sit, transfers; in standing; EO to EC, feet together, forward reach, pick object off floor, head turns, turning 360 degrees, stepping up, tandem stand, stand on one leg	Maximum score is 56, patients who score <45 are at high risk for falls; scores 54–46, a 1-point drop is associated with a 6%–8% increase in fall risk	A change of 8 points reveals genuine change in function among residential adults dependent in ADLs; may not be a predictive of function in community-dwelling adults—lacks sufficient dynamic measures. Is a valid measure of standing balance in post-stroke individuals. High validity and inter/intrarater reliability
Timed Up and Go (TUG)	Examines functional balance during rise from a chair, walk 3 m, turn, and return to chair (recommend with arm rest and 44–47 cm seat height). Performance on the Get Up and Go (GUG) is not timed.	Normal intact adults can perform the test in <10 seconds; 11–20 sec is considered normal for frail elderly or disabled patients; patients who take >20 sec are at increased risk for falls; patients who take >30 sec are at high risk for falls.	The test demonstrates good or better intra/interrater reliability, test-retest reliability. Good test for community dwelling individuals—there is some question regarding usefulness of data when assessing ADL dependent frail elderly individuals, and those with cognitive impairment
Functional Reach (FR) Modified Functional Reach Test (MFRT)	MFRT—modified to allow the individual being tested to sit (has been studied post-stroke and spinal cord injuries)	Forward reach norms: above average >12.2 in., below average <5.6 in.; forward reach <10 is considered indicative of increased fall risk.	Functional reach has been shown to be both reliable and valid to measure limits of stability in 4 directions.
Multidirectional Reach Test (MDRT)	Examines maximal distance a person can reach forward, backward, and laterally to right and left	Forward: see above. Backward: above average >7.6 in., below average <1.6 in. Lateral: above average >9.4 in., below average <3.6 in.	
Short Physical Performance Battery (SPPB)	Test to measure lower extremity function in 3 functional areas: repeated sit-stands from a chair, static balance, semi-tandem, and side-by-side stands, and gait speed—a timed 8-ft (2.44 m) walk	Tests are scored in terms of time to complete: 5 sit-to-stands, 10 sec in each of the standing conditions and an 8-ft walk. An original score is given for each section. Summary and ordinal score: 0 (worst performance) to 12 (best performance)	Is reliable in testing function in community-dwelling older adults and highly predictive of identifying those at greater risk for incidence of disability. May not be as sensitive in higher functioning individuals
Dynamic Gait Index (DGI)	Examines an individual's ability to modify balance responses during gait when there are external demands present. The test assesses (8 items) including changes in gait speed, head turns, pivot turns, obstacles, and stairs.	Ratings based on ordinal scale of 0–3 where 0 = severely impaired and 3 = normal. Normal intact adults receive a score of 21 +/−4; score of 19 or < is indicative of increased fall risk.	Most sensitive in community dwelling older adults and those with vestibular dysfunction. Good test-retest and inter/intrarater reliability, valid and predictive of risk
Balance Efficacy Scale (BES)	Examines level of self-confidence when performing functional tasks encountered in daily life; 8 questions are scored 0%–100% confidence; activities include getting out of chair, walking up/down a flight of 10 stairs, getting out of bed, getting into and out of shower, removing items from cupboard, walking on uneven ground, and standing on one leg	Total score is divided by 18 to yield mean BES score; scores <50 indicate low confidence.	

Table 3-18

Functional Balance Grades

GRADE	STATIC BALANCE	DYNAMIC BALANCE
Normal	Maintains balance without hand-hold support	Accepts maximal challenge and easily weight shifts in all directions throughout the full range
Good	Maintains balance without hand-hold support, demonstrating limited postural sway	Accepts moderate challenge (pick up item off floor without losing balance)
Fair	Maintains balance with hand-hold support, may require occasional minimal assistance	Accepts minimal challenge (maintain balance while turning head or body)
Poor	Requires hand-hold support and mod/max assistance to maintain position	Unable to accept challenge or move without loss of balance
0 Absent	Unable to maintain balance	

From: O'Sullivan S, Schmitz T, Fulk G: Physical Rehabilitation, 6th ed. Philadelphia, F.A. Davis, 2014, pg 233, with permission.

Environment and Equipment Considerations

Environmental, Home, and Work (Job/School/Play) Barriers

1. Administer a structured questionnaire to identify barriers.
2. Ask routine interview questions to determine barriers.
3. Identify common and frequently occurring barriers in home and work environments.
   a. Curbs, steps with and without railings, uneven terrain, busy streets.
   b. Inaccessible travel routes to and within environments.
   c. Throw rugs, dense carpeting.
   d. Accessibility of safety call buttons or switches.
   e. Work station, computer monitor height.

RED FLAG: Barriers present in the patient's environment must be identified to provide a comprehensive rehabilitation program ensuring safety for the patient.

Assistive and Adaptive Devices

1. Assess patient's and caregiver's safe use of the device via subjective reports regarding care, function, and benefit of device.
2. Assess alignment and fit of the device.
3. Assess proper working order of wheelchairs and ambulatory assistive devices.
   Assistive and adaptive devices are useful only if they are fit to the patient and in proper working order.

Orthotic, Protective, and Supportive Devices

1. Assess skin changes after use of an orthosis for changes signifying normal or abnormal pressure points.
2. Ability of patient and/or family member to don/doff and care for an orthosis.
3. Subjective reports from patient and caregiver regarding care, function, and benefit of orthosis.
4. Normal characteristics of function with use of orthosis.
5. Changes in function with use of orthosis.

Self-Care and Home-Management (Including Activities of Daily Living [ADL])

1. Administer standard questionnaire regarding patient's abilities with ADL.
2. Observe and report patient's use of basic adaptive skills in ADL.
3. Functional rating scales.
   a. The Functional Independence Measure (FIM). See Quick Facts 3-2.
      - Measures patient ability in six areas: self-care, sphincter control, transfers, locomotion, communication, and social cognition.
   b. Katz's index of ADL: assesses degree of assistance needed in bathing, dressing, toileting, transferring, continence, and feeding.
   c. Outcome and assessment information set (OASIS): assesses ADL/IADL such as grooming, dressing, transferring, laundry, and shopping.

QUICK FACTS 3-2 ▶ FIM SCALE

7–complete independence without assistive device.
6–complete independence with assistive device.
5–supervision or assistance with setup required.
4–minimum assistance required.
3–moderate assistance required.
2–maximum assistance required.
1–total assistance required.

Community and Work (Job/School/Play) Integration/Reintegration

1. Administer standard questionnaire to identify abilities.
2. Observe and report patient performance on IADL.

> ### Clinical Application: Functional Considerations for Intervention
>
> - Any home exercise program utilized will likely be dependent on the mentation of a patient, thereby necessitating a thorough assessment of the individual's initial and continuing status of mental functioning.
> - Feedback is used throughout therapeutic intervention. Decreased sensory functioning will limit the type of feedback that can be used. For example, an individual who is severely hard of hearing should not be given feedback solely in the form of verbal instruction but via visual and tactile cueing as well.
> - Perceptual disorders can be severely limiting to a patient's rehabilitation potential and return to function.
> - Synergies can be used to allow independent movement that otherwise would not be possible.
> - Many neurological dysfunctions lead to decreased ambulation ability and safety concerns. Gait deviations must be identified early and remediated or compensated for prior to allowing the patient being recommended for discharge.

Intervention Strategies for Patients with Neurological Dysfunction

Physical Therapist Assistant's Role and Responsibilities

Implementing Treatment

1. Understand the plan of care for the patient directed to him/her.
2. Define the indications, contraindications, and precautions of interventions delegated by the PT.
3. Use information from the data collection process to monitor patient status and progress patient toward short- and long-term goals.
4. Adjust or withhold intervention based on patient status as determined through observation and data collection.

> **RED FLAG:** The PTA must know the contraindications and precautions for each patient he/she is working with to know when it is safe to continue therapy within the plan of care and when to refer back to the physical therapist.

5. Ways to participate in patient status judgments.
   a. Report changes to supervising PT.
   b. Request reexamination or revision of plan of care.
6. Use data collection to participate in determining a patient's progress.
7. Educate the patient and significant others.
8. Participate in the discharge planning process.

General Intervention Considerations

1. Monitor heart rate and blood pressure for any patient with cardiac complications.
2. Modify the intensity of the intervention if indicated by the cardiac response.
3. Use commands and instructions consistent with the cognitive and communication abilities of the patient.
4. Demonstrating the task.
   a. From start to finish, at the appropriate speed, while identifying key components for successful task completion.
5. Examine influences of tone, the amount of resistance of muscles to passive elongation.
   a. If patient has high tone that increases during exercise, decrease the intensity of intervention, utilize inhibition techniques, and/or increase the external support.
   b. If the patient has low tone, monitor for stability to prevent unwanted stress on the joints and utilize facilitation techniques.

> **RED FLAG:** Avoid traction injuries to flaccid shoulder during upright activities; lack of adequate support (e.g., shoulder sling, manual support) can cause development of painful shoulder. Avoid use of overhead pulleys in patients with poor shoulder alignment and poor shoulder function; can cause development of a painful shoulder.

Table 3-19

Exercise/Activity Difficulty		
To decrease	Widen/broaden the base of support	• Work in supine instead of sitting • Work in bilateral stance instead of unilateral stance
	Decrease the number of segments involved	• Work in prone on elbows instead of sitting and weightbearing on an extended upper extremity • Work in tall kneeling instead of standing
	Decrease the range of movement	• Roll between ½ turn from prone and ½ turn from supine • Reach in a narrow, unilateral range in sitting instead of full range, cross midline
	Increase the stability of the support surface	• Work on sitting on a mat table instead of an exercise ball • Work on ambulation over level, tile surface instead of gravel
	Decrease stage of motor control	• Use rhythmic initiation in sidelying instead of weight shifting in sitting • Work on stepping forward and back with unaffected extremity instead of walking
To increase	Narrow the base of support	• Work in standing instead of sitting • Work in heel to toe stance instead of bilateral stance
	Increase the number of segments involved	• Work in quadruped instead of sitting • Work in standing instead of sitting
	Increase the range of movement	• Roll from supine to prone and reverse • Reach across midline in sitting
	Decrease the stability of the support surface	• Work on sitting on an exercise ball instead of on a chair • Work on ambulation over foam mats instead of level tile

> **RED FLAG:** Emphasize compensation strategies for patients with sensory and perceptual losses to prevent additional injury and functional losses.

6. When ready, the clinician should advance the difficulty of exercise/activity (Table 3-19).

Intervention Approaches

Neurodevelopmental Treatment (NDT)

1. Developed by Karel Bobath, MD, and Berta Bobath, PT. To help differentiate DNT and PNF, see Quick Facts 3-3.
2. Basic concepts.
   a. Normal movement sequences and balance reactions are the focus of therapy so an accurate analysis of the patient's movement patterns is essential.
   b. Motor learning of patterns of movement can be facilitated by repetition and experience in the environment.
   c. Abnormal tone, primitive reflex patterns, and mass synergies result in abnormal patterns of posture and movement and interfere with normal recovery and function.
   d. Inhibition of unwanted activity precedes practice of normal motor patterns.
3. Techniques.
   a. Active movements are guided or assisted.
   b. Low effort maximizes performance in the presence of tonal disorders, while high effort, maximal resistance, results in unwanted activity and is avoided.
   c. Avoid any substitution movements.
   d. Minimize verbal instructions or feedback during movement.
   e. Ensure movement success and avoid repeated failures.
   f. Normalize postural tone.
   g. Abnormal patterns of movements and reflexes are inhibited or prevented.
   h. Normalize sensory/perceptual experiences.
   i. Emphasize normal functional activities that are meaningful and goal oriented, utilizing both affected and intact body segments.

Proprioceptive Neuromuscular Facilitation (PNF)

1. Developed by Herman Kabat, MD, and Margaret Knott, PT, and later modified by Dorothy Voss, PT.

> **QUICK FACTS 3-3 ▶ NDT TO PNF COMPARISON**
>
> | NDT | PNF |
> |---|---|
> | • Focus on normal movement sequences and balance reactions.
• Movement patterns facilitated by repetition, experience in environment.
• Inhibit unwanted, abnormal tone, prior to practice of normal motor patterns. | • Focus on motor learning in synergistic muscle patterns.
• Movement patterns are spiral and diagonal.
• Incorporate proprioceptive elements, strong and weak muscles alike, into total movement patterns. |

2. Basic concepts.
   a. Facilitation of total patterns of movement focuses on motor learning in synergistic muscle patterns.
   b. Normal movements are spiral and diagonal in character.
   c. Proprioceptive elements (e.g., maximal resistance and stretch) and irradiation from strong muscles can be used to strengthen weak muscles in a pattern.
   d. Total patterns of movement and posture are important preparatory patterns for advanced functional skills (e.g., gait).
3. Techniques for facilitation (Table 3-20).
4. Diagonal patterns of movement (Table 3-21).
   a. Named for motions occurring at the proximal joint (shoulder or hip).
   b. Intermediate joint (elbow or knee) may be flexing or extending.
5. As the patient begins to regain isolated voluntary movements, begin to incorporate those and decrease the use of synergistic patterns to allow continued progression of patient movement patterns.

Movement Therapy in Hemiplegia

1. Developed by Signe Brunnstrom, PT.
   a. Some aspects of this approach are not consistent with current practice.
   b. Classification of the stages of recovery based on Brunnstrom's work is helpful to understanding recovery and outcome.
2. Basic concepts.
   a. Sensorimotor recovery occurs in a sequential pattern that can vary between and within limbs while peaking at any stage.
   b. Patients with very little recovery must first gain control of basic limb synergies.
   c. Once initial control is achieved, out-of-synergy combinations are promoted.
3. Techniques.
   a. Facilitation of volitional control movement.

Table 3-20

PNF Techniques for Facilitation

NEW TERMINOLOGY (OLD TERMINOLOGY)	DESCRIPTION	INDICATIONS
Combination of isotonics (agonist reversals)	• Combination of concentric, isometric, and eccentric contractions of one muscle	• Weak postural muscles • Poor eccentric control of body weight with movement transitions • Decreased AROM • Poor muscular control
Stabilizing reversals (alternating isometrics)	• In an alternating pattern, agonist and antagonist muscle contract isometrically.	• Decreased stability • Poor antigravity control • Weakness
Contract-relax	• Isotonic movement in rotation followed by an isometric contraction of antagonist at point of limitation with voluntary relaxation and push into new range	• Limited ROM resulting from muscle tightness or spasticity
Hold-relax	• Isometric contraction of antagonist followed by relaxation and PROM into new range	• Limited ROM resulting from muscle tightness, spasm, or pain
Rhythmic initiation	• Voluntary relaxation followed by passive movement through an increasing ROM then active assisted, active, and finally resisted movements	• Inability to initiate movement • Poorly coordinated movements • Hypertonicity • Motor learning deficits • Communication disorders
Rhythmic rotation	• Voluntary relaxation combined with slow, passive, rhythmic rotations	• Hypertonia • Limited ROM or function
Rhythmic stabilization	• Simultaneous isometric contraction (cocontraction) [cocontraction as elsewhere] of agonist and antagonist muscles	• Decreased stability in weightbearing • Poor antigravity control • Limited ROM caused by muscle tightness
Dynamic reversals (slow reversals)	• Slow isotonic contractions of agonist and then antagonist	• Decreased AROM • Weak antagonistic muscles • Poor reciprocal control • Muscular hypertonicity
Repeated stretch (repeated contractions)	• Repeated isotonic contractions induced by quick stretch and enhanced with resistance at point of weakness in range	• Weakness • Fatigue • Decreased ability to perform fucntional movement

Table 3-21

PNF Diagonal Patterns

Upper extremity

PATTERN	SHOULDER MOTIONS	VERBAL CUE
D1F	• Flexion-adduction-external rotation	• "Close your hand, turn, and pull your arm up across your face."
D1E	• Extension-abduction-internal rotation	• "Open your hand, turn, and push your arm down and out."
D2F	• Flexion-abduction-external rotation	• "Open your hand, turn, and lift your arm up and out."
D2E	• Extension-adduction-internal rotation	• "Close your hand, turn, and pull your arm down and across your body."

Lower extremity

PATTERN	HIP MOTIONS	VERBAL CUE
D1F	• Flexion-adduction-external rotation	• "Bring your foot up, turn, and pull your leg up and across your body."
D1E	• Extension-abduction-internal rotation	• "Push your foot down, turn, and push your leg down and out."
D2F	• Flexion-abduction-internal rotation	• "Lift your foot up, turn, and lift your leg up and out."
D2E	• Extension-adduction-external rotation	• "Push your foot down, turn, and pull your leg down and in."

- Reflexes: some aspects of concept regarded as inappropriate.
- Proprioceptive inputs: resistance, weight-bearing, stretching, and tapping.
- Exteroceptive inputs: rubbing, stroking.
- Eye contact and appropriate verbal commands.
- Use of unaffected side to facilitate affected side via transfer effects.
- Progress control from small range to large range and isometric to isotonic contractions.
- Fatigue, pain, and heavy resistance are avoided, as these decrease control.
- Positive reinforcement and repetition are keys to successful motor learning.

b. Patterns of movement.
- Training activities focus on the out-of-synergy combinations needed for everyday function. The patient must be able to produce out-of-synergy movements to utilize the movement therapy in hemiplegia approach.

Sensory Stimulation Techniques

1. Combines several of the treatment approaches and is based on the work of Rood.
2. Basic concepts.
    a. Indications.
        - Patients who demonstrate absent or disordered motor control and would benefit from the use of augmented feedback.
        - Most useful in the early stages of motor learning with limited movement potential.
    b. Contraindications.
        - Patients who will not benefit from a hands-on approach.
        - Patients with sufficient motor control to perform and refine a motor skill based on intrinsic feedback mechanisms. Extrinsic feedback should not be utilized with patients who have or can learn the ability to use intrinsic feedback so as not to facilitate dependence on the clinician.
    c. Response to stimulation is dependent upon multiple factors including level of intactness of CNS, initial level of arousal, and type and amount of stimulation.
    d. Early use of sensory stimulation techniques should be phased out as soon as possible in favor of active control by the learner.
    e. Multiple techniques or repeated application of the same technique may be necessary to produce the desired response in patients functioning at low levels.
3. Techniques (Table 3-22).

Compensatory Training Approach

1. General concepts.
    a. Indicated to offset or adapt to residual impairments and disabilities.
    b. Focus is on early resumption of functional independence with reliance on uninvolved segments for function.
    c. Changes are made in the patient's overall approach to tasks.
    d. Patient is made aware of movement deficiencies and alternate ways to accomplish tasks, including substitution. Compensatory strategies should not be taught until it becomes obvious the patient will not be able to rehabilitate a given skill. If used too early, compensatory mechanisms will become

Table 3-22

Proprioceptive Techniques

INHIBITORY TECHNIQUES	RESPONSE
Prolonged, slowly applied stretch	Inhibits agonist muscle, decreases tone
Inhibitory pressure (firm pressure on long tendons)	Inhibits muscle, decreases tone
FACILITATION TECHNIQUES	**RESPONSE**
Quick stretch, tapping of muscle belly or tendon	Facilitates agonist muscle, inhibits antagonist
Resistance	Recruits motor units; facilitates, strengthens agonist contraction
Joint approximation	Enhances joint awareness, facilitates co-contraction, action of postural extensors, stabilizing muscles
Joint traction	Enhances joint awareness, action of flexors; relieves muscle spasm

EXTEROCEPTIVE STIMULATION TECHNIQUES

INHIBITORY TECHNIQUES	RESPONSE
Maintained touch (maintained pressure)	Produces calming effect, generalized inhibition
Slow stroking (continuous, slow stroking to spinal posterior primary rami)	Produces calming effect, generalized inhibition
Prolonged icing	Produces inhibition of muscle tone, spasm and pain
Neutral warmth	Produces generalized inhibition of tone, relaxation, calming effect, decreased pain
FACILITATION TECHNIQUES	**RESPONSE**
Light touch, quick icing facilitation	Initiates phasic, withdrawal reactions

VESTIBULAR STIMULATION TECHNIQUES

INHIBITORY TECHNIQUES	RESPONSE
Slow, maintained vestibular stimulation (slow, repetitive rocking)	Produces generalized inhibition of tone, relaxation, calming effect
Inverted positioning (head down position)	Elicits generalized activation of postural extensors, calming effect, decreased HR and BP
FACILITATION TECHNIQUES	**RESPONSE**
Fast, irregular vestibular stimulation (spinning, fast rolling)	Produces generalized facilitation of tone, improved motor coordination, improved retinal image stability

habit, and this can slow or even prevent development of the desired skill.
2. Concerns with the compensation approach.
   a. Focus on using uninvolved segments to accomplish daily tasks may suppress recovery and contribute to learned nonuse of the impaired segments.
   b. Focus on task-specific learning may lead to the development of splinter skills that cannot be easily generalized to other tasks or environmental situations.
3. May be the only approach possible if severe motor deficits are present or no additional recovery is anticipated.
4. Strategies.
   a. Simplify activities and adapt environment to facilitate relearning of skills and enhance performance.
   b. Energy conservation and activity pacing are important to ensure completion of all daily movement requirements.
   c. Establish a new functional pattern focusing on key task elements.
   d. Repeated practice working toward consistency and efficiency.
   e. Use orthoses to support/control afflicted segments.

Motor Control/Motor Learning

Motor Control
1. Motor program.
   a. A set of prestructured muscle commands that, when initiated, result in the production of a coordinated movement sequence.
   b. A learned task that can be carried out largely uninfluenced by peripheral feedback.
2. Motor plan.
   a. An overall strategy for movement.

b. An action sequence requiring the coordination of a number of motor programs.
3. Stages of motor control.
   a. Mobility.
      - Movements in dependent postures that are poorly controlled.
      - Distal mobility.
   b. Stability.
      - The ability to maintain an antigravity posture in a weight-bearing position.
      - Proximal stability.
   c. Controlled mobility.
      - The ability to move within or between postures.
      - Distal stability with proximal mobility.
   d. Skill.
      - Highly coordinated movements.
      - Proximal stability with distal mobility.
4. Feedback.
   a. Afferent information sent by various sensory receptors to control centers.
   b. Feedback updates control centers about the correctness of movement while it progresses to shape ongoing movement.
   c. Feedback allows motor responses to be adapted to the demands of the environment.
5. Feedforward.
   a. Readies the system in advance of movement.
      - Anticipatory responses that adjust the system for incoming sensory feedback or for future movements.
6. Motor skill acquisition.
   a. Behavior is organized to achieve a goal-directed task.
   b. Active problem solving/processing is required for the development of a motor program, motor plan, or to motor learn.
   c. Adaptive to specific environmental demands.
      - Closed environment: static and controlled by the clinician.
      - Open environment: variable and changing with distracters presented.
   d. CNS recovery/reorganization is dependent upon experience.

Motor Learning

1. General concepts.
   a. A change in the capability of a person to perform a skill.
   b. Result of practice or experience.
2. Stages of motor learning (Table 3-23).
3. Measures of motor learning.
   a. Performance: level of automaticity, effort and speed of decision making.
   b. Retention: ability to demonstrate the skill after a period of no practice.
   c. Generalizability: capability to apply what has been learned to similar tasks.
   d. Resistance to contextual change: capability to apply what has been learned to other environmental contexts.
4. Feedback.
   a. Intrinsic feedback: sensory information normally acquired during performance of a task.
   b. Augmented feedback: externally presented feedback, such as verbal cueing, that is added during normally acquired task performance.
      - Knowledge of results (KR): augmented feedback about the outcome of a movement.
      - Knowledge of performance (KP): augmented feedback about the nature of the movement produced.
   c. Feedback schedules.
      - Terminal: given after task completion to facilitate long-term retention.
      - Summed: given after a set of trials is completed.
      - Fading: given frequently at first and then progressively decreased.
      - Bandwidth: given only if performance falls outside a designated margin of error.
5. Practice.
   a. Blocked practice: practice of a single motor skill repeatedly (111, 222, 333).
   b. Serial practice: practice of a group or class of motor skills in serial or predictable order (123, 123, 123).
   c. Random practice: practice of a group or class of motor skills in random order (213, 123, 312, 123).
   d. Variable practice: practice with a variety of circumstances in order to increase generalizability and long-term retention.
   e. Massed practice: relatively continuous practice with a small amount of rest time.
   f. Distributed practice: rest time is greater than practice time.
   g. Mental practice: cognitive rehearsal of a skill without physical performance.
6. Transfer.
   a. The effects, either positive or negative, of having previous practice of a skill or skills upon the learning of a new skill or upon performance in a new context.
   b. Part-whole transfer: complex motor task is broken into its component parts for separate practice before practice of the integrated whole.
   c. Bilateral transfer: improvement in movement skill performance with one limb results from practice with the opposite limb.
7. Strategies for effective learning (Quick Facts 3-4).
   a. Frequency: feedback given after every trial improves performance, while variable feedback improves learning and retention.

Table 3-23

Stages of Motor Learning and Training Strategies

COGNITIVE STAGE CHARACTERISTICS	TRAINING STRATEGIES

The learner
• develops an understanding of task, *cognitive mapping*
• assesses abilities, task demands
• identifies stimuli, contacts memory
• selects response, performs initial approximations of task
• structures motor program
• modifies initial responses
***"What to do"* decision**
	Clinician Instruction
	• Highlight purpose of task in functionally relevant terms. Demonstrate ideal performance of task to establish a *reference of correctness*
	• Have patient verbalize task components and requirements. Point out similarities to other learned tasks
	• Direct attention to critical task elements
	
	Select appropriate feedback
	• Emphasize intact sensory systems, intrinsic feedback systems
	• Carefully pair extrinsic feedback with intrinsic feedback
	• High dependence on vision: have patient watch movement
	• Provide **Knowledge of Performance (KP):** focus on errors as they become consistent; do not cue on large number of random errors
	• Provide **Knowledge of Results (KR):** focus on success of movement outcome
	  Ask learner to evaluate performance, outcomes; identify problems, solutions
	  Use reinforcements (praise) for correct performance and continuing motivation
	
	Organize feedback schedule
	• *Feedback* after every trial improves performance during early learning
	• *Variable feedback* (summed, fading, bandwidth designs) increases depth of cognitive processing, improves retention; may decrease performance initially
	
	Organize initial practice
	• Stress controlled movement to minimize errors
	• Provide adequate rest periods using *distributed practice* if task is complex, long, or energy costly or if learner fatigues easily, has short attention, or has poor concentration
	• Use manual guidance to assist as appropriate
	• Break complex tasks down into component parts, teach both parts and integrated whole
	• Use *bilateral transfer* as appropriate
	• Use *blocked (repeated) practice* of same task to improve performance
	• Use *variable practice* (serial or random practice order) of related skills to increase depth of cognitive processing and retention; may decrease performance initially
	• Use *mental practice* to improve performance and learning, reduce anxiety
	
	Assess, modify arousal levels as appropriate
	• High or low arousal impairs performance and learning
	• Avoid stressors, mental fatigue
	
	Structure environment
	• Reduce extraneous environmental stimuli, distractors to ensure attention, concentration
	• Emphasize closed skills initially gradually progressing to open skills

ASSOCIATED STAGE CHARACTERISTICS	**TRAINING STRATEGIES**
The learner practices movements, refines motor program, spatial and temporal organization; decreases errors, extraneous movements Dependence on visual feedback decreases, increases for use of proprioceptive feedback; cognitive monitoring decreases ***"How to do"* decision**	**Select appropriate feedback** • Continue to provide KP; intervene when errors become consistent • Emphasize proprioceptive feedback, "feel of movement" to assist in establishing an internal reference of correctness • Continue to provide KR; stress relevance of functional outcomes • Assist learner to improve self-evaluation, decision-making skills • Facilitation techniques, guided movements are counterproductive during this stage of learning **Organize feedback schedule** • Continue to provide feedback for continuing motivation; encourage patient to self-assess achievements • Avoid excessive augmented feedback • Focus on use of variable feedback (summed, fading, bandwidth) designs to improve retention **Organize practice** • Encourage consistency of performance • Focus on variable practice order (serial or random) of related skills to improve retention **Structure environment** • Progress toward open, changing environment • Prepare the learner for home, community, work environments

(Continued)

Table 3-23

Stages of Motor Learning and Training Strategies (Continued)

AUTONOMOUS STAGE CHARACTERISTICS	TRAINING STRATEGIES
The learner practices movements; continues to refine motor responses, spatial and temporal highly organized; movements are largely error-free; minimal level of cognitive monitoring *"How to succeed"* decision	Assess need for conscious attention, automaticity of movements **Select appropriate feedback** • Learner demonstrates appropriate self-evaluation, decision-making skills • Provide occasional feedback (KP, KR) when errors evident **Organize practice** • Stress consistency of performance in variable environments, variations of tasks (open skills) • High levels of practice (massed practice) are appropriate **Structure environment** • Vary environments to challenge learner • Ready the learner for home, community, and work environments Focus on competitive aspects of skills as appropriate; e.g., wheelchair sports

From: O'Sullivan S, Schmitz T. *Physical Rehabilitation*. 5th ed, Philadelphia, FA Davis, 2007, with permission.

QUICK FACTS 3-4 ▶ LEARNING STRATEGIES EARLY-TO-PROGRESSION

Feedback	Early Feedback	Progression
Frequency	Given every trial	Varied trials, improves learning and retention
Type of Feedback	Visual Positive and supportive	Proprioceptive Positive and supportive
Augmented Feedback	Identify success or failure, identify correct aspects of performance	Identify errors if consistent, facilitate active introspection
Environment	Closed: protected, minimal distractions	Open: more distractions, move toward typical

---

b. Type of feedback: early training should focus on visual feedback, while later training should focus on proprioceptive feedback.

c. Environment: reduce extraneous environmental stimuli (closed environment) early in learning, while later learning focuses on adaptation to environmental demands (open environment).

d. Supportive feedback can be used to shape behavior, motivate patient.

e. Assist learner in recognizing/pairing intrinsic feedback with movement responses.

f. Provide appropriate augmented feedback.
   - Knowledge of results: simply identifies success or failure of the end product.
   - Knowledge of performance early in learning provides feedback on correct aspects of performance.
   - Knowledge of performance later in learning provides feedback on errors as they become consistent.
   - Feedback dependence can be avoided by reducing augmented feedback as soon as possible and fostering active introspection and decision making by the learner.

g. Establish practice schedule based on functional goal.
   - Distributed practice is used when superior performance is desired; motivation is low; or the learner has a short attention, poor concentration or fatigues easily.
   - Massed practice is used when a task is new and the learner needs repetition to learn.
   - Use random or serial practice order, rather than blocked practice, to improve learning and retention.
   - Use mental practice when the task has a large cognitive component or to decrease fear and anxiety.

h. Use part-whole transfer when a task is complex, has highly independent parts or the learner has limited memory, attention, or difficulty with only a particular portion of a larger task.

i. Until patient develops adaptability and generalizability, transfer of learning will be optimized when tasks are highly similar.

j. With learners who have attention deficits or who mentally fatigue easily, focus on key task elements, give frequent rest periods, and limit feedback.

k. Involve learner in goal setting to make practice functionally relevant and desirable for the patient to learn.

Task-Specific Training Strategies

General Concepts
1. Emphasis is on use of the affected body segments/limbs using task-specific activities and experiences.
   a. Patients practice important functional tasks essential to independence; e.g., stand up and sit down; balance, walking and stair climbing, reaching, and manipulation.
   b. Patients practice tasks in appropriate and safe environments; focus is on anticipated environments for daily function.
   c. Repetition and extensive practice are required, including both in-therapy and out-of-therapy time.
2. Patients practice under therapist's supervision and independently.
   a. Therapists can provide initial assistance through guided movements and verbal cueing; progression is to active, independent movements as soon as possible.
   b. Therapists serve as learning coaches, encouraging correct performance.
   c. Exercise/activity logs help organize the patient's self-monitored practice.
3. Motor learning strategies are utilized, including *behavioral shaping techniques* that use reinforcement and reward to promote skill development.
4. Activity-based, task-oriented training effectively counteracts the effects of immobility and the development of indirect impairments such as muscle weakness and loss of flexibility. It prevents learned nonuse of the more involved segments while promoting recovery of the central nervous system (neuroplasticity).
5. Box 3-1 presents a summary of strategies for effect activity-based, task-oriented training.

BOX 3-1 ▷ Activity/Task-Oriented Intervention Strategies to Promote Function-Induced Recovery

- Focus on early activity as soon as possible after injury or insult to utilize specific windows of opportunity, challenge brain functions, and avoid learned nonuse: "Use it or lose it."
- Consider the individual's past history, health status, age, and experience in designing appropriate, interesting, and stimulating functional activities.
- Involve the patient in goal setting and decision-making, thereby enhancing motivation and promoting active commitment to recovery and functional training.
- Structure practice utilizing activity-based, task-oriented interventions.
- Select tasks important for independent function; include tasks that are important to the patient.
- Identify the patient's abilities/strengths and level of recovery/learning; choose tasks that have potential for patient success.
- Target active movements involving affected body segments; constrain or limit use of less involved segments.
- Avoid activities that are too difficult and result in compensatory strategies or abnormal, stereotypical movements.
- Provide adequate repetition and extensive practice as appropriate.
- Assist (guide) the patient to successfully carry out initial movements as needed; reduce assistance in favor of active movements as quickly as possible.
- Provide explicit verbal feedback to improve movement accuracy and learning and correct errors; promote the patient's own error detection and correction abilities.
- Provide verbal rewards for small improvements in task performance to maintain motivation.
- Provide modeling (demonstrations) of ideal task performance as needed.
- Increase the level of difficulty over time.
- Promote practice of task variations to promote adaptation of skills.
- Maximize practice: include both supervised and unsupervised practice; use an activity log to document practice outside of scheduled therapy sessions.
- Structure context-specific practice.
- Promote initial practice in a supportive environment, free of distracters to enhance attention and concentration.
- Progress to variable practice in real-world environments.
- Maintain focus on therapist's role as coach while minimizing hands-on therapy.
- Continue to monitor recovery closely and document progress using valid and reliable functional outcome measures.
- Be cautious about timetables and predictions, as recovery and successful outcomes may take longer than expected.

From: O'Sullivan S, Schmitz T. *Improving Functional Outcomes in Physical Rehabilitation*. Philadelphia, FA Davis, 2010, with permission.

Task Selection

1. Initial tasks are selected to ensure patient success and motivation (e.g., grasp and release of a cup, forward reach for upper extremity dressing).
2. Tasks are continually altered to increase the level of difficulty.
   a. Therapists target the functional requirements of the task, e.g., a reciprocal stepping pattern, dynamic equilibrium during propulsion, and adaptability.
   b. Verbal cueing and manual assistance are provided as needed to assist.
   c. Progression is from treadmill walking to overground walking. Community ambulation skills and adaptability are targeted.

Locomotor Training

1. Motorized treadmill training (TT) with partial body weight support (BWS): provides a means of early task training (e.g., for patients with stroke or incomplete spinal cord injury). The activity is continually adjusted to meet the needs of the patient and progress the activity.
   a. Focus is on good stepping and posture.
   b. LE movements are initially manually assisted (e.g., trunk/pelvis, LE stepping); assistance is decreased as skill and control progresses.
   c. Treadmill speeds are increased with focus on achieving normal functional walking speeds.
   d. Progression is from body weight support to no support (e.g., 40% to 30% to 20% to 10% to 0%).
   e. Training is high frequency (3–5 days/week), moderate duration (20–30 minutes), and maximum tolerated intensity (speed and slope).
2. Overground training: using BWS, progressing to no BWS.
3. Overground training with least restrictive device (LRD) to no device, as appropriate.
4. Strategies to vary locomotor task demands: practice walking forward, backward, side-stepping, crossed-stepping (braiding); stopping, starting, and turning on cue; head movements; step-ups, step-up and over, stair climbing, obstacles.
5. Strategies to promote community reintegration: practice walking in open environments; altered support surface; altered speeds; curbs, ramps, walking through doorways, elevators, dual-task walking.

Constraint-Induced (CI) Movement Therapy

1. The less-affected UE is restrained by the use of a protective hand mitt.
2. Task practice is focused on using the more affected UE.
   a. Repetitive practice of functional tasks.
   b. Shaping: a functional task is selected and is progressively made more difficult. Goal is for the participant to accomplish the task with effort.
3. Adherence-enhancing behavioral strategies are used, including use of:
   a. Daily administration of motor activity log.
   b. Home diary.
   c. Problem-solving to overcome barriers to use of the more-affected UE.
   d. Behavioral contract.
   e. Caregiver contract.
   f. Home skill assignment, home practice, and daily schedule.
4. Therapist provides feedback, coaching, modeling, and encouragement.
5. Training is high intensity (several hours/day), high frequency (daily) for a period of 2–3 consecutive weeks.
6. Modified CI therapy is less intense, using lower intensity and frequency over a longer period of time (e.g., 1 hour/day, 3 days/week for 8 weeks).
7. Progression is to functional skills performed in the home environment.

Promote Ambulation Independence

Preambulation Mat Activities, with Progression

1. Rolling: log, segmental, counterrotation. See Quick Facts 3-5.
2. Prone on elbows: PNF holding activities, active head movements, weight shifting.
3. Prone on hands: PNF holding activities, active head movements, head movements with scapular depression, forward and lateral movements.
4. Hook-lying: static holding, PNF holding activities, movements out of midline.
5. Bridging: static hold, modify BOS (feet closer, arms closer, arms crossed on trunk), slow-reversal-hold pelvic activities, active to resisted hip abduction and adduction.
6. Quadruped: static hold, PNF holding activities, weight shifting, multidirectional rocking, lifting one extremity (usually begin with arm, then leg) and progress to arm and opposite leg together.
7. Sitting: with arm support, remove arm support, static hold, PNF holding activities, active head and arm movements, weight shifting within BOS, weight shifting outside BOS.
8. Kneeling: arm support on solid surface and progress to movable support, static hold, PNF holding activities, minisquats for eccentric hip control, weight

> **QUICK FACTS 3-5 ▶ PROGRESSION OF PREAMBULATION ACTIVITIES**

shifting, balance activities, active arm activities, throw and catch ball, hip hiking.
9. Half-kneeling: static hold, PNF holding activities, weight-shifting activities, slow-reversal and slow-reversal-hold pelvis movements.
10. Modified plantigrade (standing with arm support): static hold, PNF holding activities to shoulders and pelvis, weight-shifting activities, unweighting one lower extremity.
11. Standing: tonic hold, PNF holding activities, active weight shifting with feet in parallel progressing to one forward of the other, active arm and head movements, balance activities (throw/catch ball, reaching, etc.), stepping activities.

Preambulation Parallel Bar Activities

1. Entire progression should be demonstrated and then each component reviewed prior to the patient performing the task.
2. Emphasize correct sit-to-stand procedure: scoot to edge of chair, push from the arms of the chair, and pull feet back under knees.
3. Consideration with parallel bar activities.
   a. Clinician should be positioned inside the parallel bars directly in front of the patient.
   b. Initial balance activities are modified depending on the patient's weight-bearing status and specific requirements for treatment.
   c. Monitor the patient's circulatory status closely and be aware if the patient is experiencing orthostatic hypotension.
   d. Assess the patient's limits of stability by determining how far the center of gravity can be displaced while still maintaining balance.
4. Anterior-posterior and lateral weight shifts, first with stable hand placement, then with alteration of hand placement.
5. Hip hiking: pelvic elevation by hiking one hip at a time. Resistance can be added as skill level improves.
6. Standing push-ups: hands placed on the bars just anterior to the thighs, and body weight is lifted by simultaneous elbow extension and shoulder depression.
7. Stepping forward and backward with manual resistance applied to the pelvis for increased difficulty.
8. Forward progression: patient should maintain a loose, open grip on the bars and push down rather than pull up on the bars to best mimic ambulation with use of an assistive device.
9. Turning: patient is instructed to turn toward the stronger side, stepping in a small circle, not pivoting on a single extremity.

> **RED FLAG:** Although most patients should be encouraged to turn toward the stronger side during turning, patients with an acute total hip replacement must follow the precautions outlined by the physician. This may necessitate turning toward or away from the affected side.

10. Return to seated position: cue patient to back up, release stronger hand from bar and then reach back for the wheelchair armrest.
11. Advanced parallel bar activities.
    a. Resisted forward ambulation: resistance can be applied manually to the pelvis or the shoulders.
    b. Backward ambulation: initially without resistance, then add manual resistance at the pelvis.
    c. Sidestepping: turn sideways and hold onto the bar with bilateral UE, initially without resistance, then progress to manual contacts at the pelvis.
    d. Braiding: crossed sidestep with one limb advancing alternately anteriorly and posteriorly across the other limb.

> **RED FLAG:** Braiding should not be used with patients who have total hip precautions limiting adduction past midline.

Clinical Application: Considerations for Therapeutic Intervention

- A variety of intervention techniques are available to the clinician. Selection of the appropriate approach should be based upon the patient's goals and functional status as well as the clinician's ability to apply the concepts of the given approach.
- Due to the nature of neurological dysfunction, greater length of time and practice may be required to rehabilitate the patient.
- Motor control and motor learning are the basis upon which all rehabilitation is developed. It is essential to implement rehabilitation with an understanding of these concepts to ensure success and greatest possible return to independent function.
- The PTA must be aware of the influences that increase tone (heat, stress, etc.) for a given patient and attempt to avoid such triggers.
- Activities utilized with patients should mimic functional skills to the greatest degree possible in order to facilitate generalization and adaptation to the environments the patient will be functioning in following discharge from rehabilitation.

Conditions/Pathology/Diseases with Intervention

Infectious Disorders

Physical Therapy Management
1. Includes symptomatic and supportive bed positioning, passive range of motion (PROM), skin care, and safety measures if confusion is present.
2. Clinician must know and follow standard precautions.

Meningitis
1. Basic information.
   a. Inflammation of the meninges of the spinal cord or brain.
   b. Etiology: bacterial or viral infection.
   c. Patients with bacterial infection are usually sicker and experience a more rapid time course.

   RED FLAG: If untreated, meningitis can result in seizures, coma, and death.

2. Medical management.
   a. Bacterial: treat infective organism with antibacterial therapy.
   b. Viral: treat symptoms.

Encephalitis
1. Basic information.
   a. Severe inflammation of the brain.
   b. Etiology: viral (herpes simplex) or bacterial infection.
2. Clinical picture.
   a. Headache.
   b. Nausea and vomiting.
   c. Focal signs corresponding to area of brain involved.
   d. Seizures, coma and death.
3. Medical management.
   a. Bacterial: treat infected organism with antibacterial therapy.
   b. Viral: primarily symptomatic, but antiviral medication is available for herpes simplex virus.

Brain Abscess
1. Basic information.
   a. Localized infection in the brain.
   b. Etiology: encapsulated collection of pus accumulates in the brain.
2. Clinical picture.
   a. Signs of active infection: fever, chills, and headache.
   b. Progression to focal neurological signs depending upon site of infection.
3. Medical management.
   a. Bacterial: treat infective organism with antibacterial therapy.
   b. Surgical drainage.

CNS Neoplasms

Classification
1. Primary.
   a. Originate from cells found within the brain or spinal cord.
   b. Benign: may be operable or inoperable due to location.
   c. Malignant.
2. Secondary.
   a. Originate from cells outside the brain or spinal cord.
   b. Metastatic.

Clinical Picture: Dependent upon Location of Lesion
1. Headache.
2. Mental and behavioral changes.
3. Motor, speech and/or language impairments.
4. Seizures.

Medical Management
1. Surgery, radiation therapy, chemotherapy, and/or immunotherapy

Physical Therapy Management
1. Symptomatic and supportive.
2. Bed positioning, PROM, skin care, ambulation, assistive device assessment.

Degenerative Diseases of the CNS

Amyotrophic Lateral Sclerosis (ALS)
1. Basic information.
   a. Progressive upper and lower motor neuron disease.
      - Amyotrophic: muscle fiber atrophy from peripheral nerve involvement.
      - Degeneration and scarring of the motor neurons in the lateral aspect of the spinal cord, brainstem, and cerebral cortex.
   b. Death usually results in 2–5 years due to respiratory compromise.
2. Clinical picture.
   a. Dependent upon upper and lower motor neuron and involvement.
   b. Eventually both upper motor neurons and lower motor neurons are involved.
      - Lower motor neuron signs: asymmetrical, distal weakness with eventual progressive atrophy, facial weakness that results in difficulty with swallowing.
      - Upper motor neuron signs: hyperactive tendon reflexes and spasticity.
   c. Cognition is not affected.
   d. Aerobic capacity and endurance progressively diminishes, with eventual respirator use required.
   e. Compromised cranial nerve integrity.
   f. Motor function progressively diminishes with eventual total dependency for mobility and ADL.
3. Medical management.
   a. There is no known cure.
   b. Medications to control symptoms, including drooling and spasticity.
   c. Aggressive respiratory management.
4. Physical therapy management.
   a. Symptomatic and supportive.
   b. Maintain ROM and prevent disuse atrophy.
   c. Teach energy conservation.
   d. Help patient maintain independence for as long as possible.
   e. Assess need for adaptive and assistive devices.
   f. Instruct the patient and caregiver in transfers, positioning and respiratory management (postural drainage, chest stretching).

> **RED FLAG:** Avoid overworking weakened, denervated muscles, which can lead to more rapid breakdown of musculature and further limit the patient's function.

Multiple Sclerosis (MS)
1. Basic information.
   a. Chronic, progressive demyelinating disease of the CNS with no known cure.
   b. Commonly affects young adults.
   c. Etiology is unknown, but most likely an autoimmune response to a virus.
   d. Demyelinating lesions (plaques) impair neural transmission and cause nerves to fatigue rapidly.
   e. Fluctuating periods.
      - Relapse: worsening of symptoms.
      - Remission: periods of decreased or no symptoms.
      - May progress to permanent disability.

> **RED FLAG:** During an acute relapse, exercise should be avoided. This is a direct contraindication to exercise.

   f. Categories.
      - Relapsing-remitting MS: presents with cycles of exacerbation/remission with long periods of stability; may have minimal long-term impairment.
      - Primary-progressive MS: progresses from onset with no or occasional plateaus; may experience temporary, minor improvements.
      - Secondary-progressive MS: begins as relapsing-remitting MS and turns into a progressive course.
      - Progressive-relapsing MS: progressive course with periodic acute relapses; loss of function and progressive worsening with each exacerbation.
2. Clinical picture.
   a. Dependent upon plaque sites.
   b. Early symptoms: paresthesias, diplopia, and fatigue.
   c. Emotional dysregulation, mentation, and cognition, including euphoria.
   d. Dysarthria and scanning speech.
   e. Sensory deficits: paresthesias, hyperpathia, dysesthesias, trigeminal neuralgia.
   f. Lhermitte's sign: electric shock–like sensation throughout the body produced by flexing the neck.
   g. Visual problems: diplopia, blurred vision, optic neuritis, scotoma (blind spot), and nystagmus.

> **RED FLAG:** Ensure patient safety with functional skills given the prevalence of visual problems in patients with MS.

   h. Spasticity and hyperreflexia.
   i. Paresis.
   j. Impaired coordination: ataxia, intention tremors, dysmetria, dysdiadochokinesia.

k. Vestibular dysfunction leading to impaired balance.
  l. Ataxia.
  m. Fatigue.
   - Early afternoon fatigue and exhaustion common.
   - High-energy periods in early morning.
   - Some recovery in early evening.
  n. Impaired functional mobility skills.
3. Medical management.
  a. Corticosteroids shorten recovery during exacerbations.
  b. Avoid precipitating or exacerbating factors: infections, trauma, pregnancy, and stress.
4. Physical therapy management.
  a. Minimize secondary complications.
  b. Maintain functional independence as much as possible.
  c. Manage fatigue/energy conservation.
  d. Patient and family education.
  e. Provide psychological and emotional support and encourage support group participation.
  f. Frenkel exercises.
   - Coordination exercises performed in supine, sitting, standing, and walking.
   - Primarily for the LE but concepts can be applied to develop UE exercises.
   - Progress from assisted independent and from unilateral to bilateral.

RED FLAG: Avoid factors that cause transient worsening of symptoms: heat, hyperventilation, dehydration, fatigue.

Parkinson's Disease (PD)

1. Basic information.
  a. Chronic, progressive disease of the CNS.
  b. Basal ganglia disorder.
   - Deficiency of dopamine and degeneration of the substantia nigra.
   - Loss of inhibitory dopamine results in excessive excitatory output from cholinergic system of basal ganglia.
  c. Causes: commonly idiopathic but can also be infectious, atherosclerosis, toxic, or drug induced.
2. Clinical picture.
  a. Slowly progressive with emergence of secondary impairments and permanent disability.
  b. Standardized tests/outcome measures.
   - Hoehn & Yahr Disease Stage I, II, III, IV: stages from minimal, unilateral involvement without balance involvement to bed or wheelchair confinement.
   - Unified Rating Scale for Parkinsonism (MDS-UPDRS) revision: documents the overall effects of the disease on body structure, activity, and participation.
   - The Parkinson's Disease Questionnaire (PDQ-39) is a quality-of-life questionnaire that focuses on the subjective report of the impact of Parkinson's disease on daily life.
   - Freezing of Gait Questionnaire: examines gait, freezing episodes, and community function.
   - Parkinson's Fatigue Scale: examines fatigue and its effect on activity, participation, social function, and quality of life.
   - Profile of Function and Impairment Level Experience with Parkinson's Disease (PROFILE PD): developed for patients in early or middle stages of disease; examines impairments and functional activities.
  c. Common impairments: rigidity, bradykinesia, resting tremor, impaired postural reflexes.
  d. Mentation deficits: bradyphrenia (slowing of thought processes), depression, and dementia in advanced stages.
  e. Communication.
   - Dysarthria.
   - Hypophonia (decreased speech volume) with mutism in advanced stages.
   - Masked face.
   - Micrographia: small writing.
  f. Musculoskeletal.
   - Contractures commonly present in flexors and adductors.
   - Persistent posturing in kyphosis with forward head. Contracture development can lead to impaired posture, it is essential to include a stretching and positioning component in the rehabilitation program.
   - Osteoporosis leading to high risk for fracture.
  g. Sensory impairments: abnormal cramp-like sensations that are poorly localized and perceptual deficits.
  h. Visual problems.
  i. Impaired skin integrity leading to decubitus ulcer development in later stages. Ensure good patient and family education regarding positioning to avoid skin breakdown once the patient becomes wheelchair bound or bedridden.
  j. Impaired muscle tone/reflexes.
   - Rigidity (cogwheel or leadpipe).
   - Resting tremors that progress to intention tremors in later stages.
   - Pill-rolling tremor in hands.
  k. Impaired muscle strength associated with disuse and atrophy.
  l. Impaired motor control.
   - Bradykinesia: slowed movement.
   - Akinesia: absent movement/inability to initiate movement resulting in freezing episodes.
   - Slowed reaction time and movement time.

m. Impaired balance and postural reactions.
n. Festinating gait: shortened stride, decreased speed, increased cadence, decreased arm swing and trunk rotation.
o. Impaired functional abilities.
p. Decreased muscular and general body endurance.
3. Medical management.
   a. Levadopa/Sinemet (see Table 8-2, Commonly Prescribed Medications and Associated Precautions in Chapter 8, Geriatric Physical Therapy).
   b. Anticholinergic drugs for tremor control.
   c. Surgery may be considered when medication does not control tremors and dyskinesia.

RED FLAG: Monitor closely for adverse drug effects. Patients taking Sinemet long term may experience nausea and vomiting, orthostatic hypotension, cardiac arrhythmias, involuntary movements (dyskinesias), and psychoses and abnormal behaviors (hallucinations). Be aware of drug dosing cycles and recognize signs and symptoms of on-off phenomenon (e.g., sudden changes with loss of function, immobility and severe dyskinetic movements). Notify medical and/or nursing staff; communicate with PT as appropriate.

4. Physical therapy management.
   a. Prevent/minimize secondary complications.
   b. Patient education on compensatory strategies.
   c. Therapeutic exercise.
      - Improve rotational movements (PNF strategies).
      - Reduce rigidity.
      - Facilitate appropriate posture.
      - Flexibility exercises.
   d. Functional mobility skills (i.e., rolling, supine to sit).
   e. Relaxation strategies.
   f. Improve balance, postural control and safety.
   g. Improve cardiovascular endurance.
   h. Energy conservation techniques.
   i. Promote independence with ADL.

Cerebral Vascular Accident (CVA, Stroke)

Basic Information
1. Sudden, focal neurological deficit resulting from ischemic or hemorrhagic lesions in the brain.
2. Etiologic categories.
   a. Thrombus: formation or development of a blood clot within the cerebral arteries or their branches.
   b. Embolus: traveling bits of matter (thrombi, tissue, fat, air, bacteria) that produce occlusion and infarction in the cerebral arteries.
   c. Hemorrhage: abnormal bleeding as a result of rupture of a blood vessel.
   - Subarachnoid hemorrhage.
      - Blood between the arachnoid layer and the pia mater.
      - Most common causes: aneurysm and vascular malformations.
      - Symptoms depend upon location of the hemorrhage.
   - Subdural hemorrhage.
      - Blood between the dura mater and arachnoid layer.
      - Most often caused by trauma.
      - The body can reabsorb small volumes of blood but larger amounts must be surgically evacuated.
3. Risk factors.
   a. Atherosclerosis, hypercholesterolemia, hypertension, and cardiac disease.
   b. Diabetes.
   c. Smoking, alcohol and drug abuse.
   d. Transient ischemic attacks (TIAs).
      - Brief warning episodes of dysfunction lasting less than 24 hours. This can be a precursor of stroke in more than one-third of patients.
      - Failure to educate patients on the risk factors associated with CVA could lead to an increased risk of additional insult.
4. Pathophysiology.
   a. Cerebral anoxia: lack of oxygen supply to the brain causing irreversible damage beginning 4–6 minutes after insult occurs.
   b. Cerebral infarction: irreversible cellular damage.
   c. Cerebral edema: accumulation of fluids within the brain; can result in elevated intracranial pressure and potential for herniation and death.

Clinical Picture
1. Syndromes (Table 3-24).
   a. Middle cerebral artery syndrome.
   b. Anterior cerebral artery syndrome.
   c. Posterior cerebral artery syndrome.
   d. Vertebrobasilar artery syndrome.
   e. Internal carotid artery syndrome.
2. Resting posture: initial tendency toward flaccidity, with progression to spasticity and abnormal resting postures.
3. Arousal, mentation, and cognition.
   a. Impairments in orientation, attention, memory and ability to follow commands.
   b. Left versus right hemisphere lesions (Table 3-25).
      - Patients with left hemisphere lesions (right hemiplegia) tend to be slow, cautious, insecure, and hesitant.
      - Patients with right hemisphere lesions (left hemiplegia) tend to be impulsive, quick, overestimate their ability, and use poor judgment leading to safety concerns.

Table 3-24

CVA Syndromes

Anterior cerebral artery syndrome
Supplies medial part of the frontal and parietal lobe; basal ganglia and corpus callosum
- Contralateral sensory and motor loss with LE affected more than UE
- Mental impairment (confusion, amnesia, etc.)
- Urinary incontinence
- Apraxia (deficits in motor planning) affecting the ability to imitate movement and perform bimanual tasks
- Slow, delayed movement
- Lack of spontaneous movement
- Behavioral changes

Middle cerebral artery syndrome
Supplies lateral cerebral hemispheres, including frontal, temporal, and parietal lobes
- Contralateral sensory motor loss, with face and UE affected more than LE
- Perceptual deficits
- Homonymous hemianopsia
- Broca's aphasia (expressive or motor aphasia)
- Wernicke's aphasia (receptive or sensory aphasia)
- Global aphasia

Posterior cerebral artery syndrome
Supplies occipital lobe, medial and inferior temporal lobe, thalamus, and midbrain
- Contralateral sensory and motor loss
- Homonymous hemianopsia
- Visual agnosia, prosopagnosia, and cortical blindness
- Oculomotor nerve palsy
- Involuntary movement
- Thalamic pain syndrome
- Pusher syndrome: pushing toward the paretic side in sitting, standing and when walking
- Involuntary movements (choreoathetosis, intention tremors, and hemiballismus)

Vertebrobasilar artery syndrome
Supplies medulla, pons, and cerebellum
- Wide variety of symptoms, both ipsilaterally and contralaterally
- Cranial nerve involvement (diplopia, dysphagia, dysarthria, deafness, and vertigo)
- Ataxia
- Wallenberg's Syndrome (deficits in visual disturbances [nystagmus]; deficits in balance, gait coordination, temperature, and pain sensation)
- Locked-in Syndrome (patient is awake and aware of their environment, however is unable to speak or control any muscles beyond the eyes; in complete locked-in syndrome the patient is unable to control eye movements)
- Complete basilar occlusion causes death as a result of ischemia to areas that control vital functions

Internal carotid artery syndrome
Supplies anterior cerebral artery and middle cerebral artery
- Complete occlusion results in extensive cerebral edema which causes coma and death
- Incomplete occlusion can cause a mixture of anterior and middle cerebral artery syndromes

Table 3-25

CVA Syndromes
Hemispheric Dysfunction

LEFT HEMISPHERE INJURY	STRATEGIES FOR THERAPEUTIC INTERVENTION
• Right side hemiplegia/paresis • Right side hemisensory loss • Speech-language impairments • Trouble planning/sequencing movement • Slow, cautious, anxious • Realistic in self-assessment • Communication is difficult • Can't do steps of task • Difficulty processing • Verbal cues are hard to process • Trouble expressing positive emotion	• Develop communication plan of words and gestures • Assess level of understanding • Give frequent feedback and support • Do not underestimate ability to learn

RIGHT HEMISPHERE INJURY	STRATEGIES FOR THERAPEUTIC INTERVENTION
• Left side hemiplegia/paresis • Left side hemisensory loss • Visual-perceptual deficits • Trouble sustaining movements • Quick and impulsive • Poor judgment; overestimates abilities • Safety is a concern • Can't put it all together • Abstract concepts are difficult • Visual cues are hard to process • Trouble perceiving emotions	• Use verbal cues; demonstrations or gestures may be confusing with presence of visual-perceptual deficits • Give frequent feedback • Focus on slowing down and controlling movements • Focus on safety • Avoid environmental clutter • Do not overestimate ability to learn

> **RED FLAG**: Safety is a major concern with patients who have a right-sided CVA. Patients need to be taught safety awareness techniques, and family members should be educated in proper monitoring of the patient and environment for potential safety concerns.

   c. Emotional lability: tendency to cry or laugh easily and difficulty inhibiting same behavior.
4. Speech and communication impairments.
   a. Occur with damage to parieto-occipital cortex of the dominant hemisphere.
   b. Expressive dysfunction.
     • Nonfluent aphasia (Broca's, expressive, or motor aphasia).
        ○ Occurs from damage to Broca's area.
        ○ Results in speech that requires a great deal of effort to produce.
        ○ When speech occurs, words are typically restricted, interrupted, and awkward.
     • Verbal apraxia: impairment of voluntary articulation control.

- Dysarthria.
  - Decreased ability to control movements of the jaw, tongue, and respiratory structures needed for speech control.
  - Understand spoken language and use the correct words, but spoken words are difficult to understand.
  c. Receptive dysfunction.
    - Fluent aphasia (Wernicke's or receptive aphasia).
      - Occurs from damage to Wernicke's area.
      - Spontaneous speech is preserved and fluent.
      - Auditory comprehension is severely impaired.
  d. Global aphasia: combination of expressive and receptive aphasia resulting in major difficulty with both comprehension and production of language.
5. Dysphagia: difficulty swallowing.

> **RED FLAG:** Dysphagia can lead to aspiration, which places the patient at risk of respiratory distress or pneumonia. The clinician must be aware of specific diet restrictions the patient may have, including the thickness of liquids the patient is allowed to intake. Thin liquids increase risk.

6. Sensory impairments.
7. Perceptual dysfunction.
8. Motor impairments.
   a. Muscle tone.
      - Flaccidity: transient decrease or lack of resistance to PROM occurring during a period of spinal shock immediately after injury.
      - Spasticity: increased resistance to PROM following spinal shock as function begins to return.
   b. Brunnstrom's Stages of Motor Recovery.
      - Stage 1: initial flaccidity, no voluntary movement.
      - Stage 2: emergence of spasticity, hyperreflexia, synergies (mass patterns of movement).
      - Stage 3: voluntary movement possible but only in synergies; spasticity at its peak.
      - Stage 4: voluntary control in isolated joint movements emerging, corresponding decline of spasticity and synergies.
      - Stage 5: increasing voluntary control.
      - Stage 6: control and coordination near normal.
   c. Muscle performance impairments: decreased strength, power and endurance.
   d. Voluntary movement patterns.
      - Abnormal synergy patterns associated with cerebral stroke.
      - Ataxia and hypotonia associated with cerebellar stroke.
      - Extent of upper extremity and lower extremity involvement dependent upon extent of the infarct, etiology and vascular site.
9. Gait deficits (Table 3-26).
   a. Trendelenburg's limp: lateral tilt to sound side resulting from weak hip abductors on the involved side.
   b. Scissoring: results from spastic adductors.

Table 3-26

Common Gait Deviations Seen in Patients with Stroke

HIP	
DEVIATION	POSSIBLE CAUSES
Retraction	Increased trunk and lower extremity muscle tone
Hiking	Inadequate hip and knee flexion, increased tone in the trunk and lower extremity
Circumduction	Increased extensor tone, inadequate hip and knee flexion, increased plantar flexion in the ankle or footdrop
Inadequate hip flexion	Increased extensor tone, flaccid lower extremity

KNEE	
DEVIATION	POSSIBLE CAUSES
Decreased knee flexion during swing	Increased lower extremity extensor tone, weak hip flexion
Excessive flexion during stance	Weakness or flaccidity in the lower extremity, increased flexor tone in the lower extremity
Hyperextension during stance	Hip retraction, increased extensor tone in the lower extremity, weakness in the gluteus maximus, hamstrings or quadriceps
Instability during stance	Increased lower extremity flexor tone, flaccidity, weakness of extensor muscles

ANKLE	
DEVIATION	POSSIBLE CAUSES
Footdrop	Increased extensor tone, flaccidity
Ankle inversion or eversion	Increased tone in specific muscle groups, flaccidity
Toe clawing	Increased flexor tone in the toe muscles

   c. Insufficient pelvic rotation during swing.
   d. Equinus gait: heel does not touch down.
   e. Varus foot: weight is borne on the lateral side of the foot.
   f. Unequal step lengths.
   g. Decreased cadence with uneven timing.

Medical Management

1. Anticoagulation therapy for prevention: Coumadin, clot-busting medications.
2. Surgical intervention: carotid endarterectomy.
3. Tissue plasminogen activator (tPA).
   a. Used to dissolve clots in the brain and restore blood flow.
   b. Must be administered within 3 hours of insult to be effective; if administered via catheter into the brain, it can be used later.

Physical Therapy Management

1. Prevent or minimize secondary complications.
   a. Positioning and PROM to prevent deformity and contracture development.
   b. Maintain skin integrity.
   c. Decrease shoulder pain.
      - Subluxation: caused by forces of gravity or traction and weakness of capsule and shoulder musculature.
      - Immobility can lead to adhesive capsulitis.
      - Poor dynamic stabilizers can lead to impingement syndrome.

   RED FLAG: Poor handling techniques, such as pulling on the UE during transfers and PROM without scapular mobilization, can cause cumulative microtrauma that leads to increased shoulder pain.

   d. Monitor vital signs.

   RED FLAG: Monitor heart rate and blood pressure closely during exercise or activity training; monitor for signs and symptoms of cardiovascular compromise (e.g., extension of stroke, second stroke, myocardial infarction, or deep vein thrombosis); modify or stop the intervention and notify medical and/or nursing staff and physical therapist as appropriate.

2. Promote awareness and use of hemiplegic side via tone-reducing activities (inhibition techniques) and facilitation of out-of-synergy, functional movements.
3. Improve postural control and balance.
4. Task-specific training utilizing goal-directed activities.
   a. Focus on functional mobility skills: rolling, sitting, sit-to-stand, transfers, ambulation.
   b. Develop practice schedules and utilize feedback to facilitate learning.
   c. Focus on adapting movements to specific demands of the environment.
   d. Utilize compensatory training when rehabilitation peaks.
5. Promote independence with self-care and ADL.
6. Improve respiratory and cardiovascular function.
   a. Improve chest expansion and teach diaphragmatic breathing patterns.
   b. Exercise training: cycle ergometry, walking.
7. Muscle reeducation.
   a. Biofeedback training.
      - Aids with increasing firing in paretic muscles and improving muscle control.
      - Helps to decrease firing in spastic muscles.
   b. Functional electrical stimulation to stimulate muscle action and reduce spasticity.
8. Constraint-induced movement therapy: "forced use" of the paretic extremity.

RED FLAG: Constraint-induced movement therapy should not be used until the subacute and chronic stages so as not to expand the area of injury.

9. Provide emotional support to patient and family and encourage socialization.

Traumatic Brain Injury (TBI)

Basic Information

1. Mechanism of injury is contact forces to skull and rotational acceleration forces causing varying degrees of injury to the brain.
2. May be a focal lesion with a clinical presentation resembling hemiplegia or a diffuse lesion resulting in bilateral impairments.
3. Types of head injury.
   a. Open head injury: skull fracture and torn meninges with resultant brain exposure posing a risk of infection.
   b. Closed head injury: no skull fracture or brain exposure but a risk of increased intracranial pressure exists.

RED FLAG: The clinician should be aware of the signs of increased intracranial pressure when working with a patient with a closed TBI. These include severe headache and rapid changes in level of consciousness.

4. Pathophysiology.
   a. Primary brain damage: due to forces on the brain at the time of impact.
      - Local brain damage: cerebral contusion, lacerations, swelling, and herniation.
      - Coup-contracoup injury: injury occurring at point of impact and opposite point of impact with a high-velocity impact.
      - Diffuse axonal injury.
        ○ Disruption and tearing of axons and small blood vessels from shear-strain of angular acceleration.
        ○ Results in neuronal death and petechial hemorrhages.
        ○ Common causes: high-velocity impact and shaken baby syndrome.
   b. Secondary brain damage: changes due to the brain's reaction to trauma.
      - Hypoxic-ischemic injury: results from systemic problems (cardiovascular and respiratory) that compromise cerebral circulation.
      - Swelling/edema: can result in increased intracranial pressure and brain herniation (central, uncal, or tonsilar).
   c. Concussion: loss of consciousness, either temporary or permanent; resulting from head injury.

Table 3-27

Levels of Traumatic Brain Injury (TBI)

	MILD TBI	MODERATE TBI	SEVERE TBI
Loss of consciousness	0–30 minutes	>30 minutes but <24 hours	>24 hours
Alteration of consciousness	brief; >24 hrs	>24 hours	>24 hours
Posttraumatic amnesia	<1 day	>1 but <7 days	>7 days
Glasgow Coma Scale	13–15	9–12	<9
Imaging	normal	normal or abnormal	normal or abnormal

Potential changes in HR, RR, and BP. Extent of injury:
- Mild concussion: momentary loss of consciousness; retrograde amnesia.
- Classic concussion: transient loss of consciousness; mostly reversible in 24 hours; retrograde and posttraumatic amnesia.
- Severe concussion: loss of consciousness more than 24 hours; diffuse axonal injury and coma are present.

d. Levels of brain injury. See Table 3-27.

Clinical Picture

1. Levels of arousal, mentation, cognition can be measured using various different scales.
   a. Glasgow Coma Scale (GCS).
   b. Rancho Los Amigos level of cognitive functioning (LOCF) (Table 3-28).
      - Outlines predictable sequence of cognitive and behavioral recovery.
      - Eight levels of behavior.
        ○ I = no response.
        ○ II and III = decreased response levels.
        ○ IV, V, and VI = confused levels.
        ○ VII and VIII = appropriate levels.
        ○ Usually progress through levels in sequence and can plateau at any point.
   c. Amnesia.
      - Posttraumatic amnesia: inability to remember events occurring after the injury.
      - Retrograde amnesia: inability to remember events preceding the injury.
   d. Behavioral changes.
      - Inappropriate physical, verbal, and sexual behaviors.
      - Irritable, easily frustrated.
      - Impulsivity with safety issues.
      - Depression.
2. Speech and communication impairments.
3. Sensory impairments and perceptual dysfunction.
4. Deconditioning from prolonged hospitalization.
5. Disuse atrophy, contractures, and skin breakdown.
6. Motor impairments and muscle tone.
   a. Initial transient flaccidity with subsequent long-lasting spasticity.
   b. Rigidity.
      - Decerebrate rigidity: UE and LE in extension; occurs with lesions of the brainstem.
      - Decorticate rigidity: UE in flexion and LE in extension; occurs with lesions above the brainstem.
      - The patient should always be placed out of obligatory synergy patterns in order to decrease the risk of contracture formation.
   c. Voluntary movement patterns.
      - Abnormal synergy patterns associated with cerebral lesion.
      - Ataxia and hypotonia associated with cerebellar lesion.
      - Extent of UE and LE involvement dependent upon extent of the infarct, etiology and vascular site.
7. Gait, locomotion, and balance impairments will likely be bilateral.

Medical Management

1. Monitoring of intracerebral pressure.
2. Medication.
   a. Barbiturates to control cerebral edema and increased intracerebral pressure with severe injury.
   b. Botox or baclofen for spasticity.
   c. Various medications may be used for pain management.
3. Surgical intervention: hemorrhage or hematoma evacuation and decompression of skull.

Physical Therapy Management

1. Issues to be addressed.
   a. Problems associated with acute rehabilitation.
      - Decreased arousal.
      - Development of secondary complications.
      - Poor understanding of injury and rehab by patient and family.

Table 3-28

Levels of Cognitive Functioning (LOCF) Ranchos Los Amigo

LEVEL	BEHAVIORS TYPICALLY DEMONSTRATED
I	**No responses** Patient appears to be in a deep sleep and is completely unresponsive to any stimuli.
II	**Generalized response** Patient reacts inconsistently and nonpurposefully to stimuli in a nonspecific manner. Responses are limited and often the same regardless of stimulus presented. Responses may be physiologic changes, gross body movements, and/or vocalization.
III	**Localized response** Patient reacts specifically but inconsistently to stimuli. Responses are directly related to the type of stimulus presented. May follow simple commands in an inconsistent, delayed manner, such as closing eyes or squeezing hand
IV	**Confused-agitated** Patient is in heightened state of activity. Behavior is bizarre and nonpurposeful relative to immediate environment. Does not discriminate among persons or objects; is unable to cooperate directly with treatment efforts. Verbalizations frequently are incoherent and/or inappropriate to the environment; confabulation may be present. Gross attention to environment is very brief; selective attentions often nonexistent. Patient lacks short-term and long-term recall.
V	**Confused-inappropriate** Patient is able to respond to simple commands fairly consistently. However, with increased complexity of commands or lack of any external structure, responses are nonpurposeful, random, or fragmented. Demonstrates gross attention to the environment, but is highly distractible and lacks ability to focus attention to a specific task. With structure, may be able to converse on a social-automatic level for short periods of time. Verbalization is often inappropriate and confabulatory. Memory is severely impaired; often shows inappropriate use of objects; may perform previously learned tasks with structure but is unable to learn new information.
VI	**Confused-appropriate** Patient shows goal-directed behavior, but is dependent on external input for direction. Follows simple directions consistently and shows carry-over for relearned tasks with little or no carry-over for new tasks. Responses may be incorrect due to memory problems but appropriate to the situation; past memories show more depth and detail than recent memory.
VII	**Automatic-appropriate** Patient appears appropriate and oriented within hospital and home settings; goes through daily routine automatically, frequently robotlike with minimal-to-absent confusion, but has shallow recall of activities. Shows carry-over for new learning, but at a decreased rate. With structure is able to initiate social or recreational activities; judgment remains impaired
VIII	**Purposeful and appropriate** Patient is able to recall and integrate past and recent events and is aware of and responsive to environment. Shows carryover for new learning and needs no supervision once activities are learned. May continue to show a decreased ability relative to premorbid abilities, abstract reasoning, tolerance for stress, and judgment in emergencies or unusual situations

b. Problems commonly associated with inpatient rehabilitation.
  - Decreased ROM and contracture development.
  - Posturing and increased tone.
  - Unresponsive or unaware of environment.
  - Primitive reflexes influence movement.
  - Decreased cardiovascular endurance.
  - Difficulty communicating.
2. Management with decreased response levels (LOCF I–III).
  a. Increase arousal and orientation.
    - Auditory, kinesthetic, visual, and tactile stimulation.
    - Avoid overstimulation as patient may become agitated or shut down.
    - Avoid abstract concepts (humor, slang) that could be confusing to patient.
  b. Positioning.
    - PROM and proper positioning to decrease likelihood of contracture formation.
    - Static stretching or serial casting can be used to correct deformities.
    - Utilize positioning (side-lying and semiprone) to inhibit the influence of primitive reflexes.
    - Prevent decubitus ulcer formation.
  c. Develop postural control.
    - Proximal stability (head and trunk control) before distal mobility.
    - Achieve a neutral pelvis, erect trunk, and upright head.
    - Begin with manual contacts and maintained visual contact to assist with achievement of proper posturing.
    - Completing activities hand-over-hand provides both kinesthetic and proprioceptive feedback.
    - Utilize sitting activities to help orient patient to vertical and improve visual awareness of environment.
  d. Begin transfer training.
  e. Incorporate standing activities.

- Lower extremity weight bearing helps slow development of osteoporosis.
- Increases sensory input while completing ADL and functional tasks.
- If necessary, begin with tilt table to slowly acclimate patient to upright standing.
  f. Patient and family education regarding PROM, sensory stimulation, and positioning.
3. Management with mid-level recovery (LOCF IV–VI).
  a. Prevent overstimulation.

> **RED FLAG:** Prevent overstimulation for the confused and agitated patient; reduce environmental stimulation using quiet, closed environment; provide calming stimuli; maintain calm, focused manner.

  b. Provide consistency.
   - Establish daily routine.
   - Ensure all members of the team follow the behavior modification plan.
   - Utilize clear feedback.
   - Use daily journal or memory book to communicate with family.
  c. Utilize group treatment to facilitate peer modeling and reinforce appropriate behaviors.
  d. Plan multiple activities and allow patient some choice in selecting.
  e. Emphasize safety.
  f. Educate patient and family while preparing for discharge.

> **RED FLAG:** Ensure safety of the patient and those around him/her if aggressive disinhibition (punching, biting, etc.) is present in patients at LOCF IV.

4. Management with high-level recovery (LOCF VII–VIII).
  a. Facilitate increasing independence.
   - Begin working in open environments (community outings).
   - Aid patient with reintegrating socially, cognitively, and behaviorally.
   - Patient and family education on socialization skills, behavioral control mechanisms, and available support groups.
  b. Incorporate higher level balance activities, including protective and equilibrium reactions.
  c. Encourage cardiovascular conditioning and maintenance of an active lifestyle.

Concussion

1. The most common and least serious type of traumatic injury caused by a sudden direct blow or bump to the head; movement of the brain within the skull can cause bruising, damage to blood vessels, and injury to nerves.
  a. Risk factors: falls, high-risk sports, motor vehicle collision, physical abuse, and combat injuries.
  b. Concussion signs observed (source: CDC.gov, HEADS UP):
   - Appears dazed or stunned.
   - Can't recall events prior to or after a hit or fall.
   - Forgets an instruction, appears confused.
   - Moves clumsily.
   - Answers questions slowly.
   - Loses consciousness (even briefly).
   - Shows mood, behavior, or personality changes.
  c. Concussion symptoms reported (source: CDC.gov, HEADS UP).
   - Headache or pressure in head.
   - Nausea or vomiting.
   - Balance problems, dizziness, blurry vision.
   - Bothered by light or noise.
   - Feeling sluggish, hazy, foggy, or groggy.
   - Confusion, concentration or memory problems.
   - Just not "feeling right" or "feeling down."
2. Signs and symptoms typically occur soon after injury but some may be delayed for hours or days. Check for signs and symptoms immediately after injury and a few days after injury.
3. Grades of concussion:
  a. Mild (grade 1): symptoms last less than 15 minutes; there is no loss of consciousness.
  b. Moderate (grade 2): symptoms last longer than 15 minutes; there is no loss of consciousness.
  c. Severe (grade 3): loss of consciousness lasting seconds to minutes.
4. Rest is required for the brain to heal. The individual should be closely monitored.

> **RED FLAG:** Seek immediate emergency care if the adult or child experiences any of the following:
> - Drowsiness or inability to wake up.
> - One pupil larger than the other.
> - Repeat vomiting or nausea, convulsions or seizures.
> - Loss of consciousness lasting longer than 30 seconds.
> - Headache that gets worse over time.
> - Slurred speech, numbness, or decreased coordination.
> - Changes in behavior: irritability, restlessness, agitation.
> - Confusion, disorientation, or amnesia.

5. Concussion occurring during athletic competition requires the individual to stop play; return to play or vigorous activity is contraindicated while signs or

symptoms of a concussion persist. Medical clearance is required.
6. Baseline screening: typically done by a team of specialists and consisting of:
   a. Neurocognitive testing: memory, sequencing, speed of mental processing, and executive functions.
   b. Balance and equilibrium testing: the body's reactions to different challenges and positions.
   c. Vision testing: acuity, visual scanning.
7. Teach prevention strategies.
   a. Wear protective gear during sports or recreational activities.
   b. Buckle seatbelt when in an automobile.
   c. Safety proof homes to prevent falls.
   d. Exercise regularly to strength muscles and improve balance.
   e. Educate individuals about concussions.
8. Second-impact Syndrome.
   a. A second concussion is experienced before the brain has a chance to heal from the first event.
   b. Can produce severe changes including brain swelling, massive increase in intracranial pressure and brain herniation, resulting in permanent brain damage with long-term disabilities or death.
9. Postconcussion Syndrome.
   a. Persistent post-concussion symptoms lasting three months or longer; an indicator of concussion severity.
   b. Rare after only one concussion; likely to occur with multiple concussions.
   c. Symptoms may also include post-traumatic seizures, increased risk of depression, and mild-cognitive impairment later in life.
10. Chronic Traumatic Encephalopathy (CTE).
    a. A progressive neurodegenerative brain disease resulting from repetitive head trauma. Seen in athletes and boxers with a history of multiple concussions and repeated head injury.
    b. Pathological changes: diagnosis only made at autopsy by studying brain sections; brain changes include tau-positive neurofibrillary tangles (NFTs), neuropil threads and neocortical diffuse amyloid plaques, with or without neuritic plaques.
    c. Typical signs and symptoms include:
       - Recurrent headaches and dizziness.
       - Cognitive impairments: memory loss; difficulty thinking, planning, and carrying out tasks eventually progressing to dementia.
       - Mood or behavioral disturbances: depression, apathy, anxiety, suicidal thoughts or behavior, substance abuse.
       - Impaired judgment and impulse control, aggression, irritability, anger.
       - Movement disorders (late): a small subset of individuals with CTE can develop profound weakness, atrophy, spasticity similar to patients with ALS.
    d. Teach concussion prevention strategies.

Spinal Cord Injury (SCI)

Basic Information
1. Partial or complete disruption of spinal cord resulting in paralysis, sensory loss, and altered autonomic function and altered reflex activity.
2. Spinal areas most frequently injured: C5, C7, T12, and Ll.
3. Traumatic causes: motor vehicle accident, falls, diving accidents, stab and gunshot wounds.
4. Nontraumatic causes: disc prolapsed, vascular insult, complications of osteoporosis or rheumatoid arthritis.
5. Mechanisms of injury.
   a. Flexion (most common lumbar injury).
   b. Flexion-rotation (most common cervical injury).
   c. Compression.
   d. Hyperextension.
6. Pathophysiology.
   a. Primary injury results in injury to the spinal cord and/or interruption of blood supply.
   b. Secondary sequelae: ischemia, edema, demyelination and/or necrosis of axons progressing to scar tissue formation.

Clinical Picture
1. Classification.
   a. Level of injury: UMN injury.
      - Lesion level indicates most distal uninvolved nerve root segment with normal function; muscles must have a grade of at least 3+/5 or fair+ function.
      - Tetraplegia (quadriplegia): injury occurs between C1 and C8, involves all four extremities and trunk.
      - Paraplegia: injury occurs between T1 and T12-L1, involves both lower extremities and trunk (varying levels).
   b. Degree of injury.
      - Complete: no sensory or motor function below level of lesion.
      - Incomplete: preservation of sensory or motor function below level of injury; spotty sensation, some muscle function (<3+/5 grades).
      - American Spinal Injury Association (ASIA) Impairment Scale (Quick Facts 3-6).

> **QUICK FACTS 3-6 ▶ AMERICAN SPINAL INJURY ASSOCIATION (ASIA) LEVELS**
>
> | Type of Injury | Resulting Function |
> |---|---|
> | A – Complete | No motor or sensory function is preserved in the sacral segments S4–5. |
> | B – Incomplete | Sensory but not motor function is preserved below the neurological level and includes the sacral segments S4–5. |
> | C – Incomplete | Motor function is preserved below the neurological level, and most key muscles below the neurological level have a muscle grade of less than 3. |
> | D – Incomplete | Motor function is preserved below the neurological level, and most key muscles below the neurological level have a muscle grade of 3 or more. |
> | E – Normal | Motor and sensory function is normal. |

2. Clinical syndromes. See Table 3-29.
   a. Central cord syndrome: loss of more centrally located cervical tracts/arm function, with preservation of more peripherally located lumbar and sacral tracts/leg function; typically caused by hyperextension injuries to the cervical spine.
   b. Brown-Séquard syndrome: hemisection of spinal cord typically caused by penetration wounds (gunshot or knife) with asymmetrical symptoms.
   c. Anterior cord syndrome: damage is mainly in anterior cord, resulting in loss of motor function, pain and temperature with preservation of light touch, proprioception, and position sense, typically caused by flexion injuries of the cervical spine.
   d. Posterior cord syndrome: loss of posterior columns with preservation of motor function, sense of pain and light touch; extremely rare.
   e. Cauda equina: injury below L1 results in injury to lumbar and sacral roots of peripheral nerves (LMN) with sensory loss and paralysis and some capacity for regeneration; an LMN lesion with autonomous or nonreflex bladder.
   f. Sacral sparing: sparing of tracts to sacral segments, with preservation of perianal sensation, rectal sphincter tone, or active toe flexion.

Examination

1. Vital signs. Monitor prior to and throughout intervention.
2. Respiratory function.
   a. Assess: action of diaphragm, respiratory muscles, intercostals.
   b. Monitor/assess: chest expansion, breathing pattern, cough (quality, ability), vital capacity.
   c. Respiratory insufficiency or failure occurs in lesions above C4 (phrenic nerve, C3-5 innervates diaphragm).
3. Skin condition, integrity: check areas of high pressure.
4. Muscle tone and DTRs.
5. Sensation/spinal cord level of injury: check to see if sensory level corresponds to motor level of innervation (may differ in incomplete lesions).
6. Muscle strength (MMT)/spinal cord level of injury:
   a. Lowest segmental level of innervation includes muscle strength present at a fair+ grade (3+/5).
   b. Use caution when doing MMT in acute phase with spinal immobilization.
7. Functional status: full functional assessment possible only when patient is cleared for activity and active rehabilitation.
8. Standardized tests and measures for examination of patients with spinal cord injury.
   a. FIM/FAM. See previous discussion.
   b. Wheelchair skills test provides for measurement of functional and wheelchair management skills for the patient who uses the wheelchair for primary mobility (Kirby et al., 2004; http://www.wheelchairskillsprogram.ca/eng/overview.htm).

Physical Therapy Goals, Outcomes, and Interventions

1. Monitor for changes associated with recovery. See Quick Facts Box 3-7.
2. Improve respiratory capacity.
   a. Deep breathing, exercises, strengthening exercises to respiratory muscles.
   b. Assisted coughing, respiratory hygiene (postural drainage, percussion, vibration, suctioning) as needed to keep airway clear.
   c. Abdominal support if indicated.
3. Maintain ROM, prevent contracture.
   a. PROM, positioning, splinting.
   b. Selective stretching to preserve function (e.g., tenodesis grasp).
4. Spasticity/spasms.
   a. Determine location and degree of tone.
   b. Examine for nociceptive stimuli that may trigger increased tone (e.g., blocked catheter, tight clothing or straps, body position, environmental temperature, infection, decubitus ulcers).
5. Maintain skin integrity.
   a. Frequent skin inspection and intervention to prevent decubitus ulcer or other injury.
   b. Consistent and diligent positioning program, pressure relieving devices (e.g., cushions, gel cushion, ankle boots).

Table 3-29

Spinal Cord Injury Syndromes

LESION	CHARACTERISTICS
Complete cord lesion: UMN lesion	Complete bilateral loss of all sensory modalities Bilateral loss motor function with spastic paralysis below level of lesion Loss of bladder and bowel functions with spastic bladder and bowel
Central cord lesion: UMN lesion	Cavitation of central cord in cervical section Loss of spinothalamic tracts with bilateral loss of pain and temperature Loss of ventral horn with bilateral loss of motor function: primarily upper extremities Preservation of proprioception and discriminatory sensation
Brown-Sequard syndrome: UMN lesion	Hemisection of spinal cord Ipsilateral loss of dorsal columns with loss of tactile discrimination, pressure, vibration, and proprioception Ipsilateral loss of corticospinal tracts with loss of motor function and spastic paralysis below level of lesion Contralateral loss of spinothalamic tract with loss of pain and temperature below level of lesion; at lesion level, bilateral loss of pain and temperature
Anterior cord syndrome: UMN lesion	Loss of anterior cord Loss of lateral corticospinal tracts with bilateral loss of motor function, spastic paralysis below level of lesion Loss of spinothalamic tracts with bilateral loss of pain and temperature Preservation of dorsal columns: proprioception, kinesthesia, and vibratory sense
Posterior cord syndrome: UMN lesion	Loss of dorsal columns bilaterally Bilateral loss of proprioception, vibration, pressure, and epicritic sensations (stereognosis, two-point discrimination) Preservation of motor function, pain, and light touch
Cauda equina injury: LMN lesion Dura and arachnoid mater Conus medullaris First lumber spinal nerve Cauda equina Roots of spinal nerves Posterior root ganglion Lower limit of subarachnoid space Sacrum Filum terminale Coccygeal spinal nerve Coccyx	Loss of long nerve roots at or below L1 Variable nerve root damage (motor and sensory signs); incomplete lesions common Flaccid paralysis with no spinal reflex activity Flaccid paralysis of bladder and bowel Potential for nerve regeneration; regeneration often incomplete, slows and stops after about 1 year

LMN = lower motor neuron; UMN = upper motor neuron

QUICK FACTS 3-7 ▶ SPINAL CORD INJURY – CHANGES ASSOCIATED WITH RECOVERY

Condition	Description
Spinal shock	Transient period of reflex depression and flaccidity. May last several hours or up to 24 weeks.
Spasticity/spasms	More likely to develop with incomplete lesions. Will not occur with cauda equina lesions (lower motor neuron lesions). Irritating stimuli that may increase tone. • Blocked catheter. • Tight clothing or orthotic straps. • Environmental temperature. • Infection. • Decubitus ulcers.
Heterotopic bone formation (ectopic bone)	Abnormal bone growth in soft tissues. Examine for early changes—soft tissue swelling, pain, erythema, generally near large joint. Late changes—calcification, initial signs of ankylosis.
RED FLAG: Autonomic dysreflexia (autonomic hyperreflexia, hyperreflexia)	An emergency situation in which a noxious stimulus precipitates a pathological autonomic reflex with symptoms of paroxysmal hypertension, bradycardia, headache, diaphoresis (sweating), flushing, diplopia, or convulsions; examine for irritating stimuli. Treat as a medical emergency, elevate head, check and empty catheter first. (Very common triggering event, may also be triggered by constipation)
RED FLAG: Deep venous thrombosis (DVT)	Check lower extremities for edema and tenderness.

c. Patient education: pressure relief activities (e.g., pushups) and skin inspection techniques.
d. Provide prompt treatment of pressure sores.
6. Improve strength.
   a. Strengthen all remaining innervated muscles.
   b. Use selective strengthening during acute phase to reduce stress on spinal segments.
   c. Resistive training to build muscle hypertrophy.
7. Reorient patient to vertical position.
   a. Tilt table, wheelchair.
   b. Use of abdominal binder, elastic lower extremity wraps to decrease venous pooling may be necessary.
   c. Examine for signs and symptoms of orthostatic hypotension (lightheadedness, syncope, mental or visual blurring, sense of weakness).
8. Promote early return of functional mobility skills and ADLs.
   a. Emphasis on independent rolling and bed mobility, assumption of sitting, transfers, sit-to-stand, and ambulation as indicated (see section on transfer training in Chapter 11).
   b. Improve sitting tolerance, postural control, symmetry, and balance; standing balance as indicated.

Other Clinical Considerations for SCI
1. Autonomic dysreflexia (hyperreflexia).
   a. Occurs in patients with a spinal cord lesion above T6. Noxious stimuli elicit a sympathetic response, initiating vasoconstriction and increasing the blood pressure; the normal inhibitory response is impaired.
   b. This is an emergency situation. The elevated blood pressure may lead to subarachnoid hemorrhage, seizure, or myocardial infarction.
   c. Is caused by a noxious stimulus. Noxious triggers can be full bladder, constrictive or tight clothing, full/compacted bowel, scrotal compression, kidney stones, pressure ulcers.
   d. Symptoms.
      • Paroxysmal hypertension.
      • Bradycardia.
      • Headache.
      • Diaphoresis.
      • Flushing.
      • Diplopia.
      • Convulsions.
   e. Management.
      • Elevate head.
      • Check for irritating stimuli (blocked catheter, tight ankle-foot orthosis [AFO]).

> **Clincal Application: Heterotopic Ossification**
>
> Heterotopic ossification is formation of bone in a muscle, tendon, joint capsule, or ligament. If it occurs in muscle tissue, it is often called *myositis ossificans*. While the cause is unknown, musculoskeletal trauma, spinal cord injury, traumatic brain injury, burns to the extremities, and aggressive stretching after immobilization increase the risk for patients of developing this disorder. The most commonly involved muscles are the quadriceps and brachialis. Signs of muscle involvement include muscle firmness and pain with palpation, muscle stiffness, and pain with muscle stretch or contraction. If suspected, the involved tissues should be rested until the bone is reabsorbed. Massage, stretching, and strengthening of involved muscles are contraindicated. Joint mobilization is contraindicated if the joint is involved.

> **RED FLAG:** Treat as a medical emergency. Failure to recognize the presence of autonomic dysreflexia can lead to drastic increases in blood pressure. If the patient's head is not elevated and the noxious stimuli removed, this places the patient at risk of CVA.

2. Heterotopic ossification.
   a. Abnormal bone growth in the soft tissue.
   b. Usually present in hips and knees.
   c. Initial signs: swelling, pain, erythema, and stiffness.
   d. May lead to joint ankylosis if calcification occurs.

> **RED FLAG:** Care should be taken to avoid damage to surrounding structures with PROM or stretching in the presence of heterotopic ossification.

3. Deep vein thrombosis (DVT).
   a. Previously a test called the Homan's sign may have been used by the clinician to help determine the presence of a DVT. This test has since been shown to lack specificity and sensitivity and is likely no longer widely used.

> **RED FLAG:** The clinician must know the signs of DVT to decrease the risk of a pulmonary emboli occurring. These signs include dull ache, erythema, and edema in the location of the DVT. If a DVT in the calf is suspected, the clinician should immediately notify the appropriate medical staff (inpatient—nurse; outpatient—physician, etc.).

4. Spinal cord dysesthesia.
   a. Results from noxious stimuli (urinary tract infection [UTI], spasticity, bowel impaction, smoking).
   b. TENS can be used to help decrease or resolve pain.
5. Bowel and bladder dysfunction.
   a. UTIs are the most frequent complication of SCI. Long-term maintenance of the surrounding tissues is essential.
   b. Lesions above S2–4.
      - Result in a spastic or reflexive bladder.
      - Emptying is manually triggered by cutaneous stimuli (stroking the lower abdomen or pulling the pubic hairs).
   c. Lesions of the cauda equina.
      - Result in a flaccid bladder.
      - Empty bladder by increasing intra-abdominal pressure (Valsalva's or Crede's maneuver).
   d. Reflex bowel management programs involve high-fiber diet, suppositories, and digital stimulation.
      - Initially, there is a lack, or significantly altered control, of the bowel. Prolonged digestion, constipation, and leakage can be a problem.
      - Initially, bowel regulation is managed based on the type of reflexes that return to the sphincter. The method typically includes digital stimulation or manual evacuation; individuals with dysreflexic bowels must use caution to avoid triggering a spasm, which can lead to constipation and subsequent autonomic dysreflexia.
      - Long-term management is highly individualized and best accomplished by establishing a routine that includes appropriate fiber and fluid intake, consistent time of day, and frequency for bowel evacuation.
   e. Neurogenic bladder management.
      - Initially patient will have an indwelling catheter until medically stable and ready for progression; at this point, intermittent self-catheterization (self-IC) will be taught.
      - Persons with lesions at C5–C6 may be able to perform self-IC, persons with lesions at C7 and below are typically able to perform self-IC. The individual may also need to take medications to assist with bladder spasticity and reflex control.
      - The ongoing consideration with catheterization is the potential to develop urinary tract infections.
      - Other techniques can include suprapubic tapping—the individual taps directly over the bladder to trigger bladder contraction and emptying; use of the Valsalva's maneuver or straining.
6. Sexual dysfunction.
   a. Lesions above the cauda equina allow reflexive function that responds to physical stimulation.
   b. Lesions of the cauda equina allow for psychogenic function that requires cognitive stimulation.
   c. Both men and women retain the ability to reproduce.

Medical Management

1. Medication to limit posttraumatic ischemia and address secondary complications (spasticity, DVT, etc.).

2. Fracture stabilization.
   a. Surgical stabilization.
      - Restore alignment of the bony structures.
      - Decompress neural tissue.
      - Stabilize the spine to prevent further damage.
      - Improve potential for earlier mobilization.
   b. Orthotic stabilization.
      - Cervical: halo is the most common but may see semirigid/rigid collars.
      - Thoracic/lumbar: thoracolumbosacral orthosis.
   c. Combined surgical and orthotic stabilization.

Physical Therapy Management

1. Reorient patient to vertical position using tilt table and wheelchair with use of an abdominal binder and/or elastic lower extremity wraps to decrease venous pooling.

> **RED FLAG:** Monitor for signs and symptoms of orthostatic hypotension when beginning.

2. Improve cardiovascular endurance.
   a. UE cycle ergometry.
   b. Functional wheelchair activity training.
   c. Functional electrical stimulation/LE ergometry.

> **RED FLAG:** Recognize exercise precautions for individuals with tetraplegia and high-lesion paraplegia; patients may experience blunted tachycardia, lack of pressor response, very low VO_2 peak, and substantially higher variability of most responses. Monitor heart rate and blood pressure closely during exercise and activity training.

> **RED FLAG:** Absolute contraindications to exercise (from the American College of Sports Medicine): autonomic dysreflexia, severe lesion or infected skin on weight-bearing surfaces, UTI, uncontrolled spasticity or pain, unstable fracture, insufficient ROM to perform exercises, uncontrolled hot or humid environment.

3. Improve respiratory capacity and functioning.
   a. Respiratory function improves dramatically with full intercostal innervation.
   b. Deep-breathing exercises.
   c. Respiratory muscle strengthening.
   d. Proper respiratory hygiene: assisted cough, postural drainage, percussion, vibration, and suctioning.
4. Integumentary integrity.
   a. Maintain skin free of decubitus ulcers and other injury by maintaining proper schedule for positioning changes.
   b. Pressure-relieving devices: wheelchair cushions and tilt-in-space wheelchair.
   c. Patient education on pressure relief activities (push-ups, weight shifting) and proper skin inspection.
5. Maintain ROM and limit contracture formation via PROM and positioning. Certain muscles may need strengthening, while others need to be allowed to shorten in order to preserve function via passive insufficiency (i.e., tenodesis grip, slightly hypomobile spine for support).
6. Improve strength of all remaining innervated muscles.
   a. Use selective strengthening during acute phase to reduce stress on spinal segments and increase function.
   b. Resistive training to hypertrophy muscles in rehabilitation phase.
7. Promote maximum mobility in home and community environment (Table 3-30).
   a. Promote early return of functional mobility skills.
      - Emphasis on independent rolling and bed mobility.
      - Assumption of sitting.
      - Transfers.
      - Ambulation as indicated.
   b. Improve sitting tolerance, postural control, symmetry, and balance.
   c. Promote wheelchair skills and independence in managing wheelchair parts.
   d. Community reintegration outings.
8. Facilitate ambulation ability.
   a. Nonfunctional ambulators.
      - Stand to assist with transfers and bear weight on LE.
        - Relieve pressure on buttocks.
        - Allows weight bearing through LE bones.
        - Cardiopulmonary work.
      - Lesions of upper to mid-thoracic region.
   b. Functional ambulators.
      - Ambulate independently in the home, with or without assistive device.
      - Lesions of low-thoracic region.
   c. Community ambulators.
      - Ambulate throughout home and community, with or without device.
      - Must be able to do all components of community ambulation safely (cross street in appropriate time, ascend and descend stairs/curbs).
      - Lesions of lumbar region.
9. Provide psychological and emotional support.
   a. Encourage socialization and motivation.
   b. Promote independent problem solving, self-direction.
10. Provide patient and family education with focus on strategies to prevent skin breakdown, maintaining ROM, and strengthening to increase function.

Epilepsy

Characteristics

1. A disorder characterized by recurrent seizures (repetitive abnormal electrical discharges within the brain).

Table 3-30

SCI Functional Table

NERVE ROOT LEVEL AND KEY MUSCLES INNERVATED	KEY MOVEMENTS AVAILABLE	ADL SUMMARY	W/C MOBILITY	TRANSFERS AND GAIT
C1-C3 • Face and neck	• Mouth and head	• Talking • Chewing • Sipping • Blowing	• Powered w/c with breath or chin control • Ventilator	• Total dependence • Respirator
C4 • Diaphragm • Trapezius	• Respiration • Scapular elevation	• Increased ability to use assistive devices that utilize scapular/head and mouth movement	• Power w/c with mouth or chin control	• Total dependence
C5 • Biceps • Deltoid	• Elbow flexion • Shoulder external rotation • Shoulder abduction to 90 degrees	• Self feeding • Some self care with UE assistive devices	• Powered w/c with hand controls • Limited manual w/c propulsion	• Can assist with transfers
C6 • Pectoralis major • Extensor carpi radialis • Teres major	• Shoulder flexion • Wrist extension	• Tenodesis grasp • Bed mobility with rails • Independent with pressure relief weight shifts	• Independent with manual w/c with projections • Will likely still use power w/c due to fatigue	• May be independent with sliding board transfers
C7 • Triceps • Latissimus dorsi • Extrinsic finger extensors • Flexor carpi radialis	• Elbow extension • Wrist flexion • Finger extension	• Independent living possible • Independent with: lateral push-up pressure relief • LE dressing • LE self-ROM	• Independent transfers	• Independent manual w/c propulsion
C8-T1 • Flexor carpi ulnaris • Extrinsic and intrinsic hand muscles	• Full innervation of upper extremities	• Full independence in activities requiring primarily UE use	• Negotiation of 2–4 inch curbs and wheelies in w/c	• Independent in w/c transfers
T1-T8 • Top half of intercostals	• Improved respiratory control	• Same as C8-T1 with improved respiratory and trunk control	• Negotiation of 6 inch curbs	• T6-T8 physiological standing with orthoses in parallel bars
T9-T12 • Abdominals	• Good trunk control	• Independence in all ADLs from a w/c level	• Independent	• Household ambulation with bilateral knee-ankle-foot orthosis (KAFOs) and assistive device
T12	• Same	• Same	• Will use w/c for primary means of mobility	• Community ambulation with bilateral KAFOs and assistive device • No hip flexor function
L1, L2 • Quadratus lumborum • Iliopsoas and sartorius	• Hip hiking • Weak hip flexion	• Same	• Same	• Can be independent in community ambulation with bilateral KAFOs and assistive devices
L3-L5 • L3-L4 iliopsoas strong • L4-L5 quadriceps, medial hamstrings strong	• Hip flexion • Knee extension	• Same	• Same • May continue to use w/c for efficient mobility	• Ambulation with bilateral ankle foot orthosis (AFOs) and canes possible • No gluteus maximus function
S1-S2 • Plantar flexors • Gluteus maximus	• Plantar flexion • Hip extension	• Same	• Same	• May ambulate with articulated AFOs

2. Signs and symptoms.
   a. Altered consciousness.
   b. Altered motor activity (convulsion): characterized by involuntary contractions of muscles; tonic activity (stiffening and rigidity of muscles); clonic activity (rhythmic jerking of extremities).
   c. Sensory phenomena: patient experiences somatosensory, visual, auditory, olfactory, gustatory, and vertiginous sensations.
   d. Autonomic phenomena: associated with sudden attack of anxiety, tachycardia, sweating, piloerection, abnormal sensation rising up in upper abdomen and chest.
   e. Cognitive phenomena: sudden failure of comprehension, inability to communicate, intrusion of thought, illusions, hallucinations, affective disturbances (intense feelings of fear, anger, and hate).
3. Common causes of seizures.
   a. Acquired brain disease or trauma: tumor, stroke.
   b. Degenerative brain diseases: Alzheimer's dementia, amyloidosis.
   c. Developmental brain defects, low oxygen at birth.
   d. Drug overdose: cocaine, antihistamines, cholinesterase inhibitors, methylxanthines, tricyclic antidepressants.
   e. Drug withdrawal: alcohol, benzodiazepines.
   f. Electrolyte disorders: hyponatremia, hypernatremia, hypoglycemia, hypomagnesemia.
   g. Hyperthermia.
   h. Infections; brain abscess, meningitis or encephalitis, neurocysticercosis.
   i. Pregnancy complications: eclampsia.
4. Classification of seizures.
   a. Generalized seizures: all areas of the brain (cortex) are involved. Sometimes referred to as *grand mal seizures*.
      - Symptoms include: dramatic loss of consciousness, with stiffening, then rhythmic movements of the arms and legs; eyes are generally open; breathing is altered; loss of urine is common. Typically lasts 2–5 minutes.
      - Post seizure: consciousness is gradually regained; person typically confused, drowsy, and amnesiac after the event; may last several hours.
   b. Absence or petit mal seizures: posture is maintained, repetitive blinking or other small movements may be present. Typically brief, lasting only a few seconds; may occur many times in a day.
   c. Partial or focal seizures: only one part of brain is involved; symptoms are focal (specific area of the body).
      - Complex partial seizure: person appears dazed or confused, not fully alert or unconscious.
      - Temporal lobe seizure: characterized by episodic changes in behavior, with complex hallucinations; automatisms (e.g., lip smacking, chewing, pulling on clothing); altered cognitive and emotional function (e.g., sexual arousal, depression, violent behaviors); preceded by an aura.
   d. Secondarily generalized seizures: simple or complex partial seizures evolving to a generalized seizure.
   e. Status epilepticus: prolonged seizure or a series of seizures (lasting > 30 minutes) with very little recovery between attacks; may be life threatening; medical emergency (generalized status epilepticus).

Examine/Determine
1. Time of onset, duration, type of seizure, sequence of
   a. events, frequency, duration.
2. Patient activity at onset, presence of aura.
3. Sensory elements, motor activity: type, degree, and location of involvement.
4. Presence of tongue biting, incontinence, respiratory distress.
5. Behavioral elements, changes in mood and perception.
6. Patient responses after the seizure.

Medical Management

1. Antiepileptic medications: phenytoin (Dilantin), carbamazepine (Tegretol), phenobarbital; drugs may have significant adverse side effects.
2. Surgical intervention: lobe resection, hemispherectomy.

Physical Therapy Goals, Outcomes, and Interventions

> **RED FLAG:** Recognize signs and symptoms of seizure and protect patient from injury during seizure. Remain with patient, remove potentially harmful nearby objects, loosen restrictive clothing, and do not restrain limbs. Establish airway, prevent aspiration by positioning the patient in sidelying, and wait for tonic-clonic activity to subside. Seek medical and/or nursing assistance ASAP.

1. Establish airway, prevent aspiration: turn head to side or side-lying position; check to see if airway is open, wait for tonic-clonic activity to subside before initiating artificial ventilation if needed.
2. Promote regular routines for physical activity and emotional health.

Peripheral Nervous System (PNS) Disorders

Basic Information
1. Pathology.
   a. Wallerian degeneration: degeneration of the axon and myelin sheath distal to the site of axonal interruption.

b. Segmental demyelination: axons are preserved and remyelination restores function.
   c. Axonal degeneration: degeneration of axon and myelin sheath.
2. Neuropathies (peripheral neuropathy).
   a. Overview.
      - Degenerative changes in peripheral nerves that produce sensory loss and motor weakness.
      - Caused by nutritional deficiencies, diabetes, and alcohol abuse.
   b. Mononeuropathy: involvement of a single nerve.
   c. Polyneuropathy.
      - Bilateral symmetrical involvement of peripheral nerves, usually LEs more than UEs.
      - Stocking/glove distribution: distal segments earlier and more involved than proximal.
3. Radiculopathy: involvement of nerve roots due to skeletal changes (soft tissue injuries).
4. Traumatic nerve injury. Traumatic nerve injuries fall into three main categories/classes of injury:
   a. Neurapraxia: Injury to nerve that causes a transient loss of function (e.g., compression). Nerve dysfunction may be rapidly reversed or persist a few weeks.
   b. Axonotmesis: Injury to nerve interrupting the axon and causing loss of function and degeneration distal to the lesion (e.g., crush injury). Regeneration is possible.
   c. Neurotmesis: Cutting of the nerve with severance of all structures and complete loss of function. Reinnervation typically fails without surgical intervention.
5. Entrapment syndrome.
   a. Pressure on a nerve where it passes over a bony prominence or restricted opening.
   b. Results in motor and sensory disturbances in the area distribution of the nerve.

Clinical Picture
1. Symptoms.
   a. Weakness/paresis of denervated muscle, hyporeflexia and hypotonia; rapid atrophy; fatigue.
   b. Sensory loss corresponding to motor loss.
   c. Autonomic dysfunction leading to vasodilation and loss of vasomotor tone (dryness, warm skin, edema).
   d. Hyperexcitability of remaining fibers.
      - Sensory dysesthesias (hyperalgesia, paresthesias, burning).
      - Spasms and fasiculations.
   e. Myalgia with inflammatory myopathies.

Bell's Palsy (Facial Paralysis)
1. Lower motor neuron (LMN) lesion involving the facial nerve (CNVII) resulting in unilateral facial paralysis.
2. Etiology: acute inflammatory process of unknown etiology resulting in compression of the nerve within the temporal bone.
3. Characteristics.
   a. Muscles of facial expression on one side are weakened or paralyzed.
   b. Loss of control of salivation or lacrimation.
   c. Sensation is normal.
   d. Onset is acute with maximum severity in few hours or days.
   e. Most recover fully in several weeks or months.
4. Medical management: corticosteroids and analgesics.
5. Physical therapy management.
   a. Electrical stimulation to maintain tone and support function of facial muscles.
   b. Provide active facial muscle exercises.
   c. Provide emotional support and reassurance.

RED FLAG: Instruct patient not to "overdo it," as the nerve needs to rest.

Guillain-Barré Syndrome (GBS)
1. Polyneuritis with progressive muscular weakness that develops rapidly.
2. Etiology.
   a. Unknown, but associated with an autoimmune attack.
   b. Usually occurs after recovery from an infectious illness.
   c. Evolves over a few days or weeks with slow recovery (months to a year) back to or near full functioning.
3. Pathology: acute demyelination of both cranial and peripheral nerves.
4. Clinical picture.
   a. Aerobic capacity and endurance may be severely limited, especially with pulmonary involvement.
   b. Integumentary: pain and paresthesias; typically less sensory involvement than motor.
   c. Motor function: paresis or paralysis in relative symmetrical distribution of weakness; progresses from lower extremities to upper and from distal to proximal; may produce full tetraplegia with respiratory failure; not uncommon to have residual bilateral foot drop.
   d. Potential complications: respiratory failure and risk of pneumonia, myalgia, relapse.

5. Physical therapy management throughout the ascending phase: patient is becoming weaker as the disease progresses.
   a. Monitor for signs of respiratory failure, increasing PCO_2.
   b. Use pulse oximetry for O_2 saturation monitoring.
   c. Follow standard precautions to prevent infection.
   d. Facilitate coughing and airway clearance.
   e. Prevent indirect impairments associated with immobilization.
   f. Passive range of motion within pain tolerance.
   g. Positioning.
   h. Prevent injury to denervated muscles.
6. Physical therapy management during the stabilization phase: early rehabilitation begins when patient is stable and no longer getting worse. A therapeutic pool or Hubbard's tank provides a medium to facilitate low-stress exercise.

RED FLAG: Avoid overstretching and overuse of denervated muscles.

7. Physical therapy management during the descending phase: beginning of extensive rehabilitation. Paralysis recedes and function returns.
   a. Provide muscle reeducation. PNF techniques start with active and progress to resistive exercise.
   b. Functional training as recovery progresses.
   c. Teach energy conservation techniques and activity pacing.
   d. Improve cardiovascular fitness following prolonged bed rest and deconditioning.
   e. Provide emotional support and reassurance to patient and family.

RED FLAG: Avoid overuse and fatigue, as this may prolong recovery.

Myasthenia Gravis
1. Autoimmune neuromuscular disease.
   a. Decreased acetylcholine receptors.
   b. Ineffective postsynaptic membrane stimulation and poor transmission at the neuromuscular junction.
2. Clinical picture.
   a. Fluctuating weakness that increases with repeated muscle contractions; usually affects eye movements or eyelids first; progresses to oropharyngeal, facial, proximal and respiratory muscles.
   b. More noticeable in the proximal muscles. Muscles of trunk and extremities become involved in advanced cases. Ocular, facial and bulbar muscles commonly involved.
   c. Difficulty with swallowing.
   d. Usually improves with rest and anti-cholinesterase drugs.
   e. Variable course: some rapidly progressive with early death, and others with remissions and exacerbations.

RED FLAG: Myasthenic crisis is a life-threatening weakness of the respiratory muscles and requires immediate medical attention.

   f. Functional mobility skill difficulty: climbing stairs, rising from a chair, lifting.
3. Physical therapy management.
   a. Monitor vital signs.
   b. Promote independence in functional mobility skills.
   c. Teach energy-conservation techniques.
   d. Promote optimal activity, with rest as indicated.
   e. Provide psychological and emotional support.

Postpolio Syndrome
1. New onset of weakness and severe fatigue occurring an average of 25 years after recovery from acute poliomyelitis.
2. Clinical picture.
   a. Severe long-lasting fatigue out of proportion with activity level and not relieved with rest.
   b. New onset of muscle weakness in muscles previously thought to be strong.
   c. New loss of functional abilities due to weakness.
   d. Slow, steady progression of dysfunction.
   e. Difficulty in concentration, memory, and attention.
   f. Poor aerobic capacity.
3. Physical therapy management.
   a. Address aerobic capacity and endurance: submaximal exercise can maintain and improve endurance; maintain respiratory function via deep-breathing exercises and postural drainage; instruct in energy conservation techniques; teach relaxation exercises to facilitate full relaxation periods.
   b. Strengthening exercises: overuse will increase fatigue and joint pain; partially denervated muscles will not respond to strengthening as innervated muscles would; aquatic exercises programs can minimize fatigue with strengthening.

RED FLAG: Because of the concerns with overuse, the patient should stop exercising if pain, fatigue, and/or weakness increase.

   c. Patient and family education regarding lifestyle modifications.
   d. Psychological support and reassurance.

Trigeminal Neuralgia (Tic Douloureux)
1. Neuralgia resulting from degeneration or compression of the trigeminal nerve (CNV). May also be known as tic douloureux.

2. Clinical picture.
   a. Brief periods of stabbing and/or shooting pain along the nerve distribution.
   b. Autonomical dysfunction exacerbated by stress or cold and relieved by relaxation.
   c. May see increase in pain with chewing, talking, brushing teeth, or movement of air across the face.

Medical Management

Pain medication or surgery to section or permanently anesthetize nerve.

3. Physical therapy management.
   a. TENS for pain relief.
   b. Symptomatic and supportive.

> **Clinical Application: Reinforcing the Rehabilitation Program**
>
> - The PTA will likely be called upon to provide psychological support and reassurance with a variety of patients. It is important for the clinician to develop comfort in doing so.
> - It is important for the PTA to know what type of medical management will be used with each diagnosis in order to determine the impact of such interventions on the rehabilitation of the patient.
> - When possible, activities completed in rehabilitation should be active on the part of the patient to instill a sense of independence and success.
> - The key to a successful rehabilitation program is patient education and developing functional activities based on the patient's goals.

Painful Neurological Conditions

Complex Regional Pain Syndrome (CRPS)

An Abnormal Response of a Peripheral Nerve

1. Previously known as reflex sympathetic dystrophy (RSD).
2. Painful condition that can develop following trauma to a nerve.
3. The process of the pathology is thought to facilitate or inhibit an overreaction of the sympathetic nervous system (SNS). Some studies show CNS dysfunction as well.
   a. Injury at one somatic level initiates efferent activity of the sympathetic system affecting multiple levels.

Variations

1. CRPS I: painful syndrome developing following trauma to an area, no overt nerve injury.
   a. Trauma may be planned (e.g., following shoulder surgery) or unplanned (e.g., following a fall on a knee).
2. CRPS II: painful nerve syndrome developing following trauma to a peripheral nerve; also called *causalgia*.

Etiology

1. Origin may come from a variety of conditions.
   a. Surgery.
   b. Upper motor neuron (UMN) lesion secondary to a brain injury.

> **Clinical Application: Complex Regional Pain Syndrome (CRPS) Explained**
>
> CRPS I (reflex sympathetic dystrophy) is a potential complication following musculoskeletal trauma. CRPS II (causalgia) is a potential complication following peripheral nerve injury. CPRS involves a localized malfunction of the sympathetic nervous system.
>
> Symptoms include intense pain that is out of proportion to the injury, distally located edema, warmth, redness and sweating. Early recognition is important because progression can lead to tissue changes such as osteoporosis, muscle atrophy and contractures. Treatment includes edema reduction, desensitization training and weight-bearing and/or distraction of the involved joints. Early mobility exercises and edema reduction following injury can help to prevent this disorder.

   c. Cerebrovascular accident (CVA, the shoulder-hand syndrome occasionally seen following CVA).
   d. Destructive lesion of CNS.
   e. LMN disorder following peripheral nerve injury, neuropathies, entrapments.

Clinical Picture

1. Begins with localized pain that is described as a burning sensation that occurs spontaneously; the level of pain is in excess of the stimulus.
2. The syndrome progresses in three stages (Table 3-31).

Painful Neurological Conditions   137

Table 3-31

Complex Regional Pain Syndrome: Clinical Stages

STAGE	TIME FRAME	TYPICAL SIGNS AND SYMPTOMS
Stage I	Begins up to 10–12 days following injury; lasts 1–6 months	Increasing pain that is characterized as burning or aching, is more severe than would be expected, pain response is generated by stimulus that is typically not painful. May present with edema Affected limb is cooler or warmer. Skin: dry, increased hair growth, increased nail growth
Stage II	Lasts approximately 3–6 months	Pain: worsens; is constant, burning, and aching. Abnormal painful sensations remain present; e.g. allodynia, hyperalgesia, hyperpathia. Edema spreads, causes joint stiffness. Skin: thin, glossy, cool, sweaty (hyperhydrosis); continued nail changes Osteoporosis may be starting.
Stage III	Lasts up to 12 months and may continue after that.	Pain continues, may plateau. Edema hardens and continues to limit ROM. Muscles atrophy, contractures may be present. Skin: continued altered texture and temperature; fascia thickens potentially causing contractures. Osteoporosis and ankylosis progress. Depression may be a problem.

3. Manifestations of the stages.
   a. Sensory impairments result in the perception of pain that is out of proportion to the degree of injury or insult actually present.
      - Allodynia: touch that is typically nonpainful (e.g., light touch, air movement, wearing a shirt) is interpreted as pain.
      - Hyperalgesia: increased level of sensitivity, lower pain threshold.
   b. Vasomotor/thermal changes.
   c. Tissue changes.
   d. A progression of changes in the skin from dry and warm, to moist, to cool.
      - Trophic changes begin with increased hair and nail growth and progress to thin skin, loss of hair, and thin, ridged nails.
   e. Bone demineralization and ankylosis are major concerns.
   f. Edema.

Medical Management

1. Diagnosis is made by history and clinical examination; often delayed.
2. Diagnostic tests are aimed at determining secondary changes due to the CRPS.
   a. Radiography, thermography, and Doppler flowmetry studies.
3. Limited or weak evidence for the effectiveness of:
   a. Stellate ganglion blocks or sympathectomy.
   b. Acupuncture.
   c. Corticosteroids and nonsteroidal anti-inflammatory drugs (NSAIDs).
   d. Amytriptyline to relieve depression and aid in sleep.
   e. Calcium channel blockers to help improve peripheral circulation.
4. Better evidence for the use of:
   a. Long-term intrathecal baclofen.
   b. Implanted dorsal column stimulation.
      - Has been shown to help decrease pain perception and intensity.

Physical Therapy Management

1. Education focusing on encouraging patient to use involved extremity or area as normally as possible.
2. Modalities for pain relief.
   a. Most effective when used in early stages.
   b. TENS is reported to be minimally effective.
      - May be some evidence for high- and low-frequency stimulation application to the contralateral side.
3. Pool therapy may provide a medium to encourage movement, especially when the lower extremity is involved.

Review Questions

Neuromuscular Physical Therapy

1. Describe two to three predictable deficits a clinician can expect to observe when each of the following areas of the brain is damaged: (1) frontal lobe, (2) temporal lobe and (3) cerebellum.

2. Identify what an exteroceptor is as it relates to sensory responses. Now identify two proprioceptive facilitation techniques and two proprioceptive exteroceptive inhibition techniques that can be used with patients/clients with neurological deficits.

3. A PTA is working with a patient who has a spinal cord injury (SCI). The PT has ordered a manual wheelchair with projection rims. What level of SCI is the highest-level injury a PTA should expect to be able to use this type of wheelchair?

4. Differentiate equilibrium and nonequilibrium coordination tests. Describe two equilibrium and two nonequilibrium coordination tests.

5. A PTA is working with an individual who has neurological balance deficits. The patient is able to perform static and dynamic sitting activities with little to no difficulties. Identify three ideas for progression of balance activities at this point.

4
Cardiac, Vascular, and Lymphatic Physical Therapy

SUSAN B. O'SULLIVAN, KAREN E. RYAN, KELLY MACAULEY, THOMAS SUTLIVE, and TODD SANDER

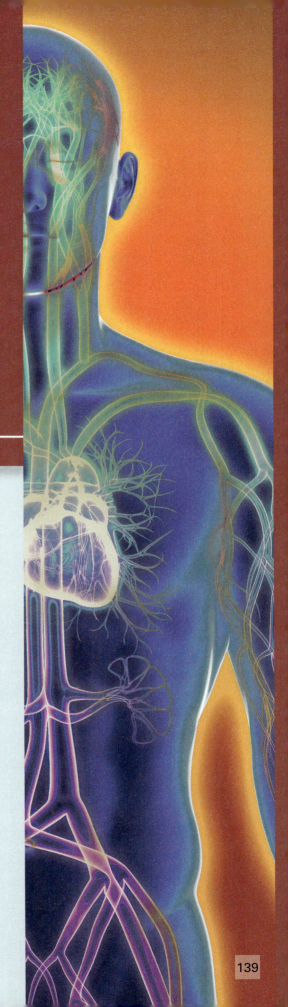

Chapter Outline

- **Anatomy and Physiology of the Cardiac, Vascular, and Lymphatic Systems, 142**
  - The Heart and Circulation, 142
  - Vascular System, 143
  - Lymphatic System, 143
  - Neurohumoral Influences, 144
- **Physical Therapy Examination and Data Collection of the Cardiovascular System, 146**
  - PTA's Role and Responsibility, 146
  - Heart Rate (HR)/Pulse Measurement, 146
  - Heart Sounds, 147
  - Electronic Measurement of Heart Rhythm, 148
  - Blood Pressure (B/P), 148
  - Respiration, 149
  - Measure Oxygen Saturation, 149
  - Assess Pain, 150
  - Physical Examination: Peripheral Vascular System, 150
  - Tests of Peripheral Venous Circulation, 152

- Tests of Peripheral Arterial Circulation, 153
- Examine Lymphatic System, 153
- Cardiovascular Diagnostic Tests, 153
- Laboratory Tests and Values, 154
- Signs and Symptoms of Cardiovascular Disease, 156
  - Chest Pain or Discomfort, 156
  - Palpitations, 156
  - Dyspnea, 156
  - Cardiac Syncope, 157
  - Fatigue, 157
  - Cyanosis, 157
  - Peripheral Edema, 157
  - Claudication, 157
- Cardiovascular Disease: Evaluation, Diagnosis, and Prognosis, 157
  - Atherosclerosis, 157
  - Acute Coronary Syndrome (ACS) (Coronary Artery Disease), 157
  - Hypertension, 159
  - Medical Management, 160
  - Medical and Surgical Management of Cardiovascular Disease, 160
- Peripheral Vascular Disease: Evaluation, Diagnosis and Prognosis, 163
  - Arterial Disease, 163
  - Venous Disease, 164
- Intervention Strategies for Patients with Cardiac Conditions, 166
  - Exercise Tolerance Testing, 166
  - Exercise Prescription, 166
  - Phase 1: Inpatient Cardiac Rehabilitation (Acute), 171
  - Phase 2: Outpatient Cardiac Rehabilitation (Subacute), 173
  - Phase 3: Community Exercise Programs (Postacute, Postdischarge from Phase 2 Program), 174

- Resistance Exercise Training, 174
- Exercise Prescription for Patients Requiring Special Considerations, 174
- Intervention: Peripheral Vascular Disease Conditions, 176
  - Rehabilitation Guidelines for Arterial Disease, 176
  - Rehabilitation Guidelines for Venous Disease, 177
- Lymphatic System, 178
  - Pathophysiology/Common Pathologies, 179
  - Examination: History, Tests, and Measures, 179
  - Intervention/Rehabilitation Guidelines for Lymphedema, 182
- Appendix 4A: Sample Exercise Programs per MET Level, 185
- Review Questions, 187

Anatomy and Physiology of the Cardiac, Vascular, and Lymphatic Systems

The Heart and Circulation

Heart Tissue
1. Pericardium: Fibrous protective sac surrounding the heart.
2. Epicardium: Inner layer of the pericardium.
3. Myocardium: Heart muscle, major portion of the heart.
4. Endocardium: Smooth lining of the inner surface and cavities of the heart.

Cardiac Cycle
1. The coordinated rhythmic pumping of the chambers of the heart, the atria, and ventricles. (See Quick Facts 4-1.)
   a. Within the chambers, the atrioventricular and semilunar valves prevent backflow of blood between chambers. (See Figure 4-1.)
2. Systole: The period of ventricular contraction. End-systole volume is the amount of blood in the ventricles after systole, about 50 mL.
3. Diastole: The period of ventricular relaxation and filling of blood. End-diastole volume is the amount of blood in the ventricles after diastole, about 120 mL.
4. Atrial contraction occurs during the last third of diastole and completes ventricular filling.

Coronary Circulation
1. Arteries. (See Figure 4-2.)
   a. Arise directly from aorta near aortic valve; blood circulates to myocardium during diastole.
   b. Four main arteries supply the different chambers of the heart.
   c. Right coronary artery (RCA): Supplies right atrium, most of right ventricle and in most individuals the inferior wall of the left ventricle, atrioventricular node (AV) and bundle of His; 60% of the time supplies the sinoatrial (SA) node.
   d. Left coronary artery (LCA): Supplies most of the left ventricle; has two main divisions.
      - Left anterior descending artery (LAD): Supplies the left ventricle and interventricular septum and in most individuals the inferior areas of the apex; it may also give off branches to the right ventricle.
      - Circumflex artery (Circ): Supplies blood to the lateral and inferior walls of the left ventricle and portions of the left atrium; 40% of the time supplies SA node.
   e. Interruption in any of the arteries can set off a cascade of cardiac events.

QUICK FACTS 4-1 ▶ HEART CHAMBERS AND CONDUCTION

Right Atrium (RA)	Left Atrium (LA)
• Receives blood from systemic circulation from superior and inferior vena cava • SA node—near superior vena cava; is pacemaker of the heart • AV—node floor of RA; receives signal from SA node, transmits signal via AV bundle/bundle of His, to depolarize and contract ventricles	• Receives oxygenated blood from lungs and four pulmonary veins

Right Ventricle	Left Ventricle
• Receives blood from RA → pumps blood through pulmonary artery to lungs for oxygenation	• Walls are thicker and stronger than the RV and form most of the left side and apex of the heart. • Receives blood from the LA and pumps blood via the aorta throughout the entire systemic circulation

HEART VALVES

Atrioventricular Valves	Semilunar Valves
• Prevent backflow of blood into the atria during ventricular systole • Close when ventricular walls contract • Right heart valve—tricuspid (three cusps or leaflets) • Left heart valve—bicuspid or mitral (two cusps or leaflets)	• Prevent backflow of blood from the aorta and pulmonary arteries into the ventricles during diastole • Pulmonary valve prevents right backflow. • Aortic valve prevents left backflow.

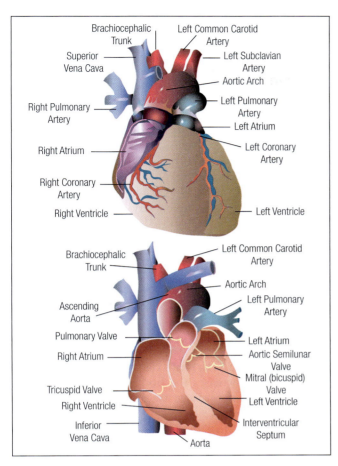

Figure 4-1 The heart.

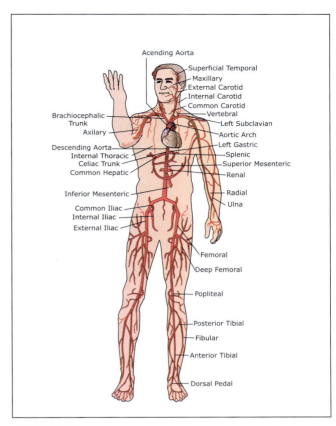

Figure 4-2 Circulatory system: Arteries.

2. Veins. See Figure 4-3.
   a. Run parallel to the arterial system; the coronary sinus receives venous blood from the heart and empties into the right atrium.

Myocardial Fibers
1. Muscle tissue: Striated muscle fibers but with more numerous mitochondria; exhibits rhythmicity of contraction; fibers contract as a unit.
2. Myocardial metabolism is essentially aerobic; sustained by continuous oxygen delivery from the coronary arteries.
3. Smooth muscle tissue is found in the walls of the blood vessels.

Hemodynamics
1. Stroke volume (SV): The amount of blood ejected with each myocardial contraction, about 70 mL.
2. Cardiac output (CO): The volume of blood discharged from the left or right ventricle per minute; approximately 4–6 L per minute in average adult.
3. Left ventricular end-diastolic pressure (LVEDP): Pressure in the left ventricle during diastole.
4. Ejection fraction (EF): Percentage of blood emptied from the ventricle during systole.
5. Atrial filling pressure: The difference between the venous and atrial pressures.
6. Diastolic filling time is decreased with increased heart rate with heart disease.
7. Myocardial oxygen demand (MVO_2) represents the energy cost to the myocardium.
   a. MVO_2 is increased with activity and increases with HR and/or B/P.

Vascular System

Structures
1. Important vascular system structures can be found in Quick Facts 4-2.

Lymphatic System

1. Drains lymph from body tissues and returns it to the venous circulation.
   a. Lymph travels from lymphatic capillaries and lymphatic vessels, through lymph nodes, to the right lymphatic and thoracic ducts before being

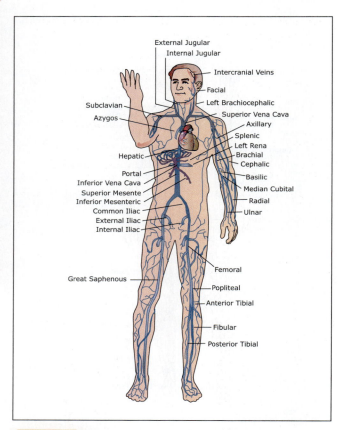

Figure 4-3 Circulatory system: Veins.

returned to the bloodstream through the subclavian veins.
- The lymph nodes contain macrophages to phagocytize (digest) bacteria and other pathogens.
- Major lymph nodes are submaxillary, cervical, axillary, mesenteric, iliac, inguinal, popliteal, and cubital.

b. Lymph vessels rely on external forces (e.g., movement, muscle contraction, respiration) to pump fluid through the system. Lymph flow is also influenced by massage and gravity.

c. Contributes to immune system response by digesting cellular debris and bacteria and producing antibodies.

Neurohumoral Influences

Sympathetic and Parasympathetic Systems
1. Control vascular responses to activity and medications; control changes in blood chemistry and volume.

Sympathetic Stimulation (Adrenergic)
1. This system increases the body's cardiovascular, respiratory, and neurologic system functions (fight-or-flight response).
2. Control located in medulla oblongata, cardioacceleratory center.

QUICK FACTS 4-2 ▶ VASCULAR SYSTEM STRUCTURES

Arteries	Veins
• Transport oxygenated blood from the heart • They decrease in size and become arterioles, eventually ending as capillaries. • Arteries have contractile abilities. • Arterial walls are thicker in order to tolerate strong blood flow pressures from the heart. • Influenced by elasticity and extensibility of vessel walls and by peripheral resistance, amount of blood in body • Change in diameter when triggered by sympathetic activity of the autonomic nervous system (ANS), vasoconstriction or vasodilation	• Transport dark, unoxygenated blood from peripheral tissues back to the heart • Veins have larger capacity and thinner, weaker walls than arteries; greater number. • Veins have a one-way valve to prevent backflow of blood because they do not have contractile abilities. • Veins rely on movement of the surrounding muscles to squeeze blood back to the heart. • Venous reflux occurs when these valves do not function properly because of veins that are enlarged or weakened. • Venous system includes both superficial and deep veins (deep veins accompany arteries, while superficial do not). • Venous circulation influenced by muscle contraction, gravity, respiration (increased return with inspiration), compliancy of right heart

Capillaries
- Minute blood vessels that connect the ends of arteries (arterioles) with the beginning of veins (venules)
- Functions for exchange of nutrients and fluids between blood and tissues
- Capillary walls are thin, permeable

3. Via cord segments T1-4, upper thoracic to superior cervical chain ganglia; innervates all but ventricular myocardium; releases epinephrine and norepinephrine.
   a. Causes: an increase in the rate and force of myocardial contraction and myocardial metabolism; coronary artery vasodilation.
4. The skin and peripheral vasculature receive only post-ganglionic sympathetic innervations, which causes vasoconstriction of cutaneous arteries. Sympathetic inhibition must occur to obtain vasodilation.
5. Drugs that are used to stimulate sympathetic activity are called *beta-adrenergic agents*; drugs that are used to decrease sympathetic activity are called *beta-adrenergic blocking agents* (beta-blockers).

Parasympathetic Stimulation
1. Causes marked decrease in heart rate.
2. Causes some decrease in muscle contractility.

Additional Control Mechanisms
1. Baroreceptors and chemoreceptors. See Quick Facts 4-3.
2. Ion concentration changes. See Quick Facts 4-4.
3. Body temperature changes impact heart rate. Increased body temperature causes heart rate to increase; decreased body temperature causes heart rate to decrease.

QUICK FACTS 4-3 ▶ RECEPTOR CONTROL MECHANISMS

Baroreceptors (pressoreceptors)
- Main mechanisms controlling heart rate
- Located in walls of aortic arch and carotid sinus, via vasomotor center
- Circulatory reflex: Respond to changes in blood pressure (B/P)
  - Increased B/P results in parasympathetic stimulation, decreased rate and force of cardiac contraction, sympathetic inhibition, and decreased peripheral resistance.
  - Decreased B/P results in sympathetic stimulation, increased heart rate and B/P, and vasoconstriction of peripheral blood vessels.
  - Increased right atrial pressure causes reflex acceleration of heart rate.

Chemoreceptors
- Located in the carotid body
- Sensitive to changes in blood chemicals: O_2, CO_2, lactic acid
  - Increased CO_2 or decreased O_2 or decreased pH (elevated lactic acid) results in an increase in heart rate.
  - Increased O_2 levels result in a decrease in heart rate.

QUICK FACTS 4-4 ▶ EFFECTS OF ION CONCENTRATION CHANGES

RED FLAG: These conditions pose a significant threat to the patient's response to and ability to participate in physical therapy interventions.

Hyperkalemia (increased potassium): Electrocardiogram (ECG) changes (widened PR interval, QRS wave, and tall T waves), tachycardia (potentially leading to bradycardia), potential cardiac arrest

Hypokalemia (decreased potassium): ECG changes (flattened T waves, prolonged PR and QT intervals), hypotension, arrhythmias may progress to ventricular fibrillation

Hypercalcemia (increased calcium): Hypertension, signs of heart block, cardiac arrest

Hypocalcemia (decreased calcium): Arrhythmias, hypotension

Hypernatremia (increased sodium): Hypertension, tachycardia, pitting edema, excessive weight gain

Hyponatremia (decreased sodium): Hypotension, tachycardia

Physical Therapy Examination and Data Collection of the Cardiovascular System

PTA's Role and Responsibility

The PTA Must be Able to
1. Perform cardiac system tests and measures to determine the patient's current cardiac condition.
2. Read and understand medical documentation. Recognize implications of test results and use this information to guide decisions for intervention.
3. Monitor cardiac response throughout physical therapy interventions.
4. Educate the patient/family throughout the rehabilitation process.
5. Use information from the data collection process to progress patient interventions within the plan of care.
6. Differentiate appropriate and adverse responses and report to the physical therapist.
7. Know cardiac risk factors (see Table 4-1).

Heart Rate (HR)/Pulse Measurement

Pulse Should be Monitored
1. Prior to initiating interventions with all patients to ensure each patient is physiologically appropriate for the intervention.
2. To identify if pulse is within normal limits for this patient. Consider age, medications, and whether there is an appropriate reaction to the intervention.
3. During the intervention to monitor the patient's physiologic response for patients with cardiovascular or pulmonary conditions and with interventions that target those systems.
4. After completion of the intervention to determine the patient's response to the intervention.

Table 4-1

Risk Factors for Cardiovascular Disease	
Non-Modifiable Risk Factors	
RISK FACTOR	**INCREASED RISK CRITERIA**
Age	Men > 45 years and women > 55 years
Family History	Cardiac event in 1st degree male relative < 55 years or 1st degree female relative < 65 years (1.5–2 fold relative risk). Risk increases further with younger age of onset, number of events, and how close genealogically the relative is.
Race	African American
Gender	Men > risk than pre-menopausal women. After menopause, the risk equalizes.
Modifiable Risk Factors	
RISK FACTOR	**GOAL TO REDUCE RISK**
Cholesterol	Total cholesterol: < 200 mg/dL LDL cholesterol: < 160 mg/dL (if low risk for cardiac disease), < 130 mg/dL (if intermediate risk for cardiac disease), < 100 mg/dL (if high risk for cardiac disease, have cardiac disease, or diabetes) HDL cholesterol: > 40 mg/dL (men) and > 50 mg/dL (women) Triglycerides: < 150 mg/dL
Diabetes	HgA1C < 7%
Diet	Low fat, salt diet with balance of vegetables, fruits, grains, and meats.
Hypertension	Normal blood pressure: less than 120/80 mm Hg
Obesity	Body Mass Index (BMI): 18.5–24.9 kg/m2 Waist circumference: < 40 inches (men) and < 35 inches (women)
Physical inactivity	At least 30 minutes of activity, 5–7 days per week
Tobacco	Smoking cessation, regardless of time smoked, reduces risk.

Adapted from Greenland et al., 2010; World Heart Federation, American Heart Association.

Physical Therapy Examination and Data Collection of the Cardiovascular System

Pulse Should be Measured
1. Via palpation of peripheral pulse; may also be monitored throughout monitoring devices if the patient is on a cardiac unit or in acute care. See Quick Facts 4-5.
2. Palpation for 30 seconds when the pulse is regular; if irregular, palpate 1–2 minutes. Please refer to Quick Facts 4-7 for best pulse locations for adults.

Heart Rate (HR) Parameters
1. Normal adult HR is 70 beats per minute (bpm); range 60–100 bpm.
2. Pediatric: Newborn average is 120 bpm; normal range 70–170 bpm.
3. Tachycardia: >100 bpm. Exercise commonly results in tachycardia. Compensatory tachycardia can be seen with volume loss (surgery, dehydration).
4. Bradycardia: <60 bpm.

Pulse Abnormalities
1. Irregular pulse: Variations in force and frequency; may be due to arrhythmias, myocarditis.
2. Weak, thready pulse: May be due to low stroke volume, cardiogenic shock.
3. Bounding, full pulse: May be due to shortened ventricular systole and decreased peripheral pressure; aortic insufficiency.

Heart Sounds

Auscultation
1. The process of listening for sounds within the body by placing a stethoscope directly on the anterior or posterior chest (see Table 4-2).

> **QUICK FACTS 4-5 ▶ MEASURING THE PULSE**
>
> The pulse is influenced by:
> - The force of cardiac contraction
> - Volume and viscosity of blood
> - Diameter and elasticity of vessels
> - Emotions
> - Exercise blood temperature
> - Hormones
>
> **SPECIAL CONSIDERATIONS** when measuring the pulse:
> - Palpate pulses only using fingertips; do not use the thumb.
> - Rate of perceived exertion scale may be more appropriate than HR as measure of actual work if the patient/client is taking beta blocking or calcium blocking medications (Quick Facts 4.6).

2. Clinician notes intensity and quality of heart sounds.
3. Performed by the PT during examination and evaluation. May also be performed by the PTA in the course of intervention.

Auscultation Landmarks
1. Aortic valve: Locate the second right intercostal space at the sternal border.
2. Pulmonic valve: Locate the second left intercostal space at the sternal border.
3. Tricuspid valve: Locate the fourth left intercostal space at the sternal border.
4. Mitral valve: Locate the fifth left intercostal space at the midclavicular area.

Table 4-2

Heart Sounds

SOUND	HEART ACTION	INDICATES
S1 Sound ("lub")	• Normal closure of mitral and tricuspid valves • Marks beginning of systole	• Will be decreased in first-degree heart block
S2 Sound ("dub")	• Normal closure of aortic and pulmonary valves • Marks end of systole	• Decreased in aortic stenosis
Murmurs: Extra Sounds	• Systolic: Falls between S1 and S2 • Diastolic: Falls between S2 and S1 • Grades of: Grade 1 (softest audible murmur) to grade 6 (audible with stethoscope off the chest)	• May indicate valvular disease (e.g., mitral valve prolapse) or may be normal • Usually indicates valvular disease
Thrill	• An abnormal tremor accompanying a vascular or cardiac murmur; felt on palpation	
Bruit	• An adventitious sound or murmur (blowing sound) of arterial or venous origin • Common in carotid or femoral arteries	• Indicative of atherosclerosis
Gallop Rhythm	• An abnormal heart rhythm with three sounds in each cycle • Resembles the gallop of a horse	• Increased fluid • May be uncomplicated, or indicate congestive heart failure

Electronic Measurement of Heart Rhythm

Continuous Monitoring
1. An inpatient is typically continuously monitored while on the unit. This is usually set up by the nursing staff or medical team.
2. An outpatient is typically monitored during cardiac rehabilitation. Typically this is set up by the physical therapist or medical team monitoring exercise training.
3. If the patient attached to an ECG, PTAs must be able to review the heart rhythm to identify the rhythm and recognize patterns that limit intervention.

Measured Electrocardiogram (ECG)
1. A 12-lead ECG provides information about:
   a. Rate.
   b. Rhythm.
   c. Conduction.
   d. Areas of ischemia and infarct.
   e. Hypertrophy.
   f. Electrolyte imbalances.

Normal Cardiac Cycle
1. Normal sinus rhythm. (See Figure 4-4.)
2. P wave: Atrial depolarization.
3. P-R interval: Time required for impulse to travel from atria through conduction system to Purkinje fibers.
4. QRS wave: Ventricular depolarization.
5. ST segment: Beginning of ventricular repolarization.
6. T wave: Ventricular repolarization.
7. QT interval: Time for electrical systole.

To Calculate Heart Rate
1. Count number of intervals between QRS complexes in a 6-second strip and multiply by 10.

Assess Rhythm
1. Regular or irregular.

Identify Arrhythmias (Dysrhythmias)
1. Abnormal, disordered rhythms.
2. Etiology: Ischemic conditions of the myocardium, electrolyte imbalance, acidosis or alkalosis, hypoxemia, hypotension, emotional stress, drugs, alcohol, caffeine.

Blood Pressure (B/P)

Performed by the PT and PTA
1. Before initiating interventions with all patients to ensure each patient is physiologically appropriate for the intervention.

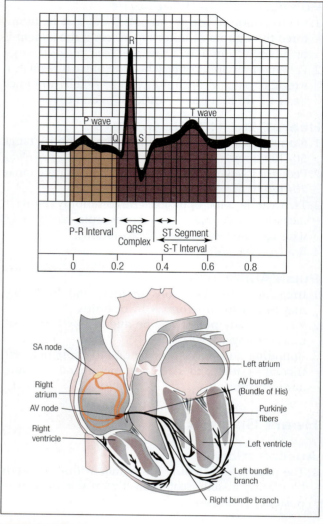

Figure 4-4 Conduction pathways of the heart.

2. During the intervention to monitor the patient's physiologic response for patients with cardiovascular or pulmonary conditions and with interventions that target those systems.
3. After completion of the intervention to determine the patient's response to the intervention.

SPECIAL CONSIDERATION: Both the PT and the PTA must recognize B/P norms as well as appropriate and inappropriate changes based upon the intervention with the patient/client. They must be prepared to react quickly to emergency situations.

Blood Pressure Measurements
1. B/P definitions and classifications for the adult and pediatric patient can be found in Table 4-3 and Table 4-4.
2. Be aware that the majority of patients with hypertension are asymptomatic.
3. Hypotension: A decrease in B/P below normal.

Table 4-3

2017 ACC/AHA Blood Pressure Guidelines*

	BP, mm Hg		
	SYSTOLIC		DIASTOLIC
Normal	< 120		< 80
Elevated	120–129	and	< 80
Stage 1	130–139	or	80–89
Stage 2	at least 140	or	at least 90
Hypertensive crisis	> 180	and/or	> 120

*2017 ACC/AHA Guideline for the Prevention, Detection, Evaluation, and Management of High Blood Pressure in Adults. J Amer C Cardiology, 71(19), May 2017.

Table 4-4

Pediatric Blood Pressure by Age (mm Hg)

AGE	SYSTOLIC BP	DIASTOLIC BP
Neonate (96 hr)	67–84	35–53
Infant (1–12 mo)	72–104	37–56
Toddler (1–2 yr)	86–106	42–63
Preschooler (3–5 yr)	89–112	46–72
School-age (6–9 yr)	97–115	57–76
Preadolescent (10–11 yr)	102–120	61–80
Adolescent (12–15 yr)	110–131	64–83

Novak C and Gill P. Pediatric Vital Signs Reference Chart. PedsCases.com. April 21, 2016.

  a. B/P is not adequate for normal perfusion/oxygenation of tissues.
  b. May be related to bed rest, drugs, arrhythmias, blood loss/shock or myocardial infarction (MI).
4. Orthostatic hypotension: Sudden drop in B/P that accompanies change in position.
  a. Common symptoms include lightheadedness, dizziness, and loss of balance.
  b. Drop in systolic B/P of >20 mm Hg or standing B/P <100 mm Hg systolic B/P is significant and should be reported.
  c. Measure by taking B/P in lying position (5 minutes). Repeat B/P at 1 and 3 minutes after moving into standing or sitting position.

Respiration

Should be Monitored
1. By the PT or PTA before initiating interventions with all patients to ensure each patient is physiologically appropriate for the intervention.
2. During the intervention to monitor the patient's physiologic response for patients with cardiovascular or pulmonary conditions and with interventions that target those systems.
3. After completion of the intervention to determine the patient's response to the intervention.

Determine Rate, Depth of Breathing
1. Normal adult respiratory rate (RR) is 12–20 breaths per minute.
2. Pediatric: Newborn RR is between 30 and 60 breaths per minute.
3. Tachypnea: An increase in rate of breathing, >20 breaths per minute.
4. Hyperpnea: An increase in depth and rate of breathing.

Dyspnea: Shortness of Breath
1. Dyspnea on exertion (DOE): Brought on by exercise or activity (see Table 4-5).
2. Orthopnea: Inability to breathe when in a reclining position.
3. Paroxysmal nocturnal dyspnea (PND): Sudden inability to breathe occurring during sleep.
4. Auscultation of the lungs: Assess respiratory sounds.
  a. Normal breath sounds.
  b. Assess for adventitious (unusual) sounds.
    • Crackles (rales): Rattling, bubbling sounds; may be due to secretions in the lungs.
    • Wheezes: Whistling sounds.
5. Assess cough: Productive or nonproductive.

Measure Oxygen Saturation

Should be Measured
1. By the PT or PTA before initiating interventions with patients who have cardiovascular and/or pulmonary conditions to ensure the patient is physiologically appropriate for the intervention.

Table 4-5

Borg Modified Dyspnea Scale (Borg 1982)	
0	Nothing at all
0.5	Very, very slight (just noticeable)
1	Very slight
2	Slight
3	Moderate
4	Somewhat severe
5–6	Severe
7–8	Very severe
9	Very, very severe (almost maximal)
10	Maximal

2. During the intervention to monitor the patient's physiologic response for patients.
3. After completion of the intervention to determine the patient's response to the intervention.

Pulse Oximetry Method
1. Is an electronic device that measures the degree of saturation of hemoglobin with oxygen (SaO_2). The device is typically clamped lightly over a finger.
2. Provides an estimate of PaO_2 based on the oxyhemoglobin desaturation curve.
   a. Normal oxygen saturation is 98%, with no change during activity or exercise.
   b. Hypoxemia: Abnormally low amount of oxygen in the blood.
   c. Hypoxia: Low oxygen level in the tissues.
3. Terminate activity if oxygen saturation drops below 90% for a healthy individual or below 86% for an individual with chronic lung disease.

Assess Pain

Should be Measured
1. By the PT and PTA before, during and after intervention.
2. Assessment method can include: Pain scale (0–10 with 10 being worst; observe facial expressions).
3. It is important to understand that chest pain may be cardiac or noncardiac in origin.

Ischemic Cardiac Pain
1. May present as diffuse, retrosternal pain, or a sensation of tightness or achiness in the chest.
2. Is often associated with dyspnea, sweating, indigestion, dizziness, syncope, anxiety.
3. Angina: Sudden or gradual onset; occurs at rest or with activity; precipitated by physical or emotional factors, hot or cold temperatures; relieved by rest or nitroglycerin. See Quick Facts 4-6.
4. Myocardial infarction pain: Sudden onset; pain lasts for more than 30 minutes; may have no precipitating factors; not relieved by medications.

QUICK FACTS 4-6 ▶ ANGINA SCALE
Anginal scale:
1+ light, barely noticeable
2+ moderate, bothersome
3+ severe, very uncomfortable
4+ most severe pain ever experienced

Referred Pain
1. Cardiac pain can refer to shoulders, arms, neck or jaw.
2. Pain referred to the back can occur from dissecting aortic aneurysm.

RED FLAG: Any complaints of pain resembling ischemic or referred symptoms should always be immediately regarded and reported to the appropriate individuals (e.g., physical therapist, nurse, physician).

Physical Examination: Peripheral Vascular System

The PTA Must be Able to
1. Perform vascular system tests and measures to determine the patient's current cardiac condition.
2. Read and understand medical documentation. Recognize implications of test results and use this information to guide decisions for intervention.
3. Monitor vascular response throughout physical therapy interventions.
4. Educate the patient/family throughout the rehabilitation process.
5. Use information from the data collection process to progress patient interventions within the plan of care.
6. Differentiate appropriate and adverse responses and report to the physical therapist.

Examine Condition of Extremities
1. Observe for changes in tissue.
   a. Diaphoresis: Excess sweating associated with decreased cardiac output.
   b. Observe skin color; use color changes to determine patient's response to intervention. See Quick Facts 4-8.
   c. Observe common skin changes associated with some cardiovascular conditions. See Quick Facts 4-9.
2. Palpate skin temperature; decrease in superficial skin temperature is associated with poor arterial perfusion.
3. Palpate and document arterial pulses.
   a. Best practice is to check bilaterally. See Quick Facts 4-7 for locations.
   b. Note appropriate pulse grade. See Quick Facts 4-10.

Monitor for Intermittent Claudication
1. Intermittent claudication (IC): pain, cramping, and lower extremity fatigue occurring during exercise and relieved by rest; associated with PAD.
2. IC pain is typically in calf; may also be in thigh, hips, or buttocks.
3. Patient may experience pain at rest with severe decrease in arterial blood supply; typically forefoot, worse at night.

Physical Therapy Examination and Data Collection of the Cardiovascular System 151

QUICK FACTS 4-7 ▶ PULSE LOCATIONS

Pulse	Pulse Location	Illustration
Apical pulse or point of maximal impulse (PMI)	Patient is supine; palpate at fifth interspace, midclavicular vertical line (apex of the heart; may be displaced upward by pregnancy or high diaphragm; may be displaced laterally in congestive heart failure, cardiomyopathy, ischemic heart disease).	
Radial	Palpate radial artery, radial wrist at base of thumb; most common monitoring site.	
Carotid	Patient is lying down with head of bed elevated; palpate over carotid artery, on either side of anterior neck between sternocleidomastoid muscle and trachea. • Assess one side at a time to reduce the risk of bradycardia through stimulation of the carotid sinus baroreceptor, which produces a reflex drop in pulse rate or B/P.	
Brachial	Palpate over brachial artery, medial aspect of the antecubital fossa; used to monitor B/P. Best in infants.	
Femoral	Palpate over femoral artery in inguinal region.	
Popliteal	Palpate over popliteal artery, behind the knee with the knee slightly flexed.	
Posterior Tibial	Palpate the posterior tibial pulse posterior, and slightly inferior, to the medial malleolus.	

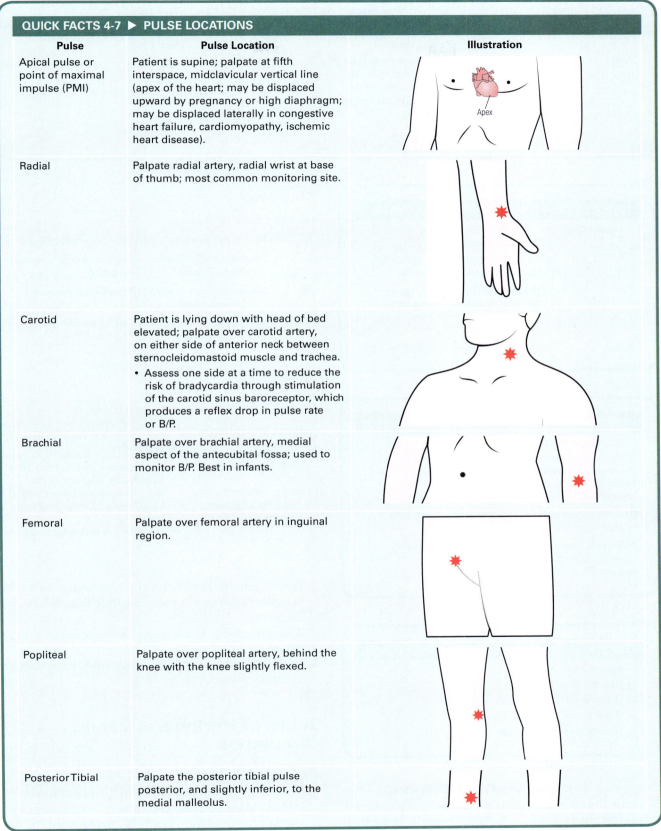

(Continued)

QUICK FACTS 4-7 ▶ PULSE LOCATIONS (Continued)

Pulse	Pulse Location	Illustration
Pedal	Palpate the dorsalis pedis artery on the dorsal surface of the foot, distal to the dorsal most prominence of the navicular bone (lateral to the extensor hallucis longus tendon).	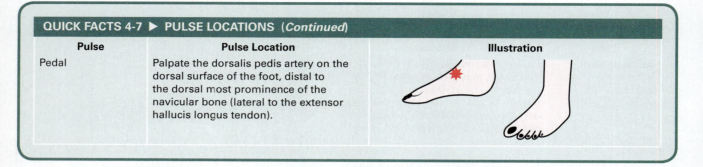

QUICK FACTS 4-8 ▶ SKIN COLOR CHANGES

Terminology	Description
Cyanosis	Bluish color related to decreased cardiac output or cold, especially lips, fingertips, nail beds
Pallor	Absence of rosy color in light-skinned individuals, associated with decreased peripheral blood flow, PVD
Rubor	Dependent redness with PVD

QUICK FACTS 4-9 ▶ CONDITIONS OBSERVED

Skin Change	Associated With
Clubbing: Curvature of the fingernails with soft tissue enlargement at base of nail	Associated with chronic oxygen deficiency, heart failure
Pale, shiny, dry skin with loss of hair	Associated with PVD
Abnormal pigmentation, ulceration, dermatitis, gangrene	Associated with PVD

QUICK FACTS 4-10 ▶ PULSE GRADING SCALE

- 4+ Bounding, very strong
- 3+ Normal, easy to palpate
- 2+ Diminished, palpable but not normal
- 1+ Weak pulse, difficult to palpate
- 0 Absent, unable to palpate

Table 4-6

Grading Scale for Edema

1+	Mild, barely perceptible indentation; < ¼ inch pitting
2+	Moderate, easily identified depression; returns to normal within 15 seconds; ¼–½ inch pitting
3+	Severe, depression takes 15–30 seconds to rebound; ½–1 inch pitting
4+	Very severe, depression lasts for > 30 seconds or more; > 1 inch pitting

Table 4-7

Guidelines for Circumferential Measurements

FOR THE BEST OUTCOMES MEASURE	TECHNIQUE
• With patient in same position • At the same time of day • Using the same rater (interrater reliability)	• Measurements must be taken using reproducible bony landmarks (e.g., "2 inches distal from head of fibula" versus "2 inches below the knee"). • Use tension-controlling tape measure.

2. Pitting edema (indentation): Depression is maintained when finger is pressed firmly into tissues. See Table 4-6.
3. Bilateral edema is associated with congestive heart failure.
4. Unilateral edema is associated with local factors, thrombophlebitis, PVD.

Tests of Peripheral Venous Circulation

Percussion Test

1. Determines competence of greater saphenous vein
    a. In standing, palpate one segment of vein while percussing vein approximately 20 cm higher.
    b. If pulse wave is felt by lower hand, the intervening valves are incompetent.

Observe for and Measure Edema

1. Check girth measurements using a tape or volumetric measurements using a volumeter (more accurate than girth measurements; useful with irregular body parts, such as hand or foot) (see Table 4-7).

Trendelenburg's Test
1. Retrograde filling test.
2. Determines competence of communicating veins and saphenous system.
3. Patient is positioned supine with legs elevated to 60 degrees (empties venous blood).
4. Tourniquet is then placed on proximal thigh (occludes venous flow in the superficial veins).
5. Patient is then asked to stand.
6. Examiner notes if veins fill in normal pattern; should take approximately 30 seconds.

Doppler Ultrasound
1. Examination using an ultrasonic oscillator connected to earphones.
   a. The physical therapist assistant would not be responsible to perform this test, though should understand what it is.
   b. Determines blood flow within a vessel; useful in both venous and arterial disease.
   c. Doppler probe placed over large vessel; ultrasound signal given transcutaneously; movement of blood causes an audible shift in signal frequency.
   d. Useful in locating nonpalpable pulses, measuring systolic B/P in extremities.

Air Plethysmography (APG)
1. Pneumatic device calibrated to measure patency of venous system; volume.

Tests of Peripheral Arterial Circulation

PTA may rarely perform these tests, however should be aware of these tests as the patient can be monitored for these conditions during therapeutic activities.

Rubor of Dependency
1. Check color changes in skin during elevation of foot followed by dependency (seated, hanging position).
2. With insufficiency, pallor develops in elevated position; reactive hyperemia (rubor of dependency) develops in dependent position.
3. Changes that take longer than 30 seconds are also indicative of arterial insufficiency.

Venous Filling Time
1. Checks time necessary to refill veins after emptying. With patient supine, leg elevated about 60° for 1 minute, then placed in dependent position. Note time for veins to refill.
2. Greater than 10–15 seconds is indicative of arterial insufficiency.

Intermittent Claudication
1. Defined: Pain or cramping in the legs that is absent at rest. This is usually calf pain, but may also occur in buttock, hip, thigh or foot.
2. Have the patient walk on level grade, 1 mile/hour (e.g., treadmill). Test is stopped with claudicatory pain.
3. Note time of test. Use subjective ratings of pain to classify degree of claudication. (See Quick Facts 4-11.)
4. Check for coldness, numbness or pallor in the legs or feet; loss of hair over anterior tibial area.
5. Leg cramps may also result from diuretic use with hypokalemia.

Examine Lymphatic System

1. Palpate superficial lymph nodes: Cervical, axillary, epitrochlear, superficial inguinal.
2. Inspect for and measure edema. The PTA may perform and record these procedures.
   a. Visual inspection: Note swelling, decreased range of motion, loss of functional mobility.
   b. Check girth measurements. (See previous section.)
3. Paresthesias may be present.
4. Lymphangiography (x-ray of lymph vessels) using radioactive agents.
   a. Medical examination, not performed by physical therapy clinicians.
   b. Provides information about lymph flow, lymph node uptake and backflow.

Cardiovascular Diagnostic Tests

1. Physical therapist assistants (PTAs) should have an understanding of diagnostic tests to understand what the physician is attempting to diagnose. This understanding should provide a basis to enhance and guide interventions while providing a background for any precautions or treatment considerations. The PTA should also be able to provide a brief explanation to the patient/client (Table 4-8).

QUICK FACTS 4-11 ▶ SUBJECTIVE PAIN RATINGS WITH INTERMITTENT CLAUDICATION

Grade I: Minimal discomfort or pain

Grade II: Moderate discomfort or pain; patient's attention can be diverted

Grade III: Intense pain; patient's attention cannot be diverted

Grade IV: Excruciating and unbearable pain

Table 4-8

Cardiovascular Diagnostic Tests

TEST	USED TO DETECT	CONSIDERATIONS
Chest X-Ray	Lung overall condition: Cancer, air around lung space (pneumothorax), emphysema, cystic fibrosis, calcium deposits Impact on lung from other condition: Pulmonary edema may be due to congestive heart failure, size of heart—increase could indicate heart stress or failure Blood vessels: Larger vessels (aorta, pulmonary arteries/veins), calcium deposits Fractures: Rib, sternum Other objects: View placement of pacemaker/defibrillator and/or associated leads, chest catheter	• While this test is noninvasive, there is some exposure to radiation.
Electrocardiogram (EKG, ECG)	Records electrical activity: Reveal rhythm (normal, arrhythmia), conduction delay, and coronary perfusion Stress test (Exercise Tolerance Test [ETT], Graded Exercise Test): Completed in a clinical setting using EKG; monitors cardiac response under increasing levels of physical activity stress. Used to detect coronary artery disease and determine safe levels of exercise stress	• Monitored in-room or via telemetry (radio transmission) • Allows continuous monitoring during intervention • Can provide exercise guidelines following cardiac procedure
Monitor or Recorder	Portable, battery powered devices worn by patients over a short period of time, several days to weeks, to monitor activity. Unit is returned to physician following assessment to be read and evaluated. Holter monitor: Records heartbeats and rhythm over 24–48 hours during normal activities Event recorder: Similar to Holter monitor, is configured with a button the patient presses as soon as possible if/when they have symptoms	• Patients may have unit affixed as PT interventions are occurring; use caution during electro-physiologic interventions.
Echocardiogram (Echo)	Utilizes ultrasound: Used to visualize internal structures of the heart: chambers, valves, septum, and heart wall movement Measures function: Visualizes and measures valve and pumping function. Measures ejection fraction (EF) of ventricle during systole	• Average EF is 55–70% (65% indicates 65% of available blood in left ventricle is pumped out during systole).
Myocardial Perfusion Imaging	Ischemic areas of the heart: Images areas of ischemia, infarct, myocardial blood flow, areas of stress-induced ischemia	• Can visualize areas of old infarct
Cardiac Catheterization (Coronary Angiogram, or Cath)	Physician conducts exam: Used to evaluate function and make treatment decisions. Small catheter inserted through a large artery to heart (via upper leg/groin, neck, upper arm). Measures pressures (central venous pressure, pulmonary artery pressure, etc.) Moving x-ray images captured to evaluate: Narrowing in arteries, size of heart chambers, pumping action of heart, valve operation, pressures within heart chambers and arteries Measures: B/P within the heart, oxygen concentrations Stent: Angioplasty with stenting may be completed during this procedure.	• Invasive exam, dye is injected into arteries • Requires insertion of a central line • 2–3 hour physician procedure

Laboratory Tests and Values

See Table 4-9

1. Enzyme changes associated with myocardial infarction (Thygesen et al, 2012).
2. Rise and fall of cardiac troponin (I or T) >99th percentile is the primary measure of myocardial infarction. It must accompany one of the following:
   a. Symptoms of ischemia.
   b. New or presumed new ST changes on ECG.
   c. Development of pathological Q waves on ECG.
   d. New loss of viable myocardium and/or new wall motion abnormality on imaging.
   e. Evidence of intracoronary thrombus via catheterization or autopsy.
3. Elevation of CK or CPK (serum creatine kinase or creatine phosphokinase) with concomitant elevation of CK-MB (serum creatine kinase MB) can also be assessed, but peaks between 12–24 hours.

Serum Lipids

1. Serum lipids panel: used to determine coronary risk. (See Table 4-1.)

Table 4-9

Laboratory Tests and Values

NORMAL VALUES	CLINICAL SIGNIFICANCE
Arterial Blood Gases (ABGs)	
SpO_2 98%–100%	SaO_2 below 88%–90% usually requires supplemental O_2
PaO_2 90–100 mm Hg	↑ in hyperoxygenation ↓ in cardiac decompensation, COPD, and some neuromuscular disorders
$PaCO_2$ 35–45 mm Hg	↑ in COPD, hypoventilation ↓ in hyperventilation, pregnancy, pulmonary embolism, and anxiety
pH, whole blood 7.35–7.45	<7.35 is acidotic, >7.45 is alkalotic ↑ in respiratory alkalosis: hyperventilation, sepsis, liver disease, fever ↑ in metabolic alkalosis: vomiting, potassium depletion, diuretics, volume depletion ↓ in respiratory acidosis: hypoventilation, COPD, respiratory depressants, myasthenia ↓ in metabolic acidosis (bicarbonate deficit): increased acids (diabetes, alcohol, starvation); renal failure, increased acid intake, and loss of alkaline body fluids
Hemostasis (Clotting/Bleeding Times)	
Prothrombin time (PT) 11–15 sec	↑ in factor X deficiency, hemorrhagic disease, cirrhosis, hepatitis drugs (warfarin)
Partial thromboplastin time (PTT) 25–40 sec	↑ in factor VIII, IX, and X deficiency
International normalized ratio (INR): Ratio of individual's PT to reference range 0.9–1.1 (ratio)	Patients with deep vein thrombosis (DVT), pulmonary embolism (PE), mechanical valves, atrial fibrillation (AF) on anticoagulation therapy will have target INRs 2–3. Patients with these conditions and/or genetic clotting disorders may have a target INR 3.5. Look for active signs of bleeding when treating these patients and use compensatory strategies to reduce fall risk.
Bleeding time 2–10 min C-reactive protein (CRP) <10 mg/L	↑ in platelet disorders, thrombocytopenia ↑ levels associated with ↑ risk of atherosclerosis >100 mg/L associated with inflammation and infection
Complete Blood Cell Count (CBC), Adult Values	
White Blood Cells (WBCs) 4300–10,800 cells/mm³	Indicative of status of immune system ↑ in infection: bacterial, viral; inflammation, hematologic malignancy, leukemia, lymphoma, drugs (corticosteroids) ↓ in aplastic anemia, B_{12} or folate deficiency With immunosuppression: ↑ risk of infection *Physical therapy considerations:* Consider metabolic demands in presence of fever and use of mask when WBCs <1000–2000 or Absolute Neutrophil Count (ANC) <500–1000
Red Blood Cells (RBCs) Male: 4.6–6.2 10^6/uL Female: 4.2–5.9 10^6/uL	↑ in polycythemia ↓ in anemia
Erythrocyte sedimentation rate (ESR) Male <15 mm/hr Female <20 mm/hr	↑ in infection and inflammation: rheumatic or pelvic inflammatory disease, osteomyelitis Used to monitor effects of treatment; e.g., RA, SLE, Hodgkin's disease
Hematocrit (Hct) % of RBC of the whole blood Male 45%–52% Female 37%–48% (age dependent)	↑ in erythrocytosis, dehydration, shock ↓ in severe anemias, acute hemorrhage *Physical therapy considerations:* Can cause ↓ exercise tolerance, ↑ fatigue, and tachycardia.
Hemoglobin (Hgb) Male: 13–18 g/dL Female: 12–16 g/dL (age dependent)	↑ polycythemia, dehydration, shock ↓ in anemias, prolonged hemorrhage, RBC destruction (cancer, sickle cell disease) *Physical therapy considerations:* Can cause ↓ exercise tolerance, ↑ fatigue, and tachycardia
Platelet count 150,000–450,000 cells/mm³	↑ chronic leukemia, hemoconcentration ↓ thrombocytopenia, acute leukemia, aplastic anemia, cancer chemotherapy *Physical therapy considerations:* Increased risk of bleeding with low levels so monitor for hematuria, petechiae, and other signs of active bleeding. <20,000: AROM, ADLs only 20,000–30,000: light exercise only 30,000–50,000: moderate exercise

Adapted from Hopkins T; Lab Notes, 2nd Ed. Philadelphia, FA Davis, 2009.

Signs and Symptoms of Cardiovascular Disease

> **RED FLAG:** When treating patients the physical therapist assistant should be aware of these general signs and symptoms of cardiovascular compromise. The PTA must observe for these signs and symptoms, recognize them as potential adverse changes, modify interventions, and notify the physical therapist as appropriate. See Table 4-10.

Chest Pain or Discomfort

1. Described as a tightness or pressure sensation in the chest.
2. Systemic complaints:
   a. May or may not be cardiac related.
   b. Can include chest pain that radiates to the neck, jaw, shoulder or upper trap area, upper back or arms (most common left arm).
3. Symptoms may also include:
   a. Nausea or vomiting.
   b. Diaphoresis (sweating).
   c. Dyspnea.
   d. Fatigue.
   e. Pallor.
   f. Some may mistake this as indigestion.
   g. May also be accompanied by weakness.

Palpitations

1. An irregular or very fast heartbeat.
2. Can indicate severe conditions such as:
   a. Coronary artery disease (CAD).
   b. Cardiomyopathy.
   c. Heart block.
   d. Ventricular aneurysm.
   e. Atrioventricular valve disease.
   f. Mitral stenosis or aortic stenosis.
   g. It should also be noted that palpitations may be the result of conditions that are not cardiac related (e.g., anxiety, caffeine intake).
3. May be described as a bump, thud, flutter, butterfly, a sensation of the heart racing.
4. The patient may complain of syncope or lightheadedness.
5. Palpation reveals a skipped beat, rapid pulse, irregular pulse.

Dyspnea

1. Shortness of breath, breathlessness.
2. Can be the result of cardiac or pulmonary conditions or other, non-life-threatening conditions.

Table 4-10

Signs and Symptoms of Cardiovascular Compromise

SIGNS AND SYMPTOMS	QUALITY
Chest pain	May be described as tightness or pressure May radiate: neck, jaw, shoulder, upper trapezius area, upper back, arms
Nausea	Vomiting may occur. Antacids may be taken to try and calm nausea.
Diaphoresis	Secondary to activation of the sympathetic nervous system
Dyspnea	May occur at rest or with exertion; termed dyspnea on exertion (DOE)
Fatigue	Is out of proportion to amount of activity or work performed
Pallor or Cyanosis	Due to decreased pumping ability of the heart
Syncope	Transient loss of consciousness due to heart's impaired pumping ability
Palpitations	May describe as a bumping, thud, flutter or a feeling of heart racing Palpation will reveal a fast heartbeat; it may be regular or irregular.
Peripheral edema	Typically seen bilaterally; secondary to failure of the right heart
Claudication	May complain of pain or cramping in the lower extremities Secondary to peripheral vascular disease

3. Dyspnea on exertion (DOE).
   a. Can be caused by left ventricular impairment, resulting in increased congestion of blood in the pulmonary system.
   b. In the case of severe involvement, dyspnea may occur at rest as well.
   c. Dyspnea increases as the severity of the pathology increases.

Cardiac Syncope

1. Lightheadedness or fainting.
2. Caused by a reduction in oxygen supply to brain secondary to impairment of the heart's pumping ability.
3. Conditions that may contribute to cardiac syncope.
   a. Arrhythmias (e.g., ventricular tachycardia).
   b. Orthostatic hypotension.
   c. CAD.
   d. Vertebral artery insufficiency.
   e. Hypoglycemia.

Fatigue

1. Tiredness out of proportion to activity or the work performed.

Cyanosis

1. The appearance of blue or purple coloration of the skin or mucous membranes.
2. Due to the tissues near the skin surface being low on oxygen.
3. Often accompanied with cardiac involvement.
4. Can also be associated with dysfunction of other systems.

Peripheral Edema

1. Commonly associated with right ventricular dysfunction or failure.
2. Typically occurs bilaterally.

Claudication

1. Cramping in the legs, leg pain.
2. Result of peripheral vascular disease (venous or arterial).
3. Can significantly limit ability to perform ADLs by limiting tolerance to standing and walking.

Cardiovascular Disease: Evaluation, Diagnosis, and Prognosis

Atherosclerosis

Characteristics
1. Disease of lipid-laden plaques (lesions) affecting moderate and large-size arteries.
2. Thickening and narrowing of the intimal layer of the blood vessel wall from focal accumulation of lipids, platelets, monocytes, plaque, and other debris.

Risk Factors (See Table 4-1)

Acute Coronary Syndrome (ACS) (Coronary Artery Disease)

Characteristics
1. Involves a spectrum of clinical entities ranging from angina to infarction to sudden cardiac death.
2. An imbalance of myocardial oxygen supply and demand resulting in ischemic chest pain.
3. Symptoms present when lumen is at least 70% occluded.
4. Three common presentations, but may also have silent ischemia diagnosed by presence of a new pathologic Q wave on ECG. Most common in patients with diabetes, patients may have ischemia without any symptoms. Subacute occlusions may also produce no symptoms.

Angina Pectoris
1. Chest pain or pressure due to ischemia; may be accompanied by Levine's sign (patient clenches fist over sternum).
2. Represents imbalance in myocardial oxygen supply and demand; brought on by:
   a. Increased demands on heart: exertion, emotional stress, smoking, extremes of temperature, especially cold, overeating, tachyarrhythmias.
   b. Vasospasm: symptoms may be present at rest.

3. Three major types of angina.
   a. Stable angina: classic exertional angina occurring during exercise or activity; occurs at a predictable rate-pressure product, RPP (HR × BP), relieved with rest and/or nitroglycerin.
   b. Unstable angina (preinfarction, crescendo angina): coronary insufficiency at any time without any precipitating factors or exertion. Chest pain increases in severity, frequency, and duration; refractory to treatment. Increases risk for myocardial infarction or lethal arrhythmia; pain is difficult to control.
   c. Variant angina (Prinzmetal's angina): caused by vasospasm of coronary arteries in the absence of occlusive disease. Responds well to nitroglycerin or calcium channel blocker long term.
4. Women more often describe sensations of discomfort, crushing, pressing, and bad ache when referring to angina.
5. With angina, patients often describe shortness of breath, fatigue, diaphoresis, and weakness as symptoms of ACS.
6. Older adults present more often with atypical symptoms (absence of chest pain): dyspnea, diaphoresis, nausea and vomiting, and syncope.

Myocardial Infarction (MI) (See Figure 4-5)

1. Prolonged ischemia, injury, and death of an area of the myocardium caused by occlusion of one or more of the coronary arteries.
2. Precipitating factors: atherosclerotic heart disease with thrombus formation, coronary vasospasm, or embolism; cocaine use.
3. Zones of infarction.
   a. Zone of infarction: consists of necrotic, noncontractile tissue; electrically inert; on ECG, see pathological Q waves.
   b. Zone of injury: area immediately adjacent to central zone, tissue is noncontractile, cells undergoing metabolic changes; electrically unstable; on ECG, see elevated ST segments in leads over injured area.
   c. Zone of ischemia: outer area, cells also undergoing metabolic changes, electrically unstable; on ECG, see T wave inversion.
4. Infarction sites.
   a. Transmural: full thickness of myocardium, which is often an ST elevated MI (STEMI) or Q wave MI.
   b. Nontransmural: subendocardial, subepicardial, intramural infarctions. Non-ST elevated MI (NSTEMI) or non-Q wave MI.
   c. Sites of coronary artery occlusion.
      - Inferior MI, right ventricle infarction, disturbances of upper conduction system: right coronary artery.
      - Lateral MI, ventricular ectopy: circumflex artery.
      - Anterior MI, disturbances of lower conduction system: left anterior descending artery.
5. Impaired ventricular function results in:
   a. Decreased stroke volume, cardiac output and ejection fraction.
   b. Increased end diastolic ventricular pressures.
6. Electrical instability: arrhythmias, present in injured and ischemic areas.

Heart Failure (HF)

1. A clinical syndrome in which the heart is unable to maintain adequate circulation of the blood to meet the metabolic needs of the body.
2. Types of heart failure. (See Quick Facts 4-12.)
   a. Left-sided heart failure (congestive heart failure, CHF): is characterized by pulmonary congestion, edema, and low cardiac output due to backup of blood from the left ventricle (LV) to the left atrium (LA) and lungs. Occurs with insult to the left ventricle from myocardial disease; excessive workload of the heart (hypertension, valvular disease or congenital defects); cardiac arrhythmias or heart damage.
   b. Right-sided heart failure: is characterized by increased pressure load on the right ventricle (RV) with higher pulmonary vascular pressures; mitral valve disease, or chronic lung disease (cor pulmonale); produces hallmark signs of jugular vein distention and peripheral edema.
   c. Biventricular failure: severe LV pathology producing back up into the lungs, increased PA pressure and RV signs of HF.

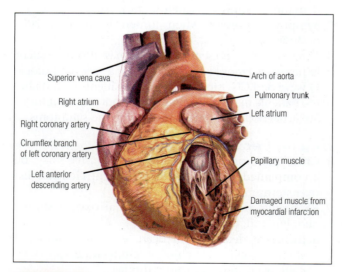

Figure 4-5 Tissue destruction in myocardial infarction.

> **QUICK FACTS 4-12 ▶ RIGHT- AND LEFT-SIDED HEART FAILURE**
>
> Left-sided heart failure (forward HF):
> - Blood is not adequately pumped into systemic circulation (pulmonary congestion); due to an inability of left ventricle to pump, increases in ventricular end-diastolic pressure and left atrial pressures
>
> Presents with:
> - Increased pulmonary artery pressures and pulmonary edema
> - Pulmonary signs and symptoms: Cough, dyspnea, orthopnea
> - Weakness, fatigue
>
> Right-sided heart failure (backward HF):
> - Blood is not adequately returned from systemic circulation to the heart; increased pressure load on the right ventricle with higher pulmonary vascular pressures
>
> Presents with:
> - Peripheral edema: Weight gain, venous stasis
> - Nausea, anorexia
> - Hallmark sign of jugular vein distension

3. Associated symptoms: muscle wasting, myopathies, osteoporosis.
4. Possible clinical manifestations of heart failure (Table 4-11).
5. Compensated heart failure: heart returns to functional status with reduced cardiac output and exercise tolerance. Control is achieved through:
   a. Physiological compensatory mechanisms: SNS stimulation, LV hypertrophy, anaerobic metabolism, cardiac dilatation, arterial vasoconstriction.
   b. Medical therapy.

Sudden Death, Usually Due to Significant Ischemia or Ventricular Arrhythmia

Hypertension

Blood Pressure

1. Measure of tension exerted against arterial walls; regulated by blood flow and peripheral vascular resistance.
2. Blood flow is determined by cardiac output.
3. B/P is determined by the resistance.
   a. Resistance is primarily determined by the diameter of blood vessels; somewhat affected by viscosity of blood.
   b. Increased peripheral resistance is the result of narrowing of arterioles.
4. Prolonged hypertension leads to decreased elasticity of arterioles.

Table 4-11

Possible Clinical Manifestations of Cardiac Failure

LEFT VENTRICULAR FAILURE	RIGHT VENTRICULAR FAILURE
Signs and symptoms of pulmonary congestion:	
Dyspnea, dry cough	Dependent edema
Orthopnea	Weight gain
Paroxysmal nocturnal dyspnea (PND)	Ascites
Pulmonary rales, wheezing	Liver engorgement (hepatomegaly)
Signs and symptoms of low cardiac output:	
Hypotension	Anorexia, nausea, bloating
Tachycardia	Cyanosis (nail beds)
Lightheadedness, dizziness	Right upper quadrant pain
Cerebral hypoxia: irritability, restlessness, confusion, impaired memory, sleep disturbances	Jugular vein distension
Fatigue, weakness	Right-sided S_3 heart sounds
Poor exercise tolerance	Murmurs of pulmonary or tricuspid insufficiency
Enlarged heart on chest x-ray	
S_3 heart sound, possibly S_4	
Murmurs of mitral or tricuspid regurgitation	

a. Elastic tissue is replaced with fibrous, collagen-based tissues that are not distensible.
b. This process increases resistance to blood flow through vessels.
c. This process also decreases blood flow to critical body tissues (kidney, heart, brain) and stimulates neurohumoral responses that increase B/P.

Clinical Manifestations
1. Hypertension is often asymptomatic, creating a significant health risk.
2. When symptoms are noticed they include:
   a. Headache.
   b. Vertigo.
   c. Flushed face.
   d. Blurred vision.
   e. Increased nocturnal urinary frequency.
   f. Increased B/P.

Medical Management

1. Prevention.
2. Diet.
   a. Follow Dietary Approaches to Stop Hypertension (DASH) diet that includes:
      - High intake of fruits, vegetables and low-fat dairy products.
      - Avoidance of processed foods (e.g., sauces, gravies, prepackaged dinners, etc.).
      - Decrease amount of sodium consumed.
3. Antihypertensive medications.
   a. These include diuretics, adrenergic blockers, vasodilators, ACE inhibitors, calcium antagonists. (See Table 4-14.)

Data Collection
1. Ongoing B/P monitoring can provide feedback regarding effectiveness of:
   a. Lifestyle modification.
   b. Medical management.
2. Use of Borg RPE Scale. (Refer to Quick Facts 4-13.)
   a. May be necessary depending upon medications used that can blunt the HR and B/P response to aerobic activity.

Physical Therapy Interventions
1. Patient education.
   a. Reinforce adherence to dietary and lifestyle modifications.
2. Initiate aerobic conditioning program gradually.
   a. Aerobic program should include exercises that primarily use the lower extremities (e.g., walking, bicycling).
      - Monitor B/P before, during and after exercise.
   b. Intensity of programs can be beneficial when started at 65%–70% of maximum heart rate and performed 3–4 times per week.
   c. Reinforce patient following medication regimen prescribed by physician.
   d. Identify possible side effects of specific medication with cardiac response.

> **QUICK FACTS 4-13 ▶ BORG RATE OF PERCEIVED EXERTION SCALE**
>
> 6 No exertion at all
> 7 Extremely light
> 8
> 9 Very light (easy walking slowly at a comfortable pace)
> 10
> 11 Light
> 12
> 13 Somewhat hard (quite an effort; patient feels tired but can continue)
> 14
> 15 Hard (heavy)
> 16
> 17 Very hard (very strenuous; patient is very fatigued)
> 18
> 19 Extremely hard (cannot continue for long at this pace)
> 20 Maximal exertion

Medical and Surgical Management of Cardiovascular Disease

Medications
1. ACE Inhibitors (e.g., captopril [capoten], enalopril [vasotec], lisinopril [zestril]): inhibit conversion of angiotension I to angiotension II, decreases Na retention and peripheral vasoconstriction in order to decrease blood pressure. (See Table 4-12.)
2. Angiotension II receptor blockers (ARBs) (e.g., losartan [cozaar]): blocks binder of angiotension II at the tissue/smooth muscle level, decreasing blood pressure.
3. Nitrates (nitroglycerin): decrease preload through peripheral vasodilation, reduce myocardial oxygen demand, reduce chest discomfort (angina); may also dilate coronary arteries, improve coronary blood flow.

Table 4-12

Medications for Cardiovascular Disease

MEDICATIONS	EFFECT
Nitrates (nitroglycerin)	• Decrease preload through peripheral vasodilation • Reduce myocardial oxygen demand • Reduce chest discomfort (angina) • May also dilate coronary arteries, improve coronary blood flow
Beta adrenergic blocking agents (e.g., propranolol/Inderal)	• Reduce myocardial demand by reducing heart rate and contractility • Control arrhythmias, chest pain • Reduce B/P
Calcium channel-blocking agents (e.g., diltiazem/Cardizem, Procardia)	• Inhibit flow of calcium ions • Decrease heart rate, decrease contractility • Dilate coronary arteries • Reduce B/P • Control arrhythmias, chest pain
Antiarrhythmics (numerous drugs, four main classes; e.g., Quinidine, Procainamide)	• Alter conductivity, restore normal heart rhythm • Control arrhythmias • Improve cardiac output
Antihypertensives (numerous drugs, four main types; [e.g., Propranolol, Reserpie])	• Control hypertension; goal is to maintain a diastolic pressure less than 90 mm Hg • Decrease afterload • Reduce myocardial oxygen demand
Digitalis (cardiac glycosides; e.g., Digoxin)	• Increases contractility and decreases heart rate • Mainstay in the treatment of CHF
Aspirin	• Decreases platelet aggregation • May prevent myocardial infarction
Tranquilizers	• Decrease anxiety • Sympathetic effects
Hypolipidemic agents (six major cholesterol-lowering drugs; e.g., Questran, Colestid, Zocor, Mevacor)	• Reduce serum lipid levels when diet and weight reduction are not effective
Thrombolytic therapy for acute myocardial infarction (e.g., Streptokinase, Tissue Plasminogen Activator [TPA], Urokinase)	• Activate the body's fibrinolytic system • Dissolve the clot • Restore coronary blood flow

4. Beta-adrenergic blocking agents (e.g., atenolol [tenormin], metoprolol [Lopressor, Toprol XL], propranolol [Inderal]): reduce myocardial demand by reducing heart rate and contractility; control arrhythmias, chest pain; reduce blood pressure.
5. Calcium channel blocking agents (e.g., diltiazem [Cardizem, Procardia], amlodipine [Norvasc]): inhibit flow of calcium ions, decrease heart rate, decrease contractility, dilate coronary arteries, reduce BP, control arrhythmias, chest pain.
6. Antiarrhythmics (numerous drugs, four main classes): alter conductivity, restore normal heart rhythm, control arrhythmias, improve cardiac output (e.g., quinidine, procainamide).
7. Digitalis (cardiac glycosides): increases contractility and decreases heart rate; mainstay in the treatment of CHF (e.g., digoxin).
8. Diuretics: decrease myocardial work (reduce preload and afterload), control hypertension, (e.g., furosemide [Lasix], hydrochlorothiazide [Esidrix]).
9. Aspirin: decreases platelet aggregation; may prevent myocardial infarction.
10. Tranquilizers: decrease anxiety, sympathetic effects.
11. Hypolipidemic agents (six major cholesterol-lowering drugs): reduce serum lipid levels when diet and weight reduction are not effective, (e.g., cholestyramine [Questran], colestipol [Colestid], simvastatin [Zocor], lovastatin [Mevacor]).

Activity Restriction

1. Acute MI: activity can be increased once the acute MI has stopped (peak in cardiac troponin levels). Activity should be limited to 5 METs or 70% of age predicted HRmax for 4–6 weeks following MI.

2. Acute heart failure: oxygen demand should not be increased in patients in acute or decompensated heart failure. Once they have been medically managed and no longer display signs of acute decompensation, their activity can be gradually increased while monitoring hemodynamic response to activity.

Surgical Interventions

1. Percutaneous transluminal coronary angioplasty (PTCA): under fluoroscopy, surgical dilation of a blood vessel using a small balloon-tipped catheter inflated inside the lumen; relieves obstructed blood flow in acute angina or acute MI; results in improved coronary blood flow, improved left ventricular function, anginal relief. (See Table 4-13.)
2. Intravascular stents: an endoprosthesis (pliable wire mesh) implanted during angioplasty to prevent restenosis and occlusion in coronary or peripheral arteries. May be coated with slow release medication to prevent more plaque buildup (drug-eluting stent, DES).
3. Coronary artery bypass graft (CABG): surgical circumvention of an obstruction in a coronary artery using an anastomosing graft (saphenous vein, internal mammary artery); multiple grafts may be necessary; results in improved coronary blood flow, improved left ventricular function, anginal relief.
4. Transplantation: used in end-stage myocardial disease; e.g., cardiomyopathy, ischemic heart disease, valvular heart disease.
   a. Heteroptics: involves leaving the natural heart and piggybacking the donor heart.
   b. Orthotopic: involves removing the diseased heart and replacing it with a donor heart.
   c. Heart and lung transplantation: involves removing both organs and replacing them with donor organs.
   d. Major problems posttransplantation are rejection, infection, complications of immunosuppressive therapy.
5. Ventricular assist device (VAD): an implanted device (accessory pump) that improves tissue perfusion and maintains cardiogenic circulation; used with severely involved patients; e.g., cardiogenic shock unresponsive to medications, severe ventricular dysfunction.

Thrombolytic Therapy

1. Administered for acute myocardial infarction.
2. Medications activate body's fibrinolytic system, dissolve clot and restore coronary blood flow, (e.g., streptokinase, tissue plasminogen activator [TPA], urokinase).

Table 4-13

Surgical Interventions for Coronary Artery Disease

SURGICAL INTERVENTION	EFFECT
Percutaneous transluminal coronary angioplasty (PTCA)	• Under fluoroscopy, surgical dilation of a blood vessel using a small balloon-tipped catheter inflated inside the lumen • Relieves obstructed blood flow in acute angina or acute MI • Results in improved coronary blood flow, improved left ventricular function, anginal relief
Intravascular stents	• An endoprosthesis (pliable wire mesh) implanted post angioplasty • Prevents restenosis and occlusion in coronary or peripheral arteries
Coronary artery bypass graft (CABG)	• Surgical circumvention of an obstruction in a coronary artery using an anastomosing graft (saphenous vein, internal mammary artery; multiple grafts may be necessary) • Results in improved coronary blood flow, improved left ventricular function, anginal relief
Transplantation	• Used in end-stage myocardial disease (e.g., cardiomyopathy, ischemic heart disease, valvular heart disease) • Heart and lung transplantation: Involves removing both organs and replacing them with donor organs • Major problems posttransplantation are rejection, infection, complications of immunosuppressive therapy
Ventricular assist device (VAD)	• An implanted device (accessory pump) that improves tissue perfusion and maintains cardiogenic circulation • Used with severely involved patients (e.g., cardiogenic shock unresponsive to medications, severe ventricular dysfunction)

Table 4-14

This table identifies common cardiac medications, their effects, and treatment considerations clinicians must keep in mind when working with patients who are taking these medications.

Common Cardiac Medications and Treatment Considerations

DRUG CATEGORY (COMMON DRUG NAMES)	EFFECTS	TREATMENT CONSIDERATIONS
ACE inhibitors • enalapril (Vasotec) • ramipril (Altace) • catopril (Capoten) • lisinopril (Prinivil, Zertril)	Decrease B/P	Watch for potential dizziness or orthostatic hypotension NSAIDs can reduce or negate the effects of these medications; monitor patients closely for elevated B/P if taking.
Anti-adrenergics • clonidine (Catapres) • guanadrel (Hylorel) • guanethidine (Ismelin) • methylodopa (Alodomet)	Decrease B/P without a selective receptor blockage	
Calcium Channel Blockers • nifedipine (Procardia, Adalat) • verapamil (Calan, Isoptin) • amlodipine (Norvasc) • diltiazem (Cardizem) • Bepridil (Vascor)	Promote vasodilation Decrease B/P and heart rate at rest and during exercise. They also help relieve anginal pain and coronary artery spasms.	Use perceived exertion scale (RPE) for monitoring physiological response to exercise May reduce blood flow to heart muscle and create ischemic response. Monitor for orthostatic hypotension
Alpha-Blockers • prazosin (Minipress) • doxazosin (Cardura) • labetalol (Trandate, Normodyne) • terazosin (Hytrin)	Decrease B/P	Monitor for signs of hypotension and reflex tachycardia; where heart rate increase to compensate for hypotension
Beta-Blockers • acebutolol (Sectral, Tenormin) • metoprolol (Lopressor, Toprol) • propranolol (Inderal) • penbutolol (Levatol)	Decrease the force of the cardiac contraction, thereby decreasing the heart rate and create decreased demands on the heart and decrease B/P	Use perceived exertion scale (RPE) for monitoring physiological response to exercise; monitoring heart rate is not useful. Watch for bradycardia and orthostatic hypotension Can worsen asthma symptoms
Diuretics • furosemide (Lasix) • digoxin (Lanoxin)	Increase B/P and heart rate at rest and during exercise to help increase cardiac contractility	Can cause fluid and electrolyte imbalances; observe patients for muscle weakness or spasms, headache, and poor coordination. Monitor for bradycardia and orthostatic hypotension
Nitrates • nitroglycerin (Nitrostat) • isosorbide dinitrate (Isordil, Diltrate)	Promote vasodilation. Increase heart rate and decrease B/P at rest	Observe for dizziness, tachycardia, and orthostatic hypotension Patients may complain of a headache.

ACE, angiotensin-converting enzyme; NSAIDs, nonsteroidal anti-inflammatory drugs; RPE, rate of perceived exertion.

Peripheral Vascular Disease: Evaluation, Diagnosis and Prognosis

Arterial Disease

Arteriosclerosis Obliterans (Atherosclerosis)

1. Chronic, occlusive arterial disease of medium and large-sized vessels.
2. The result of peripheral atherosclerosis.
3. Associated with hypertension and hyperlipidemia; patients may also exhibit CAD, cerebrovascular disease, diabetes.
4. Pulses: Decreased or absent.
5. Color: Pale on elevation, dusky red on dependency.
6. Early stages, patients exhibit intermittent claudication. Pain is described as burning, searing, aching, tightness or cramping.

7. Late stages, patients exhibit ischemia and rest pain; ulcerations and gangrene, trophic changes.
8. Affects primarily the lower extremities.
9. Differential diagnosis (see Table 4-15).

Thromboangiitis Obliterans (Buerger's Disease)

1. Chronic, inflammatory vascular occlusive disease of small arteries and also veins.
2. Occurs commonly in young adults, largely males, who smoke.
3. Begins distally and progresses proximally in both upper and lower extremities.
4. Patients exhibit paresthesias or pain, cyanotic cold extremities, diminished temperature sensation, fatigue, risk of ulceration and gangrene.

Diabetic Angiopathy

1. An inappropriate elevation of blood glucose levels and accelerated atherosclerosis.
2. Neuropathy a major problem.
3. Neurotrophic ulcers, may lead to gangrene and amputation.

Table 4-15

Wells Criteria Score for DVT

CLINICAL FINDINGS	POINTS
Active cancer (treatment ongoing, or within 6 mo or palliative)	+1
Paralysis, paresis, or recent cast immobilization of the lower extremity	+1
Bedridden recently for 3 days or longer or major surgery within 4 weeks	+1
Recently bedridden for > 3 days or major surgery < 4 wk	+1
Localized tenderness along the distribution of the deep venous system	+1
Entire leg swollen	+1
Calf swelling at least 3 cm larger than asymptomatic side	+1
Pitting edema, confined to the symptomatic leg	+1
Previously documented DVT	+1
Alternative diagnosis to DVT as likely or more likely	−2
Total Criteria Point Count	
Clinical probability of a DVT with score:	
DVT likely	≥2
DVT unlikely	<2

Wells PS, et al. *Does this patient have deep vein thrombosis?* JAMA. 2006 Jan 11; 295(2), 199–207.

Raynaud's Disease or Phenomenon

1. Episodic spasm of small arteries and arterioles.
2. Abnormal vasoconstrictor reflex exacerbated by exposure to cold or emotional stress; tips of fingers develop pallor, cyanosis, numbness and tingling.
3. Affects largely females.
4. Occlusive disease is not usually a factor.

Venous Disease

Varicose Veins

1. Distended, swollen superficial veins; tortuous in appearance.
2. May lead to varicose ulcers.

Venous Thromboembolism (VTE)

1. The formation of a blood clot in a deep vein that can lead to complications including deep vein thrombosis (DVT), pulmonary embolism (PE), or postthrombotic syndrome (PTS).
2. Mortality: incidence of 10–30% within 1 month of diagnosis.
3. Morbidity: one third experiences another VTE within 10 years.
4. Can become chronic: postthrombotic syndrome, leads to diminished quality of life.

Deep Vein Thrombophlebitis

1. Clot formation and acute inflammation in a deep vein.
2. Usually occurs in lower extremity, associated with forced immobilization (bed rest, lack of leg exercise), surgery, trauma, and hyperactivity of blood coagulation or can be unprovoked.
3. Signs and symptoms: may be asymptomatic early; progressive inflammation with tenderness to palpation; dull ache, tightness, or pain in the calf; swelling, warmth, redness, or discoloration in the lower extremity; prominent superficial veins.
4. Standardized risk assessment measure: use Wells Criteria Score for DVT (Table 4-15).
5. Medical management.
   a. Anticoagulation therapy: is used to prevent new clots from forming, prevent the existing clot from getting larger, and stabilize the clot through anti-inflammatory properties (e.g., low-molecular-weight heparin [LMWH]).
   b. LMWH is contraindicated in patients at high risk for bleeding. Patients at high risk are typically treated with unfractionated heparin [UFH].

c. Both LMWH and UFH are associated with heparin-induced thrombocytopenia (HIT) in a small percent of patients (2%–3%). HIT is associated with a paradoxical increased risk for venous and arterial thrombosis.
d. Graded compression stockings (GCS).

> **RED FLAG:** Don't use Homan's sign (dorsiflexion sign) to diagnosis DVT; though it still may be in use, it has low sensitivity and specificity and is not diagnostic of DVT.

Pulmonary Embolism
1. Presents abruptly with chest pain and dyspnea, also diaphoresis, cough, and apprehension; requires emergency treatment.
2. Life threatening: 20% with acute PE die almost immediately; 40% die within 3 months.
3. Can result in chronic thromboembolic pulmonary hypertension with reduced oxygenation and pulmonary hypertension.
4. Can lead to right heart dysfunction and failure.

Chronic Postthrombotic Syndrome
1. A combination of clinical signs and symptoms that persists after an LE DVT; thrombosis resolution is incomplete.
2. Symptoms include pain, intractable edema, limb heaviness, skin pigmentation changes, and leg ulcers.
3. Leads to reduced quality of life and impaired functional mobility.

Chronic Venous Stasis/Incompetence
1. Venous valvular insufficiency: from fibroelastic degeneration of valve tissue, venous dilation.
2. Classification:
    a. Grade I: mild aching, minimal edema, dilated superficial veins.
    b. Grade II: increased edema, multiple dilated veins, changes in skin pigmentation.
    c. Grade III: venous claudication, severe edema, cutaneous ulceration.

Differential Diagnosis of Peripheral Vascular Diseases (See Table 4-16)

Table 4-16

Differential Diagnosis: Peripheral Vascular Diseases

	CHRONIC ARTERIAL INSUFFICIENCY	CHRONIC VENOUS INSUFFICIENCY
Etiology	Atherosclerosis Thrombosis Emboli Inflammatory process	Thrombophlebitis Trauma Vein obstruction (clot) Vein incompetence
Risk factors	Age: > 60 years Smoking Diabetes mellitus Gender: slightly higher in men Dyslipidemia Hypertension Hyperhomocysteinemia Race (African American)	Venous hypertension Varicose veins Inherited trait Gender: female Age Increased BMI Sedentary lifestyle/prolonged sitting Ligamentous laxity
Signs and symptoms: determined by location and degree of vascular involvement		
Pain	Severe muscle ischemia/intermittent claudication Worse with exercise, relieved by rest Rest pain indicates severe involvement Muscle fatigue, cramping, numbness Paresthesias over time	Minimal to moderate steady pain Aching pain in lower leg with prolonged standing or sitting (dependency) Superficial pain along course of vein
Location of pain	Usually calf, lower leg, or dorsum of foot May occur in thigh, hip, or buttock	Muscle compartment tenderness
Vascular	Decreased or absent pulses Pallor of forefoot on elevation Dependent rubor	Venous dilatation or varicosity Edema: moderate to severe, especially after prolonged dependency

(Continued)

Table 4-16

Differential Diagnosis: Peripheral Vascular Diseases (*Continued*)

	CHRONIC ARTERIAL INSUFFICIENCY	CHRONIC VENOUS INSUFFICIENCY
Skin changes	Pale, shiny, dry skin Loss of hair Nail changes Coolness of extremity	Hemosiderin deposition: dark, cyanotic, thickened, brown skin Lipodermatosclerosis: fibrosing of the subcutaneous tissue May lead to stasis dermatitis, cellulitis
Acute	Acute arterial obstruction: distal pain, paresthetic, pale, pulseless, sudden onset	Acute thrombophlebitis (deep venous thrombosis, DVT): calf pain, aching, edema, muscle tenderness, 50% asymptomatic
Ulceration	May develop in toes, feet, or areas of trauma; pale or yellow to black eschar, gangrene may develop; regular in shape and may appear punched out	May develop at sides of ankles, especially medial malleolus along the course of veins; gangrene absent; painful, shallow, exudative, and have granulation tissue in the base; irregular borders

Adapted from Bickley L (2016) Bates' Guide to Physical Examination and History Taking, 12th ed. Philadelphia, Lippincott Williams & Wilkins.

Intervention Strategies for Patients with Cardiac Conditions

Exercise Tolerance Testing

1. Exercise Tolerance Test (ETT), Graded Exercise Test.
   a. Performed prior to exercise prescription to determine physiological responses during a measured exercise stress (increasing workloads); allows the determination of safe aerobic exercise levels without cardiac ischemia.
      - Serves as a basis for exercise prescription. Symptom-limited ETT is typically administered prior to the start of the Phase II outpatient cardiac rehabilitation program and following cardiac rehabilitation as an outcome measure.
      - Exercise level is set just below the level in which signs and symptoms of intolerance or ischemia begin.
   b. Testing modes.
      - Treadmill and cycle ergometry (leg or arm tests) allow for precise calibration of the exercise workload.
      - Step test (upright or sitting) can also be used for fitness screening, healthy population.
   c. ETT may be maximal or submaximal.
      - Maximal ETT: Defined by target end-point heart rate; can be determined one or two ways.
      - Submaximal ETT: Symptom-limited, used to evaluate the early recovery of patients after MI, coronary bypass, or coronary angioplasty.
   d. Continuous ETT: Workload is steadily progressed usually in 2- or 3-minute stages.
   e. Discontinuous ETT: Allows rest in between workloads/stages, used for patients with more pronounced CAD.

Exercise Prescription

Entry into Programs

1. Indications and contraindications for entry into cardiac rehabilitation programs are identified in Box 4-1.

Monitoring During Exercise and Recovery

1. Patient appearance, signs and symptoms of excessive effort and exertional intolerance; examine for:
   a. Persistent dyspnea.
   b. Dizziness or confusion.
   c. Anginal pain.
   d. Severe leg claudication.
   e. Excessive fatigue.

BOX 4-1 ▶ **Clinical Indications and Contraindications for Inpatient and Outpatient Cardiac Rehabilitation Programs**

INDICATIONS

- Medically stable postmyocardial infarction
- Stable angina
- Coronary artery bypass graft surgery
- Percutaneous transluminal coronary angioplasty (PTCA)
- Compensated congestive heart failure
- Cardiomyopathy
- Heart or other organ transplantation
- Other cardiac surgery including valvular and pacemaker insertion (including implantable cardioverter defibrillator)
- Peripheral arterial disease
- High-risk cardiovascular disease ineligible for surgical intervention sudden cardiac death syndrome
- End-stage renal disease
- At risk for coronary artery disease, with diagnoses of diabetes mellitus, dyslipidemia, hypertension, etc.
- Other patients who may benefit from structured exercise and/or patient education (based on physician referral and consensus of the rehabilitation team)

CONTRAINDICATIONS

- Unstable angina
- Resting systolic BP >200 mm Hg or resting diastolic BP >110 mm Hg
- Orthostatic BP drop of >20 mm Hg with symptoms
- Critical aortic stenosis
- Acute systemic illness or fever
- Uncontrolled atrial or ventricular dysrhythmias
- Uncontrolled sinus tachycardia (>120 bpm)
- Uncompensated congestive heart failure
- Third degree A-V heart block without pacemaker
- Active pericarditis or myocarditis
- Recent embolism
- Thrombophlebitis
- Resting ST segment displacement (>2 mm)
- Uncontrolled diabetes (resting glucose >300 mg dL or >250 mg dL with ketones present)
- Severe orthopedic problems that would prohibit exercise
- Other metabolic problems, such as acute thyroiditis, hyperkalemia, hypovolemia, etc.

Adapted from ACSMs *Guidelines for Exercise Testing and Prescription*, 10th ed, 2017.

f. Pallor, cold sweat.
g. Ataxia, incoordination.
h. Pulmonary rales.
2. Changes in HR: HR increases linearly as a function of increasing workload and oxygen uptake (VO_2), plateaus just before maximal oxygen uptake (VO_2 max).
3. Changes in BP: systolic BP should rise with increasing workloads and VO_2; diastolic BP should remain about the same.
4. Rate pressure product (RPP): the product of systolic BP and HR (the last two digits of a 5-digit number are dropped) is often used as an index of myocardial oxygen consumption (MVO_2).
   a. Increased MVO_2 is the result of increased coronary blood flow.
   b. Angina is usually precipitated at a given RPP.
5. Ratings of perceived exertion (RPE): developed by Gunnar Borg. Allows subjective rating of feelings during exercise and impending fatigue. Important to use standardized instructions to reduce misinterpretation.
   a. RPE increases linearly with increasing exercise intensity and correlates closely with exercise heart rates and work rates.
   b. RPE has intra-user reliability over time, but not inter-user reliability. Ratings can be influenced by psychological factors, mood states, environmental conditions, exercise modes, and age.
   c. RPE is an important measure for individuals who do not exhibit the typical rise in HR with exercise (e.g., patients on medications that depress HR, such as beta blockers).
   d. Category scale (original Borg scale): rates exercise intensity using numbers from 6 to 20, with descriptors from very, very light (7) to somewhat hard (13) to very, very hard (19).
   e. Category-ratio scale (Borg): rates exercise intensity using numbers from 1 to 10 with descriptors from 0 (nothing at all) to very weak (1) to moderate (3) to strong (5) to extremely strong (10).
6. Pulse oximetry: measure arterial oxygen saturation levels (SaO_2) before, during, and after exercise.
7. ECG changes with exercise: healthy individual.
   a. Tachycardia: heart rate increase is directly proportional to exercise intensity and myocardial work.
   b. Rate-related shortening of QT interval.
   c. ST segment depression, upsloping, less than 1 mm.
   d. Reduced R wave, increased Q wave.
   e. Exertional arrhythmias: rare, single PVCs.
8. ECG changes with exercise: an individual with myocardial ischemia and CAD.
   a. Significant tachycardia: occurs at lower intensities of exercise or with deconditioned individuals without ischemia.
   b. Exertional arrhythmias: increased frequency of ventricular arrhythmias during exercise and/or recovery.
   c. ST segment depression; horizontal or downsloping depression, greater than 1 mm below baseline is indicative of myocardial ischemia.
9. Delayed, abnormal responses to exercise, can occur hours later.
   a. Prolonged fatigue.
   b. Insomnia.
   c. Sudden weight gain due to fluid retention.
   d. Hypotension, especially in patients with heart failure.

Ambulatory Monitoring (Telemetry)
1. Continuous 24-hour ECG monitoring.
2. Allows documentation of arrhythmias and of ST segment depression or elevation, silent ischemia (if assessing via 12 leads only).

Transtelephonic ECG Monitoring
1. Used to monitor patients as they exercise at home.

Activity Levels: METs (Metabolic Equivalents)
1. MET: the amount of oxygen consumed at rest (sitting); equal to 3.5 mL/kg per minute.
2. MET levels (multiples of resting VO_2) can be directly determined during ETT: using collection and analysis of expired air; not routinely done.
3. MET levels can be estimated during ETT during steady state exercise; the max VO_2 achieved on ETT is divided by resting VO_2; highly predictable with standardized testing modes.
4. Can be used to predict energy expenditure during certain activities (Table 4-17).

Considerations Following Surgical Procedures
1. Restrictions following open chest procedures.
   a. The patient is not allowed to pull himself or herself up in bed, roll to side-lying position for bed transfers.
   b. Use of hand-hold assist versus assistive device may be necessary.
   c. No pushing, pulling, or lifting anything >5–10 pounds; for 6 weeks postop.
   d. Limit shoulder (flexion, abduction) and trunk motions if sternum is unstable.
      • Chest is determined to be unstable if asynchronous chest movement occurs between the two sides. Therapist can evaluate this by placing his or her hands on the two chest sides and asking the patient to cough.

Table 4-17

Metabolic Equivalent (MET) Activity Chart

INTENSITY (70-KG PERSON)	ENDURANCE PROMOTING	ACTIVITY
1.5–2 METs	Too low in energy level	Standing, walking slowly (1 mph)
2–3 METs	Too low in energy level, unless capacity is very low	Level walking (2 mph), level bicycling (5 mph)
3–4 METs	Yes, if continuous and if target heart rate reached	Level walking (3 mph), bicycling (6 mph)
4–5 METs	Recreational activities must be continuous, lasting longer than 2 minutes	Walking (3½ mph), bicycling (8 mph)
5–6 METs	Yes	Walking at brisk pace (4 mph), bicycling (10 mph)
6–7 METs	Yes	Walking at very brisk pace (5 mph), bicycling (11 mph), swimming leisurely (20 yd/min)
7–8 METs	Yes	Jogging (5 mph), bicycling (12 mph)
8–9 METs	Yes	Running (5.5 mph), bicycling (13 mph), swimming (30 yd/min)
> 10 METs	Yes	Running 6 mph = 10 METs, 7 mph = 11.5 METs, 8 mph = 13.5 METs, 9 mph = 15 METs, 10 mph = 17 METs; swimming moderate/hard (> 40 yd/min)

Adapted from: Fox, Naughton, Gorman. Mod Concepts Cardiovas Dis 1972, 4:25. American Heart Association.

2. Instruct patient in splinting sternum by "hugging a pillow" during cough.
3. Scar mobilization can begin when scar(s) are fully healed; follow typical scar mobilization techniques.
4. Typical home discharge instructions (see Quick Facts 4-14).

QUICK FACTS 4-14 ▶ TYPICAL HOME DISCHARGE INSTRUCTIONS

- No driving motorized vehicles (e.g., golf cart, car); for 8 weeks postop. Air bag precautions require sitting in rear seat.
- Avoid soaking in the bath until incision is fully healed; avoid excessively hot water
- When bypass graft in leg is present, avoid crossing the legs, prolonged positions (sit, stand), elevate LE when possible.
- Wear elastic stockings for 2 weeks following surgery when up
- Encourage walking; assists with managing edema in LE as well as helping increase development of collateral circulation
- Encourage balance between activity and rest
- Sexual relations can typically resume in 3–4 weeks following discharge when the patient feels comfortable.

Guidelines for Exercise Prescription

1. Type (exercise type).
   a. Cardiorespiratory endurance activities: Walking, jogging, or cycling recommended to improve exercise tolerance; can be maintained at a constant velocity; very low inter-individual variability.
   b. Dynamic arm exercise (arm ergometry): Uses a smaller muscle mass, results in lower VO_2 max (60%–70% lower) than leg ergometry; at a given workload, HR will be higher, stroke volume lower; systolic and diastolic B/Ps will be higher.
   c. Other aerobic activities: Swimming, cross-country skiing; less frequently used due to high inter-individual variability, energy expenditure related to skill level.
   d. Dancing, basketball, racquetball, competitive activities should not be used with high risk, symptomatic and low-fitness individuals.
   e. Early rehabilitation: Activity is discontinuous (interval training), with frequent rest periods; continuous training can be used in later stages of rehabilitation.
   f. Warm-up and cool-down activities.
      - Gradually increase or decrease the intensity of exercise, promote circulatory and muscular adjustment to exercise.
      - Type: Low intensity cardiorespiratory endurance activities, flexibility (ROM) exercises, functional mobility activities.

- Duration: 5–10 minutes.
- Abrupt beginning or cessation of exercise is not safe or recommended.

g. Resistive exercises: To improve strength and endurance in clinically stable patients.
- Usually prescribed in later rehabilitation, after a period of aerobic conditioning.
- Moderate intensities are typically used (e.g., 40% of maximal voluntary contraction).
- Monitor responses to resistive training using rate-pressure product (incorporates B/P, a safer measure).

RED FLAG: Carefully monitor HR, BP, and breathing during resistive exercise; breath holding can result in a Valsalva's maneuver (forceful exhalation against a closed airway) with a dramatic increase in BP and a reduction of stroke volume and heart output. Proper training during resistance-training is especially important (i.e., exhalation during lifting phase and inhalation during the lowering phase). Resistance training is contraindicated for patients with uncontrolled hypertension or arrhythmias.

h. Relaxation training: Relieves generalized muscle tension and anxiety.
- Usually incorporated following an aerobic training session and cool-down.
- Assists in successful stress management and lifestyle modification.

2. Intensity: Prescribed as percentage of functional capacity revealed on ETT, within a range of 40%–85% depending upon initial level of fitness; typical training intensity is 60%–70% of functional capacity; lower training intensities may necessitate an increase in training duration; most clinicians use a combination of HR, RPE and METs to prescribe exercise intensity (eliminates problems that may be associated with individual measures).

a. Heart rate.
- Percentage of maximum heart rate achieved on ETT; without an ETT, 220 minus age is used (for upper extremity work, 220 minus age minus 11 is used). 70%–85% HR max closely corresponds to 60%–80% of functional capacity or VO_2 max (Quick Facts 4-15).
- Estimated HR max is used in cases where submaximal ETT has been given.
- Heart rate range or reserve (Karvonen formula, see previous description) more closely approximates the relationship between HR and VO_2 max. Problems associated with use of HR alone to prescribe exercise intensity.

QUICK FACTS 4-15 ▶ DETERMINE MAXIMUM HEART RATE	
Age-adjusted maximum heart rate (AAMHR)	Calculate: 220 – age of individual
Heart-rate range (Karvonen formula)	Calculate: 60%–80% (HR max resting HR) + resting HR = target HR

- Beta blocking or calcium channel blocking medications: Affect ability of HR to rise in response to an exercise stress.
- Pacemaker: Affects ability of HR to rise in response to an exercise stress.
- Environmental extremes, heavy arm work, isometric exercise and Valsalva may affect HR and B/P responses.

b. Rating of Perceived Exertion, the original Borg RPE scale (6–20) (Quick Facts 4-13).
- RPE values of 12–13 (somewhat hard) correspond to 60% of HR range.
- RPE of 16 (hard) corresponds to 85% of HR range.
- Useful along with other measures of patient effort if beta-blockers or other HR suppressers are used.

c. Problems with use of RPE alone to prescribe exercise intensity.
- Individuals with psychological problems (e.g., depression).
- Unfamiliarity with RPE scale; may affect selection of ratings.

d. METs or estimated energy expenditure (VO_2) (Table 4-17).
- 40%–85% of functional capacity (maximal METs) achieved on ETT.

e. Problems associated with use of METs alone to prescribe exercise intensity.
- With high intensity activities (e.g., jogging), need to adopt a discontinuous work pattern: Walk 5 minutes; jog 3 minutes to achieve the desired intensity.
- Varying skill level or stress of competition may affect the known metabolic cost of an activity.
- Environmental stresses (heat, cold, high humidity, altitude, wind, changes in terrain such as hills) may affect the known metabolic cost of an activity.

3. Duration.
   a. Conditioning phase may vary from 15–60 minutes, depending upon intensity; the higher the intensity, the shorter the duration.
   b. Average conditioning time is 20–30 minutes for moderate intensity exercise.
   c. Severely compromised individuals may benefit from multiple, short exercise sessions spaced throughout the day (e.g., 3- to 10-minute sessions).
   d. Warm-up and cool-down periods are kept constant (e.g., 5–10 minutes each).
4. Frequency.
   a. Frequency of activity is dependent upon intensity and duration; the lower the intensity, the shorter the duration, the greater the frequency.
   b. Average: Three to five sessions/week for exercise at moderate intensities and duration (e.g., >5 METs).
   c. Daily or multiple daily sessions for low intensity exercise (e.g., <5 METs).
5. Progression.
   a. Modify exercise prescription if:
      - HR is lower than target HR for a given exercise intensity.
      - RPE is lower (exercise is perceived as easier) for a given exercise.
      - Symptoms of ischemia (e.g., angina) do not appear at a given exercise intensity.
   b. Rate of progression depends on age, health status, functional capacity, personal goals and preferences.
   c. As training progresses, duration is increased first, then intensity. (See Table 4-18.)

RED FLAGS: Consider reduction in exercise/activity with:
- Acute illness: Fever, flu.
- Acute injury or orthopedic complications.
- Progression of cardiac disease: Edema, weight gain, unstable angina.
- Overindulgence (e.g., food, caffeine, alcohol).
- Drugs (e.g., decongestants, bronchodilators, atropine, weight reducers).
- Environmental stressors (e.g., extremes of heat, cold, humidity); air pollution.

RED FLAGS: Adverse responses to inpatient exercise that lead to exercise termination (ACSM Guideliens, 2017).
- Diastolic BP equal to or greater than 110 mm Hg.
- Decrease in systolic BP >10 mm Hg during exercise.
- Significant ventricular or atrial dysrhythmias with or without associated signs/symptoms.
- Second- or third-degree heart block.
- Signs/symptoms of exercise intolerance, including angina, marked dyspnea, and ECG changes suggestive of ischemia.

6. Exercise prescription for post-PTCA (percutaneous transluminal coronary angioplasty).
   a. Wait to exercise approximately 2 weeks post-PTCA to allow inflammatory process to subside.
   b. Use post-PTCA ETT to prescribe exercise.
7. Exercise prescription post-CABG (coronary artery bypass grafting).
   a. Limit upper extremity exercise while sternal incision is healing.
   b. Avoid lifting, pushing, pulling for 4–6 weeks post-surgery.
8. Possible effects of physical training/cardiac rehabilitation can be found in Quick Facts 4-16.

Phase 1: Inpatient Cardiac Rehabilitation (Acute)

Length of stay is commonly 3–5 days for uncomplicated MI (no post-MI angina, malignant arrhythmias or heart failure) (Table 4-18).

Exercise/Activity Goals and Outcomes
1. Initiate early return to independence in activities of daily living, typically after 24 hours or until the patient is stable for 24 hours; monitor activity tolerance.
2. Counteract deleterious effects of bed rest: Reduce risk of thrombi, maintain muscle tone, reduce orthostatic hypotension and maintain joint mobility.
3. Help allay anxiety and depression.
4. Provide medical surveillance.
5. Provide patient and family education.
6. Promote risk factor modification.

Exercise/Activity Guidelines
1. Program components: ADLs, selected arm and leg exercises, early supervised ambulation.
2. Initial activities are low intensity (2–3 METs) progressing to ≥5 METs by discharge.
3. Post-MI: Limited to 70% max HR and/or 5 METs until 6 weeks post-MI.
4. Short exercise sessions, two to three times a day; gradually duration is lengthened and frequency is decreased.
5. Postsurgical patients.
   a. Typically are progressed more rapidly than post-MI, unless there as a peri-operative MI.
   b. Lifting activities are restricted, generally for 6 weeks.

Patient and Family Education Goals
1. Improve understanding of cardiac disease, support risk factor modification.

Table 4-18

Guidelines for Cardiac Rehabilitation Program

PHASE 1: INPATIENT CARDIAC REHABILITATION (ACUTE)

Length of stay is commonly 3–5 days for uncomplicated MI (no post-MI angina, malignant arrhythmias, or heart failure).

EXERCISE/ACTIVITY GOALS AND OUTCOMES	EXERCISE/ACTIVITY GUIDELINES	PATIENT AND FAMILY EDUCATION GOALS	HOME EXERCISE PROGRAM (HEP)

1. Initiate early return to independence in activities of daily living, typically after 24 hours or until the patient is stable for 24 hours; monitor activity tolerance
2. Counteract deleterious effects of bed rest: reduce risk of thrombi, maintain muscle tone, reduce orthostatic hypotension and maintain joint mobility
3. Help allay anxiety and depression
4. Provide medical surveillance
5. Provide patient and family education
6. Promote risk factor modification
	1. Program components: ADLs, selected arm and leg exercises, early supervised ambulation
	2. Initial activities: are low intensity (2–3 METs) progressing to 3–5 METs by discharge; RPE in fairly light range; HR increase of 10–20 bmp above resting, depending on medications
	3. Short exercise sessions, 2–3 times a day; gradually duration is lengthened and frequency is decreased.
	4. Post-surgical patients
	  a. Typically are progressed more rapidly than post-MI.
	  b. Greater emphasis is placed on upper extremity ROM.
	  c. Lifting activities are restricted, generally for 6 weeks.
	5. ETT (thallium scan or symptom limited ETT): may be used to determine functional capacity prior to discharge, safely progress exercise intensity greater than 5 METs.
		1. Improve understanding of cardiac disease, support risk factor modification
		2. Teach self-monitoring procedures, warning signs of exertional intolerance, e.g., persistent dyspnea, anginal pain, dizziness, etc.
		3. Teach general activity guidelines, activity pacing, energy conservation techniques; home exercise program (HEP)
		4. Teach cardiopulmonary resuscitation (CPR)
		5. Provide emotional support
			1. Low-risk patients may be safe candidates for unsupervised exercise at home.
			  a. Gradual increase in ambulation time: goal of 20–30 minutes, one to two times per day at 4–6 weeks post-MI
			  b. Upper and lower extremity mobility exercises
			2. Elderly, homebound patients with multiple medical problems may benefit from a home cardiac rehabilitation program.
			3. Patients should be skilled in self-monitoring procedures.
			4. Family training in CPR and AED (automated external defibrillator); emergency lifeline for some patients

PHASE 2: OUTPATIENT CARDIAC REHABILITATION (SUBACUTE)

Outpatient program: average of 36 visits allowed by most payers (three times a week for 12 weeks).

1. Improve functional capacity
2. Progress toward full resumption of activities of daily living, habitual and occupational activities
3. Promote risk-factor modification, counseling as to lifestyle changes
4. Encourage activity pacing, energy conservation; stress importance of taking proper rest periods

1. Outpatient program:
   a. Patients at risk for arrhythmias with exercise, angina, and other medical problems benefit from outpatient programs with availability of ECG monitoring, trained personnel, and emergency support.
   b. Group camaraderie and support of program participants may assist in risk-factor modification and lifestyle changes.
   c. Frequency: three to four sessions/week
   d. Duration: 30–60 minutes with 5–10 minutes of warm-up and cool down
   e. Programs may offer a single mode of training (e.g., walking) or multiple modes using a circuit training approach (e.g., treadmill, cycle ergometer, arm ergometer); strength training.
   f. Patients are gradually weaned from continuous monitoring to spot checks and self-monitoring.

> **QUICK FACTS 4-16 ▶ POSSIBLE EFFECTS OF PHYSICAL TRAINING/CARDIAC REHABILITATION**
> - Decreased HR at rest and during exercise; improved HR recovery after exercise
> - Increased stroke volume
> - Increased myocardial oxygen supply and myocardial contractility; myocardial hypertrophy
> - Improved respiratory capacity during exercise
> - Improved functional capacity of exercising muscles
> - Reduced body fat, increased lean body mass; successful weight reduction requires multifactorial interventions
> - Decreased serum lipoproteins (cholesterol, triglycerides)
> - Improved glucose tolerance
> - Improved blood fibrinolytic activity and coagulability
> - Improvement in measures of psychological status and functioning: self-confidence and sense of well-being
> - Increased participation in exercise; improved outcomes with adherence to rehabilitation programming
>   - Decreased angina in patients with CAD: anginal threshold is raised secondary to decreased myocardial oxygen consumption
>   - Reduced total and cardiovascular mortality in patients following myocardial infarction
>   - Decreased symptoms of heart failure, improved functional capacity in patients with left ventricular systolic dysfunction
>   - Improved exercise tolerance and function in patients with cardiac transplantation

2. Teach self-monitoring procedures, warning signs of exertional intolerance (e.g., persistent dyspnea, anginal pain, dizziness, etc.).
3. Teach concepts of energy costs, fatigue monitoring, general activity guidelines, activity pacing, energy conservation techniques; home exercise program (HEP).
4. Provide emotional support. PTA monitors need for emotional support, possibly discuss social work referral with PT.

Home Exercise Program (HEP)
1. Low-risk patients may be safe candidates for unsupervised exercise at home.
   a. Gradual increase in ambulation time: Goal of 20–30 minutes, one to two times per day at 4–6 weeks post-MI.
   b. Upper and lower extremity mobility exercises.
2. Elderly, homebound patients with multiple medical problems may benefit from a home cardiac rehabilitation program.
3. Patients should be skilled in self-monitoring procedures.
4. Discuss family training in CPR and AED (automated external defibrillator); emergency lifeline for some patients.

Phase 2: Outpatient Cardiac Rehabilitation (Subacute)

Eligible Patients
1. MI/acute coronary syndrome.
2. CABG.
3. PCI.
4. Stable angina.
5. Heart valve surgical repair or replacement.
6. Heart or heart/lung transplantation.
7. Heart failure and PAD: may not be covered by insurance but these populations benefit from supervised exercise program.

Exercise/Activity Goals and Outcomes
1. Improve functional capacity.
2. Progress toward full resumption of activities of daily living, habitual and occupational activities.
3. Promote risk-factor modification, counseling as to lifestyle changes.
4. Encourage activity pacing, energy conservation; stress importance of taking proper rest periods.

Exercise/Activity Guidelines
1. Outpatient program.
   a. Patients at risk for arrhythmias with exercise, angina and other medical problems benefit from outpatient programs with availability of ECG monitoring, trained personnel and emergency support.
   b. Group camaraderie and support of program participants may assist in risk factor modification and lifestyle changes.
   c. Frequency: Two to three sessions/week.
   d. Duration: 30–60 minutes with 5–10 minutes of warm-up and cool-down.
   e. Programs may offer a single mode of training (e.g., walking) or multiple modes using a circuit training approach (e.g., treadmill, cycle ergometer, arm ergometer); strength training.
   f. Patients are gradually weaned from continuous monitoring to spot checks and self-monitoring.

g. Suggested exit point: 9 METs functional capacity (5 METs capacity is needed for safe resumption of most daily activities).
2. Strength training is a recent addition to Phase 2 programs.
   a. Guidelines: After 3 weeks' cardiac rehab, 5 weeks' post-MI or 8 weeks' post-CABG.
   b. Begin with use of elastic bands and light weights (1–3 lb).
   c. Progress to moderate loads, 12–15 comfortable repetitions.
3. Patient and family education goals: Progression of phase 1 goals.

Phase 3: Community Exercise Programs (Postacute, Postdischarge from Phase 2 Program)

Exercise/Activity Goals and Outcomes
1. Improve and/or maintain functional capacity.
2. Promote self-regulation of exercise programs.
3. Promote life-long commitment to risk-factor modification.

Exercise/Activity Guidelines
1. Location: Community centers, YMCA, or clinical facilities.
2. Entry-level criteria: Functional capacity of 5 METs, clinically stable angina, medically controlled arrhythmias during exercise.
3. Progression is from supervised to self-regulation of exercise.
4. Progression to 50%–85% of functional capacity, three to four times/week, 45 minutes or more/session.
5. Regular medical check-ups and periodic ETT generally required.
6. Utilize motivational techniques to maintain compliance with exercise programs, lifestyle modification.
7. Continue patient and family education.
8. Progression from Phase 2 goals.
9. Discharge typically in 6–12 months.

Resistance Exercise Training

Goals and Outcomes
1. Improve muscle strength and endurance.
2. Enhance functional independence.
3. Decrease cardiac demands during daily activities.

Patient Criteria for Resistance Training
1. American Association of Cardiovascular and Pulmonary Rehabilitation Guidelines.
2. Post-MI: Resistance training permitted if remain under 70% max HR or 5 METs for 6 weeks post-MI, be cautious of Valsalva with resistance training.
3. Cardiac surgery: Lower extremity resistance training can be initiated immediately, in the absence of peri-operative MI. Upper extremity resistance training should be avoided until soft tissue and bony healing has occurred: 6–8 weeks.
4. Post-transcatheter procedure (PTCA, other): Minimum of 3 weeks following procedure and 2 weeks of consistent participation in a supervised CR endurance training program.
5. No evidence of the following conditions:
   a. Congestive heart failure.
   b. Uncontrolled dysrhythmias.
   c. Severe valvular disease.
   d. Uncontrolled hypertension.
   e. Unstable symptoms.

Exercise Prescription
1. Start with low resistance (one set of 10–15 repetitions) and progress slowly.
2. Resistance can include:
   a. Weights, 50% or more of maximum weight used to complete one repetition (1 RM).
   b. Elastic bands.
   c. Light (1- to 5-lb) cuff and hand weights.
   d. Wall pulleys.
3. Perceived exertion (Borg RPE Scale) should range from 11 to 13 ("light" to "somewhat hard"), this needs to be correlated to hemodynamic response to activity.
4. Rate-pressure product should not exceed that prescribed during endurance exercise.

Exercise Prescription for Patients Requiring Special Considerations

Heart Failure (HF)
1. Patients demonstrate significant ventricular dysfunction, decreased cardiac output, low functional capacities.
2. Classification systems (Table 4-19).
3. Criteria for exercise training.
   a. Compensated or chronic HF; no signs of acute HF.
   b. Exercise-induced ischemia and arrhythmias are poor prognostic indicators.
4. Exercise training.
   a. Assess for signs of decompensation at each visit (see Quick Facts 4-17).

Table 4-19

Classification of Heart Failure

NEW YORK HEART ASSOCIATION STAGES	FUNCTION AND SYMPTOMS
Class I: Mild HF	No limitation in physical activity (up to 6.5 METs); comfortable at rest, ordinary activity does not cause undue fatigue, palpitation, dyspnea, or anginal pain
Class II: Slight HF	Slight limitation in physical activity (up to 4.5 METs); comfortable at rest, ordinary physical activity results in fatigue, palpitation, dyspnea, or anginal pain
Class III: Marked HF	Marked limitation of physical activity (up to 3 METs); comfortable at rest, less than ordinary activity causes fatigue, palpitation, dyspnea, or anginal pain
Class IV:	Unable to carry out any physical activity (1.5 METs); without discomfort; symptoms of ischemia, dyspnea, anginal pain present even at rest; increasing with exercise
American College of Cardiology Foundation (ACCF)/ American Heart Association (AHA) Stages	
Stage A	At high risk for HF but without structural heart disease or symptoms of HF
Stage B	Structural heart disease but without signs or symptoms of HF
Stage C	Structural heart disease with prior or current symptoms of HF
Stage D	Refractory HF requiring specialized interventions.

b. Monitor at rest and during activity.
- Use RPE that is correlated with objective measures of hemodynamic response (heart rate [HR], blood pressure [B/P], respiratory rate [RR], systolic pressure [Sp]) and clinical signs of exercise intolerance.

QUICK FACTS 4-17 ▶ SIGNS OF DECOMPENSATION

- Increased shortness of breath (SOB)
- Increased LE edema or abdominal swelling
- Pronounced cough
- Sudden weight gain
- Increased pain or fatigue
- Light-headedness or dizziness

- Keep in mind HR response may be impaired (chronotropic incompetence).
- At risk for persistent post-exercise vasodilation (and hypotension) with later stages of HF.

c. Use low-level, gradual progressive aerobic training.
- Intensities: Begin with 40–60% functional capacity, increase as able.
- Gradually increasing durations, with frequent rest periods (interval training).
- Adequate warm-up and cool-down periods; may need longer than typical 5–10 minutes.

d. Use caution exercising in supine or prone positons due to orthopnea.
e. Avoid breath holding and Valsalva's maneuver.
f. Respiratory muscle training. Monitoring SaO_2 via pulse oximetry is advisable in some cases.
g. Emphasis on training in energy conservation, self-monitoring techniques.

Cardiac Transplant

1. Patients may present with:
   a. Exercise intolerance due to extended inactivity and convalescence.
   b. Side effects from immunosuppressive drug therapy: Hyperlipidemia, hypertension, obesity, diabetes, leg cramps.
   c. Decreased lower extremity strength.
   d. Increased fracture risk owing to long-term corticosteroid use.
2. Heart rate alone is not an appropriate measure of exercise intensity (heart is denervated and patients tend to be tachycardia). Use a combination of HR, B/P, RPE, METs, dyspnea scale.
3. Use longer periods of warm-up and cool-down because the physiological responses to exercise and recovery take longer.

Pacemakers and Automatic Implantable Cardioverter Defibrillators (AICDs)

1. Pacemakers are programmed to pace heart rate.
   a. Most are demand pacemakers to trigger heart to increase as workload increases.
   b. Always have a lower HR limit set; rarely have a upper limit set.
   c. HR will not change with fixed rate pacers, which will impact activity tolerance.
2. AICDs will deliver an electric shock if HR exceeds set limit and/or ventricular arrhythmia is detected.
3. Should know setting for HR limits or AICD.
4. ST segment changes may be common.
5. Avoid UE aerobic or strengthening exercise for 4–6 weeks after implant to allow the leads to scar down.

6. Electromagnetic signals may cause devices to fire (defibrillator), or slow down or speed up pacemaker.

Diabetes

1. Patients demonstrate problems controlling blood glucose, with associated cardiovascular disease, renal disease, neuropathy, peripheral vascular disease and ulceration and/or autonomic dysfunction.
2. Exercise testing.
   a. May need to use submaximal ETT tests; maximal tests precluded with autonomic neuropathy.
   b. With PVD/peripheral neuropathy, may need to shift to arm ergometry.
3. Exercise training.
   a. Use principles of exercise prescription: Intensities of 40%–85% functional capacity.
      - Insulin-dependent diabetes: Daily exercise recommended, with shorter durations (20–30 minutes).
      - Non–insulin-dependent diabetes: Five times/week recommended, with longer durations (40–60 minutes).
   b. Exercise effects include: lower blood glucose levels, overall less insulin required (see also Quick Facts 4-16).
   c. Hypoglycemia may result with too much insulin (most common response to exercise).
      - Carefully monitor for signs of hypoglycemia: Acute fatigue, restlessness, marked irritability and weakness; in severe cases, mental disturbances, delirium, coma (a life-threatening situation).
      - Control by eating carbohydrate snacks prior to or during prolonged exercise or by self–blood glucose monitoring and placing insulin in a nonexercising body part (e.g., abdominal wall).
   d. Poorly controlled diabetes: Lack adequate insulin, may lead to impaired glucose transport, ketosis, hyperglycemia (too much blood sugar).
   e. Proper footwear is important, especially with changes associated with diabetic feet.
   f. Jogging, jarring activities are contraindicated in cases of advanced diabetic retinopathy.

Intervention: Peripheral Vascular Disease Conditions

Rehabilitation Guidelines for Arterial Disease

Patient Instruction/Guidance
1. Encourage risk factor modification. (See Table 4-1.)

Limb Protection
1. Avoid excessive strain, protection of extremities from injury and extremes of temperature.
2. Bed rest may be required if gangrene, ulceration, or acute arterial disease are present.

Exercise Training for Patients with PAD
1. May result in improved functional capacity, peripheral blood flow, and muscle oxidative capacity.
2. Consider interval training (multistage discontinuous protocol) with frequent rests.
3. Walking program: Intensity such that patient reports 1 on claudication scale within 3–5 minutes, stopping if they reach a 2 (until pain subsides), total of 30–60 minutes (intervals as necessary), 3–5 days per week. (See Quick Facts 4-18.)
4. Record time of pain onset and duration.
5. Non–weight-bearing exercise (cycle ergometry, arm ergometry) may be necessary in some patients; less effective in producing a peripheral conditioning effect.

QUICK FACTS 4-18 ▶ CLAUDICATION PAIN RATING SCALE

0 – Asymptomatic, no pain
1 – Minimal discomfort, pain onset
2 – Moderate pain/discomfort (patient can be distracted)*
3 – Intense pain
4 – Unbearable pain

*Target zone for peripheral conditioning

---

6. Well-fitting shoes are essential; with insensitive feet, teach technique of proper foot inspection and care.
7. Beta-blockers for treatment of hypertension or cardiac disorders may decrease time to claudication or worsen symptoms.
8. Pentoxifylline, dipyridamole, aspirin, and warfarin may improve time to claudication.
9. High risk for CAD.

Lower Extremity Exercise
1. Modified Buerger-Allen exercises plus active plantar and dorsiflexion of the ankle; active exercises improve blood flow during and after exercise; effects less pronounced in patients with PAD.
2. Resistive calf exercises: Most effective method of increasing blood flow.

Medical Treatment
1. Medications to decrease blood viscosity, prevent thrombus formation (e.g., heparin).
2. Vasodilators are controversial.
3. Calcium channel blockers in vasospastic disease.

Surgical Management
1. Atherectomy, thromboembolectomy, laser therapy.
2. Revascularization: Angioplasty or bypass grafting.
3. Sympathectomy: Results in permanent vasodilation, improvement of blood flow to skin.
4. Amputation when gangrene is present.

Rehabilitation Guidelines for Venous Disease

Venous Thromboembolism (VTE)
1. Identification of patients who are at high risk of VTE:
   a. Requires knowledge of signs and symptoms and risk factors. See Table 4-15.
   b. PT may use standardized Risk Assessment Measure (e.g., Wells Criteria Score for DVT).
2. Initiate notification of physician, PT, and team members.
3. Physician management:
   a. Anti-coagulation (clotting) medications ordered.
   b. Inferior vena cava (IVC) filter placement.
   c. Trial of intermittent pneumatic compression pump (IPC) may be ordered for patients with severe post-thrombotic syndrome (PTS) of the leg not adequately relieved with graded compression stockings.
4. Physical therapy management:
   a. Once therapeutic levels of medication are achieved (e.g., low molecular weight heparin), initiate ambulation and leg exercises (activation of calf muscle pump).
   b. Provide education to decrease risk of recurring VTE.
   c. Assess for fall risk and institute measures to reduce fall risk.
5. Bed rest is not recommended following diagnosis of VTE once acceptable levels of medication are reached unless there are significant medical concerns.
6. Utilization of mechanical compression or graded compression stockings (GCS) with at least 30 mm Hg of pressure at the ankle.

Chronic Venous Insufficiency (CVI)
1. Positioning to manage edema.
   a. Elevate extremity a minimum of 18 cm above heart. Encourage patients to elevate leg as much as possible to avoid the dependent position.
2. Compression therapy.
   a. Bandages (elastic, tubular) applied within 20 minutes of rising.
   b. Paste bandages (Unna boot) for wound management. Gauze impregnated with zinc oxide, gelatin, and glycerin; applied for 4–7 days (less with some wounds).
   c. Graduated compression stockings with a pressure gradient of 30–40 mm Hg.
   d. Compression pump therapy, used for a 1- to 2- hour session twice daily.

> **RED FLAGS:** Contraindications of compression therapy include:
> - ABI < 0.8 in involved extremity.
> - Signs of active cellulitis or infection.
> - Systemic arterial pressure < 80 mm Hg.
> - Advanced peripheral neuropathy.
> - Uncontrolled congestive heart failure.

3. Exercise.
   a. Active ankle exercises: Focus on activation of "muscle pump" by encouraging dorsiflexion/plantarflexion, foot circles.
   b. Cycle ergometry in sitting or attached to foot of bed.
   c. Early ambulation as soon as patient is able to get out of bed, three to four times/day.
4. Patient education: Meticulous skin care.
5. Severe conditions with dermal ulceration may require surgery (ligation and vein stripping, vein grafts, valvuloplasty).

Lymphatic System

The Lymphatic System
1. A network of lymphatic vessels that withdraws excess tissue fluid (lymph) from the body's interstitial spaces, filters it through lymph nodes, and returns it to the bloodstream via the venous system.

Components (See Figure 4-6)
1. Lymphatic vessels (superficial, intermediate, deep) (see Figure 4-7).
2. Lymph fluid.
3. Lymph nodes.
   a. Submandibular.
   b. Cervical.
   c. Upper extremity (see Figure 4-8).
      - Supraclavicular.
        ○ Axillary.
        ○ Central.
        ○ Subscapular.
        ○ Pectoral.
        ○ Humeral.
      - Cubital.
   d. Parasternal.
   e. Mesenteric.
   f. Lower extremity.
      - Iliac.
      - Inguinal.
      - Popliteal.
4. Lymph tissues (mucosa associated lymphoid tissue, or MALT).
5. Organs.
   a. Spleen.
   b. Tonsils.
   c. Thymus.
   d. Bone marrow.

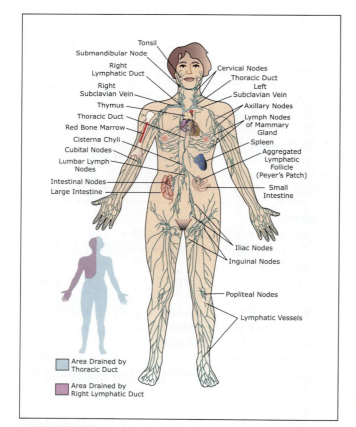

Figure 4-6 Lymphatic system.

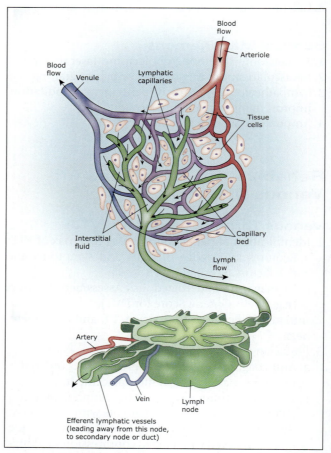

Figure 4-7 Lymph vessels and nodes.

Adapted from Moore KM, et al (2014). *Clinically Oriented Anatomy*, 7th ed. Philadelphia, Lippincott, Williams & Wilkins.

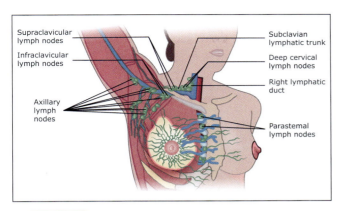

Figure 4-8 Axillary lymph nodes and lymphatic drainage of upper extremity and breast.

Adapted from Moore KM, et al (2014). *Clinically Oriented Anatomy*, 7th ed. Philadelphia, Lippincott, Williams & Wilkins.

Lymph Circulation
1. Lymph travels from the lymphatic capillaries to lymphatic vessels to large lymphatic ducts (right lymphatic duct, thoracic duct to the subclavian veins).

Lymphatic Vessel Contraction Occurs by
1. Autonomic and sensory nerve stimulation.
2. Contraction of adjacent muscles.
3. Abdominal and thoracic cavity pressure changes during normal breathing.
4. Mechanical stimulation of dermal tissues.
5. Volume changes within individual lymphatic vessels.

Pathophysiology/Common Pathologies

Lymphedema
1. Chronic disorder characterized by excessive accumulation of lymph fluid due to mechanical insufficiency of the lymphatic system (obstruction of lymph flow or removal of lymph nodes).
2. Lymph fluid volume exceeds the transport capacity/capability of lymph vessels.
3. Results in swelling of the soft tissues of the upper and lower extremities.
4. Primary lymphedema: a congenital or hereditary disorder with abnormal lymph node or lymph vessel formation.
5. Secondary lymphedema: acquired insult to the lymphatic system. Most commonly seen after surgery for breast or cervical cancer. Possible causes include:
   a. Surgery including lymph node removal.
   b. Tumors, trauma, or infection involving lymphatic system structures.
   c. Radiation therapy.
   d. Chronic venous insufficiency.
   e. Filariasis (parasitic infection of the lymphatic system; seen in tropical and subtropical regions).
6. Stages of lymphedema.
   a. Stage 0: at risk; swelling is not yet evident despite reduced transport capacity of the system. Also called the latent or pre-clinical stage.
   b. Stage 1: reversible; early accumulation of fluid with visible swelling; pitting edema that resolves with elevation (reversible pitting edema); Stemmer's sign is negative.
   c. Stage 2: spontaneously irreversible; increase in swelling; elevation does not reduce the swelling; positive Stemmer's sign.
   d. Stage 3: elephantiasis; fibrotic deep skinfolds; skin may change color; skin changes may limit mobility.
7. Differential diagnosis.
   a. Lipedema (see Figure 4-9).
      - Excessive subcutaneous fat deposition.
      - Appearance may be similar to lymphedema.
      - Normal function of the lymphatic system.
      - Symmetrical swelling of extremities.
      - Negative Stemmer's sign.
      - Seen typically in women (may be seen associated with hormonal changes during pregnancy and puberty).

Lymphadenopathy
1. Enlargement of lymph nodes, with or without tenderness.
2. Typically caused by an infection.
3. Localized lymphadenopathy: enlargement of lymph nodes in just one body region.
4. Generalized lymphadenopathy: enlargement of lymph nodes in two or more body regions.
5. Lymphadenitis describes lymphadenopathy accompanied by signs of inflammation such as redness and tenderness.

Lymphangitis
1. An acute bacterial (often streptococcus) or viral infection that spreads throughout the lymphatic system.
2. Red streaks are often seen in the skin proximal to the infection site.

Examination: History, Tests, and Measures

History
1. Presenting symptoms. In patients who are at risk for secondary lymphedema.
   a. Observable swelling.
   b. Sensation of tightness, heaviness, or fullness in the affected area.

	Lymphedema	Lipedema
Signs and symptoms	Can involve the legs, arms, trunk, genitalia or head and neck Swelling of limbs affects hands and feet Affects either sex Stemmer sign may be positive; usually not painful on pinching	Usually causes symmetrical bilateral swelling of the lower limbs; can occur in arms Swelling stops at ankles and wrists Pain and bruising are prominent features Affects mainly women In pure lipedema, Stemmer signs is negative; often painful on pinching
Etiology	Result from inadequate lymphatic drainage May be congenital or result from damage to the lymphatic system Not usually associated with hormonal imbalances	Unknown; results in excessive subcutaneous fat deposition Appears to be estrogen-related and starts at the time of hormonal change e.g. pregnancy, puberty Family history of lipedema often positive

Figure 4-9 Differential diagnosis: lymphedema vs. lipedema.

c. Tight fit of clothing or jewelry.
d. Aching sensation.
2. Known risk factors.
   a. Primary (idiopathic): congenital abnormality—hypoplasia, hyperplasia, aplasia.
   b. Secondary (acquired): caused by a known insult to the lymphatic system.
      - Cancer: seen most often in breast and cervical cancer.
        ○ Lymph node removal.
        ○ Radiation therapy.
      - Venous disease.
      - Trauma: any condition that may damage or impede lymph flow (e.g., burns, scars, wounds).
      - Cardiac disease: complications from heart failure.
      - Dependent edema.
      - Filariasis: a mosquito-borne illness and the most common cause outside of the United States.

Past Medical History
1. Other diagnoses, surgeries, infections, or cellulitis.
   a. If patient has a history of cancer, then ask:
      - Surgical history (node removal or biopsy).
      - Status of cancer diagnosis.
      - History of radiation, chemo, or hormonal therapy.
2. Medications.
3. Current use of preventive measures for previously asymptomatic patients at risk.
   a. Compressive garments.
   b. Community services and support.
4. Activities that may expose patient to risk.

Social History
1. Family and social support.
2. Living arrangements.
3. Education level/employment.
4. Impact of lifestyle on risk factors.

Quality of Life Issues
1. Impact on functional status.
2. Activities of daily living.
3. Sleep.
4. Past and present level of function.

Physical Examination
1. Assessment of swelling.
   a. Volumetric measurements—in unilateral disease lymphedema is considered present if >10% increase compared to unaffected side.
      - Water displacement.
      - Girth measurement.
      - Bioimpedance—used primarily in bilateral disease and for distinguishing between lipedema and lymphedema.
   b. Pitting edema.
2. Skin assessment: changes in appearance, dryness, scars, wounds, ulcers, skin folds, or fibrotic tissue.
   a. Lymphangiectasia: dilation of lymph vessels, may appear as blister-like protuberances.
   b. Lymphorrhea: leakage of lymph from the skin surface.
   c. Papillomatosis: development of warty growths on the skin that contain dilated lymph vessel and fibrous tissue.
   d. Lipodermatosclerosis: thickening and hardening of the subcutaneous tissue and brown skin discoloration. This is associated with chronic venous insufficiency and, when severe, can damage lymph tissue.
   e. Stemmer's sign. Stemmer's sign is a clinical sign for lymphedema indicated by the presence of a thickened fold of skin at the base of the 2nd toe or 2nd finger. The sign is positive if the skin cannot be lifted but only grasped as a lump of tissue. It is negative if the skin can be normally grasped and pulled away from the underlying tissue.
3. Vascular assessment.
   a. Ankle-Brachial Index (ABI): skin disorders may impact the accuracy of this test.
   b. Alternative assessments may include pulse oximetry, assessment of distal pulses, and tests for arterial and venous insufficiency.
   c. Blood pressure should not be assessed on the affected side.
4. Lymph node palpation.
   a. Soft, moveable, nontender lymph nodes are normal.
   b. Soft, tender lymph nodes that move easily is a sign of inflammation and/or infection. Their presence may correlate with a known illness. If not, patient should be referred to a physician.
   c. Hard, immobile lymph nodes are typically indicative of metastatic cancers and the patient should be referred to a physician.
5. Pain assessment: determine source (e.g., inflammatory, compression, entrapment).
   a. Procedural pain: pain associated with treatment of lymphedema.
   b. Incident pain: pain caused by daily activities.
   c. Background pain: intermittent or continuous pain at rest.
6. Neurological assessment: paresthesia may be present.
7. Postural assessment: changes in limb/body shape and weight may impact posture.
8. Range of motion assessment: changes in limb/body shape and weight may impact active and passive movements.
9. Compensatory movements: changes in limb/body shape and weight may impact movement.
10. Functional assessment.
    a. Changes in mobility. Important to assess suitability of footwear.
    b. Impact on ADLs.
    c. Assessment of sleep quantity and quality.
11. Nutritional status: assessment of body weight.
12. Psychosocial assessment.
    a. Screen for depression.
    b. Anxiety.
    c. Cognitive impairment.
    d. Lack of motivation.
    e. Inability to cope.
    f. Understand disease and treatment.
13. Differential diagnosis.
    a. Lipedema (see Figure 4-9).
14. Differentiate lymphedema from other disorders that affect extremities unilaterally or bilaterally.
    a. Unilateral: acute deep vein thrombosis, post-thrombotic syndrome, arthritis, Baker's cyst.
    b. Bilateral: CHF, chronic venous insufficiency, dependency or stasis edema, renal dysfunction, hepatic dysfunction, lipedema.

Diagnostic Tests
1. Imaging.
   a. Ultrasound: Assess soft tissue for thickening and fibrosis.
   b. Doppler Ultrasound: Used to exclude venous disorders (e.g., DVT).
   c. Lymphoscintigraphy: Identifies lymphatic insufficiency and performed at rest and with exercise.
   d. CT/MRI: evaluates skin thickening and traditional honeycomb patterns in soft tissue. Also differentiates between lipedema, and lymphatic obstruction by a foreign mass.
2. Laboratory tests.
   a. Most cases of lymphedema are diagnosed based on the medical history and physical examination.

b. Other lab tests are used to elucidate the cause of the swelling and to identify comorbidities: CBC, urea and electrolytes, thyroid function tests, liver function tests, fasting glucose, erythrocyte sedimentation rate, plasma total protein, and albumin.
c. See Table 4-20 for summary.

Intervention/Rehabilitation Guidelines for Lymphedema

Intervention for Asymptomatic Patients Who Are At Risk for Lymphedema

1. Meticulous skin and nail care: apply moisturizer regularly, avoid sunburn, and avoid blisters and injuries that could risk infection.
2. Lifestyle management and patient education. (See Quick Facts 4-19.)
   a. Weight management and gradual increases in activity: avoid sports that incorporate centrifugal forces (e.g., golf, tennis).
   b. Avoid sudden heavy lifting.
   c. Mosquito nets for areas where filariasis may be prevalent.

Table 4-20

Lymphedema Summary	
ETIOLOGY	Primary lymphedema: congenital Secondary lymphedema: occurs as a result of injury to lymphatic vessels (e.g., cancer surgery and/or radiation, chronic venous insufficiency) or parasitic infection (filariasis)
PROGRESSIVE OVER TIME	Without treatment, may develop into fibrosis, chronic infection (cellulitis, lymphangitis) or loss of limb function
SYMPTOMS	Heaviness, tightness or pain; swelling and persistent edema; loss of ROM and function in an arm or leg
SKIN CHANGES	Hardening and/or discoloration of skin
DIAGNOSIS	History, visual inspection and palpation, girth measurements Tests may include: MRI and CT scans; Doppler ultrasound, radionuclide imaging of the lymphatic system (lymphoscintigraphy)
STAGING	4 stage system: 0 – latent; 1 – spontaneously reversible; 2 – spontaneously irreversible; 3 – lymphostatic elephantiasis (American Society of Lymphology)
TREATMENT	Complete decongestive therapy (CDT): Manual lymph drainage, short-stretch compression bandages, exercises, functional training, skin care and lymphedema education.

QUICK FACTS 4-19 ▶ PATIENT EDUCATION FOR LYMPHEDEMA MANAGEMENT

Prevention and Maintenance Techniques

- Avoid dependent positions for extended periods of time.
- Avoid sitting cross-legged.
- When traveling, break long distances up by getting up and walking (car, plane, train). Elevate affected extremity on window ledge, dashboard, another seat when able.
- Maintain water intake.
- Maintain ideal body weight.
- Perform muscle-pumping exercises routinely.
- Avoid lifting and carrying heavy loads (e.g., carrying large brief case or suitcase, shoulder bag, or backpack).
- Avoid vigorous, repetitive tasks (e.g., lifting weights).
- Avoid wearing restrictive clothing (e.g., elastic bands on socks and sleeves). Be careful of tight jewelry (e.g., rings, wrist watch, bracelet).
- Wear compressive garments, especially when traveling.
- Monitor sodium intake in diet.

Skin Care

- Keep skin clean and moisturize. Use caution as some moisturizers have a high petroleum content and can damage or breakdown the latex fibers in compression garments.
- Pat skin dry versus rubbing dry.
- Pay careful attention to avoid infections any time integrity of skin is compromised (e.g., scrape, insect bite, blister).
- Avoid exposure to harsh chemicals (e.g., cleaning agents) by wearing gloves.
- Protect feet; wear properly fitting shoes and socks.
- Use caution with shaving; an electric razor is a good choice.
- Use caution when trimming nails.
- Avoid hot baths, whirlpools, and saunas secondary to the increase in core temperature and related superficial vasodilation.

3. Avoid limb constriction.
   a. No blood pressure checks on affected side.
   b. Loose fitting jewelry and clothing.
4. Compression garments.
   a. Ensure a good fit.
   b. Wear when exercising or flying.
5. Avoid temperature extremes.
   a. No temperatures above 102 degrees in hot tub/saunas.
   b. Avoid extreme cold.
   c. Use high factor sunscreen.

Phase I Management: Edema Secondary to Lymphatic Dysfunction

1. Complete decongestive therapy (CDT).
   a. Manual lymphatic drainage (MLD).
      - Massage (Vodder techniques, modifications by Asdonk, Leduc, and Fodi). Technique requires very low pressure effleurage strokes.
      - Emphasis is on decongesting proximal segments first at the right lymphatic duct (for right upper extremity involvement) and the thoracic duct (for left upper extremity, lower extremities and the torso).
      - Compression using multilayered padding and short-stretch bandages.
        ○ Bandages have low resting and high working pressure.
          – Bandages preserve and advance changes associated with MLD and account for 50% of improvement in symptoms.
        ○ Treatments should be applied by certified specialists: certified lymphedema therapist (CLT).
        ○ Specialized education resources for MLD and CDT.
          – National Lymphedema Network: http://www.lymphnet.org.
          – Lymphology Association of North America: https://www.clt-lana.org.

RED FLAG: Patients with significant or poorly controlled cardiopulmonary disease may become unstable if they are not able to tolerate the potential increase in plasma volume caused by lymphedema reduction.

   b. Compression bandaging/garments.
      - Short-stretch compression bandages, worn 24 hours per day.
      - Bandages have low resting and high working pressure.
      - Bandages preserve and advance changes associated with MLD and may account for 50% of improvement in symptoms.
      - Must monitor distal symptoms and swelling for excessive pressure in off-the-shelf or customized garments.

RED FLAG: Excessively high pressures will occlude superficial lymph capillaries and restrict fluid absorption.

   c. Exercise.
      - Decongestive exercises work with bandages to compress lymph between the bandage and muscles to move fluid proximally.
      - Walking and cycling program.
      - Water-based programs: water aerobics, swimming.
      - Tai chi and balance activities.
      - ADL training.

RED FLAG: Strenuous activities, jogging, ballistic movements, and rotational motions are contraindicated, as they are likely to exacerbate lymphedema.

      - Be aware of lymph overload symptoms: discomfort, aching, or pain in proximal lymph areas, change in skin color. If any are present, discontinue activity.
   d. Skin care: hygiene, skin care, nail care.
      - Protein rich fluids reduce local immune systems.
      - Bacterial infections are common: streptococcus, cellulitis.
      - Prevention of skin/nail problems.
        ○ Regular inspection: caregiver assistance if needed.
        ○ Regular cleansing.
        ○ Regular moisturizing: Maintain a pH of 5.0 on skin.
        ○ Protection: Appropriate footwear, use of appropriate socks.
   e. Patient education (regarding skin care, garment wear, and other lymphedema self-management principles).
2. Contraindicated modalities.
   a. Modalities that cause vasodilation or increase lymph load (e.g., ice, heat, hydrotherapy, saunas, contrast bath, paraffin).
   b. Electrotherapeutic modalities greater than 30 Hz.

Phase II Management

1. Continue with CDT components/principles.
2. Skin care.
3. Compression garments: may use lymphedema bandaging at night.
4. Exercise: combined with compression garments.

5. Pneumatic compression pumps used with caution.
   a. High pressures can damage lymph nodes.
   b. May move water instead of proteins.
   c. Use on lower extremity increases risk of genital lymphedema.
   d. Low pressure, sequential pumps are preferred.
   e. Use in Stage I lymphedema only: do not use if there is any change in skin or subcutaneous tissue, exacerbation of inflammation and fibrosis can occur in Stage II and Stage III patients.

RED FLAG: Pressures > 45 mm Hg are contraindicated.

6. MLD as needed.
   a. Specialized education resources for MLD and CDT.
      - National Lymphedema Network: http://www.lymphnet.org.
      - Lymphology Association of North America: https://www.clt-lana.org.
7. Patient education.
   a. Skin and nail care.
   b. Self-bandaging, garment care.
   c. Infection prevention/management.
   d. Maintain exercise while preventing lymph overload.
8. Surgery to assist in lymph drainage (severe cases).
   a. Surgical reduction: de-bulking subcutaneous tissue and skin in severe cases of those who are considerably symptomatic. Significant risk of post-surgical morbidity.
   b. Restoring lymph flow: lymphovenous anastomoses and lymphatic vessel grafting and lymph node transplantation. Successful in patients with intact distal lymph and proximal lymph obstruction.
   c. Liposuction: may be considered for patients with nonpitting lymphedema and when other conservative measures have failed. Must use compressive garments post-surgically.

Outcome Measures/Self-Report Instruments
1. Lymphoedema Quality of Life (LYMQOL).
2. Lymph-ICF.
3. Lymphedema Life Impact Scale (LLIS).

APPENDIX 4A

Sample Exercise Programs per MET Level

Exercises	Activities
LEVEL I: 1.0–1.5 METS (TABLE 4-21)	
• Passive/active assistive ROM (PROM/AAROM) to larger joints, active ROM (AROM) to smaller joints (ankles, knees, hands, wrists) • Diaphragmatic breathing • Use of incentive spirometer every hour for surgical patients	• Basic self care: Feed self, turn self, wash hands and face, use commode • Sit on edge of bed with feet supported. Perform 10–15 minutes, 1–2 times/day as tolerated; ensure 1-hour rest between activities
LEVEL II: 1.5–2.5 METS	
• May add in prone activities • Continue diaphragmatic breathing • Incorporate active exercises or larger joints (may need to limit shoulder elevation to 90 degrees) • Use of incentive spirometer every hour for surgical patients	• Sit in chair, for meals, as tolerated • May bathe entire body, with assistance for legs and back • Use commode • Sit on edge of bed with feet supported 10–15 minutes, one to two times/day • Ensure 1 hour of rest between activities
LEVEL III: 2.5–3.5 METS	
• Continue diaphragmatic breathing with surgical patients • Warm-up exercises: Active knee, ankle, and shoulder movements • Cervical AROM • Walk 100–150 feet each walk, gradually increase the distance. A minimum of three walks/day is desired.	• Use bathroom • Shave or apply makeup • May wash at sink • Up in room, as tolerated • Ensure rest between activities

(Continued)

Exercises	Activities
LEVEL IV: 3.5–4.5 METS	
Warm-up Exercises: • Continue diaphragmatic breathing exercises with surgical patients • Marching in place • Trunk rotation and side bending • Shoulder elevation to 90 degrees Exercise: • Walk 150–250 feet, three times a day	• May shower if permitted (surgical heart patients shower seventh day if incision is intact and dry and there are no stitches or staples) • Continue previous activities • Ensure rest periods between activities
LEVEL V: 4.5–5.5 METS	
Exercises (in standing) • Continue level IV warm-up • Walk 250–350 feet, three times/day • Walk up and down 10 steps slowly with a pause every fifth step. Walk should be timed and time and distance slowly increased.	• Continue previous activities, increase as tolerated within heart rate and activity guidelines

Table 4-21

Metabolic Equivalent (MET) Levels

CLASS	SIGNS AND SYMPTOMS	MAXIMUM METS AND ACTIVITIES ALLOWED
I—mild	No symptoms with ordinary physical activity No limitation in physical activity Comfortable at rest or ordinary activity does not cause undue fatigue, palpitation, dyspnea, or angina pain.	6.5 Moderate shoveling, push mower, square dancing, singles tennis, walking at 4.5 mph
II—mild	Slight limitations of physical activity. Comfortable at rest, but ordinary physical activity results in fatigue, palpitations, or dyspnea.	4.5 Painting, scrubbing floors, carrying golf clubs, foxtrot dancing, walking at 3.5 mph
III—moderate	Marked limitation of physical activities. Comfortable at rest, but minimal activity results in fatigue, palpitations, or dyspnea.	3.0 Riding lawn mower, light wood working, walking at 2 mph
IV—severe	Unable to do physical activity without discomfort. Cardiac insufficiency symptoms at rest. Angina may be present at rest.	1.5 Desk work, driving, walking <1 mph, sewing

Review Questions

Cardiac, Vascular, and Lymphatic Physical Therapy

1. List three non-modifiable and three modifiable risk factors for coronary artery disease.

2. Describe the signs and symptoms of left-sided congestive heart failure (CHF) versus right-sided CHF.

3. Differentiate these signs and symptoms of cardiovascular disease.
   Chest pain
   Dyspnea
   Claudication

4. Discuss the clinical significance of cardiovascular laboratory tests and values—SaO_2 and hematocrit percentages. Identify normal and abnormal values. Identify modifications a PTA should make during a patient treatment session when values are abnormal.

5. What effect does taking a beta blocker have on a patient who is exercising?

6. Compare and contrast Phase 1 to Phase 2 management for individuals with edema secondary to lymphatic dysfunction.

5

Pulmonary Physical Therapy

JULIE ANN STARR and KAREN E. RYAN

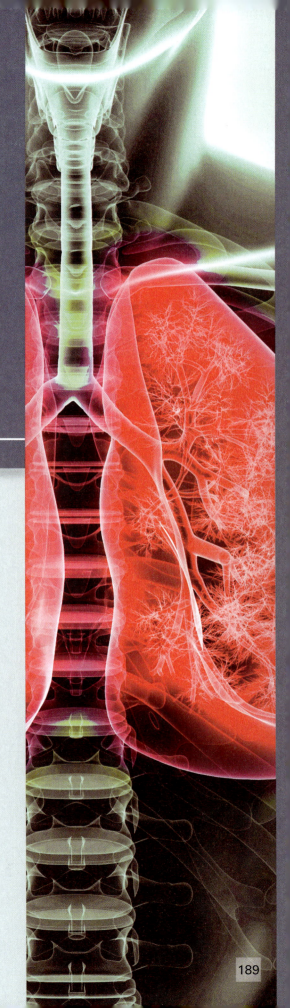

Chapter Outline

- Pulmonary Anatomy and Physiology, 191
  - Bony Thorax, 191
  - Internal Structures, 191
  - Muscles of Ventilation, 191
  - Mechanics of Breathing, 193
  - Ventilation, 193
  - Respiration, 193
  - Ventilation (V_E) and Perfusion (Blood Flow, or Q), 194
  - Control of Ventilation, 194
- Physical Therapy Examination and Data Collection, 195
  - Patient Interview, 195
  - Data Collection, 195
  - Medical Tests and Examinations, 197
- Physical Dysfunction/Impairments, 199
  - Acute Diseases, 199
  - Chronic Obstructive Diseases, 201
  - General Medical Management, 202

- General Physical Therapy Management, 202
- Chronic Restrictive Diseases, 203
- General Medical Management, 203
- General Physical Therapy Management, 203
- Bronchogenic Carcinoma, 203
- Trauma, 204
- Other Pulmonary Conditions, 204
- Physical Therapy Intervention, 206
  - Manual Secretion Removal Techniques, 206
  - Airway Clearance Techniques, 208
  - Independent Secretion Removal Techniques, 209
  - Breathing Exercises, 210
  - Postsurgical Care, 211
  - Activities for Increasing Functional Abilities, 211
  - Medical and Surgical Management of Pulmonary Disease, 212
- Intensive Care Unit Management, 214
  - Physical Therapy in the Intensive Care Unit, 214
- Review Questions, 217

Pulmonary Anatomy and Physiology

Bony Thorax

Anterior Border: The Sternum (Manubrium, Body, Xiphoid Process)
1. The lateral borders of the trachea run perpendicularly into the suprasternal notch.
2. The angle of Louis (sternal angle), the bony ridge between the manubrium and body, is the point of anterior attachment of the second rib and tracheal bifurcation.

Lateral Border: The Rib Cage
1. Ribs 1–6, termed true or costosternal ribs, have a single anterior costochondral attachment to the sternum.
2. Ribs 7–10, termed false or costochondral ribs, share costochondral attachments before attaching anteriorly to the sternum.
3. Ribs 11 and 12 are termed floating or costovertebral ribs, as they have no anterior attachment.

Posterior Border
1. The vertebral column, from T1 through T12.

Shoulder Girdle
1. Can affect the motion of the thorax.
2. Provides attachments for accessory muscles of ventilation.

Internal Structures

Upper Airways
1. Nose or mouth: entry point into the respiratory system. The nose filters, humidifies, and warms air.
2. Pharynx: common area used for both respiratory and digestive systems.
3. Larynx: connects the pharynx to trachea, including the epiglottis and vocal cords.
4. See Figure 5-1 for pulmonary anatomy.

Lower Airways
1. The conducting airways, trachea to terminal bronchioles, transport air only. No gas exchange occurs.
2. The respiratory unit: respiratory bronchioles, alveolar ducts, alveolar sacs, and alveoli. Diffusion of gas occurs through all of these structures.

Lung Structures
1. Right lung divides into three lobes by the oblique and horizontal fissure lines. Each lobe divides into segments, totaling 10 segments.

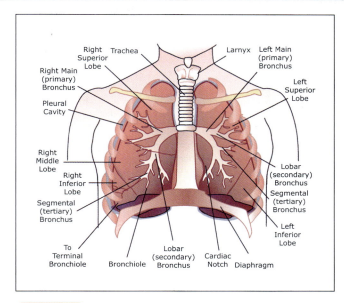

Figure 5-1 Pulmonary anatomy.

2. Left lung divides into two lobes by a single oblique fissure line. Each lobe divides into segments, totaling 8 segments.

Pleura
1. Parietal pleura covers the inner surface of the thoracic cage, diaphragm, and mediastinal border of the lung.
2. Visceral pleura wraps the outer surface of the lung, including the fissure lines.
3. Intrapleural space is the potential space between the two pleurae that maintains the approximation of the rib cage and lungs, allowing forces to be transmitted from one structure to another.

Muscles of Ventilation

Primary Muscles of Inspiration
1. Produce a normal resting tidal volume.
2. Primary muscle of inspiration is the diaphragm. The diaphragm is made of two hemidiaphragms, each with a central tendon. When the diaphragm is at rest, the hemidiaphragms are arched high into the thorax. When the muscle contracts, the central tendon is pulled downward, flattening the dome. The result is a protrusion of the abdominal wall during inhalation. See Table 5-1.
3. Additional primary muscles of inspiration are portions of the intercostals.

Table 5-1

Inspiratory and Expiratory Musculature

ACTION	MUSCLES	INNERVATION
Resting Inspiration	Diaphragm	Phrenic nerve, C3–C5 (remember "C3-4-5 stay alive")
Deep Inspiration (accessory muscles)	Muscles of resting inspiration Sternocleidomastoid, scalenes—elevate upper 2 ribs Levator costarum, scalenes—elevate remaining ribs Pectoralis major Serratus posterior superior	SCM: Accessory nerve (cranial nerve XI), cranial nerves 2, 3 Scalene: lower cervical nerve
Forced Inspiration Compensation (often assisted by fixing the shoulder girdle)	Muscles of resting and deep inspiration Trapezius Pectorals Serratus Levator scapula	Trapezius: spinal accessory (cranial nerve XI) Pectoralis: medial pectoral (C8, T1) Serratus: long thoracic, C5–7 Levator: C3–4 cervical, dorsal scapular
Resting Expiration	Normal relaxation of the muscles of inspiration and elastic recoil of the lungs Internal intercostals	Intercostal nerve T2–T6
Forced Expiration	Muscles of forced expiration Abdominal muscles (rectus abdominis, transverse abdominis, obliques) Quadratus lumborum (QL) Lower iliocostalis Serratus posterior inferior	Abdominals: 7–12th intercostal nerves, iliohypogastric, ilioinguinal QL: 12th thoracic and 1st lumbar

Accessory Muscles of Inspiration

1. Used when a more rapid or deeper inhalation is required or in disease states.
2. The upper two ribs are raised by the scalenes and sternocleidomastoid. The rest of the ribs are raised by the levator costarum and serratus. By fixing the shoulder girdle, the trapezius, pectorals, and serratus can become muscles of inspiration.
3. See Quick Facts 5-1.

Expiratory Muscles of Ventilation

1. Resting exhalation results from a passive relaxation of the inspiratory muscles and the elastic recoil tendency of the lung. Normal abdominal tone holds the abdominal contents directly under the diaphragm, assisting the return of the diaphragm to the normal high domed position.
2. Expiratory muscles are used when a quicker and/or fuller expiration is desired, as in exercise or in disease states. These are quadratus lumborum, portions of the intercostals, muscles of the abdomen, and triangularis sterni.

Patients Who Lack Abdominal Musculature (e.g., Spinal Cord Injury)

1. Have a lower resting position of the diaphragm, decreasing inspiratory reserve.
2. The more upright the body position, the lower the diaphragm and the lower the inspiratory capacity.
3. The more supine the body position, the more advantageous the position of the diaphragm.
4. An abdominal binder may be helpful in providing support to the abdominal viscera, assisting ventilation. Care must be taken not to constrict the thorax with the abdominal binder.

QUICK FACTS 5-1 ▶ MUSCLES OF RESPIRATION

Muscles	Inspiratory	Expiratory
Primary	Diaphragm Portions of the Intercostals	Passive action of relaxation after inspiration
Accessory	Scalenes Sternocleidomastoid Levator costarum, serratus (potentially, more compromised individual)	Quadratus lumborum Portions of the intercostals Muscles of the abdomen Triangularis sterni

Mechanics of Breathing

Forces Acting upon the Rib Cage
1. Elastic recoil of the lung parenchyma pulls the lungs and, therefore, visceral pleura, parietal pleura, and bony thorax into a position of exhalation (inward pull).
2. Bony thorax pulls the thorax and, therefore, parietal pleura, visceral pleura, and lungs into a position of inspiration (outward pull).
3. Muscular action pulls either outward or inward, depending on the muscles used.
4. Resting end expiratory pressure (REEP) is the point of equilibrium where these forces are balanced. Occurs at end tidal expiration.

Ventilation

Lung Volumes
1. Definition: Movement of gas in and out of the pulmonary system.
2. Tidal volume (TV): volume of gas inhaled (or exhaled) during a normal resting breath. See Figure 5-2.
3. Inspiratory reserve volume (IRV): volume of gas that can be inhaled beyond a normal resting tidal inhalation.
4. Expiratory reserve volume (ERV): volume of gas that can be exhaled beyond a normal resting tidal exhalation.
5. Residual volume (RV): volume of gas that remains in the lungs after ERV has been exhaled.

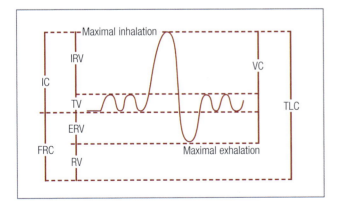

Figure 5-2 **Lung volumes and capacities.**
IRV = inspiratory reserve volume; TV = tidal volume; ERV = expiratory reserve volume; RV = residual volume; IC = inspiratory capacity; FRC = functional residual capacity; VC = vital capacity; TLC = total lung capacity.
From: O'Sullivan S, Schmidt T: *Physical Rehabilitation*, 5th ed. FA Davis, 2007, p. 562, with permission.

Capacities: Two or More Lung Volumes Added Together
1. Inspiratory capacity (IRV + TV): the amount of air that can be inhaled from REEP.
2. Vital capacity (IRV + TV + ERV): the amount of air that is under volitional control; conventionally measured as forced expiratory vital capacity (FVC).
3. Functional residual capacity (ERV + RV): the amount of air that resides in the lungs after a normal resting tidal exhalation.
4. Total lung capacity (IRV + TV + ERV + RV): the total amount of air that is contained within the thorax during a maximum inspiratory effort.

Flow Rates
1. Forced expiratory volume in 1 second (FEV_1): the amount of air exhaled during the first second of FVC. In the healthy person, at least 70% of the FVC is exhaled within the first second ($FEV_1/FVC \times 100 > 70\%$).
2. Forced expiratory flow rate (FEF 25%–75%) is the slope of a line drawn between the points 25% and 75% of exhaled volume on a forced vital capacity exhalation curve. This flow rate is more specific to the smaller airways and shows a more dramatic change with disease than FEV_1.

Respiration

Definition
1. Diffusion of gas across the alveolar membrane.

Arterial Oxygenation
1. Definition: the ability of arterial blood to carry oxygen.
2. Partial pressure of oxygen in the atmosphere (PaO_2) at sea level is 760 mm Hg (barometric pressure) × 21% = 159.6 mm Hg.
3. Partial pressure of oxygen in the arterial blood, PaO_2, depends on the integrity of the pulmonary system, the circulatory system, and the PaO_2. PaO_2 at room air is 95–100 mm Hg in a young, healthy individual. Hypoxemia: PaO_2 decreases with age, but in a young, healthy individual, mild hypoxemia would be considered at <90. Hyperoxemia: $PaO_2 > 100$.
4. Fraction of oxygen in the inspired air (FiO_2) is the percentage of oxygen in air, based on a total of 1.00. The FiO_2 of room air, approximately 21% oxygen, is written as 0.21. Supplemental oxygen increases the percentage (>21%) of oxygen in the patient's atmosphere. Supplemental oxygen is usually prescribed when the PaO_2 falls below 55 mm Hg.

Alveolar Ventilation
1. Ability to remove carbon dioxide from the pulmonary circulation and maintain pH.
2. pH indicates the concentration of free-floating hydrogen ions within the body. Normal range for pH is 7.35–7.45.
3. $PaCO_2$: the partial pressure of carbon dioxide within the arterial blood; in health, 35 to 45 mm Hg. Hypercapnea is a $PaCO_2$ >45 mm Hg. Hypocapnea is a $PaCO_2$ <35 mm Hg. Removal or retention of CO_2 by the respiratory system alters the pH of the body in an inverse relationship. An increase in the $PaCO_2$ decreases the body's pH. A decrease in the $PaCO_2$ raises the body's pH.
4. HCO_3^-: amount of bicarbonate ions within the arterial blood, normally 22–28 mEq/mL. Removal or retention of HCO_3^- alters the pH of the body in a direct relationship. An increase in bicarbonate ions increases the body's pH. A decrease in bicarbonate ions decreases the body's pH.

Ventilation (V_E) and Perfusion (Blood Flow, or Q)

Optimal Respiration
1. Occurs when ventilation and perfusion (blood flow to the lungs) are matched.
2. Different ventilation and perfusion relationships exist.

Dead Space
1. Anatomical (conducting airways) or physiological (diseases such as pulmonary emboli).
2. Dead space is a space that is well ventilated, but in which no respiration (gas exchange) occurs.

Shunt
1. No respiration occurs because of a ventilation abnormality.
2. Complete atelectasis of a respiratory unit allows the blood to travel through the pulmonary capillary without gas diffusion.

Effects of Body Position—Ventilation Perfusion Gravity Dependent
1. Upright position.
   a. Perfusion is gravity dependent (i.e., more pulmonary blood is found at the base of the lung in the upright position).
   b. Ventilation. At the static point of REEP, the apical alveoli are fuller than those at the base. During the dynamic phase of inspiration, more air will be delivered to the less-filled alveoli at the bases, causing a greater change in V_E at the bases.
   c. Ventilation perfusion ratio (V/Q ratio): the ratio of pulmonary alveolar ventilation to pulmonary capillary perfusion. In the upright position, the apices are gravity independent, with the lowest blood flow, or Q. Although relatively low, there is still more air than blood, resulting in a high V/Q ratio (dead space). Perfusion and ventilation of the middle zone of the lung are evenly matched. The bases are gravity dependent and, therefore, have the most Q. Although V_E is relatively high, there is more blood than air, resulting in a (relatively) low V/Q ratio (shunt).
2. Other body positions. Every body position creates these zones: gravity independent, middle, and gravity dependent.
   a. The gravity-independent area of the lung, despite the position of the body, acts as dead space.
   b. The gravity-dependent area of the lung acts as a shunt.
   c. Body positions can be used for a variety of treatment goals: to drain secretions, to increase ventilation, or to optimize ventilation perfusion relationships.

Control of Ventilation

Receptors
1. Baroreceptors, chemoreceptors, irritant receptors, and stretch receptors within the body assist in adjusting the ventilatory cycle by sending information to the controller.

Central Control Centers
1. Cortex, pons, medulla, and autonomic nervous system evaluate the receptors' information.
2. Send a message out to the ventilatory muscles to alter the respiratory cycle in order to maintain adequate alveolar ventilation and arterial oxygenation.

Ventilatory Muscles
1. Institute the changes deemed necessary by the central controllers.

Physical Therapy Examination and Data Collection

Patient Interview

Prior to Intervention
1. Review/obtain information from the patient, the patient's family, and the medical record.
2. Identify chief complaint.
   a. Usually involves the loss of function (decreased ability to perform activities of daily living [ADLs]) or discomfort (shortness of breath [dyspnea]).
3. Present illness.
   a. Initial onset (sudden vs. insidious) and progression of primary problem.
   b. Anything that worsens or improves condition: positions, rest, medications.
4. Review the patient's history.
   a. Occupational history. Past occupational exposures for diseases such as asbestosis, silicosis, and pneumoconiosis. Present occupational exposure to antigens within the workplace (hypersensitivity pneumonitis).
   b. Past medical history that would alter physical exam or treatment plans (e.g., heart disease, long-term steroid use).
   c. Current medications that can mask (steroids) or alter (beta blockers, bronchodilators) vital signs.
   d. Social habits.
      - Smoking in pack years (number of packs per day × number of years smoked).
      - Alcohol consumption.
      - Street drugs.
   e. Functional and exertional activity level during periods of wellness, as well as with present illness.
   f. Cough and sputum production. Record any changes from baseline because of present illness.
   g. Family history of pulmonary disease (e.g., cystic fibrosis).

Data Collection

Vital Signs
1. Temperature: normal (afebrile) 98.6°F (37°C). Core temperature increase indicates infection. See Table 5-2 for normal values.
2. Heart rate (HR): normal 60–100 bpm; tachycardia: HR >100 bpm; bradycardia: HR <60 bpm.
3. Measure and observe respirations. Note comfort with breathing, use of accessory muscles (at rest and with activity), grimacing, nasal flaring (the nares flare with inspiration).
   a. Rate: measure in breaths per minute (br/min).
   b. Rhythm: regular or irregular.

Table 5-2

Normal Values for Infants and Adults

PARAMETER	INFANT	ADULT
Heart Rate	120 bpm	60–100 bpm
Blood Pressure	75/50 mmHg	<120/80 mmHg
Respiratory Rate	40 br/min	12–20 br/min
PaO_2	75–80 mmHg	80–100 mmHg
$PaCO_2$	34–54 mmHg	35–45 mmHg
pH	7.26–7.41	7.35–7.45
Tidal Volume	20 ml	500 ml

   c. Amplitude: shallow, deep.
   d. Pattern: apnea—temporary halt to breathing; bradypnea—slowed rate, <12 br/min; dyspnea—sensation of breathlessness, rated by the patient; tachypnea—rapid, shallow breathing pattern, indicates distress. See Quick Facts 5-2.
4. Blood pressure.

> **QUICK FACTS 5-2 ▶ DYSPNEA SCALE**
> +1 Mild, noticeable to patient but no observer
> +2 Mild, some difficulty, but can continue
> +3 Moderate difficulty, but can continue
> +4 Severe difficulty, patient cannot continue

Observation
1. Symmetry or lack of: jugular veins (patients with CHF will display distention bilaterally, unilateral indicates a local condition), rib angle and chest—observe from anterior, lateral and posterior views.
   a. Rib angle: a barrel chest—ribs take on a more horizontal position and the anteroposterior (AP) diameter of the chest increases. Commonly seen in patients with COPD.
   b. Chest wall deformities: pectus excavatum/funnel chest—lower sternum is depressed, pectus carinatum/pigeon chest—upper sternum is prominent.
2. Peripheral edema seen in gravity-dependent areas and jugular venous distension indicates possible heart failure. Right ventricular hypertrophy and dilation (cor pulmonale) are common sequelae to chronic lung disease.
3. Body positions. Stabilizing the shoulder girdle (e.g., on overbed table, arm rests) places the thorax in the inspiratory position and allows the additional recruitment of muscles for inspiration (pectorals). Positional

changes, supine, sidelying, etc. affect ability to easily draw breath.
4. Color: cyanosis, an acute sign of hypoxemia, is a bluish tinge to nail beds and the areas around eyes and mouth.
5. Digital clubbing: a sign of chronic hypoxemia.
6. The configuration of the distal phalanx of fingers or toes becomes bulbous.

Auscultation with Stethoscope
1. Use of stethoscope.
   a. The diaphragm portion allows for auscultation of high-pitched sounds.
   b. The bell portion allows for auscultation of lower-pitched sounds.
2. Intensity of inspiration and expiration will be quieter at the bases than the apex.
   a. Vesicular (normal breath sound): a soft rustling sound heard throughout inspiration and expiration with no pause in between.
   b. Bronchial: a more hollow, loud, echoing sound normally found over the right superior anterior thorax; this corresponds to an area over the right main stem bronchus. All of inspiration and most of expiration are heard with bronchial breath sounds. Abnormal bronchial sounds are associated with obstruction of lung segments because of secretions—sounds become higher pitched; or by compression of the lung tissue by extrapulmonary sources, e.g., increased pleural fluid (plural effusion).
   c. Decreased or absent: sound transmission is diminished or obscured because of internal pulmonary pathology or external causes, e.g., muscular weakness, skeletal deformities (kyphosis), self-limited inspiration secondary to pain. Often associated with obstructive lung diseases.
3. Adventitious (extra) sounds. According to the American Thoracic Society, there are only two adventitious breath sounds:
   a. Crackles (also termed *rales, crepitations*): a low-pitched, discontinuous crackling sound heard usually during inspiration that indicates a condition in the peripheral airways or pathology (atelectasis, fibrosis, pulmonary edema). Sounds like: rubbing of multiple strands of hair between fingers, pulling sheets of plastic cling wrap apart.
   b. Wheezes: a musical high-pitched hissing sound, usually heard during expiration caused by airway obstruction (asthma, chronic obstructive pulmonary disease [COPD], foreign body aspiration). With severe airway constriction, as with croup, wheezes may be heard on inspiration as well.
   c. Rhonchi: a low-pitched continuous sound, heard on inspiration and expiration. Indicative of an obstructive process in the larger, more central airways. Sounds like a continuous snore.

4. Breathing patterns.
   a. Cheyne-Stokes: repeated cycles of deep breathing followed by shallow breaths or cessation of breathing. Associated with congestive heart failure, renal failure, drug overdose, meningitis; may be considered normal in infants and older people during sleep.
   b. Paradoxical breathing (reverse breathing): a portion, or all, of the chest wall depresses during inspiration; may observe abdominal expansion with exhalation; may lead to a flattened chest wall (pectus excavatum).
   c. Kussmaul's respiration: dyspnea characterized by an increased respiratory rate (>20/min) and depth of respiration, panting and labored respiration—air hunger. Associated with strenuous exercise or metabolic acidosis.

Chest Wall Excursion
1. Normal chest wall expansion occurring with inhalation should occur in a symmetrical fashion bilaterally. In a young adult, normal expansion is approximately 3.25 inches (8.5 cm) if measuring circumference of chest at xiphoid process.
   a. This measurement can be done by the therapist assistant facing the patient, placing hands bilaterally over the lateral rib area with thumb tips touching at area of xiphoid process, and upon patient inspiration assess if rib movement is felt bilaterally to an equal extent.
2. Chest wall movement will be unilaterally restricted in conditions such as lobar pneumonia and will be restricted bilaterally in conditions such as COPD.
3. Assessing chest motion via palpation. The therapist assistant stands or sits facing the patient and places their hands gently on the patient to assess rib motion as the patient inhales and exhales.
   a. Upper lobe motion: place hands so that heel of the hand is at approximately the 4th rib, fingers rest across the upper trapezius area and thumbs rest horizontally meeting at the sternum. Ask patient to inhale and assess for symmetry and extent of movement.
   b. Anterolateral and middle lobe motion: place hands so that the palms lie on the anterolateral rib area with web space between thumb and first finger resting below nipple line, thumbs rest horizontally meeting at the sternum. Ask patient to inhale and assess for symmetry and extent of movement.
   c. Posterior and lower lobe motion: (position the patient facing away from the therapist assistant) place hands so that the palms are flat on the posteriolateral chest wall at the level of the 10th rib with fingers angling toward axillary boarder of the scapula, thumbs rest horizontally meeting at the midline. Ask patient to inhale and assess for symmetry and extent of movement.

Medical Tests and Examinations

Radiographic Examination
1. Chest x-ray (CXR): a two-dimensional radiographic film to detect the presence of abnormal material (exudate, blood) or a change in pulmonary parenchyma (fibrosis, collapse).
2. Computed tomographic (CT) scan: computer-generated picture of a cross-sectional plane of the body.
3. Magnetic resonance imaging (MRI). (See Figure 5-3.)
4. Ventilation perfusion (V/Q) scan: matches the ventilation pattern of the lung to the perfusion pattern to identify the presence of pulmonary emboli.
5. Fluoroscopy: continuous x-ray beam allows observation of diaphragmatic excursion.

Laboratory Tests
1. Arterial blood gas (ABG) analysis (see Table 5-3) indicates the adequacy of:
   a. Alveolar ventilation by determining pH, bicarbonate ion, and partial pressure of carbon dioxide. Table 5-4 presents the four basic conditions of acid-base balance and the $PaCO_2$, pH, and HCO_3^- values that accompany each condition.
   b. Arterial oxygenation by determining the partial pressure of oxygen in relation to the fraction of inspired oxygen.
2. Electrocardiogram: see Chapter 4 (Cardiac, Vascular, and Lymphatic Physical Therapy) for discussion.
3. Sputum studies.
   a. Gram stain: immediate identification of the category of bacteria (gram negative or gram positive) and its appearance (e.g., pairs, chains).
   b. Culture and sensitivity: identifies the specific bacteria as well as the organism's susceptibility to various antibiotics. Results available within a few days.
   c. Cytology: reports the presence of cancer cells in sputum.
4. Pulmonary function tests (PFTs): evaluate lung volumes, capacities, and flow rates. Used to diagnose disease, monitor progression, and determine the benefits of medical management. See Figure 5-4 for changes with disease states. See Table 5-5 for classification of obstructive lung disease according to the Global Initiative for Obstructive Lung Disease (GOLD), including PFT values for each level of disease severity.
5. Blood values.
   a. White blood cell (WBC) count normal values: 4,000–11,000.
   b. Hematocrit (Hct) normal values: 35%–48%.
   c. Hemoglobin (Hgb) normal values: 12–16 g/dL.

Bronchoscopy
1. Endoscope used to view, biopsy, wash, suction, and/or brush the interior aspects of the tracheobronchial tree.

Exercise Tolerance Tests (ETT) (Graded Exercise Test)
1. Evaluates an individual's cardiopulmonary response to gradually increasing exercise.
2. Determines the presence of exercise-induced bronchospasm by testing pulmonary function, particularly FEV_1 before and after ETT.
3. Documents the need for supplemental oxygen during an exercise program by analyzing arterial blood gas values throughout the ETT. ABGs also provide a criterion for test termination. If arterial blood sampling is unavailable, pulse oximetry can be used to monitor the percent saturation of oxygen within the arterial blood. Table 5-6 presents criteria for test termination for patients with pulmonary disease.
4. See Chapter 4 (Cardiac, Vascular, and Lymphatic Physical Therapy) for additional information.

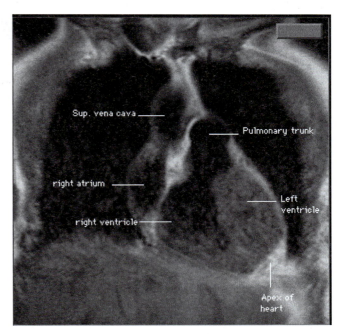

Figure 5-3 Coronal T1 MRI thoracic view of normal female.

Table 5-3

Arterial Blood Gases

BLOOD GAS	ABBREVIATION	NORMAL VALUE AT ROOM AIR	ABNORMAL VALUES
Partial pressure of oxygen (arterial concentration of oxygen in the blood)	PaO_2	80–100 mmHg (normal health, room air)	Hypoxemia = PaO_2 <90 Hyperoxemia = PaO_2 >100 Supplemental oxygen typically prescribed when PaO_2 is <55–60 mmHg
Partial pressure of carbon dioxide (levels of carbon dioxide in the blood)	$PaCO_2$	35–45 mmHg	Retention of arterial CO_2 in the blood will decrease the pH of the blood. $PaCO_2$ <35 mmHg = Hypocapnea $PaCO_2$ >45 mmHg = Hypercapnea
Concentration of free-floating hydrogen ions within the body	pH	7.35 to 7.45	pH <7.35 = respiratory acidosis pH >7.45 = respiratory alkalosis
Amount of bicarbonate ions within the arterial blood	HCO_3	23–30 mEq/mL	Retention of HCO_3 alters the pH of the body. ↑ bicarbonate ions = ↑ in body pH ↓ bicarbonate ions = ↓ in body pH

Table 5-4

Interpretation of Abnormal Acid-Base Balance

TYPE	PH	$PACO_2$	HCO_3^-	CAUSES	SIGNS AND SYMPTOMS
Respiratory alkalosis	↑	↓	WNL	Alveolar hyperventilation	Dizziness, syncope, tingling, numbness, early tetany
Respiratory acidosis	↓	↑	WNL	Alveolar hypoventilation	Early: anxiety, restlessness, dyspnea, headache Late: confusion, somnolence, coma
Metabolic alkalosis	↑	WNL	↑	Bicarbonate ingestion, vomiting, diuretics, steroids, adrenal disease	Vague symptoms: weakness, mental dullness, possibly early tetany
Metabolic acidosis	↓	WNL	↓	Diabetic, lactic, or uremic acidosis, prolonged diarrhea	Secondary hyperventilation (Kussmaul breathing), nausea, lethargy, coma

From: Roy S, Wolf S, and Scalzitti: *The Rehabilitation Specialist's Handbook*, 4th ed, Philadelphia, FA Davis, pg. 520, with permission.

Table 5-5

Classification of Obstructive Lung Disease Outlined by the Global Initiative for Obstructive Lung Disease (GOLD) with the Addition of Functional Abilities That Correspond

STAGE	FEV_1/FVC RATIO	FEV_1	SYMPTOMS	FUNCTIONAL ABILITIES
1 Mild	<70%	FEV_1 ≥80% predicted	With or without chronic symptoms	Individuals may be unaware that lung function is abnormal.
2 Moderate	<70%	50% < FEV_1 ≥80% predicted	With or without chronic symptoms	Individuals typically seek medical attention because of chronic respiratory symptoms or an exacerbation of their disease.
3 Severe	<70%	30% < FEV_1 ≥50%	With or without chronic symptoms	Individuals experience greater shortness of breath, reduced exercise capacity, fatigue, impact on quality of life.
4 Very Severe	<70%	FEV_1 <30% predicted or FEV_1 <50% with chronic respiratory failure symptoms	PaO_2 <60 $PaCo_2$ <50 Cor pulmonale Increased jugular venous distension	Quality of life is very appreciably impaired and exacerbations may be life threatening.

Retrieved 9/10/12 from http://www.goldcopd.org/guidelines-pocket-guide-to-copd-diagnosis.html

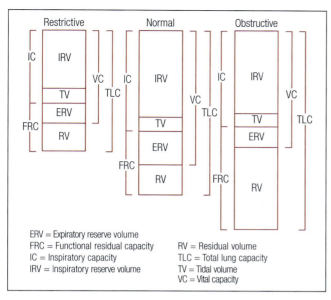

Figure 5-4 Lung volumes of a healthy pulmonary system compared with lung volumes and capacities found in restrictive and obstructive pulmonary disease.
From: Rothstein J, Roy S, and Wolf S: *The Rehabilitation Specialist's Handbook*, 3rd ed. Philadelphia, FA Davis, 2005, p. 428, with permission.

Table 5-6

Graded Exercise Test Termination Criteria

1. Maximal shortness of breath
2. A fall in PaO_2 of greater than 20 mmHg or a PaO_2 less than 55 mmHg
3. A rise in $PaCO_2$ of greater than 10 mmHg or a $PaCO_2$ greater than 65 mmHg
4. Cardiac ischemia or arrhythmias
5. Symptoms of fatigue
6. Increase in diastolic blood pressure readings of 20 mmHg, systolic hypertension greater than 250 mmHg, decrease in blood pressure with increasing workloads
7. Leg pain
8. Total fatigue
9. Signs of insufficient cardiac output
10. Reaching a ventilatory maximum

From: Brannon F, et al: *Cardiopulmonary Rehabilitation: Basic Theory and Application*, 3rd ed. Philadelphia, FA Davis, 1998, p. 300, with permission.

Physical Dysfunction/Impairments

Acute Diseases

Pneumonia
1. Three types of, see Quick Facts 5-3.

Tuberculosis (TB)
1. *Mycobacterium tuberculosis* infection spread by aerosolized droplets from an untreated infected host. Incubation period: 2–10 weeks. Primary disease lasts 10 days to 2 weeks.
2. Postprimary infection is reactivation of dormant tuberculous bacillus, which can occur years after the primary infection.
3. Two weeks on appropriate antituberculin drugs renders the host noninfectious. During the infectious stage, the patient must be isolated from others in a negative-pressure room. Anyone entering the room must wear a protective TB mask and follow universal precautions. If the patient leaves the negative-pressure room, he or she must wear a specialized mask to keep from infecting others.
4. Medication is taken for prolonged periods: 3–12 months.
5. There is an increased incidence of TB in patients with HIV.
6. Pertinent physical findings of primary disease can go unnoticed, as it causes only mild symptoms: slight nonproductive cough, low-grade fever, and possible CXR changes consistent with primary disease.
7. Pertinent physical findings of postprimary infection.
   a. Fever.
   b. Weight loss.
   c. Cough.
   d. Hilar adenopathy: enlargement of the lymph nodes surrounding the hilum.
   e. Night sweat.
   f. Crackles.
   g. Hemoptysis: blood-streaked sputum.
   h. WBC shows increased lymphocytes.
   i. CXR shows upper lobe involvement with air space densities, cavitation, pleural involvement, and parenchymal fibrosis.

QUICK FACTS 5-3 ▶ TYPES OF PNEUMONIA

Type	Description & Potential Causation	Physical Findings
Bacterial	An intra-alveolar bacterial infection. Gram-positive bacteria: typically acquired in the community. Pneumococcal: (streptococcal); most common type of gram-positive pneumonia. Gram-negative bacteria: usually develop in a host with underlying, chronic, debilitating conditions, severe acute illness, and recent antibiotic therapy. Gram-negative infections result in early tissue necrosis and abscess formation. Common infecting organisms: *Klebsiella, Haemophilus influenzae, Pseudomonas aeruginosa, Proteus, Serratia*	• Shaking chills • Fever • Chest pain if pleuritic involvement • Cough becoming productive or purulent, blood-streaked, or rusty sputum • Decreased or bronchial breath sounds and/or crackles • Tachypnea • Increased white blood cell count • Hypoxemia, hypocapnea initially, hypercapnea with increasing severity • CXR confirmation of infiltrate
Viral	An interstitial or intra-alveolar inflammatory process caused by viral agents (influenza, adenovirus, cytomegalovirus, herpes, parainfluenza, respiratory syncytial virus, measles)	• Recent history of upper respiratory infection • Fever • Chills • Dry cough • Headaches • Decreased breath sounds and/or crackles • Hypoxemia and hypercapnea • Normal white blood cell count • CXR confirmation of interstitial infiltrate
Aspiration	Aspirated material causes an acute inflammatory reaction within the lungs. Usually found in patients with impaired swallowing (dysphagia), fixed neck extension, intoxication, impaired consciousness, neuromuscular disease, recent anesthesia	• Symptoms begin shortly after aspiration event (hours). • Cough may be dry at the onset, progresses to produce putrid secretions. • Dyspnea • Tachypnea • Cyanosis • Tachycardia • Wheezes and crackles with decreased breath sounds • Hypoxemia, hypercapnea in severe cases • Chest pain over the involved area • Fever • WBC count shows varying degrees of leukocytosis. • CXR initially shows pneumonitis. Chronic aspiration shows necrotizing pneumonia with cavitation.

Pneumocystis Carinii Pneumonia (PCP)

1. Description: pulmonary infection caused by a protozoan in immunocompromised hosts. Most often found in patients who are immunosuppressed following transplantation or by chemotherapy for lymphoma or leukemia, neonates or patients infected with HIV. Has been shown to be an indicator of conversion from HIV-positive infection to the designation of AIDS.
2. Pertinent physical findings.
   a. Insidious progressive shortness of breath.
   b. Sudden, sharp onset of pleuritic chest pain; chest movement painful.
   c. Nonproductive, hacking cough.
   d. Crackles.
   e. Weakness.
   f. Fever.
   g. CRX shows interstitial infiltrates.
   h. Complete blood count (CBC) shows no evidence of infection.

SARS (Severe Acute Respiratory Syndrome)

1. An atypical respiratory illness caused by a coronovirus. Initial outbreak in southern mainland China with worldwide spread to other areas such as Singapore, Toronto, Vietnam, and Hong Kong.
2. Pertinent physical findings.
   a. High temperature.
   b. Dry cough.
   c. Decreased white blood cells, decreased platelets, decreased lymphocytes.
   d. Increased liver function tests.
   e. Abnormal CXR with borderline breath sounds changes.

Always Follow Standard Precautions
1. See Box 6-1, Standard Precautions.

Chronic Obstructive Diseases

Chronic Obstructive Pulmonary Disease (COPD)
1. According to GOLD, COPD is a disease state characterized by airflow limitation that is not fully reversible. The airflow limitation is usually both progressive and associated with an abnormal inflammatory response of the lungs to noxious particles or gases.
2. Stages.
   a. COPD is classified according to a staging system, Stage 1 (mild) to Stage 4 (very severe).
   b. Staging is based upon percentages of decreased function. In Stage 1, FEV_1 and FVC are functioning at less than 70%, FEV_1 is ≥80% predicted, and the patient/client may present with or without chronic symptoms.
   c. In Stages 2 and 3, symptoms of shortness of breath increase, exercise capacity decreases, and exacerbations of the disease occurs.
   d. In Stage 4, FEV_1 diminishes to <30–50%, symptoms of chronic respiratory failure can be observed, and exacerbations of the disease can become life-threatening.
3. Physical findings specific to COPD. Findings increase in severity as the stage of disease advances. See also Table 5-7.
   a. Cough/sputum production/hemoptysis.
   b. Increased respiratory rate (RR).
   c. Weight loss/anorexia.
   d. Increased A-P diameter of chest wall.
   e. Postures to structurally elevate shoulder girdle.
   f. CXR showing hyperinflation, flattened diaphragms, hyperlucency.
   g. ABG changes of hypoxemia, hypercapnea.
   h. PFTs showing obstructive disease, such as decreased FEV_1, decreased FVC, increased FRC and RV, and decreased FEV_1/FVC ratio.

Asthma
1. Increased reactivity of the trachea and bronchi to various stimuli (allergens, exercise, cold); reversible in nature; manifests by widespread narrowing of the airways due to inflammation, smooth muscle constriction, and increased secretions. Even during remission, some degree of airway inflammation is present.
2. Pertinent physical findings during exacerbation. See also Table 5-7.
   a. Increased secretions of variable amounts.
   b. Anxiety.

Table 5-7

Common Physical Findings in Obstructive Lung Diseases

DISEASE—OBSTRUCTIVE	COPD	ASTHMA, DURING EXACERBATION	CYSTIC FIBROSIS WITH EXACERBATION	BRONCHIECTASIS	RESPIRATORY DISTRESS SYNDROME (RDS)	BRONCHOPULMONARY DYSPLASIA
Physical Findings: X = present with this condition						
Clubbing	X		X	X		
Crackles, wheezing		X	X	X	X	X
Cyanosis	X	X	X	X	X	
Decreased breath sounds	X		X	X		X
Dyspnea	X on exertion	X	X especially on exertion	X		
Hypercapnea			X			X
Hyoocapnea		X*				
Hypoxemia		X	X	X	X	X
Increased acessory muscle use		X	X		X	
Productive cough			X			
Tachycardia		X				
Tachypnea		X	X		X	

*In response to hypoxemia

c. Hypocapnea. Responding to hypoxemia, there is an increased respiratory rate and minute ventilation. This will decrease $PaCO_2$. With severe airway constriction, an increase in minute ventilation cannot occur and hypercapnea can be found.
d. PFTs show impaired flow rates.
e. CXR shows hyperlucency and flattened diaphragms during exacerbation.

Cystic Fibrosis (CF)
1. Description: a genetically inherited disease (abnormality of chromosome 7) that affects the mucus-producing glands in the lungs, sweat glands, digestive tract, and the genitourinary system. It is characterized by thickening of secretions of all exocrine glands, leading to obstruction. Presentation can include bronchiectatic lung disease, impaired fat absorption (due to pancreatic insufficiency), malnutrition, diabetes, arthropathies, or osteoporosis. CF may present as an obstructive, restrictive, or mixed disease. Clinical signs of CF include: meconiumileus, frequent respiratory infections, especially *Staphylococcus aureus* and *Pseudomonas aeruginosa*, and inability to gain weight despite adequate caloric intake. Diagnosis is made by a positive sweat electrolyte test.
2. Pertinent physical findings during exacerbation. See also Table 5-8.
   a. Onset of symptoms usually in early childhood.
   b. Abnormal PFTs showing an obstructive pattern, restrictive pattern, or both.
   c. CXR shows increased markings, findings of bronchiectasis, and/or pneumonitis.

Bronchiectasis
1. A chronic congenital or acquired disease characterized by abnormal dilatation of the bronchi and excessive sputum production.
2. Pertinent physical findings. See also Table 5-8.
   a. Cough and expectoration of large amounts of mucopurulent secretions.
   b. Frequent secondary infections.
   c. Hemoptysis.
   d. CXR shows increased bronchial markings with interstitial changes. Bronchograms can outline bronchial dilatation, but are rarely needed.

Respiratory Distress Syndrome (RDS)
1. Alveolar collapse in a premature infant resulting from lung immaturity, inadequate level of pulmonary surfactant.
2. Pertinent physical findings within a few hours of birth. See also Table 5-8.
   a. Respiratory distress.
   b. Expiratory grunting, flaring nares.
   c. CXR shows a classic granular pattern ("ground glass") caused by distended terminal airways and alveolar collapse.
3. **SPECIAL CONSIDERATION:** Increased breathing effort caused by handling a premature infant must be carefully weighed against possible benefits of physical therapy.

Bronchopulmonary Dysplasia
1. An obstructive pulmonary disease, often a sequela of premature infants with respiratory distress syndrome; results from high pressures of mechanical ventilation, high fractions of inspired oxygen (FiO_2), and/or infection. Lungs show areas of pulmonary immaturity and dysfunction due to hyperinflation.
2. Pertinent physical findings. See also Table 5-8.
   a. Increased bronchial secretions.
   b. Hyperinflation.
   c. Frequent lower respiratory infections.
   d. Delayed growth and development.
   e. Cor pulmonale.
   f. CXR shows hyperinflation, low diaphragms, atelectasis, and/or cystic changes.

General Medical Management

Medications
1. Bronchodilators and anti-inflammatory agents to reduce airway edema, inflammation, and bronchospasm.
2. Expectorants, antihistamines, and mast cell membrane stabilizers.
3. Antidepressants, antianxiety medications as needed.

Prevention
1. Control complications, maintain good airway hygiene, avoid airway irritants or allergens.

General Physical Therapy Management

Airway
1. Implement airway clearance techniques to facilitate expectoration of secretions. See Physical Therapy Intervention section for specific techniques.

Exercise
1. Instruct in exercise to maintain posture, facilitate respiratory musculature, and include overall conditioning to improve exercise tolerance as able.
2. Instruction in controlled breathing strategies.

Chronic Restrictive Diseases

Different Etiologies
1. Typified by difficulty expanding the lungs, causing a reduction in lung volumes.
2. Restrictive disease can be due to different physical conditions or changes. See Table 5-8.

General Medical Management

Medical Interventions
1. Medications to control and reduce inflammation, corticosteroids.
2. Maintaining adequate oxygenation.
3. Weight management plans.
4. Surgical procedures.
   a. To correct orthopedic deformities, e.g., spinal surgeries.
   b. At end stages, lung transplantation for appropriate candidates.

General Physical Therapy Management

See also Physical Therapy Intervention Section for Specific Techniques
1. Exercise plan to address generalized weakness, positioning for exercise and rest.
2. Instruction in breathing strategies, airway clearance techniques.
3. Manual therapy for chest wall compliance.

Bronchogenic Carcinoma

Characteristics
1. A tumor that arises from the bronchial mucosa.
2. Smoking and occupational exposures are the most frequent causal agents.
3. Cell types: small cell carcinoma (oat cell) and non–small cell carcinoma (squamous cell, adenocarcinoma, and large cell undifferentiated).
4. Secondary changes due to the tumor: obstruction or compression of an airway, blood vessel, or nerve.
5. Local metastases in the pleura, chest wall, mediastinal structures. Common distant metastases in lymph nodes, liver, bone, brain, and adrenals.

Pertinent Physical Findings with Pulmonary Involvement
1. Unexplained weight loss.
2. Hemoptysis.
3. Dyspnea.
4. Weakness.
5. Fatigue.
6. Wheezing.
7. Pneumonia with productive cough due to airway compression.
8. Hoarseness with compression of the laryngeal nerve.
9. Atelectasis or bacterial pneumonia with nonproductive cough due to airway obstruction.

Management of Bronchogenic Cancer
1. Chemotherapy.
2. Radiation therapy.
3. Surgical resection if possible.

Table 5-8

Common Physical Findings in Restrictive Lung Diseases

COMMON PHYSICAL FINDINGS WITH RESTRICTIVE DISEASES		DYSPNEA, CRACKLES, CLUBBING, HYPOXEMIA, HYPOCAPNEA (HYPERCAPNEA WITH INCREASING SEVERITY)
Fibrotic changes or alterations in lung parenchyma and pleura	Idiopathic pulmonary fibrosis Asbestosis or radiation pneumonitis Oxygen toxicity	• PFTs reveal a reduction in vital capacity, functional residual capacity, and total lung capacity. • CXR shows reduced lung volumes, diffuse interstitial infiltrates, and/or pleural thickening.
Alterations in the chest wall; restricting motion of the bony thorax	Ankylosing spondylitis Arthritis Scoliosis Pectus excavatum Arthrogryposis Integumentary changes of the chest wall such as thoracic burns or scleroderma	• Shallow, rapid breathing • Reduced cough effectiveness • PFTs show reduced vital capacity, functional residual capacity, and total lung capacity.
Alterations in the neuromuscular apparatus; decreased muscular strength results in an inability to expand the rib cage	Multiple sclerosis Muscular dystrophy Parkinson's disease Spinal cord injury Cerebrovascular accident (CVA)	• Decreased breath sounds • Reduced cough effectiveness • PFTs show reduced vital capacity and total lung capacity. • CXR shows reduced lung volumes, atelectasis.

Physical Therapy Management Considerations

1. Pneumonias that develop behind a completely obstructed bronchus cannot be cleared with physical therapy techniques. Hold treatment until palliative therapy reduces tumor size and relieves bronchial obstruction.
2. Possible fractures from thoracic bone metastasis with chest compressive maneuvers and coughing.
3. Ecchymosis (bruising) in patients with low platelet count.
4. Fatigue that restricts necessary activities.

Trauma

Rib Fracture, Flail Chest

1. Fracture of the ribs, usually due to blunt trauma. Flail chest is two or more fractures in two or more adjacent ribs.
2. Pertinent physical findings.
   a. Shallow breathing.
   b. Splinting due to pain (especially with deep inspiration or cough).
   c. Crepitation may be felt during the ventilatory cycle over fracture site.
   d. Paradoxical movement of a flail section during the ventilatory cycle (inspiration, the flail section is pulled inward; exhalation, the flail moves outward).
   e. Confirmation by CXR.

Pleural Injury

1. Pneumothorax.
   a. Air in the pleural space, usually through a lacerated visceral pleura from a rib fracture or ruptured bullae.
   b. Pertinent physical findings all increase with severity of injury.
      - Chest pain.
      - Dyspnea.
      - Tracheal and mediastinal shift away from injured side.
      - Absent or decreased breath sounds.
      - Increased tympany with mediate percussion.
      - Cyanosis.
      - Respiratory distress.
      - Confirmation by CXR.
2. Hemothorax.
   a. Blood in the pleural space, usually from a laceration of the parietal pleura.
   b. Pertinent physical findings increase with severity of injury.
      - Chest pain.
      - Dyspnea.
      - Tracheal and mediastinal shift away from side of injury.
      - Absent or decreased breath sounds.
      - Cyanosis.
      - Respiratory distress.
      - Confirmation by CXR.
      - Possible signs of blood loss.

Lung Contusion

1. Blood and edema within the alveoli and interstitial space due to blunt chest trauma with or without rib fractures.
2. Pertinent physical findings increase with severity of injury.
   a. Cough with hemoptysis.
   b. Dyspnea.
   c. Decreased breath sounds and/or crackles.
   d. Cyanosis.
   e. Confirmation by CXR of ill-defined patchy densities.

Other Pulmonary Conditions

Pulmonary Edema

1. Excessive seepage of fluid from the pulmonary vascular system into the interstitial space; may eventually cause alveolar edema.
   a. Cardiogenic: results from increased pressure in pulmonary capillaries associated with left ventricular failure, aortic valvular disease, or mitral valvular disease.
   b. Non-cardiogenic: results from increased permeability of the alveolar capillary membranes due to inhalation of toxic fumes, hypervolemia, narcotic overdose, or adult respiratory distress syndrome (ARDS).
2. Pertinent physical findings. See also Table 5-9.
   a. Peripheral edema if cardiogenic.
   b. CXR shows increased vascular markings, hazy opacities in gravity-dependent areas of the lung in a typical butterfly pattern. Atelectasis is possible if the surfactant lining is removed by alveolar edema.

Pulmonary Emboli

1. A thrombus from the peripheral venous circulation becomes embolic and lodges in the pulmonary circulation. Small emboli do not necessarily cause infarction.

Table 5-9

Common Physical Findings in Other Lung Diseases

OTHER LUNG CONDITIONS	PULMONARY EDEMA	PULMONARY EMBOLI WITHOUT INFARCTION	PULMONARY EMBOLI WITH INFARCTION	ATELECTASIS
Physical Findings: X = present with this condition				
Clubbing				
Crackles	X			
Chest Pain			X	
Cyanosis		X		
Dyspnea	X	X Sudden Onset		X
Hemoptysis			X	
Hyoocapnea				
Hypoxemia	X	X		
Cough—pink frothy, secretions	X			
Productive cough				
Tachycardia		X		X
Tachypnea	X			

2. Pertinent physical findings without infarction. See also Table 5-9.
   a. History consistent with pulmonary emboli: deep vein thrombosis, oral contraceptives, recent abdominal or hip surgery, polycythemia, prolonged bed rest.
   b. Auscultatory findings may be normal or show crackles and decreased breath sounds.
   c. Ventilation-perfusion scan showing perfusion defects with concomitant normal ventilation.
3. Added pertinent physical findings consistent with pulmonary infarction. See also Table 5-9.
   a. CXR shows decreased vascular markings, high diaphragm, pulmonary infiltrate, and/or pleural effusion.

Pleural Effusion

1. Excessive fluid between the visceral and parietal pleura, caused mainly by increased pleural permeability to proteins from inflammatory diseases (pneumonia, rheumatoid arthritis, systemic lupus), neoplastic disease, increased hydrostatic pressure within pleural space (congestive heart failure), decrease in osmotic pressure (hypoproteinemia), peritoneal fluid within the pleural space (ascites, cirrhosis), or interference of pleural reabsorption from a tumor invading pleural lymphatics.
2. Pertinent physical findings.
   a. Decreased breath sounds over effusion; bronchial breath sounds around the perimeter. Pleural friction rub may be possible with inflammatory process.
   b. Mediastinal shift away from large effusion.
   c. Breathlessness with large effusions.
   d. CXR shows fluid in the pleural space in gravity-dependent areas of the thorax if >300 mL.
   e. Pain and fever only if the pleural fluid is infected (empyema).

Atelectasis

1. Collapsed or airless alveolar unit, caused by hypoventilation secondary to pain during the ventilatory cycle (pleuritis, postoperative pain, or rib fracture), internal bronchial obstruction (aspiration, mucus plugging), external bronchial compression (tumor or enlarged lymph nodes), low tidal volumes (narcotic overdose, inappropriately low ventilator settings), or neurologic insult.
2. Pertinent physical findings. See also Table 5-9.
   a. Decreased breath sounds.
   b. Increased temperature.
   c. CXR with platelike streaks.

Physical Therapy Intervention

Manual Secretion Removal Techniques

Indications for Manually Assisted Airway Clearance Techniques
1. Increased pulmonary secretions, e.g., cystic fibrosis, bronchiectasis.
2. Aspiration.
3. Conditions causing mucus plugs, e.g., atelectasis (collapse of alveolar segments), individuals on mechanical ventilation.
4. Weakness of respiratory musculature.

Conditions That Do Not Respond to Manual Secretion Removal Techniques
1. Conditions without large amounts of drainage:
   a. Chronic bronchitis.
   b. Pneumonia.
   c. Post-operative patients.

Postural/Bronchial Drainage
1. Placing the patient in varying positions for optimal gravity-assisted drainage of secretions and increased expansion of the involved segment (Figure 5-5).
2. Considerations prior to use of the postural drainage positions (Table 5-10). These considerations are not intended to imply absolute danger, but rather a possible need for position modification.
3. Procedure.
   a. Explain procedure to the patient.
   b. It may improve outcomes to time treatment so that it immediately follows patient use of a nebulizer (aerated bronchodilator treatment) if the patient is using one.
   c. Place patient in appropriate postural drainage position.
   d. Observe for signs of intolerance.
   e. Duration of procedure can be up to 20 minutes per postural drainage position. When used with percussion or shaking, each procedure may be applied for 3–5 minutes per lobe. Encourage the patient to take deep breaths and cough after each position.
   f. Secretions may not be dislodged immediately with treatment and can occur up to an hour following; inform the patient of this.

Percussion
1. A force rhythmically applied with the therapist's cupped hands to the specific area of the chest wall that corresponds to the involved lung segment.
2. Percussion is used to increase the amount of secretions cleared from the tracheobronchial tree; usually used in conjunction with postural drainage.
   a. See Quick Facts 5-4 for indications for use of percussion.

> **QUICK FACTS 5-4 ▶ INDICATIONS FOR PERCUSSION AND SHAKING TECHNIQUES**
> - Excessive pulmonary secretions
> - Aspiration
> - Atelectasis or collapse due to mucous plugging obstructing the airways

3. Considerations for weighing possible benefits of percussion against possible detriments prior to the application of this technique are listed in Table 5-11. Modification of the technique may be necessary for patient tolerance.
4. Procedure.
   a. Explain procedure to the patient.
   b. Place patient in the appropriate postural drainage position (increases effectiveness).
   c. Cover the area to be percussed with a lightweight cloth to avoid erythema. Avoid percussing over: a bony prominence, floating rib, breast tissue.
   d. Percuss over area of thorax which corresponds to the involved lung segment. Rate of percussion should be 100 plus times per minute. Mechanical percussors may also be used. The duration of percussion depends on the patient's needs and tolerance. Three to five minutes of percussion per postural drainage position with clinically assessed improvement is a guideline. Percussion is applied during inspiration and expiration; the patient may perform active cycle of breathing technique throughout as well.
   e. The force of percussion causes the patient's voice to quiver.

Shaking (Vibration)
1. Following a deep inhalation, shaking is a fast-paced rhythmic bouncing or shaking maneuver applied to the rib cage throughout the exhalation. Performed to

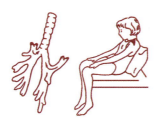

UPPER LOBES Apical Segments

Bed or drainage table flat.

Patient leans back on pillow at 30° angle against therapist.

Therapist claps with markedly cupped hand over area between clavicle and top of scapula on each side.

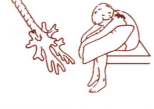

UPPER LOBES Posterior Segments

Bed or drainage table flat.

Patient leans over folded pillow at 30° angle.

Therapist stands behind and claps over upper back on both sides.

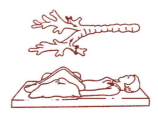

UPPER LOBES Anterior Segments

Bed or drainage table flat.

Patient lies on back with pillow under knees.

Therapist claps between clavicle and nipple on each side.

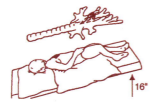

RIGHT MIDDLE LOBE

Foot of table or bed elevated 16 inches.

Patient lies head down on left side and rotates ¼ turn backward. Pillow may be placed behind from shoulder to hip. Knees should be flexed.

Therapist claps over right nipple area. In females with breast development or tenderness, use cupped hand with heel of hand under armpit and fingers extending forward beneath the breast.

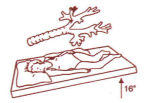

LEFT UPPER LOBE Lingular Segments

Foot of table or bed elevated 16 inches.

Patient lies head down on right side and rotates 1/4 turn backward. Pillow may be placed behind from shoulder to hip. Knees should be flexed.

Therapist claps with moderately cupped hand over left nipple area. In females with breast development or tenderness, use cupped hand with heel of hand under armpit and fingers extending forward beneath the breast.

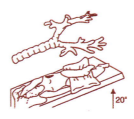

LOWER LOBE Anterior Basal Segments

Foot of table or bed elevated 20 inches.

Patient lies on side, head down, pillow under knees.

Therapist claps with slightly cupped hand over lower ribs. (Position shown is for drainage of left anterior basal segment. To drain the right anterior basal segment, patient should lie on the left side in same posture).

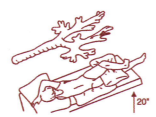

LOWER LOBES Lateral Basal Segments

Foot of table or bed elevated 20 inches.

Patient lies on abdomen, head down, then rotates ¼ turn upward. Upper leg is flexed over a pillow for support.

Therapist claps over uppermost portion of lower ribs. (Position shown is for drainage of right lateral basal segment. To drain the left lateral basal segment, patient should lie on the right side in the same posture).

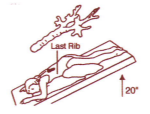

LOWER LOBES Posterior Basal Segments

Foot of table or bed elevated 20 inches.

Patient lies on abdomen, head down, with pillow under hips. Therapist claps over lower ribs close to spine on each side.

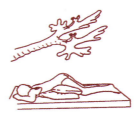

LOWER LOBES Superior Segments

Bed or table flat.

Patient lies on abdomen with two pillows under hips.

Therapist claps over middle of back at tip of scapula on either side of spine.

Figure 5-5 Bronchial drainage.

From: Rothstein J, Roy S, and Wolf S: *The Rehabilitation Specialist's Handbook*, 3rd ed., FA Davis, 2005, p. 444, with permission.

Table 5-10

Considerations Prior to the Use of Postural Drainage	
Precautions to the use of Trendelenburg position (head of bed tipped down 15 to 18 degrees)	
Circulatory system	Pulmonary edema, congestive heart failure, hypertension
Abdominal problems	Obesity, ascites, pregnancy, hiatal hernia, nausea and vomiting, recent food consumption
Neurologic system	Recent neurosurgery, increased intracranial pressure, aneurysm precautions
Pulmonary system	Shortness of breath, esophageal surgery, recent hemoptysis related to recent lung carcinoma
Precautions to the use of sidelying position	
Circulatory system	Axillo-femoral bypass graft
Musculoskeletal system	Humeral fractures, need for hip abduction brace, other situations that make sidelying uncomfortable, e.g., arthritis, shoulder bursitis
CONTRAINDICATIONS FOR ALL POSITIONS	
Circulatory	Active hemorrhage with hemodynamic instability, active hemoptysis
Neurological System	Intracranial pressure >20 mm Hg
Pulmonary System	Embolism, pulmonary edema with heart failure, large pleural effusion, empyema, flail chest
Musculoskeletal System	Recent spinal surgery or acute spinal injury, rib fracture, head or neck injury (unless satisfactorily stabilized)

hasten the removal of secretions from the tracheobronchial tree.
2. Commonly used following percussion in the appropriate postural drainage position. Modification may be necessary for patient tolerance.
   a. See Quick Facts 5-4 for indications for use of percussion.
3. Considerations prior to the application of shaking are similar to those of percussion (see Table 5-11).

Table 5-11

Considerations Prior to the Use of Percussion and Shaking	
General guidelines	Pain made worse by the technique
Circulatory system	Aneurysm precautions, hemoptysis
Coagulation disorders	Increased partial thromboplastin time (PTT), increased prothrombin time (PT), decreased platelet count (below 50,000), or medications that interfere with coagulation
Musculoskeletal system	Fractured rib, flail chest, degenerative bone disease, bone metastases

4. Procedure.
   a. Explain procedure to the patient.
   b. Place patient in appropriate postural drainage position.
   c. As the patient inhales deeply, the assistant's hands are placed side by side, or on top of each other, over the lung segment being treated so that fingers are parallel to the ribs.
   d. As the patient exhales, the assistant's hands provide a rhythmic, fast-paced bouncing motion to the ribcage. Shaking is delivered at a rate of approximately 2 times per second through the entire exhalation phase. Vibration is delivered at a rate of 12–20 vibrations per second.
   e. The duration of shaking depends on the patient's needs, tolerance, and clinical improvement. Five to 10 deep inhalations with shaking technique applied at exhalation are generally acceptable practice. Any more than 10 would risk hyperventilation (increased V_E resulting in decreased $PaCO_2$), and less than 5 may be ineffective.

Airway Clearance Techniques

Cough

1. Patient should be asked to cough in the upright sitting position, if possible, after each area of lung has been treated. Coughing clears secretions from the major central airways.
2. Teaching an effective cough:
   a. Inhale fully so that 3–5 consecutive cascading coughs can be produced.
   b. At peak of inspiration, close glottis to assist with build-up of pressure in intrathoracic area.
   c. As the intrathoracic and abdominal muscles contract, the glottis is relaxed and air is forcefully expelled through the open mouth.
   d. A manually assisted cough can be performed with the patient in supine by applying pressure with the heel of the hand at the navel and gently applying an upward thrust as the patient exhales.
   e. A manually assisted inhalation and exhalation can be performed with the patient in supine. Assistant's hands are placed at the lower ribs (costophrenic angle) with the web space and first finger aligned at the angle of the ribs and the thumbs meeting midline aligned with the ribs. Immediately preceding inhalation, the assistant applies a quick manual stretch down (toward the abdomen) and inward toward the patient's navel; the patient breaths in and holds it. Immediately preceding exhalation, the assistant applies stronger pressure toward the navel, assisting with build-up of intrathoracic pressure.

Huffing

1. More effective in patients with collapsible airways (e.g., chronic obstructive diseases); prevents the high intrathoracic pressure that causes premature airway closure.
   a. Ask patient to inhale moderately or deeply.
   b. Immediately, the patient forcibly expels the air saying, "ha, ha." An effective huff includes contraction of the abdominal muscles and an open glottis e.g., breathing out to fog the lens of eye glasses to clean them; not closed as in a cough.
   c. To clear peripheral airways—a longer and quieter huff following a medium-sized breath. To clear proximal airways—a shorter, louder huff following a deeper breath is effective.

Assisted Cough

1. Used when the patient's abdominal muscles cannot generate an effective cough (e.g., spinal cord injury).
2. The therapist's hand(s) or fist become the force behind the patient's exhaled air. The amount of force by the therapist depends on patient tolerance and abdominal sensation.
   a. Position the patient against a solid surface; supine with head of bed flat or in a Trendelenburg position, or sitting with wheelchair against the wall or against the therapist.
   b. The therapist's hand is placed below the patient's subcostal angle (similar to hand placement for the Heimlich maneuver).
   c. Patient inhales deeply.
   d. As the patient attempts to cough, the therapist's hand pushes inward and upward, assisting the rapid exhalation of air.
   e. Any secretions raised should be removed by a suction catheter if expectoration is problematic.

Tracheal Stimulation

1. Used with patients who are unable to cough on command, such as infants or patients with brain injury or stroke.
   a. The therapist's finger or thumb is placed just above the suprasternal notch, and a quick inward and downward pressure on the trachea elicits the cough reflex.

Endotracheal Suctioning

1. Used only when the above airway clearance techniques fail to adequately remove secretions.
   a. Standard precautions are employed, since contact with a patient's body fluid is expected.
   b. Equipment: suction catheters come in sizes of 14 French gauge (Fr), usually for an adult, 10 Fr for older children, 8 and 5–6 Fr for young children and infants. Suction system set at approximately 120 mm Hg of suction. Sterile glove/clean glove.
   c. Procedure: a catheter is fed through either an artificial airway, oral airway, or the nares through the pharynx, larynx to the carina. When resistance is felt at the carina, the catheter is rotated and withdrawn. Suction is applied intermittently so as not to damage the inner lining of the trachea. The usual suctioning time is 10 to 15 seconds.
   d. Complications associated with suctioning: hypoxemia, bradycardia or tachycardia, hypotension or hypertension, increased intracranial pressure, atelectasis, tracheal damage, infections.

Independent Secretion Removal Techniques

Active Cycle of Breathing Technique (ACBT)

1. An independent program used to assist in the removal of the more peripheral secretions that coughing alone may not clear. ACBT is three phases that are repeated in cycles: breathing control, thoracic expansion, forced expiratory technique (FET). Treatment is concluded when huffing becomes non-productive and is dry sounding.
2. Positioning: patient positions themself in appropriate postural drainage position; it may also be done upright.
3. Procedure. The patient:
   a. Breathes in a controlled diaphragmatic fashion.
   b. Performs thoracic expansion exercises by taking a deep breath (with or without percussion and shaking) with a hold at the top if possible. A sniff or hold at end or inspiration helps facilitate distribution of air into collapsed segments of lungs. Expiration is passive. The patient may place a hand over the area of the lungs being treated to encourage chest wall movement in that area.
   c. Forced expiration phase. The patient performs a series of huffing techniques (see huffing in previous section) and breathing control after 1–2 huffs. Repeat cycles as necessary.

Autogenic Drainage

1. An independent program used to sense peripheral secretions and clear them without the tracheobronchial irritation from coughing. The amount of time spent in each of the following phases is determined by where the patient feels the secretions. An entire treatment may take up to 30–40 minutes.
2. The unstick phase: quiet breathing (through the nose if possible) at low lung volumes to affect peripheral secretions. A 2- to 3-second breath hold at end of inhalation (allows for collateral ventilation in lung space). Then the patient performs a deep expiration

into the expiratory reserve volume of the lungs. Continue until mucus is loosened and starts to move in the upper airways.
3. The collect phase: breathing at mid lung volumes to affect secretions in the middle airways. The focus shifts to greater inspiratory reserve volume. Continue until sound of mucus decreases and mucus has moved to central airways and can be expelled.
4. The evacuation phase: breathing from mid to high lung volumes; focus is inspiration into inspiratory reserve volume to clear secretions from central airways. This phase replaces coughing as the means to clear secretions. Non-productive coughs should be avoided to prevent possible collapse of airways.
5. Repeat the steps that correspond to the area of retained secretions until all secretions are removed from the airways.

Flutter or Acapella Device
1. The patient uses an external device that vibrates the airways on exhalation to improve airway clearance with intermittent, positive expiratory pressure.
2. Patient breathes in a normal tidal volume through the nose or around the mouthpiece of the FLUTTER device.
3. Patient then exhales through the device, setting up a vibration within the airways. Experimentation in the tipped position of the device may provide the most vibration possible with exhalation.
4. Repeat between 5 and 10 times.
5. Patient then breathes in a full inhalation through the nose or around the mouthpiece.
6. This is followed by a 3-second hold at the top of inhalation and rapid, forced exhalations through the FLUTTER device.
7. Repeat 2 or 3 times.
8. Huff or cough to clear secretions.
9. Repeat steps 1–8 until all secretions are removed from the airways.

Low-Pressure Positive Expiratory Pressure (PEP) Mask
1. The patient uses positive expiratory resistance via face mask to help remove airway secretions. Low-pressure PEP measures 10–20 cm H_2O.
2. Seated, the patient breathes at tidal volumes with mask or mouth piece in place, holding inspiration for 2–3 seconds before exhalation. A nose clamp can be used with a mouthpiece to improve compliance with breathing through the device.
3. After approximately 10 breaths, the mask is removed for coughing or huffing to clear secretions.
4. The sequence is repeated until all secretions are removed from the airways.

High-Pressure Positive Expiratory Pressure (PEP) Mask
1. The patient with an unstable airway uses high expiratory pressures via face mask to assist in the removal of airway secretions. High-pressure PEP uses the point of PEP between 50 and 120 cm H_2O, where the patient is able to exhale a larger FVC with the mask than without.
2. Seated patient breathes at tidal volumes with mask in place.
3. After approximately 10 breaths, huffing from high to low lung volumes is performed with the mask in place.
4. The sequence is repeated until all secretions are removed from the airways. Treatment can last up to 15–20 minutes.

Breathing Exercises

Diaphragmatic Breathing
1. Used to increase ventilation, improve gas exchange, decrease work of breathing, facilitate relaxation, and maintain or improve mobility of chest wall.
2. Used with postoperative patients, posttrauma patients, and patients with obstructive or restrictive pulmonary lung diseases.
3. Procedure.
   a. Explain procedure to patient.
   b. Position patient in semireclined (e.g., semi-Fowler's position).
   c. Place therapist's hand gently over subcostal angle of the thorax.
   d. Apply gentle pressure throughout the exhalation phase.
   e. Increase to firm pressure at end of exhalation.
   f. Ask patient to inhale against resistance of the therapist's hand.
   g. Release pressure, allowing a full inhalation.
   h. Progress to independence of therapist's hand, in upright sitting, standing, walking, and stair climbing.

Segmental Breathing
1. Used to improve ventilation to hypoventilated lung segments, alter regional distribution of gas, maintain or restore functional residual capacity, maintain or improve mobility of chest wall, and prevent pulmonary compromise.
2. Used for patients with pleuritic, incisional, or posttrauma pain that causes decreased movement in a portion of the thorax (splinting), and those at risk of developing atelectasis.
3. Inappropriate for intractable hypoventilation until medical situation is resolved; palliative therapy to reduce bronchogenic tumor size or chest tube to reduce a pneumothorax.

4. Procedure.
   a. Explain procedure to patient.
   b. Position patient to facilitate inhalation to a certain segment, such as postural drainage positions, upright sitting.
   c. Apply gentle pressure to the thorax over area of hypoventilation during exhalation.
   d. Increase to firm pressure just prior to inspiration.
   e. Ask patient to breathe in against the resistance of therapist's hands.
   f. Release resistance, allowing a full inhalation.

Sustained Maximal Inspiration (SMI)
1. Used to increase inhaled volume, sustain or improve alveolar inflation, and maintain or restore functional residual capacity.
2. Used in acute situations; e.g., patients with post-trauma pain, postoperative pain, acute lobar collapse.
3. Procedure.
   a. Inspire slowly through nose or pursed lips to maximal inspiration.
   b. Hold maximal inspiration for 3 seconds.
   c. Passively exhale the volume.
   d. Incentive spirometers (devices used to measure and encourage deep inspiration) can help patient achieve maximal inspiration during SMI.

Pursed Lip Breathing
1. Used to reduce respiratory rate, increase tidal volume, reduce dyspnea, decrease mechanical disadvantages of impaired ventilatory pump, improve gas mixing at rest for patients with COPD, and facilitate relaxation.
2. Primarily used for patients with obstructive disease who experience dyspnea at rest or with minimal activity/exercise, or with ineffective breathing patterns during activity/exercise.
3. Procedure.
   a. Slowly inhale through nose or mouth.
   b. Passively exhale through pursed lips (position mouth as if blowing out candles).
   c. Additional hand pressure from the therapist applied to abdomen can gently prolong expiration.
   d. Abdominal muscle contraction can be used judiciously to increase exhaled volume. Care must be taken not to increase intrathoracic pressure, which may cause airway collapse.

Abdominal Strengthening
1. Used when abdominal muscles are too weak to provide an effective cough. Abdominal splinting: used when the abdominal muscles cannot provide the necessary support needed for passive exhalation, e.g., in high thoracic and cervical spinal cord injuries. It is important to ensure that the binder does not restrict inspiration.
2. Glossopharyngeal breathing (air gulping) can also be taught to assist coughing.

Postsurgical Care

Postoperative Physical Therapy Sessions
1. Decrease the number and severity of pulmonary complications.
2. Prevent postoperative pulmonary complications.
   a. Remove residual secretions.
   b. Improve aeration.
   c. Gradually increase activity.
   d. Return to baseline pulmonary functioning.
3. Pertinent physical findings of postoperative pulmonary complications.
   a. Increased temperature.
   b. Increase in white blood cell count.
   c. Change in breath sounds from the preoperative evaluation.
   d. Abnormal chest x-ray.
   e. Decreased expansion of the thorax.
   f. Shortness of breath.
   g. Change in cough and sputum production.
4. Physical therapy considerations.
   a. Determine need for pain management.
   b. Choose appropriate intervention based on patient's needs.
      - Secretion removal techniques.
      - Breathing exercises to improve aeration, incentive spirometry.
      - Early mobilization.

Activities for Increasing Functional Abilities

General Conditioning
1. A prescription for exercise can be written to improve cardiopulmonary fitness based on results of exercise tolerance test. (See Chapter 4 for discussion.)
2. Mode. Any aerobic activity that allows a graded workload; usually, a circuit program of multiple activities (e.g., bike, walking, arm ergometry) since patients with pulmonary disease may be deconditioned. Patient preference should be considered.
3. Intensity. Patients with mild or moderate lung disease will likely reach their cardiovascular endpoint with an exercise test. Using the test data in Karvonen's

formula ([maximum heart rate − resting heart rate] [40%–85%] + resting heart rate) results in safe range for exercise intensity. Patients with severe and very severe pulmonary disorders will likely reach a pulmonary end point before a cardiovascular end point. Intensity for these patients should be at or near maximum heart rate. Ratings of Perceived Exertion scale is used to monitor exercise intensity.
4. Duration. With high-intensity exercise, the patient may need an intermittent exercise program with rest periods for tolerance. Progression is directed first toward a duration of 20–30 minutes of continuous exercise before an increase in intensity is considered.
5. Frequency. The goal is 20–30 minutes of exercise three to five times per week. With durations of less than 20–30 minutes, exercise should occur more frequently (five to seven times per week).

Inspiratory Muscle Trainer (IMT)
1. Used to load muscles of inspiration by breathing through a series of graded aperture openings. By increasing strength and endurance of muscles of ventilation, the patient will develop more efficient ventilatory muscles, less effort in breathing, and decreased possibility of respiratory muscle fatigue. However, evidence is inconclusive for improved functional ability. Whether this translates into improved functional abilities has been cause for debate, and has yet to be conclusively proven.
2. IMT is appropriate for patients with decreased compliance, decreased intrathoracic volume, resistance to airflow, alteration in length tension relationship of ventilatory muscles, decreased strength of the respiratory muscles.
3. Procedure.
   a. Explain procedure to patient with emphasis on maintenance of respiratory rate and tidal volume during training sessions.
   b. Determine maximum inspiratory pressure (MIP).
   c. Choose an aperture opening that requires 30%–50% of MIP (intensity) and allows 10–15 minutes of training per session.
   d. Ask patient to inhale through device while maintaining their usual respiratory rate and tidal volume for at least 10–15 minutes.
   e. Progression initially focuses on increasing duration to 30 minutes, then increasing intensity with smaller apertures.

Paced Breathing (Activity Pacing)
1. Used to spread out the metabolic demands of an activity over time by slowing its performance.
2. Indications: patients who become dyspneic during the performance of an activity or exercise.
3. Procedure.
   a. Break down any activity into manageable components that can be performed within the patient's pulmonary system's abilities.
   b. Inhale at rest.
   c. Upon exhalation with pursed lips, complete the first component of the desired activity.
   d. Stop the activity and inhale at rest.
   e. Upon exhalation with pursed lips, complete next component of activity.
   f. Repeat steps (4) and (5) until activity is accomplished in full without shortness of breath. For example, stair climbing can be done by ascending one or more stairs on exhalation, and then resting, inhaling at rest, then more stairs on exhalation, and so on.

Energy Conservation
1. The energy consumption of many activities of daily living can be decreased with some careful thought and planning, making seemingly impossible tasks possible.
2. For example, showering is difficult for the patient with pulmonary disease, given the activity and the hot, humid environment. With a shower seat, hand-held shower, and use of a terry cloth robe after showering, the patient does not have to stand, hold his or her breath as often, or dry off in the humid environment, thus reducing the energy cost of the activity.

Medical and Surgical Management of Pulmonary Disease

Surgical Management
1. Surgeries to remove diseased lung portions. Different types include:
   a. Pneumonectomy: removal of a lung.
   b. Lobectomy: removal of a lobe of a lung.
   c. Segmental resection: removal of a segment of a lobe.
   d. Wedge resection: removal of a portion of a lung without anatomical divisions.
   e. Lung volume reduction surgery (LVRS), or pneumonectomy, removes large emphysematous, nonfunctioning areas of the lung to normalize thoracic mobility and improve gas exchange of the remaining lung.

2. Incisions types used:
   a. Midsternotomy: sternum is cut in half lengthwise and rib cage is retracted; used in most heart surgeries. The sternum is wired together at the close of surgery; therefore, physical therapy should encourage full upper-extremity range of motion postoperatively.
   b. Thoracotomy: used for most lung resections; incision follows the path of the fourth intercostal space; full range of motion should be encouraged postoperatively.

Medical Management

1. Rescue drugs.
   a. Used for immediate relief of breakthrough symptoms of tightness, wheezing, and shortness of breath.
   b. Short-acting beta-2 agonists (sympathomimetics): mimic the activity of the sympathetic nervous system that produce bronchodilation; can increase heart rate and blood pressure.
   c. Given topically through a metered-dose inhaler (MDI), unwanted systemic effects are reduced. Examples of rescue beta-2 agonists are Ventolin (albuterol), Alupent (metaproterenol), and Maxair (pirbuterol).
2. Maintenance drugs.
   a. Taken on a regular schedule to maintain optimal airway diameter.
   b. Long-acting beta-2 agonists (sympathomimetics): Mimic activity of sympathetic nervous system, allowing for bronchodilation; may decrease need for rescue drugs and inhaled anti-inflammatories. An example of this type of beta-2 maintenance drug is Serevent (salmeterol xinafoate).
   c. Anticholinergics: inhibit the parasympathetic nervous system; increase heart rate, blood pressure, and bronchodilation. Side effects can include lack of sweating, dry mouth, and delusions. Administered by MDI with minimal side effects. Should be used on a regular schedule to maintain bronchodilation. An example of this category of drug is Atrovent (ipratropium).
   d. Methylxanthines: produce smooth muscle relaxation, but use is limited due to serious toxicity, increased blood pressure, increased heart rate, arrhythmias, gastrointestinal distress, nervousness, headache, and seizures. Blood levels should be drawn to ensure medication effect without toxicity. Examples are aminophylline and theophylline.
   e. Leukotriene receptor antagonists: block leukotrienes released in allergic reactions. Inhibit airway edema and smooth muscle contraction; additive benefits when used in conjunction with other anti-inflammatories. An example of this drug is montelukast (Singulair).
   f. Cromolyn sodium: antiallergic drug; prevents release of mast cells (i.e., histamine) after contact with allergens; used prophylactically to prevent exercise-induced bronchospasm and severe bronchial asthma via oral inhalation. Not to be used as a rescue drug during acute situations. Frequent inhalation can result in hoarseness, cough, dry mouth, and bronchial irritation. Symptoms of overdosage include paradoxical bronchospasm. Brand names include Intal.
   g. Anti-inflammatory agents: used to decrease mucosal edema, inflammation, and airway reactivity. Steroids can be administered systemically or topically (MDI). Side effects of systemic administration: increased blood pressure, sodium retention, muscle wasting, osteoporosis, gastrointestinal (GI) irritation, and hypercholesteremia. The main side effect of inhaled steroids is thrush, a fungal infection of the mouth and throat. Examples are Vanceril (beclomethasone, MDI), Azmacort (triamcinolone, MDI).
   h. Vaccinations. It is recommended that patients with pulmonary disorders routinely receive the influenza and the pneumonia vaccinations.
3. Crisis drugs.
   a. May be used in a crisis situation, such as in an emergency room. Often, drugs that might be given topically are given systemically, and potentially in larger doses. For example, anti-inflammatory agents usually administered via MDI will now be prescribed as prednisone (oral) or SoluMedral (methylprednisolone, IV).
   b. Antibiotics are not recommended for maintenance, but only for treatment of infection, such as an infectious exacerbation.
      - Categories: culture and sensitivity results are used to prescribe the most effective antibiotic.
        ◦ Penicillins.
        ◦ Erythromycins.
        ◦ Tetracyclines.
        ◦ Cephalosporins.
        ◦ Aminoglycosides.
      - Side effects include allergic reactions, stomach cramps, nausea, vomiting, and diarrhea.

Intensive Care Unit Management

Physical Therapy in the Intensive Care Unit

Physical Therapy
1. Employed for pulmonary care (secretion removal or improved aeration) and early mobility (range of motion, positioning, therapeutic exercise, transfers, ambulation).
2. It is very important the physical therapist and physical therapist assistant understand the reasons for use of this equipment as well as the observations, precautions, and contraindications associated with its use. The following equipment is frequently encountered when treating patients in the ICU.

Mechanical Ventilation
1. Maintains an adequate V_E for patients who cannot do so independently.
2. Requires intubation with an endotracheal (oral), nasotracheal (nasal), or tracheal (through a tracheostomy directly into the trachea) tube. Endotracheal and nasotracheal tubes are taped in place, while tracheal tubes may be sutured in place.
3. Tubes or mechanical ventilation pose no contraindications to physical therapy treatment. A patient who is intubated can ambulate using a mechanical resuscitator bag to maintain ventilation. It is sometimes easier to use a stationary device, e.g., peddler, to exercise a patient who needs a ventilator.
4. **SPECIAL CONSIDERATION:** When moving a patient who is intubated, avoid placing excessive tension on the tube. Alteration in the placement of the tube (either a drop inward or a pull outward) could reduce optimal ventilation. If tube movement is suspected, a nurse or respiratory therapist should check tube placement. If the tube is dislodged, a physician, often an anaesthesiologist, should replace the tube.

Chest Tubes
1. Used to evacuate air or fluid trapped in the intrapleural space. Chest tubes are sutured in place to make them secure.
2. There are no contraindications to physical therapy treatment with a chest tube. If the chest tube is connected to a suction device, mobility is limited only by the length of the tubing. Portable suction machines can be used for increased mobility.

RED FLAG: If the tube is dislodged during treatment, cover the defect and seek assistance.

3. **SPECIAL CONSIDERATION:** Care must be taken during mobility activities to ensure a drainage system remains below the level of the chest to prevent the drained fluid from reentering the chest cavity.

Intravenous Lines (IVs)
1. Intravenous catheters used to deliver medications. They are typically inserted into superficial veins and the tip remains close (about 1–5 inches) to the insertion in to the tissues.
2. **SPECIAL CONSIDERATION:** There are no contraindications to physical therapy treatment with IV lines; however, the upper extremity should not be raised above the level of the IV medication for any length of time or backflow of blood may occur.
3. Rolling IV poles allow for mobility. Most IV pumps have a battery backup system to allow patient mobility.
4. **SPECIAL CONSIDERATION:** PTAs must observe tissues in the area of an IV for these common complications:
   a. Infiltrate: a leaking of the IV solution into subcutaneous tissues surrounding the IV site. Appearance-edematous around the area or limb, with possible pitting edema; tissues will feel cool to the touch and is likely painful to the patient at IV site.
   b. Phlebitis: inflammation of the vein. Appearance: red area or streak at IV site, vein may feel cord-like to palpation, patient may experience burning sensation and/or tenderness along the vein.

Central Venous Access Devices (CVAD)
1. May also be called vascular access device or central venous catheter. It is inserted into larger, more proximal veins and used when repeated injections, blood draws, or long-term IV therapy is required. CVADs are used:
   a. When medications are administered that may cause irritation to smaller vessels (e.g., chemotherapy drugs).
   b. To deliver blood or blood products, medications and parenteral nutrition.
   c. To draw blood.
2. Locations: Placed percutaneously directly into the internal or external jugular or subclavian vein. May also be tunneled just under the skin below the clavicle and inserted into the cephalic, internal or external jugular veins.
   a. Trade names of tunneled CVAD include a *Hickman* or *Broviac* catheter. All will end with the tip of the catheter in the superior vena cava.

b. Implanted central venous access ports or infusion ports are placed subcutaneously in the upper chest, typically just inferior to the clavicle with an access port that extends through the skin.
3. Complications: include occlusion, infiltrate, infection, or thrombosis.
   a. Watch for these signs and symptoms:
      - Thrombosis—arm, shoulder or neck pain.
      - Pneumothorax—chest pain, dyspnea, hypoxia, tachycardia, hypotension, nausea, or confusion.
4. Activity restrictions and precautions: There are no activity or positioning restrictions.
   a. **SPECIAL CONSIDERATION:** Ensure tubing does not become entangled, that the end cap on injection port is in place, avoid tugging on the line.

Peripherally Inserted Central Catheters (PICC Line)

1. This is a central line that is inserted peripherally versus centrally. Serves to administer medication, blood and blood products, chemotherapy drugs or parenteral nutrition; some allow for the drawing of blood as well.
   a. PICC lines are placed and meant to stay in place for extended periods of time.
2. Locations: antecubital area (basilic vein, medial cubital vein); wrist area (dorsal venous network, cephalic vein); or foot area (greater saphenous vein, dorsal plexus).
   a. The tip of the catheter is threaded through to the superior vena cava.
3. Complications: phlebitis and infiltrate. (See IVs for description.)
4. Activity restrictions and precautions: there are no activity restrictions.
5. **SPECIAL CONSIDERATION:**
   a. Caution should be taken to avoid tugging on the catheter or disconnecting (can lead to infection or air embolism), may be secured with transparent dressing or tape.
   b. Use caution, check with nursing prior to performing resisted exercise with involved extremity.
   c. Do not submerge insertion site in water.
   d. Do not use extremity with catheter for blood pressure readings.

Arterial Lines, Pulmonary Artery Catheter [Swan-Ganz Catheter], Central Line

1. Multi-lumen catheters that are placed within the arterial system, usually the radial artery. Placed to allow monitoring of the hemodymanic state of the patient.
   a. Arterial lines allow for monitoring of right arterial pressure (central venous pressure), cardiac output, and pulmonary artery pressure.
   b. Pulmonary artery catheters provide information about left ventricular function and pulmonary pressure changes.
   c. The tubing is connected to a pressure pack that exceeds arterial pressure so the line does not back up with blood.
2. Location: the catheter is inserted into the jugular vein and threaded through the superior vena cava, the right atrium and ventricle, then into the pulmonary artery.
3. Complications: watch for signs of infection at the insertion site, inaccurate readings are possible if line is pulled out of place and dislodged.

> **RED FLAG:** If this line becomes dislodged, immediate firm pressure needs to be applied to or above the arterial insertion site to stop bleeding. Call for immediate assistance.

4. Activity restrictions and precautions: no positions are contraindicated, however consult with nursing staff. When mobilizing patients, it may be appropriate to seek assistance.
5. **SPECIAL CONSIDERATION:**
   a. Avoid kinking of the line. Use positioning devices as needed.
   b. Caution should be taken, especially with elderly patients, when performing shoulder activities to avoid catheter occlusion.
   c. If blood pressure readings are gathered through the arterial line care should be taken to ensure the external transducer remains at the same level as the patient's heart.

Monitors/Oscilloscopes

1. Continuous electrocardiogram (ECG) with a reported heart rate.
2. Blood pressure reading, either periodic using noninvasive cuff (NIBP), or continuous using a transducer attached to the arterial line (ABP).
3. Continuous oxygen saturation (SaO_2) with pulse wave. SaO_2 is the percent saturation of oxygen in the arterial blood. This noninvasive measurement relates to the PaO_2 on an S-shaped curve, called the oxyhemoglobin desaturation curve. Normal levels are 98%–100% saturated. The pulse oximeter utilizes a finger sensor (or an ear sensor) to obtain a consistent reading.

Supplemental Oxygen

1. Increases the FiO_2 (up to 1) of the patient's environment. A portable oxygen cylinder attached to the oxygen delivery device (cannula, mask, or manual resuscitator bag attached to the endotracheal tube)

can be used during mobility training to provide supplemental oxygen for the patient.
2. Supplemental oxygen is indicated if SaO_2 is <88% or PaO_2 is <55 mm Hg, regardless of activity level. Monitor the patient's SaO_2 to assure adequate oxygenation with increased activity.
3. Oxygen must be prescribed by a physician, since it is considered a form of medication.
   a. Delivery modes: nasal canula—for oxygen concentration levels of approximately 24%–44% and flow rates of 2–6 liters per minute; facemask—for oxygen concentrations of 35%–60% at flow rates of 5–12 liters per minute; more sophisticated masks (rebreather, nonrebreather and Venturi) can deliver more precise regulation of oxygen to the patient, up to 60%–100% concentrations at 6–15 liters per minute.
   b. Complications: mask or cannula moving out of place, pressure sores from the cannula or mask. Monitor patient for signs of hypoxia: dizziness, fainting, tachycardia, increased respiratory depth and rate, cardiac dysrhythmia, pallor, cyanosis, dyspnea.
   c. Pulse oximetry: an external sensor device that uses infrared light to measure the level of oxygenated hemoglobin in the blood; used to detect levels of oxygenation before signs of hypoxemia present themselves. Different sensors connect to different body parts: finger, nose, ear lobe, forehead.
      - Normal levels are between 95% and 100%. Goal is typically to maintain levels of at least 85% for a patient with chronic respiratory conditions and at least 90% for those without compromise.

Review Questions

Pulmonary Physical Therapy

1. Identify normal pH levels, at normal room air. What pH value indicates a state of respiratory acidosis and alveolar hypoventilation? What signs and symptoms might a patient exhibit in the state of respiratory acidosis?

2. Define inspiratory reserve volume (IRV), expiratory reserve volume (ERV), and vital capacity.

3. Describe the active cycle of breathing technique. Describe how a clinician should instruct a patient/client to perform the technique.

4. Differentiate between the adventitious breath sounds—crackles, wheezes, and rhonchi. Which portion of the stethoscope should be used for each?

5. Describe the palpation method used to assess chest wall excursion of the apical segments of the right upper lobe and the right middle lobe of the lung. When assessing chest wall excursion, should palpation be performed unilaterally or bilaterally? What type of pathological condition might cause a unilateral restriction in chest wall expansion?

6. What is a central venous catheter? Describe where it might be located on a patient and what type of patient may have a central venous catheter. What activity restrictions and precautions apply to physical therapy intervention?

6

Other Systems

SUSAN B. O'SULLIVAN, KAREN E. RYAN and JODI CUSACK

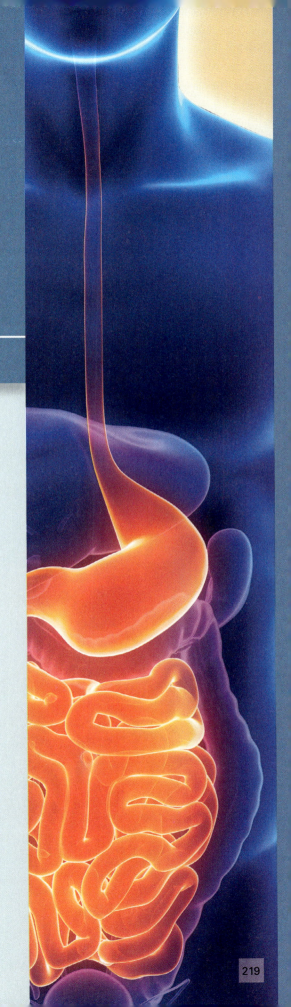

Chapter Outline

- Immune System, 222
    - Overview, 222
    - Acquired Immunodeficiency Syndrome (AIDS), 223
    - Medical Interventions HIV, 224
    - Chronic Fatigue Syndrome (CFS), 224
    - Medical Interventions, 225
    - Fibromyalgia Syndrome (FMS), 229
    - Medical Management, 229
- Infectious Diseases, 230
    - Staphylococcal Infections, 230
    - Streptococcal Infections, 230
    - Hepatitis, 232
    - Medical Interventions, 232
    - Tuberculosis (TB), 233
    - Medical Interventions, 234
- Centers for Disease Control and Prevention (CDC) Standard Precautions, 234
    - Infection Precautions, 234
    - Physical Therapy–Related Infection Control, 234

- **Hematological System, 235**
  - Overview, 235
  - Anemia, 237
  - Medical Intervention, 237
  - Sickle Cell Disease, 237
  - Medical Interventions, 238
  - Hemophilia, 238
  - Medical Interventions, 238
- **Cancer, 239**
  - Overview, 239
  - Medical Interventions, 240
  - Considerations for Physical Therapy Intervention, 241
  - Physical Therapy Goals, Outcomes, and Interventions, 241
- **Gastrointestinal System, 243**
  - Overview, 243
  - Esophagus, 245
  - Stomach, 246
  - Intestines, 246
  - Rectum, 248
- **Genital/Reproductive System, 248**
  - Overview: Female Reproductive System, 248
  - Pregnancy: Normal, 248
  - Pregnancy-Related Pathologies, 250
  - Disorders of the Female Reproductive System, 251
  - Overview: Male Reproductive System, 251
  - Disorders of the Male Reproductive System, 252
- **Renal and Urological Systems, 252**
  - Overview, 252
  - Urinary Regulation of Fluids and Electrolytes, 253
  - Renal and Urological Disorders, 255

- Endocrine and Metabolic Systems, 257
  - Overview of the Endocrine System, 257
  - Overview of the Metabolic System, 258
  - Diabetes Mellitus (DM), 258
  - Medical Goals and Interventions, 260
  - Obesity, 262
  - Surgical Intervention, 263
  - Thyroid Disorders, 265
  - Adrenal Disorders, 265
- Vestibular System, 266
  - Overview of the Vestibular System, 266
  - Etiology, 266
  - Medical Evaluation and Testing, 266
- Psychiatric Conditions, 269
  - Psychiatric States/Mechanisms, 269
  - Pathologies, 269
  - Grief Process, 270
  - Death and Dying, 271
  - Interventions, 271
- Review Questions, 272

Immune System

Overview

Anatomy and Physiology of the Immune System

1. The immune system consists of immune cells, central immune structures where immune cells are produced (the bone marrow and thymus), and the peripheral immune structures (lymph nodes, spleen, and other accessory structures).
2. There are several different types of immune cells.
   a. An antigen (immunogen) is a foreign molecule that elicits the immune response. Antibodies or immunoglobulins are the proteins that are engaged to tag antigens.
   b. Lymphocytes (T and B lymphocytes) are the primary cells of the immune system.
   c. Macrophages are the accessory cells that process and present antigens to the lymphocytes.
   d. Cytokines are molecules that link immune cells with other tissues and organs.
   e. CD molecules (e.g., CD4 helper cells) serve as master regulators of the immune response by influencing the function of all other immune cells.
   f. Recognition of foreign threat from self (autoimmune responses) is mediated by major histocompatibility complex (MHC) membrane molecules.
3. The thymus is the primary central gland of the immune system. It is located behind the sternum above the heart and extends into the neck region to the lower edge of the thyroid gland.
   a. It is fully developed at birth and reaches maximum size at puberty. It then decreases in size and is slowly replaced by adipose tissue.
   b. It produces mature T lymphocytes.
4. The lymph system is a vast network of capillaries, vessels, valves, ducts, nodes, and organs that function to produce, filter, and convey various lymph and blood cells.
   a. Lymph nodes are small areas of lymphoid tissue connected by lymphatic vessels throughout the body. High concentrations are found in the axillae, in the groin, and along the great vessels of the neck, thorax, and abdomen.
   b. Lymph nodes function to filter the lymph and trap antigens. Lymphocytes, monocytes, and plasma cells are formed in lymph nodes.
5. The spleen is a large lymphoid organ located in the upper left abdominal cavity between the stomach and the diaphragm.
   a. It functions to filter antigens from the blood and produce leukocytes, monocytes, lymphocytes, and plasma cells in response to infection.
   b. In the embryo, the spleen produces red and white blood cells; after birth, only lymphocytes are produced unless severe anemia exists.

The Immune Response

1. A coordinated response of the body's cells and molecules that provides protection from infectious disease (bacteria, viruses, fungi, parasites) and foreign substances (plant pollens, poison ivy resin, insect venom, transplanted organs). It also defends against abnormal cells produced by the body (cancer cells).
2. Provides natural resistance to disease and consists of rapidly activated phagocytes (macrophages, neutrophils, natural killer cells, dendritic cells). Barriers also provide a natural defense (skin, mucous membranes) as do inflammation and fever (antimicrobial molecules).
3. The adaptive immune response includes the slower acting defenses mediated by the lymphocytes.
4. Repeat exposure activates immunological memory, producing more rapid and efficient responses.
5. Excessive immune response causes allergies or autoimmune reactions.

Immunodeficiency Diseases

1. Characterized by depressed or absent immune responses.
2. Primary immunodeficient disorders result from a defect in T cells, B cells, or lymphoid tissues.
   a. Congenital disorders are a failure of organs to develop and produce mature lymphocytes.
   b. Severe combined immunodeficiency disease (SCID).
3. Secondary immunodeficiency disorders are caused by underlying pathology or treatment that depresses the immune system, resulting in failure of the immune response.
   a. Diseases include leukemia, bone marrow tumor, chronic diabetes, renal failure, cirrhosis, cancer treatment (chemotherapy, radiation therapy).
   b. Organ transplant, graft-versus-host disease.

Autoimmune Diseases

1. Characterized by immune system responses directed against the body's normal tissues; self-destructive processes impair body function.
2. Can be organ-specific: Hashimoto's thyroiditis.

3. Can be systemic (non–organ specific): systemic lupus erythematosus (SLE), fibromyalgia.
4. Etiology is unknown; possible factors include genetic predisposition, hormonal changes, environment, viral infection, and stress.

Acquired Immunodeficiency Syndrome (AIDS)

Characteristics
1. AIDS is caused by the human immunodeficiency virus (HIV-1 or HIV-2); is a blood-borne pathogen.
2. The virus can exist in the system for several weeks undetected and may not produce symptoms for longer periods of time.
3. With the AIDS virus the body fails to produce antibodies to fight off infection thus weakening the immune system and leaving the body susceptible to opportunistic infections. The body fails to recognize, thus defend against, infectious agents that a healthy body would be able to defend against.

Loss of Immune System Function Leads to Secondary Infections
1. Opportunistic infections: most common is *Pneumocystis carinii* pneumonia; also oral and esophageal candidiasis (fungal infection–thrush), cytomegalovirus infection, cryptococcus, atypical mycobacteriosis, chronic herpes simplex, toxoplasmosis, *Mycobacterium tuberculosis*.
2. Malignancies: most common is Kaposi's sarcoma (malignant blood vessel and skin condition); also non-Hodgkin's lymphoma; primary brain lymphoma.
3. Neurological disease: focal encephalitis (central nervous system [CNS] toxoplasmosis); cryptococcal meningitis; AIDS dementia complex; herpes zoster.

Pathophysiology
1. HIV is an RNA retrovirus which attaches itself to the CD4+ receptor on the T-lymphocytes, resulting in CD4+ T lymphocytopenia, a major defect in the immune system. A retrovirus: replicates in reverse fashion, i.e., the RNA code is transcribed into DNA.
2. T-lymphocytes, sometimes called helper T cells, are white blood cells of the immune system that are responsible for destroying unrecognized cells, e.g., those infected with viruses, cancer cells.
3. A latency period between the onset of infection with the HIV virus and full-blown AIDS can be between 10–15 years.

Stages of HIV
1. Stage 1 acute HIV infection: flulike illness within 2–4 weeks after infection.
2. Stage 2 clinical latency: asymptomatic HIV infection or chronic HIV infection; can last a decade or longer.
3. Stage 3 AIDS: the most severe phase; over time, HIV destroys so many cells that the body cannot fight off infections and disease, resulting in opportunistic illnesses.

Transmission
1. Through contact with infected body fluids (blood, saliva, semen, pre-seminal fluids, cerebrospinal fluid, breast milk, vaginal/cervical secretions, rectal fluids). Fluid must come in contact with mucous membrane, damaged tissue, or be directly injected into the blood stream (needle or syringe).
2. High-risk behaviors for HIV transmission.
   a. Unprotected anal or vaginal sex with someone who has HIV.
   b. Sharing needles or syringes, rinse water, or other equipment used to prepare drugs for injection with someone who has HIV.
   c. Maternal-fetal transmission in utero or at delivery; contaminated breast milk.
3. Low-risk behaviors for HIV transmission.
   a. Occupational transmission: needle sticks.
   b. Casual contact: kissing (open-mouth kissing if both partners have sores or bleeding gums).
4. HIV is not spread by saliva, tears, or sweat that is not mixed with the blood of an HIV-positive person; touching, hugging, shaking hands; sharing toilets, sharing dishes; or closed-mouth "social" kissing.
5. AIDS cannot be contracted through respiratory inhalation, skin contact, or human waste (urine, feces, sweat, or vomit).

Diagnosis of HIV Requires Positive Results from Two HIV Tests
1. CD4 cell count: 500–1200 cells/mm.
2. Testing with HIV-1/HIV-2 antigen/antibody combination immunoassays.
3. Medical evaluation and laboratory evaluation including plasma HIV viral load, blood cell and CD4 count, antiretroviral resistance assay, drug-resistance testing, and testing for sexually transmitted infections (STDs).

Diagnosis of AIDS
1. CD4 cell count drops below 200 cells/mm or if they develop certain opportunistic illnesses. People with AIDs have a high viral load and are very infectious.
2. AIDS-related complex (ARC): presence of acute symptoms secondary to immune system deficiency.

HIV Signs and Symptoms
1. Includes flu-like symptoms: recurrent fever and chills, night sweats, swollen lymph glands, sore throat, rash,

and muscle aches. Symptoms usually disappear after a few weeks.
2. Getting tested is the only way to tell if HIV is present.

AIDS Signs and Symptoms
1. Infected person exhibits some or all of the symptoms along with a general failure to thrive.
2. Opportunistic infections: AIDS-defining conditions include pneumocystis pneumonia, candidiasis, cytomegalovirus, and toxoplasmosis.
3. Malignancies: most common is Kaposi's sarcoma; also non-Hodgkin's lymphoma; primary brain lymphoma.
4. Neurological conditions: focal encephalitis (central nervous system [CNS] toxoplasmosis); cryptococcal meningitis; AIDS dementia complex; herpes zoster.
5. Deconditioning, anxiety, and depression are common.

Clinical Course
1. May exhibit brief, early, nonspecific viral HIV infection, and then remain asymptomatic for many years.
2. There is no cure for HIV infection. Without treatment nearly every person will progress to AIDS.

Medical Interventions HIV

1. Antiretroviral therapies (ARTs): antiviral drugs (ARVs) are used to reduce the amount of virus (viral load) in the system and are always given in combination (usually three or more drugs); recommended for everyone infected with HIV, starting immediately.
2. ART does not not cure HIV, but does keep people with HIV healthy for many years if taken consistently and correctly.

> **RED FLAG:** common adverse effects of ART include rash, nausea and vomiting, diarrhea, headaches, dizziness, fatigue, and pain.

3. Symptomatic treatment.
   a. Education to prevent the spread of infection and disease.
   b. Treat opportunistic infections; prophylactic vaccinations.
   c. Maintain nutritional status.
   d. Provide supportive care for management of fatigue, e.g., energy-conservation techniques, self-care.
   e. Respiratory management as needed.
   f. Provide skin care.
   g. Maintain functional mobility and safety; prevent disability.
   h. Provide supportive care, e.g., emotional support for patients and families.

Physical Therapy Goals, Outcomes, and Interventions
1. Observe standard AIDS/HIV precautions for healthcare workers (see Box 6-1).
2. Exercise has a positive effect on the immune system; reduces stress level and pain; improves cardiovascular endurance and strength (disuse effects common).
3. Exercise recommendations.
   a. Moderate aerobic exercise training.
   b. Strength training, coordination, balance, endurance (when appropriate), gait training, functional mobility training.
   c. Instruction in use of assistive and adaptive devices and equipment.
   d. Avoid exhaustive exercise with symptomatic individuals.
   e. During acute stages of opportunistic infections: reduce exercise to mild levels.
4. Teach activity pacing: balancing rest with activity; scheduling strenuous activities during periods of high energy.
5. Teach energy conservation: analysis and modification of daily activities to reduce energy expenditure.
6. Teach stress management, relaxation training (e.g., meditation and mindfulness, tai chi chuan, yoga).
7. Neurological rehabilitation for patients with involvement of the CNS (see Chapter 3).

Chronic Fatigue Syndrome (CFS)

Pathophysiology and Clinical Characteristics
1. Etiology: unknown; theories include multiple triggers (e.g., viral infection), immune dysfunction, or a combination of factors.
   a. May also be referred to as myalgic encephalomyelitis (ME).
2. Symptoms: significantly lower level of tolerance for activity than previously—extreme exhaustion that sleep doesn't help improve, general flu-like symptoms, problems with sleep, persistent muscle pain, joint pain (without signs of inflammation), headache, tender lymph nodes in neck or armpit, sore throat. Additional problems can include: a "mental fog," irritable bowel, difficulty tolerating an upright position, dizziness or fainting, visual disturbances (light sensitivity, blurring, eye pain), depression or mood problems (irritability, anxiety, panic attacks).
3. Potentially present: immunological abnormalities neuroendocrine changes.

Diagnosis and Prognosis
1. There is no single test to confirm a diagnosis of CFS. The CDC criteria include severe fatigue lasting longer

than 6 months as well as the presence of at least four other symptoms. Exclusion of other chronic conditions.
2. The cluster of criteria required for a diagnosis of CFS:
   a. New or definite onset of severe chronic fatigue that has been present for at least 6 or more consecutive months, is not due to ongoing exertion and is not substantially alleviated by rest.
   b. Fatigue level significantly interferes with work and daily activities.
   c. Presence of 4 or more of the following symptoms:
      - Malaise or inability to recover from exertion lasting >24 hours.
      - Unrefreshing sleep.
      - Sore throat that is frequent or recurring—nonexudative.
      - Lymph node pain and tenderness (cervical and axillary).
      - Muscle pain.
      - Multi-joint pain without signs of inflammation.
      - Significant impairment of short-term memory or concentration.
      - Headaches of a new type, pattern or severity.
3. More common in women than men and in younger ages (20s and 30s).
4. Limited recovery: only 5%–10% recover completely.

Medical Interventions

1. A team approach, including multiple medical disciplines, that is directed at managing symptoms that are more disruptive or disabling at the time for each patient is suggested.
2. Cytokines, produced by our body to help fight infection are being studied; specifically IFN-alpha

BOX 6-1 ▶ Standard Precautions*

Standard Precautions combine the major features of Universal Precautions (UP) and Body Substance Isolation (BSI) and are based on the principle that all blood, body fluids, secretions, excretions except sweat, nonintact skin, and mucous membranes may contain transmissible infectious agents. Standard Precautions include a group of infection prevention practices that apply to all patients, regardless of suspected or confirmed infection status, in any setting in which health care is delivered. These include hand hygiene; use of gloves, gown, mask, eye protection, or face shield, depending on the anticipated exposure; and safe injection practices. Also, equipment or items in the patient environment likely to have been contaminated with infectious body fluids must be handled in a manner to prevent transmission of infectious agents (e.g., wear gloves for direct contact, contain heavily soiled equipment, properly clean and disinfect or sterilize reusable equipment before use on another patient). The application of Standard Precautions during patient care is determined by the nature of the health care worker (HCW)–patient interaction and the extent of anticipated blood, body fluid, or pathogen exposure. For some interactions (e.g., performing venipuncture), only gloves may be needed; during other interactions (e.g., intubation), use of gloves, gown, and face shield or mask and goggles is necessary. Education and training on the principles and rationale for recommended practices are critical elements of Standard Precautions because they facilitate appropriate decision-making and promote adherence when HCWs are faced with new circumstances. An example of the importance of the use of Standard Precautions is intubation, especially under emergency circumstances when infectious agents may not be suspected, but later are identified (e.g., severe acute respiratory syndrome [SARS]–coronavirus [CoV], *Neisseria meningitidis*). Standard Precautions are also intended to protect patients by ensuring that health care personnel do not carry infectious agents to patients on their hands or via equipment used during patient care.

A.1. New Elements of Standard Precautions Infection control problems that are identified in the course of outbreak investigations often indicate the need for new recommendations or reinforcement of existing infection control recommendations to protect patients. Because such recommendations are considered a standard of care and may not be included in other guidelines, they are added here to Standard Precautions. Three such areas of practice that have been added are Respiratory Hygiene/Cough Etiquette, safe injection practices, and use of masks for insertion of catheters or injection of material into spinal or epidural spaces via lumbar puncture procedures (e.g., myelogram, spinal or epidural anesthesia). While most elements of Standard Precautions evolved from Universal Precautions that were developed for protection of health care personnel, these new elements of Standard Precautions focus on protection of patients.

A.1.a. Respiratory Hygiene/Cough Etiquette The transmission of SARS-CoV in emergency departments by patients and their family members during the widespread SARS outbreaks in 2003 highlighted the need for vigilance and prompt implementation of infection control measures at the first point of encounter within a health care setting (e.g., reception and triage areas in emergency departments, outpatient clinics, and physician offices). The strategy proposed has been termed Respiratory Hygiene/Cough Etiquette and is intended to be incorporated into infection control practices as a new component of Standard Precautions. The strategy is targeted at patients and accompanying family members and friends with undiagnosed transmissible respiratory infections, and applies to any person with signs of illness including cough, congestion, rhinorrhea, or increased production of respiratory secretions when entering a health care facility. The term cough etiquette is derived from recommended source control measures for *Mycobacteria tuberculosis*. The elements of Respiratory Hygiene/Cough Etiquette include (1) education of health care facility staff, patients, and visitors; (2) posted signs, in language(s) appropriate to the population

(Continued)

BOX 6-1 ▷ Standard Precautions* (Continued)

served, with instructions to patients and accompanying family members or friends; (3) source control measures (e.g., covering the mouth/nose with a tissue when coughing and prompt disposal of used tissues, using surgical masks on the coughing person when tolerated and appropriate); (4) hand hygiene after contact with respiratory secretions; and (5) spatial separation, ideally >3 feet, of persons with respiratory infections in common waiting areas when possible. Covering sneezes and coughs and placing masks on coughing patients are proven means of source containment that prevent infected persons from dispersing respiratory secretions into the air. Masking may be difficult in some settings (e.g., pediatrics, in which case the emphasis by necessity may be on cough etiquette. Physical proximity of <3 feet has been associated with an increased risk for transmission of infections via the droplet route (e.g., *N. meningitidis* and group A streptococcus) and therefore supports the practice of distancing infected persons from others who are not infected. The effectiveness of good hygiene practices, especially hand hygiene, in preventing transmission of viruses and reducing the incidence of respiratory infections both within and outside health care settings is summarized in several reviews.

These measures should be effective in decreasing the risk of transmission of pathogens contained in large respiratory droplets (e.g., influenza virus, adenovirus, *Bordetella pertussis*, and *Mycoplasma pneumoniae*. Although fever will be present in many respiratory infections, patients with pertussis and mild upper respiratory tract infections are often afebrile. Therefore, the absence of fever does not always exclude a respiratory infection. Patients who have asthma, allergic rhinitis, or chronic obstructive lung disease also may be coughing and sneezing. While these patients often are not infectious, cough etiquette measures are prudent.

Health care personnel are advised to observe Droplet Precautions (i.e., wear a mask) and hand hygiene when examining and caring for patients with signs and symptoms of a respiratory infection. Health care personnel who have a respiratory infection are advised to avoid direct patient contact, especially with high-risk patients. If this is not possible, then a mask should be worn while providing patient care.

Recommendations

IV. Standard Precautions
Assume that every person is potentially infected or colonized with an organism that could be transmitted in the health care setting and apply the following infection control practices during the delivery of health care.

IV.A. Hand Hygiene
IV.A.1. During the delivery of health care, avoid unnecessary touching of surfaces in close proximity to the patient to prevent both contamination of clean hands from environmental surfaces and transmission of pathogens from contaminated hands to surfaces.
IV.A.2. When hands are visibly dirty, contaminated with proteinaceous material, or visibly soiled with blood or body fluids, wash hands with either a nonantimicrobial soap and water or an antimicrobial soap and water.
IV.A.3. If hands are not visibly soiled, or after removing visible material with nonantimicrobial soap and water, decontaminate hands in the clinical situations described in IV.A.3.a–f. The preferred method of hand decontamination is with an alcohol-based hand rub. Alternatively, hands may be washed with an antimicrobial soap and water. Frequent use of an alcohol-based hand rub immediately following hand washing with nonantimicrobial soap may increase the frequency of dermatitis. Perform hand hygiene:
IV.A.3.a. Before having direct contact with patients.
IV.A.3.b. After contact with blood, body fluids or excretions, mucous membranes, nonintact skin, or wound dressings.
IV.A.3.c. After contact with a patient's intact skin (e.g., when taking a pulse or blood pressure or lifting a patient).
IV.A.3.d. If hands will be moving from a contaminated body site to a clean body site during patient care.
IV.A.3.e. After contact with inanimate objects (including medical equipment) in the immediate vicinity of the patient.
IV.A.3.f. After removing gloves.
IV.A.4. Wash hands with nonantimicrobial soap and water or with antimicrobial soap and water if in contact with spores (e.g., *Clostridium difficile* or *Bacillus anthracis*) is likely to have occurred. The physical action of washing and rinsing hands under such circumstances is recommended because alcohols, chlorhexidine, iodophors, and other antiseptic agents have poor activity against spores.
IV.A.5. Do not wear artificial fingernails or extenders if duties include direct contact with patients at high risk for infection and associated adverse outcomes (e.g., those in intensive care units [ICUs] or operating rooms).
IV.A.5.a. Develop an organizational policy on the wearing of nonnatural nails by health care personnel who have direct contact with patients outside of the groups specified above.

IV.B. Personal protective equipment (PPE)
IV.B.1. Observe the following principles of use:
IV.B.1.a. Wear PPE, as described in IV.B.2–4, when the nature of the anticipated patient interaction indicates that contact with blood or body fluids may occur.

(Continued)

BOX 6-1 ▷ Standard Precautions* (Continued)

IV.B.1.b. Prevent contamination of clothing and skin during the process of removing PPE.

IV.B.1.c. Before leaving the patient's room or cubicle, remove and discard PPE.

IV.B.2. Gloves

IV.B.2.a. Wear gloves when it can be reasonably anticipated that contact with blood or other potentially infectious materials, mucous membranes, nonintact skin, or potentially contaminated intact skin (e.g., of a patient incontinent of stool or urine) could occur.

IV.B.2.b. Wear gloves with fit and durability appropriate to the task.

IV.B.2.b.i. Wear disposable medical examination gloves for providing direct patient care.

IV.B.2.b.ii. Wear disposable medical examination gloves or reusable utility gloves for cleaning the environment or medical equipment.

IV.B.2.c. Remove gloves after contact with a patient and/or the surrounding environment (including medical equipment) using proper technique to prevent hand contamination. Do not wear the same pair of gloves for the care of more than one patient. Do not wash gloves for the purpose of reuse since this practice has been associated with transmission of pathogens.

IV.B.2.d. Change gloves during patient care if the hands will move from a contaminated body site (e.g., perineal area) to a clean body site (e.g., face).

IV.B.3. Gowns

IV.B.3.a. Wear a gown that is appropriate to the task to protect skin and prevent soiling or contamination of clothing during procedures and patient-care activities when contact with blood, body fluids, secretions, or excretions is anticipated.

IV.B.3.a.i. Wear a gown for direct patient contact if the patient has uncontained secretions or excretions.

IV.B.3.a.ii. Remove gown and perform hand hygiene before leaving the patient's environment.

IV.B.3.b. Do not reuse gowns, even for repeated contacts with the same patient.

IV.B.3.c. Routine donning of gowns upon entrance into a high-risk unit (e.g., ICU, neonatal intensive care unit [NICU], hematopoietic stem cell transplantation [HSCT] unit) is not indicated.

IV.B.4. Mouth, nose, eye protection.

IV.B.4.a. Use PPE to protect the mucous membranes of the eyes, nose, and mouth during procedures and patient-care activities that are likely to generate splashes or sprays of blood, body fluids, secretions, and excretions. Select masks, goggles, face shields, and combinations of each according to the need anticipated by the task performed.

IV.B.5. During aerosol-generating procedures (e.g., bronchoscopy, suctioning of the respiratory tract [if not using in-line suction catheters], endotracheal intubation) in patients who are not suspected of being infected with an agent for which respiratory protection is otherwise recommended (e.g., *M. tuberculosis*, SARS, or hemorrhagic fever viruses), wear one of the following: a face shield that fully covers the front and sides of the face, a mask with attached shield, or a mask and goggles (in addition to gloves and gown).

IV.C. Respiratory Hygiene/Cough Etiquette

IV.C.1. Educate health care personnel on the importance of source control measures to contain respiratory secretions to prevent droplet and fomite transmission of respiratory pathogens, especially during seasonal outbreaks of viral respiratory tract infections (e.g., influenza, respiratory syncytial virus [RSV], adenovirus, parainfluenza virus) in communities.

IV.C.2. Implement the following measures to contain respiratory secretions in patients and accompanying individuals who have signs and symptoms of a respiratory infection, beginning at the point of initial encounter in a health care setting (e.g., triage, reception and waiting areas in emergency departments, outpatient clinics, and physician offices).

IV.C.2.a. Post signs at entrances and in strategic places (e.g., elevators, cafeterias) within ambulatory and inpatient settings with instructions to patients and other persons with symptoms of a respiratory infection to cover their mouths/noses when coughing or sneezing, use and dispose of tissues, and perform hand hygiene after hands have been in contact with respiratory secretions.

IV.C.2.b. Provide tissues and no-touch receptacles (e.g., foot pedal–operated lid or open, plastic-lined waste basket) for disposal of tissues.

IV.C.2.c. Provide resources and instructions for performing hand hygiene in or near waiting areas in ambulatory and inpatient settings; provide conveniently located dispensers of alcohol-based hand rubs and, where sinks are available, supplies for hand washing.

IV.C.2.d. During periods of increased prevalence of respiratory infections in the community (e.g., as indicated by increased school absenteeism, increased number of patients seeking care for a respiratory infection), offer masks to coughing patients and other symptomatic persons (e.g., persons who accompany ill patients) upon entry into the facility or medical office and encourage them to maintain special separation, ideally a distance of at least 3 feet, from others in common waiting areas.

IV.C.2.d.i. Some facilities may find it logistically easier to institute this recommendation year-round as a standard of practice.

(Continued)

BOX 6-1 ▸ Standard Precautions* (Continued)

IV.D. Patient placement

IV.D.1. Include the potential for transmission of infectious agents in patient placement decisions. Place patients who pose a risk for transmission to others (e.g., uncontained secretions, excretions or wound drainage, infants with suspected viral respiratory or gastrointestinal infections) in a single-patient room when available.

IV.D.2. Determine patient placement based on the following principles:
- Route(s) of transmission of the known or suspected infectious agent
- Risk factors for transmission in the infected patient
- Risk factors for adverse outcomes resulting from a hospital-acquired infection (HAI) in other patients in the area or room being considered for patient placement
- Availability of single-patient rooms
- Patient options for room sharing (e.g., cohorting patients with the same infection)

IV.E. Patient-care equipment and instruments/devices

IV.E.1. Establish policies and procedures for containing, transporting, and handling patient-care equipment and instruments/devices that may be contaminated with blood or body fluids.

IV.E.2. Remove organic material from critical and semicritical instruments/devices, using recommended cleaning agents before high-level disinfection and sterilization to enable effective disinfection and sterilization processes.

IV.E.3. Wear PPE (e.g., gloves, gown), according to the level of anticipated contamination, when handling patient-care equipment and instruments/devices that are visibly soiled or may have been in contact with blood or body fluids.

IV.F. Care of the environment

IV.F.1. Establish policies and procedures for routine and targeted cleaning of environmental surfaces as indicated by the level of patient contact and degree of soiling.

IV.F.2. Clean and disinfect surfaces that are likely to be contaminated with pathogens, including those that are in close proximity to the patient (e.g., bed rails, over-bed tables) and frequently touched surfaces in the patient-care environment (e.g., doorknobs, surfaces in and surrounding toilets in patients' rooms) on a more frequent schedule compared to that for other surfaces (e.g., horizontal surfaces in waiting rooms).

IV.F.3. Use Environmental Protection Agency (EPA)–registered disinfectants that have microbiocidal (i.e., killing) activity against the pathogens most likely to contaminate the patient-care environment. Use in accordance with manufacturer's instructions.

IV.F.3.a. Review the efficacy of in-use disinfectants when evidence of continuing transmission of an infectious agent (e.g., rotavirus, *C. difficile*, norovirus) may indicate resistance to the in-use product and change to a more effective disinfectant as indicated.

IV.F.4. In facilities that provide health care to pediatric patients or have waiting areas with child play toys (e.g., obstetric/gynecology offices and clinics), establish policies and procedures for cleaning and disinfecting toys at regular intervals.

Use the following principles in developing this policy and procedures:
- Select play toys that can be easily cleaned and disinfected.
- Do not permit use of stuffed furry toys if they will be shared.
- Clean and disinfect large stationary toys (e.g., climbing equipment) at least weekly and whenever visibly soiled.
- If toys are likely to be mouthed, rinse with water after disinfection; alternatively wash in a dishwasher.
- When a toy requires cleaning and disinfection, do so immediately or store in a designated labeled container separate from toys that are clean and ready for use.

IV.F.5. Include multiuse electronic equipment in policies and procedures for preventing contamination and for cleaning and disinfection, especially those items that are used by patients, those used during delivery of patient care, and mobile devices that are moved in and out of patient rooms frequently (e.g., daily).

IV.F.5.a. No recommendation for use of removable protective covers or washable keyboards. Unresolved issue.

IV.G. Textiles and laundry

IV.G.1. Handle used textiles and fabrics with minimum agitation to avoid contamination of air, surfaces, and persons.

IV.G.2. If laundry chutes are used, ensure that they are properly designed, maintained, and used in a manner to minimize dispersion of aerosols from contaminated laundry.

IV.H. Safe injection practices: see CDC website.

IV.I. Infection control practices for special lumbar puncture procedures: see CDC website.

IV.J. Worker safety. Adhere to federal and state requirements for protection of health-care personnel from exposure to bloodborne pathogens.

*Excerpted with modifications from Centers for Disease Control and Prevention, Guideline for Isolation Precautions: Preventing Transmission of Infectious Agents in Healthcare Settings, 2007. PDF (1.33MB/219 pages), downloaded 9.15.08. http://www.cdc.gov/ncidod/dhqp/gl_isolation_standard.html
**Date last modified: October 12, 2007.

which has been shown to cause problems sleeping and change the secretion of cortisol. Cortisol is an important hormone that helps the body regulate metabolism and the immune system. Antiviral agents are now being explored in clinical trials.
3. Supportive and symptomatic treatment; symptoms may persist for months or years.
   a. Medications to manage pain; analgesics and non-steroidal anti-inflammatory medications for myalgia and arthralgia; narcotics are not recommended. Antidepressants are only recommended if true depression exists.
   b. Nutritional support and lifestyle changes—prevent overexertion, stress management.
   c. Cognitive behavior therapy and graded exercise appear to be the most beneficial interventions.

Physical Therapist Assistant Assessment
1. Assess exercise tolerance levels. Vital signs may reveal fluctuations in HR and BP; orthostatic hypotension is common. If deconditioned, dyspnea with exercise.
2. Assess posture. Postural stress syndrome (poor posture) and movement adaptation syndrome (inefficient movement patterns) may be present and can contribute to chronic pain.
3. Assess activity levels and degree of fatigue. Objective measure: Modified Fatigue Impact Scale.
4. Monitor for depression and degree of emotional support present.

Physical Therapy Goals, Outcomes and Interventions
1. Activities are reduced when fatigue is maximal; bed rest contraindicated other than for sleep.
2. Exercise recommendations (ACSM's Exercise Management for Persons with Chronic Diseases and Disabilities Human Kinetics, 2009):
   a. Overall goal to prevent deconditioning.
   b. Aerobic exercise (e.g., walking).
      - Intensity: low to moderate levels of intensity (RPE 9–12/20), progress very gradually.
      - Frequency: 3–5 days/week.
      - Duration: to tolerance, 5 min/session initially progressing to 40–60 minutes.
3. Avoid overexertion. Provide education that individuals may experience increased fatigue in the first few weeks of an exercise program. Individuals should reduce exercise when symptoms are increased or they are not feeling well.
4. Teach activity pacing: balancing rest with activity; scheduling strenuous activities during periods of high energy.
5. Teach energy conservation: analysis and modification of daily activities to reduce energy expenditure.
6. Provide education on good sleep habits (e.g., get up same time each day, avoid electronic devices/television 60 minutes before bed time, cool temperature, dark room, etc.).
7. Teach stress management, relaxation training (e.g., meditation and mindfulness, tai chi chuan, yoga).
8. Refer to support group.

Fibromyalgia Syndrome (FMS)

Pathophysiology
1. Etiology: unknown; multifactorial; viral cause suspected. May develop after a triggering event: trauma, surgery, infection, or significant psychological stress.
2. Immunological and neurohormonal abnormalities are present. More common in individuals with rheumatic disease.
3. Genetic factor: tends to run in families.
4. More common in women (75%–80% of cases) than men.

Signs and Symptoms
1. Myalgia (muscle pain), generalized aching, persistent fatigue (mental and physical), sleep disturbances with generalized morning stiffness, and multiple tender points (trigger points).
2. Different from CFS in that patients with CFS tend to experience more fatigue and patients with FMS tend to experience more pain. To a greater degree, FMS is associated with perpetuating circumstances, e.g., psychologically traumatic event, primary sleep disorder, inflammatory rheumatic arthritis.
3. Additional signs and symptoms: visual problems, mental and physical fatigue, spasm, cold intolerance, headaches, irritable bladder or bowel, gastrointestinal disturbances, cognitive problems (impaired memory, decreased attention and concentration), restless legs, atypical patterns of numbness and tingling (sensitivity amplification).
4. Anxiety and depression are common.

Medical Management
1. Diagnosis—two criteria:
   a. Widespread pain lasting at least 3 months and presence of 11 positive tender points out of total 18 (Copenhagen Fibromyalgia Syndrome definition).

2. Medical management is approached from a multidisciplinary, holistic approach including: modification of pain, increase tolerance for ADLs, improve sleep. Patient education regarding nutrition, lifestyle modification, cognitive behavioral therapy (pain response behaviors), graded exercise program.
3. Medication management includes symptom management. Pregabalin (Lyrica, for pain and sleep), duloxetine (Cymbalta), or milnacipran (Savella) for pain, fatigue.
4. Psychological support and counseling; antidepressants if necessary.
5. Prognosis: FMS is a chronic condition—however, it is not progressive and does not cause tissue or joint destruction.

Physical Therapy Goals, Outcomes, and Interventions

1. See recommendations for chronic fatigue syndrome.
2. May initially demonstrate exercise intolerance, a slow steady progression to increase tolerance, without creating a pain response, is key to a successful exercise program. Daily exercise is important. Focus is on aerobic training, mild to moderate intensities, potentially for only 2–20 minute duration initially, progressing to 30–40 minutes, 2 times/week. Recognize a patient with FMS will respond painfully to stimuli that are not typically painful. Exercise may have to be broken into 2–3 exercise sessions of 10–15 minutes each and may take weeks to months to reach identified goals.
3. Teach protection strategies to avoid overuse syndromes; histology of tissues in persons with FMS reveal they may be at greater risk than general population.
4. Aquatic therapy is ideal to decrease pain and increase cardiovascular conditioning and strength.
5. Teach techniques for taking control: self-responsibility for health, education, coping strategies, keeping a journal. Tai chi and yoga have been shown to be beneficial.
6. Work and work environment adjustments.
7. Refer to support group.

Infectious Diseases

Staphylococcal Infections

Staphylococcus Aureus (SA)
1. A common bacterial pathogen.
2. Pathophysiology.
   a. Typically begins as localized infection; entry is through skin portal, e.g., wounds, ulcers, burns.
   b. Bacterial invasion and spread is through bloodstream or lymphatic system to almost any body location, e.g., heart valves, bones (acute staphylococcal osteomyelitis), joints (bacterial arthritis), skin (cellulitis, furuncles and carbuncles, ulcers), respiratory tract (pneumonia), bowel (enterocolitis).
   c. Infection produces suppuration (pus formation) and abscess.
3. Medical interventions.
   a. Laboratory diagnosis to confirm pathogen.
   b. Antibiotic therapy; determine antibiotic sensitivity. Antibiotic resistance is common.
   c. Drainage of abscesses. Follow standard precautions for infection control procedures.
   d. Skin infections that are untreated can become systemic; sepsis can be lethal.

Methicillin-Resistant *Staphylococcus Aureus* (MRSA)
1. An antibiotic-resistant strain.
2. MRSA is resistant to all penicillins (especially methicillin) and cephalosporins.
3. It is found in about 1% of the population.
4. Hospitalized patients with MRSA infections are isolated and standard mask-gown-gloves precautions required (Tables 6-1 and 6-2.)

Vancomycin-Resistant *Staphylococcus Aureus* (VRSA)
1. Resistant to vancomycin.
2. Can be a life-threatening infection.

Streptococcal Infections

Characteristics
1. A common bacterial pathogen.
2. Types.
   a. Group A streptococcus (*S. pyogenes*): pharyngitis, rheumatic fever, scarlet fever, impetigo, necrotizing fasciitis (gangrene), cellulitis, myositis.

Table 6-1

Modes of Transmission and Protective Measures

MODE OF TRANSMISSION	EXAMPLE	POSSIBLE PATHOGEN	PROTECTIVE MEASURE
Direct Contact Microorganism transferred from one infected person to another—without a contaminated object or person	Blood, or blood fluid enters HCW via skin break or mucous membrane. HCW has unprotected contact with HSV while providing care. Fecal-oral route via hands or food	Herpes simplex virus Norovirus Hepatitis A	Hand washing Glove
Indirect Contact Transfer of infectious agent through a contaminated intermediate object	HCW transmits pathogen from host to another individual via contaminated hands, gait belt, or surgical instruments	Bacteria—pseudomonas aeruginosa Viral MRSA VRE C. difficile	Glove Gown Mask
Droplet (technically a contact transmission) An infection droplet (respiratory) travels from host to another individual; typically thought to be ≤3 feet	Infected individual sneezes or coughs—producing infected droplets Suctioning of endotracheal fluids may produce droplets	Influenza SARS A Streptococcus Mycoplasma pneumonia Smallpox (variola virus) GI viruses, e.g., norovirus, rotavirus	Mask Utilize Standard Precautions + Contact Precautions
Airborne Microorganism that is small enough (droplet nuclei) to be carried via the air currents, capable of traveling long distances	Infected individual talks, coughs/sneezes	Mycobacterium tuberculosis Aspergillis spp Measles (rubeola virus) SARS (severe acquired respiratory syndrome)	Special air handling and ventilation systems Specifically designed mask required—typical mask is ineffective

Abbreviations: HCW—health care worker; HSV—herpes simplex virus; GI—gastrointestinal.

Table 6-2

Select Healthcare-Associated Infections

INFECTIOUS AGENT	SYMPTOMS	TRANSMISSION	INFECTION CONTROL MEASURES
Norovirus (known as stomach flu or viral gastroenteritis)	Causes inflammation of stomach and intestines S&S—diarrhea, emesis, nausea, fever, stomach pain, body aches, headache Seen in all age groups, of most concern in very young and elderly	Virus can be found in stool or vomit of infected person; contact transmission occurs by coming into contact with infected body fluid (aerosolized vomit) or a contaminated object. Virus may also be found on contaminated food (has been handled by infected individual). Spreads rapidly in confined populations, short incubation time and low doses needed for infection; of particular concern in schools, daycare centers, long term care, hospitals	Frequent hand washing Gown and mask Effectively disinfecting equipment, clothing, and utensils Isolating infected individuals/wards Staffing replacements
Rotavirus	Causes inflammation of stomach and intestines S&S—fever, vomiting, diarrhea, abdominal pain Common in infants and young children, can occur in older children and adults	Primarily via fecal-oral route Ingesting contaminated water, food Contact with contaminated surface or object	CDC recommends vaccination of infants. Hand washing Effectively disinfecting toys, surfaces, clothing, and utensils

(Continued)

Table 6-2

Select Healthcare-Associated Infections (Continued)

INFECTIOUS AGENT	SYMPTOMS	TRANSMISSION	INFECTION CONTROL MEASURES
MRSA	In community—appear as skin pustule or boil, occur at site of visible skin trauma (cut, abrasion) and areas covered by hair (back of neck, groin, armpit) Susceptible individuals: patients and visitors to healthcare facilities with weakened immune systems	MRSA is a bacteria found on healthy human skin, poses infection concern for those with weakened immune system Transmission can occur via: contact with tissue or body fluid where bacteria can live, e.g., nose, wound or skin abrasion; contact with bacteria on an object or surface; hands of HCW that have come in contact with MRSA.	Standard Precautions Contact Precautions Keep sores covered. Do not share personal care items, e.g., razor, towels, bed linens.
VRE	Bacteria normally present in human intestines and the female genital tract, also found in environment Can cause infection in urinary tract, bloodstream, in existing wounds Susceptible individuals: those with weakened immune system, long term use of antibiotics, following surgical procedure, those colonized with VRE	Spread on contaminated hands of HCW Contact with contaminated surface or object	Hand washing Contact Precautions Effectively disinfecting toys, surfaces, clothing, and utensils
C. difficile (clostridium difficile; often called "C-diff")	Most cases occur in individuals taking antibiotics; typically does not infect those who are not S&S: diarrhea, fever, abdominal pains, nausea, loss of appetite	C. difficile is a bacteria that can live in the environment for a long time. Transmission most commonly occurs via: contact with contaminated surfaces, hands, bathrooms and bathroom equipment.	Contact Precautions Hand washing Patient placement—with others who have C. diff

Abbreviations: S&S—signs and symptoms; MRSA—methicillin-resistant staphylococcus aureus; HCW—healthcare worker; VRE—vancomycin-resistant enterococci.

b. Group B streptococcus (*S. agalactiae*): neonatal and adult streptococcal B infections.
c. Group C streptococcus (*S. pneumoniae*): pneumonia, otitis media, meningitis, endocarditis.

Medical Interventions
1. Laboratory diagnosis to confirm pathogen.
2. Antibiotic therapy; antibiotic resistance common.
3. Skin infections that are untreated can become systemic.

Hepatitis

Characteristics
1. Inflammation of the liver; may be caused by viral or bacterial infection; chemical agents (alcohol, drugs, toxins).

Types and Symptoms
1. There are three types of hepatitis: A, B and C. See Quick Facts 6-1.

a. During the first weeks after infection, which is the acute phase, there may be no symptoms. For all types, when patients are symptomatic, symptoms may include fatigue, nausea, poor appetite, belly pain, mild fever, yellow skin, or eyes (jaundice).
b. Hepatitis A is typically a short-term infection. Hepatitis B and C can become chronic. When hepatitis B and hepatitis C virus become chronic, the individual may have no symptoms for years; when symptoms present themselves, liver damage be unavoidable or has already happened.

Medical Interventions
1. No specific treatment for acute viral hepatitis; treatment is symptomatic (e.g., IV fluids, analgesics).
2. Chronic hepatitis: direct acting antivirals are the main therapy.
3. Viral hepatitis is the leading cause of liver cancer and a common reason for liver transplant.

QUICK FACTS 6-1 ▶ HEPATITIS REVIEW

Type	Transmission	Clinical Factors	Prevention
Hepatitis A (HAV)	Is HIGHLY contagious! Transmitted primarily through fecal-oral route; contracted through contaminated food or water, or person-to-person contact (infected food handlers)	An acute illness (not chronic) Symptoms can range from mild to severe; the virus will dissipate and not cause long-term liver damage	Good personal hygiene, hand washing Wash fruits, vegetables prior to consumption Cook foods thoroughly Sanitation Immunization (vaccine)
Hepatitis B (HBV)	Transmitted from blood or body fluids/tissues Oral or sexual contact (unprotected) with a person infected with HBV Contaminated needles, needle sharing (sharing razors, toothbrushes) Blood transfusion (prior to 1992) Infected mother can pass virus to baby during childbirth	Symptoms can range from mild (acute, lasting a few weeks) to severe (chronic, lifelong) HBV can lead to liver damage, failure or cancer	Education, use of disposable needles, avoid needle sharing Screening of blood donors Precautions for health care workers Immunization (vaccine)
Hepatitis C (HCV)	Transmitted from blood or body fluids/tissues Most commonly transmitted via contaminated needles, needle sharing; health care setting needle stick; born to a mother who has HCV Less commonly spread via sharing personal items (razors, toothbrushes), sexual contact with person infected with HCV, getting tattoo or piercing in unregulated setting Blood transfusion (prior to 1992)	Symptoms generally mild and flu-like (fatigue, muscle soreness, joint pain, fever, nausea, stomach pain) Can be acute or chronic	Education, use of disposable needles, avoid needle sharing Screening of blood donors No vaccine available

Tuberculosis (TB)

Characteristics

1. An airborne infectious disease caused by the bacillus *Mycobacterium tuberculosis*. Spread by aerosolized droplets from untreated infected host. Incubation period: 2–10 weeks.
   a. Primary disease lasts 10 days to 2 weeks.
   b. Postprimary infection is reactivation of dormant tubercle bacilli, which can occur years after the primary infection.

RED FLAG: Two weeks on appropriate antituberculin drugs renders the host noninfectious. During the infectious stage, the patient must be isolated from others in a negative-pressure room. Anyone entering the room must wear a protective TB mask and follow universal precautions. If the patient leaves the negative-pressure room, he or she must wear a specialized mask to keep from infecting others.

2. Most commonly affects the respiratory system; may also affect the gastrointestinal and genitourinary systems, bones, joints, the nervous system, and skin. May lie dormant in the body for years. At risk individuals: elderly, infants, individuals with weakened immune systems; also associated with crowded or unsanitary living conditions.
3. Course: may be acute, generalized or chronic, localized.

Signs and Symptoms

1. Pulmonary: productive cough, crackles, dyspnea, pleuritic pain, and hemoptysis (blood-streaked sputum).
2. Physical findings postprimary infection: fatigue or weakness, low-grade fever, chills, night sweats, anorexia, and unintentional weight loss. WBC shows increased lymphocytes, enlargement of the lymph nodes surrounding the hilum (hilar adenopathy).

Diagnosis

1. Physical signs: may include swollen or tender lymph nodes in neck, clubbing of the fingers or toes (with advanced disease).
2. Medical tests: chest CT or x-ray, detection of unusual breath sounds (crackles), blood and sputum tests, tuberculin skin test (Mantoux, PPD, TST).

Medical Interventions

1. TB disease: chemotherapy—a combination of daily drugs typically lasting 6–9 months. There is a slight potential for isolation or hospitalization. If hospitalized patient will be placed in a specially ventilated hospital room. Adequate diet.
2. Latent TB infection (bacteria present in the body but they are not active, the individual is not sick and cannot spread the TB bacteria—unless the bacteria become active): treatment may be prescribed to prevent the bacteria from becoming active and developing TB disease. A medication regimen is prescribed and adhered to for 3–9 months. Is especially important for individuals with weakened immune systems.
3. It is important for individuals to complete the full course of TB medications. Stopping treatment too soon or skipping doses can allow the bacteria that are still alive to become resistant to those medications.

Pulmonary Precautions
1. Instruct patient in infection control measures.
2. Transmission is through:
   a. Respiratory droplets or sputum: use tissues to cover nose and mouth when coughing or sneezing; disposable containers for sputum, tissues.
   b. Soiled dressings.

Centers for Disease Control and Prevention (CDC) Standard Precautions

Infection Precautions

Standard Precautions
1. Apply to all patient care, regardless of suspected or confirmed infection status. See Box 6-1.

Universal Precautions
1. Techniques used by healthcare workers to reduce/prevent exposure to bloodborne pathogens from infected individuals. Intended to prevent parenteral (injection, needle delivered), mucous membrane, and nonintact skin exposure.
2. All human blood, body fluids containing visible blood, other body fluids (pleural, peritoneal, etc.), secretions (semen, vaginal), nonintact skin, and mucous membranes may contain transmissible infectious agents.
   a. Does NOT include feces, nasal secretions, sputum, sweat, tears, urine, or vomitus—unless they contain visible blood.
3. Techniques include education, standard precautions, hand hygiene, personal protective equipment (PPE), needle-stick and sharps injury prevention techniques, cleaning and disinfection, and safe handling/disposal of contaminated material.

Physical Therapy–Related Infection Control

Purpose
1. Destroy bacteria and infectious organisms, prevent transmission of such.

Sterilization
1. The total destruction of all microorganisms by exposure to chemical or physical agents; required for all objects introduced to the body; e.g., scalpels, catheters.
2. Methods:
   a. Autoclaving: sterilization of instruments by heat (250°F–270°F) and water pressure; contraindicated with heat-sensitive articles.
   b. Boiling water (212°F): kills organisms that do not form spores.
   c. Ionizing radiation: used to sterilize some medications, plastics, or sutures.
   d. Dry heat: prolonged exposure to high heat in ovens.
   e. Gaseous: ethylene oxide, formaldehyde gas.

Disinfection
1. The reduction of the number of microorganisms; typically used on surfaces or equipment, e.g., respiratory and hydrotherapy equipment.
2. Methods:
   a. Ultraviolet light: used for air and surface disinfection; harmful to unprotected skin and eyes.
   b. Filtration: used for water or air purification.
   c. Physical cleaning.
      - Ultrasonic: disinfects instruments.
      - Washing with an antimicrobial product: used to disinfect hands and surfaces.
   d. Chemicals.
      - Chlorination: used for water disinfection, filtration systems; also used for food surface sanitizing.

- Iodines: used in hydrotherapy when filtering system not possible; provides full bactericidal activity when organic matter (skin, feces, urine) is present.
- Phenols: general disinfectants.
- Quaternary ammonia compounds, e.g., benzalkonium chloride (Zephiran).
- Formaldehyde (5%).

e. Hydrotherapy disinfection.
  - Drain and clean tanks after every patient.
  - Scrub pumps and equipment (e.g., drains, agitator unit) with a germicidal detergent, e.g., sodium hypochlorite (bleach), povidoneiodine, chloramine-T (Chlorazene).
  - Rinse before refilling.

Hematological System

Overview

Composition of Blood

1. Plasma makes up about 55% of total blood volume and is the liquid part of blood and lymph; it carries the cellular elements of blood through the circulation.
   a. Plasma is composed of about 91% water, 7% proteins, and 2%–3% other small molecules.
   b. Electrolytes in plasma determine osmotic pressure and pH balance and are important in the exchange of fluids between capillaries and tissues.
   c. Carries nutrients, waste products, and hormones.
   d. Plasma proteins include albumin, globulins, and fibrinogen.
   e. Serum is plasma without the clotting factors.
2. Erythrocytes or red blood cells (RBCs), make up about 45% of the total blood volume and contain the oxygen-carrying protein hemoglobin responsible for transporting oxygen and assists with maintenance of acid-base balance.
   a. RBCs are produced in the marrow of the long bones and controlled by hormones (erythropoietin). RBCs are time-limited, surviving for approximately 120 days.
   b. Normal RBC count is $4.2–5.4 \times 10^6/mm^3$ for men and $3.6–5.0 \times 10^6/mm^3$ for women. RBC count varies with age, activity and environmental conditions.
3. Leukocytes, or white blood cells (WBCs), make up about 1% of total blood volume and circulate through the lymphoid tissues.
   a. Leukocytes function in immune processes as phagocytes of bacteria, fungi, and viruses. They also aid in capturing toxic proteins resulting from allergic reactions and cellular injury.
   b. Leukocytes are produced in the bone marrow.
   c. There are five types of leukocytes: lymphocytes and monocytes (agranulocytes) and neutrophils, basophils, and eosinophils (granulocytes).
   d. Normal WBC is $4.4–11.3$ cells/mm^3
4. Platelets (PLT) are produced in bone marrow and essential for initiating the clotting mechanism of blood. Normal platelet values in adults = $140–450/mm^3$.

Hematopoiesis

1. The normal function and generation of blood cells in the bone marrow.
2. Production, differentiation, and function of blood cells is regulated by cytokines and growth factors (chemical messengers) acting on blood-forming cells (pluripotent stem cells).
3. Disorders of hematopoiesis include aplastic anemia and leukemias.

Blood Screening Tests

1. Complete blood count (CBC) determines the number of red blood cells, white blood cells, and platelets per unit of blood (see Table 6-3).
2. White cell differential count determines the relative percentages of individual white cell types.
3. Erythrocyte sedimentation rate (ESR) is the rate that red blood cells settle out in a tube of unclotted blood; expressed in millimeters per hour.
   a. Elevated ESR indicates the presence of inflammation.

Hemostasis

1. The termination or arrest of blood flow by mechanical or chemical processes. Mechanisms include vasospasm, platelet aggregation, and thrombin and fibrin synthesis.
2. Blood clotting requires platelets produced in bone marrow, von Willebrand's factor produced by the endothelium of blood vessels, and clotting factors produced by the liver using vitamin K.
3. Fibrinolysis is clot dissolution that prevents excess clot formation.
4. Prothrombin time (PT) and partial thromboplastin time (PTT) are measures of the bloods' ability to clot via different pathways, or mechanisms, in the body.

Table 6-3

Complete Blood Count Lab Values—Clinical Significance

BLOOD COMPONENT	NORMAL VALUE WOMEN	NORMAL VALUE MEN	CLINICAL SIGNIFICANCE
Red Blood Count (RBC, erythrocytes) Comprise 45% of blood volume	$3.6–5.0 \times 10^6/mm^3$	$4.2–5.4 \times 10^6/mm^3$	Increased levels (polycythemia) could indicate dehydration or chronic heart disease; observe for irritability, blurred vision, fainting, cyanosis. Decreased levels indicate anemia; observe for pallor, dyspnea on exertion with rapid pulse, decreased diastolic blood pressure.
White Blood Count (WBC, leukocytes) Comprise 1% of blood volume	4400–11300 cells/mm^3		Significantly elevated counts (as occurs in leukemia) will restrict activity if levels are such that the body cannot supply blood flow to vital organs; observe for signs of inflammation or infection. Decreased WBC counts (leukopenia) place the individual at risk for infection and potentially placed in isolation; exercise is not contraindicated unless WBC drop below 5000 cells/mm^3 and fever exists, take infection control precautions—hand washing, masks, disinfect equipment prior to use
Hemoglobin (Hb, Hgb)	12–16 g/dL	13–18 g/dL	Decreased hemoglobin levels of 8–10 g/dL can result in fatigue, decreased exercise tolerance and tachycardia. Exercise recommendations: No exercise: <8 g/dL; Light exercise: 8–10 g/dL; Resistive exercise: >10 g/dL
Hematocrit (hct)	36–48%	42–52%	Elevated levels may indicate dehydration in older, postoperative individuals or increase a risk of thrombus; observe for signs of pulmonary embolism or deep vein thrombosis. Exercise recommendations: No exercise: <25%; Light exercise: 25–30%; Resistive exercise: 30–32%
Platelets	140000–450000 cells/mm^3		Increased levels (thrombocytosis) >400000/mm^3 may indicate inflammation or infection, cancer; observe for signs of thrombi or infection. Decreased levels (thrombocytopenia) <140000/mm^3 may indicate anemia, adverse drug reaction, infection or cancer; observe for signs of bleeding or bruising, use caution to avoid falls and with joint ROM activities, avoid valsalva maneuver. Exercise recommendations: No exercise: <20000 cells/mm^3; Light exercise: 20000–30000 cells/mm^3; Moderate exercise: 30000–50000 cells/mm^3; Resistive exercise: 50000–150000 cells/mm^3

a. PT measures the extrinsic pathway of the clotting cascade and how long it takes to form a clot, normal is between 11 and 15 seconds.
b. PTT measures the intrinsic and common pathways of clot formation. This requires the blood to be separated in plasma and cells, then substances are added to activate the intrinsic pathway; if this process is speeded up, an "activator" substance is added and the test is then called an activated partial thromboplastin time (APTT). Normal APTT is between 25–40 seconds.
c. INR (Internal Normalization Ratio) is used as a measurement to adjust for the different reagents used to test prothombin time. Normal INR is 0.9–1.1. Persons on blood thinning agents, e.g., warfarin, are monitored so that the normal values are about 1.5–2.5 times the normal value for an adjusted INR of 2.0–3.0.

Hypercoaguability Disorders

1. Increased platelet function as seen in atherosclerosis, diabetes mellitus, elevated blood lipids, and cholesterol.
2. Accelerated activity of the clotting system as seen in congestive heart failure, malignant diseases, pregnancy and use of oral contraceptives, immobility.

Hypocoagulopathy (Bleeding)

1. Platelet defects as seen in bone marrow dysfunction, thrombocytopenia, thrombocytopathia.

2. Coagulation defects as seen in hemophilia and von Willebrand's disease.
3. Vascular disorders as seen in hemorrhagic telangiectasia, vitamin C deficiency, Cushing's disease; senile purpura.

Shock
1. An abnormal condition of inadequate blood flow to the body tissues. It is associated with hypotension, inadequate cardiac output, and changes in peripheral blood flow resistance.
2. Hypovolemic shock is caused by hemorrhage, vomiting, or diarrhea. Loss of body fluids also occurs with dehydration, Addison's disease, burns, pancreatitis, or peritonitis.
3. Orthostatic changes may develop, characterized by a drop in systolic blood pressure of 10–20 mm Hg/HGB or more. Pulse and respiration increase.
4. Progressive shock is associated with restlessness and anxiety, weakness, lethargy, pallor with cool, moist skin, and fall in body temperature.
5. Vital functions must be carefully monitored and restored as quickly as possible. The patient should be placed supine or in a modified Trendelenburg position to aid venous return.
6. Signs and symptoms of hematological disorders
   a. Easy bruising with spontaneous petechiae and purpura of the skin.
   b. External hematomas may also be present (e.g., thrombocytopenia).
7. Medications
   a. Long-term use of certain drugs (steroids, nonsteroidal anti-inflammatory drugs [NSAIDs]) can lead to bleeding and anemia.

> **RED FLAGS:** Physical therapy interventions
> - Use extreme caution with manual therapy and use of some modalities (e.g., mechanical compression).
> - Strenuous exercise is contraindicated due to the risk of increased hemorrhage.

Anemia

Characteristics
1. Decrease in hemoglobin levels in the blood.
2. Normal range (see Table 6-3).

Etiology
1. Decrease in RBC production: nutritional deficiency (iron, vitamin B, folic acid); cellular maturation defects, decreased bone marrow stimulation (hypothyroidism), bone marrow failure (leukemia, aplasia, neoplasm), and genetic defect.
2. Destruction of RBCs: autoimmune hemolysis, sickle cell disease, enzyme defects, parasites (malaria), hypersplenism, chronic diseases (rheumatoid arthritis, tuberculosis, cancer).
3. Loss of blood (hemorrhage): trauma, wound, bleeding, peptic ulcer, excessive menstruation.
4. Anemia values for women = <12 g/100 mL; for men = <14 g/100 mL.

Clinical Symptoms
1. Fatigue and weakness with minimal exertion.
2. Dyspnea on exertion.
3. Pallor or yellow skin of the face, hands, nail beds, and lips.
4. Tachycardia.
5. Bleeding of gums, mucous membranes, or skin in the absence of trauma.
6. Severe anemia can produce hypoxic damage to liver and kidney, heart failure.

Medical Intervention
1. Variable, depends on causative factors.
2. Transfusion.
3. Nutritional supplements.

Physical Therapy Intervention

> **RED FLAGS:** Patients with anemia exhibit decreased exercise tolerance.
> - Exercise should be instituted gradually with physician approval.
> - Perceived exertion levels should be used (rate of perceived exertion [RPE] ratings).

Sickle Cell Disease

Characteristics
1. Group of inherited, autosomal recessive disorders; erythrocytes, specifically hemoglobin S (Hb S), are abnormal. RBCs are crescent or sickle-shaped instead of biconcave.
2. Sickle cell trait: heterozygous form of sickle cell anemia characterized by abnormal red blood cells. Individuals are carriers and do not develop the disease. Counseling is important, especially if both parents have the trait.
3. Chronic hemolytic anemia (sickle cell anemia): hemoglobin is released into plasma with resultant reduced oxygen delivery to tissues; results from bone marrow aplasia, hemolysis, folate deficiency, or splenic involvement.

4. Vaso-occlusion from misshapen erythrocytes: results in ischemia, occlusion, and infarction of adjacent tissue.
5. Chronic illness that can be fatal.

Sickle Cell Crisis
1. Acute episodic condition occurring in children with sickle cell anemia.
2. Symptoms.
   a. Pain: acute and severe from sickle cell clots formed in any organ, bone, or joint.
      - Acute abdominal pain from visceral hypoxia.
      - Painful swelling of soft tissue of the hands and feet (hand-foot syndrome).
      - Persistent headache.
   b. Bone and joint crises: migratory, recurrent joint pain; extremity and back pain.
   c. Neurological manifestations: dizziness, convulsions, coma, paresthesias, cranial nerve palsies, blindness, nystagmus.
   d. Coughing, dyspnea, tachypnea may occur.
   e. Vascular complications: stroke, chronic leg ulcers, bone infarcts, avascular necrosis of femoral head.
   f. Renal complications: enuresis, nocturia, hematuria, renal failure.
   g. Anemic crisis: characterized by rapid drop in hemoglobin levels.
   h. Aplastic crisis: characterized by severe anemia; associated with acute viral, bacterial, or fungal infection. Increased susceptibility to infection.
   i. Splenic sequestration crisis: liver and spleen enlargement, spleen atrophy.

Medical Interventions
1. Immediate transfusion of packed red cells in acute anemic crisis.
2. Analgesics or narcotics as needed for pain.
3. Short-term oxygen therapy in severe anoxia.
4. Hydration, electrolyte replacement.
5. Antibiotics for infection control.
6. Oral anticoagulants to relieve pain of vaso-occlusion; associated with increased risk of bleeding.
7. Splenectomy may be considered.
8. Bone marrow transplant in severe cases.
9. Uremia may require renal transplantation or hemodialysis.

Physical Therapy Goals, Outcomes, and Interventions
1. Pain control: application of warmth is soothing (e.g., hydrotherapy).

> **RED FLAG:** Cold is contraindicated, as it increases vasoconstriction and sickling.

2. Relaxation techniques.
3. Emotional support and counseling of family.
4. Patient and family education: avoidance of stressors that can precipitate a crisis.

Hemophilia

Pathophysiology. A Group of Hereditary Bleeding Disorders
1. Inherited as a sex-linked recessive disorder of blood coagulation; affects males, females are carriers.
2. Clotting factor VIII deficiency (hemophilia A) is most common; classic hemophilia.
3. Clotting factor IX deficiency (hemophilia B or Christmas disease).
4. Level of severity and rate of spontaneous bleeds varies by percentage of clotting factor in blood: mild, moderate, severe.
5. Bleeding is spontaneous or a result of trauma; may result in internal hemorrhage and hematuria.
6. Hemarthrosis (bleeding into joint spaces) most common in synovial joints: knees, ankles, elbows, hips.
   a. Joint becomes swollen, warm, and painful with decreased range of motion (ROM).
   b. Long-term results can include chronic synovitis and arthropathy leading to bone and cartilage destruction.
7. Hemorrhage into muscles often affects forearm flexors, gastrocnemius/soleus, and iliopsoas.
   a. Produces pain.
   b. Decreases movement.

Medical Interventions
1. Blood infusion, factor replacement therapy.
2. Use of acetaminophen (Tylenol), not aspirin, for pain management.
3. Rest, ice, elevation, functional splinting, and no weight-bearing during an acute bleed.
4. HIV or hepatitis transmission was a possible transfusion result prior to current purification techniques.

Complications
1. Joint contractures.
   a. Hip, knee, elbow flexion; ankle plantar flexion.
2. Muscle weakness around affected joints.
3. Leg length discrepancies.
4. Postural scoliosis.
5. Decreased aerobic fitness.

6. Gait deviations.
   a. Equinus gait.
   b. Lack of knee extensor torque.
7. Activities of daily living (ADL) deficiencies, e.g., elbow contractures could affect dressing ability.

Physical Therapy Examination
1. Clinical signs and symptoms of acute bleeding episodes: decreased ROM, stiffening, pain, swelling, tenderness, heat, prickling, or tingling sensations.
2. Goniometry.
3. Joint deformities, e.g., genu valgum, rearfoot/forefoot.
4. Muscle strength; girth.
5. Functional mobility skills, gait.
6. Pain.
7. Activities of daily living.

Physical Therapy Interventions, Acute Stage
1. RICE: rest, ice, compression, elevation.
2. Maintain position, prevent deformity.

Physical Therapy Interventions, Subacute Stage After Hemostasis
1. Factor replacement best done just before treatment.
2. Isometric exercise and aquatic therapy early.
3. Pain management: transcutaneous electrical nerve stimulation (TENS), massage, relaxation techniques, ice, biofeedback.
4. Active assistive exercise progressing to active, isokinetic, and open chain resistive exercises.
   a. Passive ROM rarely, if ever, used.
   b. Closed chain exercise may put too much compressive force through joint.
   c. Important to strengthen hip, knee, elbow extensors, and ankle dorsiflexors.
5. Contracture management.
   a. Manual traction, mobilization techniques, serial casting, dynamic splinting during the day, resting splints at night.

> **RED FLAG:** Passive stretching is rarely used, due to risk of myositis ossificans.

6. Functional and gait training as needed.
   a. Protective use of helmets or pads for very young boys during ambulation and play.
   b. Temporary use of ambulatory aids as needed.
   c. Foot orthoses, shoe inserts, and adhesive taping for ankle or foot problems.

Physical Therapy Interventions, Chronic Stage
1. Daily home exercise program to maintain or increase joint function, aerobic fitness, and strength.
2. Outpatient physical therapy as necessary.
3. Appropriate recreational activities or adaptive physical education if at school.
4. Emotional support for patients and families.

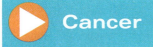

Cancer

Overview

Characteristics
1. Cancer is a broad group of diseases characterized by rapidly proliferating anaplastic cells.
2. Involves all body organs; is invasive.
3. Etiology: unknown; multiple factors are implicated.
   a. Carcinogens: chemical (e.g., asbestos, smoking or oral tobacco), radiation (e.g., x-rays, sun exposure), or viral (e.g., herpes simplex, AIDS/immune system depression).
   b. Genetic factors: hereditary.
   c. Dietary factors: obesity, high-fat diet, diet low in vitamins A, C, E.
   d. Psychological factors: chronic stress.
4. Early warning signs.
   a. Unusual bleeding or discharge.
   b. A lump or thickening of any area, e.g., breast, testicles.
   c. A sore that does not heal.
   d. A change in bladder or bowel habits.
   e. Hoarseness or persistent cough.
   f. Indigestion or difficulty swallowing.
   g. Change in size/thickness or appearance of a wart, mole, or mouth sore.
   h. Unexplained weight loss.
   i. Persistent low-grade fever (constant or intermittent), fatigue, nausea, vomiting.
5. Classification (staging): delineates extent and prognosis of disease.

6. Incidence: second leading cause of death in United States.
7. Prognosis: aggressive treatments have resulted in higher cure rates, increased survival times.
8. Quality of life (maintaining normal function and lifestyle) is an important issue.

Pathophysiology

1. Tumor or neoplasm: an abnormal growth of new tissue that is nonfunctional and competes for vital blood supply and nutrients.
2. Benign tumor (neoplasm): localized, slow-growing, usually encapsulated; not invasive.
3. Malignant tumor (neoplasm): invasive, rapid growth giving rise to metastasis; can be life-threatening.
   a. Carcinoma: a malignant tumor originating in epithelial tissues, e.g., skin, stomach, colon, breast, rectum. Carcinoma in situ is a premalignant neoplasm that has not invaded the basement membrane.
   b. Sarcoma: a malignant tumor originating in connective and mesodermal tissues, e.g., muscle, bone, fat.
   c. Lymphoma: affecting the lymphatic system, e.g., Hodgkin's disease, lymphatic leukemia.
   d. Leukemias and myelomas: affecting the blood (unrestrained growth of leukocytes) and blood-forming organs (bone marrow).
4. Metastasis: movement of cancer cells from one body part to another; spread is via lymphatic system or bloodstream.

Cancer Staging

1. Stages describe the extent or severity of a person's cancer. Based on primary tumor (T), regional lymph node involvement (N), and metastasis (M).
   a. Stage 0: carcinoma in situ.
   b. Stage I: tumor is localized, equal to or less than 2 cm; has not spread to lymph nodes.
   c. Stage II: tumor is locally advanced; 2 cm to 5 cm with or without lymph node involvement.
   d. Stage III: tumor is locally more advanced; spread to lymph nodes; cancer is designated stage II or III depending upon specific type of cancer.
   e. Stage IV: the tumor has metastasized, or spread to other organs throughout the body.
2. Cancer grades.
   a. Grade I (low-grade): cancer cells resemble normal cells (well differentiated) and are slow growing.
   b. Grade II (intermediate-grade): cancer cells look more abnormal (moderately differentiated) and are slightly faster growing.
   c. Grade III (high-grade): cancer cells are abnormal (poorly differentiated); grow or spread more aggressively.
   d. Grade IV (high-grade): cancer cells are abnormal (undifferentiated).

Medical Interventions

1. Curative versus palliative (relief of symptoms, e.g., pain); can be used alone or in combination.
2. Surgery.
   a. Can be curative (tumor removal following biopsy) or palliative (to relieve pain, correct obstruction).
   b. Often used in combination with chemotherapy or radiation therapy.
   c. Can result in significant functional deficits, e.g., weakness and/or edema.
3. Radiation therapy (see Table 6-4).
   a. Destroys cancer cells, inhibits cell growth and division.
   b. Can be used preoperatively to shrink tumors, prevent spread.
   c. Can be used postoperatively to kill/prevent residual cancer cells from metastasizing.
4. Chemotherapy.
   a. Drugs can be given orally, subcutaneously, intramuscularly, intravenously, intrathecally (within the spinal canal).
   b. Usually intermittent doses to allow for bone marrow recovery.
5. Biotherapy (immunotherapy).
   a. Strengthens host's ability to fight cancer cells.
   b. Agents can include interferons, interleukin-2, and cytokines.
   c. Bone marrow (stem cell) transplant; follows high doses of chemotherapy or radiation that destroys both cancer cells and bone marrow cells.
   d. Monoclonal antibodies.
   e. Hormonal therapy.

> **RED FLAGS:** Local and systemic effects of cancer therapy.
> - With radiation therapy, can see radiation sickness, immunosuppression, fibrosis, burns, delayed wound healing, edema, hair loss, lymph flow disruption and central nervous system effects (radiation encephalopathy, demyelination).
> - With chemotherapy, can see gastrointestinal symptoms (anorexia, nausea, vomiting, diarrhea, ulcers, hemorrhage), bone marrow suppression, skin rashes, neuropathies, phlebitis, and hair loss.
> - With immunotherapy, can see fatigue, weight loss, flu-like symptoms (fever, chills), nausea, vomiting, anorexia, fluid retention.
> - With hormonal therapy, can see gastrointestinal symptoms, hypertension, steroid-induced diabetes and myopathy, weight gain, hot flashes and sweating, altered mental status, impotence.

Table 6-4

Side Effects of Treatment for Cancer & Clinical Considerations		
TREATMENT	COMMON SIDE EFFECTS	SIDE EFFECTS—CLINICAL CONSIDERATIONS
Radiation Site-specific administration	Fatigue, radiation sickness, CNS or PNS effects, hair loss, diarrhea	Immunosuppression (decreased WBC count), decreased platelet count, tissue damage with potential for tissue restrictions and scar tissue, potential for scarring to affect lymphatic flow
Chemotherapy Systemic administration	Fatigue, nausea and vomiting, GI effects, hair loss, sterilization, sexual dysfunction	Fluid and electrolyte imbalance possible, decreased bone density, muscle weakness, bone marrow suppression, leukopenia
Biotherapy	Nausea, vomiting, fatigue, fever, chills, altered taste, fluid retention	CNS effects, memory problems, slowed thinking
Bone marrow or stem cell transplant	Nausea, vomiting, infertility, cataract formation, thyroid dysfunction	Immunosuppression, delayed healing, osteoporosis, bone marrow suppression

Hospice Care for the Terminally Ill Patient and Family

1. Multidisciplinary focus.
2. Palliative care provided at home or in a hospice center.
3. Provision of supportive services: emotional, physical, social, spiritual, financial.

Considerations for Physical Therapy Intervention

Pain

1. Cancer pain syndrome: cancer-related pain is a common experience, e.g., nerve or nerve root compression, ischemic response to blockage of blood supply, bone pain. Sympathetic signs and symptoms may accompany moderate to severe pain, e.g., tachycardia, hypertension, tachypnea, nausea, vomiting.
2. Pain at site distal to initial tumor site may suggest metastasis.
3. Iatrogenic pain may result from surgery, radiation, or chemotherapy.

Metastasis

1. Lung, breast, prostate, thyroid, and lymphatic cancers commonly metastasize to bone.
2. Pathological fractures, pain, and muscle spasms may result.

Cancer-Related Fatigue

1. Most common symptom reported by patients with all cancers.
2. Multiple causative factors: physical and emotional. Can use Brief Fatigue Inventory (BFI).
3. Need to assess impact on Quality of Life (QOL).

RED FLAGS: Adverse side effects of cancer treatment.
- With immunosuppressed patient, monitor vital signs, physiological responses to exercise carefully; may see elevated HR and BP, dyspnea, pallor, sweating, fatigue. Patient is easily fatigued with minimal exertion.
- Muscle atrophy and weakness: secondary to high doses of steroids in many chemotherapy protocols; weakness may also result from disuse or tumor compression/invasion.
- ROM deficits: particularly with high-dose radiation around joints.
- Hematological disruptions.
  - White blood suppression (leukopenia).
  - Platelet suppression and increased bleeding (thrombocytopenia).
  - Red blood cell suppression (anemia) with diminished aerobic capacity.

Physical Therapy Goals, Outcomes, and Interventions

Patient and Family

1. Educate patient and family about disease process, rehabilitation goals, process, and expected outcomes.
   a. Assist in coping mechanisms.
   b. Assist through the grieving process.

Positioning

1. Provide for proper positioning to prevent or correct deformities, maintain skin integrity.
2. Provide for overall patient comfort.

Edema Control

1. Elevation of extremities, active ROM.
2. Massage.

3. Postoperative compression (elastic bandages, pressure garments).

Pain Control
1. TENS stimulation: may not control deep cancer pain; effective for postoperative pain.
2. Massage.

Maintain or Correct Loss of ROM
1. Active-assisted/stretching.
2. Active ROM exercises.

Maintain or Correct Loss of Muscle Mass and Strength
1. Isometric and lightweight isotonic strengthening exercises safe for most patients with cancer.

> **RED FLAGS:** Patients with significant bony metastases, osteoporosis, or low platelet counts (<20,000).
> - AROM, ADL exercise only.
> - Weight bearing may be restricted; provide appropriate ambulatory aids, orthoses.
> - High risk of vertebral compression and other fractures with metastatic disease. Use light exercise only.

Improve Aerobic Capacity
1. Formal exercise testing should be individualized: based on history of diagnosis, treatment, adverse effects, and comorbidities.
2. Exercise prescription should be individualized and matched to patient's level of function (see ACSM Guidelines, 2017).
   a. Generally low to moderate intensities (40%≤ 60% oxygen uptake reserve or heart rate reserve; 11–13/20 Borg RPE scale; 3–5 days/wk, for 20–60 minutes/session.
   b. Utilize a warm-up and cool-down before and after each session.
3. Functional (activity) training includes activities of daily living and functional mobility skills, e.g., bed mobility, transfers, and ambulation.
4. Monitor fatigue levels closely. Start slowly, progress incrementally, avoid exhaustion. Assess fatigue levels 12 hours later.
   a. Encourage self-monitoring of fatigue level.
   b. Use activity pacing, carefully balance activity and rest periods; use short sessions throughout the day.
   c. Teach energy-conservation techniques.

Exercise Contraindications/Precautions
1. Exercise recommendations will vary based on individual patients and their past and present medical history.
2. Review lab values prior to beginning each examination or treatment session. Table 6-1 presents exercise guidelines based on lab values.

> **RED FLAGS:** Contraindications to exercise:
> - Day of intravenous chemotherapy or within 24 hours of treatment.
> - Severe reaction to radiation therapy.
> - Acute infection or febrile illness (temp. > 100°F).
> - Severe nausea, vomiting, or diarrhea within 24–36 hours, dehydration, poor nutrition.
> - Unusual or extreme fatigue, muscular weakness, recent bone pain.
> - Chest pain, rapid or slow HR, elevated BP, swelling of ankles.
> - Severe dyspnea, pain on deep breath, cough/wheezing.
> - Dizziness/lightheadedness, disorientation, confusion, blurred vision, ataxia.

3. Patients with low PLT may experience shortness of breath, excessive fatigue, possibly angina. Patients may develop petechiae, purpura, ecchymoses, hematuria, anemia, and hematochezia. Patients with critically low PLT (< 10,000/mm) may experience spontaneous bleeding.
4. Patients with neutropenia (decreased neutrophils in blood) are at increased risk for infection. Adhere to infection control guidelines.
5. Patients with bony metastases have increased risk of pathological fractures. Manual muscle testing, progressive resistive exercises, and high stress activities should be avoided.
6. Recognize cancer-specific emergencies (sudden loss of limb function, spinal cord compression, fever in immune-compromised patients, superior vena cava syndrome). Initiate plan for emergency situation.

Specific Considerations for Exercise Programs
1. Postmastectomy.
   a. Focus is on restoration of pain-free full ROM of the shoulder, prevention/reduction of edema, restoration of function.
   b. Early postoperative exercise is stressed: some protocols as early as Day 1.
2. Post–bone marrow transplant.
   a. Experience prolonged hospitalization and inactivity: average is 30 days; prolonged chemotherapy and radiotherapy, strict isolation.
   b. Focus is on restoration of function, overcoming the effects of deconditioning.

> **RED FLAG:** Exercise is contraindicated in patients with platelet counts 20,000 or less; use caution with counts 20,000–50,000. See Table 6-3.

Physical Agents

1. Thermal agents (hot packs, paraffin baths, fluidotherapy, infrared lamps) and deep heating agents (ultrasound, diathermy) (see Chapter 10).

> **RED FLAGS:**
> - Do not use directly over tumor.
> - Do not use over dysvascular tissue: tissue exposed to radiation therapy.
> - Do not use with individuals with decreased sensitivity to temperature or pain in affected area.
> - Do not use in areas of increased bleeding or hemorrhage, typically the result of corticosteroid therapy.
> - Do not use with acute injury, inflammation, open wounds.

2. Cryotherapy.

> **RED FLAGS:** Do not use with patients with insensitivity to cold or delayed wound healing.
> - Do not use over dysvascular tissue: tissue exposed to radiation therapy.

3. Hydrotherapy with agitation.

> **RED FLAGS:** Do not use over dysvascular tissue: tissue exposed to radiation therapy.
> - Do not use with individuals with decreased sensitivity to temperature or pain in affected area.
> - Do not use in areas of increased bleeding or hemorrhage or open wounds.
> - Risk of cross infection is high with immunosuppressed patients.

Clinical Application: Modalities, to Use or Not to Use—That Is the Question

In learning to use therapeutic modalities, students are taught that "cancer" is a contraindication to their use. With the diagnosis of cancer, the health care team needs to be aware of the expected journey of the patient: will modalities be used to decrease discomfort because the patient is expected to make a recovery? Or are modalities being used to decrease discomfort as a palliative measure because the patient is not expected to make a recovery?

The use of modalities as identified in this section outlines precautions necessary when the patient is expected to make a recovery. Both the physician and physical therapist must make the decision to use the modality with long-term benefits in mind. If a patient is not expected to recover and modalities are being used palliatively, a clinician still has to "cause no harm" but is not overly concerned with the contraindicated use of the modality.

Gastrointestinal System

Overview

Anatomy/Physiology

1. The gastrointestinal (GI) tract is a long hollow tube extending from the mouth to the anus. Ingested foods and fluids are broken down into molecules that are absorbed and used by the body, while waste products are eliminated (Figure 6-1).
   a. The upper GI tract consists of the mouth, esophagus, and stomach and functions for ingestion and initial digestion of food.
   b. The middle GI tract is the small intestine (duodenum, jejunum, and ileum). The major digestive and absorption processes occur here.
   c. The lower GI tract consists of the large intestine (cecum, colon, and rectum), with primary functions that include absorption of water and electrolytes, storage, and elimination of waste products.
   d. Accessory organs aid in digestion by producing digestive secretions and include the salivary glands, liver, and pancreas.
2. GI motility propels food and fluids through the GI system and is provided by rhythmic, intermittent contractions (peristaltic movements) of smooth muscle (except for pharynx and upper one-third of the esophagus).
3. Neural control is achieved by the autonomic nervous system (ANS). Both sympathetic and parasympathetic plexuses extend along the length of the GI wall. Vagovagal (mediated by the vagus nerve) reflexes control the secretions and motility of the GI tract.
4. Major GI hormones include cholecystokinin, gastrin, and secretin.

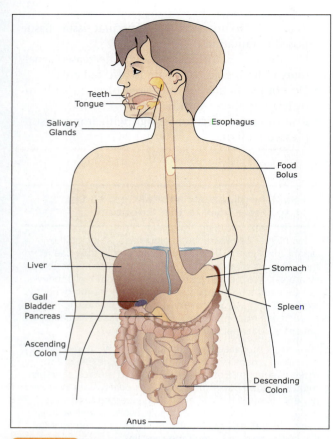

Figure 6-1 Gastrointestinal system anterior view.

Signs and Symptoms Common to Many Types of GI Disorders

1. Nausea and vomiting. Nausea is an unpleasant sensation that signals stimulation of medullary vomiting center and often precedes vomiting. Vomiting is the forceful oral expulsion of abdominal contents.
    a. Nausea and vomiting can be triggered by many different causes including food, drugs, hypoxia, shock, inflammation of abdominal organs, distention, irritation of the GI tract, and motion sickness.
    b. Prolonged vomiting can produce fluid and electrolyte imbalance, and can result in pulmonary aspiration and mucosal or GI damage.
2. Diarrhea is the passage of frequent, watery, unformed stools. The amount of fluid loss determines the severity of the illness.
    a. Dehydration, electrolyte imbalance, dizziness, thirst, and weight loss are common complications of prolonged diarrhea.
    b. Numerous conditions can trigger diarrhea including infectious organisms (*Escherichia coli*, rotavirus, *Salmonella*), dysentery, diabetic enteropathy, irritable bowel syndrome, hyperthyroidism, neoplasm, and diverticulitis. Diet, medications, and strenuous exercise can also cause diarrhea.
3. Constipation is a decrease in normal elimination with excessively hard, dry, stools and difficult elimination.
    a. Constipation causes increased bowel pressure and lower abdominal discomfort.
    b. Many different factors can trigger constipation, including a diet lacking in bulk and fiber, inadequate consumption of fluids, sedentary lifestyle, increasing age, and drugs (opiates, antidepressants, calcium channel blockers, anticholinergics).
    c. Numerous conditions can cause constipation including hypothyroidism, diverticular disease, irritable bowel syndrome, Parkinson's disease, spinal cord injury, tumors, bowel obstruction, and rectal lesions.
    d. Obstipation is intractable constipation with resulting fecal impaction, the retention of hard, dry stools in the rectum and colon. Impaction can cause partial or complete bowel obstruction. The patient may exhibit a history of watery diarrhea, fecal soiling, and fecal incontinence. Removal of the fecal mass is indicated. Can be seen in post-surgical patients, those taking long-term opiates, or individuals with spinal cord injuries.

> **RED FLAG:** Constipation can cause abdominal pain and tenderness in the anterior hip, groin, or thigh regions.

    e. Constipation may develop as a result of muscle guarding and splinting; e.g., in the patient with low back pain.
4. Anorexia is the loss of appetite with an inability to eat. It is associated with anxiety, fear, and depression along with a number of different disease states and drugs.
    a. Anorexia nervosa is a disorder characterized by prolonged loss of appetite and inability to eat. Individuals exhibit emaciation, emotional disturbance concerning body image, and fear of gaining weight. It is common in adolescent girls, who may also exhibit amenorrhea.
5. Dysphagia refers to difficulty in swallowing.
    a. Patients experience choking, coughing, or abnormal sensations of food sticking in the back of the throat or esophagus.
    b. Numerous conditions can cause dysphagia, including lesions of the CNS (stroke, Alzheimer's disease, Parkinson's disease), strictures and esophageal scarring, swelling, cancer, and scleroderma.
    c. Achalasia is a condition in which the lower esophageal sphincter fails to relax and food is trapped in the esophagus.

6. Heartburn is a painful burning sensation felt in the esophagus, in the midepigastric area behind the sternum or in the throat.
   a. It is typically caused by reflux of gastric contents into the esophagus.
   b. Certain foods (fatty foods, citrus foods, chocolate, peppermint, alcohol, coffee, caffeine), increased abdominal pressure (food, tight clothing, back supports, pregnancy), and certain positions/movements (bending over or lying down after a large meal) can aggravate heartburn.
7. Abdominal pain is common in GI conditions. It is the result of inflammation, ischemia, and mechanical stretching. Visceral pain can occur in the epigastric region (T3–T5 sympathetic nerve distribution), the periumbilical region (T10 sympathetic nerve distribution), and the lower abdominal region (T10–L2 sympathetic nerve distribution).

> **RED FLAGS:** Referred GI pain patterns:
> - Visceral pain from the esophagus can refer to the midback.
> - Midthoracic spine pain (nerve root pain) can appear as esophageal pain.
> - Visceral pain from the liver, diaphragm, or pericardium can refer to the shoulder.
> - Visceral pain from the gallbladder, stomach, pancreas, or small intestine can refer to the midback and scapular regions.
> - Visceral pain from the colon, appendix, or pelvic viscera can refer to the pelvis, low back, or sacrum.

8. GI bleeding is evidenced by blood appearing in vomitus or feces.
   a. It can result from erosive gastritis, peptic ulcers, prolonged use of NSAIDs, and chronic alcohol use.
   b. Occult or hidden blood can be revealed only by stool testing.
9. Abdominal pain is generally aggravated by coughing, sneezing, or straining.
10. Medical management: many gastrointestinal symptoms can be managed with prescription medications. See Table 6-5.

Esophagus

Gastroesophageal Reflux Disease (GERD)

1. Caused by reflux or upward movement of gastric contents of the stomach into the esophagus, producing heartburn.
2. Results from failure of the lower esophageal sphincter to regulate flow of food from the esophagus into the stomach and increased gastric pressure.
3. The diaphragm that surrounds the esophagus and oblique muscles also contribute to antireflux function.
4. Over time, acidic gastric fluids (pH <4) damage the esophagus, producing reflux esophagitis.
5. Heartburn commonly occurs 30–60 minutes after eating and at night when lying down (nocturnal reflux).

Table 6-5

Commonly Prescribed Medications and Associated Precautions—Gastrointestinal System

MEDICATION	PRESCRIBED FOR	SIDE EFFECTS	INTERACTIONS	PHYSICAL THERAPY CONSIDERATIONS*
Omeprezole (Prilosec)	GERD (Gastroesophageal Reflux Disease)	Malabsorption of certain drugs Decrease absorption of Ca, Mg and other nutrients	Citolapram, Clopidogrel (Plavix), Methotrexate and many others that need acid in stomach for absorption	Increased risk of fractures from osteoporosis
Dicyclomine (Bentyl)	Stomach cramps, Irritable bowel symdrome	Dizziness, fatigue, constipation, blurred vision	Potassium supplements, topiramate, zonisamide	Fatigue and lack of focus during PT
Loperamide (Imodium)	Diarrhea	Stomach pain, worsening or ongoing diarrhea, severe skin reaction	Saquinavir and most medications because of fast transit through gut	Dehydration, bowel control and weakness

*Medications used in the medical management of diseases and conditions are included in the NPTE. PTAs should be familiar with categories of medications and their indications for use. PTAs should be acutely aware of potential effects on tolerance to physical therapy intervention.
Note: Generic drug names appear first followed by brand names in parenthesis; brand names may be trademarked or registered.

> **RED FLAGS:**
> - Atypical pain may present as head and neck pain.
> - Chest pain is sometimes mistaken for heart attack; it is unrelated to activity.
> - Respiratory symptoms can occur, including wheezing and chronic cough due to microaspiration, laryngeal injury, and vagus-mediated bronchospasm. Hoarseness can also result from chronic inflammation of the vocal cords.

6. Complications include strictures and Barrett's esophagus (a precancerous state).
7. Physical therapy interventions.
   a. Positional changes from full supine to modified, more upright positions are indicated.
   b. Valsalva's maneuver is contraindicated.
8. Lifestyle modifications include avoiding large meals and certain foods; sleeping with head elevated; medications include acid-suppressing proton pump inhibitors (PPIs) (e.g., Prilosec), H_2 blockers (e.g., ranitidine [Zantac], cimetidine [Tagamet]), and antacids (e.g., Tums). In severe cases, surgery is an option.

Hiatal Hernia
1. Protrusion of the stomach upward through the diaphragm (rolling hiatal hernia) or displacement of both the stomach and gastroesophageal junction upward into the thorax (sliding hiatal hernia).
2. May be congenital or acquired.
3. Symptoms include heartburn from GERD.
4. Conservative or symptomatic treatment is the same as for GERD. Surgery may be indicated.

Stomach

Gastritis
1. Inflammation of the stomach mucosa. Gastritis can be acute or chronic.
2. Acute gastritis is caused by severe burns, aspirin or other NSAIDs, corticosteroids, food allergies, or viral or bacterial infections. Hemorrhagic bleeding can occur.
3. Symptoms include anorexia, nausea, vomiting, and pain.
4. Chronic gastritis occurs with certain diseases such as peptic ulcer, bacterial infection caused by *Helicobacter pylori*, stomach cancer, pernicious anemia, or with autoimmune disorders (thyroid disease, Addison's disease).

> **RED FLAG:** Patients taking NSAIDs long-term should be monitored carefully for stomach pain, bleeding, nausea, or vomiting.

5. Management is symptomatic and includes avoiding irritating substances (caffeine, nicotine, alcohol), dietary modification, and medications that include acid-suppressing PPIs, H_2 blockers, and antacids.

Peptic Ulcer Disease
1. Refers to ulcerative lesions that occur in the upper GI tract in areas exposed to acid-pepsin secretions. It can affect one or all layers of the stomach or duodenum.
2. Caused by a number of factors, including bacterial infection (*H. pylori*), acetylsalicylic acid (aspirin) and NSAIDs, excessive secretion of gastric acids, stress, and heredity.
3. Symptoms include epigastric pain, which is described as a gnawing, burning, or cramp-like. Pain is aggravated by change in position and absence of food in the stomach and relieved by food or antacids.

> **RED FLAG:**
> - Pain from peptic ulcers located on the posterior wall of the stomach can present as radiating back pain; may also radiate to right shoulder.
> - Stress and anxiety can increase gastric secretions and pain.

4. Complications include hemorrhage. Bleeding may be sudden and severe or insidious with blood in vomitus or stools. Symptoms can include weakness, dizziness, or other signs of circulatory shock.
5. Management includes use of antibiotics for treatment of *H. pylori* along with acid-suppressing drugs (PPIs, H_2 blockers, and antacids). Dietary modification including avoidance of stomach irritants is indicated. Surgical intervention is indicated for perforation and uncontrolled bleeding.

Intestines

Malabsorption Syndrome
1. A complex of disorders characterized by problems in intestinal absorption of nutrients (fat, carbohydrates, proteins, vitamins, calcium, and iron).
2. Can be caused by gastric or small bowel resection (short-gut syndrome) or a number of different diseases including cystic fibrosis, celiac disease, Crohn's disease, chronic pancreatitis, and pernicious anemia. Malabsorption can also be drug-induced (NSAID gastroenteritis).
3. Deficiencies of enzymes (pancreatic lipase) and bile salts are contributing factors.
4. Symptoms can include anorexia, weight loss, abdominal bloating, pain and cramps, indigestion, and steatorrhea (abnormal amounts of fat in feces). Diarrhea can be chronic and explosive.

> **RED FLAG:** Can produce iron-deficiency anemia and easy bruising and bleeding due to lack of vitamin K.

   a. Muscle weakness and fatigue due to lack of protein, iron, folic acid, and vitamin B.
   b. Bone loss, pain, and predisposition to develop fractures from lack of calcium, phosphate, and vitamin D.
   c. Neuropathy including tetany, paresthesias, numbness, and tingling from lack of calcium, vitamins B and D, magnesium, potassium.
   d. Muscle spasms from electrolyte imbalance and lack of calcium.
   e. Peripheral edema.

Inflammatory Bowel Disease (IBD)

1. Refers to two related chronic inflammatory intestinal disorders, Crohn's disease (CD) and ulcerative colitis (UC). Both diseases result in inflammation of the bowel and are characterized by remissions and exacerbations.
2. Symptoms include abdominal pain, frequent attacks of diarrhea, fecal urgency, and weight loss.

> **RED FLAGS:**
> - Joint pain (reactive arthritis) and skin rashes can occur. Pain can be referred to the low back.
> - Complications can include intestinal obstruction and corticosteroid toxicity (low bone density, increased fracture risk).
> - Intestinal absorption is disrupted and nutritional deficiencies are common.
> - Chronic IBD can lead to anxiety and depression.

3. Crohn's disease involves a granulomatous type of inflammation that can occur anywhere in the GI tract. Areas of adjacent normal tissue called skip lesions are present.
4. Ulcerative colitis involves an ulcerative and exudative inflammation of the large intestine and rectum. It is characterized by varying amounts of bloody diarrhea, mucus, and pus. Skip lesions are absent.

Irritable Bowel Syndrome (IBS)

1. Characterized by abnormally increased motility of the small and large intestines. IBS is also known as spastic, nervous, or irritable colon.
2. IBS is associated with emotional stress and certain foods (high fat content or roughage, lactose intolerance). No structural or biochemical abnormalities have been identified.
3. Symptoms include persistent or recurrent abdominal pain that is relieved by defecation. Patients may experience constipation or diarrhea, bloating, abdominal cramps, flatulence, nausea, and anorexia.
4. Stress reduction and medications to reduce anxiety or depression are important components of treatment.
5. Regular physical activity is effective in reducing stress and improving bowel function.

Diverticular Disease

1. Characterized by pouch-like herniations (diverticula) of the mucosal layer of the colon through the muscularis layer.
2. Diverticulosis refers to pouch-like herniations of the colon, especially the sigmoid colon.
   a. Symptoms are minimal but can include rectal bleeding.
   b. Dietary factors (lack of dietary fiber), lack of physical activity, and poor bowel habits contribute to its development.
   c. Diverticulosis can lead to diverticulitis.
3. Diverticulitis refers to inflammation of one or more diverticula. Fecal matter penetrates diverticula and causes inflammation and abscess.
   a. Symptoms include pain and cramping in the lower left quadrant, nausea and vomiting, slight fever, and an elevated WBC.
   b. Complications include bowel obstruction, perforation with peritonitis, and hemorrhage.

> **RED FLAG:** Patients may complain of back pain.

4. Regular exercise is an important component of treatment.

Appendicitis

1. An inflammation of the vermiform appendix. As the condition progresses, the appendix becomes swollen, gangrenous, and perforated. Perforation can be life threatening and lead to the development of peritonitis.
2. Pain is abrupt at onset, localized to the epigastric or periumbilical area, and increases in intensity over time.
3. Rebound tenderness (Blumberg's sign) is present in response to depression of the abdominal wall at a site distant from the painful area.
4. Point tenderness is located at McBurney's point, the site of the appendix located 1½ to 2 inches above the anterior superior iliac spine in the right lower quadrant.

> **RED FLAG:** Immediate medical attention is required with positive signs. Elevations in WBC count ($>20,000/mm^3$) are indicative of perforation; surgery is indicated.

Peritonitis

1. Inflammation of the peritoneum, the serous membrane lining the walls of the abdominal cavity.
2. Peritonitis results from bacterial invasion and infection of the peritoneum. Common agents include *E. coli, Bacteroides, Fusobacterium,* and streptococci.
3. A number of different factors can introduce infecting agents, including penetrating wounds, surgery, perforated peptic ulcer, ruptured appendix, perforated diverticulum, gangrenous bowel, pelvic inflammatory disease, and gangrenous gallbladder.
4. Symptoms include abdominal distension, severe abdominal pain, rigidity from reflex guarding, rebound tenderness, decreased or absent bowel sounds, nausea and vomiting, and tachycardia.
5. Elevated WBC count, fever, electrolyte imbalance, and hypotension are common.
6. Peritonitis can lead to toxemia and shock, circulatory failure, and respiratory distress.
7. Treatment is aimed at controlling inflammation and infection and restoring fluid and electrolyte imbalances. Surgical intervention may be necessary to remove an inflamed appendix or close a perforation.

Rectum

Rectal Fissure
1. A tear or ulceration of the lining of the anal canal.
2. Constipation and large, hard stools are contributing factors.

Hemorrhoids (Piles)
1. Varicosities in the lower rectum or anus caused by congestion of the veins in the hemorrhoidal plexus.
2. Hemorrhoids can be internal or external (protruding from the anus).
3. Symptoms include local irritation, pain, rectal itching.
4. Prolonged bleeding can result in anemia.
5. Straining with defecation, constipation, and prolonged sitting contribute to discomfort.
6. Pregnancy increases the risk of hemorrhoids.
7. Treatment includes topical medications to shrink the hemorrhoid, dietary changes, sitz baths, local hot or cold compresses, and ligation or surgical excision.

Genital/Reproductive System

Overview: Female Reproductive System

Anatomy/Physiology
1. External genitalia, located at the base of the pelvis, consist of the mons pubis, labia majora, labia minora, clitoris, and perineal body (Figure 6-2).
2. The urethra and anus are in close proximity to the external genital structures, and cross-contamination is possible.
3. The internal genitalia consist of the vagina, the uterus and cervix, the fallopian tubes, and paired ovaries.

Sexual and Reproductive Functions
1. The ovaries store female germ cells (ova) and produce female sex hormones (estrogens and progesterone) under control of the hypothalamus (gonadotropin-releasing hormone) and the anterior pituitary gland (gonadotropic follicle-stimulating and luteinizing hormones).
2. Sex hormones influence the development of secondary sex characteristics, regulate the menstrual cycle (ovulation), maintain pregnancy (fertilization and implantation, gestation), and influence menopause (cessation of the menstrual cycle).
   a. Estrogens decrease the rate of bone resorption.
   b. Estrogens increase production of the thyroid and increase high-density lipoproteins (a protective effect against heart disease).

RED FLAG: Osteoporosis and risk of bone fracture increase dramatically after menopause. Heart disease and stroke risk increases after menopause.

Breasts
1. Mammary tissues located on the anterior chest wall between the 3rd and 7th ribs.
2. Breast function is related to production of sex hormones and pregnancy, producing milk for infant nourishment.

Pregnancy: Normal

Weight Gain
1. Average weight gain during pregnancy is 20–30 lbs.

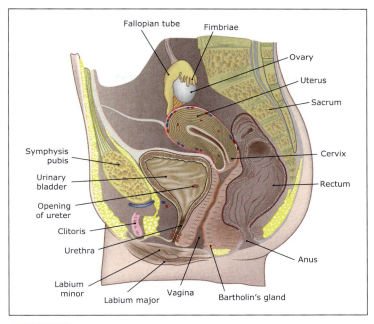

Figure 6-2 Female Reproductive System.

Physical Therapists Teach Childbirth Education Classes

1. Relaxation training: e.g., Jacobsen's progressive relaxation, relaxation response, mental imagery, yoga.
2. Breathing management: slow, deep, diaphragmatic breathing; Lamaze techniques; avoidance of Valsalva's maneuver.
3. Provide information about pregnancy and childbirth.

Common Changes with Pregnancy and Physical Therapy Interventions

1. Postural changes: kyphosis with scapular protraction, cervical lordosis and forward head; lumbar lordosis; postural stress may continue into postpartum phase with lifting and carrying the infant.
   a. Postural evaluation.
   b. Teach postural exercises to stretch, strengthen, and train postural muscles.
   c. Teach pelvic stabilization exercises, e.g., posterior pelvic tilt.
   d. Teach correct body mechanics, e.g., sitting, standing, lifting, ADLs.
   e. Limit certain activities in the third trimester, e.g., supine position to avoid inferior vena cava compression, bridging.
2. Balance changes: center of gravity shifts forward and upward as the fetus develops; with advanced pregnancy, there will be a wider base of support, increased difficulty with walking and stair climbing, rapid challenges to balance.
   a. Teach safety strategies.
3. Ligamentous laxity secondary to hormonal influences (relaxin).
   a. Joint hypermobility (e.g., sacroiliac joint), pain.
   b. Predisposition to injury especially in weight-bearing joints of lower extremities and pelvis.
   c. May persist for some time after delivery; teach joint protection strategies.
4. Muscle weakness: abdominal muscles are stretched and weakened as pregnancy develops; pelvic floor weakness with advanced pregnancy and childbirth. Stress incontinence secondary to pelvic floor dysfunction (experienced by 80% of women).
   a. Teach exercises to improve control of pelvic floor, maintain abdominal function.
   b. Stretching exercises to reduce muscle cramping.
   c. Avoid Valsalva's maneuver: may exacerbate condition.
5. Urinary changes: pressure on bladder causes frequent urination; increased incidence of reflux, urinary tract infections.
6. Respiratory changes: elevation of the diaphragm with widening of thoracic cage; hyperventilation, dyspnea may be experienced with mild exercise during late pregnancy.
7. Cardiovascular changes: increased blood volume; increased venous pressure in the lower extremities; increased heart rate and cardiac output, decreased blood pressure due to venous distensibility.
   a. Teach safe progression of aerobic exercises.
      - Exercise in moderation, with frequent rests.
      - Stress use of familiar activities; avoidance of unfamiliar.

- Postpartum: emphasize gradual return to previous level of activity.
b. Stress gentle stretching, adequate warm-ups and cool-downs.
c. Teach ankle pumps for lower extremity edema (late-stage pregnancy); elevate legs to assist in venous return.
d. Wear loose, comfortable clothing.
8. Altered thermoregulation: increased basal metabolic rate; increased heat production.

Pregnancy-Related Pathologies

Diastasis Recti Abdominis
1. Lateral separation or split of the rectus abdominis; separation from midline (linea alba) greater than 2 cm is significant; associated with loss of abdominal wall support, increased back pain.
2. Physical therapy interventions.
   a. Teach protection of abdominal musculature: avoid abdominal exercises, e.g., full sit-ups or bilateral straight leg raising.
   b. Resume abdominal exercises when separation is less than 2 cm: teach safe abdominal strengthening exercises, e.g., partial sit-ups (knees bent), pelvic tilts; utilize hands to support abdominal wall.

Pelvic Floor Disorders
1. The result of weakening of pelvic floor muscles (pubococcygeal [PC] muscles).
2. PC muscles normally function to support the vagina, urinary bladder, and rectum and help maintain continence of the urethra and rectum.
3. Weakness or laxity of PC muscles typically results from overstretching during pregnancy and childbirth. Further loss of elasticity and muscle tone during later life can result in partial or total organ prolapse. Examples include:
   a. Cystocele: the herniation of the bladder into the vagina.
   b. Rectocele: the herniation of the rectum into the vagina.
   c. Uterine prolapse: the bulging of the uterus into the vagina.
4. PC muscles can also go into spasm.
5. Symptoms include pelvic pain (perivaginal, perirectal, lower abdominal quadrant), urinary incontinence, and pain with sexual intercourse.

> **RED FLAG:** Pain can radiate down the posterior thigh.

6. Surgical correction is often required, depending on degree of prolapse.

Pelvic Floor Exercises
1. Indications: women and men with urinary and/or bowel incontinence; women who have started menopause or have cancer treatments causing early menopause; women who are pregnant or who have previously given birth, middle aged, and older women.
2. Contraindications: individuals with recent surgery, urinary catheter in place, or excessive pelvic pain.
3. Teaching pelvic floor exercises (Kegel exercises).
   a. Patient assumes comfortable position, typically lying down with knees bent to start; can also be done in sitting or standing; make sure bladder is empty before beginning.
   b. Tighten pelvic floor muscles: imagine sitting on a toilet and peeing. Then imagine stopping the flow of urine midstream. The muscles around the vaginal/anal area should tighten. Hold for 5–10 seconds. Relax for 10 seconds.
   c. Repeat 5 times to start, progress to 10 times, 3 times/day.
   d. Finding the pelvic muscles can be facilitated by briefly stopping the flow of urine midstream once while urinating.

> **RED FLAG:** Stopping and starting urine while emptying the bladder is not part of Kegel exercises and can be harmful; can interfere with urinary reflexes and contribute to bladder infection.

4. Postural education and muscle reeducation, pelvic mobilization, and stretching of tight lower extremity (LE) muscles are also important components.

Low Back and Pelvic Pain
1. Physical therapy interventions
   a. Teach proper body mechanics.
   b. Balance rest with activity.
   c. Emphasize use of a firm mattress.
   d. Massage, modalities for pain (no deep heat).

Sacroiliac Dysfunction
1. Secondary to postural changes, ligamentous laxity.
2. Symptoms include posterior pelvic pain; pain in buttocks, may radiate into posterior thigh or knee.
3. Associated with prolonged sitting, standing, or walking.
4. Physical therapy interventions.
   a. External stabilization, e.g., sacroiliac support belt, may help reduce pain.
   b. Avoid single-limb weight bearing: may aggravate sacroiliac dysfunction.

Varicose Veins
1. Physical therapy interventions.
   a. Elevate extremities; avoid crossing legs, which may press on veins.
   b. Use of elastic support stockings may help.

Preeclampsia
1. Pregnancy-induced, acute hypertension after the 24th week of gestation.
2. May be mild or severe.

3. Evaluate for symptoms of hypertension, edema, sudden excessive weight gain, headache, visual disturbances, or hyperreflexia.
4. Initiate prompt physician referral.

Cesarean Childbirth
1. Surgical delivery of the fetus by an incision through the abdominal and uterine walls; indicated in pelvic disproportion, failure of the birth process to progress, fetal or maternal distress, or other complications.
2. Physical therapy interventions.
   a. Postoperative TENS can be used for incisional pain; electrodes are placed parallel to the incision.
   b. Prevent postsurgical pulmonary complications: assist patient in breathing, coughing.
   c. Postcesarean exercises.
      - Gentle abdominal exercises; provide incisional support with pillow.
      - Pelvic floor exercises: labor and pushing is typically present before surgery.
      - Postural exercises; precautions about heavy lifting for 4–6 weeks.
   d. Ambulation.
   e. Prevent incisional adhesions: friction massage.

Disorders of the Female Reproductive System

Endometriosis
1. Characterized by ectopic growth and function of endometrial tissue outside of the uterus. Common sites include ovaries, fallopian tubes, broad ligaments, uterosacral ligaments, pelvis, vagina, or intestines.
   a. The ectopic tissue responds to hormonal influences but is not able to be shed as uterine tissue during menstruation.
   b. Endometrial tissue can lead to cysts and rupture, producing peritonitis and adhesions as well as adhesions and obstruction.
2. Symptoms include pain, dysmenorrhea, dyspareunia (abnormal pain during sexual intercourse), and infertility.

> **RED FLAG:** Patients may complain of back pain. Endometrial implants on muscle (e.g., psoas major, pelvic floor muscles) may produce pain with palpation or contraction.

3. Treatment involves pain management, endometrial suppression, and surgery.

Pelvic Inflammatory Disease (PID)
1. An inflammation of the upper reproductive tract involving the uterus (endometritis), fallopian tubes (salpingitis), or ovaries (oophoritis).
2. PID is caused by a polymicrobial agent that ascends through the endocervical canal.
3. Symptoms include lower abdominal pain that typically starts after a menstrual cycle, purulent cervical discharge, and painful cervix. Fever, elevated WBC count, and increased ESR are present.
4. Complications can include pelvic adhesions, infertility, ectopic pregnancy, chronic pain, and abscesses.
5. Treatment involves antibiotic therapy to treat the infection and prevent complications.

Overview: Male Reproductive System

Anatomy/Physiology
1. The male reproductive system is composed of paired testes, genital ducts, accessory glands, and penis (Figure 6-3).
2. The testes, or male gonads, are located in the scrotum, paired egg-shaped sacs located outside the abdominal cavity. They produce male sex hormones (testosterone) and spermatozoa (male germ cells).
3. The accessory glands (seminal vesicles, prostate gland, and bulbourethral glands) prepare sperm for ejaculation.
4. The ductal system (epididymides, vas deferens, and ejaculatory ducts) stores and transports sperm.
5. The urethra, enclosed in the penis, functions in the elimination of urine and semen.
6. Sperm production requires an environment that is 2°C–3°C lower than body temperature.
7. Testosterone and other male sex hormones (androgens).
   a. During development, induce differentiation of the male genital tract.
   b. Stimulate development of primary and secondary sex characteristics during puberty and maintain them during life.

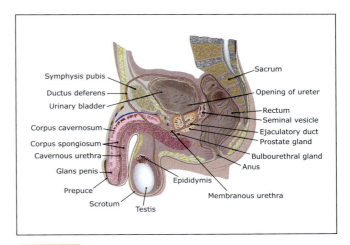

Figure 6-3 Male Reproductive System.

c. Promote protein metabolism, musculoskeletal growth, and subcutaneous fat distribution (anabolic effects).
8. The hypothalamus and anterior pituitary gland maintain endocrine system function via gonadotropic hormones (follicle-stimulating hormone [FSH] and luteinizing hormone [LH]).
   a. FSH initiates spermatogenesis.
   b. LH regulates testosterone production.

Disorders of the Male Reproductive System

Erectile Dysfunction (ED) (Impotence)
1. The inability to achieve and maintain erection for sexual intercourse.
2. Organic causes.
   a. Neurogenic causes: stroke, cerebral trauma, spinal cord injury, multiple sclerosis, Parkinson's disease.
   b. Hormonal causes: decreased androgen levels with hypogonadism, hypothyroidism, and hypopituitarism.
   c. Vascular causes: hypertension, coronary heart disease, hyperlipidemia, cigarette smoking, diabetes mellitus, pelvic irradiation.
   d. Drug-induced: antidepressants, antipsychotics, antiandrogens, antihypertensives, amphetamines, alcohol.
   e. Aging increases risk of ED.
3. Psychogenic causes.
   a. Performance anxiety.
   b. Depression and psychiatric disorders (schizophrenia).
4. Surgical causes.
   a. Transurethral procedures.
   b. Radical prostatectomy.
   c. Proctocolectomy.
   d. Abdominoperineal resection.
5. Treatment requires accurate identification and remediation of specific causes of ED.
6. Medications are available to improve function (e.g., sildenafil [Viagra]).

Prostatitis
1. Infection and inflammation of the prostate gland.
2. Types include acute bacterial, chronic prostatitis, and nonbacterial.
   a. Acute bacterial prostatitis involves bacterial urinary tract infection (UTI) and is associated with catheterization and multiple sex partners. Symptoms include urinary frequency, urgency, nocturia, dysuria, urethral discharge, fever and chills, malaise, myalgia and arthralgia, and pain.

> **RED FLAG:** Dull, aching pain may be found in the lower abdominal, rectal, lower back, sacral, or groin regions.

   b. Chronic prostatitis can also be bacterial in origin and is associated with recurrent UTI. Symptoms include urinary frequency and urgency, myalgia and arthralgia, and pain in the low back or perineal region.
   c. Nonbacterial inflammatory prostatitis produces pain in the penis, testicles, and scrotum; painful ejaculation; low back pain or pain in the inner thighs; urinary symptoms; decreased libido; and impotence.
3. Because the prostate encircles the urethra, obstruction of urinary flow can result.

Renal and Urological Systems

Overview

Anatomy
1. Kidneys are paired, bean-shaped organs located outside of the peritoneal cavity (retroperitoneal) in the posterior upper abdomen on each side of the vertebral column at the level of T12–L2 (Figure 6-4).
2. Each kidney is multilobular; each lobule is composed of more than 1 million nephrons (the functional units of the kidney).
3. Each nephron consists of a glomerulus that filters the blood and nephron tubules. Water, electrolytes, and other substances vital for function are reabsorbed into the bloodstream, while other waste products are secreted into the tubules for elimination.
4. The renal pelvis is a wide, funnel-shaped structure at the upper end of the urethra that drains the kidney into the lower urinary tract (bladder and urethra).
5. The bladder is a membranous sac that collects urine and is located behind the symphysis pubis.
6. The ureter extends from the renal pelvis to the bladder and moves urine via peristaltic action.
7. The urethra extends from the bladder to an external orifice for elimination of urine from the body.

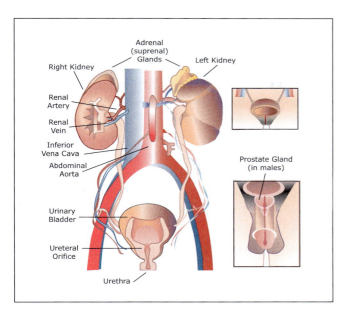

Figure 6-4 Renal and urological system anterior view.

8. In females, proximity of the urethra to vaginal and rectal openings increases the likelihood of UTI.

Functions of the Kidney
1. Regulates the composition and pH of body fluids through reabsorption and elimination; controls mineral (sodium, potassium, hydrogen, chloride, and bicarbonate ions) and water balance.
2. Eliminates metabolic wastes (urea, uric acid, creatinine) and drugs/drug metabolites.
3. Assists in blood pressure regulation through rennin-angiotensin-aldosterone mechanisms and salt and water elimination.
4. Contributes to bone metabolic function by activating vitamin D and regulating calcium and phosphate conservation and elimination.
5. Controls the production of red blood cells in the bone marrow through the production of erythropoietin.
6. The glomerular filtration rate (GFR) is the amount of filtrate that is formed each minute as blood moves through the glomeruli and serves as an important gauge of renal function.
   a. Regulated by arterial blood pressure and renal blood flow.
   b. Measured clinically by obtaining creatinine levels in blood and urine samples.
   c. Normal creatinine clearance is 115–125 mL/min.
7. Blood urea nitrogen (BUN) is urea produced in the liver as a by-product of protein metabolism that is eliminated by the kidneys.
   a. BUN levels are elevated with increased protein intake, gastrointestinal bleeding, and dehydration.
   b. BUN-creatinine ratio is abnormal in liver disease.

Normal Values of Urine (Urinalysis Findings)
1. Color: yellow-amber.
2. Clarity: clear.
3. Specific gravity: 1.010–1.025 with normal fluid intake.
4. pH: 4.6–8.0; average is 6 (acid).
5. Protein: 0–8 mg/dL.
6. Sugar: 0.

Urinary Regulation of Fluids and Electrolytes

Homeostasis
1. Regulated through thirst mechanisms and renal function via circulating antidiuretic hormone (ADH)

Fluid Imbalances
1. Daily fluid requirements vary based on presence or absence of such factors as sweating, air temperature, and fever.
2. Dehydration: excessive loss of body fluids; fluid output exceeds fluid intake.
   a. Causes: poor intake; excess output: profuse sweating, vomiting, diarrhea, and diuretics; closely linked to sodium deficiency.
   b. Observe for poor skin turgor, dry mucous membranes, headache, irritability, postural hypotension, incoordination, lethargy, disorientation.
   c. May lead to uremia and hypovolemic shock (stupor and coma).
   d. Decreased exercise capacity, especially in hot environments.
3. Edema: an excess of body fluids with expansion of interstitial fluid volume.
   a. Causes.
      • Increased capillary pressure: heart failure, kidney disease, premenstrual retention, pregnancy, environmental heat stress; venous obstruction (liver disease, acute pulmonary edema, venous thrombosis).
      • Decreased colloidal osmotic pressure: decreased production or loss of plasma proteins (protein-losing kidney disease, liver disease, starvation, malnutrition).
      • Increased capillary permeability: inflammation, allergic reactions, malignancy, tissue injury, burns.
      • Obstruction of lymphatic flow.

b. Observe for swelling of the ankles and feet, weight gain; headache, blurred vision; muscle cramps and twitches.
- Edema can be restrictive, producing a tourniquet effect.
- Tissues are susceptible to injury and delayed healing.
- Pitting edema occurs when the amount of interstitial fluid exceeds the absorptive capacity of tissues.

Potassium
1. Normal serum level is 3.5–5.5 mEq/L.
2. Hypokalemia.
   a. Causes: deficient potassium or excessive loss due to diarrhea, vomiting, metabolic acidosis, renal tubular disease, alkalosis.
   b. Observe for muscle weakness, aches, fatigue; cardiac arrhythmias; abdominal distention; nausea and vomiting.
3. Hyperkalemia.
   a. Causes: inadequate secretion with acute renal failure, kidney disease, metabolic acidosis, diabetic ketoacidosis, sickle cell anemia, SLE.
   b. Often symptomless until very high levels. Observe for muscle weakness, arrhythmias, electrocardiogram (ECG) changes (tall T wave, prolonged P-R interval and QRS duration).

Sodium
1. Normal serum level is 135–146 mEq/L.
2. Hyponatremia
   a. Causes: water intoxication (excess extracellular water) associated with excess intake or excess ADH (tumors, endocrine disorders).
   b. Observe for confusion; decreased mental alertness can progress to convulsions; signs of increased intracerebral pressure; poor motor coordination; sleepiness; anorexia.
3. Hypernatremia.
   a. Causes: occurs with water deficits (not salt excesses) with dehydration, insufficient water intake.
   b. Observe for: circulatory congestion (pitting edema, excessive weight gain); pulmonary edema with dyspnea; hypertension, tachycardia; agitation, restlessness, convulsions.

Calcium
1. Normal total calcium in blood is 8.4–10.4 mg/dL.
2. Hypocalcemia.
   a. Causes: reduced albumin levels, hyperphosphatemia, hypoparathyroidism, malabsorption of calcium and vitamin D, alkalosis, acute pancreatitis, vitamin D deficiency.
   b. Observe for muscle cramps, tetany, spasms; paresthesias; anxiety, irritability, twitching convulsion; arrhythmias, hypotension.
3. Hypercalcemia.
   a. Causes: hyperparathyroidism, tumors, hyperthyroidism, vitamin A intoxication.
   b. Observe for fatigue, depression, mental confusion, nausea/vomiting, increased urination, occasional cardiac arrhythmias.

Magnesium
1. Normal serum level is 1.8–2.4 mg/dL.
2. Hypomagnesemia.
   a. Causes: hemodialysis, blood transfusions, chronic renal disease, hepatic cirrhosis (alcoholism), chronic pancreatitis, hypoparathyroidism, malabsorption syndromes, severe burns, excess loss of body fluid.
   b. Observe for hyperirritability, confusion; leg and foot cramps.
3. Hypermagnesemia.
   a. Causes: renal failure, diabetic acidosis, hypothyroidism, Addison's disease, with dehydration and with use of antacids.
   b. Observe for hyporeflexia, muscle weakness, drowsiness, lethargy, confusion, bradycardia, hypotension.

Acid-Base Balance
1. Balance of acids and bases in the body (normally a ratio of 20 base to 1 acid; normal serum pH is 7.35–7.45 [slightly alkaline]); regulated by blood buffer systems (the lungs and the kidneys).
2. Metabolic acidosis: a depletion of bases or an accumulation of acids; blood pH falls below 7.35.
   a. Causes: diabetes, renal insufficiency or failure, diarrhea.
   b. Observe for hyperventilation (compensatory), deep respirations; weakness, muscular twitching; malaise, nausea, vomiting and diarrhea; headache; dry skin and mucous membranes, poor skin turgor.
   c. May lead to stupor and coma (death).
3. Metabolic alkalosis: an increase in bases or a reduction of acids; blood pH rises above 7.45.
   a. Causes: excess vomiting, excess diuretics, hypokalemia; peptic ulcer, and excessive intake of antacids.
   b. Observe for hypoventilation (compensatory), depressed respirations; dysrhythmias; prolonged vomiting, diarrhea; weakness, muscle twitching; irritability, agitation, convulsions, and coma (death).
4. Respiratory acidosis: CO_2 retention, impaired alveolar ventilation (see Table 5-4).
   a. Causes: hypoventilation, drugs/oversedation, chronic pulmonary disease (e.g., emphysema, asthma, bronchitis, pneumonia) or hypermetabolism (sepsis, burns).
   b. Observe for dyspnea, hyperventilation cyanosis; restlessness, headache.
   c. May lead to disorientation, stupor and coma, death.

5. Respiratory alkalosis: diminished CO_2, alveolar hyperventilation.
   a. Causes: anxiety attack with hyperventilation, hypoxia (emphysema, pneumonia), impaired lung expansion, congestive heart failure (CHF), pulmonary embolism, diffuse liver or CNS disease, salicylate poisoning, extreme stress (stimulation of respiratory center).
   b. Observe for tachypnea, dizziness, anxiety, difficulty concentrating, numbness and tingling, blurred vision, diaphoresis, muscle cramps, twitching or tetany, weakness, arrhythmias, convulsions.

Renal and Urological Disorders

Urinary Tract Infections (UTIs)
1. Infection of the urinary tract with microorganisms.
2. Lower UTI: cystitis (inflammation and infection of the bladder) or urethritis (inflammation and infection of the urethra).
   a. Usually secondary to ascending urinary tract infections; may also involve kidneys and ureters.
   b. Associated with symptoms of urinary frequency, urgency, burning sensation during urination. Urine may be cloudy and foul smelling. Pain is noted in suprapubic, lower abdominal, or groin area, depending on site of infection.
3. Upper UTI: pyelonephritis (inflammation and infection of one or both kidneys).
   a. Associated with symptoms of systemic involvement: fever, chills, malaise, headache, tenderness and pain over kidneys (back pain), tenderness over the costovertebal angle (Murphy's sign). Symptoms also include frequent and burning urination; nausea and vomiting may occur.
   b. Palpitation or percussion over the kidney typically causes pain.
   c. Can be acute or chronic; generally more serious than lower UTI.
4. Increased risk of UTI in persons with autoimmunity, urinary obstruction and reflux, neurogenic bladder and catheterization, diabetes, and kidney transplantation. Older adults and women are also at increased risk for UTI.
5. Medical management of urinary tract infections, painful urination, and incontinence may include medications. See Table 6-6.

Renal Cystic Disease
1. Renal cysts are fluid-filled cavities that form along the nephron and can lead to renal degeneration or obstruction.
2. Types include polycystic, medullary sponge, acquired, and simple renal cysts.
3. Symptoms can include pain, hematuria, and hypertension. Fever can occur with associated infection, Cysts can rupture producing hematuria. Simple cysts are generally asymptomatic.

Obstructive Disorders
1. Developmental defects, renal calculi, prostatic hyperplasia or cancer, scar tissue from inflammation, tumors, and infection.
2. Pressure build-up backward from site of obstruction; can result in kidney damage. Dilation of ureters and renal pelvis may be used to reduce obstruction. Observe for pain, signs and symptoms of UTI, and hypertension.
3. Renal calculi (kidney stones): crystalline structures formed from normal components of urine (calcium,

Table 6-6

Commonly Prescribed Medications and Associated Precautions—Genitourinary System

MEDICATION	PRESCRIBED FOR	SIDE EFFECTS	INTERACTIONS	PHYSICAL THERAPY CONSIDERATIONS*
Sulfamethoxazole/ Trimethoprim (Bactrim DS)	UTI (urinary tract infection)	Very serious skin reaction: Steven-Johnson Syndrome, allergic reactions	Alcohol (increases effect through enzyme inhibition), folate deficiency, colitis	Watch for skin problems
Oxybutynin (Ditropan)	Urinary incontinence	Dry skin, stomach pain, painful urination, dizziness	Alcohol increases mental impairment so driving could be dangerous, potassium supplements	Evaluate mental state and recommend something for dry skin
Phenazopyridine (Pyridium)	Painful urination	Fever, confusion, weakness, dizziness, infrequent or stopped urination, discolored urine or tears (orange-red)	Hemolytic anemia or hepatitis (both rare), leflunomide (medication used to treat RA, rejection of organ transplant)	Pyrdium is OTC but does not cure a UTI and may mask symptoms, watch for confusion and weakness

*Medications used in the medical management of diseases and conditions are included in the NPTE. PTAs should be familiar with categories of medications and their indications for use. PTAs should be acutely aware of potential effects on tolerance to physical therapy intervention.
Note: Generic drug names appear first followed by brand names in parenthesis; brand names may be trademarked or registered.

magnesium ammonium phosphate, uric acid, and cystine).
   a. Etiological influences include concentration of stone components in urine and a urinary environment conducive to stone formation.
   b. Symptoms include renal colic pain (pain from a stone lodged in the ureter made worse by stretching the collecting system). Pain may radiate to the lower abdominal quadrant, bladder area, and perineal area (scrotum in the male and labia in the female). Nausea and vomiting are common and the skin may be cool and clammy.
   c. Extracorporeal shock wave lithotripsy (ESWL) is used to break up stones into fragments to allow for easy passage.
   d. Treatment/prevention can also include increased fluid intake, thiazide diuretics, dietary restriction of foods high in oxalate, acidification or alkalinization of urine depending on type of stone.

Renal Failure

1. Acute renal failure: sudden loss of kidney function with resulting elevation in serum urea and creatinine.
   a. Etiology: may be due to circulatory disruption to kidneys, toxic substances, bacterial toxins, acute obstruction, or trauma.
2. Chronic renal failure: progressive loss of kidney function leading to end-stage failure.
   a. Etiology: may result from prolonged acute urinary tract obstruction and infection, diabetes, SLE, uncontrolled hypertension.
   b. Uremia: an end-stage toxic condition resulting from renal insufficiency and retention of nitrogenous wastes in blood; symptoms can include anorexia, nausea, and mental confusion.

RED FLAGS: May lead to multisystem abnormalities and failure.

3. Dialysis: process of diffusing blood across a semipermeable membrane for the purposes of removal of toxic substances; maintains fluid, electrolyte, and acid-base balance in presence of renal failure; peritoneal, or renal (hemodialysis).
   a. Dialysis disequilibrium: symptoms of nausea, vomiting, drowsiness, headache, and seizures; the result of rapid changes after beginning dialysis.
   b. Dialysis dementia: signs of cerebral dysfunction (e.g., speech difficulties, mental confusion, myoclonus, seizures, eventually death); the result of long-standing years of dialysis treatment.

RED FLAG: Taking BP on the vascular access arm of a patient who is on dialysis is contraindicated. Avoid trauma to the area of the peritoneal catheter (peritoneal dialysis is used with patients in kidney failure).

   c. Examine for multisystem dysfunction: vital signs, strength, sensation, ROM, function, and endurance.
4. Transplantation is a major treatment choice (renal allograft).

Urinary Incontinence

1. Inability to retain urine; the result of loss of sphincter control; may be acute (due to transient causes, e.g., cystitis) or persistent (e.g., stroke, dementia).
2. Types.
   a. Stress incontinence: sudden release of urine due to:
      - Increases in intra-abdominal pressure, e.g., coughing, laughing, exercise, straining, obesity.
      - Weakness and laxity of pelvic floor musculature, sphincter weakness, e.g., postpartum incontinence, menopause, damage to pudendal nerve.
   b. Urge incontinence: bladder begins contracting and urine is leaked after sensation of bladder fullness is perceived; an inability to delay voiding to reach toilet due to:
      - Detrusor muscle instability or hyperreflexia, e.g., stroke.
      - Sensory instability: hypersensitive bladder.
   c. Overflow incontinence: bladder continuously leaks secondary to urinary retention (an overdistended bladder or incomplete emptying of bladder) due to:
      - Anatomical obstruction, e.g., prostate enlargement.
      - Acontractile bladder, e.g., spinal cord injury, diabetes.
      - Neurogenic bladder, e.g., multiple sclerosis, suprasacral spinal lesions.
   d. Functional incontinence: leakage associated with inability or unwillingness to toilet due to:
      - Impaired cognition (dementia); depression, e.g., Alzheimer's disease.
      - Impaired physical functioning, e.g., stroke.
      - Environmental barriers.
3. Management.
   a. Dietary management: control of food and beverages that aggravate the bladder or incontinence (e.g., citrus fruit or juices, caffeine, chocolate); control fluid intake.
   b. Medical management.
      - Identify and treat acute, reversible problems, e.g., cystometry.
      - Drug therapy for urge, stress, and overflow incontinence, e.g., estrogen with phenylpropanolamine (see Table 6-6).

- Control of medications that may aggravate incontinence, e.g., diuretics for CHF, anticholinergic or psychotropic drugs.
- Catheterization: used for overflow incontinence and other types if unresponsive to other treatments and skin integrity is threatened; associated with high rates of urinary tract infection.
- Surgery: bladder neck suspension, removal of prostate obstructions; suprapubic cystostomy.

c. Bladder training: prompted voiding to restore a pattern of voiding.
- Involves toileting schedule: taking patient to bathroom at regular intervals.
- May also include intermittent catheterization, e.g., for patients with overdistention, persistent retention (e.g., multiple sclerosis).

4. Examination.
   a. Symptoms of incontinence: onset and duration, urgency, frequency, timing of episodes/causative factors.
   b. Strength of pelvic floor muscles using a perineometer.
   c. Functional mobility, environmental factors.

5. Physical therapy goals, outcomes, and interventions for stress and urge incontinence.
   a. Teach pelvic floor muscle exercises (pubococcygeus muscle): used to treat stress incontinence.
   - Kegel's exercises: active, strengthening exercises; type 1 works on holding contractions, progressing to 10-second holds, rest 10 seconds between contractions; type 2 works on quick contractions to shut off flow of urine, 10–80 repetitions a day. Avoid squeezing buttocks or contracting abdominals (bearing down).
   - Functional electrical stimulation: for muscle reeducation if patient is unable to initiate active contractions.
   - Biofeedback: uses pressure recordings to reinforce active contractions, relax bladder.
   - Progressive strengthening: use of weighted vaginal cones for home exercises or pelvic floor exerciser.
   - Incorporating Kegel's exercise into everyday life: e.g., with lifting, coughing, changing positions.

   b. Provide behavioral training.
   - Record keeping: patients are asked to keep a history of their voiding (voiding diary).
   - Education: regarding anatomy, physiology, reasons for muscle weakness, incontinence; avoidance of Valsalva's maneuver, heavy resistance exercises.

   c. Functional mobility training as needed. Ensure independence in sit-to-stand transitions, ambulation, and safe toilet transfers.
   d. Environmental modifications as needed: e.g., toilet rails, raised toilet seat, or commode.
   e. Maintain adequate skin condition.
   - Teach appropriate skin care, maintain toileting schedule.
   - Adequate protection: adult diapers, underpads.

   f. Provide psychological support: emotional and social consequences of incontinence are significant.

Endocrine and Metabolic Systems

Overview of the Endocrine System

Hormonal Regulation

1. The endocrine system uses hormones (chemical messengers) to relay information to cells and organs and regulate many of the body functions (digestion, use of nutrients, growth and development, electrolyte and water balance, and reproductive functions) (Figure 6-5).
2. The hypothalamus and pituitary gland, along with the nervous system, make up the central network that exerts control over many other glands in the body with wide-ranging functions. Endocrine functions are also closely linked with the immune system.
3. Hormones bind to specific receptor sites that are linked to specific systems and functions.
4. The hypothalamus controls release of pituitary hormones (corticotropin-releasing hormone [CRH], thyrotropin-releasing hormone [TRH], growth hormone–releasing hormone [GHRH], and somatostatin).
5. The anterior pituitary gland controls the release of growth hormone (GH), adrenocorticotropic hormone (ACTH), follicle-stimulating hormone (FSH), luteinizing hormone (LH), and prolactin.
6. The posterior pituitary gland controls the release of antidiuretic hormone (ADH) and oxytocin.
7. The adrenal cortex controls the release of mineral corticosteroids (aldosterone), glucocorticoids (cortisol), adrenal androgens (dehydroepiandrosterone [DHEA]), and androstenedione.

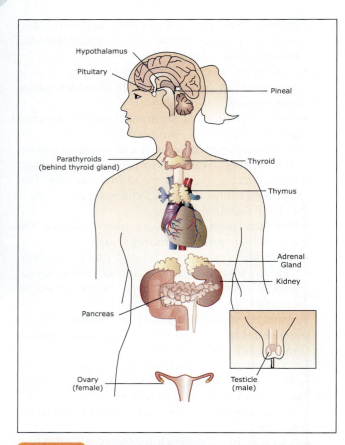

Figure 6-5   Endocrine system anterior view.

Hormones Released by Islets of Langerhans in Pancreas

1. Insulin: allows uptake of glucose from the bloodstream; suppresses hepatic glucose production, lowering plasma glucose levels. Secreted by the beta cells.
2. Glucagon: stimulates hepatic glucose production to raise glucose levels, especially in fasting state. Secreted by the alpha cells.
3. Amylin: modulates rate of nutrient delivery (gastric emptying); suppresses release of glucagon. Secreted by the beta cells.
4. Somatostatin: acts locally to depress secretion of both insulin and glycogen; decreases motility of stomach, duodenum, and gallbladder; decreases secretion and absorption of GI tract. Secreted by the delta cells.

Diabetes Mellitus (DM)

Characteristics
1. A complex disorder of carbohydrate, fat, and protein metabolism caused by deficiency or absence of insulin secretion by the beta cells of the pancreas or by defects of the insulin receptors resulting in increased blood sugar levels that are unhealthy.
2. May be acquired, familial, idiopathic, neurogenic, or nephrogenic. Possible viral/autoimmune and genetic etiology. Represents 5%–10% of DM.

Types
1. Prediabetes.
   a. Prediabetes is a "pre-diabetic" condition in which individuals have impaired glucose tolerance. Prediabetes is reversible through lifestyle modification (healthy diet, active lifestyle-exercise).
   b. Commonly occurs prior to the individual developing type 2 diabetes.
   c. It does not present with any symptoms and typically occurs in:
      • Individuals with a family history of type 2 diabetes who are overweight or inactive.
      • Individuals who have high cholesterol or triglycerides.
      • Elderly individuals.
2. Type 1 diabetes mellitus (T1DM); also known as insulin-dependent, juvenile-onset diabetes.
   a. Characteristics include:
      • Decrease in size and number of islet cells resulting in absolute deficiency in insulin secretion.
      • Usually occurs in children and young adults. Long preclinical period, often with abrupt onset of symptoms around the age of puberty.
      • Insulin-dependent: requires insulin delivery by injection, insulin pump, or inhalation.

8. The adrenal medulla controls the release of epinephrine and norepinephrine.
9. The thyroid controls the release of triiodothyronine and thyroxine. Thyroid C cells control the release of calcitonin.
10. The parathyroid glands control the release of parathyroid hormone (PTH).
11. The pancreatic islet cells control the release of insulin, glucagons, and somatostatin.
12. The kidney controls the release of 1,25-dihydroxy-vitamin D.
13. The ovaries control the release of estrogen and progesterone.
14. The testes control the release of androgens (testosterone).

Overview of the Metabolic System

Glucose Control
1. Normal glucose control is the result of nutrient, neural and hormonal regulation.

b. Etiology: caused by autoimmune abnormalities, genetic causes, or environmental causes.
c. Prone to ketoacidosis. Presence of ketone bodies in the urine, the by-products of fat metabolism (ketonuria).
3. Type 2 diabetes mellitus (T2DM) results from inadequate utilization of insulin (insulin resistance) and progressive beta cell dysfunction; also known as adult-onset or non-insulin dependent diabetes. Represents 90%–95% of DM cases.
   a. Characteristics include:
      - Gradual onset; may have familial pattern.
      - Usually not insulin dependent.
      - Individual is not prone to ketoacidosis (may form ketones with stress).
   b. Etiology: a progressive disease caused by a combination of factors, including:
      - Insulin resistance in muscle and adipose tissue.
      - Progressive decline in pancreatic insulin production.
      - Excessive hepatic glucose production.
      - Inappropriate glucagon secretion.
   c. Risk factors include:
      - Linked to obesity and older adults (typically over the age of 40). Can occur in nonobese individuals with increased percentage of body fat in the abdominal region.
      - Family history of diabetes.
      - Unhealthy eating patterns.
      - Lack of physical activity.
4. Insulin resistance and metabolic syndrome (insulin resistance syndrome, syndrome X).
   a. A group of risk factors that increase the likelihood of developing heart disease, stroke, and type 2 diabetes. Criteria for diagnosis include three or more of the following:
      - Abdominal obesity: waist circumference >40 inches in men or >35 inches in women.
      - Elevated triglycerides: triglyceride level of 150 mg/dL or higher.
      - Low HDL cholesterol or being on medicine to treat low HDL: HDL level lower than 40 mg/dL in men or 50 mg/dL in women.
      - Elevated blood pressure: systolic BP 130 mm Hg or higher and/or diastolic pressure 85 mm Hg or higher.
      - Fasting plasma glucose level >110 mg/dL. A level between 100 and 125 mg/dL is considered prediabetes.
   b. Lifestyle changes can reverse or reduce the chance of developing metabolic syndrome: weight loss, exercise, medications to control triglycerides, cholesterol, blood pressure, or glucose.
5. Secondary diabetes: associated with other conditions (pancreatic disease or removal of pancreatic tissue), endocrine disease (e.g., acromegaly, Cushing's syndrome, pheochromocytoma), drugs (e.g., some diuretics, diazoxide, glucocorticoids, levodopa), and chemical agents.
6. Impaired glucose tolerance (IGT): asymptomatic or borderline diabetes with abnormal response to oral glucose test; 10%–15% of individuals will convert to type 2 diabetes within 10 years.
7. Gestational diabetes mellitus (GDM): glucose intolerance associated with pregnancy; most likely in third trimester.

Signs and Symptoms
1. Elevated blood sugar (hyperglycemia).
2. Elevated sugar in urine (glycosuria).
3. Excessive excretion of urine (polyuria).
4. Excessive thirst (polydipsia).
5. Excessive hunger (polyphagia) and unexplained weight loss (usually type 1).

Complications of DM
1. Microvascular disease.
   a. Retinopathy.
   b. Renal disease.
   c. Polyneuropathy.
2. Macrovascular disease: dyslipidemia (accelerated atherosclerosis).
   a. Cerebrovascular accident (CVA, stroke).
   b. Myocardial infarction (MI).
   c. Peripheral arterial disease (PAD).
3. Integumentary impairments: including degenerative connective tissue changes; anhidrosis; increased risk of ulcers and infections.
4. Musculoskeletal impairments.
   a. Joint stiffness and increased risk of contractures.
   b. Increased risk of adhesive capsulitis of shoulder, tenosynovitis, plantar fasciitis.
   c. Increased risk of osteoporosis.
5. Neuromuscular impairments.
   a. Diabetic polyneuropathy.
      - Symmetrical; stocking and glove distribution.
      - Distal (long nerves first) progressing to proximal.
      - Altered sensations; paresthesias, shooting pain; loss of protective sensations.
      - Motor weakness: foot/ankle weakness initially with balance and gait impairments.
   b. Diabetic autonomic neuropathy (DAN).
      - Cardiovascular autonomic neuropathy (CAN): resting tachycardia; exercise intolerance with abnormal HR, BP, and cardiac output responses; exercise-induced hypoglycemia; postural hypotension.
      - Integumentary: anhidrosis, abnormal sweating, dry skin, heat intolerance.

- Gastrointestinal: gastroparesis, GERD, diarrhea, constipation.
- Metabolic: abnormal or delayed responses to hypoglycemia; lack of awareness of hypoglycemia.

c. Mononeuropathies: focal nerve damage resulting from vasculitis with ischemia and infarction.
d. Entrapment neuropathies: resulting from repetitive trauma to superficial nerves.

6. Kidney impairments, including kidney failure.
7. Vision impairments, including diabetic retinopathy (associated with chronic hyperglycemia) and diabetic macular edema.
8. Liver impairments, including fatty liver disease (steatosis).

Diagnostic Criteria for DM

1. Symptoms of diabetes plus casual plasma glucose concentration ≥200 mg/dL (11.1 mmol/L). "Casual" is defined as any time of day, without regard to time since last meal (Table 6-7).
2. Fasting plasma glucose (FPG) ≥126 mg/dL (7 mmol/L). Fasting is defined as no caloric intake for at least 8 hours.
3. 2-hour postload glucose ≥200 mg/dL (11.1 mmol/L) during an oral glucose tolerance test (OGTT). OGTT, as described by the World Health Organization, uses a glucose load containing the equivalent of 75 g anhydrous glucose dissolved in water.

Medical Goals and Interventions

1. Maintain insulin glucose homeostasis.
   a. Frequent monitoring of blood glucose levels.
   b. Dietary control: weight reduction, control of carbohydrate, protein, fat, and calorie intake.
   c. Oral hypoglycemic agents to lower blood glucose; indicated for type 2 diabetes.
   d. Insulin to lower blood glucose via injections, infusion pump, or intraperitoneal dialysis for patients with renal failure. Indicated for type 1 diabetes or for more severe type 2 diabetes.
   e. Maintenance of normal lipid levels.
   f. Control of hypertension.
2. Blood sugar monitoring can be completed using a variety of tests.
   a. Blood glucose testing: provides information about blood sugar levels at the time testing is performed; may be performed multiple times per day, before/after meals, and before bed time. Individuals taking insulin should check blood sugar levels more often.
   b. A1C Test: provides information about blood sugar levels over the last 2–4 months. Target levels for persons with diabetes is below 7, higher levels increase long-term risk factors, e.g., eye, kidney, nerve and heart problems.
3. Medical management of diabetic conditions may include medications. See Table 6-8.
4. Exercise and physical fitness.
5. Health promotion.

Physical Therapy Goals, Outcomes, and Interventions

1. Exercise.
   a. Outcomes of exercise include improved glucose tolerance, increased insulin sensitivity, decreased glycosylated hemoglobin, and decreased insulin requirements. Additional outcomes include improved lipid profiles, BP reduction, weight management, increased physical work capacity, and improved well-being.
   b. Response to exercise is dependent upon adequacy of disease control.
2. Exercise testing is recommended prior to exercise due to increased cardiovascular risk.
3. Exercise prescription—Cardiovascular training (American College of Sports Medicine [ACSM] Guidelines, 2017).
   a. Intensity: 50%–80% of maximal oxygen uptake (VO_2 max) or heart rate reserve (HRR) corresponding

Table 6-7

Blood Sugar Levels

CONDITION	A1C PERCENT*	FASTING PLASMA GLUCOSE (FPG)**	ORAL GLUCOSE TOLERANCE TEST (OGTT)***
Normal	~ 5.6% or <	100 mg/dL or <	140 mg/dL or <
Pre-Diabetes	5.7–6.4%	100–125 mg/dL	140–199 mg/dL
Diabetes	6.5% or >	126 mg/dL or >	200 mg/dL or >

*A1C (hemoglobin A1C test): reflects the average blood sugar levels over past 2–4 months.
**Fasting plasma glucose: blood glucose is measured after an 8 hour fast.
***Oral glucose tolerance test: blood glucose is measured after a fast then again 2 hours after consuming a beverage containing a large amount of sugar; if glucose is higher than normal it identifies "impaired glucose tolerance."
Note: Target range/meals: before-between 70 and 130, 2 hours after meal starts-below 180.

Table 6-8

Commonly Prescribed Medications and Associated Precautions—Diabetes Management

MEDICATION	PRESCRIBED FOR	SIDE EFFECTS	INTERACTIONS	PHYSICAL THERAPY CONSIDERATIONS*
Metformin (Glucophage)	Diabetes	Lactic acidosis, muscle pain or weakness, stomach pain, hypoglycemia	Alcohol, gatifloxacin, diatrizoate, and many others	Watch for muscle weakness as lactic acidosis has slow onset
Liraglutide (Victoza)	Diabetes	Headache, loss of appetite, nausea, vomiting, diarrhea or constipation	Delays gastric emptying which decreases effectiveness of antibiotics and pain meds	Effectiveness of pain med and weight loss
Pioglitazone (Actos)	Diabetes	Stomach pain, painful urination, muscle pain, shortness of breath	Warfarin, gemfibrozil, insulin, and rifampin	Be aware of shortness of breath in exertion, potential for new or worsening vision problems (blurred vision)

*Medications used in the medical management of diseases and conditions are included in the NPTE. PTAs should be familiar with categories of medications and their indications for use. PTAs should be acutely aware of potential effects on tolerance to physical therapy intervention.
Note: Generic drug names appear first followed by brand names in parenthesis; brand names may be trademarked or registered.

---

to rating of perceived exertion (RPE) of 12–16 on the 6–20 Borg scale.
   b. Frequency: 3–7 days/week.
   c. Duration: 20–60 minutes.
   d. Type: rhythmic, large muscle activity (e.g., biking, treadmill walking, overground walking).
4. Exercise prescription: resistance training (ACSM Guidelines, 2017).
   a. Frequency: 2–3 days/week.
   b. Intensity: resistance 60%–80% of one repetition max, 2–3 sets of 8–10 repetitions.
   c. Type: multijoint exercises of major muscle groups.
   d. Proper technique: minimize sustained gripping, static work, and Valsalva's maneuver (essential to decrease risk of hypertensive response).
5. Flexibility exercises.
6. Balance exercises.
7. Exercise precautions. See Box 6-3 and Box 6-4.

RED FLAGS: Monitor glucose levels prior to and following exercise.

- Hypoglycemia is the most common problem for patients with diabetes who exercise.
  - Observe for signs and symptoms of hypoglycemia (Box 6-2). Do not exercise if blood glucose is <70 mg/dL. Provide carbohydrate snack initially (15 g of carbohydrate); have readily available during exercise (15 g carbohydrate for every hour of intense activity).
  - Hypoglycemia associated with exercise may last as long as 48 hours after exercise. To prevent postexercise hypoglycemia, monitor plasma glucose levels and ingest carbohydrates as needed (Box 6-2).

BOX 6-2 ▸ Signs and Symptoms of Hypoglycemia (Low Blood Sugar)

Glucose is low: <70 mg/dL or a rapid drop in glucose. Onset is rapid (minutes)

Early signs and symptoms:

Pallor

Shakiness/trembling

Sweating

Excessive hunger

Tachycardia and palpitations

Fainting or feeling faint

Dizziness

Fatigue and weakness

Poor coordination and unsteady gait

Late signs and symptoms:

Nervousness and irritability

Headache

Blurred or double vision

Slurred speech

Drowsiness

Inability to concentrate, confusion, delusions

Loss of consciousness and coma

Response: If patient is awake, provide sugar (juice, candy bar, glucose tablets and gel).

If patient unresponsive, seek immediate medical treatment; glucagon injection or intravenous glucose is required.

BOX 6-3 ▷ Signs and Symptoms of Hyperglycemia (Abnormally High Blood Sugar)

Glucose is high: >300 mg/dL. Gradual onset (days)

Weakness

Increased thirst

Dry mouth

Frequent, scant urination

Decreased appetite, nausea/vomiting, abdominal tenderness

Dulled senses, confusion, diminished reflexes, paresthesias

Flushed, signs of dehydration

Deep, rapid respirations

Pulse: rapid, weak

Fruity odor to the breath (acetone breath)

Hyperglycemic coma

Response: Seek immediate medical treatment.

BOX 6-4 ▷ Exercise Precautions for Individuals with Diabetes Mellitus

Monitor glucose levels prior to and following exercise.

Hypoglycemia is the most common problem for patients with diabetes who exercise.

- Observe for signs and symptom of hypoglycemia (Box 6-2). Do not exercise if blood glucose is < 70 mg/dL. Provide carbohydrate snack initially (15 g of carbohydrate); have readily available during exercise (15 g carbohydrate for every hour of intense activity).
- Hypoglycemia associated with exercise may last as long as 48 hours after exercise. To prevent postexercise hypoglycemia, monitor plasma glucose levels and ingest carbohydrates as needed.

Hyperglycemia: Do not exercise when blood glucose levels are high (fasting glucose > 300 mg/dL) or poorly controlled (ketosis is present with urine test) (Box 6-3).

Do not exercise without eating at least 2 hours before exercise.

Do not exercise without adequate hydration. Maintain hydration during exercise session.

Do not exercise alone. Exercise with a partner or under supervision.

Do not inject short-acting insulin in exercising muscles or sites close to exercising muscles as insulin is absorbed more quickly. Abdominal injection site is preferred.

Use caution or do not exercise patients with poorly controlled complications.

- Cardiovascular disease, hypertension. May see chronotropic incompetence, blunted HR and systolic BP response, blunted oxygen uptake, and anhidrosis. RPE may be used to regulate exercise intensity.
- Retinopathy. Avoid activities that dramatically increase BP (> 170 mm Hg systolic BP); avoid pounding or jarring activities.

BOX 6-4 ▷ Exercise Precautions for Individuals with Diabetes Mellitus (*Continued*)

- Neuropathy, nephropathy. Limit weight-bearing exercise for patients with significant neuropathy. There is increased fall risk with balance and gait abnormalities.
- Autonomic neuropathy is associated with sudden death and silent ischemia. Monitor for signs and symptoms of silent ischemia due to patient's inability to perceive angina.
- Nephropathy. Limit exercise to low to moderate intensities; discourage strenuous intensities.

Do not exercise in extreme environmental temperatures (very hot or cold due to impaired thermoregulation).

8. Emphasize proper diabetic foot care: good footwear, hygiene.
9. Patient and family education.
   a. Control of risk factors (obesity, physical inactivity, prolonged stress, and smoking).
   b. Dietary intervention strategies.
   c. Injury prevention strategies.
   d. Self-management strategies.

Obesity

Body Mass Index (BMI)

1. Formula for determining obesity (a condition characterized by excess body fat).
2. BMI is calculated by dividing an individual's weight in kilograms by the square of the person's height in meters.
3. Criteria: World Health Organization classification (adopted by National Institutes of Health).
   a. Overweight is defined as BMI ranging from 25 to 29.9 kg/m^2.
   b. Obesity is defined as BMI ≥30 kg/m^2.
   c. Morbid obesity is defined as BMI ≥40 kg/m^2.
4. Measurement by skin calipers using a fold of skin and subcutaneous fat from various body locations (mid biceps, midtriceps, and subscapular or inguinal areas). Greater than 1 inch is indicative of excess body fat.

Medical Problems Associated with Obesity

1. Obesity is associated with many complications, including three of the leading causes of death: cardiovascular disease, diabetes mellitus, osteoarthritis, sleep apnea, liver disease, stroke and cancer.
2. Other complications include: thromboembolic disorders, digestive tract disorders (reflux, gallstones), obstructive sleep apnea and pulmonary compromise, menstrual irregularities and infertility.
3. Obesity also increases the risk of cancer (endometrium, breast, prostate, colon).

Physical Problems Associated with Obesity

1. Impaired functional mobility, ADL limitations, difficulty climbing stairs, difficulty walking.
2. Increased risk for falls.
3. Shortness of breath.
4. Fatigue.
5. Increased occurrence of back, hip and knee pain.
6. Potential for skin breakdown and/or pressure ulcers, neuropathic ulcers and foot ulcerations.
7. Knee osteoarthritis (OA).
   a. Evidence supports an increased risk of knee OA in persons with obesity; there is not conclusive evidence of increased OA at other joints.

Surgical Intervention

1. Multiple surgical gastric reduction procedures exist to assist individuals with weight loss (see Table 6-9).
2. Individuals seeking gastric reduction procedures go through extensive medical and psychological assessment prior to medical approval to receive the procedure.
3. Each gastric reduction procedure has its specific post-op protocol. Of specific concern are:
   a. Water intake: dehydration is a significant concern, water intake is limited to sips at a time—not glasses at a time and may be more water than typically recommended for healthy individuals
   b. Food: the kind of foods that may be consumed is very specific and will likely include some foods to avoid, e.g., those that tend to produce gas. Food may have to be blended prior to consumption.
   c. Lifting and resistance exercise may be restricted for up to 4–6 weeks post-op.
4. Clinicians working with individuals who are post-op must work closely with the physician and the patient to adhere to and facilitate success with the rehabilitation process. It is also very likely the individual is also working with a dietitian; a multidisciplinary approach is beneficial.

Prevention and Management

1. Lifestyle modification: combination of dietary changes to reduce body weight combined with increased physical activity.
   a. Personalized diet with reduced caloric intake: fat intake of < 30% of total energy intake, emphasis on fruits, vegetables, whole grains, and lean protein.
   b. Personalized exercise program, including stretching exercises, resistance exercises, and aerobic exercises.
   c. Instruction in self-monitoring of exercise responses (heart rate, perceived exertion).
2. Behavior therapy: self-monitoring of eating habits and physical activity (use of a food and exercise diary); stress management, relapse prevention, and social support.
3. Pharmacology: over-the-counter (OTC) and prescriptive weight loss therapy (e.g., sibutramine, orlistat).
4. Surgery (bariatric surgery): usually limited to persons with BMI over 40 (or individuals with comorbid conditions and BMI over 35). Procedures include gastric banding and gastric bypass.

Table 6-9

Selected Gastric Reduction Procedures

PROCEDURE	POST-OP CARE	CONSIDERATIONS FOR REHABILITATION
Lap Band Frequent adjustments: stomach opening can be tightened or loosened over time to change the size of passage Adjustable for each pt, can be reversed, less expensive and less restrictive diet Frequent adjustments	Hospital <24 hours, return to work about 1 week Dietary restrictions Can begin walking upon discharge home	May have been sedentary and need to begin exercise program slowly. May have lifting restrictions 4 weeks
Vertical Sleeve Gastrectomy Remove a large part of the stomach leaving a much smaller stomach	Hospital 2–4 days Laparoscopic procedure Return to work depends on the type of job, healing of the stomach that has been removed and stapled back together, takes 4–6 weeks	Have often been sedentary for years, need to consider previous level of activity Can begin walking for clot prevention while in the hospital, need clearance from surgeon to lift restrictions, Walking is main activity for 2 weeks to 3 months, Lifting restrictions for 6 weeks
Gastric Bypass Most invasive, and most common for the last 15 years Can have major complications Changes to stomach are lifelong and difficult to reverse or adjust	Hospital 3–5 days. Invasive surgery, surgeon will have restrictions for activity as well as dietary. Can begin their walking program when they go home. Suggest short distances 6 times a day. Give them a progression to gradually increase, with signs and symptoms to monitor.	Often have been sedentary, need to assess prior level of activity, and may need a lot of encouragement as they may have never been physically active. Often multiple other medical history you will need to monitor.

Physical Therapy Interventions and Considerations

1. Gain "buy in" from individual for continued participation in activity modification.
   a. Stress the overall health benefits of sticking with a consistent exercise program versus emphasizing weight loss.
      - Studies indicate that regular physical activity reduces cardiovascular morbidity for obese individuals even if they remain overweight.
      - Studies indicate that in obese individuals more fat and less lean body tissue is lost when diet and exercise are combined.
      - Studies show that exercise decreases visceral fat even if weight loss does not occur.
      - Resistance exercise can increase lean body mass as well as improve ability to perform ADL.
   b. Assist the individual to identify potential barriers to a regular exercise program; develop strategies to mitigate.
   c. Seek input from individual regarding what type of aerobic and strengthening activity they would prefer to use; identify availability and incorporate into their program.
   d. Provide written program that includes pictures.
   e. Provide exercise flow sheet for tracking, monitoring and encouragement.
      - Encourage the use of an exercise journal/diary; record successes, struggles and barriers.
      - The journal/diary can be reviewed by both the patient and clinician providing a great mechanism to visualize progress, provide encouragement, and open a door to assist overcoming hurdles.
   f. Bariatric equipment and patient management options. Refer to Chapter 11 for further detail.
2. Potential complications during exercise:
   a. Increased risk for heat intolerance; carefully observe for signs of heat stroke or heat exhaustion.
   b. Angina pectoris or myocardial infarction.
   c. Excessive rise in blood pressure.
   d. Difficulty with blood sugar regulation.
   e. Hypohydration and reduced circulating blood volume.
   f. Joint problems: irritation of degenerative arthritis, ligamentous injuries.
   g. Excessive sweating; skin chafing.
3. Baseline and follow up exercise testing.
   a. Physician clearance should be gained prior to any exercise testing or to beginning an exercise program.
   b. Consider any medications the individual is taking for concomitant conditions, e.g., beta blockers, insulin, etc.
   c. There is a likelihood of lowered exercise tolerance; typical starting point and termination criteria may need adjusting.
   d. Musculoskeletal considerations may necessitate the use of a recumbent bicycle rather than a treadmill to enable participation.
   e. Ensure you have appropriate size BP cuff.

Exercise Evaluation (ACSM Guidelines, 2017)

1. Individuals are typically sedentary with low physical work capacities. See Quick Facts 6-2.
2. Interviews should include goals, past exercise history, perceived barriers to exercise participation, and exercise likes and dislikes.
3. Exercise testing: submaximal, low initial workload (typically 2–3 METs), small workload increments per test stage (0.5–1.0 METs).
4. Use of leg or arm ergometry may enhance testing performance.
5. Use of proper size equipment: wide seat ergometer, large-size BP cuff.

Exercise Prescription (ACSM Guidelines, 2017)

1. Start slowly, provide adequate warm-ups and cool-downs. Initial exercise intensity should be moderate (40%–60% oxygen uptake reserve [VO_2R] or HRR).
2. Increase intensity gradually in order to prevent injury: moderate-intensity activity (50%–70% VO_2R or HRR).
3. Frequency: 5–7 days/week.
4. Duration: 30–60 minutes.
5. Type: aerobic physical activities. Use of circuit training in order to combine resistive training with aerobic training activities. Provide with short rests between activities/exercise bouts.
6. Involve the patient in activity selection, incorporating individual preferences.

QUICK FACTS 6-2 ▶ EXERCISE PRECAUTIONS FOR INDIVIDUALS WHO ARE OVERWEIGHT OR OBESE

Typically exhibit cardiopulmonary compromise: shortness of breath, elevated blood pressure, and angina.

Typically exhibit altered biomechanics affecting hips, knees, ankle/foot; back and joint pain; and increased risk of orthopedic injury.

Increased risk of skin breakdown due to shear forces.

Increased heat intolerance, risk of hyperthermia and heat exhaustion.

Increased risk of therapist injury: poor body mechanics, inadequate assistance during transfers and lifts.

7. Select adequate footwear and orthotic devices as needed.
8. Aquatic exercise programs can assist in reducing musculoskeletal strain and injury.
9. Use of special bariatric equipment: wide seats on ergometers, bariatric lifts.

Thyroid Disorders

Hypothyroidism
1. An underactive thyroid gland with deficient thyroid secretion (thyroxine); lower than normal T4 levels.
2. Results in slowed metabolic processes, affecting body temperature, heartbeat, and slowing of body processes.
3. Etiology: decreased thyroid-releasing hormone secreted by the hypothalamus or by the pituitary gland; atrophy of the thyroid gland; chronic autoimmune thyroiditis (Hashimoto's disease); overdosage with antithyroid medication.
4. Symptoms include weight gain or difficulty losing weight, mental and physical lethargy, depression, dry skin and hair, low blood pressure, constipation, intolerance to cold, and goiter.
5. If untreated, leads to myxedema (severe hypothyroidism) with symptoms of swelling of hands, feet, face. Can lead to coma and death.
6. Treatment: life-long thyroid replacement therapy.

> **RED FLAG:** Can result in exercise intolerance, weakness, apathy; exercise-induced myalgia; reduced cardiac output.

Hyperthyroidism
1. Hyperactivity of the thyroid gland.
   a. Etiology is unknown.
2. Thyroid gland is typically enlarged and secretes greater than normal amounts of thyroid hormone (thyroxine), e.g., Graves' disease, thyroid storm, thyrotoxicosis.
3. Metabolic processes are accelerated.
4. Symptoms include nervousness, hyperreflexia, tremor, hunger, weight loss, fatigue, heat intolerance, palpitations, tachycardia, and diarrhea.
5. Treatment: antithyroid drugs.
6. Radioactive iodine may also be prescribed; surgical ablation may be necessary.

> **RED FLAG:** Can result in exercise intolerance; fatigue is associated with hypermetabolic state.

Adrenal Disorders

Primary Adrenal Insufficiency (Addison's Disease)
1. Partial or complete failure of adrenocortical function; results in decreased production of cortisol and aldosterone.
2. Etiology: autoimmune processes, infection, neoplasm, or hemorrhage.
3. Signs and symptoms.
   a. Increased bronze pigmentation of skin.
   b. Weakness, decreased endurance.
   c. Anorexia, dehydration, weight loss, gastrointestinal disturbances.
   d. Anxiety, depression.
   e. Decreased tolerance to cold.
   f. Intolerance to stress.
4. Medical interventions.
   a. Replacement therapy: glucocorticoid, adrenal corticoids.
   b. Adequate fluid intake, control of sodium and potassium.
   c. Diet high in complex carbohydrates and protein.

Secondary Adrenal Insufficiency
1. Can result from prolonged steroid therapy (ACTH); rapid withdrawal of drugs; and hypothalamic or pituitary tumors.

Cushing's Syndrome
1. Metabolic disorder resulting from chronic and excessive production of cortisol by the adrenal cortex.
2. From drug toxicity (overadministration of glucocorticoids).
3. Etiology: most common cause is a pituitary tumor with increased secretion of ACTH.
4. Signs and symptoms.
   a. Decreased glucose tolerance.
   b. Round "moon" face.
   c. Obesity: rapidly developing fat pads on chest and abdomen; buffalo hump.
   d. Decreased testosterone levels or decreased menstrual periods.
   e. Muscular atrophy.
   f. Edema.
   g. Hypokalemia.
   h. Emotional changes.
5. Medical interventions.
   a. Goal is to decrease excess ACTH: irradiation or surgical excision of pituitary tumor or control of medication levels.
   b. Monitor weight, electrolyte, and fluid balance.

Vestibular System

Overview of the Vestibular System

The vestibular system is a system of organs of the inner ear and nerves providing feedback related to the effects of gravity and movement. It is responsible for providing feedback for appropriate reactions of the eye and head in response to position changes to orient the body in space. The semicircular canals are particularly important in orienting the head and body in space. Each canal contains sensory hair cells that are activated as the fluid in the canals moves. This movement generates nerve impulses that travel along the vestibular portion of cranial nerve VIII to the brainstem and the cerebellum.

The vestibular system works together with the visual and somatosensory systems to regulate appropriate postural strategies for balance and upright postures. Improper functioning of the vestibular system can lead to balance disturbances, mild to severe nausea, complaints of dizziness (lightheaded, rocking sensation) and vertigo (feeling of movement).

Etiology

Dysfunction can occur at any age or gender. External factors that may trigger an episode may include whiplash, a fall, recent airplane flight (air pressure changes). Internal factors that may trigger an episode may include infection (vestibular neuronitis, labyrinthitis), use of medications such as sedatives or aspirin, high doses of ototoxic medication, a stroke or migraine that blocks blood flow to the inner ear. Often the underlying cause is unidentifiable.

Causes for vestibular dysregulation can be peripheral or central. Etiology may be unilateral or bilateral. See Box 6-5 Peripheral and Central Causes of Vertigo.

Characteristics

1. Dizziness: sensation of lightheadedness, faintness, or giddiness.
2. Vertigo: sensation of movement of self or objects around the person, tends to come in episodes, may be accompanied by nausea and vomiting.
3. Visual changes.
    a. Nystagmus: involuntary, cyclical movement of the eyeball, can be horizontal or rotary.
    b. Blurred vision: gaze instability secondary to dysfunction of the vestibular ocular reflex (VOR—eye movement that stabilizes images on the eye).

BOX 6-5 ▷ Peripheral and Central Causes of Vertigo

Peripheral Causes—individual will present with unilateral symptoms

- Episodic Conditions: benign positional paroxysmal vertigo (BPPV)—episode of vertigo brought on by stimulation of the vestibular sense organs (e.g., lying down or rolling over in bed, certain head positions; Meniere's disease—episodes of vertigo, hearing loss, tinnitus caused by increased volume of endolymph in semicircular canals, potentially edema of membranous labyrinth
- Space occupying lesion: cholesteatoma—cyst-like lesion filled with keratin debris, typically found in middle ear; otosclerosis—abnormal growth of bone in middle ear, acoustic neuroma, gliomas/brainstem or cerebellar meduloblastoma
- Fistula—an inappropriate opening between the middle and inner ear

Peripheral Causes—individual will present with bilateral symptoms

- Infection: Labyrinthitis—inflammation of the labyrinth organs (viral or bacterial); vestibular neuritis—inflammation of the vestibular nerve (typically viral)

Central Causes

- Neuroma: vestibular schwannoma, ependymoma, neurofibromatosis
- Disease/Condition: cerebrovascular vascular accident causing ischemia to the vertebrobasilar system; demylinazion of white matter in CNS, e.g., multiple sclerosis

4. Dysequilibrium or postural instability: dysfunction of the vestibular spinal reflex (VSR—stabilize the head and neck on the body), ataxia, gait disturbances.

Medical Evaluation and Testing

1. Eye movement: tests for eye movement and ability to focus during head movement may include electronystagmography (ENG), videostagmography (VNG), rotary-chair testing, caloric testing (flushing the ear with warm and cool water).
2. Balance testing: the vestibular evoked myogenic potential (VEMP) test is used to evaluate the saccule and inferior vestibular nerve function; balance responses may be measured using computerized dynamic posturography (CPD).
3. Neuroimaging studies may be performed if the individual presents with neurologic signs and

symptoms, or has risk factors, e.g., for cerebrovascular disease or progressive unilateral hearing loss.
4. Medical management: signs and symptoms of vertigo may be related to internal fluid levels and regulation. Medications (diuretics) may be prescribed to decrease the overall amount of fluid in the body. In addition if headaches or migraines are triggered by, or in response to vestibular disorders medications may be ordered to manage these symptoms as well.
5. Diet: dietary measures such as decreasing or eliminating salt intake can help with fluid levels in the body, thus help manage symptoms.

Physical Therapy Evaluation
1. Physical therapist diagnosis: the PT must determine if the disturbance is central or peripheral.
2. Factors indicating peripheral cause include: symptoms brought on by position changes, symptoms associated with migraine, symptoms including nausea, horizontal and rotational nystagmus that is triggered by movement (or other provocation) that disappears when the patient focuses gaze, episodic vertigo with a more sudden onset.
3. Factors indicating central cause include: nystagmus is pure horizontal or vertical or rotational and does not diminish with focusing gaze, vertigo is more long-lasting, vertigo that is accompanied by changes in motor or sensory function, weakness, vision or hearing changes.

Examination Should Include
1. History of onset to help determine type, nature, and duration of symptoms, triggering stimuli/activity.
2. Subjective assessment may include administration of the Dizziness Handicap Inventory (DHI, see description below).
3. Systems function tests: VOR—examine for saccades (jumping of the eye as it moves) or blurred vision with head and total body movements. VSR—examine posture and balance, instability in sitting and in stance, during functional and gait activities.
4. Musculoskeletal: examine upper thoracic and particularly cervical spine ROM and mobility, tissue tension in upper cervical musculature as well as suboccipital area; should include assessment of vertebral artery.
5. Current functional status: evaluate for intact vision and proprioception (especially feet and ankles) and assess any compensatory postural adjustments.
6. Standardized tests and measures for patients with dizziness and vestibular disorders.
   a. The DHI is a 25 item questionnaire to determine the individuals self-perceived level of handicap, asks questions across three domains of dizziness and unsteadiness to determine the level of functional impairment—functional, emotional, physical.
   b. The Clinical Test of Sensory Interaction for Balance (CTSIB) tests sensory interaction in balance and identifies which system the patient relies on to maintain balance. The patient is instructed to stand with feet together and arms crossed at waist and to maintain balance for 30 seconds at a time. Produces excellent test-retest as well as inter/intrarater reliability. The administrator (PT or PTA) manipulates the conditions in which the individual stands by introducing challenges:
      - Somatosensory input: assessing ability to maintain balance on different support surfaces for stance, e.g., soft foam surface or firm.
      - Visual input: assessing changes in balance based on eyes open vs. eyes closed.
      - Vestibular input: provide vestibular disturbances e.g., sway platform, dome, moving lights and objects.
7. Predictive tests (performed by MD, PT, or PTA as evaluation or as habituation treatment): the Dix-Hallpike test is helpful to predict BPPV with a positive predictive value of 83% and negative predictive value of 53% for the anterior and posterior semicircular canals. A roll test can be performed to assess the horizontal canal. If after repeated testing the patient response diminishes, the test is also indicative of peripheral vertigo, symptoms do not tend to diminish with vertigo secondary to a central cause.
   a. Dix-Hallpike maneuver is performed by the PT during evaluation of the patient and is followed by the Eply maneuver or CRT (Canalith Repositioning Technique) performed by either the PT or PTA for intervention of vertigo (Box 6-6).

Physical Therapy Goals, Outcomes, and Intervention
1. Patient comfort and safety: encourage patient to limit triggering stimuli (e.g., grocery shopping, bright lights, moving head into triggering positions, driving, walking up/down stairs), use compensatory strategies; encourage use of assistive devices if necessary for safety.
2. Perform habituation training: repetition of movements (head and body) provoking symptoms. Specific movements are identified based on the canal (anterior, horizontal, posterior) affected and are meant to "recalibrate" the system. These are part of in-clinic intervention as well as home exercise.
   a. Brandt-Daroff habituation exercise (Box 6-7): designed to stimulate specific semicircular canals by positioning the head in multiple planes. This abundance of signal (movement processing) affects the CNS in two ways. 1) The CNS must recalibrate after the CRT is performed to appropriately process

BOX 6-6 ▷ Vestibular System Test

Dix-Hallpike Test

a. Starting Position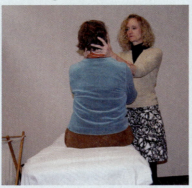

b. Ending Position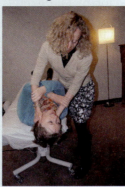

The patient begins in a sitting position facing the clinician; clinician should instruct patient this maneuver is likely to trigger vertigo. The patient turns their head to 30–45 degrees to the side being tested (a), is asked to keep eyes open and not focus on anything specific (focusing may suppress nystagmus). While holding the patients head, the clinician quickly lies the patient down into a supine position with the neck extended 20–30 degrees beyond neutral (b). After a slight latent period (2–20 seconds) clinician observes for the onset of nystagmus; a torsional nystagmus is a positive sign for BPPV with the direction of fast phase indicating side of dysfunction.

BOX 6-7 ▷ Vestibular System Exercise

Brandt-Daroff Habituation Exercises

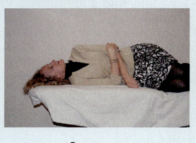 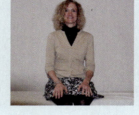 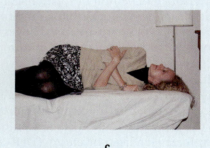

a   b   c

a. From a seated position lie down toward affected side (or as directed by PT) facing upward. Remain in this position for 30 seconds or until symptoms subside.
b. Return to a seated position for 30 seconds or until symptoms subside.
c. Lie down to opposite side facing upward. Remain in this position for 30 seconds or until symptoms subside.

the new information. 2) The CNS is desensitized to the remaining mismatch and the noxious response to the stimuli decreases.
  b. Modifications of the Brandt-Daroff exercises exist to address canalith repositioning as well.
3. Engagement of VOR and VSR: performance of activities that are designed to promote enhanced function of poorer functioning areas of the vestibular system; activities must be initiated slowly with attention to limiting severity of symptoms provoked. Activities can be part of a home or in-clinic exercise program; progress exercises from exercising one system to multisystem interaction. Example: maintain head position as performing eye movements (up-down, side-side), maintain focus on one spot as head turns standing still. Then with walking or other external movement, stand on firm surface with eyes open, then head turns, then eyes closed, then with head motions, balance ball activities, etc.
4. Address any accompanying musculoskeletal symptoms or limitations. Relaxation training may be necessary.
5. Provide psychological support and reassurance, patients may become very emotional.

Psychiatric Conditions

Psychiatric States/Mechanisms

Anxiety
1. Feelings of apprehension, worry, uneasiness; a normal reaction to tension, conflict, or stress.
2. Degree of anxiety is related to degree of perceived threat and capacity to engage behaviors that can reduce anxiety.
3. Anxiety can be constructive, stimulate an individual toward purposeful activity, or neurotic (pathological).
4. Sympathetic responses (fight or flight) generally accompany anxiety, e.g., increased heart rate, dyspnea, hyperventilation, dry mouth, GI symptoms (nausea, vomiting, diarrhea); palpitations.

Depression
1. Altered mood characterized by morbid sadness, dejection, sense of melancholy. Can be a chronic, relapsing disorder.
2. Management.
   a. Treatment is pharmacological: tricyclic antidepressant drugs.

   RED FLAG: Patients on these medications may exhibit disturbed balance, postural hypotension, falls and fractures, increased HR, dysrhythmias, ataxia, seizures.

   b. Cognitive therapy may help.
3. Physical therapy interventions.
   a. Maintain a positive attitude, consistently demonstrate warmth and interest.
   b. Acknowledge depression, provide hope.
   c. Use positive reinforcement, build in successful treatment experiences.
   d. Involve the patient in treatment decisions.
   e. Avoid excessive cheerfulness.
   f. Take all suicidal thoughts and acts seriously.

Coping and Adapting Mechanisms
1. Typically unconscious behaviors by which the individual resolves or conceals conflicts or anxieties.
2. Compensation: covering up a weakness by stressing a desirable or strong trait, e.g., a learning disabled child becomes an outstanding athlete.
3. Denial: refusal to recognize reality, e.g., refusal to acknowledge a fatal disease.
4. Repression: refusal or inability to recall undesirable past thoughts or events.
5. Displacement: the transferring of an emotion to a less dangerous substitute, e.g., yelling at your child instead of your boss.
6. Reaction formation: a defensive reaction in which behavior is exactly opposite what is expected, e.g., a messy individual becomes neat.
7. Projection: the attributing of your own undesirable behavior to another, e.g., "He made me do it."
8. Rationalization: the justification of behaviors using reasons other than the real reason, e.g., presenting an attitude of not caring.
9. Regression: resorting to an earlier, more immature pattern of functioning, e.g., in traumatic brain injury; common under high stress situations.

General Adaptation Syndrome (GAS)
1. Total body coping/adaptation to a catastrophic event (illness, trauma).
2. Alarm stage, or "fight-or-flight" response: activation of the sympathetic system.
3. Sustained resistance.
4. Chronic resistance, exhaustion leading to stress-related illnesses.

Pathologies

Anxiety Disorders (Anxiety Neurosis)
1. Excessive anxiety not associated with realistically threatening specific situations, e.g., generalized anxiety.
2. Panic attacks: acute, intense anxiety or terror; may be uncontrollable, accompanied by sympathetic signs, loss of mental control, sense of impending death.
3. Phobias: excessive and unreasonable fear leads to avoidance behaviors, e.g., agoraphobia (fear of being alone or in public places).
4. Obsessive-compulsive behavior: persistent anxiety is manifested by repetitive, stereotypic acts; behaviors interfere with social functioning, e.g., hand washing, counting, and touching.

Posttraumatic Stress Disorder (PTSD)
1. Exposure to a traumatic event produces a variety of stress-related symptoms.
2. PTSD symptoms.
   a. Reexperiencing the traumatic event.
   b. Psychic numbing with reduced responsiveness.
   c. Detachment from the external world; survival guilt.
   d. Exaggerated autonomic arousal, hyperalertness.

    e. Disturbed sleeping.
    f. Ongoing irritability.
    g. Impaired memory and concentration.
3. PTSD can be acute (symptoms last <3 months) or chronic (3 months or longer); onset can also be delayed.
4. Symptoms should not be ignored. A mental health consultation is indicated.

Psychosomatic Disorders (Somatoform Disorders)

1. Physical signs or diseases that are related to emotional causes, e.g., psychosocial stress.
2. Characteristics.
    a. Cannot be explained by identifiable disease process or underlying pathology.
    b. Not under voluntary control; provides a means of coping with anxiety and stress.
    c. Patient is frequently indifferent to symptoms.
3. Types.
    a. Conversion disorder (hysterical paralysis): loss of or altered physical functioning representing psychosocial conflict or need, e.g., can result in paralysis, hemiplegia.
    b. Hypochondria: abnormal or heightened concerns about health or body functions; false beliefs about suffering from some disease or condition.
4. Management.
    a. Physical symptoms are real: treat the patient as you would any other patient with similar symptoms.
    b. Provide a supportive environment.
    c. Identify primary gain (internal conflicts); assist patient in learning new, alternative methods of stress management.
    d. Identify secondary gains (additional advantages, e.g., attention, sympathy); do not reinforce.
    e. Provide encouragement and support for the total person.

Schizophrenia

1. A group of disorders characterized by disruptions in thought patterns; of unknown etiology; a biochemical imbalance in the brain.
2. Symptoms.
    a. Disordered thinking: fragmented thoughts, errors of logic, delusions, poor judgment, memory.
    b. Disordered speech: may be coherent but unintelligible, incoherent, or mute.
    c. Disordered perception: hallucinations and delusions.
    d. Inappropriateness of affect: withdrawal of interest from other people and from the outside world; loss of self-identity, self-direction; disordered interpersonal relations.
    e. Functional disturbances: inability to function in daily life, work.
    f. Little insight into problems and behavior.
3. Paranoia: a type of schizophrenic disorder characterized by feelings of extreme suspiciousness, persecution, grandiosity (feelings of power or great wealth), or jealousy; withdrawal of all emotional contact with others.
4. Catatonia: a type of schizophrenic disorder characterized by mutism or stupor; unresponsiveness; catatonic posturing (remains fixed, unable to move or talk for extended periods).

Bipolar Disorder (Manic-Depressive Illness)

1. A disorder characterized by mood swings from depression to mania; a biochemical dysfunction.
2. Often intense outbursts, high energy and activity, excessive euphoria, decreased need for sleep, unrealistic beliefs, distractibility, poor judgment, denial.
3. Followed by extreme depression (see depression symptoms).
4. Treatment is pharmacological, e.g., lithium carbonate.

Perseveration

1. The continued repetition of a movement, word, or expression, e.g., patient gets stuck and repeats the same activity over and over again; often accompanies traumatic brain injury or stroke.

Grief Process

Grief

1. Emotional process by which an individual deals with loss, e.g., loss of a significant other, body part, or function.

Characteristics

1. Somatic symptoms: e.g., fatigue, sighing, hyperventilation, anorexia, insomnia.
2. Psychological symptoms: e.g., sorrow, discomfort, regret, guilt, anger, irritability, depression.
3. Resolution may take months or years.

Stages

1. Shock and disbelief; inability to comprehend loss.
2. Increased awareness and anguish; crying or anger is common.
3. Mourning.
4. Resolution of loss.
5. Idealization of lost person or function.

Management

1. Provide support and understanding of the grief process.
2. Encourage expression of feelings, memories.
3. Respect privacy, cultural, or religious customs.

Death and Dying

Characteristics
1. Decreasing physical and mental functioning, gradual loss of consciousness.

Stages (Kübler-Ross)
1. Denial: patients insist they are fine, joke about themselves, are not motivated to participate in treatment.
    a. Allow denial: denial is a protective compensatory mechanism necessary until such time as the patient is ready to face his/her illness.
    b. Provide opportunities for patient to question, confront illness and impending death.
2. Anger, resentment: patients may become disruptive, blame others.
    a. Be supportive: allow patient to express anger, frustration, resentment.
    b. Encourage focus on coping strategies.
3. Bargaining: patients bargain for time to complete life tasks; turn to religion or other individuals, make promises in return for function.
    a. Provide accurate information, honest, truthful answers.
4. Depression: patients acknowledge impending death, withdraw from life; demonstrate an overwhelming sense of loss, low motivation.
    a. Observe closely for suicidal ideation.
    b. Allay fears and anxieties, especially loneliness and isolation.
    c. Assist in providing for comfort of the patient.
5. Acceptance and preparation for death: acceptance of their condition; relate more to their family, make plans for the future.

Management
1. Support patient and family during each stage.
2. Maintain hope without supporting unrealistic expectations.

Interventions

Physical Therapist Assistant's Role
1. Motivate patients, manage the human side of rehabilitation.
2. Establish boundaries of the professional relationship: identify problems, expectations, purpose, roles, and responsibilities.
3. Provide empathic understanding: the capacity to understand what your patient is experiencing from that patient's perspective.
    a. Recognize losses; allow opportunity to mourn "old self."
    b. Ask open-ended questions that reflect what the patient is feeling.
        - Empathetic response; e.g., "It sounds like you are worried and anxious about your pain and are trying your best."
        - Nonempathetic response; e.g., "Don't worry about your pain" or "You're overreacting."
    c. Sympathy is not helpful or therapeutic; care-giver is closely affected by the patient's behaviors, e.g., therapist cries when the patient cries.
4. Set realistic, meaningful goals; involve the patient and family in the goal-setting process; self-determination is important.
5. Set realistic time frames for the rehabilitation program; recognize symptoms, stages of the grief process, or death and dying and adjust accordingly.
6. Recognize and reinforce healthy, positive, socially appropriate behaviors; allow the patient to experience success.
7. Recognize secondary gains, unacceptable behaviors; do not reinforce (e.g., malingering behaviors such as avoidance of work).
8. Provide an environment conducive to the patient's emotional state, learning, and optimal function.
    a. Provide a message of hope tempered with realism.
    b. Keep patients informed.
    c. Lay adequate groundwork or preparation for expected changes or discharge.
    d. Help to reestablish personal dignity and self-worth; acknowledge whole person.
9. Help patients identify feelings, successful coping strategies, recognize successful conflict resolution, and rehabilitation gains.
    a. Stress ability to overcome major obstacles.
    b. Stress that recovery is unique and highly individual.

Review Questions

Other Systems

1. Name the primary immune and helper cells the body deploys in reaction to infectious agents. How are these affected when an individual has an immune deficient disease?

2. Identify secondary infections or complications that may be a result of the compromised immune system of a patient who has acquired immunodeficiency syndrome.

3. Describe the clinical presentation/characteristics of a patient with chronic fatigue versus fibromyalgia syndrome. Describe physical therapy intervention for each.

4. Compare the mode of transmission and protective measures for norovirus, hepatitis A, and measles.

5. Describe physical therapy management for the conditions of sacroiliac dysfunction, varicose veins, and post-cesarean childbirth.

6. What is the difference between stress, urge, and functional incontinence? Describe different methods of management of incontinence.

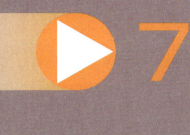

7

Integumentary Physical Therapy

SUSAN B. O'SULLIVAN and LAURA A. SAGE

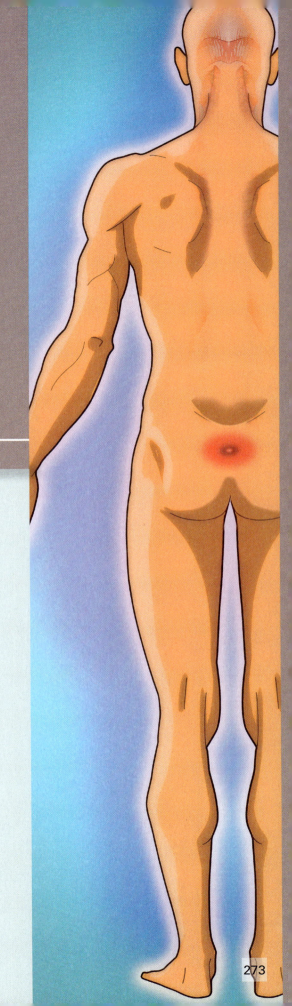

Chapter Outline

- Integumentary System, 275
  - Skin or Integument, 275
  - Circulation, 275
- Conditions/Pathology/Diseases with Intervention, 276
  - Dermatitis (Eczema), 276
  - Medical Management, 276
  - Bacterial Infections, 276
  - Viral Infections, 276
  - Other Infections, 277
  - Parasitic Infections, 278
  - Immune Disorders of the Skin, 278
  - Skin Cancer, 279
  - Skin Trauma, 280
- Physical Therapy Examination and Data Collection, 280
  - Role of the PTA, 280
  - Tissue Assessment, 280
  - Other Systems, 281

- Physical Therapy Intervention for Impaired Integumentary Integrity, 283
  - Interventions, 283
- Burns, 284
  - Pathophysiology, 284
  - Complications of Burn Injury, 284
  - Burn Healing, 285
  - Burn Management, 285
  - Medical Management, 285
  - Physical Therapy Goals, Outcomes, and Interventions, 286
- Skin Ulcers, 287
  - Venous Ulcer (also known as Stasis Ulcers), 287
  - Arterial Ulcer, 288
  - Diabetic Ulcer, 288
  - Pressure Injury (also known as Decubitus Ulcer or Bed Sore), 288
  - Assessment of Wounds, 289
  - Wound Care, 291
- Review Questions, 296

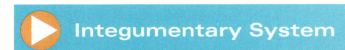
Integumentary System

Skin or Integument

External Covering of the Body
1. It is recognized as the largest organ system of the human body and accounts for approximately 15–20% of the body weight.
2. It is arranged in layers. See Table 7-1.

Functions of Skin
1. Protection of underlying body structures against injury or invasion.
2. Insulation of body.
3. Maintenance of homeostasis: fluid balance, regulation of body temperature.
4. Aids in elimination: small amounts of urea and salt are excreted in sweat.
5. Synthesizes vitamin D.
6. Receptors in dermis give rise to cutaneous sensations.

Appendages of the Skin
1. Hair.
   a. Terminal hair: coarse, thick, pigmented; e.g., scalp, eyebrows.
   b. Vellus hair: short, fine; e.g., arms, chest.
2. Nails: nail plate, lunula (whitish moon), proximal nail fold/cuticle, lateral nail folds.

Table 7-1

Layers of Skin	
Epidermis	Outer, most superficial layer; contains no blood vessels
	Composed of two layers of stratified epithelium:
	1. Stratum corneum is outermost, horny layer, composed of nonliving cells
	2. Stratum lucidum, composed of living cells; produces melanin responsible for skin color
Dermis (corium)	Inner layer composed primarily of collagen and elastin fibrous connective tissues
	Mucopolysaccharide matrix and elastin fibers provide elasticity, strength to skin
	Contains lymphatics, blood vessels, nerves and nerve endings, sebaceous and sweat glands
Subcutaneous tissues	Underneath dermis
	Consists of loose connective and fat tissues
	Provides insulation, support, and cushion for skin; stores energy for skin
	Muscles and fascia lie underneath subcutaneous layer

3. Sebaceous glands: secrete fatty substance through hair follicles; on all skin surfaces except palms and soles.
4. Sweat glands.
   a. Eccrine glands: widely distributed, open on skin; help control body temperature.
   b. Apocrine glands: found in axillary and genital areas, open into hair follicles; stimulated by emotional stress.

Circulation

Blood Flow to Capillaries of the Skin
1. Increased blood flow with an increase in oxyhemoglobin to skin capillaries causes reddening of the skin.
2. Peripheral cyanosis is due to reduced blood flow to skin and loss of oxygen to tissues (changes to deoxyhemoglobin) and results in a darker, somewhat blue color.
3. Central cyanosis is due to reduced oxygen level in the blood; causes include advanced lung disease, congenital heart disease, and abnormal hemoglobins.

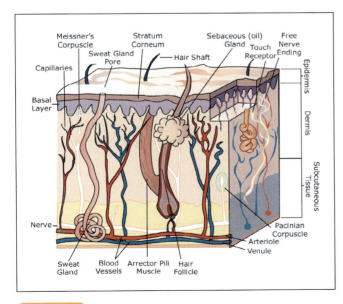

Figure 7-1 Cross-section of the skin.

Conditions/Pathology/Diseases with Intervention

Dermatitis (Eczema)

Inflammation
1. Causes itching, redness, skin lesions.

Etiology
1. Allergic or contact dermatitis; e.g., poison ivy, harsh soaps, chemicals, adhesive tape.
2. Actinic: photosensitivity, reaction to sunlight, ultraviolet.
3. Atopic: etiology unknown, associated with allergic, hereditary, or psychological disorders.

Stages
1. Acute: red, oozing, crusting rash; extensive erosions, exudate, pruritic vesicles.
2. Subacute: erythematous skin, scaling, scattered plaques.
3. Chronic: thickened skin, increased skin marking secondary to scratching; fibrotic papules, and nodules; postinflammatory pigmentation changes. Course can be relapsing.

Precautions or CONTRAINDICATIONS
1. Some physical therapy modalities (e.g., paraffin and electrical stimulation).
2. Avoid use of alcohol.

Daily Care
1. Includes hydration and lubrication of skin.

Medical Management
1. Aimed at inflammation. Topical or systemic therapy.

Bacterial Infections

Entry Point(s)
1. Bacteria enter the body through portals in the skin; e.g., abrasions or puncture wounds.

Impetigo
1. Superficial skin infection caused by staphylococci or streptococci.
2. Associated with inflammation, small pus-filled vesicles, itching.
3. Contagious; common in children and the elderly.

Cellulitis
1. Suppurative inflammation of cellular or connective tissue in or close to the skin.
2. Tends to be poorly defined and widespread.
3. Streptococcal or staphylococcal infection common; can be contagious.
4. Skin is hot, red, and edematous.
5. Management: antibiotics; elevation of the part; cool, wet dressings.
6. If untreated, lymphangitis, gangrene, abscess, and sepsis can occur.
7. The elderly and individuals with diabetes, wounds, malnutrition, or on steroid therapy are at increased risk.

Abscess
1. A cavity containing pus and surrounded by inflamed tissue.
2. The result of a localized infection.
3. Commonly a staphylococcal infection.
4. Healing typically facilitated by draining or incising the abscess.

Viral Infections

Warts

> **RED FLAG**: Common, benign infection by human papilloma viruses (HPVs). May be contagious, use skin care precautions.

1. Transmission is through direct contact; autoinoculation is possible.
2. Common warts: on skin, especially hands and fingers.
3. Plantar wart: on pressure points of feet.
4. Management: cryotherapy, acids, electrodessication, and curettage; over-the-counter medications.

Herpes Infections
1. See Quick Facts 7-1.

Herpes Zoster (Shingles)
1. Caused by varicella-zoster virus (chickenpox); reactivation of virus lying dormant in cerebral ganglia or ganglia of posterior nerve roots.
2. Pain and tingling affecting spinal or cranial nerve dermatome; progresses to red papules along distribution of infected nerve; red papules progressing to vesicles develop along a dermatome.

QUICK FACTS 7-1 ▶ HERPES INFECTIONS

	Herpes Simplex Virus Type-1	Herpes Simplex Virus Type-2	Herpes Zoster (Shingles)
Causes Persons become more susceptible with general illness, fatigue, immunosuppression, trauma to area	Exposure to virus through casual contact, e.g., sharing lip balm or eating utensils	Exposure to virus through sexual contact	Reactivation of varicella-zoster virus (chickenpox), which was lying dormant in cerebral ganglia or ganglia of posterior nerve roots
Transmission	Oral–oral contact, saliva contact. Can be spread even when sores are not present	Sexual contact. Can be spread even when sores are not present	Virus is spread through direct contact with fluid from rash blisters. Note: A person with a shingles rash in the blister phase is infectious. Not infectious before blister phase and after rash crusts
Presentation	Itching and soreness, cold sore, fever blister	Vesicular genital blisters or sores (called ulcers)	Pain and tingling blisters or rash affecting spinal or cranial nerve dermatome. Red papules on skin surface along affected nerve, dermatome
Complications	Severe immunocompromise may cause more severe symptoms, rarely resulting in encephalitis or keratitis	In newborns: may cause meningo-encephalitis; can be fatal. Increases risk of acquiring new HIV infection. Severe immunocompromise may cause more severe symptoms, rarely resulting in meningoencephalitis, esophagitis, hepatitis, pneumonitis	Ocular complications with cranial nerve (CN) III involvement: eye pain, corneal damage; loss of vision with CN V involvement. Postherpetic neuralgic pain: may be intermittent or constant; lasts weeks; occasionally, intractable pain lasts months or years. Can cause birth defects in certain trimesters
Treatment	No cure; antiviral medications (cream, pills, or shot) used to shorten healing time		Prevention: Adults who have never had chickenpox should be vaccinated. No curative agent; antiviral drugs slow progression. Symptomatic treatment for itching and pain; e.g., systemic corticosteroids

3. Usually accompanied by fever, chills, malaise, gastrointestinal (GI) disturbances.
4. Ocular complications with cranial nerve (CN) III involvement: eye pain, corneal damage; loss of vision with CN V involvement.
5. Postherpetic neuralgic pain: may be intermittent or constant; lasts weeks; occasionally, intractable pain lasts months or years.
6. Management: no curative agent, antiviral drugs slow progression; symptomatic treatment for itching and pain; e.g., systemic corticosteroids.

RED FLAGS:
- Contagious to individuals who have not had chickenpox.
- Heat or ultrasound contraindicated: can increase severity of symptoms.

Other Infections

Ringworm (Tinea Corporis)
1. Fungal infection involving the hair, skin, or nails.
2. Forms scaly, crusted rash, which often appears in ring-shaped patches on the skin.
3. Itchy; transmission is through direct contact.
4. Treated with topical or oral antifungal drugs (e.g., griseofulvin). See Quick Facts 7-2.

Athlete's Foot (Tinea Pedis)
1. Fungal infection of foot, typically between the toes.
2. Causes erythema, inflammation, pruritus, itching, and pain.
3. Treated with antifungal creams.
4. Can progress to bacterial infections, cellulitis if untreated.

QUICK FACTS 7-2 ▶ PARASITIC AND FUNGAL INFECTIONS

FUNGAL INFECTIONS

Condition	Cause/Presentation	Treatment	Transmission
Ringworm (tinea corporis)	Ring-shaped patches with vesicles or scales	Topical or oral antifungal drugs	Through direct contact
Athlete's foot (tinea pedis)	Fungal infection of foot, typically between the toes	Antifungal creams	Person-to-person or animal-to-person

PARASITIC INFECTIONS

Condition	Cause/Presentation	Treatment	Transmission
Scabies (mites)	Inflammation, itching due to burrowing of mites under skin	Scabicide ointment	Insect and animal contacts
Lice (pediculosis)	Bite marks, redness	Special soap or shampoo	Person-to-person or sexually transmitted

Transmission
1. Person-to-person or animal-to-person.
2. Observe standard precautions (see Box 6-1).

Parasitic Infections

Cause
1. Caused or transmitted by insect and animal contacts.

Scabies (Mites)
1. Burrow into skin, causing inflammation, itching, and possibly pruritus.
2. Treated with scabicide.

Lice (Pediculosis)
1. A parasite that can affect head, body, and genital area with bite marks, redness, and nits.
2. Treatment with special soap or shampoo.

Transmission
1. Person-to-person or sexually transmitted.
2. Avoid direct contact; observe standard precautions.

Immune Disorders of the Skin

Psoriasis
1. Chronic disease of skin characterized by erythematous plaques covered with a silvery scale; common on ears, scalp, knees, elbows, and genitalia.
2. Common complaints: itching and pain from dry, cracked lesions.
3. Variable course: exacerbations and remissions are common.
4. May be associated with psoriatic arthritis, joint pain, particularly of small distal joints.
5. Etiological factors: hereditary, associated immune disorders, certain drugs.
6. Precipitating factors: trauma, infection, pregnancy and endocrine changes; cold weather, smoking, anxiety, and stress.
7. Management: no cure; topical preparations (corticosteroids, occlusive ointments, coal tar); systemic drugs (methotrexate).
8. Physical therapy intervention: long-wave ultraviolet (UV) light; combination UV light with oral photosensitizing drugs (psoralens).

Lupus Erythematosus
1. Chronic, progressive inflammatory disorder of connective tissues; characteristic red rash with raised, red, scaly plaques.
2. Discoid lupus erythematosus (DLE): affects only skin; flare-ups with sun exposure; lesions can resolve or cause atrophy, permanent scarring, hypopigmentation, or hyperpigmentation.
3. Systemic lupus erythematosus (SLE): chronic, systemic inflammatory disorder affecting multiple organ systems, including skin, joints, kidneys, heart, nervous system, mucous membranes; can be fatal; commonly affects young women. Symptoms can include fever, malaise, characteristic butterfly rash across bridge of nose, skin lesions, chronic fatigue, arthralgia, arthritis, skin rashes, photosensitivity, anemia, hair loss, Raynaud's phenomenon.
4. Management: no cure; topical treatment of skin lesions (corticosteroid creams); salicylates, or indomethacin with fever and joint pain; immunosuppressive agents (cytotoxic agents) with life-threatening disease.
5. Observe for side effects of corticosteroids: edema, weight gain, acne, hypertension, bruising, purplish stretch marks; long-term use of corticosteroids is

QUICK FACTS 7-3 ▶ PHYSICAL THERAPY INTERVENTIONS FOR IMMUNE DISORDERS OF THE SKIN

Condition	Interventions	Complications and Special Considerations
Psoriasis	Long-wave ultraviolet light (UV) UV in combination with oral photosensitizing drugs (psoralens)	Consider pain level
Systemic lupus erythematosus (SLE)	Medical management includes: • Topical treatments (ointment) • Medications for pain, fever	Observe for side effects of corticosteroids Patient/client may be immunosuppressed
Scleroderma	Physical therapy interventions to slow development of contracture and deformity Medical management includes corticosteroids, vasodilators, analgesics, immunosuppressive agents	Use caution with sclerosed skin: may be sensitive to pressure Acute hypertension may occur; stress regular blood pressure checks

associated with increased susceptibility to infection (immunosuppressed patient); osteoporosis, myopathy, tendon rupture, diabetes, gastric irritation, low potassium (see Quick Facts 7-3).

Scleroderma
1. Chronic, diffuse disease of connective tissues causing fibrosis of skin, joints, blood vessels, and internal organs (GI tract, lungs, heart, kidneys). Usually accompanied by Raynaud's phenomenon. Progressive systemic sclerosis (PSS) is a relatively rare autoimmune form.
2. Skin is taut, firm, edematous, firmly bound to subcutaneous tissues.
3. Limited disease/skin thickening: symmetrical skin involvement of distal extremities and face; slow progression of skin changes; late visceral involvement.
4. Diffuse disease/skin thickening: symmetrical, widespread skin involvement of distal and proximal extremities, face, trunk; rapid progression of skin changes with early appearance of visceral involvement.
5. Management: no specific therapy; supportive therapy can include corticosteroids, vasodilators, analgesics, immunosuppressive agents.
6. Physical therapy slows development of contracture and deformity.
7. Precautions with sclerosed skin, sensitive to pressure; acute hypertension may occur, stress regular blood pressure checks.

Polymyositis (PM)
1. A disease of connective tissue characterized by edema, inflammation, and degeneration of the muscles; dermatitis is associated with some forms.
2. Affects primarily proximal muscles: shoulder and pelvic girdles, neck, pharynx; symmetrical distribution.
3. Etiology unknown; autoimmune reaction affecting muscle tissue with degeneration and regeneration, fiber atrophy; inflammatory infiltrates.
4. Rapid, severe onset: may require ventilatory assistance, tube feeding.
5. Cardiac involvement: may be fatal.
6. Management: medication (corticosteroids and immunosuppressants).
7. Precautions: additional muscle fiber damage with too much exercise; contractures and pressure ulcers from inactivity, prolonged bed rest.

Skin Cancer

Benign Tumors
1. Seborrheic keratosis: proliferation of basal cells leading to raised lesions, typically multiple lesions on trunk of older individuals; untreated unless causing irritation, pain; can be removed with cryotherapy.
2. Actinic keratosis: flat, round or irregular lesions, covered by dry scale on sun-exposed skin. Precancerous: can lead to squamous cell carcinoma.
3. Common mole (benign nevus): proliferation of melanocytes, round or oval shape, sharply defined borders, uniform color, <6 mm, flat or raised. Can change into melanoma: signs include new swelling, redness, scaling, oozing, or bleeding.

Malignant Tumors
1. Basal cell carcinoma: slow-growing epithelial basal cell tumor, characterized by raised patch with ivory appearance; has rolled border with indented center. Rarely metastasizes, common on face in fair-skinned individuals. Associated with prolonged sun exposure.
2. Squamous cell carcinoma: has poorly defined margins; presents as a flat red area, ulcer, or nodule. Grows more quickly, common on sun-exposed areas,

Table 7-2

Clinical Examination of Malignant Melanoma "ABCDEs"	
Asymmetry	Uneven edges, lopsided
Border	Irregular, poorly defined edges, notching
Color	Variations, especially mixtures of black, blue, or red
Diameter	Larger than 6 mm
Evolution	Change in appearance over time

face and neck, back of hand. Can be confined (in situ) or invasive to surrounding tissues; can metastasize.
3. Malignant melanoma: tumor arising from melanocytes (cells that produce melanin); superficial spreading melanoma (SSM) most common type.
   a. Clinical manifestations of melanoma (see Table 7-2).
   b. Melanoma risk factors: family history, intense year-round sun exposure, fair skin and freckles, nevi that are changing or atypical, especially if >50.
   c. Lesions may have swelling or redness beyond the border, oozing or bleeding, or sensations of itching, burning, or pain.

RED FLAG: Suspicious lesions should be referred to a dermatologist for further evaluation and biopsy. Treatment is surgical resection. Prognosis depends on extent of invasion.

4. Kaposi's sarcoma (KS): lesions of endothelial cell origin with red or dark purple/blue macules that progress to nodules or ulcers; associated with itching and pain.
   a. Common on lower extremities; may involve internal structures producing lymphatic obstruction.
   b. Increased incidence in individuals of central European descent and with AIDS-associated immunodeficiency.

Skin Trauma

1. Contusion.
   a. Injury in which skin is not broken; a bruise.
   b. Characterized by pain, swelling, and discoloration.
   c. Immediate application of cold may limit effects.
2. Ecchymosis.
   a. Bluish discoloration of skin caused by extravasation of blood into the subcutaneous tissues.
   b. The result of trauma to underlying blood vessels or fragile vessel walls.
3. Petechiae.
   a. Tiny red or purple hemorrhagic spots on the skin.
4. Abrasion.
   a. Scraping away of skin due to injury or mechanical abrasion (e.g., dermabrasion).
5. Laceration.
   a. An irregular tear of the skin that produces a torn, jagged wound.

Physical Therapy Examination and Data Collection

Role of the PTA

Review Patient History
1. Age, sex, race/ethnicity, social/health habits, work, living, general health status, medical/surgical, nutritional status.

Observe
1. Be aware of changes in the appearance of tissues over the course of working with patients or clients.
2. Report changes (as appropriate) to supervising physical therapist.

Tissue Assessment

PTA Responsibilities
1. The physical therapist assistant should understand skin conditions and the possible causes of such skin conditions.
2. The physical therapist assistant is responsible for monitoring skin conditions and reporting changes (as appropriate) to supervising physical therapist.

Techniques for Tissue Inspection
1. Include: observation, palpation, photographic assessment, and thermography.

Inspect Tissues for
1. Presence of lesions, unusual growths.
   a. Determine/document anatomical location and distribution; i.e., generalized or localized, exposed or non-exposed surface, symmetrical or asymmetrical.
   b. Type.
      - Flat spot: macule (small, up to 1 cm), patch (1 cm or greater).
      - Palpable elevated solid mass: papule (small, up to 1 cm), plaque (elevated, 1 cm or larger), nodule (marble-like lesion), wheal (irregular, localized skin edema; e.g., hives).
      - Elevated lesions with fluid cavities: vesicle (up to 1 cm, contains serous fluid; e.g., herpes simplex); bulla or blister (1 cm or larger, contains serous fluid; e.g., second-degree burn); pustule (contains pus; e.g., acne).
   c. Color.
   d. See Table 7-3 for description of different skin conditions.

Other Systems

Body Composition
1. Height, weight.
2. Body mass index; skinfold thickness.

Circulation (Arterial, Venous, Lymphatic)
1. Heart rate, rhythm, sounds.
2. Blood pressures and flow.
3. Superficial vascular responses.

Respiratory
1. Respiratory rate.
2. Respiratory pattern.

Sensory
1. Superficial sensations: sharp/dull discrimination, temperature, light touch, pressure.
2. Deep sensations: proprioception, kinesthesis.
3. Pain and soreness.

Musculoskeletal
1. Gross range of motion (ROM) including muscle length.
2. Gross strength.

Neuromuscular
1. Coordination.
2. Gait, locomotion, balance.

Functional
1. Activities, positions, postures that produce or reduce trauma to skin.
2. Safety during functional activities.
3. Assistive, adaptive, protective, orthotic, or prosthetic devices that produce or reduce skin trauma.
4. Likelihood of trauma to skin.

Table 7-3

Skin Conditions and Descriptions

CONDITION	PRESENTATION	POTENTIALLY INDICATIVE OF	INSPECTION/MEASUREMENT
Pruritus	Itching	Diabetes Drug hypersensitivity Hyperthyroidism	Observation
Urticaria	Smooth, red, elevated patches of skin, hives	Allergic response to drugs or infection	Observation
Rash	Local redness and eruption on the skin, typically accompanied by itching, inflammation, and skin irritation	Skin diseases, chronic alcoholism, vasomotor disturbances, pyrexia, and medications; e.g., diaper rash, heat rash, drug rash.	Observation
Xeroderma	Excessive dryness of skin with shedding of epithelium	Deficiency of thyroid function, diabetes	
Edema	Increased girth, may be soft (pitting) or firm	Anemia, venous or lymphatic obstruction, inflammation; cardiac, circulatory, or renal decompensation.	Determine activities and postures that aggravate or relieve edema. Palpation, volume, and girth measurements

(Continued)

Table 7-3

Skin Conditions and Descriptions (*Continued*)

CONDITION	PRESENTATION	POTENTIALLY INDICATIVE OF	INSPECTION/MEASUREMENT
Changes in nails	Clubbing: thickened and rounded nail end with spongy proximal fold White spots seen with trauma to nails	Chronic hypoxia secondary to heart disease, lung disease or cancer, cirrhosis, inflammatory bowel disease, liver disease, AIDS	Condition is observed visually Measured in grades and determined by amount of fluctuation of the nail bed
Changes in skin pigmentation, tissue mobility, skin turgor, and texture	Wrinkling dehydration Blistering	May be due to aging or prolonged immersion in water (maceration) Pressure, rubbing	Observe for source of moisture (i.e., drainage, incontinence) or pressure/rubbing (i.e., shoes that are too tight)
Changes in skin color	Cherry red	Indicative of carbon monoxide poisoning	
	Cyanosis: slightly bluish, grayish, slate-colored discoloration	Lack of oxygen (hemoglobin); can indicate congestive heart failure, advanced lung disease, congenital heart disease, venous obstruction	Examine lips, oral mucosa, tongue for blue color (central causes) or nails, hands, feet (peripheral causes).
	Pallor (lack of color, paleness)	Anemia, internal hemorrhage, lack of exposure to sunlight. Temporary pallor seen with arterial insufficiency and syncope, chills, shock, vasomotor instability, or nervousness	Take vital signs.
	Yellow (jaundice)	Liver disease	Look for yellow color in sclera of eyes, lips, skin. With increased carotene intake (carotenemia), look for yellow color of palms, soles, and face.
	Liver spots: brownish yellow spots	Aging, uterine and liver malignancies, pregnancy	
	Brown (Hemosiderin staining)	Venous insufficiency	Edema, increased firmness of skin
Changes in skin temperature	Warmer or cooler than other side or surrounding skin	Abnormal heat can indicate febrile condition, hyperthyroidism, mental excitement, excessive salt intake	Examine with backs of fingers for generalized warmth or coolness.
	Correlate with internal temperature, unless skin is exposed to local heat or cold	Abnormal cold can indicate poor circulation or obstruction; e.g., vasomotor spasm, venous or arterial thrombosis, hypothyroidism	Examine temperature of reddened areas: local warmth may indicate inflammation or cellulitis.
Hidrosis	Moist skin (hyperhidrosis)	Increased perspiration: can indicate fevers, pneumonic crisis, drugs, hot drinks, exercise	May be measured by provider or researcher; it is not applicable for physical therapy measurement
	Dry skin (hypohidrosis)	Can indicate dehydration, ichthyosis, or hypothyroidism	
	Cold sweats	Great fear, anxiety, depression, or disease (AIDS)	
Changes in hair	Alopecia: hair loss	Hypothyroidism: thinning hair; hyperthyroidism sees silky hair	Examine quality, texture, distribution.

Physical Therapy Intervention for Impaired Integumentary Integrity

Interventions

Plan of Care
1. Physical therapist–directed interventions found within the plan of care will typically follow the Preferred Practice Patterns for the Integument. See Table 7-4.

Patient/Client-related Instruction
1. Enhance disease awareness, healthy behaviors.
2. Assist patient to avoid harsh soaps, known irritants, temperature extremes, exacerbating factors, or triggers.
3. Enhance activities of daily living (ADLs), functional mobility, and safety.
4. Enhance self-management of symptoms.

Infection
1. See Box 6-1 for infection control practices.

Therapeutic Exercise
1. Strengthening and ROM exercises.
2. Aerobic conditioning.
3. Body mechanics, postural awareness training.
4. Gait, locomotion, and balance training.
5. Aquatic therapy.

Functional Training
1. ADL training (basic and instrumental).
2. Activity pacing and energy conservation; stress management.
3. Skin and joint protection techniques.
4. Instruction in safe use of assistive and adaptive devices.
5. Prescription, application, and training in use of orthotic, protective, or supportive devices.

Tissue Congestion
1. See Chapter 4 for descriptions of manual lymphatic drainage and therapeutic massage.

Wounds
1. See wound care section and Table 7-7 for dressings and topical agents used to manage.

Electrotherapeutic Modalities
1. Electrical muscle stimulation (EMS). See Chapter 10 for further description.
2. High-voltage pulsed current (HVPC).
3. Transcutaneous electrical nerve stimulation (TENS): relief of pain.
4. Sound agents: ultrasound, phonophoresis.
5. Hydrotherapy: aquatic therapy, whirlpool tanks.
6. Light agents: ultraviolet.
7. Mechanical modalities: compression therapies.

Table 7-4

Preferred Practice Patterns: Integumentary	
PATTERN 7A	Primary Prevention/Risk Reduction for Integumentary Disorders
PATTERN 7B	Impaired Integumentary Integrity Associated with Superficial Skin Involvement
PATTERN 7C	Impaired Integumentary Integrity Associated with Partial-Thickness Skin Involvement and Scar Formation
PATTERN 7D	Impaired Integumentary Integrity Associated with Full-Thickness Skin Involvement and Scar Formation
PATTERN 7E	Impaired Integumentary Integrity Associated with Skin Involvement Extending into Fascia, Muscle, or Bone and Scar Formation

From: Practice Patterns. American Physical Therapy Association, 2014.
Note: On the APTA website, each practice pattern includes:
- Inclusion criteria: risk factors or consequences of pathology/pathophysiology, impairments of body functions and structures, activity limitations, or participation restrictions
- Exclusion or Multiple-Pattern Classification
- Examination: relevant tests and measures
- Evaluation, Diagnosis and Prognosis (including Plan of Care) factors
- Intervention categories

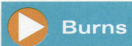

Burns

Pathophysiology

Burn Injury
1. Results from thermal, chemical, electrical, or radioactive agents.
2. Burn wound, consists of three zones.
   a. Zone of coagulation: cells are irreversibly injured, cell death occurs.
   b. Zone of stasis: cells are injured; may die without specialized treatment, usually within 24–48 hours.
   c. Zone of hyperemia: minimal cell injury; cells should recover.

Degree of Burn
1. Burns are classified by severity, layers of skin damaged (see Table 7-5).
2. Extent of burned area. Rule of Nines for estimating burn area (estimates are for adult patients).
   a. Head and neck: 9%.
   b. Anterior trunk: 18%.
   c. Posterior trunk: 18%.
   d. Arms: 9% each.
   e. Legs: 18% each.
   f. Perineum: 1%.
   g. Percentages vary by age (growth) for children: use Lund-Browder charts for estimating body areas.
3. Classification by percentage of body area burned.
   a. Critical: 10% of body with third-degree burns and 30% or more with second-degree burns; complications common (e.g., respiratory involvement, smoke inhalation).
   b. Moderate: less than 10% with third-degree burns and 15%–30% with second-degree burns.
   c. Minor: less than 2% with third-degree burns and 15% with second-degree burns.

Complications of Burn Injury

Infection
1. Leading cause of death; gangrene may develop.
2. Sepsis, life threatening infection, may cause shock.

Table 7-5

Burn Wound Classification				
THICKNESS	**DEGREE**	**SKIN LAYER AFFECTED**	**CHARACTERIZATION**	**HEALING**
Superficial	First-degree	Epidermis	• Blisters • Inflammation • Severe pain	3–7 days
Superficial partial thickness	Second-degree	Epidermis Upper layers of dermis	• Blisters • Inflammation • Severe pain	7–21 days
Deep partial thickness	Second-degree	Epidermis Dermis Nerve endings Hair follicles Sweat glands	• Red or white in appearance • Edema • Blisters • Severe pain	21–28 days Scar formation and reepithelialization
Full-thickness	Third-degree	Epidermis Dermis Subcutaneous tissue	• White, gray or black • Dry surface • Edema • Eschar • Little pain	Removal of eschar Grafting
Subdermal	Fourth-degree	Epidermis Dermis Subcutaneous Muscle Bone	• White, gray or black • Dry surface • Edema • Eschar • Little pain	Extensive surgery Amputation

Pulmonary Complications
1. Smoke inhalation injury from inhalation of hot gases, smoke poisoning; results in pulmonary edema and airway obstruction; suspect with burns of the face, singed nose hairs.
2. Restrictive lung disease from burns of the trunk.
3. Pneumonia.

Metabolic Complications
1. Increased metabolic and catabolic activity results in weight loss, negative nitrogen balance, and decreased energy.

Cardiac and Circulatory Complications
1. Fluid and plasma loss results in decreased cardiac output; hypovolemic shock.
2. Systemic inflammatory response, release of vasoactive mediators.
   a. Can cause local vasoconstriction, systemic vasodilation, and capillary leak leading to shock.

Burn Healing

Epidermal Healing
1. Retention of viable cells allows for epithelialization to occur (epithelial cells grow and proliferate, migrate to cover the wound).
2. Protection of epithelial cells is critical.
3. Loss of sebaceous glands can result in drying and cracking of wound; protection with moisturizing creams is important.

Dermal Healing
1. Results in scar formation (injured tissue is replaced by connective tissue).
2. Scars are initially red or purple, later become white.
3. Phases.
   a. Inflammatory phase: characterized by redness, edema, warmth, pain, decreased range of motion; lasts 3–5 days.
   b. Proliferative phase: fibroblasts form scar tissue (deeper tissues); characterized by wound contraction; reepithelialization may occur at wound surface if viable cells remain.
   c. Maturation phase: scar tissue remodeling lasts up to 2 years.
      - Hypertrophic scar may result: a raised scar that stays within the boundaries of the burn wound and is characteristically red, raised, firm.
      - Keloid scar may result: a raised scar that extends beyond the boundaries of the original burn wound and is red, raised, firm. More common in young women and those with dark skin.

Burn Management

Emergency Care
1. Immersion in cold water if less than half the body is burned and injury is immediate; cold compresses may also be used.
2. Cover burn with sterile bandage or clean cloth; no ointments or creams.

Burn Wound Healing
1. Factors that affect healing include nutrition, infection, associated illnesses (e.g., diabetes, malignancy, vascular insufficiency), cytotoxic treatments.
2. Significant burn injury more likely in very young or the elderly who have very thin skin.

Medical Management

Asepsis and Wound Care
1. Removal of charred clothing.
2. Wound cleansing.
3. Topical medications (antibacterial agents): can be applied without dressings (open technique); reapplied daily.
   a. Silver nitrate: acts only on surface organisms; applied with wet dressings; requires frequent dressing changes.
   b. Silver sulfadiazine: common topical agent.
   c. Sulfamylon (mafenide acetate): penetrates through eschar.
4. Occlusive dressings (closed technique): dressings are applied on top of a topical agent.
   a. Prevents bacterial contamination, prevents fluid loss, and protects the wound.
   b. May additionally limit ROM.

Establish and Maintain Airway
1. Maintain adequate oxygenation and respiratory function.
2. Monitor.
   a. Arterial blood gases, serum electrolyte levels, urinary output, vital signs.
   b. Gastrointestinal function: provide nutritional support.

Pain Relief
1. For example, morphine sulfate, oxycodone, nonsteroidal anti-inflammatories.

Prevention and Control of Infection
1. Tetanus prophylaxis.
2. Antibiotics.
3. Isolation, sterile techniques.

Fluid Replacement Therapy
1. Prevention and control of shock.
2. Post-shock fluid and blood replacement.

Surgery
1. Primary excision: surgical removal of eschar.
2. Grafts: closure of the wound.
   a. Allograft (homograft): use of other human skin; e.g., cadaver skin; temporary grafts for large burns, used until autograft is available.
   b. Xenograft (heterograft): use of skin from other species; e.g., pigskin; a temporary graft.
   c. Biosynthetic grafts: combination of collagen and synthetics.
   d. Cultured skin: laboratory grown from patient's own skin.
   e. Split-thickness graft: contains epidermis and upper layers of dermis from donor site.
   f. Full-thickness graft: contains epidermis and dermis from donor site.
3. Surgical resection of scar contracture; e.g., Z-plasty (surgical incision in the form of the letter Z used to lengthen a burn scar).

Physical Therapy Goals, Outcomes, and Interventions

Burn Wound Care

> **RED FLAG:** Infection control techniques must be implemented at all times.

1. Maintain temperature of burn wound by warming cleansing solutions, maintaining ambient temperature, and avoiding lengthy exposure of wet wound surfaces.
2. Cleansing with disinfectant soap and warm water.
   a. Some wounds or dressings benefit from soaking, wet removal of dressings.
   b. Excessive immersion is contraindicated. Risks include auto-contamination and electrolyte imbalance.
3. Wound debridement: removal of loose, charred, dead skin tissues.
   a. Autolytic dressings: use of moist dressings such as hydrogels or hydrocolloids to help remove eschar.
   b. Surgical or sharp debridement: excision of eschar using sterilized surgical instruments (forceps, scalpel, scissors). (NOTE: This is typically performed by the physician.)
   c. Enzymatic: e.g., fibrinolysins.
   d. Mechanical: wet to dry dressings, pulsed lavage, gently washing.

Rehabilitation
1. Overall goal is to limit loss of ROM to prevent or reduce the complications of immobilization through positioning and splinting, reduce edema. Provide emotional support.
2. Include exercises to promote deep breathing and chest expansion; ambulation to prevent pneumonia.
3. Stretching and early mobilization, taking all joints through full passive full ROM. This typically includes twice-daily therapy sessions.
   a. Schedule therapy and dressing changes/wound cleansing to coincide with optimal pain medication (typically 30–45 minutes before session).
   b. Postgrafting: discontinue exercise for 3–5 days to allow grafts to heal.
4. Edema control: elevation of extremities, active ROM.

Anti-contracture Positioning and Splinting
1. Used to prevent or correct deformities. This begins day one and continues for many months.
2. See Quick Facts Box 7-4 for common deformities and positioning.

Rehabilitation (Post-acute)
1. Continued active and passive exercise to promote full ROM, increase full active ROM as able.
2. Progressive strengthening exercises to correct loss of muscle mass and strength.
3. Minimize edema. Elastic supports to control edema.
4. Scar management.
   a. Massage and application of moisturizer.
   b. Regular massage and desensitization to aid with hypersensitive scars.
   c. Pressure garments to help prevent hypertrophic scarring or keloid formation.
5. Progressive ambulation to improve activity tolerance and cardiovascular endurance.
6. Promote independence in ADLs and functional mobility skills. Prepare for home, work, play, or school.
7. Management of chronic pain.
8. Provide ongoing education and emotional support.

QUICK FACTS 7-4 ▶ POSITIONING TO PREVENT CONTRACTURE DEVELOPMENT

Anatomical Area	Common Deformity	Positioning
Anterior neck	Flexion	Stress hyperextension
		Position with firm (plastic) cervical orthosis
Shoulder	Adduction	Stress abduction, flexion, and external rotation
	Internal rotation	Position with an axillary splint (airplane splint)
Elbow	Flexion	Stress extension and supination
	Pronation	Position in extension with posterior arm splint
Hand	Claw hand (intrinsic minus position)	Stress wrist extension (15°), MP flexion (70°), PIP, and DIP extension, thumb abduction (intrinsic plus position)
		Position in intrinsic plus position with resting hand splint
Hip	Flexion	Stress hip extension and abduction
	Adduction	Position in extension, abduction, and neutral rotation
Knee	Flexion	Stress extension
		Position in extension with posterior knee splint
Ankle	Plantar flexion	Stress dorsiflexion
		Position with foot-ankle in neutral with splint or plastic ankle-foot orthosis

Abbreviations: MP = metacarpophalangeal joint, PIP = proximal interphalangeal joint, DIP = distal interphalangeal joint

Skin Ulcers

Venous Ulcer (also known as Stasis Ulcers)

Etiology
1. Associated with chronic venous insufficiency; valvular incompetence, history of deep venous thrombosis (DVT), venous hypertension.

Clinical Features
1. Can occur anywhere in lower leg; common over "gaiter area," medial lower leg. See Table 7-6.
2. Pulses: normal.
3. Pain: none to aching pain in dependent position.
4. Color: normal or cyanotic in dependent position. Dark pigmentation, "hemosiderin staining," is common.
5. Liposclerosis (thick, tender, indurated, fibrosed tissue). Lipodermatosclerosis: fibrous tissue replaces fat, resulting in up-side-down wine bottle appearance of the leg.
6. Temperature: normal.
7. Edema: often marked and is firm.
8. Skin changes: pigmentation, stasis dermatitis may be present; thickening of skin as scarring develops.

Table 7-6

Differentiation of Arterial Venous and Diabetic Wounds

	ARTERIAL	VENOUS	DIABETIC
Location	Toes, dorsum of foot, lateral malleolus	Medial malleolus	Dorsum of foot
Depth	Often full thickness	Typically partial thickness	Often full
Wound Edges	Well demarcated, "punched-out" lesion	Irregular, uneven	Regular with callus
Base	Pale, no granulation	Yellow fibrous covering (fibrin) with granulating tissue	Pink
Blood Flow	Decreased pulses	Good	Fair
Painful	Yes	No	No

9. Ulceration: may develop, especially medial ankle; wet, with large amount of exudate.
10. Gangrene: absent.
11. Wound edges (margins) are irregular.

Degrees of Severity
1. Venous, arterial, and diabetic ulcers are measured using the partial- and full-thickness classifications as found in Table 7-5.

Arterial Ulcer

Etiology
1. Associated with chronic arterial insufficiency, arteriosclerosis obliterans; atheroembolism; history of minor nonhealing trauma.

Clinical Features
1. Can occur anywhere in lower leg; common on small toes, feet, bony areas of trauma (shin).
2. Preceded by signs of arterial insufficiency; pulses poor or absent.
3. Pain: often severe, intermittent claudication, progressing to pain at rest.
4. Color: pale on elevation; dusky rubor on dependency.
5. Temperature: cool.
6. Skin changes: trophic changes (thin, shiny, atrophic skin); loss of hair on foot and toes; nails thickened.
7. Ulceration: of toes or feet; can be deep.
8. Dry Gangrene: black, gangrenous skin adjacent to ulcer can develop.
9. Even, regular wound margins.
10. Minimal exudate.

Diabetic Ulcer

Etiology
1. Diabetes is associated with arterial disease and peripheral neuropathy.
2. Caused by repetitive trauma on insensitive skin.

Clinical Features
1. Occurs where arterial ulcers usually appear; or where peripheral neuropathy appears (plantar aspect of foot). See Figure 7-2.
2. Pain: typically not painful; sensory loss usually present.
3. Pulses: may be present or diminished.
4. Absent ankle jerks with neuropathy.
5. Sepsis common; gangrene may develop.

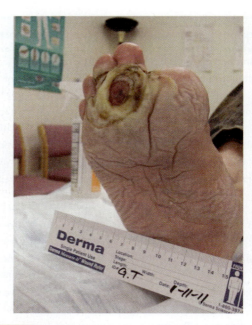

Figure 7-2 Full-thickness diabetic wound at base of second metatarsal head. Wound edge has callus and periwound skin is macerated. Note amputation of great toe.

Pressure Injury (also known as Decubitus Ulcer or Bed Sore)

Etiology
1. Lesions caused by unrelieved pressure resulting in ischemic hypoxia and damage to underlying tissue.

Risk Factors
1. Prolonged pressure, shear forces, friction, repetitive stress.
2. Nutritional deficiency.
3. Maceration (softening associated with excessive moisture).
4. Common in:
   a. Elderly, debilitated, or immobilized individuals.
   b. Decrease blood flow from hypotension or microvascular disease: diabetes, atherosclerosis.
   c. Neurologically impaired skin: decreased sensation.
   d. Cognitive impairment.

Clinical Features
1. Location: occurs over bony prominences; i.e., sacrum, heels, trochanter, lateral malleoli, ischial areas, elbows.
2. Color: red, brown/black, or yellow.
3. Localized infection.

4. Pain: can be painful if sensation intact.
5. Inflammatory response with necrotic tissue: hyperemia, fever, increased white blood cell count (WBC).
6. If left untreated, will progress from superficial simple erosion to involvement of deep layers of skin and underlying muscle and bone.

Grading
1. Graded by stages of severity (tissue damage).[1]
   a. Stage 1 pressure injury: nonblanchable erythema of intact skin.
      - Intact skin with a localized area of nonblanchable erythema, which may appear differently in darkly pigmented skin. Presence of blanchable erythema or changes in sensation, temperature, or firmness may precede visual changes.
   b. Stage 2 pressure injury: partial-thickness skin loss with exposed dermis.
      - The wound bed is viable, pink or red, moist, and may also present as an intact or ruptured serum-filled blister. Adipose (fat) and deeper tissues are not visible. Granulation tissue, slough and eschar are not present. These injuries commonly result from adverse microclimate and shear in the skin over the pelvis and shear in the heel.
   c. Stage 3 pressure injury: full-thickness skin loss.
      - Adipose (fat) is visible in the ulcer and granulation tissue and epibole (rolled wound edges) are often present. Slough and/or eschar may be visible. The depth of tissue damage varies by anatomical location. Undermining and tunneling may occur. Fascia, muscle, tendon, ligament, cartilage, and/or bone are not exposed. If slough or eschar obscures the extent of tissue loss, this is an unstageable pressure injury.
   d. Stage 4 pressure injury: full-thickness skin and tissue loss.
      - Exposed or directly palpable fascia, muscle, tendon, ligament, cartilage, or bone in the ulcer. Slough and/or eschar may be visible. Epibole (rolled edges), undermining, and/or tunneling often occur. Depth varies by anatomical location. If slough or eschar obscures the extent of tissue loss this is an unstageable pressure injury.
   e. Unstageable pressure injury: obscured full-thickness skin and tissue loss.
      - Full-thickness skin and tissue loss in which the extent of tissue damage within the ulcer cannot be confirmed because it is obscured by slough or eschar. If slough or eschar is removed, a Stage 3 or Stage 4 pressure injury will be revealed. Stable eschar (i.e., dry, adherent, intact without erythema or fluctuance) on the heel or ischemic limb should not be softened or removed.
   f. Deep tissue pressure injury: persistent nonblanchable deep red, maroon, or purple discoloration.
      - Intact or nonintact skin with localized area of persistent nonblanchable deep red, maroon, purple discoloration or epidermal separation revealing a dark wound bed or blood filled blister. Pain and temperature change often precede skin color changes. Discoloration may appear differently in darkly pigmented skin. This injury results from intense and/or prolonged pressure and shear forces at the bone-muscle interface. The wound may evolve rapidly to reveal the actual extent of tissue injury, or may resolve without tissue loss.

Assessment of Wounds

Review History
1. Review history and risk factors identified in physical therapist evaluation.

Physical Examination
1. Determine location of wound: use anatomical landmarks.
2. Assess size: (length, width, depth, wound area).
   a. Use clear film grid superimposed on wound for size.
   b. Insert sterile cotton tip applicator into deepest part of wound for depth; indicate gradations of depth from shallow to deep.
3. Examine wound edges.
   a. Assess for undermining: where the wound edge is not in contact with the wound bed.
   b. Evaluate for tunneling (communication with deeper structures); associated with unusual or irregular borders.
   c. Assess for epibole (wound edges have rolled under and communicated with healthy tissue), which delays or prevents healing. See Figure 7-3.
   d. Sinogram (radiographic imaging studies) can be used to assess extent.
4. Determine wound exudate (drainage).
   a. Type: serous (watery serum), purulent (containing pus), sanguineous (containing blood).
   b. Amount: dry, moderate, or high exudate.
   c. Odor (either present or absent).
   d. Consistency: e.g., macerated periwound skin due to high fluid environment. Appears whiter than unaffected skin.

---

[1] Adapted from the National Pressure Ulcer Advisory Panel definition, http://www.npuap.org/national-pressure-ulcer-advisory-panel-npuap-announces-a-change-in-terminology-from-pressure-ulcer-to-pressure-injury-and-updates-the-stages-of-pressure-injury/.

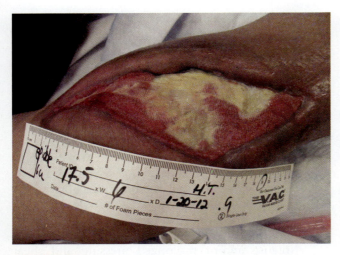

Figure 7-3 This incision is healing by secondary intention. The progress is slowed by marked epibole at the top of the wound and yellow slough. Note the shiny periwound skin.

5. Identify color and tissues involved.
   a. Clean red wounds: healthy granulating wounds (in need of protection); absence of necrotic tissue.
   b. Yellow wounds: include slough (necrotic or dead tissue), fibrous tissue.
   c. Black wounds: covered with eschar (dried necrotic tissue).
   d. Indolent ulcer: ulcer that is slow to heal; is not painful.
   e. Check to see if fascia, muscle, tendons, or bone involved are visible in the wound bed.
6. Determine temperature: indicative of inflammation. Use temperature probe (thermistor) to detect surface temperature.

Determine Girth
1. Use circumferential measurements of both involved and noninvolved limbs; referenced to bony landmarks.
2. Use volumetric measurements: measure water displacement from filled volumeter.

Examine Viability of Periwound Tissue
1. Halo of erythema, warmth, and swelling may indicate infection (cellulitis).
2. Maceration of surrounding skin due to moisture (urine, feces) or wound drainage increases risk for wound deterioration and enlargement.
3. Trophic changes may indicate poor arterial nutrition.
4. Cyanosis may indicate arterial insufficiency.

Determine Sensory Integrity
1. This assists with risk assessment for trauma or pressure breakdown.
   a. Use monofilament testing for protective sensation on diabetic feet.

Examine for Signs of Infection
1. Bacterial culture: to identify colonization and infection; culture wound site only.
2. Observations, palpation.

Wound Scar Tissue Characteristics
1. Assess for banding, pliability, texture.

Documentation
1. Photographic records of wound appearance aid narrative descriptions.
2. Use marker pen to outline wound edges on transparent dressing with a calibrated grid to provide a measuring scale.
3. Weekly documentation of wound size (length, width, and depth), using clock method or the greatest length × greatest width method

Ankle Brachial Index (ABI)
1. Compares lower extremity to upper extremity blood pressure. See Quick Facts 7-5.
2. Divide the ankle BP/brachial, which is documented as a decimal.
   a. Low numbers indicate impaired circulation. Numbers greater than 1.0 are due to calcification (hardening) of arteries.

QUICK FACTS 7-5 ▶ MEANING OF ANKLE BRACHIAL INDEX MEASURES

ABI	Implication	Treatment	Precaution/contraindication
1.0–1.4	Normal	None	Possible false-negative results
0.9	Early arterial disease	Monitor circulation	Compression okay
0.8–0.5	Moderate blockage		Compression not advised, no elevation
<0/.5	Significant blockage	Bypass surgery	NO compression or elevation

Wound Care

Infection Control
1. Wounds are cultured; antibiotic treatment regimen prescribed.
   a. Topical antimicrobial agents: e.g., silver nitrate, silver sulfadiazine, erythromycin, gentamicin, neomycin, triple antibiotic, medical-grade honey (Manuka).
   b. Anti-inflammatory agents: e.g., corticosteroids, hydrocortisone, ibuprofen, indomethacin.
   c. Topical anesthetics and analgesics: e.g., lidocaine, lignocaine.
2. Hand washing of health care practitioners.
3. Sterile technique for debridement, clean technique for dressing changes.

Surgical Intervention
1. Indicated for excising of ulcer, enhancing vascularity and resurfacing wound (grafts), and preventing sepsis and osteomyelitis.
2. May be indicated for stage III and IV pressure injuries.

Hyperbaric Oxygen Therapy (HBO)
1. Patient breathes 100% oxygen in a sealed, full-body chamber with elevated atmospheric pressure (between 2.0 and 2.5 atmospheres absolute, ATA).
2. Hyperoxygenation reverses tissue hypoxia and facilitates wound healing due to enhanced solubility of oxygen in the blood.
3. Contraindicated in untreated pneumothorax and some antineoplastic medications (e.g., doxorubicin, disulfiram, cisplatin, mafenide acetate).

Wound Cleansing
1. See Quick Facts 7-6 for wound cleansing agents and systems.
2. **TREATMENT CONSIDERATION:** The use of hydrotherapy whirlpool is not supported for wound care.
   a. Adverse events can include: contamination and associated infection from pathogen found in WP equipment, excess pressure may damage granulation tissue, limbs are placed in dependent position and can increase vascular congestion.

Wound Debridement
1. Removal of necrotic or infected tissue that interferes with wound healing. See Table 7-7 for methods of wound debridement.
2. Allows examination of ulcer, determination of extent of wound.
3. Decreases bacterial concentration in wound; improves wound healing.
4. Decreases spread of infection; i.e., cellulitis or sepsis.

QUICK FACTS 7-6 ▶ WOUND CLEANSING AGENTS AND DELIVERY SYSTEMS

Purpose	Removal of loose cellular debris, metabolic wastes, bacteria, and topical agents that retard wound healing Typically completed initially and at each dressing change
Cleansing agents	Normal saline (0.9% NaCl) recommended for most ulcers; nontoxic effects in wound Cleansing agents: contain surfactants that lower surface tension. Limited use, may be toxic to healing tissues; e.g., povidone-iodine solution, sodium hypochlorite solution, Dakin's solution, acetic acid solution, hydrogen peroxide. **TREATMENT CONSIDERATION:** Avoid harsh soaps, alcohol-based products, or harsh antiseptic agents; may erode skin.
Delivery Systems	Irrigation: Using syringe, squeezable bottle with tip, or battery-powered irrigation device (pulsatile lavage) • Loosens wound debris and removes it by suction • Safe and effective irrigation pressures range from 4 to 15 psi

Wound Dressings
1. Topical products: protect the wound from contamination and trauma; permit application of medications; absorb drainage; debride necrotic tissue; and enhance healing (see Table 7-8).
2. Moisture-retentive (occlusive) wound dressings: maintain a moist environment; wound tissue fluid is maintained in contact with tissues and cells; facilitates autolytic debridement, wound healing (re-epithelialization) with less pain.
   a. Alginate dressings: e.g., Sorbsan, Kaltostat.
   b. Transparent film dressings: e.g., Bioclusive, OpSite.
   c. Foam dressings: e.g., LYOfoam, Flexzan.
   d. Hydrogel dressings: e.g., Second Skin, Clearsite.
   e. Hydrocolloid dressings: e.g., DuoDerm, Curaderm.
3. Gauze dressings.
   a. Standard gauze (not impregnated).
   b. Impregnated gauze: e.g., Telfa pad, Vaseline Petroleum Gauze.
4. Semirigid dressings: Unna boot is a pliable, non-stretchable dressing impregnated with ointments; e.g., zinc oxide, calamine, and gelatin.

Edema Management
1. Leg elevation (contra-indicated with arterial wounds) and exercise (ankle pumps).

Table 7-7

Methods of Wound Debridement

METHOD	DEFINITION	INDICATIONS	CONTRAINDICATIONS
Autolytic	A selective method of natural debridement promoted under occlusive or semiocclusive moisture-retentive dressings that results in solubilization of necrotic tissue only by phagocytic cells and by proteolytic and collagenolytic enzymes inherent in the tissues.	• Individuals on anticoagulant therapy • Individuals who cannot tolerate other forms of debridement • All necrotic wounds in people who are medically stable	• Infected wounds • Wounds of immunosuppressed individuals • Dry gangrene or dry ischemic wounds
Enzymatic	A selective method of chemical debridement that promotes liquefication of necrotic tissue by applying topical preparations of proteolytic or collagenolytic enzymes to those tissues. Proteolytic enzymes help loosen and remove slough or eschar while collagenolytic enzymes digest denatured collagen in necrotic tissue.	• All moist necrotic wounds • Eschar after cross-hatching • Homebound individuals • People who cannot tolerate surgical debridement	• Ischemic wounds unless adequate vascular status has been determined • Dry gangrene • Clean, granulated wounds
Mechanical	A nonselective method of debridement that removes foreign material and devitalized or contaminated tissue by physical forces (wet-to-dry gauze dressing, dextranomers, pulsatile lavage with suction or whirlpool), and may remove healthy tissue as well.	• Wounds with moist necrotic tissue or foreign material present	• Clean, granulated wounds
Sharp	A selective method of debridement using sterile instruments (scalpel, scissors, forceps, silver nitrate stick) that sequentially removes only necrotic wound tissue without anesthesia and with little or no bleeding induced in viable tissue.	• Scoring and/or excision of leathery eschar • Excision of moist necrotic tissue	• Clean wounds • Advancing cellulitis with sepsis • When infection threatens the individual's life • Individual on anticoagulant therapy or has coagulopathy
Surgical	For deep (stage III or IV) or complicated pressure ulcer, the most efficient method of debridement. It is selective and is performed by a physician or surgeon using sterile instruments (scalpel, scissors, forceps, hemostat, silver nitrate sticks) in a one-time operative procedure. The procedure usually removes most, if not all, necrotic tissue, but may also remove some healthy tissue in what is termed wide excision. Because there may be associated pain and/or bleeding, the individual may require anesthesia, and the procedure will likely require an operating or special procedures room.	• Advancing cellulitus with sepsis • Immunocompromised individuals • When infection threatens the individual's life • Clean wounds as a preliminary procedure to surgical wound closure line • Granulation and scar tissue may be excised	• Cardiac disease, pulmonary disease, or diabetes • Severe spasticity • Individuals who cannot tolerate surgery • Individuals with a short life expectancy • Quality of life cannot be improved

From: Consortium for Spinal Cord Medicine: Pressure Ulcer Prevention and Treatment Following Spinal Cord Injury, Paralyzed Veterans of America, August 2000, with permission.

Table 7-8

Characteristics of Some Major Dressing Categories

DRESSING CATEGORY AND DEFINITION	INDICATIONS	ADVANTAGES
Transparent Films Clear, adhesive, semipermeable membrane dressings. Permeable to atmospheric oxygen and moisture vapor yet impermeable to water, bacteria, and environmental contaminants.	• Stage I and II pressure ulcers • Secondary dressing in certain situations • For autolytic debridement • Skin donor sites • Cover for hydrophilic powder and paste preparations and hydrogels	• Visual evaluation of wound without removal • Impermeable to external fluids and bacteria • Transparent and comfortable • Promote autolytic debridement • Minimize friction
Hydrocolloids Adhesive wafers containing hydroactive/absorptive particles that interact with wound fluid to form a gelatinous mass over the wound bed. May be either occlusive or semi-occlusive. Available in paste form that can be used as a filler for shallow cavity wounds.	• Protection of partial-thickness wounds • Autolytic debridement of necrosis or slough • Wounds with mild exudate	• Maintain a moist wound environment • Nonadhesive to healing tissue • Conformable • Impermeable to external bacteria and contaminants • Support autolytic debridement • Minimal to moderate absorption • Waterproof • Reduce pain • Easy to apply • Time-saving • Thin forms diminish friction
Hydrogels Water- or glycerine-based gels. Insoluble in water. Available in solid sheets, amorphous gels, or impregnated gauze. Absorptive capacity varies.	• Partial- and full-thickness wounds • Wounds with necrosis and slough • Burns and tissue damaged by radiation	• Soothing and cooling • Fill dead space • Rehydrate dry wound beds • Promote autolytic debridement • Provide minimal to moderate absorption • Conform to wound bed • Transparent to translucent • Many are nonadherent • Amorphous form can be used when infection is present
Foams Semipermeable membranes that are either hydrophilic or hydrophobic. Vary in thickness, absorptive capacity, and adhesive properties	• Partial- and full-thickness wounds with minimal to moderate exudate • Secondary dressing for wounds with packing to provide additional absorption • Provide protection	• Insulate wounds • Provide some padding • Most are nonadherent • Conformable • Manage light or moderate exudate • Easy to use • Some newer products are designed for deep cavities
Alginates Soft, absorbent, nonwoven dressings derived from seaweed that have a fluffy cottonlike appearance. React with wound exudate to form a viscous hydrophilic gel mass over the wound area. Available in ropes and pads.	• Wounds with moderate to large amounts of exudate • Wounds with combination exudate and necrosis • Wounds that require packing and absorption • Infected and noninfected exuding wounds	• Absorb up to 20 times their weight in drainage • Fill dead space • Support debridement in presence of exudate • Easy to apply
Gauze Dressings Made of cotton or synthetic fabric that is absorptive and permeable to water and oxygen. May be used wet, moist, dry, or impregnated with petrolatum, antiseptics, or other agents. Come in varying weaves and with different size intersticies.	• Exudative wounds • Wounds with dead space, tunneling, or sinus tracts • Wounds with combination exudate or necrotic tissue WET TO DRY • Mechanical debridement of necrotic tissue and slough CONTINUOUS DRY • Heavily exudating wounds CONTINUOUS MOIST • Protection of clean wounds • Autolytic debridement of slough or eschar • Delivery of topical needs	• Readily available • Can be used with appropriate solutions such as gels, normal saline, or topical antimicrobials to keep wounds moist • Can be used on infected wounds • Good mechanical debridement if properly used • Cost-effective filler for large wounds • Effective delivery of topicals if kept moist

(Continued)

Table 7-8

Characteristics of Some Major Dressing Categories (*Continued*)

DISADVANTAGES	CONSIDERATIONS
Transparent Films • Nonabsorptive • Application can be difficult • Channeling or wrinkling occurs • Not to be used on wounds with fragile surrounding skin or infected wounds	• Allow 1- to 2-inch wound margin around bed • Shave surrounding hair • Secondary dressing not required • Dressing change varies with wound condition and location • Avoid in wounds with infection, copious drainage, or tracts
Hydrocolloids • Nontransparent • May soften and change shape with heat or friction • Odor and yellow drainage on removal (melted dressing material) • Not recommended for wounds with heavy exudate, sinus tracts, or infections; wounds that expose bone or tendon; or wounds with fragile surrounding skin • Dressing edges may curl	• Characteristic odor with yellow exudate similar to pus; normal when dressing is removed • Allow 1- to 1½-inch margin of healthy tissue around wound edges • Taping edges will help prevent curling • Frequency of changes depends on amount of exudate • Change every 3–7 days and as needed with leakage • Avoid in wounds with infection or tracts
Hydrogels • Most require a secondary dressing • Not used for heavily exudating wounds • May dry out and then adhere to wound bed • May macerate surrounding skin	• Sheet form works well on partial-thickness ulcers • Do not use sheet form on infected ulcers • Sheet form can promote growth of *Pseudomonas* and yeast • Dressing changes every 8–48 hours • Use skin barrier wipe on surrounding intact skin to decrease risk of maceration
Foams • Nontransparent • Nonadherent foams require secondary dressing, tape, or net to hold in place • Some newer foams have tape on edges • Poor conformability to deep wounds • Not for use with dry eschar or wounds with no exudate	• Change schedule varies from 1–5 days or as needed for leakage • Protect intact surrounding skin with skin sealant to prevent maceration
Alginates • Require secondary dressing • Not recommended for dry or lightly exudating wounds • Can dry wound bed	• May use dry gauze pad or transparent film as secondary dressing • Change schedule varies (with type of product used and amount of exudate) from every 8 hours to every 2–3 days
Gauze Dressings • Delayed healing if used improperly • Pain on removal (wet to dry) • Labor-intensive • Require secondary dressing	• Change schedule varies with amount of exudate • Pack loosely into wounds; tight packing compromises blood flow and delays wound closure • Use continuous roll of gauze for packing large wounds (ensures complete removal) • If too wet, dressings will macerate surrounding skin • Use wide mesh gauze for debridement and fine mesh gauze for protection • Protect surrounding skin with moisture barrier ointment or skin sealant as needed

From: Consortium for Spinal Cord Medicine: Pressure Ulcer Prevention and Treatment Following Spinal Cord Injury, Paralyzed Veterans of America, August 2000, with permission.

2. Compression therapy: to facilitate movement of excess fluid from lower extremity (contra-indicated in arterial wounds).
   a. Compression wraps: elastic or tubular bandages.
   b. Paste bandages; e.g., Unna boot.
   c. Compression stockings; e.g., Jobst.
   d. Compression pump therapy.

Electrical Stimulation for Wound Healing
1. Uses capacitive coupled electrical current to transfer energy to a wound, improve circulation, facilitate debridement, enhance tissue repair.
   a. See Chapter 10 for full description and settings.
2. Continuous waveform application with direct current.
3. High-voltage pulsed current.
4. Microcurrent electrical stimulation (MENS).
5. Alternating/biphasic current.

Nutritional Considerations
1. Delayed wound healing associated with malnutrition and poor hydration. Tested with albumin and pre-albumin blood tests.
2. Albumin: normal is 3.5–5.5 mg/dl; less than 3.5 = malnutrition.
3. BMI ≤ 21 with weight loss increased risk for pressure ulcer.
4. Provide adequate hydration: individuals with wounds require approximately 3 or more liters of water a day.
5. Provide adequate nutrition: frequent high-calorie/high-protein meals; energy intake (25–35 kcal/kg/body weight) and protein (1.5–2.5 gm/kg body weight).
6. Patients with trauma stress and burns require higher intakes.

Injury Prevention or Reduction
1. Daily, comprehensive skin inspection, paying particular attention to bony prominences (e.g., sacrum, coccyx, trochanter, ischial tuberosities, medial or lateral malleolus).
2. Techniques to relive pressure and/or protect skin. See Quick Facts 7-7.
3. Patient and caregiver education.
   a. Mechanisms of pressure ulcer development.
   b. Daily skin inspection.
   c. Avoidance of prolonged positions.
   d. Repositioning, weight shifts, lifts.
   e. Safety awareness during self-care.
   f. Safety awareness with use of devices and equipment.
   g. Importance of ongoing activity/exercise program.

QUICK FACTS 7-7 ▶ INJURY REDUCTION TECHNIQUES

Therapeutic positioning	• In bed: turn or reposition every 2 hours during acute and rehabilitation phases • In wheelchair: wheelchair push-ups every 15 minutes
Skin protection techniques	• Lift, not drag, during transfers • Use turning and draw sheets; trapeze, manual, or electric lifts • Use transfer boards for sliding wheelchair transfers • Use of cornstarch, lubricants, pad protectors, thin film dressings, or hydrocolloid dressings over friction risk sites
Pressure-relieving devices (PRDs)	• Static devices for use if patient can assume a variety of positions; examples include foam, air, or gel mattress overlays; water-filled mattresses; pillows or foam wedges, protective padding (heel relief boots) • Dynamic devices for use if patient cannot assume a variety of positions; examples include alternating pressure air mattresses, fluidized air or high-air-loss bed • Seating supports for use with chair-bound or wheelchair-bound patients; examples include cushions made out of foam, gel, air, or some combination
Clothing	• AVOID: restrictive clothing, e.g., with rough textures, hard fasteners, and studs • AVOID: tight-fitting shoes, socks, splints, and orthoses
Avoid maceration injury	• Prevent moisture accumulation and temperature elevation where skin contacts support surface • Incontinence management strategies: use of absorbent pads, brief, or panty pad; scheduled toileting and prompted voiding; ointments, creams, and skin barriers prophylactically in perineal and perianal areas

Review Questions

Integumentary Physical Therapy

1. Name four different assessments performed during inspection of a wound.

2. What viral infection produces pain and tingling along a spinal or cranial nerve dermatome? It often appears as raised red papules and vesicles that follow along a nerve path. What causes this condition and is it contagious? Identify the following: (a) describe associated signs and symptoms, (b) describe management of the condition.

3. Differentiate between these two immune disorders of the skin—systemic lupus erythematosus (SLE) and scleroderma. Describe the condition, symptoms, management and precautions for each.

4. What type of wound may appear as a partial-thickness wound with shaggy edges and present with good blood flow, granulation tissue, and a yellow fibrous covering on it?

5. Compare and contrast between a foam and a hydrocolloid wound dressing.

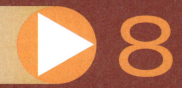

8

Geriatric Physical Therapy

SUSAN B. O'SULLIVAN and KAREN E. RYAN

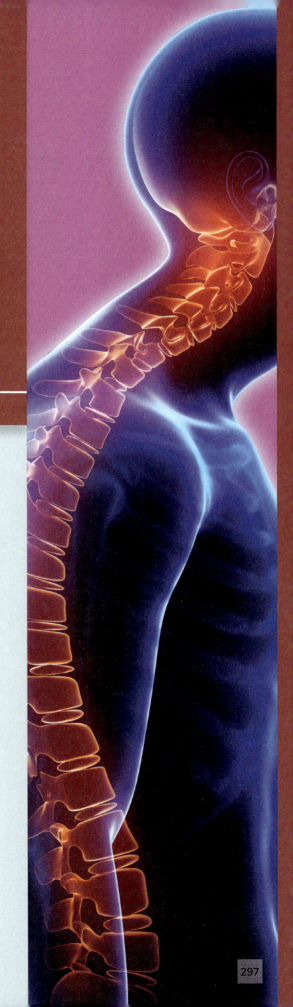

Chapter Outline

- **Definitions and Theories of Aging, 299**
  - General Concepts and Definitions, 299
- **Demographics and Socioeconomic Costs, 299**
  - Demographics, Mortality, and Morbidity, 299
  - Socioeconomic Factors, 300
- **Patient Care Concepts, 300**
  - Principles of Geriatric Rehabilitation, 300
  - Reimbursement Issues, 301
  - Ethical and Legal Issues, 301
- **Physiological Changes and Adaptations Associated with Aging, 302**
  - Cellular Changes, 302
  - Soft Tissue Changes, 302
  - Skeletal System, 303
  - Body Fat Composition, 303
  - Neurological System, 303
  - Sensory Systems, 304
  - Cognitive Changes, 307
  - Medical Management, 307
  - Cardiovascular System, 308
  - Pulmonary System, 308

- Integumentary System, 309
- Gastrointestinal System, 309
- Hepatic, Renal, and Genitourinary Systems, 310
- Endocrine System, 310
- **Musculoskeletal System Conditions Associated with the Aging Adult, 310**
  - Osteoporosis, 310
  - Medical Management, 311
  - Paget's Disease (Osteitis Deformans), 316
  - Medical Management and Tests, 316
  - Fractures, 317
  - Degenerative Arthritis/Osteoarthritis (OA), 317
  - Medical Management, 318
  - Rheumatoid Arthritis (RA), 318
  - Medical Management, 319
- **Neurological Disorders and Diseases Affecting Aging Adults, 320**
  - Intervention Considerations for Neurological Rehabilitation, 320
  - Cerebrovascular Accident (Stroke, CVA), 320
  - Parkinson's Disease, 322
  - Medical Diagnosis and Management, 322
- **Cognitive Disorders Affecting Aging Adults, 323**
  - Delirium, 323
  - Dementia, 324
  - Depression, 326
  - Medical Management, 326
  - Cardiopulmonary and Integumentary Disorders and Diseases, 327
  - Metabolic Pathologies, 327
- **Common Problem Areas for Aging Adults, 327**
  - Immobility-Disability, 327
  - Falls and Instability, 328
  - Medication Errors, 329
  - Nutritional Deficiency, 330
- **Review Questions, 331**

Definitions and Theories of Aging

General Concepts and Definitions

Aging
1. The progressive and cumulative physiological, biological, and functional changes in the body systems. A complex and variable process from individual to individual; common to all members of a given species; evidenced by a decline in homeostatic efficiency; increasing probability that reaction to injury will not be diminished or unsuccessful.
2. Categories of elderly.
   a. Young elderly, ages 65–74 (60% of elderly population).
   b. Old elderly, ages 75–84.
   c. Old, old elderly or frail elderly, ages >85.

Terminology, Definitions
1. Gerontology.
   a. The scientific study of the factors impacting the normal aging process and the effects of aging.
2. Geriatrics.
   a. The branch of medicine concerned with the illnesses of old age and their care.
3. Life span.
   a. Maximum survival potential, the inherent natural life of the species.
4. Life expectancy.
   a. The number of years of life expectation from year of birth.
   b. 77.7 years in United States, 2006.
   c. Women live 6.6 years longer than men.
5. Senescence.
   a. The last stages of adulthood through death.
6. Ageism.
   a. Discrimination and prejudice leveled against individuals on the basis of their age.

Theories of Aging
1. Developmental—genetic theories.
   a. Concepts include: aging is intrinsic in the organism; there are preprogrammed biological changes of tissues and cells that lead to aging; there are limits in the number of cell divisions that can be performed; cell damage results from free radicals, poor nutrition or hydration.
2. Nongenetic theories.
   Concepts include: environmental factors damage DNA; genetic mutation or changes in genes occur over time; accumulation of cross-linked proteins damage tissues and cells.
3. New theories.
   a. Include theories related to sleep and sleep pattern changes, imbalances and changes at the hormonal and cellular levels, and genetic influences.

Demographics and Socioeconomic Costs

Demographics, Mortality, and Morbidity

Demographics
1. Persons over 65.
   a. Represent a rapidly growing segment of the population.
   b. They represented more than 40 million in 2010 which is a little more than 1 in 8 individuals. By year 2030, it is expected that there will be over 69 million (21% of total population) elderly Americans.
   c. Minority populations are projected to represent 25% of those aged 65 or older by year 2020.
2. Reasons for increased life expectancy, aging of the population
   a. Advances in health care include improved infectious disease control.
   b. Advances in infant/child care resulting in decreased mortality rates.
   c. Improvements in nutrition and sanitation.

Mortality and Morbidity
1. Leading causes of death (mortality) in persons over 65, in order of frequency (2012 U.S. Department of Health & Human Services).
   a. Coronary heart disease (CHD).
   b. Cancer.
   c. Stroke.

d. Chronic pulmonary disease.
e. Unintentional injuries, motor vehicle accident (MVA).
f. Diabetes.
2. Leading causes of morbidity and risk factors in persons over 65, in order of frequency (2012 U.S. Department of Health & Human Services).
   a. Heart disease.
   b. Cancer.
   c. Hypertension.
   d. High serum cholesterol.
   e. Obesity.
   f. Cigarette smoking.
   g. Inactivity, lack of exercise.
   h. Persons over 65 reporting fair or poor health - 26.9%.

Socioeconomic Factors

1. Most elderly Americans live on fixed incomes.
2. About half of older persons have completed high school.
3. Noninstitutionalized elderly.
   a. Slightly more than half lived with a spouse in 2010, about 30% live alone.
   b. Almost 50% of women >75 years of age live alone. Only about 4% live in institutional settings. As the person ages, this statistic increases.
4. Almost 3.5 million elderly individuals had an income below the poverty level in 2010.
   a. In 2009 the major source of income reported was Social Security.
5. Institutionalized elderly.
   a. About 5% of persons >65 reside in nursing homes. Percentage increases dramatically with age (22% of persons >85).
6. Percentage of population of older persons.
   a. 12% of population and 36% of total health care expenditures.
   b. 33% of all hospital stays and 44% of all hospital days of care.

Patient Care Concepts

Principles of Geriatric Rehabilitation

Recognize Variability of Older Adults
1. Uniqueness of the individual.
2. Developmental issues unique to the elderly.

Focus on Careful and Accurate Clinical Assessments
1. Determined by physical therapist at time of initial evaluation.
2. Ongoing assessment by physical therapist assistant.
   a. Determine capacity for safe function.
   b. Determine effects of inactivity versus activity.
   c. Determine effects of normal aging versus disease pathologies.

Focus on Functional Goals
1. Determine priorities, remediable problems.
2. Implement plan of care in conjunction with patient/caregiver.

Promote Optimal Health

RED FLAG: Strength training programs yield positive results with older adults; failure to prescribe adequate frequency, intensity, and duration of exercise matched to the individual's abilities and strengths will negatively impact functional abilities and outcomes.

1. Focus on increasing health-conducive behaviors, prevention of disability.
2. Minimize and compensate for health-related losses and impairments of aging.

Promote Maximal Function
1. Restore/maintain the individual's highest level of function and independence within the care environment.
2. Determine how patient autonomy can be maximized by appropriate assistance and environmental manipulations.
3. Empower elders: ensure they are in control of their own decisions whenever possible.
4. Be sensitive to cultural and ethnicity issues, losses, fears, and insecurities; provide comfort and sustenance.
5. Enhance coping skills; seek/provide resources for social networking.
6. Recognize functional abilities, limitations of caregivers; enhance function and support caregivers.

Holism
1. Consider the whole patient; integrate all facets of an individual's life.
2. Determine social support systems, effects of social isolation.
3. Determine effects of losses.
4. Determine effects of depression, dementia.

Recognize Demands
1. Enhance continuity of care, interactions in a complex health care delivery system.
2. Advocate for needed services.
3. Provide effective documentation.

Reimbursement Issues

Benefits from Government Programs
1. Cover about two-thirds (63%) of health care expenditures of older persons.
2. Medicare: federal government–sponsored insurance for persons over age 65, disabled persons of all ages.
   a. Part A (Hospital Insurance) covers inpatient hospital care, skilled nursing facility care, home health care provided by agencies, hospice care.
      - No premiums; eligibility under social security.
      - Must pay deductibles and coinsurance.
   b. Part B (Medical Insurance) covers physician services, eligible home health services, outpatient services, durable medical equipment.
      - Must pay premiums to be eligible.
      - Must pay deductibles and coinsurance.
3. Medicaid (federal-state funding): covers long-term care of frail and aged patients in nursing homes, impoverished adults, and children.
   a. Must spend down or exhaust income to qualify for low-income status.
   b. Administered by individual states that set qualification guidelines; specific requirements vary by state.

Supplemental Insurance
1. May be purchased from private insurance companies.
2. Copayments that elderly must pay under Medicare (Medex), termed Medigap policies.
3. Long-term care insurance.
4. Enrollment in health maintenance organizations (HMOs).

Documentation and Reimbursement
1. Requirements specific to type of insurance program.
   a. Medicare requirements for physical therapy services.
      - Must be under the care of a physician; plan of care established and reviewed regularly by M.D.
      - Must include a determination of need: reasonable and necessary for individual's illness or injury according to acceptable standards of practice.
      - Requires the skilled services of a licensed physical therapist.
         ○ Condition must be expected to improve in a reasonable and generally predictable period of time.
         ○ A skilled therapist is needed to safely and effectively establish the plan of care (POC) for a patient.
         ○ A skilled therapist is needed to safely and effectively do maintenance therapy for a patient's condition.
      - The physician should review and sign and date the POC (certification). The POC should be certified for the first 30 days of treatment and recertified every 30 days (signed and dated).
      - If the service is not covered under Medicare statutes (e.g., exceeds the therapy cap), the patient can be billed directly.
   b. Private insurance requirements: vary by specific carrier; most adopt Medicare requirements (e.g., physician certification).
2. Baseline data must be described in functional and measurable terms.
3. Goals and outcomes should be measurable, objective, specific to patient, and indicate a predicted time frame.
4. Plan of care (POC).
   a. Address findings, relate impairments to functional performance.
   b. Include frequency and duration of treatment, projected end date, and disposition.
5. Progress report.
   a. Focuses on objective changes; subjective statements by patient.
   b. Documents remaining deficits, lack of progress, or declining status.
   c. Must be completed at least once during each Progress Report period.

Ethical and Legal Issues

Professional Practice
1. Affirms patient rights and dignity (professional ethical standards, APTA Code of Ethics).

Informed Consent
1. Respect for personal autonomy.
   a. Competent patients have the right to refuse treatment (e.g., do not resuscitate [DNR] orders).
2. Legal right to self-determination.
   a. Information must be provided to patient that outlines:
      - The nature and purpose of treatment.
      - Treatment alternatives.
      - Risks and consequences of treatment.
      - Likelihood of success or failure of treatment.
3. Consent must be obtained from a legal guardian if the individual is judged incompetent.
   a. Older adults with fluctuating mental abilities must be carefully evaluated for periods of lucidity.
   b. Documentation with a mental status exam is essential.

Advance Care Medical Directive (Living Will)

1. Established by federal Patient Self-Determination Act of 1990.
2. Health care proxy (durable power of attorney).
   a. Identifies a valid agent who is granted the authority to make health care decisions for an individual should that individual become incapacitated.
3. Requirements:
   a. Regulated by individual states; specific requirements vary by state.
   b. Must be in writing.
      • Signed by principal; witnessed by two adults.
   c. Empowers health care agent.
      • Includes specific guidelines as to which treatment options will be allowed, which will not (e.g., artificial life support, feeding tubes).
   d. Defines conditions/scope of agent's authority.

Physiological Changes and Adaptations Associated with Aging

Cellular Changes

Cell Number
1. The total number of cells decreases with age. Cells are less organized in function and have more variation.

Apoptosis
1. Aging interferes with apoptosis (the preprogrammed cell death that does not release harmful substances into surrounding tissues).
2. Apoptosis slowed; programmed cell death does not occur, leads to cancers such as leukemia. Cancer cells do not die but rather they invade surrounding healthy tissue.
3. Apoptosis accelerated, killing healthy good cells, leads to tissue damage and disorders such as Parkinson's, Alzheimer's, and Huntington's diseases.

Soft Tissue Changes

Cartilage
1. Relies on blood flow from adjacent bones and movement of synovial fluid for nutrients.
2. Normally thins with age; degenerative changes are not reversible; decreased hydration and increasing fibrous growth around bony prominences can contribute to stiffness at joints.
3. Cellular changes in the matrix of cartilage decrease the ability of cartilage to maintain hydration and nutrition.
4. Regular weight-bearing exercise is critical to maintain hyaline cartilage; with inactivity, hyaline cartilage is converted to fibrocartilage.
5. Compressive forces (weight bearing, contraction of muscle with exercise) followed by release are necessary for movement of nutrients and waste products into and out of cartilage.
6. Implications for Intervention
   a. Activity that reinforces alternate compressive (weight-bearing) and relaxing forces can help maintain health of cartilage.
   b. Maintenance of strength around joints can help decrease joint stress.

Muscular System
1. Changes in muscle may be due more to decreased activity levels and disuse than directly from aging.
   a. Mild loss of strength and muscle mass is part of the normal aging process (sarcopenia); decreased activity levels can lead to weakness resulting in increased prevalence of falls; dietary changes such as decreased intake of food (energy) and protein can negatively affect muscle loss.
   b. Muscular endurance: muscles fatigue more readily due to decreased muscle tissue oxidative capacity and decreased peripheral blood flow.
   c. Muscle strength: will be less than that of a younger person; however, it can be increased and maintained in the elderly; girth measurements are not a reliable measure of improved strength in the elderly.
      • Strength peaks at age 30 and remains relatively constant until age 50.
      • After age 50, there is accelerating loss of strength (15%–20% per decade) in the sixth to seventh decade and increases to 30% per decade after that in the nonexercising adult.
   d. Muscle power: significant declines due to losses in speed of contraction secondary to changes in nerve conduction and synaptic transmission.
2. Intervention implications.
   a. Muscle strength can be increased and maintained in the aging individual.
   b. Norms for muscle strength testing will be less than those of a younger individual and are best judged on ability to perform functional and recreational activities rather than on strength testing.

c. Girth measurements are not reliable measures of improved strength; both the size and number of muscle fibers decrease with age.

Skeletal System

Effects of Normal Aging
1. Bone mass and density loss.
2. Decreasing levels of activated vitamin D circulating in bloodstream causes less calcium to be absorbed.
3. Imbalance in osteoblast (bone building) and osteoclast (bone breakdown) activity.
4. Osteoclast activity is stronger and leads to bone loss.
5. Women who are postmenopausal have decreased estrogen levels that influence parathyroid hormone and calcitonin to increase bone reabsorption.
6. Other contributing factors to bone loss can include: hyperthyroidism, steroid therapy, decreased progesterone.
7. Peak bone mass is acquired in the late teens and twenties; bone loss begins after that.
   a. Between ages 45–70, bone mass decreases by approximately 25% in women and 15% in men.
   b. Bone mass decreases another 5% by age 90.
   c. Calcium absorption diminishes with aging, leading to loss of bone strength, especially trabecular bone. Age-related trabecular bone loss starts at age 35, cortical bone loss starts around age 40.
8. Postural changes: forward head, increased kyphosis of the thoracic spine, flattening of lumbar lordosis, hip and knee flexion contractures secondary to increased sitting.
9. Intervention implications
   a. Weight-bearing exercise can help maintain and improve bone strength.
   b. Muscles contracting and relaxing as well as progressive resistive exercise have been shown to improve bone strength.

> **RED FLAG:** Persons with weaker bones are more prone to fracture; fall risk assessment should be performed.

Body Fat Composition

Body Fat
1. In mid-life, body fat increases: women until late 60s, men until late 50s. After this, fat levels decrease; women's decreases more slowly than men's.
2. Body fat distribution changes so that it moves from under the skin to deeper areas of the body. Women tend to store fat in the lower body (hips, thighs); men tend to store in the abdomen.

Evidence
1. Supports that regular physical activity helps minimize age-related body composition changes.
2. Physical activity can help maintain ability to participate in exercise and can promote physiological as well as psychological well-being.

Neurological System

Age-Related Changes
1. Atrophy of nerve cells in cerebral cortex: overall loss of cerebral mass/brain weight of 6%–11% between ages of 20 and 90; accelerating loss after age 70.
2. Changes in brain morphology.
   a. Generalized cell loss in cerebral cortex: especially frontal and temporal lobes' association areas (prefrontal cortex, visual).
   b. Presence of lipofuscins, senile or neuritic plaques and neurofibrillary tangles (NFTs): significant accumulations associated with pathology (e.g., Alzheimer's dementia).
   c. More selective cell loss in basal ganglia (substantia nigra and putamen), cerebellum, hippocampus, locus ceruleus; brain stem minimally affected.
3. Decreased cerebral blood flow and energy metabolism.
4. Changes in synaptic transmission.
   a. Decreased synthesis and metabolism, as well as delay in impulse conduction and synaptic transmission of major neurotransmitters (e.g., serotonin, catecholamines, and dopamine). (Dopamine loss is associated with Parkinson's disease.)
   b. Slowing of many neural processes, especially in polysynaptic pathways.
5. Changes in spinal cord/peripheral nerves.
   a. Neuronal loss and atrophy: 30%–50% loss of anterior horn cells, 30% loss of posterior roots (sensory fibers) by age 90.
   b. Loss of motoneurons results in increase in size of remaining motor units (development of macromotor units).
   c. Loss of sympathetic fibers may account for: diminished autonomic stability, increased incidence of postural hypotension in older adults.
6. Age-related tremors (essential tremors [ETs]).
   a. Occur as an isolated symptom, particularly in hands, head, and voice.
   b. Characterized as postural or kinetic, rarely resting.
   c. Benign, slowly progressive; in late stages may limit function.
   d. Exaggerated by movement and emotion.

Clinical Implications
1. Effects on movement:
   a. Overall speed and coordination are decreased; increased difficulties with fine motor control.

b. Slowed recruitment of motoneurons contributes to loss of strength.
c. Both reaction time and movement time are increased.
d. Older adults are affected by the speed/accuracy trade-off.
- The simpler the movement, the less the change.
- More complicated movements require more preparation, longer reaction and movement times.
- Faster movements decrease accuracy, increase errors.
e. Older adults typically shift in motor control processing from open to closed loop (e.g., demonstrate increased reliance on visual feedback for movement).
f. Demonstrate increased cautionary behaviors; an indirect effect of decreased capacity.
2. General slowing of neural processing: learning and memory may be affected.
3. Problems in homeostatic regulation: stressors (heat, cold, excess exercise) can be harmful, even life threatening.

> **RED FLAG:** Older adults may exhibit impairments in homeostatic regulation; stressors (heat, cold, excess exercise) can be harmful, even life-threatening.

Intervention, Implications, and Compensatory Strategies

1. Increase levels of physical activity: encourages neuronal branching, slows rate of neural decline, improves cerebral circulation.

> **Clinical Application: Considerations for Intervention Provided to the Elderly Patient/Client**
>
> - Allow additional reaction time: overall movements and reaction times become slower; there may be decreased functional mobility and movement limitations; movements may be stiffer, fewer automatic movements.
> - Approach tissue-stretching activities carefully: connective tissues become more dense and stiff and less elastic; increased risk for strains/strains/tears; increased tendency for fibrinous adhesions and contractures.
> - Recognize normal gait changes: slower cadence, shorter steps, wider base of support, increased double-support phase (safety, compensate for balance disturbance), decreased trunk rotation and arm swing; less steady gait.
> - Provide strength training: significant increases in strength can be achieved through isometric and progressive resistive programs; higher intensity training (70%–80% max) produces changes more quickly and more predictably than moderate-intensity programs (both, however, are successful). Decreases in muscle function are typically more related to decreased levels in activity than to the aging process itself.

2. Correction of medical problems.
3. Improve health: diet, smoking cessation.
4. Provide effective strategies to improve motor learning and control.
   a. Allow for increased reaction and movement times: will improve motivation, accuracy of movements.
   b. Allow for limitations of memory: avoid long sequences of movements.
   c. Allow for increased cautionary behaviors: provide adequate explanation and/or demonstration when teaching new movement skills.
   d. Stress familiar, well-learned skills: incorporate repetitive movements.

Sensory Systems

Vision

1. Aging causes a general decline in visual acuity; gradual prior to sixth decade, more rapid decline between ages 60 and 90; visual loss may be as much as 80% by age 90.
   a. Presbyopia: visual loss in middle and older ages characterized by inability to focus properly and blurred image; due to loss of accommodation, elasticity of lens.
   b. Decreased reaction time to adapt to changes of dark and light; reduced ability to quickly change focus from far to near.
   c. Increased sensitivity to light and glare.
   d. Loss of color discrimination, especially for blues and greens.
   e. Decreased pupillary responses; size of resting pupil increases.
   f. Decreased sensitivity of corneal reflex; less sensitive to eye injury or infection.
   g. Oculomotor responses diminished: restricted upward gaze; reduced pursuit eye movements; ptosis may develop.
2. Medication induced vision changes: antihistamines, tranquilizers, antidepressants, or steroids have the potential to cause fuzzy or impaired vision.
3. Pathological conditions impacting vision that can occur in the elderly population. See Quick Facts 8-1.
4. Interventions and compensatory strategies can assist individuals with vision limitations. See Quick Facts 8-2.

Hearing

1. Aging changes: occur as early as fourth decade; affects a significant number of elderly (23% of individuals aged 65–74 have hearing impairments and 40% over age 75 have hearing loss; rate of loss in men is twice the rate of women; also starts earlier).
   a. Outer ear: buildup of cerumen (ear wax) may result in conductive hearing loss; common in older men.

QUICK FACTS 8-1 ▶ PATHOLOGICAL VISION PROBLEMS IN THE GERIATRIC POPULATION

Condition	Description
Cataracts	Opacity; clouding of lens due to changes in lens proteins; results in gradual loss of vision: central first, then peripheral; increased problems with glare; general darkening of vision: loss of acuity, distortion.
Glaucoma	Increased intraocular pressure, with degeneration of optic disc; atrophy of optic nerve; results in early loss of peripheral vision (tunnel vision), progressing to total blindness.
Senile Macular Degeneration	Loss of central vision associated with age-related degeneration of the macula compromised by decreased blood supply or abnormal growth of blood vessels under the retina; initially patients retain peripheral vision, may progress to total blindness.
Diabetic Retinopathy	Damage to retinal capillaries, growth of abnormal blood vessels, and hemorrhage lead to retinal scarring and finally retinal detachment; central vision impairment; complete blindness is rare.
Due to CVA	Homonymous hemianopsia: loss of one-half visual field in each eye (nasal half of one eye and temporal half of other eye); produces an inability to receive information from right or left side; corresponds to side of sensorimotor deficit.
Medication	Impaired or fuzzy vision may result with antihistamines, tranquilizers, antidepressants, or steroids.

QUICK FACTS 8-2 ▶ VISUAL AND AUDITORY LOSS COMPENSATORY ADAPTATIONS

Visual Compensations	Adaptation
Visual Deficits	Assess for visual deficits (e.g., acuity, peripheral vision). Light and dark adaptation, depth perception, diplopia.
Glasses	If applicable, be sure individual is wearing glasses when appropriate. Assist to clean glasses when necessary.
Adequate Lighting	Reduce glare, avoid abrupt changes in light or moving from light to dark or dark to light quickly.
Peripheral Vision	Peripheral vision may be reduced—limits social interactions and physical function. Stand directly in front of individual at eye level when communicating.
Color Discrimination	Use warm colors (yellow, orange, red) for identification and color coding.
Sensory Clues	When vision is limited provide additional sensory clues (e.g., verbal descriptions to new environments, touching to communicate you are listening).
Safety Education	Provide safety education, reduce fall risks.
Auditory/Hearing Compensations	**Adaptation**
Hearing Aids	Encourage use; determine if working.
Auditory Distractions	Minimize auditory distractions; work in quiet environment, speak directly in front of individual.
Verbal communication	Speak slowly and clearly; face individual when communicating.
Nonverbals	Use nonverbal communication (e.g., gestures, demonstrations) to reinforce your message.
Provide Orientation	Orient individuals to topics of conversation that cannot be heard to reduce isolation, paranoia, confusion.

b. Middle ear: minimal degenerative changes of bony joints.
c. Inner ear: significant changes in sound sensitivity, understanding of speech and maintenance of equilibrium may result with degeneration and atrophy of cochlea and vestibular structures, loss of neurons.

2. Types of hearing loss.
   a. Conductive: mechanical hearing loss from damage to external auditory canal, tympanic membrane, or middle ear ossicles; results in hearing loss (all frequencies); tinnitus (ringing in the ears) may be present.

b. Sensorineural: central or neural hearing loss from multiple factors (e.g., noise damage, trauma, disease, drugs, arteriosclerosis).
   c. Presbycusis: sensorineural hearing loss associated with middle and older ages; characterized by bilateral hearing loss, especially at high frequencies at first, then all frequencies; poor auditory discrimination and comprehension, especially with background noise; tinnitus.
3. Additional hearing loss with pathology.
   a. Otosclerosis: immobility of stapes results in profound conductive hearing loss.
   b. Paget's disease.
   c. Hypothyroidism.
4. Intervention and compensatory techniques.
   a. Determine if patient/client uses hearing aids and encourage their use.
   b. Minimize auditory distractions: work in quiet environment.
   c. Speak slowly and clearly; face patient/client.
   d. Use nonverbal communication to reinforce your message (e.g., gesture, demonstration).
   e. Orient person to topics of conversation that cannot be heard to reduce paranoia, isolation.

Vestibular/Balance Control
1. Aging changes: vestibular system functions to monitor head position and detect movements of the head. Degenerative changes in otoconia of utricle and saccule; vestibular ocular reflex (VOR) gain decreases; begins at age 30, accelerating decline at ages 55–60 resulting in diminished vestibular sensation. See Chapter 6.
   a. Diminished acuity, delayed reaction times, longer response times.
   b. Reduced function of VOR; affects retinal image stability with head movements, produces blurred vision.
   c. Altered sensory organization: older adults more dependent upon somatosensory inputs for balance.

RED FLAG: Less able to resolve sensory conflicts when presented with inappropriate visual or proprioceptive inputs due to vestibular losses.

   d. Postural response patterns for balance are disorganized: characterized by diminished ankle torque, increased hip torque, increased postural sway.
2. Additional loss of vestibular sensitivity with pathology.
   a. Ménière's disease: episodic attacks characterized by tinnitus, dizziness, a sensation of fullness or pressure in the ears; may also experience sensorineural hearing loss.
   b. Benign paroxysmal positional vertigo (BPPV): brief episodes of vertigo (less than 1 minute) associated with position change; the result of degeneration of the utricular otoconia that settle on the cupula of the posterior semicircular canal; common in older adults.
   c. Medications: antihypertensives (postural hypotension), anticonvulsants, tranquilizers, sleeping pills, aspirin, nonsteroidal anti-inflammatory drugs (NSAIDs).
   d. Cerebrovascular disease: vertebrobasilar artery insufficiency (transient ischemic attack [TIAs], strokes), cerebellar artery stroke, lateral medullary stroke.
   e. Cerebellar dysfunction: hemorrhage, tumors (acoustic neuroma, meningioma); degenerative disease of brain stem and cerebellum; progressive supranuclear palsy.
   f. Migraine headaches.
   g. Cardiac disease.
3. Intervention, implications, and compensatory strategies.

RED FLAG: Increased incidence of falls in older adults.
- See section on falls and instability.

Somatosensory
1. Aging changes: decline in sensitivity to touch, temperature, and vibration due to decline in sensibility of peripheral sensory receptors, Meissner's corpuscles (touch, texture receptors), pacinian's corpuscles (pressure, vibration receptors) and Krause's corpuscles (temperature receptors).
   a. Lower extremities may be more affected than upper.
   b. Proprioceptive losses: increased thresholds in vibratory sensibility, beginning around age 50; greater in lower extremities than upper extremities; greater in distal extremities than proximal.
   c. Loss of joint receptor sensitivity; losses in lower extremities; cervical joints may contribute to loss of balance.
   d. Cutaneous pain thresholds increased: greater changes in upper body areas (upper extremities, face) than for lower extremities.
2. Additional loss of sensation with pathology.
   a. Diabetes, peripheral neuropathy, cerebrovascular accident (CVA), central sensory losses, peripheral vascular disease, peripheral ischemia.
3. Intervention, implications, and compensatory strategies.
   a. Allow extra time for responses with increased thresholds.
   b. Use touch to communicate: maximize physical contact (e.g., rubbing, stroking).

c. Highlight or enhance naturally occurring intrinsic feedback during movements (e.g., stretch, tapping).
d. Provide augmented feedback through appropriate sensory channels (e.g., walking on carpeted surfaces may be easier than on smooth floor).
e. Teach compensatory strategies to prevent injury to anesthetic limbs, falls.
f. Provide assistive devices as needed for fall prevention.
g. Utilize biofeedback devices as appropriate (e.g., limb load monitor).

Taste and Smell

1. Changes: gradual decrease in taste sensitivity; decreased smell sensitivity.
2. Additional loss of sensation with:
   a. Smoking.
   b. Chronic allergies, respiratory infections.
   c. Wearing dentures.
   d. CVA, involvement of hypoglossal nerve.
3. Clinical implications/compensatory strategies:
   a. Decreased taste, enjoyment of food leads to poor diet and nutrition.
   b. Older adults frequently increase use of taste enhancers (e.g., salt or sugar).
   c. Decreased home safety (e.g., gas leaks, smoke).

Cognitive Changes

Age-Related Changes

1. No uniform decline in intellectual abilities throughout adulthood.
   a. Changes do not typically show up until mid 60s; significant declines affecting everyday life do not show up until early 80s.
   b. Most significant decline in measures of intelligence occurs in the years immediately preceding death (termed terminal drop).
2. Tasks involving perceptual speed: show early declines (by age 39); require longer times to complete tasks.
3. Numeric ability (tests of adding, subtracting, and multiplying): abilities peak in mid 40s; well maintained until 60s.
4. Verbal ability: abilities peak at age 30; well maintained until 60s.
5. Memory: impairments are typically noted in short-term memory; long-term memory retained; most difficulty noted with novel or new learning conditions; use of memory tools (e.g., notes, reminder calls) beneficial.
6. Learning: the ability to learn is not lost; new learning may take longer. Affected by increased cautiousness, anxiety, fast pace, interference from prior learning.

Medical Management

1. Improve health.
   a. Correction of medical problems: imbalances between oxygen supply and demand to central nervous system (CNS) (e.g., cardiovascular disease, hypertension, diabetes, hypothyroidism).
   b. Pharmacological changes: drug reevaluation; decreased use of multiple drugs; monitor closely for drug toxicity; reduction in chronic use of tobacco and alcohol; correction of nutritional deficiencies.

Intervention, Implications, and Compensatory Strategies

1. Use context-based strategies (e.g., practice stair climbing, perform many transfers in same situation) versus memorization (young adults); stress relationship, importance for function; decrease pace as appropriate, incorporate repetition; use memory tools.
2. Increase physical activity.
3. Increase mental activity.
   a. Keep mentally engaged ("Use it or lose it") (e.g., chess, crossword puzzles, high level of reading, math games/puzzles).
   b. Encourage engaged lifestyle: socially active (e.g., clubs, travel, work).
   c. Cognitive training activities.
4. Auditory processing may be decreased; provide written instructions.

Clinical Application: Considerations for Elderly Persons with Sensory or Cognitive Changes

- Compensate for possible vestibular changes and balance difficulties
- Provide additional time for responses with new learning
- Use repetition
- Use and encourage use of memory tools
- Provide additional feedback: walking surface, touch, etc.
- Provide written instructions
- Speak slowly, clearly, enunciating clearly, use appropriate volume for individual's abilities
- Ensure well-lighted treatment and home environments; minimize glare
- Limit moving from well-lit to dark areas quickly
- Use visual markers, warm colors (yellows, oranges and reds)

5. Provide stimulating, "enriching" environment; avoid environmental dislocation (e.g., hospitalization or institutionalization may produce disorientation and agitation in some elderly).
6. Stress support systems for remaining active: family and friends, senior groups supporting participation, activity, travel, and sports.

Cardiovascular System

Age-Related Changes
1. Changes more due to inactivity and disease than aging; no significant alteration in the work capacity of the heart.
2. Degenerative changes: slight increased heart size; mild increased thickness of ventricular wall; mild thickening of endocardium and valves (due to increased tissue density, cross-linking); nodular thickening at atrioventricular valves (due to repeated mechanical stress).
3. Heart rate (HR): resting HR and cardiac output show minimal changes; max HR decreases; HR response typically not affected at sub-max levels.
    a. Rate at which HR peaks is increased: can lead to lower cardiac output and stroke volume, creating increased possibility of orthostatic hypotension.
    b. Exercise response: aging heart will increase cardiac output by increasing stroke volume to meet demands.
    c. Maximum exercise heart rate lower.
4. Decline in neurohumoral control: baroreceptors less responsive to position changes; can lead to orthostatic hypotension.
5. Changes in conduction system: loss of pacemaker cells in sinoatrial node (SA) node.
6. Changes in blood vessels: arteries thicken, less distensible; slowed exchange capillary walls; increased peripheral resistance.
7. Resting blood pressure rises: systolic greater than diastolic.
8. Decreased blood volume, hemopoietic activity of bone.
9. Increased blood coagulability.

Implications for Intervention
1. Changes at rest are minor: resting heart rate and cardiac output relatively unchanged; resting blood pressures increase.
2. Cardiovascular responses to exercise: blunted, decrease in heart rate acceleration, decrease maximal oxygen uptake and heart rate, reduced exercise capacity, increased recovery time.
3. Decreased stroke volume due to decreased myocardial contractility.
4. Maximum heart rate declines with age (HR max = 220 – age).
5. Cardiac output decreases 1% per year after age 20; due to decreased heart rate and stroke volume.

> **RED FLAG:** Orthostatic hypotension: common problem in elderly due to reduced baroreceptor sensitivity and vascular elasticity. Avoid quick position changes.

6. Increased fatigue; anemia common in elderly.
7. Systolic ejection murmur common in elderly.
8. Possible electrocardiographic (ECG) changes: loss of normal sinus rhythm; longer PR and QT intervals; wider QRS; increased arrhythmias.

Pulmonary System

Age-Related Changes
1. Chest wall stiffness, changes in spinal curvature and declining strength of intercostal muscles results in increased work of breathing.
2. Loss of lung elastic recoil, decreased lung compliance.
3. Changes in lung parenchyma: alveoli enlarge, become thinner; fewer capillaries for delivery of blood; less effective oxygen uptake.
4. Changes in pulmonary blood vessels: thicken, less distensible.
5. Decline in lung capacity: residual volume increases (amount of air remaining in lungs after maximum expiration), vital capacity (volume of air that can be forcibly exhaled) decreases.
6. Forced expiratory volume (airflow) decreases.
7. Altered pulmonary gas exchange: oxygen tension falls with age, at a rate of 4 mm Hg/decade; PaO_2 at age 70 is 75 versus 90 at age 20.
8. Blunted ventilatory responses of chemoreceptors in response to respiratory acidosis: decreased homeostatic responses.
9. Blunted defense/immune responses: decreased ciliary action to clear secretions, decreased secretory immunoglobulins, alveolar phagocytic function.

Implications for Intervention
1. Respiratory responses to exercise: similar to younger adult at low and moderate intensities; at higher intensities, responses include increased ventilatory cost of work, greater blood acidosis, increased likelihood of breathlessness, increased perceived exertion.
2. Clinical signs of hypoxia are blunted; changes in mentation and affect may provide important cues.
3. Cough mechanism is impaired.
4. Gag reflex is decreased; increased risk of aspiration.
5. Recovery from respiratory illness prolonged in the elderly.
6. Significant changes in function with chronic smoking, exposure to environmental toxic inhalants.

Intervention, Implications, and Compensatory Strategies

1. Complete cardiopulmonary assessment by the physical therapist prior to commencing an exercise program is essential in older adults due the high incidence of cardiopulmonary pathologies.
   a. Selection of appropriate exercise tolerance testing protocol (ETT) is important.
   b. Absence of standardized test batteries and norms for elderly.
   c. Many elderly cannot tolerate maximal testing; submaximal testing commonly used.
2. Individualized exercise prescription essential.
   a. Choice of training program is based on fitness level, presence or absence of cardiovascular disease, musculoskeletal limitations, individual's goals and interests.
   b. Prescriptive elements (frequency, intensity, duration, and mode) are the same as for younger adults; developed by the physical therapist.
   c. Walking, chair, and floor exercises, modified strength/flexibility calisthenics well tolerated by most elderly.
   d. Consider aquatic programs (exercises, walking, and swimming) for aging adults with bone and joint impairments.
   e. Consider multiple modes of exercise (circuit training) on alternate days to reduce likelihood of muscle injury, joint overuse, pain, fatigue.
3. Aerobic training programs can significantly improve cardiopulmonary function in the elderly. Benefits of aerobic training programs:
   a. Decreased heart rate at a given submaximal power output.
   b. Improved maximal oxygen uptake (VO_2max).
   c. Greater improvements in peripheral adaptation, muscle oxidative capacity, than central changes; major difference from training effects in younger adults.
   d. Improved recovery heart rates.
   e. Decreased systolic blood pressure; may produce a small decrease in diastolic blood pressure.
   f. Increased maximum ventilatory capacity: vital capacity.
   g. Reduced breathlessness, lowers perceived exertion.
   h. Psychological gains: improved sense of well-being, self-image.
   i. Improved functional capacity.
4. Improve overall daily activity levels for independent living.
   a. Lack of exercise is an important risk factor in the development of cardiopulmonary diseases.
   b. Lack of exercise contributes to problems of immobility and disability in the elderly.

Integumentary System

Changes in Skin Composition
1. Dermis thins with loss of elastin.
2. Decreased vascularity; vascular fragility results in easy bruising.
3. Decreased sebaceous activity and decline in hydration.
4. Appearance: skin appears dry, wrinkled, yellowed, inelastic, aging spots appear (clusters of melanocyte pigmentation); increased with exposure to sun.
5. General thinning and graying of hair due to vascular insufficiency and decreased melanin production.
6. Nails grow more slowly, become brittle and thick.

Loss of Effectiveness as Protective Barrier
1. Skin grows and heals more slowly; less able to resist injury and infection.
2. Inflammatory response is weakened.
3. Decreased sensitivity to touch, perception of pain and temperature; increased risk for injury from concentrated pressures or excess temperatures.
4. Decreased sweat production with loss of sweat glands results in decreased temperature regulation and homeostasis.

Gastrointestinal System

Age-Related Changes
1. Decreased salivation, taste, and smell along with inadequate chewing (tooth loss, poorly fitting dentures); poor swallowing reflex may lead to poor dietary intake, nutritional deficiencies.
2. Esophagus: reduced motility and control of lower esophageal sphincter.
   a. Lower esophageal sphincter hesitant to relax may result in feeling of fullness at substernal area; lower esophageal sphincter weakens which may result in acid reflux and heartburn.
3. Stomach: reduced motility, delayed gastric emptying; decreased digestive enzymes and hydrochloric acid; decreased digestion and absorption of nutrients;

Clinical Application: Exercise Implications When Working with the Elderly

- Monitor exercise response carefully using a variety of tools (observation of patient, verbal responses, rate of perceived exertion)
- Blood pressure (BP) and HR changes may be blunted by medication requiring the use of alternative indicators of exercise level (e.g., rate of perceived exertion)
- Changes in rib cage excursion and postural changes can diminish effectiveness of respiration.
- Recovery time following exertion is prolonged which requires lengthened cool-down phase of aerobic activity.

indigestion common. Avoid exercise following a moderate meal.
4. Liver: decreased blood flow; diminished capacity to regenerate cells; changes in medication metabolism.
5. Small intestine: generally maintains ability to absorb nutrients; however, reduced blood supply can hinder absorption; changes in metabolism and absorption of lactose, calcium, and iron.

> **RED FLAG:** Decrease in calcium necessitates increased calcium intakes.

6. Large intestine: decreased motility, decreased mobility, and dehydration can all lead to constipation; can be offset with increased physical activity, higher fiber intake, increased water consumption.

Hepatic, Renal, and Genitourinary Systems

Age-Related Changes
1. Renal system: loss of kidney mass and total weight with nephron (filtering unit) atrophy, decreased renal blood flow (by as much as 10% per decade), decreased filtration.
   a. Blood urea rises.
   b. Decreased excretory and reabsorptive capacities.
   c. Reduced hormonal response (vasopressin): leads to impaired ability to conserve salt and contribute to increased risk for dehydration.

2. Pancreas: beta cells possess decreased ability to increase insulin production in response to increases in blood glucose levels.
3. Bladder: muscle weakness; decreased capacity causing urinary frequency; difficulty with emptying causing increased retention; increased incidence of urinary tract infections due to reflux of urine into ureters.
   a. Urinary incontinence common: affects over 10 million adults; over half of nursing home residents and one-third of community dwelling elders; affects older women with pelvic floor weakness and older men with bladder or prostate disease.
   b. Inadequate hydration: causes concentrated urine which irritates the lining of bladder wall, which causes involuntary contractions and leakage; increased water intake can assist.

Endocrine System

Age-Related Changes
1. Insulin (secreted by pancreas): muscle cells may become less responsive to insulin; after age 50, normal fasting blood glucose levels rise 6–14 mg/dL every 10 years.
2. Adrenal glands: aldosterone (important in regulating electrolyte and fluid balance) levels decrease; can cause problems with orthostatic hypotension.

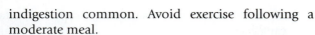

Musculoskeletal System Conditions Associated with the Aging Adult

Osteoporosis

Disease Process
1. Results in a reduction of bone mass. It is a metabolic disease that depletes bone mineral density/mass, predisposing individual to fracture. Senile osteoporosis occurs due to a decrease in bone cell activity (osteoblast activity) secondary to genetics or acquired abnormalities.

Diagnostic Criteria
1. The World Health Organization (WHO) has established diagnostic criteria. See Table 8-1.
   a. Osteopenia (systemic, evenly distributed, decrease in bone loss): defined by bone mineral density (BMD) between 1.0 and 2.5 standard deviations (SDs) below the young normal mean reference population. One standard deviation is equal to a 10%–12% difference in bone mass.
   b. Osteoporosis: defined by BMD at the hip or spine that is 2.5 SDs below the young normal mean reference population. One standard deviation is equal to a 10%–12% difference in bone mass.

Etiological Factors
1. Hormonal deficiency associated with menopause and hypogonadism: loss of estrogens or androgens.
2. Nutritional deficiency, inadequate calcium, impaired absorption of calcium; excessive alcohol, caffeine consumption.
3. Decreased physical activity: inadequate mechanical loading.
4. Additional risk factors: family history, white/Asian race, early menopause, thin/small build, smoking.

Table 8-1

Bone Mineral Density and Treatment Recommendations

CATEGORY	TREATMENT RECOMMENDATIONS
WHO (World Health Organization) Criteria for Bone Mineral Density	
Normal	
BMD −1 to +4 *Presents average or below average risk of fracture	Weight-bearing exercise Trunk extension activities and exercise Resistance exercise
Osteopenia	
BMD −1 to −2.5 *Presents increased risk for fracture	Weight-bearing exercise Trunk extension activities and exercise Functional activities Resistance exercise Postural/balance training Safety education/fall prevention
Osteoporosis	
BMD ≤2.5 * Presents significantly increased risk of fracture	Same as above—also add: Deep breathing exercise; more severe cases may need environmental modification or protective clothing

BMD, bone mineral density.

QUICK FACTS 8-3 ▶ BONE LOSS – DISEASES AND MEDIATIONS AFFECTING

Diseases Affecting	Medications Affecting
Hyperthyroidism	Corticosteroids
Hyperparathyroidism	Thyroid hormone
Rheumatic disease (lupus)	Anticonvulsants
Celiac disease	Catabolic drugs (e.g., hormones such as cortisol, glucagon, adrenaline)
Gastric bypass	
Pancreatic disease	Estrogen antagonists (some)
Multiple myeloma	
Sickle cell disease	Chemotherapeutic drugs
End-stage renal disease	
Paget's disease	
Cancer	
Chemotherapeutic drugs	

5. Diseases and medications can also affect bone loss. See Quick Facts 8-3.

Characteristics

1. Estimated 10 million Americans with osteoporosis; will affect about one in two women.
2. Bone loss is about 1% per year (starting for women at ages 30–35, for men ages 50–55); accelerating loss in postmenopausal women, approximately 5% per year for 3–5 years.
3. Structural weakening of bone.
4. Decreased ability to support loads.
5. High risk of fractures.
6. Trabecular bone more involved than cortical bone.
   a. Common areas affected: vertebral column, femoral neck, distal radius/wrist, humerus.
   b. Potential for deformity: feet—hammer toes, bunions lead to antalgic gait; postural kyphosis, forward head position; hip and knee flexion contractures.

Assessment

1. Medical tests: BMD testing; x-rays for known or suspected fractures.
   a. BMD score can be reported as a "T score," which is bone density compared to that of a healthy young woman, or a "Z score," which is bone density compared to that of people of the patient's age, gender, and race. Normal T score is −1.0 or above.
   b. A negative number indicates thinner bones; the greater the negative number, the higher the risk of fracture.
2. Physical therapist examination will include: physical activity/fall history, history, physical exam, nutritional history.
3. Physical therapist assistant ongoing assessments.
   a. Assess dizziness: may use Dizziness Handicap Inventory.
   b. Sensory integrity: vision, hearing, somatosensory, vestibular, sensory integration.
   c. Motor function: strength, endurance, motor control.
   d. Range of motion (ROM)/flexibility.
   e. Postural hypotension.
   f. Gait and balance assessment.

Medical Management

1. Medical therapy: initiated with BMD T-scores −2.5 at femoral neck or spine (obtained by dual-energy x-ray absorptiometry [DXA]) or individuals >50 years with low bone mass (T-score between 1.0 and 2.5, osteopenia). Current Food and Drug Administration (FDA)–approved pharmacological options include medications (Table 8-2).
2. Promote health; provide counseling on risk of osteoporosis and related fractures, health behaviors.
   a. Daily calcium intake, individuals age 50 or older: 1200 mg per day.
   b. Daily vitamin D intake, individuals age 50 or older: 800–1000 IU per day.
   c. Diet: low in salt, avoid excess protein: inhibits body's ability to absorb calcium.
   d. Avoid tobacco smoking and excessive alcohol intake.

Table 8-2

Commonly Prescribed Medications and Associated Precautions*

MEDICATION**	PRESCRIBED FOR	SIDE EFFECTS	INTERACTIONS	PHYSICAL THERAPY CONSIDERATIONS
Medications Used for Bone Disorders				
alendronate (Fosamax) calcitonin (Miacalcin, Calcimar) raloxifene (Evista)	Bone disorders (e.g., osteoporosis and Paget's disease)	Constipation Indigestion Diarrhea Abdominal pain Deterioration (osteonecrosis) of the jaw Muscle cramps Headaches Calcitonin: nasal spray can cause irritation in nose (e.g., sores, dryness, itching, bleeding). Injectable can cause: stomach pain, diarrhea, nausea or vomiting, flushing (face, ears, hands, feet), loss of appetite.	Can cause increases in abdominal distress if combined with use of aspirin. Calcium or antacids taken with medication can interfere with uptake of medication. Calcium intake should be monitored by MD. Calcitonin: may interfere with other meds taken for Paget's disease. Calcium intake should be monitored by MD. Raloxifene: may affect blood clotting (an increased risk of blood clots with this medication); individuals on warfarin (Coumadin). Calcium intake should be monitored by MD as levels could become too high.	Alendronate: patient should take the medication on an empty stomach, should not lie down within 30 minutes of taking the medication; increased chance of irritation of esophagus. Raloxifene: monitor carefully for bruising. Ensure the patient is getting blood test for clotting times (prothrombin time, international ratio).
Medications Used to Treat Inflammatory Disorders				
Nonsteroidal Antiinflammatory Drugs (NSAIDs) aspirin ibuprofen (Motrin, Advil) naproxen (Aleve, Naprosyn)	Inflammatory conditions and pain Rheumatoid arthritis Osteoarthritis	Stomach and gastrointestinal irritation Can cause symptoms of dizziness, fatigue, dyspnea, tinnitus, headache		
COX-2 inhibitors Celecoxib (off the market: Vioxx)	Inflammatory conditions and pain Rheumatoid arthritis	Produce less stomach and gastrointestinal irritation than NSAIDs; however, increased risk for potential heart problems Liver dysfunction, contributes to declining kidney function. Fluid accumulation mimicking congestive heart failure	When taken with anticoagulants, aspirin, corticosteroids or SSRIs, may cause increased risk of stomach bleeding Effectiveness of ACE inhibitors or diuretics may be decreased by this medication.	
Corticosteroid Injections	Arthritis inflammation and other painful inflammatory conditions	Weakens tissues, especially with repeated use		Be cautious of weakened tissues and cartilage in the case of multiple injections
Disease-Modifying Antirheumatic Drugs (DMARDs) Gold therapy compounds	Rheumatoid arthritis		Modifies the immune system response to the inflammatory process and stops or slow its progress	
Steroids, methylprednisolone (Medrol) Prednisone	Rheumatoid arthritis	Significant weakening of tendon, muscle, and bone can occur May weaken the immune system	Prednisone may increase or decrease effects of anticoagulant medications.	Clinician should pay careful attention to posture, monitor for changes that may reflect weakening of the spine or other support structures.

(Continued)

Table 8-2

Commonly Prescribed Medications and Associated Precautions* *(Continued)*

MEDICATION**	PRESCRIBED FOR	SIDE EFFECTS	INTERACTIONS	PHYSICAL THERAPY CONSIDERATIONS
Medications Used to Treat Ischemic Conditions of the Heart				
Cholesterol-Lowering Medications Lovastatin, colestipol (Colestid), fluvastatin (Lescol), pravastatin (Pravachol), atorvastatin ((Lipitor), cholestyramine (Questran), fenofibrate (Antara, Fenoglide, Lipofen), gemfibrozil (Lopid), rosuvastatin calcium (Crestor)	Hyperlipidemia Atherosclerosis Ischemic heart disease	Nausea, fatigue, diarrhea, weakness, myalgia, myositis		
Fish Oil (Lovaza)	Hyperlipidemia. Fish oil helps to lower triglyceride levels; may help decrease risk of heart disease, may help lower blood pressure,	May cause belching, bad breath, loose stools, heartburn, nausea, rash, nosebleeds May reduce immune system activity	May lower blood pressure in persons who are taking blood pressure lowering medications May cause slow blood clotting; potential for increased bruising or bleeding, especially if combined with medications such as aspirin, naproxen, ibuprofen, warfarin May increase symptoms of depression	Monitor for hypotension
Beta-Blockers atenolol (Tenormin) Carvedilol (Coreg) metoprolol (Lopressor) propranolol (Inderal)	Atherosclerosis Ischemic heart disease Angina pectoris • Slows heart rate and decreases the force needed to contract the heart muscle • Decreases blood pressure and myocardial oxygen demand	Nausea, fatigue, slow pulse, weakness, increased blood glucose levels, nightmares, depression, asthmatic attacks, sexual dysfunction		Use RPE scale to monitor patient tolerance to exercise • Blood pressure and heart rate are not good indicators of the work being done as they are being artificially controlled by the medication
Calcium Channel Blockers nifedipine (Procardia) verapamil (Calan, Verelan) Nicardipine (Cardene) diltiazem (Cardizem)	Atherosclerosis Ischemic heart disease Angina pectoris • Medications cause vasodilation of the coronary arteries, lower blood pressure, and can suppress some arrhythmias.	Hypotension, postural hypotension, dizziness, headache, fluid retention—peripheral edema, palpitations, flushes		Be aware of possibility of postural hypotension. Warrants MD notification. Use RPE scale to monitor patient tolerance to exercise • Blood pressure and heart rate are not good indicators of the work being done as they are being artificially controlled by the medication.
aspirin	Atherosclerosis Ischemic heart disease • Decreases the risk of a blood clot forming in the coronary arteries			
Nitrates (Vasodilators) nitroglycerine (Nitrostat, Nitro-Bid)	Atherosclerosis Ischemic heart disease Angina pectoris • Act to cause vasodilation of coronary arteries	Nausea, vomiting, tachycardia, transient headache, hypotension, weakness, flush on face and neck		Orthostatic hypotension and tachycardia warrant notification of MD and PT.

(Continued)

Table 8-2

Commonly Prescribed Medications and Associated Precautions* (Continued)

MEDICATION**	PRESCRIBED FOR	SIDE EFFECTS	INTERACTIONS	PHYSICAL THERAPY CONSIDERATIONS
Medications Used to Treat Congestive Conditions of the Heart				
Diuretics hydrochlorothiazide (HydroDIURIL, Aquazide H) spironolactone (Aldactone) furosemide (Lasix) bumetanide (Bumex)	Congestive heart conditions • Work to increase excretion of sodium and water, thus decrease amount of fluid in the body	Potential electrolyte imbalances, muscle cramps, weakness, joint pains, drowsiness, dehydration, gout, nausea, blood glucose abnormalities		Dizziness and lightheadedness warrants notification of the MD and PT.
Digitalis Compounds digoxin (Lanoxin, Digitek)	Congestive heart conditions • Increases force of the heart's contractions • Slows heart rate to allow chambers to fill completely	Nausea, vomiting, diarrhea, confusion, loss of appetite, heartbeat irregularities		
Ace Inhibitors (Angiotensin-Converting Enzyme Inhibitors) enalapril maleate (Vasotec) ramipril (Altace) Captopril (Capoten) lisinopril (Prinivil, Zestril)	Congestive heart conditions • Decreases how hard the heart has to work to pump blood through the heart by decreasing pressure in vessels of heart • Prevents constrictions of blood vessels and retention of sodium and fluid	Persistent dry cough, weakness, headache, palpitations, swelling of feet or abdomen, dizziness, fainting, numbness or tingling of hands, feet or lips	May cause congenital defects if taken during the first trimester of pregnancy	May cause postural hypotension Swelling of feet or abdomen, dizziness, or fainting warrant notification of MD.
Beta-blockers atenolol (Tenormin) carvedilol (Coreg) metoprolol (Lopressor, Toprol-XL) propranolol (Inderal)	Congestive heart conditions • Reduces the output of blood and heart rate by counteracting a hormone called norepinephrine • Relaxes blood vessels of the heart muscle by blocking sympathetic conduction of B-receptors on the SA node and myocardial cells; reduces force of contraction and decreases heart rate	Nausea, fatigue, slow pulse, weakness, increased blood glucose levels, nightmares, depression, asthmatic attacks, sexual dysfunction		Dizziness warrants contacting MD and PT. Can cause postural hypotension
Medications Used to Treat Arrhythmias of the Heart				
Digitalis Drugs digoxin *Antiarrhythmics* quinidine (Cardioquin) Procainamide HCl (Procanbid, Procan Sr)	Atrial fibrillation • Work to slow or alter the electrical conduction patterns of the heart • Increases heart muscle's ability to contract and pump correctly	Nausea, palpitations, vomiting, insomnia, dizziness, symptoms of CHF, shortness of breath, swollen ankles, coughing up blood		If symptoms of CHF develop immediately contact MD, supervising PT and document.
Medications Used to Treat Cognitive Disorders				
Tricyclics amitriptyline (Elavil)	Depression • Meds work on chemical imbalances in brain	Dry mouth or eyes, weight gain, drowsiness, constipation, nausea, sweating		Tricyclic antidepressants can cause postural hypotension.

(Continued)

Table 8-2

Commonly Prescribed Medications and Associated Precautions* (*Continued*)

MEDICATION**	PRESCRIBED FOR	SIDE EFFECTS	INTERACTIONS	PHYSICAL THERAPY CONSIDERATIONS
nortriptyline (Pamelor, Aventyl HCl) Desipramine (Norpramin) *Serotonin and Norepinephrine Reuptake Inhibitors (SNRIs)* venlafaxine (Effexor, Effexor XR) duloxetine HCl (Cymbalta) *Selective Serotonin Reuptake Inhibitors (SSRIs)* fluoxetine (Prozac, Sarafem) paroxetine (Paxil) escitalopram (Lexapro) sertraline (Zoloft) citalopram (Celexa)	• SSRIs increase brain serotonin levels	SSRIs: symptoms that will likely diminish: anxiety, restlessness, increased sleepiness, heartburn; symptoms that may not resolve unless SSRI is stopped: sexual problems		
Symptom Modifying Medications Levodopa (Sinemet, Stalevo) *Dopamine Agonists* *COMT Inhibitors* Selegiline (Eldepryl, Zelapar)	Parkinson's disease • Body works to turn levodopa into dopamine • Dopamine agonists increase effect of levodopa • COMT inhibitors block the enzyme that breaks down levodopa; prolong its effect when taken at same time • Selegiline agents prevent breakdown of dopamine	Mental confusion, hallucinations, abnormal movements, restlessness, heart rhythm disturbances, insomnia, mouth sores, constipation, back pain, nausea and vomiting Note: dopamine agonists can increase the side effects of levodopa.	Narcotic painkillers, antidepressants, decongestants, alcohol, foods high in tyramine (aged meats, aged cheese, sausage, herring, and more)	Levodopa may cause postural hypotension. With selegiline agents, notify MD immediately if any of the following occur: lightheadedness, restlessness, irritability, twitching, or muscle movement, painful or difficult urination.
Anticholinergic	Parkinson's disease • Works to decrease tremors	Dry mouth, constipation, urine retention, blurred vision In elderly patients, can cause confusion and hallucinations		
Acetyl cholinesterase inhibitors donepezil (Aricept) rivastigmine (Exelon) Galantamine (Razadyne) memantine (Namenda)	Alzheimer's disease • Increases the availability of acetylcholine • Namenda may regulate glutamate through its action on the NMDA receptors in the brain			
Medications Used to Inhibit Blood Clotting				
Warfarin: inhibits formation of vitamin K (Coumadin) Heparin: inactivates thrombin	Anticoagulation of the blood (treat blood clot or prevent blood clot)	Bleeding, stomach/abdominal pain, chest pain	Antibiotics, aspirin, NSAIDS (cream or oral), leafy green vegetables, cranberry, soy, herbal products	Patient must have INR consistently monitored; clinicians should know the current INR levels; protect against possible cuts, falls, potential bleeds; manual therapy.
Lovenox SubQ	Anticoagulation of the blood (treat blood clot or prevent blood clot)	Bleeding, fever, fluid retention, decreased blood platelets, confusion	Other anticoagulants	
dabigatran etexilate (Pradaxa) Rivaroxaben (XARELTO)	Anticoagulation, DVT prophylaxis	Bleeding; discontinuing medication places patient at risk for thrombotic event	NSAIDS, aspirin DO NOT interact with food, illness, vitamin K as warfarin does	

*Medications used in the medical management of diseases and conditions are included in the licensure exam. PTAs should be familiar with categories of medications and their indications for use. PTAs should also be acutely aware of potential effects on tolerance to physical therapy intervention.

**Generic drug names appear first followed by brand names in parentheses; brand names may be trademarked or registered.

ACE, angiotensin-converting enzyme; CHF, congestive heart failure; COMT, catecholamine O-methyl transferase; NMDA, *N*-methyl-D-aspartate; RPE, rate of perceived exertion; SSRIs, selective serotonin reuptake inhibitors.

Intervention, Implications, and Compensatory Strategies

1. Promote maintenance of bone mass by including regular weight-bearing exercise:
   a. Walking (30 min/day); stair-climbing; use of weight belts to increase loading.
   b. Muscle strengthening (resistance exercises) reduces risk of falls and fractures.
2. Postural/balance training.
   a. Postural reeducation, postural exercises to reduce kyphosis, forward head position.
   b. Flexibility exercises.
   c. Functional balance exercise (e.g., chair rises), standing/kitchen sink exercises (e.g., toe raises, unilateral stance, hip extension, hip abduction, partial squats).
   d. Tai chi.
   e. Gait training.
3. Safety education/fall prevention.

> **RED FLAG:** Advise individuals to avoid movements that can result in spinal fractures, including: forward bending, twisting motions, lifting heavy objects, sudden forceful movements involving spinal stability.

   a. Avoid long-term bed rest.
   b. Proper shoes: flat shoes enhance balance abilities (no heels).
   c. Assistive devices to decrease fall risk: cane, walker as needed.
   d. Hip protectors for patients with significant risk for falls or who have previously fractured a hip.
   e. Include home assessment for fall risk.

Paget's Disease (Osteitis Deformans)

Description and Etiology

1. Progressive metabolic bone disease: characterized by increased bone resorption and excessive, unorganized new bone formation (new bone lacks structural stability of normal bone); eventual replacement of bone marrow with vascular fibrous tissue.
2. Affects both men and women with slight increased prevalence in men; often familial.
3. Etiology: often inherited in an autosomal dominant pattern; genetic basis not well understood.

Musculoskeletal Manifestations

1. Primarily affects axial skeleton; lesions occur in multiple sites in the spine, pelvis, femur, tibia, as well as the skull.
2. Can cause pathological fractures; affected bones change shape and size.

Clinical Presentation/Symptoms

1. Pain; if periosteum is irritated, pain may be described as "deep, boring."
   a. Pain is likely worse at night; pain can be reduced (not eliminated) with activity.
2. Other symptoms can include fatigue, lightheadedness, general stiffness, headache, and muscular aches.
3. Active disease process can cause increased release of calcium (due to overactive osteoclasts) in the blood to cause hypercalcemia state; results in fatigue, weakness, loss of appetite, abdominal pain, constipation.
4. Clinical findings: increased kyphosis, bowing of femurs or tibias; waddling gait due to femoral neck causing coxa vara; pain from altered mechanical stresses if joint deformities exist.

Medical Management and Tests

1. Diagnostics: may take years; often made incidentally through radiographic or laboratory tests looking for other pathology; laboratory tests assessing alkaline phosphatase levels; bone scan.
2. Treatment: bone resorption inhibitors oral alendronate or risedronate (nitrogen-containing bisphosphonates); treatment can induce remission of the disease process; pain control through use of non-steroidal anti-inflammatory; surgical intervention in cases of potential compromise to vital structures or if severe degenerative joint exists (see Table 8-2).

Physical Therapy Screening

1. Condition can be difficult to diagnose.
2. The PT must be aware of symptomatic complaints (e.g., vague diffuse headache, hearing loss, tinitus, incontinence, diplopia, swallowing difficulties).

Intervention and Implications

1. Interventions include:
   a. Regular cardiovascular and strengthening activity; postural exercises.
   b. Weight-bearing and strengthening exercises to maintain joint alignment and ROM.
   c. Coordination and balance exercises.

> **RED FLAG:** Avoid high-impact activities such as jogging, running, and jumping (particularly in cases of spinal involvement); avoid forward bending and twisting exercises.

Fractures

Risks
1. There is a high risk of fractures in the elderly; associated with low bone density and multiple risk factors (e.g., age, comorbid diseases, dementia, psychotropic medications).

Hip Fracture
1. Common orthopedic problem of older adults with a mortality rate of 20% and is associated with complications.
2. About 50% will not resume their premorbid level of function (e.g., walk independently).
3. May result in dependency; continued institutionalization occurs in as many as one-third of hip fracture patients.
4. Majority of hip fractures are treated surgically; 95% are femoral neck or intertrochanteric fractures; remaining 5% are subtrochanteric fractures.
5. Intensive interdisciplinary rehabilitation program with early mobilization may improve outcome.
6. Treatment protocols are based on the type of fracture and surgical procedure used; internal fixation versus prosthetic replacement.

Vertebral Compression Fractures
1. Usually occur in lower thoracic, lumbar regions (T8-L3).
2. Typically result from routine activity: bending, lifting, rising from chair.
3. Chief complaints: immediate, severe local spinal pain, increased with trunk flexion.
4. Lead to shortening of spine, progressive loss of height; spinal deformity (kyphosis); can progress to respiratory compromise.
5. Intervention, implications, and compensatory strategies.
   a. Acute phase: horizontal bed rest; out of bed 10 minutes every hour; isometric extension exercises in bed.
   b. Emphasis on extension postures (sleeping, sitting, standing) and exercises; avoid flexion activities; postural training.
   c. Modalities for relief of pain.
   d. Safety education/modify environment.
   e. Decrease vertebral loading; use soft-soled shoes.
   f. Surgical repair: kyphoplasty or vertebroplasty can be performed for individuals with painful vertebral fractures.

RED FLAG: Use caution when patient/client is taking pain medications that can cause disorientation or sedation that can result in falls.

Stress Fractures
1. Fine, hairline fractures, also called insufficiency fractures, without soft tissue injury.
2. In the aging adult, commonly found in spine, pelvis, proximal tibia, distal fibula, metatarsal shafts, foot.
   a. May be an unsuspected source of pain.
   b. Observe for signs of local tenderness and swelling (e.g., post exercise).
3. Interventions and goals.
   a. Rest.
   b. Reduction of vertical loading (e.g., soft-solder shoes, postural correction [supportive device]).
   c. Correction of exercise excesses or faulty exercise posture or program. Avoid spinal flexion exercise or position if spine involved.
4. For discussion of fracture assessment and management, see Chapter 2 on Musculoskeletal Physical Therapy.

Clinical Implications
1. Fractures heal more slowly.
2. Older adults are prone to complications: pneumonia, decubitus ulcers, mental status complications with hospitalization.
3. Rehabilitation may be complicated or prolonged by lack of support systems, comorbid conditions, decreased vision, poor balance.

Degenerative Arthritis/Osteoarthritis (OA)

Description
1. A noninflammatory, progressive, degenerative process affecting articular cartilage of synovial joints.
2. Eventually produces bony remodeling and overgrowth (spurs, lipping), synovial and capsular thickening, and joint effusion.
3. Typically affects weight-bearing joints such as hips, knees, the cervical and lumbar spine, the distal interphalangeal joints of the fingers, and carpometacarpal joints of the thumb.

Risk Factors
1. Genetic link especially in hands, hips; smaller incidence in knees.
2. Obesity; weak quadriceps muscle.
3. Joint impact; repetitive impact and twisting (e.g., sports activities).
4. Occupational activities involving kneeling and squatting with heavy lifting.

Clinical Manifestations
1. Tissue degradation: thinning and splitting of cartilage; decreased ability to withstand stress of use; eventual exposure of subchondral bone.

2. Characterized by: pain, swelling, and stiffness, worse early morning (usually <30 minutes); increased pain with weight-bearing and strenuous activity; muscle spasm; loss of ROM and mobility; bony deformity, crepitus; muscle weakness secondary to disuse.
3. Bony deformities.
   a. Herberden's nodes: enlargement of distal interphalangeal joints of fingers.
   b. Bouchard's nodes: enlargement of proximal interphalangeal joints.

Medical Management

NSAIDs, corticosteroid injections, topical analgesics, joint replacements (see Table 8-2).

Intervention

1. Reduction of pain and muscle spasm; modalities, relaxation training, medical intervention; NSAIDS.
2. Maintain or improve ROM: stretch muscle; manage joint restrictions with joint play and mobilization techniques.
3. Correct muscle imbalances; strengthening exercises to promote neuromuscular control of joint; improve balance and ambulation.
4. Balance training exercises—tai chi.
5. Aerobic conditioning: low-impact (walking, biking, swimming) and low, moderate, or high-intensity aerobic conditioning programs.
6. Aquatic programs (e.g., pool walking, Arthritis Foundation program) produce beneficial effects similar to aerobic conditioning, enhance ease of movement.

Clinical Application: Using Evidence to Enhance Patient Outcomes

- Evidence supports aerobic conditioning and strengthening exercise programs can help to decrease joint symptoms, decrease disability, decrease pain, and improve overall sense of well-being in patients/clients with OA.
- Evidence supports hip joint mobilizations to improve arthrokinematics which can have a greater clinical effect on muscle function and joint motion than active exercise alone in patients/clients with OA.
- Evidence supports that patients with medically controlled rheumatoid arthritis (RA) respond favorably to carefully supervised exercise programs. Benefits of exercise program include improved function and muscle strength, decreased number of clinically active joints and decreased disease activity. Long-term adherence to these programs can lead to improved aerobic capacity, improved strength and functional ability, improved psychological well-being.

Patient Education and Empowerment

1. Teach patients about disease, taking an active role in care, symptom management.
2. Teach joint protection, safe exercise for strength and muscle performance, ROM and endurance.
3. Provide assistive devices for ambulation and activities of daily living (e.g., canes, walkers, shoe inserts, reachers).
4. Promote healthy lifestyle: weight reduction to relieve stress on joints.

Rheumatoid Arthritis (RA)

Description

1. Chronic systemic autoimmune disorder of unknown etiology thought to have a genetic basis. Diffuse connective tissue disease resulting in inflammation of synovial membrane, release of proteolytic enzymes that perpetuate inflammation and joint damage; inflammatory changes in tendon sheaths (tenosynovitis); pannus formation (granulation tissue) covers and erodes articular cartilage, bone, ligaments, and the joint capsule.
   a. Individuals with RA produce antibodies to their own immunoglobulins, such as rheumatoid factor (RF) and anti-citrullinated protein antibody (ACPA). The disease is commonly characterized by periods of exacerbation and remission.
2. Affects women at a two to four times greater incidence than men, with onset between 40 and 60 years of age.

Characteristics

1. Systemic manifestations include weight loss, fever, and extreme fatigue. May also include morning stiffness, which is more pronounced and lasts longer than with OA.
2. Symmetrical, bilateral joint involvement; joint erythema and swelling; elevated serum rheumatoid factor.
3. Periods of exacerbation and remission.
4. Eventual rheumatoid nodules and joint malalignment. Deformities are typically bilateral and symmetrical.
5. Patients may develop limited mobility and present with signs of inflammation (pain, swelling, redness, and increased tissue temperature).

Joints Impacted

1. The most commonly affected joints include the hands, feet, and cervical spine.
   a. Upper cervical spine (C1–C2) involvement can be life threatening.
   b. May also involve costovertebral joints, spinal facet joints, and sacroiliac joint.

2. Shoulder joints: glenohumeral, sternoclavicular, or acromioclavicular.
3. Elbow, wrist, or hand joints.

Common Joint Deformities
1. Swan neck deformity: proximal interphalangeal (PIP) hyperextension with distal interphalangeal (DIP) flexion.
2. Boutonniere deformity: DIP extension with PIP flexion.
3. Thumb deformities: termed types I–III; affect all joints.
4. Foot deformities: splayed foot with weakening of the transverse arch from synovitis; hallux valgus and bunions may exist; hammer toes—volar subluxation of metatarsophalangeal joints combined with flexion of the PIP and hyperextension of the DIP joints; claw toes—volar subluxation of metatarsal head with flexion of the PIP and DIP joints.

Other Tissues
1. Muscle involvement can include atrophy (unknown if result of disuse or other unknown mechanism).
   a. In long-standing disease, atrophy of intrinsic hand musculature and quadriceps may be observed.
2. Tendon involvement: inflammation of synovial lining of tendon sheaths leading to tenosynovitis.

Medical Management
1. Laboratory testing: for elevated erythrocyte sedimentation rate (ESR) or C-reactive protein (CRP), elevated rates are indicative of active inflammation; laboratory testing for rheumatoid factor (RF) does not confirm or rule out diagnosis of RA. Complete blood count (CBC), red blood cells often decreased, white blood cell count typically normal, thrombocytosis (high platelet count) not uncommon.
2. Synovial fluid analysis: enhances differential diagnosis; will be cloudy, less viscous, and will clot; increase in fluid; presence of crystals can confirm diagnosis of gout.
3. Radiographic imaging: PT or MD will review for joint alignment, bone density, and condition of joint surface, cartilaginous spacing, soft tissue swelling evidence.
4. Medications: NSAIDS and disease-modifying antirheumatic drugs (DMARDS), including biological response modifiers (BRMs) and corticosteroids (see Table 8-2).
5. Surgical management: selectively chosen for appropriate individuals.
   a. Soft tissue surgeries: synovectomy, soft tissue release, tendon transfer.
   b. Bone and joint surgeries: osteotomy, arthroplasty, arthrodesis.

Intervention
1. Decrease pain: modalities (use caution with cold applications due to Raynaud's phenomenon with RA); gentle massage, relaxation techniques.
2. Increase or maintain ROM sufficient for functional activities: active or passive ROM within pain limits; manual techniques, grades I and II oscillations, teach self ROM; implement appropriate neurological stretching techniques.

> **RED FLAG:** Do not stretch swollen joints. Avoid exercise-induced pain that lasts greater than an hour following treatment.

3. Joint protection: use orthoses or splints to support joints when appropriate, specially designed shoes to decrease forces through foot.
4. Resistance exercises: include isometric exercise (submaximum effort); use concentric and eccentric muscle contractions; do not cause pain with resistance.
5. Establish regular exercise and physical activity routine: include endurance, crucial to long-term quality of life.
6. Implementation of aerobic and endurance conditioning or reconditioning, such as aquatic programs.
7. Gait: improve safety, improve efficiency of pattern.
8. Teach joint protection principles (see Table 8-3).

Table 8-3

Joint Protection Principles for Rheumatoid Arthritis

- Respect fatigue: alternate activities; stop activity when fatigue begins to develop
- Conserve energy: work or exercise in short episodes, several times/day rather than long episodes; balance work and rest activities
- Work postures: avoid performing work/exercise in deforming positions; avoid prolonged positions—change every 20–30 minutes throughout day
- Avoid pain: decrease activity level, or omit, if pain persists following activity that lasts >1 hour
- Maintain joint alignment: use appropriate adaptive equipment to decrease joint forces and workload

Neurological Disorders and Diseases Affecting Aging Adults

Intervention Considerations for Neurological Rehabilitation

Implications for Intervention
1. Older adults are prone to complications/indirect impairments (e.g., contracture and deformity, decubitus ulcers, mental status complications).
2. Rehabilitation may be complicated or prolonged by lack of support systems, comorbid conditions, decreased sensorimotor function, poor balance.
3. With irreversible neurologic disease, it is important to address the impairments and functional limitations responsive to interventions; overall focus should be on improved function and safety.
4. Compensatory treatment strategies should be utilized when impairments cannot be remediated; strategies can include environmental modifications, assistive devices, use of home health aides.

Cerebrovascular Accident (Stroke, CVA)

Stroke
1. Stroke occurs when the blood supply to the brain is interrupted or reduced. This can result from ischemia or from hemorrhagic lesions in the brain.
2. Early diagnosis is critical to minimize brain damage.
3. Stroke syndromes and presenting signs and symptoms depend on the specific location of the insult. (See Table 8-4.)

Etiological Categories
1. Ischemic stroke. Occurs in 80% of cases.
   a. Cerebral thrombosis: formation or development of a blood clot or thrombus within the cerebral arteries or their branches.
   b. Cerebral embolism: traveling bits of matter (thrombi, tissue, fat, air, bacteria) that produce occlusion and infarction in the cerebral arteries.
2. Hemorrhagic stroke: abnormal bleeding as a result of rupture of a blood vessel (estradural, subdural, subarachnoid, intracerebral). Occurs in 20% of cases.
3. Transient ischemic attack (TIA): a temporary period of symptoms resulting from decreased blood supply to the brain; there is no permanent damage.

Risk Factors
1. Atherosclerosis.
2. Hypertension.
3. Cardiac disease (rheumatic valvular disease, endocarditis, arrhythmias, cardiac surgery).
4. Diabetes, metabolic syndrome.
5. Transient ischemic attacks: brief warning episodes of dysfunction (<24 hours); a precursor of major stroke in more than one-third of patients.
6. Medical diagnosis and management.
   a. Doppler ultrasound studies of blood flow through arteries; neuroimaging (CT, computed tomography; MRI, magnetic resonance imaging; DWI, diffusion-weighted [magnetic resonance] imaging; PET, positron emission tomography).
7. Medical Treatment.
   a. Embolic stroke: maintaining cerebral perfusion, maintain appropriate blood pressure levels through diuretics, beta-blockers, or angiotensin-converting enzymes; control edema through use of water restriction or agents that increase serum osmolarity.
   b. Ischemic stroke: thrombolytic and antithrombotic agents; emergent care includes use of recombinant tissue plasminogen activator (tissue plasminogen activator activates plasmin which, in turn, actively digests fibrin strands and aids in dissolving thrombosis or clots); when administered within 3 hours of initial stroke, tissue plasminogen activator results in a 30% greater chance of recovery.
   c. Intracerebral hemorrhage: reduction of elevated blood pressures through rapid-acting antihypertensive medications; control edema; hyperventilation and diuretics (mannitol) to move fluid from the intracranial compartment can be used; however, it has rebound effects and can worsen the condition; surgical draining most appropriate for cerebellar hemorrhage.
   d. Subarachnoid hemorrhage: consists of management of secondary complications of rebleeding, vasospasm, hydrocephalus, hyponatremia, and seizures; increase fluids; avoid antihypertensive drugs.

Clinical Signs, Symptoms, and Interventions
1. See Table 8-4.
2. For a complete discussion of interventions, refer to Chapter 3 on Neuromuscular Physical Therapy.

Pathophysiology
1. Cerebral anoxia: lack of oxygen supply to the brain (irreversible anoxic damage to the brain begins after 4–6 minutes).
2. Cerebral infarction: irreversible cellular damage.

Table 8-4

Neurovascular Syndromes: Stroke

LESION LOCATION	CHARACTERISTICS	OTHER LOCALIZING FEATURES (NOT ALWAYS PRESENT)
Hemisphere lesion: cortex and internal capsule	Contralateral hemiplegia face, UE, LE Contralateral hemisensory loss Homonymous hemianopsia *MCA syndrome:* LE more spared *ACA syndrome:* UE more spared	Impairment of consciousness Motor speech involvement—nonfluent aphasia (dominant hemisphere) Perceptual deficit (nondominant hemisphere) Loss of conjugate gaze to the opposite side Sensory ataxia Apraxia Akinetic mutism
Hemisphere lesion: primary visual cortex, occipital lobe	*PCA syndrome:* Contralateral sensory loss Involuntary movements—choreoathetosis, tremor, hemiballismus Transient contralateral hemiparesis Homonymous hemianopsia	Visual agnosia Memory defect Dyslexia Central (thalamic) pain Weber's syndrome Oculomotor n. palsy
Internal capsule lesion-posterior limb	*Lacunar (pure motor) stroke* Contralateral hemiplegia UE and LE	No aphasia Visual field deficit rare
Midbrain lesion	Contralateral hemiplegia	Contralateral CN III palsy
Pontine lesion	*Medial inferior pontine syndrome:* Ipsilateral to lesion: Cerebellar ataxia, nystagmus Paralysis of conjugate gaze to side of lesion Diplopia Contralateral to lesion: Hemiparesis UE, LE Impaired sensation *Lateral inferior pontine syndrome:* Ipsilateral to lesion: Cerebellar: ataxia, nystagmus, vertigo Facial paralysis Paralysis of conjugate gaze to the side of the lesion Deafness, tinnitus Impaired facial sensation Contralateral to lesion: Impaired pain and temperature sensation half of body *Locked-in syndrome:* Tetraplegia Lower bulbar paralysis (CN V–XII) Mutism (anarthria) Preserved consciousness Preserved vertical eye movements and blinking	

(Continued)

Table 8-4

Neurovascular Syndromes: Stroke (Continued)

LESION LOCATION	CHARACTERISTICS	OTHER LOCALIZING FEATURES (NOT ALWAYS PRESENT)
Medullary lesion CONTRALATERAL MEDULLARY LESION	*Medial medullary syndrome:* Ipsilateral to lesion: paralysis of half of tongue Contralateral to lesion: Hemiplegia UE and LE Impaired sensation *Lateral medullary (Wallenberg's) syndrome:* Ipsilateral to lesion: Cerebellar symptoms (ataxia, vertigo, nystagmus) Loss of pain and temperature to face Sensory loss UE, trunk, or LE Contralateral to lesion: Loss of pain and temperature to body and face	 Horner's syndrome (miosis, ptosis, decreased sweating) Dysphagia Impaired speech

ACA = anterior cerebral artery; CN = cranial nerve; LE = lower extremity; MCA = middle cerebral artery; PCA = posterior cerebral artery; UE = upper extremity

3. Cerebral edema: accumulation of fluids within brain; causes further dysfunction; elevates intracranial pressures; can result in herniation and death.

Parkinson's Disease

Overview
1. A chronic progressive disease of the CNS with degeneration of the dopaminergic substantia nigra neurons and nigrostriatal pathways.

Etiology
1. Cause is unknown. Some causes identified include infections/postencephalitic, atherosclerosis, ideopathic, toxic drugs included; certain gene variations or exposure to certain environmental toxins or factors may increase risk; however, this is relatively small.

Signs and Symptoms
1. Characterized by rigidity/stiffness (leadpipe or cogwheel), slowing of movement (bradykinesia, hypokinesia), resting tremor and impaired postural reflexes (postural instability, impaired movement initiation, impaired reflexive or automatic movements).
2. Individuals may demonstrate little/no facial expression; speech may become affected.
3. Slowly progressive with emergence of secondary impairments an dpermanent dysfunction.
4. Stages (Hoehn and Yahr classification). See Quick Facts 8-4.

Medical Diagnosis and Management

1. Diagnosis: assessment of the triad of tremor, rigidity, and akinesia coupled with asymmetry of symptoms and presence of resting tremor and good response to levodopa can best differentiate PD from parkinsonism from other causes. Functional brain imaging is also sensitive to changes in brain metabolism and receptor binding.
2. Medical treatment: drug administration to treat symptoms; patients develop tolerance for medications with resultant increases in doses and decreased time frame for relief of symptoms; common medications: levodopa, carbidopa, catechol-O-methyl (COMT); dopamine agonists (bromocriptine), anticholinergic drugs to improve motor functions (see Table 8-2).

RED FLAG: Monitor closely for adverse drug effects. Patients taking sinemet long-term may experience nausea, vomiting, orthostatic hypotension, cardiac arrhythmias, involuntary movements (dyskinesias), and psychoses and abnormal behaviors (hallucinations). Monitor closely drug dosing cycles and recognize signs and symptoms of on-off phenomenon (e.g., sudden changes with loss of function, immobility, and severe dyskinetic movements). Notify medical and/or nursing staff as appropriate.

QUICK FACTS 8-4 ▶ PARKINSON'S STAGES (HOEHN AND YAHR CLASSIFICATION)	
Stage	**Description**
Stage One	Minimal or absent disability. Unilateral symptoms. May include tremor, rigidity, or unilateral impairment in facial expression.
Stage Two	Minimal bilateral or midline involvement, no balance involvement, general slowness in ADLs, stiffness or rigidity of trunks muscles, stooped posture. May develop months or years after stage one. Facial involvement may involve loss of facial expression bilaterally, decreased blinking, speech abnormalities may be present (soft speech, monotone, fading volume, slurring).
Stage Three	Impaired balance (inability to make rapid, automatic involuntary balance adjustments), slowness of movement. Falls may be common at this stage. Individual may still be fully independent at this stage.
Stage Four	Significantly impaired, symptoms become severe. Standing and walking require assistance, unable to live independently.
Stage Five	Severely impaired, confinement to bed or wheelchair. Inability to rise from chair or bed without help, may fall when standing or turning, may freeze or stumble during gait. Assistance with all ADLs. May experience hallucinations or delusions.

Physical Therapy Goals, Outcomes, and Interventions

1. Monitor changes associated with disease progression and pharmacological interventions; revise intervention accordingly; follow established maintenance program.
2. Prevent or minimize secondary impairments associated with disuse and inactivity.
3. Teach compensatory strategies to initiate movement and unlock freezing episodes (e.g., repetitive auditory stimulation/music).
4. See Chapter 3 on Neuromuscular Physical Therapy for further discussion and interventions.

Cognitive Disorders Affecting Aging Adults

Delirium

Description
1. Fluctuating attention state causing temporary confusion and loss of mental function, disorientation to place and time; an acute disorder, potentially reversible (Table 8-5).

Etiology
1. Drug toxicity and/or systemic illness, oxygen deprivation to brain; environmental changes, and sensory deprivation (e.g., recent hospitalization, institutionalization).

Characteristics
1. Acute onset, often at night; fluctuating course with lucid intervals; worse at night.
2. Duration; hours to weeks.
3. May be hypo- or hyperalert, distractible; fluctuates over course of day.
4. Orientation and memory impaired; difficulty with concentration; easily distracted.
5. Illusions/hallucinations, periods of agitation.
6. Memory deficits: immediate and recent.
7. Disorganized thinking, incoherent speech.
8. Sleep/wake cycles always disrupted; sundowning (increased agitation late in day and early evening) may be present.

Treatment Principles
1. Environment: keep calm and quiet environment; low-level lighting without shadows; exposure to natural light; keep familiar objects nearby; having familiar individuals involved is beneficial.
2. Physical therapy implications: include reorientation activities; use clear explanations; ensure that patient has eyeglasses and hearing aids in place if appropriate.

Table 8-5

Differential Diagnosis: Organic Brain Syndromes

	MULTI-INFARCT DEMENTIA	SENILE DEMENTIA ALZHEIMER'S TYPE (SDAT)	PRESENILE DEMENTIA ALZHEIMER'S TYPE (PDAT)
Age of onset	55–70	60+	40–60
Gender distribution	M:W = 3:1	M:W = 2:3	M:W = 2:3
Duration	varies: days > years	varies: months > years; mean survival 7–11 yr	rapid mean survival 4 years
Mode of onset	sudden	gradual	less gradual than SDAT
Course	intermittent step-wise	slowly or rapidly progressive	rapidly progressive
Prognosis	varies	poor: mod. or severe cases	very poor
Outcome	death from CVA, CAD, or infection	death from general system failure, infection	
Hereditary precipitating factors	atherosclerosis; some familial tendency	multifactorial: age genetic: chromosome 21 abnormality; APOE4 gene; traumatic brain injury, Down Syndrome	
Neuropathology	small or large areas of infarction; secondary gliosis, senile plaques not common	neuronal degeneration, neurofibrillary tangles, amyloid deposits, senile plaques, decreased cholinergic neuronal activity	
Clinical signs of brain damage	diffuse or focal, areas of preserved function	diffuse, generalized	diffuse, generalized, more severe than SDAT
Impairment of higher cortical functions	isolated impairments, focal signs, episodes of confusion with lucid intervals, some insight	progressive dementia, progressive disorientation, memory loss, impaired cognition, judgment, abstract thinking, visuospatial deficits, apraxia, delusions, hallucinations; late stages: disorders of sleep, eating, sexual behavior, no insight	
Affect	emotional lability, anxious, depressed	variable: depressed, anxious, paranoid, hostile, restlessness, agitation, wandering, "sundowning" late: apathy personality changes: egocentricity, impulsivity, irritability, inappropriate social behaviors	
Neuromuscular	focal signs: may see hemiparesis, hemisensory loss	occasional tremors, generalized weakness, unsteady gait, increased tone: rigid postures, decreased postural reflexes, increased fall risk, repetitive behaviors	
Seizures	yes	rare	occasional
Medical	TIAs, CVA, hypertension, headaches	infections, contractures, fractures, decubitus ulcers, urinary and fecal incontinence	

Dementia

Description
1. Acquired disorder of cognitive and behavioral impairment causing dysfunction in daily living (see Table 8-5).
2. Incidence rates of dementia.
   a. Reversible dementias: between 10% and 20% of the population, multiple causes.
   b. Alzheimer's type dementia: between 60% and 80% of dementias, most common cause of dementia.

Criteria for Dementia
1. Deterioration of intellectual functions: impoverished thinking; impaired judgment; disorientation, confusion, impaired social functioning.
2. Disturbances in higher cortical functions: language (aphasia); motor skills (apraxia); perception (agnosia).
3. Memory impairment; recent and remote.
4. Personality changes: alteration or accentuation of premorbid traits; behavioral changes.
5. Alertness (consciousness) usually normal.
6. Sleep often fragmented.

Types of Dementia
1. Reversible dementia: 10%–20% of dementias, multiple causes.
   a. Drugs: sedatives, hypnotics, antianxiety agents, antidepressants, antiarrhythmics, antihypertensives, anticonvulsants, antipsychotics, drugs with anticholinergic side effects.

b. Nutritional disorders: B_6 deficiency, thiamine deficiency, B_{12} deficiency/pernicious anemia, folate deficiency.
c. Metabolic disorders: hyper/hypothyroidism, hypercalcemia, hyper/hyponatremia, hypoglycemia, kidney or liver failure, Cushing's syndrome, Addison's disease, hypopituitarism, carcinoma.
d. Psychiatric disorders: depression, anxiety, psychosis.
e. Toxins: air pollution, alcohol.
f. Primary degenerative dementia, Alzheimer's type, 50%–70% of dementias.
   - Third costliest disease in United States; fourth leading cause of death.
   - Etiology unknown: evidence of chromosomal abnormalities; predisposing factors: family history, Down's syndrome, traumatic brain injury, aluminum toxicity.
   - Pathophysiology.
     - Generalized atrophy of brain with decreased synthesis of neurotransmitters, diffuse ventricular dilation.
     - Histopathological changes: neurofibrillary tangles; neuritic senile plaques, build-up of beta-amyloid protein.
   - Types (see Table 8-5).
   - Characteristics.
     - Dementia: insidious onset with generally progressive deteriorating course; irreversible; mean survival time postdiagnosis is 4 years.
     - May have periods of agitation, restlessness, wandering.
     - Sundowning syndrome: confusion and agitation increases in late afternoon.
g. Multi-infarct dementias (MIDs), 20%–25% of dementias.
   - Etiology: large and small vascular infarcts in both gray and white matter of brain, producing loss of brain function.
   - Characteristics.
     - Sudden onset rather than insidious: stepwise progression.
     - Spotty and patchy distribution of deficits: areas of preserved ability along with impairments.
     - Focal neurological signs and symptoms: e.g., gait and balance abnormalities, weakness, exaggerated deep tendon reflexes (DTRs).
     - Emotional liability common.
     - Associated with history of stroke, cardiovascular disease, hypertension.
h. Other types of dementias.
   - Parkinson's disease: dementia is sometimes found in late stages of the disease.
   - Alcohol-related; chronic alcoholism with prolonged nutritional (B1) deficiency (e.g., Korsakoff's psychosis).

Examination
1. The examination is performed by physical therapist on evaluation. The physical therapist assistant should be aware of information gathered at initial evaluation and assess for changes throughout treatment sessions and throughout the episode of care.
2. History: determine onset of symptoms, progression, triggering events; common problems, social history.
3. Examine cognitive functions: orientation, attention, calculation, recall, language. Standardized test: Mini-Mental State Exam (MMSE); score of <24 of a possible 30 is indicative of mental decline/dementia.
4. Examine for impairments in higher cortical functions; inability to communicate, perceptual dysfunction.
5. Examine for behavioral changes: restless, agitated, distracted, paranoid, wandering, inappropriate social behaviors, repetitive behaviors.
6. Examine self-care: ability to carry out ADLs (e.g., limitations in grooming and hygiene, continence).
7. Examine motor abilities: dyspraxia, gait, and balance instability.
8. Examine environment for safety, optimal function.

Interventions, Implications, and Compensatory Strategies
1. Environment.
   a. Provide safe environment: prevent falls, injury or further dysfunction, safety from wandering, utilize safety monitoring devices as needed (e.g., alarm device).
   b. Provide soothing environment with reduced environmental distractions; reduces agitation, increases attention.
2. Support individual's remaining function.
   a. Approach the patient in a friendly, supportive manner; model calm behavior.
   b. Use consistent, simple commands; speak slowly.
   c. Use nonverbal communication: sensory cues, gesture, demonstration.
   d. Provide reorienting information: use prompts, wall calendars, daily schedules, memory aids whenever possible.
   e. Avoid stressful tasks, emphasize familiar, well-learned skills; provide redirection.
   f. Approach learning in a simple, repetitious way; proceed slowly, provide adequate rest time.
   g. Provide mental stimulation; utilize simple, well-liked activities, games.
3. Provide regular physical activity: safe walking program, balance activities for fall prevention, activities to promote body awareness and sensory stimulation.
4. Participate in restraint reduction program.
5. Educate/support family, caregivers.
6. Present a realistic, consistent team approach to management.

Depression

Description
1. Depression is a disorder characterized by depressed mood and lack of interest or pleasure in all activities and associated symptoms for a period of at least 2 weeks.
2. Incidence.
   a. Community-dwelling elderly: 5% have clinically diagnosed major depression (exhibit at least 5 symptoms); another 10-20% have depressive symptoms. See Quick Facts 8-5.
   b. Institutionalized elderly: 12% have major depression; another 15-20% have depressive symptoms.

Predisposing Factors
1. The physical therapist will asses the individual for predisposing factors. These may include, but are not limited to:
   a. Family history, prior episodes of depression.
   b. Illness, drug side effects; hormonal.
   c. Chronic condition; loss of physical functions, pain (e.g., stroke).
   d. Sensory deprivation (loss of vision or hearing).
   e. History of losses: death of family and friends, job, income, independence.
   f. Social isolation, lack of family support.
   g. Psychological losses; memory, intellectual functions.
2. Standardized testing that may be administered.
   a. Mini-Mental State Exam (MMSE) may be used to assess changes/decline in cognitive function. This is an 11-item measure of 5 areas of cognitive function; maximum score = 30. (Score of: 20-24 suggests mild dementia, 13-20 suggests moderate dementia, <12 indicates severe dementia).
   b. Geriatric Depression Scale. There is a short form (15 questions) and a long form (30 questions), both used to indicate severity of depressive symptoms. Long form: 0-9 suggests normal, 10-19 mild depression, 20-30 suggests severe depression. Short form: >5 suggestive of depression, ≥ 10 indicative of depression. Scores >5 warrant medical follow up.

Medical Management

Medications
1. Primary treatment option for depression typically includes medication management.
2. Medications often take 1-2 weeks to begin to improve symptoms and can take several weeks to begin to fully work. Individuals should be advised of this lag-time. Medications for depression are typically prescribed for daily administration and not "as needed"; individuals should be reminded to take even when "feeling better."
3. Concerns for the aging adult include drug interactions with other medications, missing doses or overdosing. Aging individuals may be more sensitive to medications and should be monitored closely.

Psychotherapy
1. Psychotherapy is often combined with medication management.
2. May be just as effective in the aging population, especially when the individual is concerned about taking more mediations.

Complementary Therapies
1. Therapies such as yoga, exercise, social interaction, and certain dietary supplements have been beneficial.

Electroconvulsive Therapy (ECT)
1. ECT may be used with severe depression when medication or psychotherapy has been unsuccessful.

Interventions, Implications, and Compensatory Strategies
1. Avoid excessive cheerfulness; provide support and encouragement.
2. Assist patient in adjustment process to losses, coping strategies.
3. Encourage activities, exercise program; aerobic training is associated with increased feelings of well-being.

QUICK FACTS 8-5 ▶ DEPRESSION - SYMPTOMS OF

Symptoms of Depression (Note: A medical provider must diagnose depression.)

- Nutritional problems: digestive, appetite changes with weight gain or loss, dehydration.
- Sleep disturbances: insomnia, hypersomnia, early-morning wakefulness.
- Psychomotor changes: inactivity with resultant functional impairments, weakness or agitation; aches, pains, headaches, or cramps that won't go away.
- Fatigue, loss of energy.
- Irritability, restlessness.
- Inability to concentrate, remembering details, making decisions.
- Feelings of guilt, worthlessness, helplessness, or low self-esteem.
- Withdrawal from family and friends, self-neglect.
- Suicidal thoughts or attempts.

4. Assist in improving/maintaining independence; emphasize mastery by patient, achievement of short-term goals rather than long-term goals.

Cardiopulmonary and Integumentary Disorders and Diseases

Cardiovascular Diseases
1. Hypertension.
   a. Significant risk factor in cardiovascular disease, stroke, renal failure, and death.
2. Coronary artery disease (CAD)
   a. Affects 40% of individuals aged 65–74 and 50% over age 75.
   b. Angina.
      - Angina pain not always a consistent indicator of ischemia in elderly; shortness of breath, ECG ST segment depression may be more reliable indicators.
   c. Acute myocardial infarction.
      - Clinical presentation may vary from younger adults: may present with sudden dyspnea, acute confusion, syncope.
      - Clinical course often more complicated in the elderly, mortality rates twice that of younger adults.
   d. Congestive heart failure.
   e. Conduction system diseases: pacemaker dysfunction results in low cardiac output.
3. Peripheral vascular disease.
4. Clinical signs and symptoms; examination and intervention; see Chapter 4.

Pulmonary Diseases
1. Chronic bronchitis.
2. Chronic obstructive pulmonary disease (COPD).
3. Asthma.
4. Pneumonia.
   a. Initial symptoms may vary: instead of high fever and productive cough, may see altered mental status, tachypnea, dehydration.
5. Lung cancer.
6. Clinical signs and symptoms; examination and intervention; see Chapter 5.

Integumentary Conditions
1. Pressure ulcers (decubitus ulcers).
   a. Characteristics.
      - Affects 10%–25% of hospitalized, ill elderly patients.
      - Risk factors: immobility and inactivity, sensory impairment, cognitive deficits, decreased circulation, poor nutritional status, incontinence, and moisture.
      - Common over bony prominences: ischial tuberosities, sacrum, greater trochanter, heels, ankles, elbows, and scapulae.

> **RED FLAG:** If not treated promptly, ulcers can progress to infection and damage of deep tissues; can be potentially fatal in the frail elderly and chronically ill.

   b. Clinical signs and symptoms; examination and intervention. See Chapter 7.

Metabolic Pathologies

Diabetes Mellitus
1. Aging is associated with deteriorating glucose tolerance; type 2 diabetes affects as many as 10%–20% of individuals over age of 60.
2. Associated with obesity and sedentary lifestyle.
3. Clinical signs and symptoms; examination and intervention. See Chapter 6.

Common Problem Areas for Aging Adults

Immobility-Disability

Considerations
1. Impaired mobility and disability can result from a host of diseases and problems.
2. Limitations in function increase with age.
   a. Include difficulty with personal care activities and home management activities.
3. Immobility can result in additional problems.
   a. Immobility can lead to complications in almost every major organ system (e.g., pressure sores, contractures, bone loss, muscular atrophy, deconditioning).
   b. Metabolic changes can include: negative nitrogen and calcium balance, impaired glucose tolerance, decreased plasma volume, altered drug pharmacokinetics.

c. Psychological changes can include loss of positive self-image, depression.
   d. Behavioral changes can include confusion, dementia secondary to sensory deprivation, egocentricity.
   e. Loss of independence and dependency.
4. Physical therapist examination to identify source of immobility or disability.

Interventions, Goals, and Outcomes
1. Establishment of a supportive relationship and promotion of self-determination of goals.
2. Focus on optimal function, gradual progression of physical daily activities.
3. Prevent further complications or injury.
4. A team approach of health professionals to address all aspects of the patient's problems; patient participation in decision making.

Falls and Instability

Incidence / Impact of
1. Falls and fall injury are a major public health concern for the elderly.
   a. Each year approximately 30% of persons over the age of 65 fall.
   b. Falls often result in soft tissue injuries and fractures; are a factor in 40% of admissions to nursing homes.
   c. Falls result in: increased caution and fear of falling, loss of confidence to function independently, reduced motivation and levels of activity, increased risk of recurrent falls.

Fall Etiology
1. Most falls are multifactorial, the result of multiple intrinsic and extrinsic factors and their cumulative effects on mobility (e.g., disease states, age-related changes).
2. Intrinsic/physiological factors.
   a. Age: incidence of falls increases with age.
   b. Sensory changes.
      - Reduced vision, hearing, cutaneous proprioceptive, vestibular function.
      - Altered sensory organization for balance, reduced resolution of sensory conflict situations, increased dependence on support surface somatosensory inputs.
   c. Musculoskeletal changes: weakness; decreased ROM; altered postural synergies.
   d. Neuromotor changes: dizziness, vertigo common.
      - Timing and control problems: impaired reaction and movement times, slowed onset.
   e. Cardiovascular changes: orthostatic hypotension; hyperventilation, coughing, arrhythmias.
   f. Drugs.
      - Strong evidence linking psychotropic agents.
      - Some evidence linking certain cardiovascular agents, especially those that cause peripheral vasodilation.
      - Conflicting evidence linking analgesics, hypoglycemics.
3. Intrinsic/psychosocial factors.
   a. Mental status/cognitive impairment.
   b. Depression.
   c. Denial of aging.
   d. Fear of falling, associated with self-imposed activity restriction.
   e. Relocation.
4. Extrinsic/environmental factors.
   a. Setting: three times as many falls for institutionalized or hospitalized elderly than for community dwelling.
   b. Consider ground surfaces, lighting, doors/doorways, stairs.
   c. At home most falls occur in bedroom (42%), bathroom (34%).
5. Activity-related risk factors.
   a. Most falls occur during normal daily activity: getting up from bed/chair, turning head/body, bending, walking, climbing/descending stairs.
   b. Some falls are caused by improper use of assistive device: walker, cane, wheelchair.

Fall Prevention
1. Examination, performed by PT.
   a. Accurate fall history: location, activity, time, symptoms, previous falls.
   b. Physical examination of patient: cognitive, sensory, neuromuscular, cardiopulmonary.
   c. Standardized tests and measures for functional balance and instability. See Table 3-17.
2. Identify fall risk; determine all intrinsic and/or extrinsic factors.
3. Interventions, goals, and outcomes as established by physical therapist. Followed up by the physical therapist assistant.
   a. Eliminate or minimize all fall risk factors; stabilize disease states, medications.
   b. Improve functional mobility.
   c. Provide exercise to increase strength, flexibility.
   d. Provide sensory compensation strategies.
   e. Balance and gait training.
   f. Functional training.
      - Focus on sit-to-stand transitions, turning, walking, stairs.
      - Modify ADL; provide assistive devices, adaptive equipment as appropriate.
      - Allow adequate time for activities; instruct in gradual position changes.

g. Safety education.
      - Identify risks.
      - Provide instructions in writing.
      - Communicate with family and caregivers.
   h. Modify environment to reduce falls and instability.
      - Use environmental checklist.
      - Ensure adequate lighting.
      - Use contrasting colors to delineate hazardous areas.
      - Simplify environment, reduce clutter.
4. When the patient falls:
   a. Do not attempt to lift patient by yourself: get help, provide first aid and call emergency services if necessary.
   b. Check for dizziness that may have preceded the fall.
   c. Provide reassurance.
   d. Contact supervising physical therapist.
   e. Solicit witnesses of fall event.
   f. Document event.

Medication Errors

Scope of the Problem
1. Most elderly (60%–85%) utilize prescription drugs to address a chronic medical problem.
2. One-third have three or more medical problems requiring multiple medications and complex dosage schedules.
3. Average older person takes between four and seven prescription drugs each day.
   a. Also, an additional 3.2 over-the-counter drugs.
4. Adverse drug reactions are associated with:
   a. Hospital admissions.
   b. High incidence of falls/hip fracture (e.g., effects of psychotropic agents).
   c. Motor vehicle accidents.

Increased Risk for Drug Toxicity
1. Factors include age-related changes in pharmacokinetics:
   a. Alterations in drug absorption, distribution to tissues, oxidative metabolism.
   b. Altered sensitivity to the effects of drugs.
      - Increased with certain drugs (e.g., narcotic analgesics, benzodiazepines).
      - Decreased with certain drugs (e.g., drugs mediated by beta-adrenergic receptors, isoproterenol, propranolol).
   c. Alterations in excretion associated with a decline in hepatic and renal function: decreased clearance in certain drugs (e.g., digoxin, lithium).
   d. Drugs may interfere with brain function, cause confusion (e.g., psychoactive drugs, sedatives, hypnotics, antidepressants, anticonvulsants, antiparkinsonism agents).
   e. Older adults have less homeostatic reserve (e.g., more susceptible to orthostatic hypotension with vasodilating drugs due to dampened compensatory baroreceptor response).
   f. Drug-processing effects: multiple drugs compete for binding sites.
      - Drug-to-drug interactions (e.g., levadopa combined with monoamine oxidase inhibitors [MAOIs] may result in hypertensive response).
      - Most drugs exert more than one specific action in the body (polypharmacological effects: e.g., prednisone prescribed for anti-inflammatory action may benefit arthritic symptoms but will aggravate a coexisting diabetic state (augments blood glucose levels).
2. Physicians may prescribe medications that are inappropriate for use with some elderly persons (e.g., those causing hypotension or dizziness).
3. Most patients are not knowledgeable about drug actions, drug side effects.
4. Drug-food interactions can interfere with effectiveness of medications (e.g., efficacy of levadopa is compromised if ingested too soon before or after a high-protein meal); potential vitamin/drug interactions.
5. Polypharmacy phenomena: multiple drug prescriptions.
   a. Exacerbated by elderly who visit multiple physicians, use different pharmacies.
   b. Lack of integrated care (e.g., computerized system of drug monitoring).
6. Health status influences/socioeconomic factors.
   a. Older adults have a high rate of medication dosage errors: associated with memory impairment, visual impairments, uncoordination, low literacy.
   b. Financial issues: due to high costs and/or fixed incomes the elderly may skip dosages or stop taking medications.
7. Common adverse effects.
   a. Confusion/dementia (e.g., tranquilizers, barbiturates, digitalis, antihypertensives, anticholinergic drugs, analgesics, antiparkinsonians, diuretics, beta-blockers).
   b. Sedation/immobility (e.g., psychotropic drugs, narcotic analgesics).
   c. Weakness (e.g., antihypertensives, vasodilators, digitalis, diuretics, oral hypoglycemics).
   d. Postural hypotension (e.g., antihypertensives, diuretics, tricyclic antidepressants, tranquilizers, nitrates, narcotic analgesics).
   e. Depression (e.g., antihypertensives, anti-inflammatory, antimycobacterial, antiparkinsonians, diuretics, sedative-hypnotics, vasodilators).

f. Drug-induced movement disorders.
- Dyskinesias: involuntary, stereotypic and repetitive movements (e.g., lip smacking, hand movements) associated with long-term use of neuroleptic drugs and anticholinergic drugs, levadopa.
- Akathisia (motor restlessness) associated with antipsychotic drugs.
- Essential tremor associated with tricyclic antidepressants, adrenergic drugs.
- Parkinsonism: associated with antipsychotics, sympatholytics.

g. Incontinence: caused by or exacerbated by a variety of drugs (e.g., barbiturates, benzodiazapines, antipsychotic drugs, anticholinergic drugs).

Interventions, Goals, and Outcomes

1. Assess in adequate monitoring of drug therapy.
   a. Recognize drug-related side effects.
      - Adverse reactions to drugs.
      - Potential drug interactions in the elderly.
   b. Carefully document patient responses to medications, exercise and activity.
2. Assist in patient and family drug education/compliance (e.g., understanding of purpose of drugs, dosage, potential side effects).
3. Encourage centralization of medications through one pharmacy.
4. Assist in simplification of drug regimen and instructions.
   a. Administration of drugs (e.g., daily pill box, drug calendar).
   b. Check to see if patient is taking medications on schedule.
   c. Time doses in conjunction with daily routine.
5. Coordinate physical therapy with drug schedule/optimal dose (e.g., exercise during peak dose with individual on Parkinson's medications).
6. Recognize potentially harmful interaction effects: modalities that cause vasodilatation in combination with vasodilating drugs.

Nutritional Deficiency

Many Older Adults Have Primary Nutritional Problems

1. Nutritional problems in elderly are linked to health status and poverty rather than to age itself.
   a. Chronic diseases alter the overall needs for nutrients/energy demands, the abilities to take in and utilize nutrients, and overall activity levels (e.g., Alzheimer's disease, CVA, diabetes).
   b. Limited, fixed incomes severely limit food choices and availability.
2. Both undernourishment and obesity exist in the elderly and contribute to decreased levels of vitality and fitness.
3. Contributing factors to poor dietary intake:
   a. Decreased sense of taste and smell.
   b. Poor teeth or poorly fitting dentures.
   c. Reduced gastrointestinal function: decreased saliva, gastromucosal atrophy, reduced intestinal mobility, reflux.
   d. Loss of interest in foods.
   e. Lack of social support, socialization during meals.
   f. Lack of mobility: inability to get to grocery store, shop; inability to prepare foods.
4. There is an age-related slowing in basal metabolic rate and a decline in total caloric intake. Most of the decline is associated with a concurrent reduction in physical activity.
5. Dehydration is common in the elderly, resulting in fluid and electrolyte disturbances.
   a. Thirst sensation is diminished.
   b. May be physically unable to acquire/maintain fluids.
   c. Environmental heat stresses may be life threatening.
6. Diets are often deficient in nutrients, especially vitamins A and C, B12, thiamine, protein, iron, calcium/vitamin D, folic acid, zinc.
7. Increased use of taste enhancers (e.g., salt and sugar or alcohol) influences nutritional intake.
8. Drug/dietary interactions influence nutritional intake (e.g., reserpine, digoxin, antitumor agents, excessive use of antacids).

Dietary Status Assessment

1. Dietary history: patterns of eating, types of foods.
2. Psychosocial: mental status, desire to eat/depression, social isolation.
3. Body composition: weight/height measures; skin fold measurements (triceps/subscapular skin fold thickness); upper arm circumference.
4. Sensory function: taste and smell.
5. Dental and periodontal disease, fit of dentures.
6. Ability to feed self: mastication, swallowing, hand/mouth control, posture, physical weakness, fatigue.
7. Integumentary: skin condition, edema.
8. Compliance to special diets.
9. Functional assessment: basic ADL, feeding, overall exercise/activity levels.

Interventions, Goals, and Outcomes

1. Assist in monitoring adequate nutritional intake.
2. Assist in health promotion.
   a. Maintain adequate nutritional support.
      - Nutritional consults as necessary.
      - Nutritional educational programs.
      - Assistance in grocery shopping, meal preparation; e.g., recommendations for home health aides.
      - Elderly food programs: home delivered/"meals on wheels"; congregate meals/senior center daily meal programs; federal food stamp programs.
   b. Maintain physical function, adequate activity levels.

Review Questions

Geriatric Physical Therapy

1. Summarize changes in the following systems as a result of aging:
   Muscular system
   Skeletal system
   Vestibular system

2. Identify what a normal T-score is and what a lower T-score indicates. Identify medical management of an individual who has low T-scores.

3. Identify three physical therapy interventions each for osteoarthritis and rheumatoid arthritis that have good evidence supporting their use in treatment programs.

4. Differentiate modifiable and non-modifiable risk factors for stroke/cerebrovascular accident.

5. Which balance assessment test is more appropriately used for a community-dwelling older adult—the Dynamic Gait Index (DGI) or the Performance Oriented Mobility Assessment (POMA) test? Compare and contrast these two balance assessments.

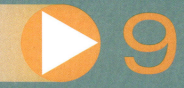

Pediatric Physical Therapy

TIFFANY BOHM and SUZANNE GIUFFRE

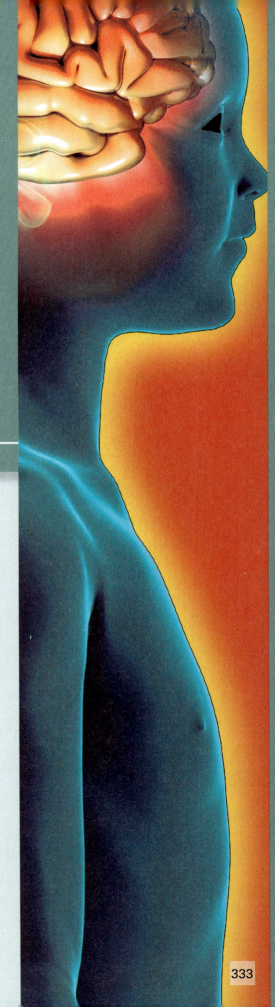

Chapter Outline

- The Typically Developing Child, 335
  - Human Development and Learning/Development Theories, 335
  - Effect of Motor Control and Motor Learning on Development, 335
  - Neonatal Development, 335
  - Developmental Milestones by Age and Domain, 336
  - Posture and Gait, 338
- Physical Therapy Examination and Data Collection, 344
  - Basic Assessments, 344
  - Screening Tests, 344
  - Standardized Developmental Tests Commonly Used by Therapists, 344
  - Performance Scales Measuring Function and Outcomes of Therapy, 344
- Intervention, 345
  - Overview, 345
  - Intervention Approaches, 345
  - Physical Therapy Tools for Working with Children, 345
  - Adaptive Equipment, 346

- Conditions/Pathology/Diseases: Orthopedic Disorders, 348
  - Developmental Dysplasia of the Hip (DDH), 348
  - Medical Intervention, 348
  - Legg-Calvé-Perthes Disease (LCPD), 348
  - Medical Intervention, 349
  - Slipped Capital Femoral Epiphysis (SCFE), 349
  - Medical Intervention, 350
  - Juvenile Rheumatoid Arthritis (JRA), 350
  - Medical Interventions, 350
  - Osteogenesis Imperfecta (OI), 351
  - Medical Intervention, 351
  - Arthrogryposis Multiplex Congenita, 351
  - Medical Intervention, 352
  - Pediatric Fractures, 352
  - Medical Intervention, 352
  - Foot and Ankle Deformities, 352
  - Medical Intervention, 353
  - Brachial Plexus Injury, 353
  - Medical Intervention, 353
- Conditions/Pathology/Diseases with Intervention: Pediatric Neurological and Genetic Disorders, 353
  - Cerebral Palsy (CP), 353
  - Medical Intervention, 355
  - Traumatic Brain Injury (TBI), 356
  - Spina Bifida, 356
  - Down Syndrome (Trisomy 21), 358
  - Duchenne Muscular Dystrophy (Pseudohypertrophic Muscular Dystrophy), 358
  - Pervasive Developmental Disorder (PDD), 359
  - Intellectual Disability/Developmental Disability/Developmental Delay, 360
  - Sickle Cell Anemia, 360
- Special Considerations when Working with the Pediatric Population, 361
  - Team Members, 361
  - Environments of Care, 361
  - Legislation Guiding the Provision of Services, 361
- Review Questions, 363

The Typically Developing Child

Human Development and Learning/Development Theories

Definition
1. Human development: the growth, change, evolution, or maturation of an individual over time.

Learning/Development Theories
1. Maturational. Human behavior is innate and determined by a combination of genetic and biological factors.
2. Empirical: The environment provides the greatest influence on human development.
3. Behavioral.
   a. Environmental reinforcement influences learned behavior.
   b. Behavior management.
      - Consistent or intermittent reinforcement can cause behaviors to be learned.
      - Ignoring behaviors can extinguish them.
4. Social cognitive and sociocultural.
   a. Social learning and reinforcement help a child develop new skills by building new behaviors and skills related to existing knowledge.
   b. Learning is accomplished through partnerships with more mature members of the learning community.
5. Social maturational.
   a. A child's readiness for learning particular skills is primarily biological, with modifications based on subsequent environmental experiences.
   b. Pattern of learning is sequential.
   c. The child will experience periods of equilibrium (mastery) and disequilibrium (lack of mastery).

Effect of Motor Control and Motor Learning on Development

Motor Development
1. Motor control and motor learning are necessary for motor development to occur.
2. Refer to Chapter 3 for full explanation of motor control and motor learning.

Maturation
1. Neural maturation determines motor development.
2. Earliest movements, including reflexes, are determined by primitive neural structures.
3. Mature movements are directed by advanced neural structures that differentiate complex movements.

Learning
1. Motor programs.
   a. Intrinsic and automatic patterns of movement.
   b. Can be modified to adapt to a situation based on sensory feedback and conditions.
2. Generalization of skills occurs and child is able to use previously learned skills to decrease the time and effort necessary to learn a similar task.

Variables Influencing Development
1. Motivation.
2. Muscle strength.
3. Body weight.
4. Level of arousal.
5. Complexity and maturation of neural networks.
6. Environmental forces.

Neonatal Development

Prematurity
1. Birth at less than 37 weeks of gestation.
2. A fetus is considered viable at 22 to 23 weeks of gestation.

Reflexes
1. Basic unit of movement in the hierarchical theory of motor control.
2. Involve the combination of a sensory stimulus and a motor response (Table 9-1).

Neonatal (Primitive) Reflexes
1. Normal for young infants and typically present at birth (Table 9-2).
2. Usually integrated in the first 9 months of life.
   a. Persistent, absent, or asymmetrical reflexes usually indicate early brain damage and affect normal development.

Postural Control
1. Definition: the ability to maintain alignment of the body.
2. Development: directional concepts.
   a. Cephalocaudal: head control followed by upper extremity use followed by lower extremity use.

Table 9-1

Normal Reflexes & Responses
Primitive Reflexes

REFLEX	STIMULUS	RESPONSE
Suck-swallow	Object touches roof of the mouth	• Sucking
Rooting	Stroke or brush on the cheek	• Turns head toward touch and opens mouth
Flexor withdrawal	Noxious stimuli to sole of foot or palm of hand	• Flexion of knee or elbow to withdrawal from stimulus
Crossed extension	Noxious stimulus to sole of foot	• Flexion and then extension of contralateral leg
Traction response	Traction on upper extremities (as in pull-to-sit)	• Flexion of upper extremities with the appearance of "helping" into sitting position
Moro	Rapid neck extension	• Initially, arms abduct and extend followed quickly by arms flexing in as if grasping for parent and crying
Plantar grasp	Pressure on ball of the foot or toes	• Foot will dorsiflex and toes will curl
Positive support	Child is supported under the arms and feet bounce on a flat surface	• Extends legs for 20 to 30 seconds to support self in standing followed by flexion of legs and entering a sitting position
Stepping/walking	Infant held upright (slightly tilted forward) with solid surface under feet	• Reciprocal stepping motion of legs
Galant	Stroke is made on the paravertebral area from neck to low back	• Lateral flexion of trunk toward the side being stroked with hips and legs moving toward side of stimulus
Asymmetrical tonic neck reflex (ATNR)	Head turned to one side	• Arm and leg on the face side extend, arm and leg on the skull side flex
Tonic labyrinthine reflex (TLR)	Supine or prone position	• In supine, trunk and extremities extend • In prone, trunk and extremities flex
Placing reaction (proprioceptive placing)	Firm touch of dorsum of foot or hand on solid surface such as a table	• Flexion and subsequent extension of extremity resulting in hand or foot being placed on surface (table)
Palmar grasp	Object placed in open hand	• Grasping of object
Babinski	Stroke to lateral plantar surface of foot	• Great toe extension and fanning of the other toes
Symmetrical tonic neck reflex (STNR)	Neck placed in flexion or extension	• When neck extends, arms extend and legs flex • When neck flexes, arms flex and legs extend

b. Proximal to distal: midline control must develop first to provide a stable base upon which the head and extremities may move.
c. General to specific: whole body movements develop before disassociation occurs.
d. Gross to fine: large muscle movements usually occur before small muscle movements.
3. Development: kinesiological concepts (in order of development).
   a. Physiological flexion: position in which babies are born.
   b. Antigravity extension: active movements into extension occur first, as the extensors have been in a lengthened position and are prepared to move before flexors.
   c. Antigravity flexion: as infant spends more time in supine, flexors are lengthened and strengthened by moving to overcome gravity.
   d. Lateral flexion.
   e. Rotation.

Postural Reactions
1. Assist child with orienting the world in an upright position. Table 9-3.
2. Develop in infancy to early childhood.
3. Includes righting reactions, protective responses, and equilibrium responses (see Quick Facts 9-1).

Developmental Milestones by Age and Domain

First Year Milestones
1. Table 9-4. During the first year, even months are typically the significant milestone months (see Quick Facts 9-2).
2. The two most significant milestones.
   a. Head control.
   b. Sitting.

Table 9-2

Primitive Reflexes

REFLEX	AGE OF ONSET	AGE OF INTEGRATION	PROBLEMS IF REFLEX PERSISTS
Suck-swallow	28 weeks gestation	2–5 months	• Feeding • Releasing objects from mouth
Rooting	28 weeks gestation	3 months	• Oral motor development • Developing midline head control • Optical righting • Social interaction • Visual tracking
Flexor withdrawal	28 weeks gestation	1–2 months	• Standing and walking • Upper extremity functional activities
Crossed extension	28 weeks gestation	1–2 months	• Standing and walking
Traction response	28 weeks gestation	4–5 months	• Grading upper extremity response to traction
Moro	28 weeks gestation	4–6 months	• Sitting balance • Protective reactions in sitting • Eye-hand coordination • Visual tracking
Plantar grasp	28 weeks gestation	9 months	• Ability to stand with feet flat on a surface • Balance reactions and weight shift in standing
Positive support	35 weeks gestation	1–2 months	• Standing and walking • Balance reactions and weight shift in standing • *Can lead to plantar flexion contractures*
Stepping/walking	Birth	2 months	• Balance and controlled ambulation when accommodating to uneven surfaces
Galant	Birth	3–6 months	• Development of sitting balance • *Can lead to scoliosis*
ATNR	Birth	4–6 months	• Feeding • Visual tracking • Bilateral hand use • Midline use of hands • Rolling • Development of crawling • *Can lead to muscular shortening and a variety of skeletal deformities (scoliosis, hip dislocation, etc.)*
TLR	Birth	4–6 months	• Initiating rolling • Propping on elbows with extended hips (in prone) • Flexing trunk and hips to sit from supine • Full body extension • Sitting and standing balance
Placing reaction (proprioceptive placing)	Birth	6 months	• Organizing sensory input and motor output • Developing proprioception in extremities
Palmar grasp	Birth	9 months	• Voluntary grasp and release • Weight bearing on open hand • Crawling • Protective extension responses
Babinski	Birth	12 months	• Weight bearing on feet • Standing balance • Ambulation • *If present in a child over 2 years old, damage to the corticospinal tract may be present*
STNR	4–6 months	8–12 months	• Propping on arms in prone • Attaining and maintaining quadruped position • Reciprocal crawling • Sitting balance when head is moving • Using hands when looking at objects in sitting

Table 9-3

Postural Reactions

Righting Reactions

REACTION	AGE OF ONSET	AGE OF INTEGRATION	BEHAVIOR ACHIEVED
Neonatal neck righting (neck on body: NOB)	Birth	4–6 months	• Rolling (log rolling and then segmental rolling)
Body righting on body (BOB)	4–6 months	5 years	
Optical righting labyrinthine righting	Birth–2 months	Persist	• Maintaining head in upright position (head control)
Body righting on head (BOH)	4–6 months	5 years	
Landau	3–4 months	18–24 months	• Aligning head and body against gravity

Protective Responses

Parachute or forward	5–6 months	Persist	• Protection in sitting
Lateral	7–8 months		
Posterior	9–10 months		• Protection against falling when standing or walking
Stepping	15–18 months		

Equilibrium and Tilting Responses

Prone	6 months	Persist	• Realigning the center of gravity in the base of support
Supine	7–8 months		
Sitting	7–8 months		
Quadruped	9–12 months		
Standing	12–24 months		

QUICK FACTS 9-1 ▶ POSTURAL REACTIONS

Righting reactions	Responsible for orienting head and body in space Involve head and trunk movements
Protective responses	Utilized with rapid body displacement in response to an outside force Involve movement of extremities in the direction of displacement
Equilibrium responses	Utilized when slow changes occur between the center of gravity and base of support Degree of displacement determines the response used, beginning with movement of the head, then trunk and, if large enough, shoulder and/or hip abduction.

RED FLAG: Failure of the child to develop postural reactions can pose a safety risk to the child (Table 9-3).

QUICK FACTS 9-2 ▶ FIRST YEAR MILESTONES

Month	Milestone
4 months	Head control
6–8 months	Log roll between 4–6 months Segmental roll between 6–8 months Rolling prone → supine usually occurs first, after developing antigravity extension
8 months	Sitting
10 months	Cruising
12 months	Walking

Posture and Gait

Postural Flexibility

1. Infants under 1 year have normal physiological flexion.
2. Younger children are usually more flexible than older children.
3. Girls exhibit more flexibility than boys at all ages.

Table 9-4

Developmental Milestones by Age and Domain

	GROSS MOTOR DEVELOPMENT	FINE MOTOR DEVELOPMENT
Birth to 1 month	• Physiological flexion • Head held to the side in prone • Full head lag in pull-to-sit	• Visually tracks objects to midline or beyond • Fisted hands
2–3 months	• Lifts head in prone 45–90 degrees • Can bear some weight through forearms in prone • Head to side in supine • Variable head lag in pull-to-sit • Head bobs in supported sitting • Hips in flexion in supported standing	• Hands begin to open more • Visually tracks objects 180 degrees • Reflexive palmar grasp
4–5 months	• Rolls prone to side or supine • Bears weight through forearms in prone • Rolls supine to side • Head steady in supported sitting • Scapular adduction with upper trunk extension in supported sitting • Bears most weight through flexed hips in supported standing	• Grasps toys • Ulnar-palmar grasp (fingers opposing ulnar side of palm, thumb adducted and flexed) • Bilateral reaching with forearms pronated
6–7 months	• Rolls from supine to prone • Holds weight on one hand in prone to reach for toy • Holds weight on extended arms in prone • Lifts head in supine • Sits without support • Stands holding on • Bounces in standing	• Radial-palmar grasp (rakes objects into palm with adducted thumb and flexed fingers) • Voluntary release to transfer objects between hands • Approaches objects unilaterally • Arm in neutral when approaching toy
8–9 months	• Gets into hands and knees position • Creeps on hands and knees • Moves from hands and knees to sitting • Sits without hand support for longer periods • Pulls-to-stand • Walks along furniture, "cruising" • Stands alone briefly	• Develops active supination in arms • Points and pokes with index finger • Takes objects out of containers • Develops more refined release of objects • Develops more variation in grasping including radial-digital grasp (thumb opposing side of index finger) • Radial-palmar grasp (fingers raking object into palm) • Three-jaw-chuck grasp (first two fingers opposing thumb)
10–11 months	• Pulls to stand using half-kneel intermediate position • Stands without support for longer • Picks up object from floor while holding on • Bear walks on hands and feet • Walks with two hands held • Walks with one hand held • May walk a few steps without help	• Inferior pincer grasp (thumb opposing ventral surface of index finger) • Fine pincer grasp (tips of fingers oppose tip of thumb) • Puts objects into containers • Grasps crayon
12–15 months	• Walks alone • Walks backward and sideways • Bends over to look between legs • Creeps upstairs • Throws ball in sitting position • Runs/fast-walks with wide-based gait	• Builds tower of two cubes • Marks paper with crayon • Uses neat pincer grasp
16–23 months	• Squats in play • Propels ride-on toys • Kicks ball in standing with minimum control • Throws ball in standing • Ascends and descends stairs with one hand held • Jumps off bottom step • Runs with more coordination	• Holds paper • Strings beads • Stacks six cubes • Imitates vertical and horizontal strokes with crayon on paper

(Continued)

Table 9-4

Developmental Milestones by Age and Domain (Continued)

	GROSS MOTOR DEVELOPMENT	FINE MOTOR DEVELOPMENT
24–36 months	• Rides tricycle • Walks on tiptoe • Runs well • Catches large ball • Uses reciprocal gait pattern on stairs • Jumps with both feet • Hops on one foot • Cultural factors may influence development of movement skills (e.g., riding tricycle, ball play, hopping)	• Cuts with scissors • Builds tower using eight cubes • Opens and closes jar • Completes 3- to 4-piece puzzles • Folds clothes • Buttons clothes
3–4 years	• Throws ball overhand • Hops two to ten times on one foot • Stands on tiptoes • Walks on a line 10 feet • Runs fast and avoids obstacles • Jumps over 12 inch obstacles	• Copies a circle or cross • Draws a recognizable human figure with head and two extremities • Draws squares
5–8 years	• Skips on alternate feet • Gallops • Balances on one foot • Jumps with rhythm • Bounces large ball • Greater speed and control in running • Kicks ball with skill	• Hand preference is clear • Prints well • Starts to learn cursive writing • Able to fasten small buttons and hooks
9–12 years (pre-adolescent)	• More mature patterns of throwing and jumping • Able to run faster with more efficiency • Enjoys competitive games • Improved balance and coordination • Girls may develop pubescent body changes • Boys may develop preadolescent fat spurt	• Handwriting is well developed • Can do more skilled hand tasks such as those involved in art
13–18 years (adolescent)	• Rapid growth • Pubescent changes leading to increased size and strength; especially boys • Improved balance skills • Coordination • Endurance	• Greater dexterity developed for fine motor tasks • Develops skills in knitting, sewing, art, crafts, etc.
	SOCIAL DEVELOPMENT	LANGUAGE DEVELOPMENT
Birth to 1 month	• Eye contact • Molds body when held	• Monotonous cry to indicate needs
2–3 months	• Enjoys physical contact • Responds with smile	• Coos open vowel sounds like "aaa" • Laughs • Cries vary in pitch to communicate different emotions/needs • Vocalizes in response to conversation
4–5 months	• Socializes with strangers/others • Lifts arms to mother	• Reacts to music • Reacts to own name
6–7 months	• Recognizes mother visually • Anxious about strangers • Yells to get attention • Enjoys vigorous play • Anxious about separating from mother	• Waves bye-bye • Uses simple gestures • Babbles double consonants "baba" • Produces more consonant sounds when babbling
8–9 months	• Explores environment • Lets only mother meet needs • Enjoys social games	• Babbles single consonants • Uses "mama" or "dada" nonspecifically • Uses more mature pattern of inflection
10–11 months	• Tests parental reactions • Extends object to show	• Says "dada" and "mama" purposefully • Repeats sounds or gestures if laughed at • Babbles when alone • Language skills plateau while learning to walk

Table 9-4

Developmental Milestones by Age and Domain (Continued)

	SOCIAL DEVELOPMENT	LANGUAGE DEVELOPMENT
12–15 months	• Displays tantrum behaviors • Resists adult control • Easily distracted • Enjoys imitating adult behaviors	• Has one- to three-word vocabulary • Says "no" meaningfully • Uses words or approximations to express self • Uses exclamatory sentences ("uh-oh")
16–23 months	• Expresses affection • Plays alone for short time • Gets frustrated easily • Demonstrates parallel play • Interacts with peers	• Uses two-word sentences • Has a vocabulary of up to 50 words • Imitates sounds ("woof-woof") • Tries to sing songs • Uses own name
24–36 months	• Values own property ("Mine") • Talks loudly • Obeys simple rules • Has trouble with changes • May have tantrums • May develop fears of unfamiliar things such as animals or clowns	• Uses three- to five-word sentences • Uses expressive vocabulary of 50 to 200 words • Gives full name on request • Uses plurals and past tense • Frustrated if not understood • Recites nursery rhymes
3–4 years	• Plays cooperatively • Enjoys making friends • Enjoys helping with adult activities, like setting the table • Needs praise and guidance from adults	• Has expressive vocabulary of up to 1000 words • Talks to self during play • Uses rhythmic language • Loves to talk • Learns entire songs
5–8 years	• Prefers to play with peers rather than adults • Learns to give and receive • Shares • Cares what others think of him/her	• Has vocabulary of 2000 to 4000 words • Uses tenses correctly • Uses pronouns correctly • Interested in new words • Recites songs and rhymes
9–12 years (pre-adolescent)	• Interested in organized sports • Enjoys group activities • Develops motivation and discipline to practice skills	• Increasing vocabulary and maturity of language skills • Improved self-expression
13–18 years (adolescent)	• Orientation changes away from family to peers • Self-conscious • Usually interested in the opposite sex • More sophistication in social skills • Able to manage schedule	• Expressive skills in speaking and writing improve
	COGNITIVE DEVELOPMENT	**ADAPTIVE DEVELOPMENT**
Birth to 1 month	• Quiets when picked up • Consoles self by sucking	• Coordinates sucking, swallowing, and breathing
2–3 months	• Looks for sound • Plays with own hands • Shows active interest in person for 1 minute	• Hands to mouth • Stays awake longer during day • Sleeps longer at night
4–5 months	• Looks for hidden voice • Plays for 2–3 minutes with one toy	• Eats pureed or strained foods • Naps two to three times per day
6–7 months	• Plays peek-a-boo • Plays with paper • Looks for familiar people when named • Shakes toys to hear sound	• Mouths solid food • Bites and chews toys • Feeds self a cracker • Very messy
8–9 months	• Throws and drops objects • Enjoys looking at books • Stacks and unstacks ring toy	• Finger feeds self • Holds spoon • Chews using munching pattern • Up/down with jaw • Sleeps up to 14 hours at night
10–11 months	• Guides action toy manually • Dances	• Holds spoon • Helps with dressing

(Continued)

Table 9-4

Developmental Milestones by Age and Domain (*Continued*)

	COGNITIVE DEVELOPMENT	ADAPTIVE DEVELOPMENT
12–15 months	• Enjoys messy play including finger painting and feeding self • Helps to turn pages of books	• Brings spoon to mouth • Holds cup • Drinks with some spilling • Shows pattern of elimination behavior • Expresses discomfort with dirty diaper
16–23 months	• Names up to six body parts • Sorts objects • Puts things away • Understands personal pronouns • Turns pages one at a time	• Turns knob to open door • Feeds self with spoon • Some spilling • Helps with washing hands • Begins toilet training • Uses rotary movements to chew food
24–36 months	• Matches colors • Plays house • Loves being read to • Sorts shapes • Matches simple pictures • Matches pictures and objects • Engages in simple make-believe activities • Obeys two-part commands	• Recognizes common dangers • Uses spoon and fork • Uses napkin • Uses toilet consistently • Insists on doing things without help • Blows nose with help • Washes and dries hands • Dresses with help
3–4 years	• Identifies colors and shapes • Able to do at least a 30-piece puzzle • Identifies money • May confuse fantasy with reality	• Uses toilet without help • Uses eating utensils independently • Brushes teeth with supervision • May eliminate naps
5–8 years	• Learns to read • Learns addition and subtraction • Learns to write • Enjoys table games	• Learns to tie shoes • Can bathe independently • Washes hair with supervision • Takes role in household tasks • Can manage chores with supervision • Definite likes and dislikes with food • May have stomachaches related to school attendance
9–12 years (pre-adolescent)	• Increased attention span • Able to think more abstractly • Curious • Reads a variety of printed materials	• Independent in self-care activities • Learns to cook • Independent in simple household chores
13–18 years (adolescent)	• Formal thinking skills develop • Able to develop hypotheses, theories • Interests expand beyond self and local environment to world issues	• Learns to drive • Develops independence in most household tasks

4. During growth spurts, children lose flexibility.
   a. Bone to muscle length ratio changes.
   b. Usually regain flexibility as muscles elongate to catch up to bone length.

Typical Pediatric Posture and Alignment

1. Birth–12 months.
   a. Spine changes from flexible rounded posture at birth to beginning lordosis in neck and lower spine. This helps provide greater stability in the back and neck.
   b. Lower extremities change from physiological flexion to greater range in extension. Additionally LEs transition from a more varus position of the hip and knee toward a more neutral position.
2. 1–6 years.
   a. Spine develops greater lordosis in neck and low back.
   b. 1–2 years: Child learns to stand and walk. Stands with a wide base of support and high guard position of the arms. Hips decrease angle of anteversion.
   c. 3–4 years: Flexor tightness continues to decrease allowing full hip extension.
   d. 3 years: Hips and knees develop greater valgus angles, sometimes having a "knock-kneed" appearance at age 3 years (maximum physiological genu valgum).
3. 6–12 years.
   a. Boys lose flexibility throughout childhood.
   b. Children continue to grow and to develop strength and coordination.

c. Major postural changes do not typically occur during this stage.
4. Adolescence.
   a. Girls have slight genu valgum while boys have slight genu varum.
   b. Final growth spurt occurs earlier in girls (8–14 years) than boys (11–16 years).
   c. Full height and strength are achieved during adolescence.
   d. Growth plates fuse in late adolescence to early 20s.

Typical Pediatric Gait

1. Typically, developing children walk between the ages of 9–15 months. See Quick Facts 9-3.
2. Standing.
   a. Begin with bilateral upper extremity support and transition to unilateral support.
   b. Initially stand using a wide base of support. Hips positioned in abduction, flexion, and external rotation. Upper extremities positioned in abduction and external rotation for balance. See Quick Facts 9-4.
3. Early ambulation is characterized by:
   a. 8–9 months: Cruising sideways using furniture for support emerges.
   b. 9–10 months: Walking forward using support (hands held or holding a moving object) occurs.
   c. Development of more mature gait pattern. See Quick Facts 9-5.

QUICK FACTS 9-3 ▶ GAIT ACHIEVEMENTS

Median age of gait achievement	10.5 months—stand independently 11 months—take first steps 11.5 months—walk independently
Prerequisite skills for standing	Adequate body proportions Sufficient range of motion (ROM) Adequate strength and motor control Coordination of visual, proprioceptive, and vestibular systems for balance

Clinical Application

- Typical development requires the integration of a variety of intrinsic and extrinsic factors.
- Reflexes are the basis upon which a child develops and matures.
- Children require an extended period of practice and constant repetition to learn new skills.
- Although typical developmental stages and sequence are known, each child is different.
- Assessment of a child's early posture and gait should not be conducted using adult standards.

QUICK FACTS 9-4 ▶ EARLY AMBULATION CHARACTERISTICS

Location	Positioning and Gait Characteristics Typically Noted
Lower extremity positioning	• Wide base of support • Excessive hip and knee flexion • Full-foot contact
Gait deviations	• Short stride • Longer stance phase • Increased cadence • Heel eversion in stance • Relative foot drop in swing phase
Upper extremity positioning	• Initially held in 'high guard' position (arms in abduction, elbows flexed) • As gait matures, arms move to mudguard then low guard position

Note: Electromyographic (EMG) studies show cocontraction of antagonistic muscle groups to support stability.

QUICK FACTS 9-5 ▶ MATURING GAIT PATTERN

Timeframe	Clinical Observations
By 18 months	Legs are closer together Cadence is slower Stride is longer
By 2 years	Consistent heel strike has emerged. Center of gravity lowering allows for improved balance and stability. Duration of the stance phase decreases as balance and coordination improve.
By 3 years	More mature gait pattern is seen. Joint angles in the hip and knee are similar to those of an adult. Although continued heel eversion is seen in the stance phase, cocontraction of antagonists is more mature. Balance and coordination have improved significantly by this point.
By 7 years	Gait patterns can be assessed by adult standards

Physical Therapy Examination and Data Collection

Basic Assessments

Strength
1. Young children cannot cooperate with typical manual muscle tests.
2. Usually assessed through observation and participation in play and functional skills.

ROM
1. Normal ROM changes through infancy, toddlerhood, childhood, and adolescence.
2. Growth spurts affect muscle length and, in turn, ROM.

Developmental Skills
1. The *sequence* of developmental skills is similar for typically developing children.
2. The *timing* of skill development is unique to each child within a normal range of time.

Functional/Adaptive Skills
1. Includes development of functional/adaptive skills such as dressing, eating, and toileting.
2. Dependent not only on individual maturation, but on environmental factors such as culture, parenting styles, environment, and opportunities for practice.

Screening Tests

Completed By
1. Usually administered by physicians or nurse practitioners.

Apgar
1. Administered to newborn infants at 1 and 5 minutes after birth and again at 10 minutes if concerns are present.
2. Measures heart rate, respiratory effort, muscle tone, reflex irritability, and color.
3. Each area has a score between 0 and 2 with a maximum total score of 10.
4. Scores between 7 and 10 are considered normal.
5. Low scores may indicate a lack of oxygen prior to or during birth.

Denver Developmental Screening Test II (DENVER II)
1. Screening tool most commonly used in pediatrician's offices during well-baby checks.
2. Assesses the need for further developmental testing on children up to 6 years of age.
3. Tests personal-social, fine motor, gross motor, and language skills.

Standardized Developmental Tests Commonly Used by Therapists

Neonatal Behavioral Assessment Scale (NBAS)
1. Used with typically developing infants from 37–48 weeks' gestational age.
2. Assesses habituation, oral-motor, truncal, vestibular, and social-interactive domains.

Movement Assessment of Infants (MAI)
1. Used with infants birth to 12 months.
2. Assesses muscle tone, reflexes, automatic reactions, and volitional movement.

Bayley Scales of Infant Development, 3rd Edition (Bayley-III)
1. Used with children from birth to 42 months of age.
2. Assesses adaptive, cognitive, language, motor, and social-emotional development.

Peabody Developmental Motor Scales
1. Second edition: PDMS-2.
2. Used with children from birth to 5 years of age.
3. Measures gross and fine motor function.

Performance Scales Measuring Function and Outcomes of Therapy

Gross Motor Function Measure
1. Second edition: GMFM-2.
2. Used for children with cerebral palsy and related disorders through acquisition of advanced gait activities.
3. Measures gross motor skills including lying and rolling, sitting, crawling and kneeling, standing, walking, running, and jumping.

Functional Independence Measure for Children (WeeFIM)
1. For children between 6 months and 7 years for typically developing children; may be used up to age 21 for those with developmental disabilities.
2. Measures self-care, mobility, locomotion, communication, and cognitive skills.

Pediatric Evaluation of Disability Inventory (PEDI)
1. Useful for children from 6 months to 7 years.
2. Measures functional skills in the areas of self-care, mobility, and social function, including notation of caregiver modifications.

Clinical Application
- While standard developmental timelines have been presented, it is important to remember development of such skills is dependent on both nature and nurture.
- Most assessments by the physical therapist or physical therapist assistant will take place while they are assessing the individual's completion of functional activities; standard manual muscle testing and goniometric techniques may be difficult to obtain accurately.
- A variety of assessments and performance scales are available based upon what information is desired.

Intervention

Overview

Best Practice
1. Most clinicians achieve success by using an assortment of therapeutic techniques.
2. Intervention techniques for adult and pediatric neurologically impaired patients/clients are similar. See Chapter 3.
3. *Remember*: Play is the work of children, so therapy has to be fun!

Intervention Approaches

Neurodevelopmental Treatment (NDT)
1. Developed by Karel and Berta Bobath.
2. Normal movement sequences are facilitated and substitution/compensation is not permitted.
3. Promote the use of involved body segments.
4. Address innate postural and reflex responses to affect functional motor skills.
5. Utilize sensory input to influence motor output.
   a. Substitution or compensation should not be permitted with NDT intervention.

Sensorimotor Integration (SI)
1. Developed by A. Jean Ayres.
2. Attributes problems with learning, attention, behavior, and visual perception to faulty integration of sensory input.
3. Treatment focuses on providing systematic sensory input to help organize a child's motor output.

Motor Control Approaches
1. A number of approaches to therapy build on theories of motor control and motor learning.
2. Refer to previous discussion and Chapter 3 regarding more information on motor control and motor learning.

Physical Therapy Tools for Working with Children

Handling and Environmental Stimuli
1. Use of sensory input to produce changes in motor output.
2. Responses to sensory input can be affected by environment, health, and emotions of child.
3. For a child with low muscle tone, the goal is to increase motor output.
   a. Handling techniques: tapping, brushing, vibrating, quick movements, deep pressure, spinning, swinging, and bouncing.
   b. Environmental stimuli: loud music, fast rhythms, loud voice, bright colors, and changing activities frequently.
4. For a child with high muscle tone or dystonia, the goal is to decrease motor output.
   a. Handling techniques: rocking, firm touch, rhythmic movements, slow movements, stroking, warm water, and wrapping/swaddling.
   b. Environmental stimuli: consistent sensory input, relaxing music, singing, quiet voice.
      - It is essential that the clinician correctly identify hypotonia or hypertonia.

- Use of inhibition techniques with hypotonia or facilitation techniques with hypertonia can lead to undesired increases or decreases in tone, thereby decreasing the benefits of future therapeutic interventions provided during that session.

Adaptive Equipment

Positioning for Function
1. Helps maintain alignment of trunk and limbs.
2. Prevents or minimizes contractures.
3. Promotes strengthening, balance, and postural reflexes.
4. Facilitates functional skills.
5. Allows optimal mobility and participation in age-appropriate activities.

Floor Positioning and Mobility Devices
1. Mat: allows free floor mobility and provides a safe, cushioned surface.
2. Wedge: allows a variety of positions for child to visually access environment, promotes weight bearing through extremities, and facilitates postural reactions.
3. Sidelyer: gives child visual access to hands, keeps head in midline to decrease asymmetrical tonic neck reflex (ATNR), and allows flexion of hips and knees to decrease extensor tone.
4. Bolster: stimulates balance and postural reflexes and aids with development of dynamic postural control.
5. Ball: used to stimulate postural reflexes and to complete strengthening and coordination activities.
6. Scooter board: used to promote floor-level mobility in prone, supine, or quadruped position.

Seated Positioning and Mobility Devices
1. Adapted chairs.
   a. Allow access to typical environments (e.g., dining room table, classroom desks).
   b. Provide child the needed support and stability that typical chairs do not have.
2. Adapted tricycle.
   a. Foot pedals with straps.
   b. Built-up handlebars.
   c. Greater contour in seat.
   d. Seat back: improves trunk alignment and provides greater stability in sitting.
3. Manual and power wheelchair benefits:
   a. Allow custom positioning and mobility.
   b. Can be used in multiple environments.
   c. Allow independent mobility.
   d. Available positioning components can be used in any wheelchair depending on specific postural needs of child (Table 9-5).

Table 9-5

Wheelchair Positioning Components

Head support	Provides posterior, lateral, or anterior support for head and for safety during transportation
Lateral trunk supports	Provide postural support for upright positioning and for supporting scoliosis
Lateral hip guides	Promotes neutral positioning of lower extremities, neutral position of the pelvis
Medial thigh supports (pommel)	Provides for neutral positioning of thighs. Not to be used as a weight-bearing surface for groin to keep pelvis back in chair
Foot supports	Supports lower extremities, provides neutral positioning for lower extremities
Lap tray	Provides upper extremity positioning and support to assist with trunk extension. Provides a surface for upper extremity activities
Pelvic belt	Maintains pelvic positioning in chair. Provides a measure of safety to prevent falls out of the chair
Chest strap	Maintains trunk positioning and prevents falling forward. Used as a supplement to a posterior and lateral positioning aid
Butterfly strap	Provides a broad surface to promote anterior chest support for upright positioning
Thigh strap	Promotes pelvic alignment during seating. Supplements the pelvic belt
Sub ASIS bar	Promotes pelvic alignment while seated. Potential for skin breakdown if not fitted correctly. Could be viewed as a restraint

4. Stroller-type chair benefits: lighter than wheelchairs and usually foldable to provide portability.
5. Power scooter benefits: less expensive than power wheelchairs but provide less trunk support and require greater balance and upper extremity skill to use.

Standing Positioning and Mobility Devices
1. Benefits.
   a. Child has standing-level view of environment.
   b. Weight bearing through long bones to decrease effects of osteoporosis.
   c. Facilitate postural reflex mechanisms.
   d. Allow use of arms and hands for functional tasks.

e. Dynamic standers can have wheels added to allow the child to move in a standing position through manual or powered propulsion.
2. Supine stander: provides posterior support for head control and encourages passive weight bearing with full posterior support.
3. Prone stander: provides anterior support and stimulates postural activation to hold up head and upper trunk.
4. Parapodium: allows child to move in a standing position at the same visual height as peers; can initially be used as a standing device and then child progresses to using it for pregait and gait activities.
5. Anterior rolling walker: promotes upright posture, active weight bearing through lower extremities, strengthening, endurance, and independent mobility skills.
6. Posterior rolling walker: promotes trunk extension with more erect posture than an anterior walker, which may help decrease abnormal movements (i.e., poor reciprocal movement, lack of disassociation between lower extremities) during gait.
7. Gait trainers: provide greater support through trunk and may attach hip-knee-ankle-foot orthosis (HKAFO) for lower extremity positioning.
8. Axillary or forearm support crutches: require greater balance, trunk strength, and postural control than walkers.
   a. Adaptive equipment must be continually monitored for correct fit as the child grows in order to maximize its usefulness.

Orthoses

1. Benefits.
   a. Provide external support to maintain or correct alignment of extremities or trunk.
   b. Improve postural stability to allow greater mobility and functional skills.
   c. Reduce the effects of spasticity through alignment of joints and muscles.
2. Submalleolar or University of California Biomechanics Laboratory (UCBL) shoe insert.
   a. Closely molded around the calcaneus to hold or prevent excessive calcaneal inversion or eversion.
   b. Helpful for children with foot posture problems.
3. Supramalleolar orthosis (SMO).
   a. Provides support and alignment at the foot and medial/lateral ankle support.
   b. Provides added stability during standing and walking activities.
4. Ankle-foot orthosis (AFO).
   a. Maintains distal limb in optimal alignment and provides a stable base of support.
   b. Decreases the effects of abnormal muscle tone.
   c. Made of plaster or polypropylene and are bivalved, one piece, or articulating.
   d. May be useful for children with cerebral palsy, sacral levels of spina bifida, or general low muscle tone.
5. Knee-ankle-foot orthosis (KAFO).
   a. Provides support and alignment of the foot, ankle, and knee.
   b. Used for children who require greater external support because of significant weakness.
6. HKAFO.
   a. Provides greater external stability for children with significant weakness at hips as well as knee and ankle.
   b. Allows standing and walking with assistive device.
   c. May be useful for children with high lumbar or low thoracic levels of spina bifida or spinal cord injury.
7. Reciprocating gait orthosis (RGO).
   a. Allows children with significant weakness through lower extremities and trunk to walk with support.
   b. A body jacket with HKAFOs bilaterally and a cable system to facilitate reciprocal gait (2-point or 4-point gait pattern).
   c. May be useful for young children with T8-12 levels of spina bifida or traumatic spinal cord injury.
8. Thoracolumbosacral orthosis (TLSO). For types of, see Quick Facts 9-6.
   a. Provides stability through the trunk to prevent or minimize spinal deformity and allow greater function.
   b. May be useful for children with no more than 40 degrees of scoliosis.

QUICK FACTS 9-6 ▶ TYPES OF THORACOLUMBOSACRAL ORTHOSES

Brace	Use
Milwaukee orthosis (cervicothoracolumbosacral orthosis [CTLSO])	Used for all levels of scoliotic or kyphotic curves
Boston orthosis (thoracolumbosacral orthosis [TLSO])	Used with midthoracic or lower scoliosis curves

RED FLAGS:
- Areas of redness that do not disappear within 20 minutes following removal of the orthotic device indicate a dangerous area of pressure.
- A trained individual should be consulted to adapt or refit an orthotic.

Clinical Application

- Play is the work of children and, therefore, it should be the basis for therapeutic interventions when working with pediatric patients.
- Many of the intervention approaches utilized with adult patients with neurological dysfunction can also be used with children presenting with neurological dysfunction.
- Adaptive equipment and orthoses should be used to increase function and facilitate quality of movement and body alignment.
- When selecting adaptive equipment, the needs of the family and their environment should be considered.

Conditions/Pathology/Diseases: Orthopedic Disorders

Developmental Dysplasia of the Hip (DDH)

Basic Information
1. A group of disorders involving poor alignment of the acetabulum and the head of the femur in the developing hip.
2. Usually develops in the last trimester of pregnancy and may result from elevated levels of the female hormone relaxin, tight in utero positioning, or breech positioning.
3. Affects girls more than boys and left hip twice as often as the right hip.
4. Exacerbated by swaddling and carrying infants with hips in extension and adduction.

Clinical Picture
1. Nonambulatory child.
   a. Asymmetrical hip abduction in flexion.
   b. Asymmetrical groin or buttock skinfolds.
   c. Pistoning of affected hip with manual traction.
   d. Apparent femoral shortening on the affected side.
2. Ambulatory child.
   a. Trendelenburg's gait.
   b. Decreased hip abduction.
   c. Thigh pistoning.
   d. Bilateral DDH presents with lordosis and swaying gait typical of a bilateral Trendelenburg.

Physical Therapy Intervention
1. Assessments.
   a. Barlow's test: hip click felt when manually moving flexed hip from abduction to adduction.
   b. Ortolani's test: hip click felt with passive movement of adducted and flexed hip into abduction with traction.
2. Measuring and fitting brace.
3. Parent education: brace application and positioning of hips in flexion and abduction.
4. Direct intervention: strengthen, maintain, or increase ROM and promote developmental skills.

Medical Intervention
1. Bracing and splinting of hip in flexion and abduction.
   a. Pavlik harness.
      - Typically used with infants under 9 months of age.
      - Allows active kicking to facilitate lower extremity strength and mobility and to decrease the complication of avascular necrosis of the hip.
   b. Children over 9 months will need an abduction orthosis that allows walking.
2. Traction and/or surgery (usually done after 18 months of age).

> **RED FLAG:** Failure to correctly address the dysplasia can increase the risk of developing avascular necrosis of the hip.

Legg-Calvé-Perthes Disease (LCPD)

Basic Information
1. Self-limiting degeneration of the femoral head due to a disturbance in blood supply.
2. Due to genetic predisposition, trauma, anatomical variations, or disorder of epiphyseal cartilage.
3. Most commonly occurs in boys 4–7 years of age.
4. Occurs less frequently in girls with onset at older ages and poorer rehabilitation potential.

5. The younger the onset, the more positive the outcome.
6. Approximately 20% occur bilaterally.

Clinical Picture
1. 2- to 4-year progression of the disease with four stages.
   a. Initial stage: failure of femoral head to grow due to decreased blood supply.
   b. Fragmentation stage: fragmented epiphysis and revascularization of the femoral head.
   c. Reossification stage: bone density returns to normal with changes in shape and structure of femoral head and neck.
   d. Healed stage: femoral head and neck retain deformity from the repair process.
2. Signs and symptoms.
   a. Initial sign is a limp with ambulation, typically a Trendelenburg gait.
   b. Mild pain in groin, medial knee, or thigh.
   c. Decreased ROM most noticeable in hip abduction and internal rotation.
   d. Thigh, calf, or buttock atrophy from disuse.
   e. Limb length discrepancy.

Physical Therapy Intervention
1. Ongoing assessment of ROM, strength, and functional skills.
2. Patient and family education: gait training, ROM, strengthening exercises, transfers, and functional skills training.
3. Consultation with school staff to encourage and support inclusion and mobility.

Medical Intervention

1. Some physicians recommend no treatment, allowing condition to heal on its own.
2. Most physicians advocate treatment.
   a. Observation and monitoring course of disease via radiographs.
   b. Avoid participation in contact sports in favor of non–weight-bearing exercise, such as swimming.
   c. If condition is more vigorous, avoid weight bearing with use of crutches.
   d. For advanced condition, splinting in abduction and internal rotation or surgery to contain the femoral head in the acetabulum may be necessary.
      - **SPECIAL CONSIDERATION:** Failure to follow the necessary precautions can slow the recovery process.

Slipped Capital Femoral Epiphysis (SCFE)

Basic Information
1. Hip deformity related to slippage of the femoral epiphysis.
2. May result from a genetic predisposition or hormonal influences leading to weak growth plates.
3. Occurs in children who are tall, with delayed skeletal maturity, obese, near the onset of puberty (9–16 years of age).
4. More common in boys than girls and children of African American or Polynesian ethnicity.
5. Bilateral slips may occur in 25%–30% of cases.

Clinical Picture
1. Onset.
   a. Chronic slip: most common with a gradual onset and progression of symptoms for 3 weeks or more.
   b. Acute slip: sudden onset of severe pain and is usually precipitated by trauma.
   c. Acute-on-chronic slip: gradual symptoms that build up over a period of time and a traumatic episode causes an onset of severe symptoms.
2. Grades of slippage.
   a. Preslip: mild changes in the x-ray including a widened growth plate.
   b. Grade 1 (mild slip): femoral head slipped less than 1/3 the width of the femoral neck.
   c. Grade 2 (moderate slip): femoral head slipped 1/3–1/2 the width of the femoral neck.
   d. Grade 3 (severe slip): femoral head slipped greater than 1/2 the width of the femoral neck.
3. Signs/symptoms.
   a. Intermittent limp and pain in groin, buttock, knee, or thigh.
   b. Antalgic and/or Trendelenburg's gait.
   c. Leg held in external rotation and hip flexion is accompanied by external rotation.
   d. Limitations of hip internal rotation, abduction, and sometimes flexion.

Physical Therapy Intervention
1. Aim to minimize or reduce slippage, maintain hip ROM and function, and prevent or minimize degenerative changes in later years.
2. Order adaptive equipment (crutches, wheelchair).
3. Patient and family education: home exercise program for strength and ROM, proper use of adaptive equipment and transfers, mobility and/or gait training.
4. Home evaluation for accessibility.
5. Consultation with school staff regarding mobility issues.

Medical Intervention

1. With early changes but no slip, conservative measures may help avoid surgery until skeletal maturity is reached.
   a. Vigilant monitoring by radiograph.
   b. Non–weight-bearing using crutches.
   c. Weight loss.
   d. Forbidding athletics.
2. Surgery is usually required to pin the hip and prevent further slippage in mild or moderate cases.
3. Varus osteotomy may be required to change the angle of the femoral neck to shaft for more severe cases.
   a. When early changes are apparent but no slip exists, conservative measures must be followed. This allows surgery to be withheld until skeletal maturity and likely decreases the number of surgeries the child will require.

Juvenile Rheumatoid Arthritis (JRA)

Basic Information
1. Group of disorders characterized by inflammation of connective tissue including joints and other systems.
2. Occurs in children under 16 years of age where arthritis is present for 6 weeks or more.
3. Cause is unknown but may be a genetic predisposition or due to a viral or bacterial infection triggering an autoimmune response.

Clinical Picture and Classification
1. Classifications of JRA, see Table 9-6.
2. Signs/symptoms.
   a. Joint pain, swelling, and stiffness.
   b. Decreased ROM in affected joints.
   c. Myalgia (muscle pain).

Physical Therapy Intervention
1. Splinting to maintain joint ROM.
2. Stretching to maintain soft tissue flexibility.
3. Modalities for pain control.
4. Activities to improve strength and endurance.
5. Patient and family education.
   a. Avoidance of joint trauma, especially during inflammation flares.
   b. Facilitating appropriate developmental skills for age and ability.
   c. Instruction, assistance, and adaptations for functional skills such as mobility and self-help skills.

> **RED FLAG:** Failure to identify disease flares and make the necessary accommodations in intervention approach can ultimately lead to a more rapid onset of joint damage.

Medical Interventions

1. Pharmaceutical management.
   a. Aspirin and nonsteroidal anti-inflammatory drugs (NSAIDS) (e.g., ibuprofen, naproxen, and indomethacin).
   b. Slow-acting antirheumatic drugs (SAARDs) (e.g., gold salts, hydroxychloroquine, and penicillamine).
   c. Corticosteroids (e.g., prednisone).
   d. Immunosuppressive and cytotoxic agents (e.g., cyclosporine, methotrexate).
2. Surgical management.
   a. Synovectomy.
   b. Soft tissue release.
   c. Osteotomy or epiphyseodesis (joint fusion).
   d. Total joint replacement.

Table 9-6

Juvenile Rheumatoid Arthritis		
Classification	Oligoarticular or pauciarticular	Characterized by arthritis in fewer than five joints. Affected joints usually have asymmetrical distribution
	Polyarticular	Characterized by arthritis in five or more joints. Affected joints have a symmetrical distribution. Slow onset with gradual joint pain developing or acute onset with low-grade fever
	Systemic	Characterized by acute onset with high spiking fevers, rash on trunk and proximal extremities, and possible organ inflammation (pericardium, heart, lungs). Causes joint destruction and potential disability

Osteogenesis Imperfecta (OI)

Basic Information
1. Abnormality in the collagen gene causing problems with the amount and quality of collagen in the body.
2. Equal likelihood in boys and girls with a genetic predisposition.

Clinical Picture
1. Characterized by fragile bones that break easily and often for no apparent reason.
2. Other common symptoms: dental problems, scoliosis, kyphosis, short stature, and hearing loss.
3. Four types (see Quick Facts 9-7).

Physical Therapy Intervention
1. Aim to minimize fractures through joint protection, maximize activity and weight bearing for bone and muscle strength, and facilitate maximum functional skills.
2. Active exercise for strengthening with positioning and stretching to maintain ROM.

> **RED FLAG:** Passive stretching is not recommended due to risk of fracture or joint subluxation.

3. Assistive devices such as walkers, crutches, or wheelchairs to improve mobility.
4. For some children with type IV, weight training with a very low amount of weight can be indicated.
5. Low-impact endurance activities such as swimming and walking.
6. Parent education including supporting child at the head and trunk region, not at long bones, and rolling child during diaper changes, not lifting at the ankles.

QUICK FACTS 9-7 ▶ TYPES OF OSTEOGENESIS IMPERFECTA (OI)

Type I	Most common; usually have triangular-shaped face, thin, smooth skin, and hearing loss beginning in teens or 20s
Type II	Most severe form with newborns often suffering fractures before birth and dying shortly after birth
Type III	Least common; involves progressive deformity of the long bones, skull, and spine resulting in very small stature, dental and hearing problems, barrel-shaped rib cage, and respiratory compromise secondary to severe kyphoscoliosis
Type IV	Relatively rare; presents with loose, easily overstretched joints, dental problems, and mild short stature

Medical Intervention
1. Orthotic devices such as splints, lower extremity orthotics, or body jackets for protection, to allow weight bearing, and to prevent deformity.
2. Assurance of adequate calcium intake.
3. Assess for and treat fractures.

Arthrogryposis Multiplex Congenita

Basic Information
1. Nonprogressive neuromuscular disorder causing multiple joint contractures at birth.
2. Etiology is usually unknown but may result from lack of fetal movement, trauma or insult during first trimester of pregnancy, maternal history of fevers during pregnancy, or maternal multiple sclerosis, myasthenia gravis, or myotonic dystrophy.

Clinical Picture
1. Variability in clinical picture usually includes severe joint contractures and absence of muscle development.
   a. Contractures with severity increasing distally.
   b. Joint dislocation at hips or knees.
   c. Thin subcutaneous tissue.
   d. Absence or decreased size of muscle groups.
2. Typically affected body parts in order of prevalence.
   a. Foot: clubfoot.
   b. Hip: flexion or abduction and external rotation deformities.
   c. Wrist: flexion, ulnar deviation.
   d. Knee: extension or flexion.
   e. Elbow: extension or flexion.
   f. Shoulder: internal rotation and extension or flexion.
3. Children with distal involvement have a good prognosis for being community ambulators, while children with systemic joint involvement may be household ambulators or use wheelchairs.

Physical Therapy Intervention
1. Strengthening of neck, trunk, and extremity muscles using developmental activities (i.e., prone on elbows, sitting, rolling, kneeling, and standing).
2. Functional mobility training: rolling, crawling/creeping, ambulation, and/or power wheelchair training.
3. Use of assistive devices: cane, walker, gait trainer, adapted stroller, or wheelchair.
4. Parent instruction in daily stretching and positioning to maintain and increase ROM.

Medical Intervention

1. Lower and upper extremity splints and orthotic devices.
2. Body jackets and other braces to prevent formation of scoliosis; development of scoliosis can lead to decreased lung capacities.
3. Surgical intervention.
   a. Clubfoot surgery may be deferred until the child is ready to stand.
   b. Hip dislocation.
      - If one hip is dislocated, surgery is done to prevent pelvic obliquity and scoliosis.
      - If bilateral dislocation, surgical intervention may be withheld because painless dislocated hips are better than stiff located hips.
   c. Knee flexion contractures: usually addressed when child is ambulatory, involving hamstring lengthening or posterior capsulotomy of knee joint.
   d. Knee extension contractures: quadriceps lengthening is performed when knee position interferes with sitting or ambulation.
   e. Scoliosis may be managed via surgical fusion.

Pediatric Fractures

Basic Information
1. Multiple causes: trauma, child abuse, motor vehicle accident, and genetics.
2. Fracture patterns are different than adults due to bones that are more flexible, more porous, and less dense than adult bones.
3. Children's periosteum is thicker than adults, leading to better blood supply and faster rate of healing (2–4 weeks).
4. Active epiphyseal plates are affected in 30% of pediatric fractures.

Clinical Picture
1. Common fracture sites include distal radius, tibial shaft, clavicle, and elbow.
2. Signs and symptoms: redness, swelling, pain, heat, muscle spasm, deformity, and nonuse of extremity.
3. Types of fractures.
   a. Buckle fracture (torus fracture): compression of long bone on one side.
   b. Greenstick fracture: compression on one side of long bone with distraction on other side.
   c. Bending fracture (plastic deformation): bending of long bone in the direction of force.
   d. Epiphyseal fracture: fracture involving the epiphyseal plate.
   e. Spiral fracture: caused by twisting force on long bone.

Physical Therapy Intervention
1. Instructing patient and family in use of assistive device.
2. Strengthening exercises.
3. Balance exercises.
4. Endurance exercises.

Medical Intervention
1. Splinting or casting.
2. Analgesics for pain control.

Foot and Ankle Deformities

Basic Information
1. Causes of congenital deformity include the following.
   a. In utero positioning.
   b. Neuromuscular disorders.
   c. Genetic disorders.

Clinical Picture
1. Classification.
   a. Metatarsus adductus: metatarsals deviated medially.
   b. Talipes equinovarus (clubfoot): adduction of forefoot, varus position of hindfoot, and equinus at ankle.
   c. Calcaneovalgus: foot dorsiflexion, eversion or valgus of hindfoot, and abduction of metatarsals.
2. Signs/symptoms: visual deformity, gait disturbances, and delays in development of gross motor and mobility skills.

Physical Therapy Intervention
1. Stretching to counter deformity and supplement splinting or bracing.

> **RED FLAG:** It is essential to stretch the gastrocnemius/soleus muscles while avoiding breakdown of the midfoot ligaments.

2. Serial casting.
   a. Splints or casts are applied to counter the deformity (e.g., for clubfoot).
   b. The cast is applied in the direction of forefoot abduction, hindfoot valgus, and ankle dorsiflexion.
   c. Casts are changed every 1–2 weeks for several months until bones have remodeled.
3. Gait training.
4. Promote normal developmental skills through play.
5. Sensory input.
   a. Casted limbs may need sensory stimulation during periods of time out of the cast.
   b. Sensory stimulation includes rubbing with textured material, water and sand play, massage, and weight bearing.

c. **SPECIAL CONSIDERATION:** Failure to provide the necessary sensory stimulation can lead to difficulties with ambulation if the child is not able to tolerate sensory input on the soles of the feet.

Medical Intervention

1. Casting.
2. If not successful, surgery to fuse the ankle joint in a functional position.

Brachial Plexus Injury

Basic Information
1. Damage to all or some of the nerve roots from C5 through T1.
2. Commonly caused by a traction or compression injury.
3. Degree of injury.
   a. Avulsion: nerve is torn from the spinal cord.
   b. Rupture: nerve sheath or nerve fibers are torn, but not at the spinal attachment.
   c. Neuroma: nerve was torn and healed, but scar tissue prevents nerve conduction to the tissues.
   d. Neuropraxia or stretch: most common type of injury when nerve is damaged but not torn.

Clinical Picture
1. See Chapter 2 for a clinical picture.

Physical Therapy Intervention
1. Initial positioning.
   a. Infant swaddled with arm across upper abdomen.
   b. Arm across the body (shoulder adduction and internal rotation).
   c. Utilized for 1–2 weeks to allow nerve to rest and recover.
2. After initial recovery.
   a. Gentle ROM to prevent contractures.
   b. Facilitate awareness of involved extremity.
   c. Facilitate motor output through sensory inputs (i.e., stroking, approximation).
   d. Facilitate muscle activity via hand-overhand activities and weight bearing.
3. As child grows, teach strategies to accomplish age-appropriate tasks and introduce assistive devices to increase functional skills.

Medical Intervention

1. Surgery may be necessary to repair avulsion injuries.
2. With onset of spasticity, oral muscle relaxers or Botox may be used.

Clinical Application

- A number of the pediatric orthopedic conditions utilize non–weight-bearing, aquatic exercise, and other conservative approaches to decrease the risk of further damage.
- It is important to address the child's mobility and assistive device needs with the educational staff to ensure appropriate inclusion in the academic environment.
- Once medical restrictions are lifted, therapeutic intervention should focus on facilitating achievement of developmental mobility and other age-appropriate skills.
- Positioning plays a very important part in prevention of further deformity and increasing the child's rehabilitation potential.

Conditions/Pathology/Diseases with Intervention: Pediatric Neurological and Genetic Disorders

Cerebral Palsy (CP)

Basic Information
1. Insult to the brain during development, at birth, or within the first few years resulting in permanent, non-progressive damage.

Etiology
1. Prenatal causes: maternal infections, diabetes, malnutrition, seizures, or radiation exposure.
2. Perinatal causes: prematurity, low birth weight, multiple births, prolapsed umbilical cord, intraventricular hemorrhage, and asphyxia.
3. Postnatal causes: infection (meningitis, encephalitis), asphyxia, traumatic brain injury (TBI) (falls, shaken baby syndrome), stroke, near drowning, and brain tumor.

Clinical Picture
1. Distribution of motor involvement may take one of three different types (see Quick Facts 9-8).
2. Classification of muscle tone.
   a. Hypotonia (floppy, rag doll, or low tone). Muscle tone lower than normal, usually throughout the body. Characteristics include:
      - Excessive ROM.
      - Weak deep tendon reflexes and primitive reflexes.

QUICK FACTS 9-8 ▶ DISTRIBUTION OF MOTOR INVOLVEMENT WITH CP			
	Diplegia	**Hemiplegia**	**Quadriplegia/ Tetraplegia**
Extremities impacted	Both legs affected while trunk and arms may be affected to a lesser degree	One arm and leg on the same side affected	All four extremities and trunk involved
Typical standing posture	• Hip flexion, adduction, and internal rotation • Knee flexion • Ankle plantar flexion	• Shoulder adduction and internal rotation • Elbow and wrist flexion • Hip internal rotation • Knee extension • Ankle plantar flexion	With greater levels of trunk involvement the child may demonstrate head involvement.
Typical gait	• Poor disassociation between legs, noted trunk rotation, and high guard positioning of arms for balance • May use wheelchair, walker, or crutches	• Asymmetrical gait with circumduction of lower extremity • May use cane or crutch for balance	

- Child is usually overweight due to deficient energy output.
- Impaired speech due to poor oral motor control.
- Gait characterized by wide base of support, short stride length, and poor balance.

b. Hypertonia (tight, spastic, stiff or rigid). Muscle tone higher than normal with location determined by area of motor cortex involved. Characteristics include:
- ROM of motion may be limited.
- Common contractures: hip adduction, internal rotation and flexion; knee flexion; ankle plantar flexion.
- Hyperreflexive deep tendon reflexes.
- Persistence of primitive reflexes (asymmetrical neck reflex [ATNR], symmetrical tonic neck reflex [STNR], tonic labyrinthine reflex [TLR]) limiting the development of normal movements.
- Child usually thin due to excessive energy output.
- Speech usually impaired due to poor oral motor control.
- Gait characterized by poor muscle control and decreased balance with variations related to the distribution of muscle tone.

c. Athetosis or dystonia. Poor stability in midline resulting from a lesion in the basal ganglia or cerebellum. Identified by writhing movements, fluctuating tone, and constantly moving between end ranges. Characteristics include:
- Distribution throughout body, including face.
- ROM usually normal but may be excessive due to constant movement throughout range.
- Hyperreflexive deep tendon reflexes.
- Hypotonia in infancy changes to athetosis as child matures.
- Persistence of primitive reflexes (ATNR, STNR, TLR) limiting the development of normal movements.
- Child usually thin due to excessive energy output.
- Speech usually impaired due to poor oral motor control.
- Many children are unable to obtain enough stability to stand and walk; those who do have excessive movements and poor balance and likely require a walker, crutches, or wheelchair for mobility.

d. Ataxia. Results from a lesion in the cerebellum. Identified by wide base of support and high guard position of the upper extremities during gait, poor balance, tremors, low postural tone, and poor visual tracking. Characteristics include:
- Distribution throughout body.
- Poor balance.
- ROM usually normal or excessive due to low tone.
- Hyporeflexivity of deep tendon reflexes.
- Weak primitive reflexes.

e. Mixed.
- More than one type of muscle tone.
- Hypertonicity and athetosis is the most common form of mixed CP.

3. Physical therapy interventions for CP based on tone classification. See Table 9-7.
4. Classification based on severity.
   a. Mild: independent functional skills including feeding and walking; develop at least some language skills.
   b. Moderate: independent mobility (crawling or walking with support), need assistance for some functional skills such as feeding, may develop a few words of language.
   c. Severe: needs help for most functional tasks including mobility and feeding, does not develop language skills.

Table 9-7

	Interventions Based on Tone Classification
Hypotonia	• Support all limbs to prevent injury • Use care to prevent hyperextension at elbows and knees • Use vigorous passive and active movement to stimulate increased muscle output • Promote active weight bearing to stimulate postural reflexes
Hypertonia	• Position hips and knees in greater than 90 degrees of flexion to inhibit strong reflexive extension • Use midline symmetrical positioning to inhibit abnormal reflexes • Use gentle, rhythmic movement to encourage controlled movement • Promote active weight bearing with aligned limbs and trunk to allow optimal independence in motor skills
Athetosis	• Encourage midline, symmetrical posture to minimize effects of abnormal reflexes • Use gentle, rhythmic movements to encourage controlled motor output • Allow abnormal movements if they contribute to functional skills • Encourage child to problem solve motor difficulties
Ataxia	• Encourage midline, symmetrical posture for maximum function • Provide sensory input (tactile, proprioceptive, auditory, visual) to help the child orient in space • Weighted vest or belts to increase proprioceptive feedback and improve balance • Use aids to assist with balance (e.g., weighted walker, crutches, and canes)

Related Problems

1. Mental retardation (50%–75%).
2. Visual impairment (50%).
3. Speech/language deficits or delays and oral-motor problems (50%).
4. Seizures (30%).
5. Hearing impairment (10%).
6. Visual-motor and perceptual disorders.
7. Behavior disorders.
8. Orthopedic disorders: joint contracture, hip subluxation or dislocation, scoliosis, kyphosis, or lordosis, tibial torsion, and clubfoot.

RED FLAG: It is essential to be aware of related problems children present with in order to safely provide intervention, including seizure and oral-motor problems.

Physical Therapy Intervention

1. Intervention is individualized, working as a team with the child and family in setting goals.
2. Benefits of positioning and adapted equipment.
   a. Allow visual access to the environment.
   b. Facilitate functional use of extremities.
   c. Encourage mobility.
   d. May allow standing when otherwise impossible. Standing:
      • Improves weight bearing through long bones.
      • Improves visceral function (bowel and bladder elimination, respiratory function, venous return).
      • Decreases risk of developing lower extremity flexion contractures.
   e. Good positioning promotes:
      • Symmetrical posture.
      • Aligned trunk, pelvis, and extremities.
      • Head in midline to minimize persistent primitive reflexes.
      • Hips and knees at 90 degrees when sitting.

Medical Intervention

1. Medications for seizures.
   a. Seizures: Tegretol, Dilantin, Depakote, phenobarbital, Clonazepam.
2. Medications for spasticity.
   a. Botulinum toxin A (Botox) injections.
      • Prevents release of acetylcholine at the neuromuscular junction.
      • Lasts 1–4 months.
      • Common muscles of injection: gastrocnemius/soleus, hamstrings, hip flexors, and hip adductors.
   b. Baclofen.
      • Decreases excitatory input into alpha motor neurons.
      • May be given orally or by intrathecal injection (through lumbar puncture or catheter).
      • Children who have Botox injections must be given extensive therapy to stretch tight agonist muscles and strengthen the antagonist muscles.
      • Following administration of any muscle relaxant, loss of spasticity may present difficulty with previously acquired functional mobility skills and ambulation.
3. Surgical procedures.
   a. Dorsal rhizotomy: cutting of dorsal nerve rootlets supplying the affected muscles to decrease spasticity and increase function.
   b. Z-plasty: release of a muscle or tendon to reverse contractures.

> **RED FLAG:** It is imperative to utilize proper positioning to increase functioning and to avoid further limitations of the child.

   f. Special considerations for positioning.
      - If strong extensor tone is present, hips and knees can be positioned in more than 90 degrees.
      - Posterior tilt-in-space wheelchair can be used if gravity needed to help keep trunk and head aligned in upright position.
      - Prompts can be used and reduced as child improves stability and mobility skills.
      - Serial casting may be necessary to obtain optimal positioning for use of equipment.
   g. Positioning examples: corner seat, molded seat, sidelyer, wheelchair with appropriate supports, and prone or supine stander.
3. Orthoses.
4. Dynamic positioning supports.
5. Optimizing functional skills.
   a. Handling: elongate shortened muscle groups, facilitate dynamic movement, inhibit primitive reflexes, and facilitate optimal muscle tone.
   b. Promote weight bearing.
   c. Provide postural challenges to improve balance, muscle tone, and strength.
   d. Utilize principles of motor learning to help a child learn new skills.

Traumatic Brain Injury (TBI)

Refer to Chapter 3
1. For full discussion of TBI.

Special Considerations in the Pediatric Patient
1. Length of time of unconsciousness (coma), especially in the pediatric population, is a predictor of outcome.
2. Behavioral scales that assess a child's recovery.
   a. Pediatric Glasgow Coma Scale.
      - Same areas of assessment and scoring as with Adult Glasgow Coma Scale.
      - Indicators given for both infant and pediatric patients.
3. Glasgow Coma Scale.
4. Rancho Los Amigos Scale.
5. Educate family members and caregivers to provide sensory stimulation and, when appropriate, facilitate return of functional mobility.

Spina Bifida

Basic Information
1. Group of congenital malformations of the spine, including the vertebrae and the spinal cord.
2. Caused by a genetic predisposition, maternal deficiency of folic acid, and maternal exposure to alcohol or valproic acid during the first 4 weeks of pregnancy.

Clinical Picture
1. Spina bifida is classified different ways based on structures involved.
   a. Occulta (not visible).
      - Results from incomplete fusion of the posterior vertebral arch with no protrusion of neurological or superficial tissues.
      - May be indicated by a hair tuft, fat pad, dimple or sinus at base of spine.
      - No disability usually results from this disorder.
   b. Acculta or cystica (visible).
      - Meningocele. Cerebrospinal fluid and superficial tissue protrudes from the spine in a sac at the level of lesion but neurological tissue is rarely involved. If disability is present, impaired bowel and bladder function and foot weakness are most likely.
      - Myelomeningocele. Meninges and parts of the spinal cord protrude from the abnormally formed spine in a sac at the level of lesion. Disability includes paralysis and loss of sensation below the level of the lesion. Extent of disability depends on level of lesion and scope of neurological involvement.

Signs/Symptoms
1. Meningitis may result due to infection of exposed tissue if lesion is not closed soon after birth.
2. Hydrocephalus. Increased accumulation of cerebrospinal fluid within the ventricles of the brain occurs in 60%–90% of children with myelomeningocele. It is treated with a ventriculoperitoneal shunt.
   a. Shunt precautions.
      - Avoid placing pressure on the shunt.
      - Avoid stretching the neck.
      - Do not place child in Trendelenburg's position.

> **RED FLAG:** The clinician must be aware of the signs of shunt malfunction: irritability, vomiting, fontanel bulging, lethargy, headache, and changes in behavior, coordination, or seizure activity.

3. Arnold-Chiari malformation, type II.
   a. Common in children with myelomeningocele.
   b. Brain stem and cerebellum protrude into the spinal canal through the foramen magnum.
   c. Can result in compression of spinal cord with resulting symptoms.
      - Dysphagia.
      - Feeding difficulties.
      - Trouble breathing.
      - Choking.
      - Arm stiffness.

4. Tethered cord.
   a. Congenital anomaly or scarring/adhesion of the spinal cord tissue to overlying dura or skin.
   b. May result in increased neurological problems as child grows and traction of spinal nerves results in damage to the nerves.

> **RED FLAG:** Older children who demonstrate a rapid decline in function or increase in and development of new symptoms may be experiencing a tethered cord and further medical evaluation is warranted.

5. Level of disability. See Table 9-8 for functional skills based on level of involvement of myelomenigocele.
6. Orthopedic deformities from lack of movement in utero.
   a. Clubfeet.
   b. Bowed long bones.
   c. Hip flexion contractures.
   d. Dislocated hips.
   e. Scoliosis or kyphosis.
7. Additional complications of spina bifida.
   a. Obesity.
   b. Osteoporosis.
   c. Incontinence of bowel and bladder (with lesion at or above S2).
   d. Skin breakdown due to lack of sensation.
   e. Learning problems.
   f. Visual-perceptual problems.
   g. Seizures.
   h. Developmental delays.
   i. Latex allergy.

> **RED FLAG:** Latex allergy can range from a rash to severe pulmonary crisis. Inspect all items that will come in contact with the child for the presence of latex. Common items include medical gloves, balloon, rubber toys, adhesive tape, and pacifiers.

Physical Therapy Intervention
1. Family education.
   a. Positioning to prevent/minimize joint deformities, especially hip, knee, and ankle flexion contractures.
   b. Handling to support flaccid lower limbs and reduce risk of fracture due to osteoporosis.
   c. Activities to promote development.
   d. Use of assistive devices to promote optimal development in all areas.
   e. Awareness of potential shunt malfunction.
2. Maximize functional skills.
   a. Strengthening through play.
   b. Stretching tight joints and muscles.
   c. Fit and teach use of appropriate assistive devices to promote normal developmental activities.

Table 9-8

Level of Functional Skills for Myelomeningocele

LEVEL OF LESION	INNERVATED MUSCLES	FUNCTIONAL PROGNOSIS	ASSISTIVE DEVICES
Thoracic	Neck, upper limbs, shoulder girdle, trunk muscles	No lower limb movements. Trunk muscles may be weak. Arms may be weak due to lack of trunk stability. Will use wheelchair for most mobility. No bowel or bladder control	Power wheelchair, manual wheelchair, reciprocating gait orthosis, standing frame and body jacket for spinal stability
High lumbar (L1–2)	As above, plus hip flexors	Weak hip flexion. May develop dislocated hips. May ambulate short distances with assistive devices. No bowel and bladder control. At risk for hip flexion contractures	Power wheelchair, manual wheelchair, reciprocating gait orthosis, standing frame, HKAFO, rollator walker, forearm crutches
Mid lumbar (L3–4)	As above, plus hip adductors, knee extensors and flexors, may have some ankle dorsiflexion (L4)	No sensation in lower legs or feet. Walks short distance with aids while young. No bowel or bladder control	KAFO, AFO, walker, forearm crutches, wheelchair for longer distances
Low lumbar (L4–5)	As above, plus weak hip extension and abduction, weak plantar flexion against gravity with eversion	Sensation impaired in lower legs and feet. Can walk without orthoses, but needs aids due to fatigue. Can ride a bicycle. No bowel and bladder control	AFO, crutches
Sacral	As above, plus increased strength in ankle plantar flexion and dorsiflexion, more control of intrinsic foot muscles	Sensation impaired in feet. Good hip strength and function. Can walk without support. Bowel and bladder control may be impaired	AFO

d. Fit and teach use of proper orthotic devices.
e. Facilitation of functional motor development.

Down Syndrome (Trisomy 21)

Basic Information
1. Results from malformation of the 21st chromosome and can result in different types.
2. Types of Down Syndrome. See Quick Facts 9-9.
3. Increasing maternal and, in a small percentage, paternal age has been linked to increased incidence of Down syndrome.

Clinical Picture
1. Characteristic features.
    a. Upward slant to eyes.
    b. Small ears and mouth with protruding tongue.
    c. Palmar crease on feet or hands.
    d. Microcephaly with flattened occiput.
    e. Short stature (average height is under 5 feet).
2. Hypotonia leading to decreased strength and joint hypermobility.
3. Congenital heart defects.
4. Visual and hearing deficits.
5. Mental retardation.
6. Speech and articulation disorders.
7. Feeding difficulties, especially in the early years.
8. Developmental delays in all areas, including delayed postural reactions and motor development.
9. Other related problems.
    a. Hypothyroidism.
    b. Vertebral instability at the atlantoaxial (C1-2) joint.
        - Acute or gradual spinal cord injury, especially with a sudden incident of hyperflexion.
        - Important to identify as early symptoms as these indicate a medical emergency.

> **RED FLAGS:** Early symptoms indicating a medical emergency:
> - Weakness and loss of functional skills, including ambulation.
> - Change in deep tendon reflexes and sensation.

c. **SPECIAL CONSIDERATION:** If a screening radiograph demonstrates instability, activities to avoid include diving, tumbling, headstands, contact sports, and any other activities that could cause a hyperflexion injury to the neck.

Physical Therapy Intervention
1. Facilitate gross motor skill development.
    a. Encourage postural control and movement.
    b. Promote activities that facilitate increasing strength, motor control, and gross and fine motor development.
2. Support oral-motor skills: facilitate lip closure and inhibit tongue protrusion.
3. Patient and family education.

Duchenne Muscular Dystrophy (Pseudohypertrophic Muscular Dystrophy)

Basic Information
1. Most common form of congenital, degenerative sex-linked disease of muscle tissue.
2. Almost all affected are boys.
3. Lack of dystrophin increases muscle cell membrane permeability: calcium infiltrates cells and muscle tissue breaks down.

Clinical Picture
1. Progressive muscle weaknesses from proximal to distal muscles.
    a. Gower's sign. The child pushes up from the floor on his hands, walking hands up legs to stand. This is due to weak knee and hip extensors. Typically occurs by 4–7 years of age.
    b. Waddling gait and falls are typical.
2. Pseudohypertrophic muscles: muscles appear hypertrophied as fat and connective tissue replace muscle tissue in calves, deltoids, quadriceps, and tongue.
3. Contractures: result from significant muscle imbalances, most commonly in heel cords, tensor fascia latae, hip flexors, and hamstrings.
4. Lumbar lordosis, thoracic kyphosis, and scoliosis.

QUICK FACTS 9-9 ▶ TYPES OF DOWN SYNDROME

Nondisjunction	Translocation	Mosaic
• Nondisjunction: Extra chromosome present on the 21st pair	• Translocation: Third copy of the 21st chromosome is attached to another pair of chromosomes.	• Mosaic: Some cells in the body exhibit normal chromosomes, others exhibit abnormal chromosomes in the 21st pair.
• More than 90% of individuals with Down syndrome have this type.	• In 25% of cases, it results from one or both parents being carriers.	• Degree of disability is dependent on the percent of cells exhibiting abnormal chromosomes.

> **QUICK FACTS 9-10 ▶ PROGRESSION OF DUCHENNE MUSCULAR DYSTROPHY**
>
> | Age | |
> |---|---|
> | Age 3–5 | Weakness, tripping, Gower's sign |
> | Age 6–8 | Gait deviations (toe walking, wide base of support), lordosis, unable to ascend stairs, poor endurance |
> | Age 9–11 | Walks with braces or may lose ambulation skills |
> | Age 12–14 | Loss of ambulation skills, increased obesity, development of spinal deformities, increasing contractures at hips, knees, and elbows |
> | Age 15–17 | Increased respiratory compromise may lead to assisted ventilation, dependent in most ADLs |
> | Young adulthood | Increased dependence, death in early 20s due to increasing respiratory compromise |

5. Cardiac muscle myopathy.
6. Mild to moderate intellectual impairment becomes evident as child gets older.
7. Progression. See Quick Facts 9-10.

Physical Therapy Intervention
1. Work with family, child, and team of providers to determine how to best support child as functional skills diminish.
2. Maintain range of motion via positioning, splinting, and stretching.
3. Maintain ambulation and standing skills.
4. Utilize assistive devices: braces, crutches, standing frames, and dynamic standers.
5. Maintain functional skills, including communication and mobility, by utilizing power wheelchairs and augmentative and alternative communication devices.
6. Maintain cardiorespiratory function and strength via spontaneous, active motion through normal recreation and ADL.

> **RED FLAG:** The clinician should avoid strengthening exercises in order to preserve muscle tissue. Aquatic therapy may be a good alternative as it can build strength and endurance while not increasing rate of tissue breakdown.

Pervasive Developmental Disorder (PDD)

Basic Information
1. Spectrum of neurobiological disorders related to specific abnormalities in brain function, of which autism is the most common.
2. Causes of autism are largely unknown but some genetic factors have been identified.
3. Other common disorders in the PDD spectrum.
    a. Rett's syndrome: onset 6–18 months, only in girls, with severe apraxia, seizures, lack of speech, and hand flapping.
    b. Asperger's disorder: milder form of autism with social isolation, eccentric behavior, and differences in speech inflection and patterns.
    c. PDD-NOS (not otherwise specified): marked impairment of social interaction, communication, and stereotyped behavior patterns but does not meet the full definition for a diagnosis of autism.
    d. Childhood disintegrative disorder: period of at least 2 years of typical development followed by loss of previously acquired skills occurring before the age of 10.

Clinical Picture of Autism
1. Symptoms usually become apparent between 2 and 3 years of age.
2. Impairments in communication.
    a. Delays or abnormalities in expressive and receptive language skills.
    b. Nonverbal communication.
    c. Echolalic (immediate, involuntary repetition of words heard from another person) speech.
    d. Flat and monotonous, or high pitched and loud voice.
3. Impairments in socialization.
    a. Difficulty maintaining eye contact.
    b. Do not understand gestures and social cues.
    c. Prefer to be alone.
4. Impairments in imagination.
    a. Prefer predictable events and objects.
    b. Play with objects in stereotypical ways rather than imaginative (spinning car wheels instead of making car "drive").
5. Abnormal relationships to objects and events.
    a. Routine is essential and changes to routine can lead to behavior issues.
    b. Difficulty with new situations, objects, people.
    c. Stereotypical mannerisms and behaviors (hand flapping, head banging, rocking).
6. May have abnormalities in muscle tone (usually low), decreased strength, poor balance, clumsiness, and delays in gross motor skills.
7. Difficult behaviors including temper tantrums and social withdrawal.

Physical Therapy Considerations
1. Use familiar objects and routines.
2. Prepare the child for changes in routine.
3. Follow behavioral protocols.
4. Speak clearly and keep instructions simple.

5. Encourage eye contact with child during communication.
6. Structure environment to teach appropriate social skills with peers.
7. Use daily activities to increase strength and functional skills (e.g., climbing stairs, running on the playground).
   a. Each child will likely follow a different behavior plan. The clinician must know the guidelines of the plan and follow it every day in order to help the child develop appropriate behaviors.
   b. Consistency in approach and daily schedule is necessary.

Intellectual Disability/ Developmental Disability/ Developmental Delay

Basic Information
1. Intellectual disability: subaverage intellectual functioning that manifests before age 18.
2. Developmental disability: manifests before age 22 and likely continues through life.
3. Developmental delay: usually diagnosed in children less than 3 years of age; can be used with children as old as 9 years in order to qualify for special education under the Individuals with Disabilities Education Act (IDEA).

Clinical Picture
1. Mental retardation is decreased intellectual functioning with concurrent limitations in two or more adaptive skill areas: communication, self-care, home living, social skills, community use, self-direction, health and safety, functional academics, leisure, and work.
2. Developmental disability substantially limits functioning in three or more areas: self-care, receptive and expressive language, learning, mobility, self-direction, capacity for independent living, economic self-sufficiency; requires individualized interdisciplinary services for extended duration.
3. Developmental delay in one or more of the following areas: gross motor skills, fine motor skills, language skills, and social skills.
   a. May result in later diagnosis of developmental disability or resolve with intervention or maturation.

Physical Therapy Intervention
1. Services utilized are dependent on strengths and needs of the child and family.
2. Common goals of intervention: gait, strength, endurance, flexibility, balance, and motor planning.
3. Treatment focuses on play to increase strength, endurance, and functional activities.
4. Utilize orthoses, adaptive equipment, and assistive technology.
5. Work with the child as part of a team that includes the child and family.

Sickle Cell Anemia

Basic Information
1. Autosomal recessive genetic trait.
2. Found in people of African or Mediterranean descent.

Clinical Picture
1. Abnormally shaped red blood cells cause health impairments.
   a. Sickled cells cannot pass through small capillaries and cause blockages resulting in poor oxygen supply to some tissues.
   b. Cells break down faster than normal, causing jaundice.
   c. Lack of adequate red blood cells causes anemia.
2. Symptoms (vary with each child).
   a. Fatigue due to anemia.
   b. Organ enlargement, necrosis, scarring, and pain due to occluded blood vessels in highly vascularized organs such as spleen, liver, bones, and kidneys.
   c. Stroke.
   d. Skin ulcers.

Physical Therapy Intervention
1. Dependent on needs of the child and must occur as part of a team effort.
2. Encourage general exercise to maintain strength and endurance.
3. Strengthening exercises to address orthopedic needs.
4. Intervention considerations.
   a. Developmental therapy for children with motor delays due to pain, fatigue, multiple surgeries, or stroke.
   b. Orthopedic intervention for children with fractures due to osteoporosis.
   c. Wound care (including debridement) for children with skin ulcers.

Clinical Application

- Contracture formation is present in a variety of the congenital pediatric disorders. While not totally preventable, the PTA can play a major role in limiting contractures by providing appropriate patient and family education on positioning and stretching.
- Persistence of primitive reflexes (ATNR, STNR, TLR) often limits the development of normal movements. The PTA should work to decrease the influence of these reflexes prior to implementing functional activity training.
- Physical therapy will often focus on increasing functional mobility and independence in the school and home environments. The PTA should remember this when working with the patient and family to determine goals and therapeutic activities.
- Because many of these disorders have a genetic component or are related to a maternal issue during pregnancy, the PTA should be prepared to face family members taking or placing blame for the child's condition. Additionally, many family members will be going through the grieving process in the early stages following diagnosis. If not comfortable dealing with these issues, the PTA should consult with a social worker.

Special Considerations when Working with the Pediatric Population

Team Members

Family
1. Family is the primary context for the child and, as such, PTs and PTAs must collaborate with family members as full members of any team servicing a child.
2. Family members are constant in a child's life, whereas medical and educational personnel change.

Teamwork
1. Intradisciplinary: involves collaborating with colleagues in the same discipline about a particular child or problem.
2. Multidisciplinary: many disciplines work with the same child, each writing separate reports and developing discipline-specific goals and treatment activities.
3. Interdisciplinary: many disciplines work with the same child and collaborate with each other in some aspects of care, including assessment, report writing, planning goals, and providing intervention.
4. Transdisciplinary: requiring "role release" between disciplines, it is most likely to occur in early intervention settings where multiple service providers would be inefficient, intrusive, and confusing to the child and family.

Environments of Care

Medical Systems
1. Usually address acute and chronic health issues.
2. Settings include hospitals, rehabilitation centers, outpatient clinics.
3. May assist a child and family with the transition to community care systems such as early intervention programs and schools.

Educational Systems
1. Usually address educational and vocational issues.
2. Settings include early intervention programs, schools, and vocational programs.
3. Services for children are tailored to the system of care that is providing the service and therefore may vary according to the setting.

Legislation Guiding the Provision of Services

IDEA
1. Initially authorized in 1975 as the Education for All Handicapped Children's Act (Public Law 94-142) and most recently reauthorized in 2004 (Public Law 108-446).
2. A federal program overseen by the states and implemented at the district level.
3. Part C provides services for children birth to 3 years of age and their families.
   a. Includes public awareness, child find activities (identification of children in need of services), and service to eligible children.
   b. Providers deliver services that are family directed and occur in natural environments whenever possible.
   c. An Individualized Family Service Plan (IFSP) is developed by providers and the child's family to address the needs of the child and the family.
4. Part B provides services for individuals between 3 and 21 years of age.

a. Services are child-centered and mandated to support the individual's educational (not medical) needs.
b. FAPE: all children are guaranteed a *free and appropriate public education*.
c. LRE: educational services must be provided in the *least restrictive environment*.
d. IEP: an Individualized Educational Plan is devised for each child. The plan is developed by all individuals working with the child, including classroom staff and parents. It includes present levels of performance, goals and objectives, services to be provided, and evaluation criteria.
e. Special education is provided to meet the unique and individual needs of the child.
f. Related services, including physical therapy, are provided when necessary to allow the child to benefit from the special education services provided.
g. Vocational programs.
   - Schools are required to have transition plans in place in the IEP by the time a child is 16 years of age.
   - Adult vocational service systems may be part of this plan.
   - Children must be eligible to receive services.

The Rehabilitation Act of 1973, Section 504

1. Civil rights legislation that addresses the rights of all children with disabilities, whether or not they qualify for special education.
2. Includes appropriate accommodations, educational, and related services needed by the child.

The Americans with Disabilities Act (ADA)

1. Legislation passed in 1990 that addresses civil rights for all Americans with disabilities, including children.

Clinical Application

- Play is what children are about and, in turn, should be the focus of pediatric therapy.
- Multidisciplinary teams are the most beneficial when working with children and families but take a great deal of trust and coordination on the part of the team members.
- All children, regardless of ability or disability, have the right to receive an education that is appropriate for their level of functioning.
- While many parents will desire services, all related services (including physical therapy) can only be provided in the school district when they are limiting the child's ability to benefit from their special education.

Review Questions

Pediatric Physical Therapy

1. What does the IDEA (Public Law 108-446) require?

2. What impairments are expected in a child with Duchenne muscular dystrophy? Identify three physical therapy interventions/goals for a child with Duchenne muscular dystrophy.

3. In what position should a splint for an infant with congenital hip dysplasia position the hips?

4. What characteristic impairments should a PTA working with a child who has a Pervasive Developmental Disorder (PDD) expect the child to present with?

5. A PTA is working with a teenager with spina bifida at S1 level to address increased lower extremity weakness that is limiting walking. During treatment, the PTA notes the teenager appears fatigued. The teenager reports a headache, recent sleep disturbances, and recent problems with bowel and bladder control. What should the PTA suspect is the problem and report immediately to the supervising physical therapist?

10

Therapeutic Modalities

JOHN CARLOS, JR, ELIZABETH OAKLEY and KAREN E. RYAN

Chapter Outline

- Physical Agents, 367
  - Superficial Thermotherapy, 367
  - Methods of Application-Superficial Heat Agents, 368
  - Hydrotherapy, 369
  - Nonimmersion Irrigation, 371
  - Cryotherapy, 371
  - Methods of Cryotherapy Application, 372
- Deep Thermotherapy, 374
  - Biophysics Related to Ultrasound, 374
  - Methods of Application, 376
  - Electromagnetic Energy: Diathermy, 377
- Mechanical Agents and Massage, 378
  - Mechanical Spinal Traction (Intermittent Traction), 378
  - Methods of Application for Intermittent Traction, 379
  - Intermittent Pneumatic Compression, 380

- Methods of Application for Intermittent Pneumatic Compression, 380
- Continuous Passive Motion (CPM), 381
- Tilt Table, 382
- Massage, 382

• Concepts of Electricity for Treatment, 383
- Electrical Stimulation (ES), 383
- Guidelines for Applying ES, 385

• Specific Electrical Stimulation Treatments, 387
- Iontophoresis, 387
- Transcutaneous Electrical Nerve Stimulation (TENS), 387
- High-Voltage Pulsed Galvanic Stimulation, 389
- Interferential Current (IFC), 390
- Neuromuscular Electrical Stimulation (NMES), 391
- Electromyographic (EMG) Biofeedback, 391

• Review Questions, 393

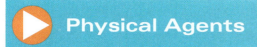
Physical Agents

Superficial Thermotherapy

Physics Related to Heat Transmission
1. Conduction: heat transfer from a warmer object to a cooler object by means of direct molecular interaction of objects in physical contact. Conductive modalities: hot packs, paraffin.
2. Convection: heat transfer by movement of air or fluid from a warmer area to a cooler area or moving past a cooler body part. Convective modalities: whirlpool, Hubbard tank.

Physiological Effects
1. General heat application.
   a. Large areas of the body surface area are exposed to heat modality resulting in systemic changes in the body; e.g., whirlpool (hip and knee immersed), Hubbard tank (lower extremities and trunk immersed). (See Table 10-1.)
2. Small surface area application.
   a. Heat modality applied to small, specific area of body; e.g., low back, hamstring, neck.
3. Indications and goals for use of superficial thermotherapy. See Quick Facts 10-1.
4. Precautions and contraindications for the use of superficial thermotherapy. See Quick Facts 10-2.

Body Tissue Responses to Superficial Heat
1. Skin temperature rises rapidly and exhibits greatest temperature change.
2. Superficial tissue temperature will rise more rapidly and exhibit greater change.
3. Subcutaneous tissue temperature rises less rapidly and exhibits smaller change.
4. Muscles and joints show least temperature change, depending on size of structure.
5. Physiological effects on body systems and structures in response to heat modalities are listed in Tables 10-2 and 10-3.
6. Electrical stimulation may be used in preparation for electrical stimulation (ES); massage; passive and active exercise.

General Treatment Preparation for Thermotherapy and Cryotherapy
1. The application of physical agents must be performed by a qualified physical therapist or personnel supervised by a physical therapist (physical therapist assistant, affiliating physical therapist, physical therapist

Table 10-1

Physiological Effects of General Heat Application

INCREASED	DECREASED
Cardiac output	Blood pressure
Metabolic rate	Muscle activity (sedentary effect)
Pulse rate	Blood to internal organs
Respiratory rate	Blood flow to resting muscle
Vasodilation	Stroke volume

QUICK FACTS 10-1 ▶ GOALS AND INDICATIONS FOR SUPERFICIAL THERMOTHERAPY

Modulate pain	Accelerate rate of tissue healing
Increase connective tissue extensibility	Reduce or eliminate soft tissue and joint restriction
Reduce or eliminate soft-tissue inflammation and swelling	Reduce muscle spasm

QUICK FACTS 10-2 ▶ PRECAUTIONS AND CONTRAINDICATIONS FOR SUPERFICIAL THERMOTHERAPY

Precautions for Use of Superficial Thermotherapy

Cardiac insufficiency	Impaired thermal regulation
Edema	Metal in treatment site
Impaired circulation	Pregnancy
In areas where topical counterirritants have recently been applied	Demyelinated nerves
Open wounds	

CONTRAINDICATIONS TO THE USE OF SUPERFICIAL THERMOTHERAPY

Acute and early subacute traumatic and inflammatory conditions	Impaired cognitive function
Decreased circulation	Malignant tumors
Decreased sensation	Tendency toward hemorrhage or edema
Deep vein thrombophlebitis	Very young and very old patients

Table 10-2

INCREASED Physiological Responses of Body Systems and Structures to Local Heat Application	
SYSTEM/STRUCTURE	MECHANISM
Blood flow	Dilation of arteries and arterioles
Capillary permeability	Increased capillary pressure
Elasticity of nonelastic tissues	Increased extensibility of collagen tissue
Metabolism	For every 10°C increase in tissue temperature, the rate of cellular oxidation increases by two to three times (van't Hoff's law)
Vasodilation	Activation of axon reflex and spinal cord reflex, release of vasoactive agents (bradykinin, histamine, prostaglandin)
Edema	Increased capillary permeability

Table 10-3

DECREASED Physiological Responses of Body Systems and Structures to Local Heat Application	
SYSTEM/STRUCTURE	MECHANISM
Joint stiffness	Increased extensibility of collagen tissue and decreased viscosity
Muscle strength	Decreased function of glycolytic process
Muscle spasm	Decreased firing of II afferents of muscle spindle and increased firing of Ib golgi tendon organ (GTO) fibers reduces alpha motor neuron-activity, and thus decreases tonic extrafusal activity
Pain	Presynaptic inhibition of A delta and C fibers via activation of A beta fibers (gate theory), disruption of pain-spasm cycle

assistant student, or doctoral physical therapist student). The treatment and expected sensations must be explained to the patient.
2. Place patient in comfortable position.
3. Expose treatment area and drape patient properly.
4. Inspect skin and check temperature sensation prior to treatment.
5. If patient has good cognitive function, a call bell or other signaling device should be given to patient to alert personnel of any untoward effects of treatment. Check patient frequently during treatment.
6. Dry and inspect skin at conclusion of treatment.
7. Specific procedures for each physical agent are listed separately.

Methods of Application-Superficial Heat Agents

Hot Packs

1. Hot packs are canvas pack filled with silica gel, heated by immersion in water between 165°F and 170°F.
2. Method of heat transmission: conduction.
3. Add 6–8 layers of toweling between the hot pack and the patient. This can be accomplished in the following ways:
4. Place pack(s) into a terry cloth cover, which usually equals 4–6 layers of toweling. Place one folded towel between patient and pack for hygienic purposes.
   a. Towel folded width-wise method:
      - Fold four towels in half, width-wise.
      - Place each towel on top of the other, forming eight layers of toweling.
      - Place towels on treatment area.
      - Place pack on towels and cover pack with folded towel to retard heat loss.
   b. Towel folded length-wise method:
      - This method is appropriate only for the standard-size pack. Typical towels used in the clinic are not wide or long enough for a full-size pack.
        ○ Fold two towels lengthwise and place one perpendicular over the other, forming a cross.
        ○ Place pack in the center of the towels.
        ○ Fold the ends of the towels over the pack, forming eight layers of toweling on top of the pack. Invert pack, placing the eight layers of toweling on patient.
        ○ Place pack on patient.
5. **TREATMENT CONSIDERATION:** Use additional towels to minimize excessive heating of treatment area caused by weight of patient on pack and to protect bony prominences. Additional pillows may be necessary to support and make the patient comfortable when lying on top of the pack.
   a. Secure the pack to the patient with towels or straps, if needed.
   b. Cover pack with folded towel to retard heat loss.
6. **TREATMENT CONSIDERATION:** The hot pack reaches peak heat within the first 5 minutes of application; during this time, the patient is at the greatest risk for a burn. Thus, the physical therapist or physical therapist assistant should check the skin within the first 5 minutes of treatment and periodically thereafter, especially if the patient is lying on top of the pack.
7. Treatment time: 20–30 minutes.

Paraffin

1. Paraffin bath is the therapeutic application of liquid paraffin to a body part for the transmission of heat. Paraffin bath is a thermostatically controlled unit that contains a paraffin wax and mineral oil mixture in a 6:1 or 7:1 ratio. The paraffin/mineral oil mixture melts between 118°F and 130°F and is normally self-sterilizing at temperatures of 175°F and 180°F. Paraffin is primarily applied to small, irregularly shaped areas such as the wrist, hand, and foot.
2. Method of heat transmission: conduction.
3. Glove method (dip and wrap).
   a. Remove jewelry, or cover jewelry with several layers of gauze, if jewelry cannot be removed.
   b. Wash the part and check for infection and open areas.
   c. The part is dipped several times to apply 6–12 layers of paraffin.
   d. After the paraffin has solidified, the part is wrapped with plastic wrap or waxed paper, and covered with several layers of toweling, and secured with tape or rubber bands.
   e. The patient places the part in a comfortable or elevated position for 15–20 minutes.
4. Dip and immersion method: the procedure follows the steps above, except that the part remains comfortably in the bath after the final dip.
5. Treatment temperature of paraffin: 125°F–127°F.
6. Treatment time: 15–20 minutes.
7. Indications and goals for use of paraffin. See Quick Facts 10-3.
8. Contraindications for use of paraffin. See Quick Facts 10-4.

Hydrotherapy

Principles of Hydrotherapy

1. Specific heat is the heat-absorbing capacity of water, representing the amount of heat a gram of water absorbs or gives off to change the temperature 1°C. The specific heat of water is about four times that of air.
2. Buoyancy is the upward force of water on an immersed or partially immersed body or body part that is equal to the weight of the water that it displaced (Archimedes' principle).
3. Viscosity is the ease at which fluid molecules move with respect to one another. High temperature lowers the viscosity of the fluid. An increase in viscosity creates resistance.
4. Hydrostatic pressure is the circumferential water pressure exerted on an immersed body part. A pressure gradient is established between the surface water and deeper water caused by the increase in water density at deeper levels.
5. Cohesion is the tendency of water molecules to adhere to one another. The resistance encountered while moving through water is partially caused by the cohesion of water molecules and the force needed to separate them.
6. **TREATMENT CONSIDERATIONS:**
   a. Hydrostatic pressure can assist in venous return, heart rate reduction, and centralization of blood flow.
   b. Buoyancy causes a relative "weightlessness." The amount the body is submerged in water determines the weightlessness. The more the body is submerged, the less stress there is on joints, muscle, and connective tissue.
   c. Resistance created by viscosity can increase strength and cardiovascular output. The speed of movement affects resistance.
      - Moving the body and/or limbs slowly in the water creates less resistance to movement; can provide strengthening for weakened muscles.
      - Moving the body and/or limbs more quickly in the water creates more resistance; develops greater strength.
7. Indications for use of hydrotherapy. See Quick Facts 10-5.
8. Precautions and contraindications for use of hydrotherapy. See Quick Facts 10-6.

Method of Application for Whirlpool

1. Hydrotherapy (whirlpool and Hubbard tank).
   a. Partial or total immersion baths in which the water is agitated and mixed with air to be directed against or around the affected part. Patients can move the extremities easily because of the buoyancy and therapeutic effect of the water.
2. Method of heat transmission: convection.
3. Fill the tank with water to the proper level and to the desired temperature. See Table 10-4. Whirlpool liners may be used for patients with burns or wounds, or those who are infected with blood-borne pathogens (human immunodeficiency virus [HIV] or hepatitis-B virus).
   a. Add disinfectant if open wounds are present. Common antibacterial agents: sodium hypochlorite (bleach), dilution of 200 parts per million (ppm); Chloramine-T, 100–200 ppm.
   b. Standard precautions (gowns, goggles, masks, and gloves) should be applied when working in infected

---

QUICK FACTS 10-3 ▶ GOALS AND INDICATIONS FOR PARAFFIN USE

Painful joints caused by arthritis or other inflammatory conditions in the late subacute or chronic phase	Joint stiffness

QUICK FACTS 10-4 ▶ CONTRAINDICATIONS FOR PARAFFIN

Allergic rash	Recent scars and sutures
Open wounds	Skin infections

environment, particularly when working with possibility of splashing. (See Box 6-1.)
   c. Assist patient in immersing his or her body or body part into the tank.
   d. Pressure points should be padded for patient comfort and to minimize compression of blood vessels and nerves. Keep towels out of water.
   e. Adjust agitator to desired position.
   f. Turn on agitator and adjust the force, direction, depth, and aeration.
   g. Monitor patient's response and tolerance to the whirlpool.
   h. At end of treatment, dry and inspect skin.

Method of Application for Hubbard Tank

1. Fill the tank with water to the proper level and to the desired temperature. See Table 10-4.
2. Add disinfectant if open wounds are present.
3. Position and secure patient supine on stretcher or pneumatic lift.
4. Lift patient over edge of tank and slowly lower to water line to enable patient to get accustomed to the water temperature.
5. Continue to lower patient into the water with head elevated. Secure head end of stretcher to bracket in the tank. Remove the suspended hoist when stretcher is resting on bottom of tank or halt descent of lift at desired level.
6. Turn on agitator and adjust the force, direction, depth, and aeration.
7. Monitor patient's response and tolerance to the Hubbard tank.
8. At end of treatment, remove patient onto stretcher or lift. Dry and inspect skin.
9. Treatment time for hydrotherapy: 20 minutes, or up to 30 minutes if other therapeutic procedures are also being performed.
10. Indications for use of hydrotherapy. See Quick Facts 10-5.
11. Precautions and contraindications for use of hydrotherapy. See Quick Facts 10-6.

Table 10-4

Treatment Temperature for Hydrotherapy	
VARIES WITH SIZE AND STATUS OF AREA TREATED	
103°F–110°F	Whirlpool
100°F	Hubbard tank
95°F–100°F	Peripheral vascular disease
92°F–96°F	Open wounds

QUICK FACTS 10-5 ▶ INDICATIONS FOR HYDROTHERAPY

Decubitus ulcers	Postsurgical conditions of hip
Open burns and wounds	Subacute and chronic musculoskeletal conditions of neck, shoulders, and back
Post-hip fractures	Rheumatoid arthritis

QUICK FACTS 10-6 ▶ PRECAUTIONS AND CONTRAINDICATIONS FOR IMMERSION HYDROTHERAPY

Precautions for Local Immersion Hydrotherapy	
Decreased temperature sensation	Impaired cognition
Recent skin graft	Deconditioned state
Precautions for Full Body Immersion Hydrotherapy	
Decreased strength, endurance, balance or ROM	Impaired cognition
Hydrophobia	Urinary incontinence
Alcohol ingestion	Respiratory problems
Precautions for Full Body Immersion Hydrotherapy in Hot or Very Warm Water	
Pregnancy	Multiple sclerosis
Impaired thermal regulatory system	
CONTRAINDICATIONS FOR LOCAL IMMERSION HYDROTHERAPY	
Bleeding	Wound maceration
CONTRAINDICATIONS FOR FULL-BODY IMMERSION HYDROTHERAPY	
Cardiac instability	Profound epilepsy
Suicidal patients	Bowel incontinence
Infections that can be spread by water	

> **RED FLAG:** Electrical safety considerations with hydrotherapy:
> Safety precautions must be taken with any modality that potentially exposes the patient to electrical hazards from faulty electrical connections. A ground fault circuit interrupter should be installed at the circuit breaker of receptacle of all whirlpools and Hubbard tanks. The electrical circuit is broken if current is diverted to the patient (macroshock) who is grounded rather than to a grounded modality. All whirlpool turbines, tanks, and motors, and motors used to lift patients should be checked for current leakage (broken or frayed connections).

Principles for Consideration with Application of Aquatic (Pool) Therapy

1. **Aquatic therapy** is a form of hydrotherapy used primarily for weight-bearing activities, active exercise, or horizontal floating activities. Swimming pools or walking tanks may be used; some incorporate treadmill units or forced water flow to regulate resistance.
2. Movement horizontal to or upward toward the water surface (active assistive exercise) is facilitated by the buoyancy of the water. A flotation device may be used as well.
3. Movement downward is more difficult. A flotation device increases resistance.
4. Increasing speed of movement increases resistance because of turbulence and cohesion of water. Use of hand-held paddles, held width-wise, increases resistance. Streamlining can be achieved by turning the paddle and slicing through the water.
5. Amount of weight bearing can be determined by water depth. The greater the depth, the less is the load on the extremities because of buoyancy.
6. Water temperature for aquatic therapy is 92°F–98°F.
7. Treatment time for aquatic therapy varies with patient tolerance.
8. Open wounds and skin infections must be covered.
9. Goals and indications for aquatic (pool) therapy. See Quick Facts 10-7.
10. Precautions and contraindications for aquatic (pool) therapy. See Quick Facts 10-8.

Nonimmersion Irrigation

Pulsed Lavage

1. A small device, typically a hand-held electric water pump that produces a water jet to create a shearing force to loosen tissue debris.
2. Some devices produce a pulsed lavage and include suction to remove debris.

Method of Application for Pulsed Lavage

1. Treatment should take place in an enclosed area.
2. Face and eye protection, gloves, and waterproof gown are required.
3. Sterile, warm saline is used. Antimicrobials may be added.
4. Select appropriate treatment pressure, usually 4–8 pounds per square inch (psi). Pressure may be increased in presence of large amounts of necrotic tissue or tough eschar. Pressure should be decreased with bleeding, near a major vessel, or if a patient complains of pain.
5. Treatment time for nonimmersion irrigation device (pulsed lavage) is usually 5–15 minutes, once a day. Wound size and amount of necrotic tissue may increase treatment parameters.

QUICK FACTS 10-7 ▶ GOALS AND INDICATIONS FOR AQUATIC THERAPY

Improve standing balance	Improve ROM
Partial weight-bearing ambulation	Increase muscle strength via active assistive, active, or resistive exercise.
Aerobic exercise	

QUICK FACTS 10-8 ▶ PRECAUTIONS AND CONTRAINDICATIONS FOR AQUATIC THERAPY

Unprotected open wounds	Unstable blood pressure

Cryotherapy

Physics Related to Cryotherapy Energy Transmission

1. Abstraction: the removal of heat by means of conduction or evaporation.
2. Conduction: transfer of heat from a warmer object to a cooler object by means of direct molecular interaction of objects in physical contact. Conductive modalities: cold pack, ice pack, ice massage, cold bath.
3. Evaporation (heat of vaporization): highly volatile liquids that evaporate rapidly on contact with warm object. Evaporative modality: vapocoolant sprays (Fluori-Methane). Continued use questionable due to environmental concerns.

Table 10-5

Physiological Effects of General Cold Application	
DECREASED	**INCREASED**
Metabolic rate	Blood flow to internal organs
Pulse rate	Cardiac output
Respiratory rate	Stroke volume
Venous blood pressure	Arterial blood pressure
	Shivering (occurs when core temperature drops)

Table 10-6

Decreased Physiological Responses of Body Systems and Structures to Local Cold Application	
SYSTEM/STRUCTURE	**MECHANISM**
Blood flow	Sympathetic adrenergic activity produces vasoconstriction of arteries, arterioles, and venules
Capillary permeability	Decreased fluids into interstitial tissue
Elasticity of nonelastic tissues	Decreased extensibility of collagen tissue
Metabolism	Decreased rate of cellular oxidation
Muscle spasm	Decreased firing of II afferents of muscle spindle, increased firing of Ib GTO fibers reduces alpha motor neuron activity and thus decreases tonic extrafusal activity
Muscle strength	Decreased blood flow, increased viscous properties of muscle (long duration: >5–10 min)
Spasticity	Decreased muscle spindle discharge (afferents: primary, secondary), decreased gamma motor neuron activity
Vasoactive agents	Decreased blood flow

Table 10-7

Increased Physiological Responses of Body Systems and Structures to Local Cold Application	
SYSTEM/STRUCTURE	**MECHANISM**
Joint stiffness	Decreased extensibility of collagen tissue and increased tissue viscosity
Pain threshold	Inhibition of A delta and C fibers via activation of A beta fibers (gate theory), interruption of pain-spasm cycle, decreased sensory and motor conduction, synaptic transmission slowed or blocked
Increased blood viscosity	Decreased blood flow in small vessels facilitates red blood cells adhering to one another and vessel wall, impeding blood flow
Muscle strength	Facilitation of alpha motor neuron (short duration: 1–5 min)

Physiological Effects of Cold Application

1. General (large surface area) cold application.
   a. Decreases: metabolic rate, pulse rate, respiratory rate, and venous blood pressure. See Table 10-5.
2. Local (small surface area) cold application. See Table 10-6 and Table 10-7 for increased and decreased responses.
3. Effects of cold application on body tissues.
   a. Skin temperature falls rapidly and exhibits greatest temperature change.
   b. Subcutaneous temperature falls less rapidly and displays smaller temperature change.
   c. Muscles and joints show least temperature changes, requiring longer cold exposure.
4. Vasoconstriction of skin capillaries that results in blanching of skin in the center of contact area and hyperemia due to a decreased rate in oxygen-hemoglobin dissociation, around the edge of contact area in normal tissue.
5. Cold-induced vasodilation: cyclic vasoconstriction and vasodilation following prolonged cold exposure (>15 minutes). Occurs mostly in hands, feet, and face, where arteriovenous anastomoses are found. Called the "hunting" reaction. Recent studies have questioned the clinical significance of this reaction.

> **RED FLAGS:** Adverse physiological effects of cold due to hypersensitivity:
> - Cold urticaria: erythema of the skin with wheal formation, associated with severe itching due to histamine reaction.
> - Facial flush, puffiness of eyelids, respiratory problems, and in severe cases, anaphylaxis (decreased blood pressure, increased heart rate) with syncope are also related to histamine release.

Methods of Cryotherapy Application

Cold Packs

1. Vinyl casing filled with silica gel or sand-slurry mixture.
2. Method of cold transmission for cold pack: conduction.
3. Method of application for cold pack.
   a. Keep patient warm throughout treatment.
   b. Dampen a towel with warm water, wring out excessive water, fold in half width-wise, and place cold pack on towel.
   c. Place pack on patient and cover with dry towel to retard warming.
   d. Secure pack.
4. Treatment temperature for cold pack: packs are maintained in refrigerated unit at 0°F–10°F.
5. Treatment time for cold pack: 10–20 minutes.

Physical Agents 373

> **QUICK FACTS 10-9 ▶ GOALS AND INDICATIONS FOR CRYOTHERAPY**
>
> | | |
> |---|---|
> | Modulate pain | Reduce or eliminate soft-tissue inflammation or swelling |
> | Reduce muscle spasm | Reduce spasticity |
> | Cryokinetics | Cryostretch |
> | Management of symptoms in multiple sclerosis | |

> **QUICK FACTS 10-10 ▶ PRECAUTIONS AND CONTRAINDICATIONS FOR CRYOTHERAPY**
>
> **Precautions for Use of Cryotherapy**
>
> | | |
> |---|---|
> | Hypertension | Open wound |
> | Impaired temperature sensation | Over superficial nerve |
> | Very old or young | Cognitive changes |
>
> **CONTRAINDICATIONS for Use of Cryotherapy**
>
> | | |
> |---|---|
> | Cold hypersensitivity (urticaria) | Cold intolerance |
> | Cryoglobulinemia | Peripheral vascular disease |
> | Impaired temperature sensation | Raynaud's disease |
> | Paroxysmal cold hemoglobinuria | Over regenerating peripheral nerves |

6. Goals and indications for use of cryotherapy. See Quick Facts 10-9.
7. Precautions and contraindications for use of cryotherapy. See Quick Facts 10-10.

Ice Packs
1. Ice Packs are the use of crushed ice folded in moist towel or placed in plastic bag covered by moist towel.
2. Method of cold transmission for ice packs: conduction (abstraction).
3. Method of application for ice packs.
   a. Apply the ice pack to body part.
   b. Cover pack with dry towel.
4. Treatment time for application of ice pack: 10–20 minutes.

Ice Massage
1. Ice massage uses an ice cylinder formed by freezing water in a paper or Styrofoam cup. Salt may be added to create a colder slush mixture. A lollipop stick or wooden tongue depressor may be placed in water during freezing process. During the application of ice massage, the patient will usually experience the following sequence of physiological response stages: cold, burning, aching, and numbness.
2. Method of cold transmission for ice massage: conduction.
3. Method of application for ice massage.
   a. Remove ice from container.
   b. Wrap ice with towel or washcloth, if ice has no lollipop stick. If ice is retained in container, tear off bottom half and hold top half.
   c. Apply the ice massage to an area no larger than 4 × 6 inches in slow (2 inches/second) overlapping circles or overlapping longitudinal strokes, each stroke covering one-half of previous circle or stroke. If treating a large area, divide into smaller areas.

   RED FLAG: Do not massage over bony area or superficial nerve (e.g., peroneal/fibular).

   d. Use a towel to dab excess water from treatment area. Ice will melt rapidly at first, but rate of melting will slow as skin cools.
   e. Continue treatment until anesthesia is achieved.
4. Treatment time for ice massage: 5–10 minutes, or until analgesia occurs.

Contrast Baths
1. Alternating immersion of a body part in warm and cold water to produce vascular exercise through active vasodilation and vasoconstriction of the blood vessels.
2. The effectiveness of this method to raise deep tissue temperature via increased circulation of deep vessels has been questioned. It may be useful in promotion of pain modulation.
3. For Indications and Contraindications see See Quick Facts 10-11 and Quick Facts 10-12 respectively.
4. Method of heat/cold transmission for contrast bath: conduction.
5. Method of application for contrast bath.
   a. Treatment usually begins in warm to hot water (100°F–111°F).

> **QUICK FACTS 10-11 ▶ INDICATIONS FOR CONTRAST BATH**
>
> | | |
> |---|---|
> | Any condition requiring stimulation of peripheral circulation in limbs | Peripheral vascular disease |
> | Sprains | Strains |
> | Delayed onset muscle soreness | Trauma (after acute condition abates) |

> **QUICK FACTS 10-12 ▶ CONTRAINDICATIONS FOR CONTRAST BATH**
>
> | | |
> |---|---|
> | Advanced arteriosclerosis | Arterial insufficiency |
> | Loss of sensation to heat and cold | |

b. Place part in warm water for 4 minutes, and then transfer to cold water for 1 minute.
c. Immerse part in warm water for 4 minutes.
d. Continue sequence of 4:1, usually ending in warm water.
e. Patient's condition may determine the ending temperature. Ending in cold water may be more beneficial if reducing edema is the goal.
6. Treatment temperature for contrast bath.
   a. Warm to hot water: 98°F–111°F.
   b. Cold water: 50°F–65°F.
7. **TREATMENT CONSIDERATION:** During initial treatment, you may wish to begin with the upper end of the cold range and the lower end of the hot range.
8. Treatment time for contrast bath: 20–30 minutes.

Cryo-cuff

1. A cryo-cuff is a portable mechanical/or gravity driven device with a sleeve or cuff attached, via tubing, to a cooler containing ice water.
2. Applied to inflamed area or joints following injury or surgical intervention to minimize edema via a combination of compression and cold simultaneously.
3. Indications for Cryo-cuff: pain and edema following surgical intervention or injury.
4. Contraindications for Cryo-cuff: refer to Quick Facts 10-10.
5. Methods of application for Cryo-cuff.
   a. Attach the sleeve or cuff to affected area. Elevate and support affected area.
   b. Mechanical unit: turn unit on, water circulates automatically to maintain temperature.
   c. Gravity driven unit: raise unit above cuff (allows cooled water to flow into cuff), when water warms lower unit below cuff (allows warm water to remix with ice water in unit), repeat.
6. Treatment time with Cryo-cuff: 10–20 minutes, 1–2 times per hour or as needed to minimize edema and pain.

Deep Thermotherapy

Biophysics Related to Ultrasound

Conversion
1. Mechanical energy produced by sound waves at frequencies between 85 KHz and 3 MHz are delivered at intensities between 1 w/cm^2 and 3 w/cm^2. The mechanical energy is absorbed by body tissues and changed to thermal energy.

Ultrasound Applicator
1. The applicator contains a piezoelectric crystal (transducer) that converts electrical energy into acoustical energy by means of reverse piezoelectric effect. Alternating voltage causes mechanical deformation of the crystal. The crystal resonates (vibration) at current frequency. Oscillating crystal produces sound waves with little dispersion of energy (collimated beam). Oscillating sound wave produces mechanical pressure waves in the tissue fluid medium. The molecules within the tissue vibrate, and the resulting friction produces heat.

Transducer Size
1. US transducers come in a variety of sizes, from 1 cm^2 to 10 cm^2. The most commonly used is 5 cm^2.
2. Treatment consideration: Transducer size should be selected relative to the size of the treatment area (1 cm^2 = wrist; 5 cm^2 = shoulder, leg).
3. Effective radiating area (ERA) is the area of the faceplate (crystal size), which is smaller than the soundhead.

Spatial Characteristics of US
1. Continuous US is applied to achieve thermal effects (e.g., chronic conditions).
2. Treatment consideration: Uneven intensity produces a high level of energy in the center of the US beam relative to the surrounding areas. This effect produces a "hot spot" (peak spatial intensity) in the beam. Moving the soundhead or using pulsed US tends to reduce the effect of the hot spot.
   a. Spatial average intensity is the total power (watts) divided by the area (cm^2) of the transducer head. This is typically the measurement used to document US treatments.
   b. Beam nonuniformity ratio (BNR) is the ratio of spatial peak intensity to spatial average intensity. The lower the BNR, the more uniform the energy distribution, and the less risk of tissue damage. BNR should be between 2:1 and 6:1.

Temporal Characteristics of US
1. During pulsed US, temporal characteristics of the US are important.
   Pulsed US is applied when nonthermal effects are desired (e.g., acute soft tissue injuries).

a. Duty cycle is the fraction of time the US energy is on over one pulse period (time on + time off). For example, a 20% duty cycle could have an on-time of 2 msec and an off-time of 8 msec. A duty cycle of ≤50% is considered pulsed US. A duty cycle of 51%–99% produces less acoustic energy and less heat.
b. Temporal peak intensity is the peak intensity of US during the on-time phase of the pulse period.
c. Temporal average intensity is the US power averaged over one pulse period.
d. Attenuation is the reduction of acoustical energy as it passes through soft tissue. Absorption, reflection, and refraction affect attenuation.
2. Treatment consideration: Absorption is highest in tissues with high collagen and protein content (muscles, tendons, ligaments, capsules). The scattering of sound waves that result from reflection and refraction produces molecular friction that the sound wave must overcome to penetrate tissues.
3. Depth of penetration is 3–5 cm. Depth of penetration is influenced by the frequency of US.
    a. A frequency of 3 MHz will cause greater heat production in superficial layers. This is caused by greater scatter (attenuation) of sound waves in superficial tissue; e.g., temporomandibular joint (TMJ).
    b. A frequency of 1 MHZ will cause an increased heat production in deep layers of tissue by less scatter in superficial tissues; thus, more US energy is able to penetrate to deeper tissues.

Physiological Effects of Ultrasound

1. Thermal effects are produced by continuous sound energy of sufficient intensity. Intensity may range from 0.5–3 w/cm². US intensity will vary depending upon tissue type and pathology.
    a. **TREATMENT CONSIDERATION:** There may be an increased temperature at tissue interfaces due to reflection and refraction. Tissue interfaces could be bone/ligament, bone/joint capsule, and bone/muscle.
    b. **TREATMENT CONSIDERATION:** Excessively high temperatures may produce a sudden, strong ache caused by overheating of periosteal tissue (periosteal pain). Reduce intensity or increase surface area of treatment if periosteal pain is expressed by patient.
    c. **TREATMENT CONSIDERATION:** Insufficient coupling agent may produce discomfort caused by a "hot spot," which is the uneven distribution of the acoustical energy through the sound head. However, this is a greater problem if the stationary technique is used.
2. Goals and indications for use of thermal ultrasound. See Quick Facts 10-13.

> **QUICK FACTS 10-13 ▶ GOALS AND INDICATIONS FOR USE OF THERMAL ULTRASOUND**
>
> | | |
> |---|---|
> | Increased tissue temperature | Increased pain threshold |
> | Increased collagen tissue extensibility | Alteration of nerve conduction velocity |
> | Increased enzymatic activity | Increased tissue perfusion |

3. Nonthermal effects of ultrasound are generated by very low intensity or pulsed (intermittent) sound energy. Pulsed US is related to duty cycle. Typical duty cycles are 20%–50% for nonthermal intervention.
    a. Treatment considerations: Cavitation is the alternating compression (condensation phase) and expansion (rarefaction phase) of small gas bubbles in tissue fluids caused by mechanical pressure waves.
    b. Stable cavitation occurs when gas bubbles resonate without tissue damage. Stable cavitation may be responsible for diffusional changes in cell membranes.
    c. Unstable cavitation occurs when there is a severe collapse of gas bubbles during compression phase of US can result in local tissue destruction due to high temperatures.
    d. Acoustic streaming is the movement of fluids along the boundaries of cell membranes resulting from mechanical pressure wave. Acoustic streaming may produce alterations in cell membrane activity, increased cell wall permeability, increased intracellular calcium, increased macrophage response, and increased protein synthesis; may accelerate tissue healing.
4. Goals and indications for the use of non-thermal ultrasound. See Quick Facts 10-14.
5. Precautions and contraindications for the use of Ultrasound. See Quick Facts 10-15.

> **QUICK FACTS 10-14 ▶ GOALS AND INDICATIONS FOR USE OF NON-THERMAL ULTRASOUND**
>
> | | |
> |---|---|
> | Modulate pain | Increase connective tissue extensibility |
> | Reduce or eliminate soft-tissue inflammation | Accelerate rate of tissue healing |
> | Wound healing | Reduce or eliminate soft-tissue and joint restriction and muscle spasm |

QUICK FACTS 10-15 ▶ PRECAUTIONS AND CONTRAINDICATIONS FOR ULTRASOUND	
Precautions for Use of Ultrasound	
Acute inflammation in area of treatment	Breast implants if treating in pectoral area
Open bone epiphyses	Healing fractures in area of treatment
CONTRAINDICATIONS FOR USE OF ULTRASOUND	
Impaired circulation	Impaired cognitive function
Impaired sensation	Malignant tumor
Joint cement	Over or near an area with thrombophlebitis
Directly over plastic components	Over vital areas such as brain, ear, eye, heart, cervical ganglia
Reproductive organs	Exposed or unprotected spinal cord
Over or in the area of cardiac pacemakers	Over the abdomen, low back, uterus, or pelvis during pregnancy

Methods of Application

Direct Contact
1. Transducer-to-skin interface; moving sound head in contact with relatively flat body surface.
   a. Apply generous amount of coupling medium (gel/cream) to skin.
   b. US requires a homogenous medium (mineral oil, water, commercial gel) for effective sound wave transmission and acts as a lubricating agent.
   c. Select sound head size (ERA one-half the size of the treatment area). Place sound head at right angle to skin surface.
   d. Move sound head slowly (~1.5 inches/sec) in overlapping circles or longitudinal strokes, maintaining sound head to body surface angle.
   e. Each motion covers one-half of previous circle or stroke.
   f. Do not cover an area greater than two to three times the size of the ERA per 5 minutes of treatment. To cover an area greater than twice the ERA, apply US in two or more sections.
   g. While sound head is moving and in firm contact, turn up intensity to desired level.
2. Treatment intensity: 0.5–2.5 w/cm^2, depending on treatment goal.
3. **TREATMENT CONSIDERATIONS:** Lower intensities for acute conditions or thin tissue (wrist joint); for chronic conditions or thick tissue (low back), higher intensities should be considered.

RED FLAG: Periosteal pain occurring during treatment may be caused by high intensity, momentary slowing, or cessation of moving head. If this occurs, stop treatment and readjust US intensity or add more coupling agent.

4. Treatment time for ultrasound: 3–10 minutes, depending on size of area, intensity, condition, and frequency.

Indirect Contact
1. Water immersion is used over irregular body surface areas.
   a. Fill container with water high enough to cover treatment area. A plastic container is preferred because it will reflect less acoustic energy than a metal container.
   b. Place body part in water.
   c. Place sound head in water, keeping it 1 cm from skin surface and at right angle to body part.
   d. Move sound head slowly, as in direct contact.
2. Treatment consideration: If applying stationary technique, reduce intensity or use pulsed US.
   a. Turn up intensity to desired level.
   b. Periodically wipe off any air bubbles that may form on sound head or body part during treatment.
3. Indirect contact (using a fluid-filled/thin-walled bag) is used with irregular body parts.
4. Use a balloon, condom, or surgical glove applied over irregular bony surfaces. Not widely used, but may be an alternative to immersion technique.
   a. Place bag around side of sound head, squeeze out fluid until all air is removed and sound head is immersed in water.
   b. Apply coupling agent to skin and place bag over treatment area.
   c. Move sound head slowly within bag to maintain a right angle between sound head and treatment area. Do not slide bag on skin.
   d. Increase intensity to desired level.

Phonophoresis
1. The use of US to drive medications through the skin into the deeper tissues. See Quick Facts 10-16.

> **QUICK FACTS 10-16 ▶ GOALS AND INDICATIONS FOR USE OF PHONOPHORESIS**
>
> Pain modulation | Decrease inflammation in subacute and chronic musculoskeletal conditions.

> **QUICK FACTS 10-17 ▶ GOALS AND INDICATIONS FOR USE OF SWD**
>
> Increase blood flow | Increase deep tissue heating
> Increase cellular activity

2. Local analgesics (lidocaine) and anti-inflammatory drugs (dexamethasone, salicylates) are often used.
3. Method of application is similar to direct contact technique of US, except that a medicinal agent, typically a cream, is used as part of coupling medium.
4. Mode: pulsed 20%.
5. Treatment intensity: 1–3 w/cm^2.
6. Treatment time: 5–10 minutes.
7. Intensity: 0.5–0.75 w/cm^2, using a medication that is prepared in a medium that will allow transmission of the US. Gel mediums or transdermal patches have good transmissivity; avoid pastes and creams.

> **QUICK FACTS 10-18 ▶ CONTRAINDICATIONS FOR USE OF SWD**
>
> Decreased sensation | Peripheral vascular compromise
> Over tumors/testes/open inflamed tissues, active bleeding, over eye, metallic objects | Pregnancy
> Implanted electrical devices

Electromagnetic Energy: Diathermy

Biophysics of Short-wave Diathermy

1. Diathermy utilizes high-frequency, short-wave, electromagnetic energy applied to the body where it is converted to heat. It is applied in the form of continuous (SWD) or pulsed short-wave (PSWD). SWD preferentially heats skeletal muscle, blood, and synovial fluid (low impedance tissues). SWD provides deep heat (up to 4 cm) to large tissue areas versus the small tissue areas treated by ultrasound.
2. Frequencies: 27.12 MHz (most commercial machines) with wavelength of 11 meters, 13.56 MHz with wavelength of 22 meters, and, rarely, 40.68 MHz with wavelength of 7.5 meters.

Physiological Effects of SWD

1. Produces increased blood flow (providing increased oxygen and nutrients and waste product removal), speeds rate of metabolism in area, and increases rate of ion diffusion across cellular membranes in treatment area, thus increasing tissue temperature and extensibility and decreasing pain.
   a. See Quick Facts 10-17.
2. **TREATMENT CONSIDERATIONS:** Evidence shows that SWD can produce tissue heating that occurs as deep as 1 MHz of ultrasound. Tissues heated with SWD maintain extensibility 2–3 times longer than tissues heated with US.
   a. See Quick Facts 10-18.
3. Treatment times: generally 15–30 minutes in length.

Dosing for Continuous SWD

1. Based on patient's report of heat sensation, four levels of heating with first being athermal.
   a. Dose I = just below sensation of heat.
   b. Dose II = mild perception of heat.
   c. Dose III = moderate, comfortable sensation of heat.
   d. Dose IV = vigorous heating sensation, no pain or burning sensation.

Methods of Application for SWD

1. Capacitor electrodes create stronger electrical field.
   a. Air spaced electrodes contain metal plate encased in plastic guard; plate can be moved within 3 cm of guard; patient becomes part of the circuit.

> **RED FLAG:** Capacitor heating must be used carefully in areas with high fat content to prevent tissue damage.

   b. Treatment consideration: Heat sensation is proportionate to electrode distance from skin—closer to the skin produces more superficial heat, farther from the tissue surface produces heat in deeper tissues. Placing electrodes closer together results in higher tissue temperatures; tissues at the center of electrical field receive greater current density. Tissues most resistant to current flow develop the most heat, e.g. muscle, blood, fat.
2. Pad electrodes: patient is part of circuit. Must have uniform contact between pad, patient, and toweling. Better to treat superficial soft tissues.
   a. Treatment consideration: Depth of penetration diminishes with pads placed closer together; farther apart results in deeper penetration BUT diminished

current density. Pads should not be placed closer together than the diameter of one pad.
3. Inductance electrodes produce electromagnetic field by generating eddy currents to generate heat. These electrodes heat tissues with least resistance—blood, muscle, fat; tissues high in electrolytic content respond best to magnetic field. Inductance electrodes can be applied using a coil/cable or drum method.

Coil/Cable Method of Application
1. A coil or cable is wrapped around treatment limb or on top of treatment area, may also be contained in an electrode.
2. Coils placed in a "pancake" shape on top of patient must have a 6 inch open center and be evenly spaced (5–10 cm apart); coils placed around a limb must be evenly spaced 5–10 cm apart around the treatment area.
3. Toweling must be used between the cable and the patient; at least 1 cm of toweling should be used.

Drum Method of Application
1. With SWD drum uses coil is pre-spaced and enclosed within drum type housing. This method may allow for a maximum heat penetration of 3 cm.
   a. A light towel must be used between drum and treatment tissues to absorb perspiration;
   b. Drum is placed directly on top of toweling.

RED FLAG: Droplets can overheat and cause hot spots resulting in burns.

Dosing PSWD
1. PSWD delivers pulsed energy between 1 and 7000 Hz with pulse duration between 20–400 μsec; intensity up to 1000 watts per pulse. Produces athermal effects with minimal physiologic heating.
2. Heating does occur; however, it dissipates during off time, therefore reducing overall tissue heating. Mean power is the measure of heat production for the treatment.
   a. Pulse period (pulse on time + pulse off time): peak pulse power (w)/pulse repetition frequency (Hz).
   b. Percentage on time: pulse duration (msec)/pulse period (msec).
   c. Mean power: peak pulse power (w)/percentage on time.

Mechanical Agents and Massage

Mechanical Spinal Traction (Intermittent Traction)

Intermittent Traction
1. Creates a distraction force applied to the spine to separate articular surfaces between vertebral bodies and elongate spinal structures. This force is applied to multiple spinal segments in the cervical and lumbar region.

Effects of Intermittent Traction
1. Joint distraction: a separation of the facet joints occurs with sufficient force. This opens up the intervertebral foramen, relieves pressure on the nerve root and decreases compressive forces on the facets. See Quick Facts 10-19.
   a. For the lumbar region, a force of 50% of the patient's body weight is required to cause separation. In the cervical region, 7% of the patient's body weight or about 20–30 lbs results in separation.
   b. **TREATMENT CONSIDERATION:** Lower traction forces (lumbar: 30–40 lbs; cervical: 8–10 lbs) are recommended for initial treatment to decrease reactive muscle spasm and determine patient tolerance. In follow-up treatments, force can be gradually increased to achieve a maximal decrease in symptoms, but not to exceed 7% of body weight in the cervical region and 50% in the lumbar region.
2. Reduction of disc protrusion: separation of vertebral bodies occurs at higher forces, causing a decrease in intradiscal pressure that creates a suction-like effect

QUICK FACTS 10-19 ▶ GOALS AND INDICATIONS FOR USE OF INTERMITTENT TRACTION	
Decrease joint stiffness (hypomobility)	Muscle spasm
Degenerative disc or joint disease	Disc protrusion
Discogenic pain	Subacute or chronic joint pain
Reduce nerve root impingement	

on the nucleus, drawing it back in centrally. The surrounding ligamentous structures are stretched taut, which also helps to push the disc in centrally.
   a. Treatment consideration: For the lumbar region, 60–120 lbs or up to 50% of a patient's body weight, and for the cervical region, 12–15 lbs is recommended to achieve these desired effects.
3. Soft-tissue stretching: The surrounding spinal muscles, ligaments, tendons, and discs can be stretched, decreasing the pressure on the facet joints, nerve roots, vertebral bodies, and discs without achieving joint separation.
   a. **TREATMENT CONSIDERATION:** Lower traction forces are sufficient to achieve this effect (lumbar region: 25% of body weight; cervical region: 12–15 lbs).
4. Muscle relaxation: Both intermittent and static traction can decrease muscle tone. Traction can interrupt the pain-muscle spasm cycle by stimulating mechanoreceptors through the motion caused by interrupted traction, and by inhibiting motor neuron firing with static traction.
   a. Treatment consideration: The forces recommended for soft-tissue stretching are also used for muscle relaxation.
5. Joint mobilization: At lower forces, intermittent traction stimulates the mechanoreceptors to inhibit pain and decrease spasm, while high force traction causes decreased pressure on the joints and stretches the surrounding soft tissue. Unlike manual joint mobilization, traction cannot be isolated to a particular segment and provides general mobilization in the cervical or lumbar region.

Methods of Application for Intermittent Traction

Cervical Traction
1. Can be seated or supine. Supine position is generally preferred.
2. Cervical halter.
   a. Head halter is placed under the occiput and the mandible.
   b. Head halter is attached to the traction cord directly or to the traction unit through the spreader bar.
   c. Slack is removed from the traction cord. The neck should be maintained in 20–30 degrees of flexion; a pillow may be used to achieve this angle.
   d. Some target area specificity may be achieved by varying the neck angle approximately 0–5 degrees of cervical flexion to increase intervertebral space and joint separation at C1 through C5; up to 25–30 degrees for C5 through C7; neutral spine (approximately 20 degrees of flexion) for disc dysfunction.
   e. **TREATMENT CONSIDERATION:** Traction force should be applied to the occipital region and not on the chin. If patient expresses discomfort in the temporomandibular joint area, treatment should stop, and head halter should be readjusted to ensure that the force is properly applied.
3. Cervical sliding device.
   a. The head is placed on padded headrest, which positions the neck in 20–30 degrees of flexion.
   b. Adjustable neck yoke is tightened to firmly grip just below the mastoid process.
   c. Head strap is secured across the forehead.
   d. Traction rope is then attached to the gliding platform of the device.
4. Traction force is determined by treatment goals and patient tolerance.
   a. Acute phase.
      - Disc protrusion, elongation of soft tissue, muscle spasm, 10–15 pounds or 7%–10% of body weight.
      - Joint distraction 20–30 pounds.
5. Treatment time: Five to 10 minutes for acute conditions and disc protrusion, 15–30 minutes for other conditions.
6. Duty cycle.
   a. Static traction is recommended for disc protrusions or when symptoms are aggravated by motion.
   b. Intermittent traction can also be used for disc protrusions and joint distraction, but a 3:1 hold/rest ratio is recommended. A 1:1 ratio is recommended when mobility is desired, i.e., joint mobilization.
7. Precautions and contraindications for use of intermittent traction. See Quick Facts 10-20.

Lumbar Traction
1. Technique.
   a. A split table is usually used to minimize friction between the body and the table.
   b. Supine position, with pillow under the knee or small bench under lower leg, is recommended when the goal is to open up the intervertebral foramen, separate the facet joints, or elongate the muscles. The prone position may be preferable in the case of a posterior herniated lumbar disc. Some target area specificity may be achieved by varying the angle of pull (i.e., to increase intervertebral space at L5 to S1 up to 45–60 degrees of hip flexion, or at L3 to L4 up to 75–90 degrees).
   c. Apply the pelvic harness so that the top edge is above the iliac crest.
   d. Attach the thoracic harness so that the inferior margin is slightly below lower ribs.
   e. Secure the harness around the pelvis and attach it to the traction rope or spreader bar.
   f. Thoracic harness provides countertraction to the pull on the pelvis, and is secured at the top of the table.

QUICK FACTS 10-20 ▶ PRECAUTIONS AND CONTRAINDICATIONS FOR INTERMITTENT TRACTION	
Precautions for Use of Intermittent Traction	
Claustrophobia	Hiatal hernia
Vascular compromise	Pregnancy
Impaired cognition	Any disease or condition that can compromise the structure of the spine, such as: osteoporosis, tumor, infection, rheumatoid arthritis
TMJ (with use of cervical traction)	Disc extrusion
Medial disc protrusion	Complete resolution of severe pain with traction
CONTRAINDICATIONS for Use of Intermittent Traction	
Acute strains, sprains, and inflammation	Spondylolisthesis
Fractures	Postop spinal surgery
Spinal joint instability or hypermobility	Spinal cord compression
Uncontrolled hypertension	Increased peripheralization of pain, numbness, or tingling
Decreased myotomal strength	Decreased reflex response

2. Treatment force.
    a. Acute phase, 30–40 pounds.
    b. Disc protrusion, spasm; elongation of soft tissues, 25% of body weight.
    c. Joint distraction, 50 pounds or 50% of body weight.
3. Treatment time: 5–10 minutes for herniated disc, 10–30 minutes for other conditions.

Intermittent Pneumatic Compression

1. Use a mechanical device that applies external pressure to an extremity through an inflatable appliance (sleeve). Sleeves are designed in a variety of sizes and lengths to fit either the upper or lower extremity (ankle, ankle and lower leg, or full extremity). The compression units and sleeves are designed to inflate a single compartment to produce uniform, circumferential pressure on the extremity, or multiple compartments by applying pressure in a sequential manner. Pressure is greater in the distal compartments and lesser in the proximal compartments. Cold can be applied simultaneously with intermittent compression in which a coolant (50°F–77°F) is pumped through an inflatable sleeve.

Physiological Effects of Intermittent Pneumatic Compression

1. External pressure on the extremity increases the pressure in the interstitial fluids, forcing the fluids to move into the lymphatic and venous return systems, thus reducing the fluid volume in the extremity. In addition to mechanical compression, some conditions may require the daily use of compression stockings to counteract the effect of gravity on the vascular and lymph systems in the lower extremities.
2. Goals and indications for intermittent pneumatic compression. See Quick Facts 10-21.
3. Precautions and contraindications for intermittent pneumatic compression. See Quick Facts 10-22.

Methods of Application for Intermittent Pneumatic Compression

1. Check patient's blood pressure. See Red Flag.

> **RED FLAG:** Inflation pressure should not exceed diastolic blood pressure.

2. Place patient in comfortable position, with limb supported and elevated approximately 45 degrees and abducted 20–70 degrees.

QUICK FACTS 10-21 ▶ GOALS AND INDICATIONS FOR PNEUMATIC COMPRESSION	
Amputation	Decrease chronic edema
Postmastectomy lymphedema	Stasis ulcer
Venous insufficiency	

QUICK FACTS 10-22 ▶ PRECAUTIONS AND CONTRAINDICATIONS FOR PNEUMATIC COMPRESSION

Precautions for Use of Intermittent Pneumatic Compression

Impaired sensation	Malignancy
Uncontrolled hypertension	Over an area where there is a superficial peripheral nerve, such as the fibular nerve

CONTRAINDICATIONS FOR USE OF INTERMITTENT PNEUMATIC COMPRESSION

Acute inflammation, trauma, or fracture	Acute deep venous thrombosis (DVT) and thrombophlebitis
Obstructed lymph or venous return	Arterial disease/insufficiency
Arterial revascularization	Acute pulmonary edema
Decreased sensation	Cancer
Edema with cardiac or renal impairment	Impaired cognition
Infection in treatment area	Hypoproteinemia (<2 g/dL)
Very old or young patients	

3. Apply stockinet over extremity. Be sure all wrinkles are removed.
4. Place the sleeve over the extremity and attach the rubber tube to both the appliance and the compression unit.
5. Set the inflation and deflation ratio to ~3:1. Generally, for edema reduction, 45–90 seconds on/15–30 seconds off. To shape residual limb, a 4:1 ratio is often used.

RED FLAG: Inflation pressure should not exceed diastolic blood pressure.

6. Turn the power on and slowly increase the pressure to the desired level.
7. The patient's blood pressure determines the setting of the device. See Red Flag.
   a. Treatment consideration: Inflation pressures are fairly low: 30–60 mmHg for the upper extremity and 40–80 mmHg for the lower extremity.

RED FLAG: Numbness, tingling, pulse, or pain should not be felt by the patient during the treatment.

8. At the end of the treatment, turn off the unit, remove the appliance and stockinet. Inspect skin.
9. Usually an elastic bandage or compression stocking is placed on the extremity to retain the reduction before a dependent position is allowed.

RED FLAGS:
- Inflation pressure should not exceed diastolic blood pressure.
- Numbness, tingling, pulse, or pain should not be felt by the patient during the treatment.

10. Treatment time.
    a. The duration may vary, depending on the patient's tolerance and condition.
       - Lymphedema: 2 hours progressing to two 3-hour sessions daily.
       - Traumatic edema: 2 hours daily.
       - Venous ulcers: 2.5 hours three times per week progressing to 2 hours daily.
       - Residual limb edema: 1 hour progressing to three 1-hour sessions daily.
    b. Some conditions may warrant shorter treatment times initially.

Continuous Passive Motion (CPM)

1. A mechanical device that provides uninterrupted passive motion of the joint through controlled ROM extended periods of time.

Physiological Effects of CPM
1. Accelerate rate of interarticular cartilage regeneration, tendon and ligament healing.
2. Decrease edema and joint effusion. Minimize contractures. Decrease postoperative pain.
3. Increase synovial fluid lubrication of the joint. Improve circulation. Prevent adhesions.
4. Improve nutrition to articular cartilage and periarticular tissues. Increase joint ROM.

Goals and Indications for CPM
1. Postimmobilization fracture, tendon or ligament repair; total knee or hip replacement.

Precautions and Contraindications for CPM

1. Precaution: intracompartmental hematoma from anticoagulant.
2. **CONTRAINDICATION:** increases in pain, edema, or inflammation following treatment.

Method of Application for CPM (Postoperative Knee)

1. CPM applied immediately postoperatively, with carriages appropriately measured and adjusted.
   a. Rate of Motion: set at 1- to 4-minute cycles.
   b. ROM Setting: If applied at the knee, ROM may be 20–40 degrees of knee flexion initially and increased 5–10 degrees, as tolerated, until optimal range is reached. Usually a goal of 110–120 degrees is acceptable.
   c. Treatment time: as little as 1-hour sessions, three times a day, up to 24 continuous hours. This is generally directed by physician protocol. Patient's limb may be removed periodically for active or active assistive exercise, or activities of daily living (ADL) activities.
   d. Duration of treatment: 1 to 3 weeks or until therapeutic goals are attained.

Tilt Table

1. A tilt table is a mechanical or electrical table designed to elevate patient from horizontal (0 degrees) to vertical (90 degrees) position in a controlled, incremental manner.

Physiological Effects of Tilt Table

1. Stimulate postural reflexes to counteract orthostatic hypotension.
2. Facilitate postural drainage.
3. Gradual loading of one or both lower extremities.
4. Begin active head or trunk control.
5. Provide positioning for stretch of hip flexors, knee flexors, and ankle plantar flexors.
6. Goals and indications for use of the Tilt Table. See Quick Facts 10-23.
7. Contraindications for use of the Tilt Table. See Quick Facts 10-24.

Methods of Application for Tilt Table

1. Patient is placed in supine position.
2. Abdominal binder, long elastic stockings, or tensor bandaging to counteract orthostatic hypotension (venous pooling) may be used.
3. Patient secured to table by straps. Knee (just proximal to patella), hip (over pelvis), and trunk (over chest just under the axilla).
4. Take baseline vitals (blood pressure, heart rate, respiratory rate).
5. Table raised gradually to given angle. Incremental rise to 30 degrees, 45 degrees, 60 degrees, 80 degrees, or 85 degrees, or as tolerated. Position can be maintained for as long as 30–60 minutes.
   a. Treatment consideration: Vital signs (blood pressure, heart rate, respiratory rate) need to be monitored to assess the patient's tolerance to treatment.

RED FLAG: Cyanotic lips or fingernail beds may indicate compromised circulation.

6. Treatment time: Initially, the duration of treatment depends on the patient's tolerance, but should not exceed 45 minutes, once or twice daily.

Massage

Definition

1. Mechanical and rhythmical manipulation of soft tissues by use of the hands.

QUICK FACTS 10-23 ▶ GOALS AND INDICATIONS FOR TILT TABLE

Prolonged bed rest	Immobilization
Spinal cord injury	Traumatic brain injury
Orthostatic hypotension	Spasticity

QUICK FACTS 10-24 ▶ CONTRAINDICATIONS FOR MASSAGE

Acute inflammation in area	Acute febrile condition
Severe atherosclerosis	Severe varicose veins
Phlebitis/thrombophlebitis	Areas of recent surgery
Cardiac arrhythmia	Malignancy
Hypersensitivity	Severe rheumatoid arthritis
Hemorrhage in area	Edema secondary to kidney dysfunction
Heart failure	Venous insufficiency

Physiological Effects of Massage
1. Increased venous and lymphatic flow.
2. Stretching and loosening of adhesions.
3. Edema reduction.
4. Sedation.
5. Muscle relaxation.
6. Modulate pain.

Description of Selected Massage Techniques
1. Stroking (effleurage): gliding movements of hands over surface of skin. Superficial stroking: light contact. Deep stroking: heavy pressure.
2. Kneading (petrissage): grasping and lifting of tissues. Similar to kneading bread.
3. Friction: compression of tissue using small circular or long stroking movements, usually with the palmar surface of hand or fingers. Pressure may be light (superficial) initially, progressing to heavy (deep), moving superficial tissues over deeper tissues.
4. Tapping (tapotement): rapid striking with palmar surface of hand and/or fingers, cupped hand (clapping, percussion), or ulnar edge of hand and fingers (hacking) in an alternating manner.
5. Vibration: shaking of tissue using short, rapid quivering motion with hands in contact with the body part.

Method of Application for Massage
1. Stroking: usually initiates and ends treatment. Hand is molded over body part and movement is usually distal to proximal. Stroking is used to move from one area to another and between other strokes. Superficial strokes make no attempt to move deep tissue. Some passive muscle stretching is performed with deep stroking.
2. Kneading: milking effect of kneading aids in loosening adhesions and increasing venous return. Technique can be done with one or both hands, fingers, or the thumb and first finger. Wring and lift tissues to break down adhesions. Direction of strokes may vary, depending on body structure; however, to increase venous return, strokes should move from distal to proximal along the extremity.
3. Friction: heavy compression over soft tissues will stretch scars and loosen adhesions. Ball of fingers or thumb should move in small circular or stroking manner, pressing and moving superficial tissues over deep structures. Pressure gradually increases to the patient's tolerance as technique moves up and down or around the targeted structures. Pressure never abruptly released. Cross-fiber friction consists of deep strokes across the muscle fiber rather than along longitudinal axis of the fibers.
4. Tapotement: used when stimulation is desired treatment effect.
5. Cupping: applied to the chest to mobilize bronchial secretions (postural drainage).
6. Vibration: often used in conjunction with cupping for postural drainage to loosen adherent secretions.

General Considerations for the Application of Massage
1. Place patient in comfortable, relaxed position with treatment part in gravity-eliminated position, or position in which gravity will assist in venous flow.
2. Body part exposed and well supported, with no clothing restricting circulation.
3. Begin with superficial stokes. May move to deep stroking.
4. Deep stroking may be followed by kneading. May alternate between stroking and kneading.
5. Stroking or kneading should follow friction massage.
6. Massage should begin in the proximal segment of the extremity, move distally, and return to proximal region. All stroking movements are directed distal to proximal, especially for edema.
7. Complete treatment with stroking, moving from deep to superficial stroking.

Concepts of Electricity for Treatment

Electrical Stimulation (ES)

Characteristics of Electrical Stimulation
1. See Table 10-8.
2. Current: movement or flow of charged particles in response to a stimulus. Current is measured in ampere (A).
3. Voltage: force of electrical current. Voltage is measured in volts (V).
4. Resistance: opposition to the flow of electrical current. Resistance is measured in Ohms (Ω).

Wave Forms
1. Monophasic wave (direct or galvanic current): a unidirectional flow of charged particles. A current

Table 10-8

Basic Concepts of Electricity

Electrical current	The movement of electrons through a conducting medium
Amperage	The rate of flow of electrons
Voltage	The force that drives electrons through the conductive medium
Resistance	The property of a medium that opposes the flow of electrons. A substance with a high resistance (e.g., rubber) is an insulator, and a substance with a low resistance (e.g., metal) is a conductor.
Ohm's Law	Expresses the relationship between amperage, voltage, and resistance. The current is directly proportional to the voltage and inversely proportional to the resistance. The inverse of resistance is called conductance.

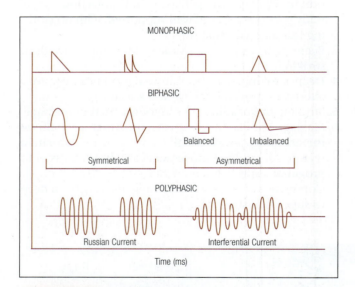

Figure 10-1 Basic waveform characteristics.

flow in one direction for a finite period of time is a phase (upward or downward deflection from and return to baseline). It has either a positive or negative charge. See Figure 10-1.
2. Biphasic wave (alternating current): a bidirectional flow of charged particles. This type of wave form is illustrated as one-half of the cycle above the baseline and the second phase below the baseline. One complete cycle (two phases) equals a single pulse. It has a zero net charge if symmetrical.
3. Polyphasic wave (biphasic current): modified to produce three or more phases in a single pulse. This waveform in medium frequency may be Russian or interferential current.

Treatment Parameters

1. Amplitude (intensity): described by neuroexcitation (i.e., subsensory, sensory, motor, or pain). The higher the amplitude the stronger the excitatory response; therefore, a higher amplitude is required for a motor response, and a lower amplitude is required for a sensory response.
2. Frequency (pulse rate): determine the type of muscle response elicited from electrical stimulation. Increased frequency will increase muscle fatigue. Impedance decreases as frequency increases.
   a. Low-frequencies (1–10 pulses per second [pps]) can produce brief twitch contractions. May be used for brief-intense TENS or muscle fatigue in the case of spasm.
   b. Frequencies of 20–50 pps are most common for muscle strengthening. See the strength-duration curve section that follows.
   c. Lower frequencies produce more noxious, tapping effect; higher frequencies are generally more comfortable as they produce a tingling effect.
3. Pulse duration: increased pulse duration increases recruitment of motor units resulting in improved muscle contraction. To facilitate a contraction, pulse duration should be between 150 and 300 ms. Lower pulse duration is recommended for smaller muscle groups.
   a. Denervated muscle requires longer pulse durations to achieve muscle contraction.
4. Strength-duration curve.
   a. This describes the relationship between pulse duration and intensity of the electrical stimulation.
   b. As the pulse duration increases, less amplitude is required to achieve a motor response. This concept can be useful for patients/clients who are particularly sensitive to electrical stimulation.

Current Modulation

1. Continuous mode: uninterrupted flow of current.
2. Interrupted mode: intermittent cessation of current flow for ≥1 second.
3. Surge mode: a gradual increase and decrease in the current intensity over a finite period of time.
4. Ramped mode: a time period with a gradual rise of the current intensity, which is maintained at a selected level for a given period of time, followed by a gradual or abrupt decline in intensity.

> **RED FLAGS:** Safety considerations:
> - Do not use any electrical modality if there is evidence of broken or frayed wires or if the unit is not connected to a ground fault circuit interrupter (see Hydrotherapy section).
> - Electrodes that are too small, have uneven contact, or are self-adhesive and no longer stick or conduct well can cause skin irritation or burns.
> - Electrical stimulation should not be used while playing sports, driving, operating heavy machinery, near a diathermy device, or in conjunction with other electronic monitoring equipment.

Goals and Indications for ES

1. Pain modulation: through activation of the Gate Theory.
2. Decrease muscle spasm via differing mechanisms.
   a. Muscle fatigue: mild-moderate tetanic contraction sustained for several minutes through continuous modulation.
   b. Muscle pump: interrupted or surge modulation to produce rhythmic contraction and relaxation of the muscle to increase circulation. This method can be combined with thermal ultrasound for the added benefit of increased tissue temperature. See Table 10-9.
3. Impaired joint range of motion (ROM).
   a. Electrical stimulation can supplement deficient muscle strength; assist to overcome spasticity.
   b. Decrease pain associated with movement to encourage joint motion.
   c. Decrease edema if it is impeding motion.
4. Neuromuscular reeducation: train muscle to respond to volitional effort.
   a. Acts as active-assistive exercise. Prevents disuse atrophy.
   b. Provides proprioceptive feedback.
   c. Assists in coordinated muscle movement.
5. Soft tissue healing and repair (wound healing).
   a. Pulsed currents (monophasic, biphasic, polyphasic) with interrupted modulations. Improved circulation via the muscle pump helps to improve tissue nutrition and hasten metabolic waste removal.
   b. Monophasic currents (low-volt continuous, high-volt pulsed currents). Assists in producing bactericidal and biochemical effects in the wound area for restoration of electrical charges in wound area.
   c. Galvanotaxic effect: attraction of tissue repair cells via electrode polarity.
      - Inflammation phase: macrophages (positive), mast cells (negative), neutrophils (positive or negative).
      - Proliferation phase: fibroblasts (positive).
      - Wound contraction phase: alternating positive/negative.
      - Epithelialization phase: epithelial cells (positive).
6. Edema reduction through muscle pump action to increase lymph and venous flow.
   a. Use electrical field phenomenon for acute edema. By electrostatic repulsion, a monophasic waveform with a negative polarity is set up to surround the injured area and repel the negatively charged proteins attempting to accentuate in the interstitium.
7. Spasticity/reduce hypertonicity.
   a. Fatigue of the agonist.
   b. Reciprocal inhibition (stimulate antagonist/inhibit agonist).
8. Denervated muscle.
   a. Controversy exists relative to the use of ES for denervated muscle. Previous studies (animal, clinical) indicated denervated muscle can be stimulated by mono or biphasic currents with long pulse durations. Goals of stimulation are to retard effects pf disuse atrophy and shorten recovery time.
   b. More recent animal studies suggest ES may be deleterious to denervated muscle.

Precautions and Contraindications for ES

1. See Quick Facts Box 10-25.

Guidelines for Applying ES

General Guidelines

1. Explain procedure and effects to patient.
2. Place patient in comfortable position with treatment area properly exposed.
3. Support body part to be treated.
4. Assess skin condition and sensation prior to each treatment.
   a. This is especially important for long-term or repeated use of ES, and skin breakdown can become a concern.
5. Reduce skin resistance, if necessary (hot pack, alcohol rub, gentle abrasion).

Table 10-9

Specific Treatment Goals and Indications for Use of ES

GOAL: MUSCLE STRENGTHENING, DECREASE MUSCLE SPASM OR EDEMA (MUSCLE PUMP), OR INCREASE ROM

Intensity	Slowly increase intensity until a muscular contraction is observed. 10–25 muscle contractions is sufficient to obtain treatment goal.
Duty Cycle	Interrupted/ramped modulation of current allows the muscle to recover between stimulation periods. It has been shown that stimulation on/off ratios of ≥1:3 minimize the fatigue effects of ES.

QUICK FACTS 10-25 ▶ PRECAUTIONS AND CONTRAINDICATIONS FOR ES

General Precautions for Electrical Stimulation

Cardiac disease	Impaired cognitive function
In areas of impaired sensation, malignant tumors, skin irritation, or open wounds	Applying iontophoresis in the area after the application of another physical agent
Patients with hypotension or hypertension, excessive adipose tissue, or edema	Bleeding disorders
In area of uterus during menstruation	Pregnancy: during labor and delivery
Impaired sensation	Severe edema

General CONTRAINDICATIONS for Use of Electrical Stimulation

Anywhere in the body for patients with demand-type pacemakers, unstable arrhythmias, suspected epilepsy, or seizure disorder	Over or in the area of the carotid sinus, thrombosis or thrombophlebitis, eyes, thoracic region, phrenic nerve, urinary bladder stimulators, and abdomen or low back during pregnancy
Transcerebrally or transthoracically	In the presence of active bleeding or infection
Over superficial metal implants	Over pharyngeal or laryngeal muscles
Motor-level stimulation should not be applied in conditions that prohibit motion	Over active bleeding
Over malignancies or phlebitis in treatment area	Over healing fractures (unless specifically used for bone stimulation)

6. Check to confirm that all controls are in proper starting position before turning on the modality.
7. **Secure electrodes** to body part.
8. **Set parameters:** frequency, waveform, and modulation rate.
9. **Adjust intensity** to achieve the optimal treatment effect.
10. **At end of treatment**, slowly decrease intensity to zero before lifting the active electrode from skin. Turn all controls to beginning position.

Electrode Selection Considerations

1. Two electrodes (leads) are required to complete the current circuit. One electrode is generally called the active (stimulating) electrode and is often placed on the motor point; the second, larger electrode is called the dispersive or inactive electrode. The active electrode is usually placed over the treatment site (motor point), in order to produce a stimulation effect. The dispersive electrode may be placed on the treatment site or at a remote site (see electrode placement).
2. Current density (the amount of current that is dispersed under the electrode) is relative to the electrode size. A given current intensity passing through the smaller active electrode produces high current density and thus a strong stimulus, while the same current is perceived as less intense under the larger dispersive electrode because of the lesser current density.
3. Electrode size should be relative to the size of the treatment site. Large electrodes in a small treatment area (i.e., forearm) could result in current overflowing to surrounding muscles and produce undesired effects.
4. Conversely, small electrodes applied to a large muscle (i.e., quadriceps) could result in high current density under the electrodes that make ES uncomfortable to the patient.

Electrode Preparation

1. Metal plate/sponge: moisten sponge, then remove sponge from water and remove excess water.
2. Carbonized rubber: place small amount of gel in center of electrode. Spread gel to cover entire surface.
3. Pregelled electrode: remove protective cover and place a small amount of gel (metal mesh, foil electrode) or water (Karaya electrode) on electrode.

Electrode Placement

1. A motor point is an area of greatest excitability on the skin surface in which a small amount of current generates a muscle response. In innervated muscle, the motor point is located at or near where the motor nerve enters the muscle, usually over the muscle belly. In denervated muscle, the area of greatest excitability is located over the muscle distally toward the insertion.

a. **Unipolar/monopolar placement:** one single electrode or multiple (bifurcated) active electrodes placed over treatment area. Usually larger dispersive electrode (inactive) placed ipsilaterally away from treatment area.
b. **Bipolar placement:** equal-sized active and dispersive electrodes on same muscle group or in same treatment area. Smaller, bifurcated treatment electrodes may be used to better conform to small treatment areas.

2. The space between the active and dispersive electrodes should be at least the diameter of the active electrode. The distance between the electrodes should be as great as is practicable. The greater the space between electrodes, the lesser the current density in the intervening superficial tissue, thus minimizing the risk of skin irritation and burns. If deep penetration causes contraction of undesired muscles, move the electrodes closer together.

Specific Electrical Stimulation Treatments

Iontophoresis

Definition
1. Iontophoresis is the application of a continuous direct current to transport medicinal agents through the skin or mucous membranes for therapeutic purposes.

Physics Principles Related to Iontophoresis
1. The application of iontophoresis is based on the concept of electrical "poles." Like charges repel like charges, and unlike charges attract unlike charges.
2. Positive ions move toward the negative pole (cathode).
3. Negative ions move toward the positive pole (anode).
4. The number of ions transferred through the skin is directly related to the:
   a. Duration of treatment.
   b. Current density.
   c. Concentration of ions in the solution.

Method of Application for Use of Iontophoresis
1. Clean and inspect skin.
2. Position patient and support treatment area.
3. Place appropriate-sized active electrode on treatment area. The active electrode should be the same polarity as the medicinal ion. To reduce the alkaline effect on the skin, the negative electrode should be twice as large as the positive regardless of which is the active electrode.
4. Dispersive electrode placed at either proximal or distal distant site about 4–6 inches away.
5. The space between the active and dispersive electrodes should be at least the diameter of the active electrode. However, commercial electrode sets have a fixed distance that limits the spacing between electrodes.
6. Determine dose. Dosage is product of time and current intensity. Safe limit for active electrode: anode, 1 mA/cm^2, cathode, 0.5 mA/cm^2. Duration is 10–40 minutes.
7. Turn intensity up slowly to selected level unless apparatus automatically adjusts parameters.
8. Observe treatment area every 3–5 minutes. Report any adverse reactions.
9. Turn intensity down slowly to zero at completion of treatment. Some units have an automatic cut off.

Uses for Iontophoresis
1. For indications, see Table 10-10.
2. For contraindication, see Quick Facts 10-26.

Transcutaneous Electrical Nerve Stimulation (TENS)

Description
1. TENS is designed to provide afferent stimulation for pain management.
2. Pain is modulated through activation of central inhibition of pain transmission (gate theory, Figure 10-2). Large diameter A-beta fibers activate inhibitory interneurons (substantia gelatinosa) located in the dorsal horn (primarily laminae II and III) of the spinal cord, producing inhibition of smaller A-delta and C-fibers (pain fibers). Presynaptic inhibition of the T-cells closes the "gate" and modulates pain. The gating mechanism also includes release of enkephalins, which combine with opiate receptors to depress release of substance P from the A-delta and C-fibers.
3. TENS can modulate pain through descending pathways generating endogenous opiates (Figure 10-3). Noxious stimuli generate endorphin production from the pituitary gland and other central nervous system (CNS) areas. Endogenous opiate-rich nuclei,

Table 10-10

Indications for the Use of Iontophoresis and Ions Commonly Used

INDICATIONS	ION	POLARITY	SOURCE
Analgesia	Lidocaine, Xylocaine Salicylate	Positive Negative	Lidocaine, Xylocaine Sodium salicylate
Calcium deposits	Acetate	Negative	Acetic acid
Dermal ulcers	Zinc	Positive	Zinc oxide
Edema reduction	Hyaluronidase	Positive	Wyadase
Fungal infections	Copper	Positive	Copper sulfate
Hyperhidrosis	Water	Positive/Negative	Tap water
Muscle spasm	Calcium Magnesium	Positive Positive	Calcium chloride Magnesium sulfate
Musculoskeletal inflammatory conditions	Dexamethasone Hydrocortisone	Negative Positive	Dexamethasone phosphate Hydrocortisone sodium succinate

QUICK FACTS 10-26 ▶ CONTRAINDICATIONS FOR IONTOPHORESIS*

Impaired skin sensation	Allergy or sensitivity to medicinal agent or direct current
Denuded area or recent scars	Cuts, bruises, or broken skin
Metal in or near treatment area	

*Refer to general rules for use of ES.

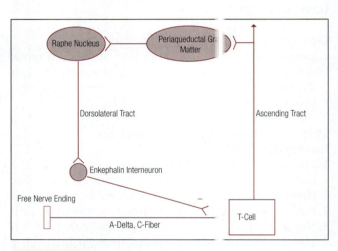

Figure 10-3 Schematic of descending inhibition mechanisms.

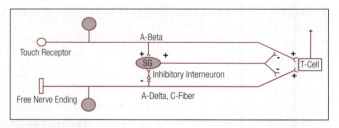

Figure 10-2 Schematic of gate control theory. (Adapted from Melzack and Wall.)

periaqueductal gray matter (PAG) in the midbrain and thalamus are also activated by strong stimuli. Neurotransmitters from the PAG facilitate the cells of the nucleus raphe magnus (NRM) and reticularis gigantocellularis (RGC). Efferents from these nuclei travel through the dorsal lateral funiculus, terminating on the enkephalinergic interneurons in the spinal cord and presynaptically inhibiting the release of substance P from the A-delta and C-fibers.

ES Characteristics of TENS

1. Wave form: typically, asymmetrical biphasic with a zero net direct current component. Other variations including pulsed monophasic current have been used.
2. Current: continuous pulsatile or burst.

Electrode Placement

1. Several options should be considered with use of TENS. Acupuncture site, dermatome distribution of involved nerve, over painful site, proximal or distal to pain site, segmentally related myotomes, or trigger points are all possible electrode placement options.

Goals and Indications for Use

1. Acute and chronic pain modulation.

Contraindications for Use
1. Patient with demand-type pacemaker or over chest of patient with cardiac disease.
2. TENS not applied over eyes, laryngeal or pharyngeal muscles, head and neck of patient following cerebral vascular accident, or with epilepsy.
3. TENS not applied to mucosal membranes.

Conventional TENS
1. Sometimes called "high-rate" TENS, this is the most common mode of TENS can be applied during the acute or chronic phase of pain. Modulation of pain via inhibition of pain fibers by large-diameter fiber activation (gate mechanism). Onset of pain relief is relatively fast and duration of relief is relatively short.
2. Treatment parameters
   a. Amplitude: comfortable tingling sensation, paresthesia. No muscle response.
   b. Pulse rate (frequency): 50–80 pps.
   c. Pulse duration: 50–100 msec.
   d. Mode: continuous.
   e. Duration of treatment: 20–60 minutes.
   f. Duration of pain relief: temporary.

Acupuncture-like (Strong Low-Rate) TENS
1. Can be applied during the chronic phase of pain. Analgesia produced through stimulation-evoked production of endogenous opiates. Onset of pain relief may be as long as 20–40 minutes. Duration of relief may be long-lasting (≥1 hour).
2. Treatment parameters.
   a. Amplitude: strong, but comfortable rhythmic muscle twitches.
   b. Pulse rate (frequency): 1–5 pps.
   c. Pulse duration: 150–300 msec.
   d. Mode: continuous.
   e. Duration of treatment: 30–40 minutes.
   f. Duration of pain relief: long-lasting.

Brief Intense TENS
1. This mode is used to provide rapid-onset, short-term pain relief during painful procedures (wound debridement, deep friction massage, joint mobilization, or passive stretching).
2. Treatment parameters.
   a. Amplitude: to patient's tolerance.
   b. Pulse rate (frequency): 80–150 pps.
   c. Pulse duration: 50–250 msec.
   d. Mode: continuous.
   e. Duration of treatment: 15 minutes.
   f. Duration of pain relief: temporary (30–60 minutes).

Burst-mode (Pulse Trains) TENS
1. Combines characteristics of both high- and low-rate TENS. Stimulation of endogenous opiates, but current is more tolerable to patient than low-rate TENS. Onset of analgesia similar to low-rate TENS.
2. Treatment parameters.
   a. Amplitude: comfortable, intermittent paresthesia.
   b. Pulse rate (frequency): 50–100 pps delivered in packets or bursts of 1–4 pps.
   c. Pulse duration: 50–200 msec.
   d. Mode: continuous.
   e. Duration of treatment: 20–30 minutes.
   f. Duration of pain relief: long-lasting (hours).

Hyperstimulation (Point Stimulation) TENS
1. Use of a small probe to locate and noxiously stimulate acupuncture or trigger points. Multiple sites may be stimulated per treatment. Onset of pain relief is similar to acupuncture-like TENS.
2. Treatment parameters.
   a. Amplitude: strong, to patient's tolerance
   b. Pulse rate (frequency): 1–5 pps
   c. Pulse duration: 150–300 msec
   d. Duration of treatment: 15- to 30-second increments
   e. Duration of pain relief: long-lasting

Modulation Mode TENS
1. A method of modulating the parameters of the above TENS modes to prevent neural or perceptual adaptation due to constant ES. Frequencies, intensities, or pulse durations can be altered by ≥10%, one or two times per second.

High-Voltage Pulsed Galvanic Stimulation

Description
1. High-voltage pulsed current (HVPC) is typically delivered using monophasic, twin-peaked pulses of short duration. The waveform is typically paired monophasic, with instantaneous rise and exponential fall.
   a. The current can be continuous, surged, or interrupted pulsatile current.

Wound Healing Concepts
1. Intact skin surface negative with respect to deeper epidermal layers.
2. Injury to skin develops positive potentials initially and negative potentials during healing process.
3. Absent or insufficient positive potentials retard tissue regeneration.

4. Addition of positive potentials, initially through anode, may promote or accelerate healing.

Wound Healing Parameters
1. Amplitude: comfortable tingling sensation, paresthesia, no muscle response.
2. Pulse rate (frequency): 50–200 pps.
3. Pulse duration: 20–100 msec.
4. Mode: continuous.
5. Duration of treatment: 20–60 min.

Methods of Application Wound Healing
1. Inspect wound area.
2. Position patient and support treatment area.
3. Clean and debride wound site. Pack with sterile saline-soaked gauze.
4. Both high-volt pulsed current and low-intensity continuous low-volt direct current can be used for wound healing. Although current characteristics differ, treatment parameters are similar in current intensity and treatment duration.
5. Place active electrode over gauze.
6. For bactericidal effect, active electrode should have negative polarity. For culture-free wound, active electrode should be positive.
7. Turn the intensity up slowly to selected level.
8. At conclusion of treatment, turn intensity down slowly to zero.

Goals and Indications for Wound Healing
1. Inflammation phase: free from necrosis and exudates. Promote granulation.
2. Proliferation phase: reduce wound size, including depth, diameter, and tunneling.
3. Epithelialization phase: stimulate epidermal proliferation and capillary growth.

Contraindications for Use of HVPC for Wound Healing
1. See general contraindications for ES.

Interferential Current (IFC)

Description
1. Interferential current (IFC) is characterized by the crossing of two sinusoidal waves with similar amplitudes, but different carrier frequencies that interfere with one another to generate an amplitude-modulated beat frequency. The consequent beat frequency is the net difference between the two superimposed frequencies. The wave form is polyphasic, sinusoidal (amplitude-modulated) beats. The current is amplitude-modulated continuous (pain); interrupted (muscle exercise).

Physics Related to IFC
1. Constructive interference: When the two waves are in phase, the sum of the superimposed wave is large (Figure 10-4, represented by line A).
2. Destructive interference: The sum of the two waves is zero when the waves are 180 degrees out of phase (Figure 10-4, represented by line B).
3. Beat frequency (amplitude-modulated): Resultant frequency produced by the two frequencies going into and out of phase (Figure 10-4, represented by pattern C).
4. Constant beat frequency: Both carrier frequencies are fixed. Beat frequency is net difference between both frequencies.
5. Variable beat frequency: One carrier frequency is fixed and the other varies in frequency, generating a variable or sweep frequency. Sweep used to minimize accommodation.

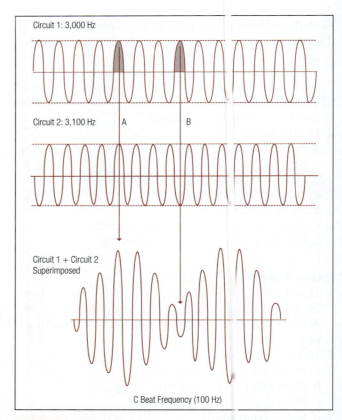

Figure 10-4 Interferential current. Amplitude modulated polyphasic waveform.

6. Premodulated IFC occurs when two carrier frequencies are crossed in the ES unit. The interference occurs in the unit, and the current can then be delivered through one circuit. This is ideal for small areas that would be amply covered with two electrodes.

Methods of Application for IFC
1. Electrode placement.
    a. Bipolar (premodulated IFC): Active and dispersive electrodes placed over or around small area.
    b. Quadripolar: Two sets of electrodes placed diagonally to one another over large area.
    c. Ensure that area of greatest pain, or area of pain generation, is centered between electrodes.

Treatment Parameters
1. Pain protocol is similar to high- or low-rate TENS.
2. Muscle contraction protocol is similar to low- or medium-frequency ES.

Contraindications for Use of IFC
1. See general contraindications for ES.

Neuromuscular Electrical Stimulation (NMES)

Description
1. Encompasses a wide range of stimulator units and techniques for disuse atrophy, impaired ROM, muscle spasm, muscle reeducation, and spasticity management. Treatment parameters are similar for each with the on:off ratio being the primary difference. NMES is also called functional electrical stimulation and functional neuromuscular electrical stimulation. NMES has a wave form that is asymmetric biphasic square.
2. This type of electrical stimulation is often used during rehabilitation to assist with gait; e.g., dorsiflexion assist during gait, plantar flexor assist to assist push-off phase, hamstring assist to prevent knee hyperextension, etc.

Muscle Strengthening Parameters
1. Amplitude: motor contraction.
2. Pulse rate (frequency): 35–50 pps.
3. Pulse duration: 150–200 msec for small muscles; 200–350 msec for large muscles.
4. On/off times and ratio: dependent on treatment goal.
5. Ramp time: at least 2 seconds.
6. Duration of treatment: dependent on treatment goal.

Electromyographic (EMG) Biofeedback

Description
1. Electromyographic (EMG) biofeedback uses an electronic instrument used to measure motor unit action potentials (MUAP) generated by active muscles. The signals are detected, amplified, and converted into audiovisual signals that are used to reinforce voluntary control. The signal is processed through amplification, rectification (positive and negative components of the signal are made unidirectional), and integration (area under curve is computed). The integrated signal provides readings in microvolt-seconds and is displayed as the EMG biofeedback signal. The EMG biofeedback signals, in conjunction with the patient's voluntary effort, are used to either increase or decrease muscle activity to achieve a functional goal.
2. A motor unit is the functional unit of the neuromuscular system that consists of the anterior horn cell, its axon, the neuromuscular junction, and all the muscle fibers innervated by the axon. Motor unit potentials (MUP) are measured in microvolts (mV). The signals generated by the MUP, which contain both positive and negative phases, are also called compound action potentials (CAP) because the sensors pick up signals from multiple motor units.

Biofeedback Electrodes
1. Surface electrode.
    a. Global detection: signals from more than one muscle.
    b. Detection from mostly superficial muscles.
    c. Advantages: easy to apply, acceptable to patient/client.
    d. Disadvantages: detection from mostly superficial muscles, frequently from more than one muscle group.
2. Types of surface electrodes/sensors.
    a. Metal electrodes (silver/silver chloride): cup-shaped to accommodate conducting gel.
    b. Disposable electrodes: pregelled center with surrounding adhesive backing.
    c. Carbonized rubber electrodes (reusable): flexible to conform to body part.
3. Needle electrodes/sensors.
    a. Local detection: signals from specific muscle or muscle group.
    b. Detection of deep muscles.
    c. Used for EMG diagnosis or research. Rarely used for EMG biofeedback.
    d. Advantages: detection of specific muscles.
    e. Disadvantages: requires skill to apply, less acceptable to patient/client.

Electrode Application

1. Electrode selection: Select small electrodes (0.02 cm) for specific muscles (hand, forearm, face); large electrodes (1 cm) for large muscles or muscle groups.
2. Electrode placement
   a. Bipolar technique: two active (positive and negative) and one reference (ground) electrode. The reference electrode may be placed between or adjacent to active electrodes. This minimizes or eliminates extraneous electrical activity (noise or cross-talk).
   - Active electrodes are placed on or near motor point of targeted muscle or muscle group.
   - Generally, active electrodes are placed 1–5 cm apart and parallel to muscle fibers. Reference electrode is placed near treatment site.
   - Active electrodes are placed close together; minimizes cross-talk; yields small, more precise signals.
   - Active electrodes are placed further apart; yields large signals, detection from more than one muscle.

Methods of Application for Biofeedback

1. Begin treatments in quiet setting, if possible.
2. Clean treatment site with alcohol (slight abrasion, if necessary) to remove dirt and oils from skin to reduce skin impedance.
3. Apply conductive gel, if needed.
4. Secure the electrodes.
5. Protocol for increasing muscle activity (motor recruitment).
6. For weak muscles, begin with electrodes widely spaced and biofeedback instrument sensitivity high, to increase detection.
7. For a single weak muscle, begin with electrodes close together if a more precise signal is desired.
8. Instruct patient to try and contract muscle (isometrically for 6–10 sec) to produce an audiovisual signal.
9. As patient's motor recruitment ability improves, decrease the sensitivity, making it more difficult to produce an audiovisual signal.
10. Use facilitation techniques (tapping, cross-facilitation, vibration) to encourage motor unit recruitment, if necessary.
11. Progress from simple to more complex/functional movements as patient gains motor control.
12. Treatment sessions may be from 5–10 minutes to ≥30 minutes, depending on patient tolerance.
13. At end of session, clean patient's skin and electrodes.

Protocol for Decreasing Muscle Activity (Muscle Relaxation)

1. Begin with electrodes closely spaced and bio-feedback instrument sensitivity low to minimize cross-talk.
2. Instruct patient to relax, using deep breathing or visual imagery to help lower the audiovisual signal.
3. Progress from low to high sensitivity as patient gains ability to relax muscle and perform functional activities.
4. Treatment sessions may be from 5–10 minutes to ≥30 minutes, depending on patient tolerance.
5. At end of session, clean patient's skin and electrodes.

Criteria for Patient Selection for Biofeedback Training

1. Good vision, hearing, and communication abilities.
2. Good comprehension of simple commands, concentration.
3. Good motor planning skills.
4. No profound sensory or proprioceptive loss.

Review Questions

Therapeutic Modalities

1. When is a patient/client who is receiving a hot pack treatment at greatest risk for burn? What is the correct temperature range for a hydrocollator unit containing hot packs? How is this different when using canvas versus plastic hot packs?

2. Describe how to best manage tissue heating when using a capacitor heating unit with a short-wave diathermy device. What type of tissue responds best to short-wave diathermy?

3. How would the application of cervical traction change when used to treat a patient/client who has a degenerative joint condition versus a protruding disc in the cervical spine at the C5–C6 level?

4. What type of nerve and motor tissue response will an electrical current that is 0.5 msec in duration and applied at 80 pulses per second achieve?

5. Zinc oxide may be used to treat dermal ulcers. What lead should be attached to the active electrode to drive ions of zinc oxide into the tissues?

6. Name five contraindications to the use of electrical stimulation with a patient/client.

11

Functional Training, Equipment, and Devices

SUSAN B. O'SULLIVAN

Chapter Outline

- **Gait, 397**
    - Phases of the Gait Cycle, 397
    - Swing Phase, 399
    - Common Gait Deviations, 400
- **Ambulatory Aids, 402**
    - Canes, 402
    - Crutches, 403
    - Walkers, 403
    - Additions to Gait Devices, 403
    - Bariatric Equipment, 403
    - Gait Patterns: Use of Assistive Devices, 404
    - Guarding, 405
    - Locomotor Training, 405
- **Orthotics, 406**
    - General Concepts, 406
    - Lower-Limb Orthoses: Components/Terminology, 406
    - Spinal (Trunk) Orthoses: Components/Terminology, 410

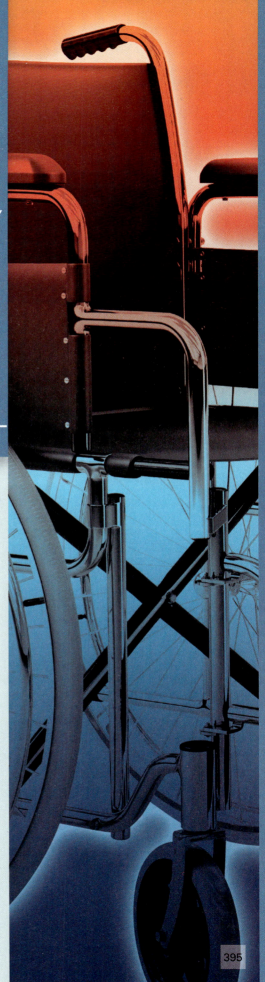

- Upper-Limb Orthoses or Splints: Components/Terminology, 411
- Physical Therapy Intervention, 412
- Adhesive Taping, 413
  - General Concepts, 413
- Prosthetics, 414
  - General Concepts, 414
  - Lower-Limb Prosthetics (LLPs), 414
  - Upper-Limb Prosthetics (ULPs), 417
  - Physical Therapy Intervention, 417
- Wheelchairs, 421
  - Components, 421
  - Wheelchair Measurements, 423
  - Wheelchair Training, 424
- Transfer Training, 425
  - Dependent Transfers, 425
  - Assisted Transfers, 425
  - Training, 425
- Bariatric Specific Equipment, 426
  - Equipment, 426
  - Assistive Devices for Transferring, 426
  - Lift Devices, 427
  - Facility Modifications, 427
- Environmental Considerations, 427
  - Environmental Modification, 427
- Appendix 11A: Ergonomics, 429
- Review Questions, 433

Gait

Phases of the Gait Cycle

Traditional terminology appears first and refers to points in time in the gait cycle; Rancho Los Amigos (RLA) terminology follows and refers to lengths of time in the gait cycle. Because both are in clinical use, readers should be familiar with both. These two types of terminologies do not always coincide exactly when describing the gait cycle.

Stance Phase

1. Heel strike: the point when the heel of the reference or support limb contacts the ground at the beginning of stance phase.

   Initial contact (RLA): the instant that the foot of the lead extremity strikes the ground.

   Muscle activation patterns (Figure 11-1, Table 11-1): knee extensors (quadriceps) are active at heel strike through early stance to control small amount of knee flexion for shock absorption; ankle dorsiflexors (anterior tibialis, extensor hallucis longus, extensor digitorum longus) decelerate the foot, slowing the plantarflexion from heel strike to foot flat.

2. Foot flat: the point when the sole of the foot of the reference or support limb makes contact with the ground; occurs immediately after heel strike.

   Loading response (RLA): the first period of double support immediately after initial contact until the contralateral leg leaves the ground.

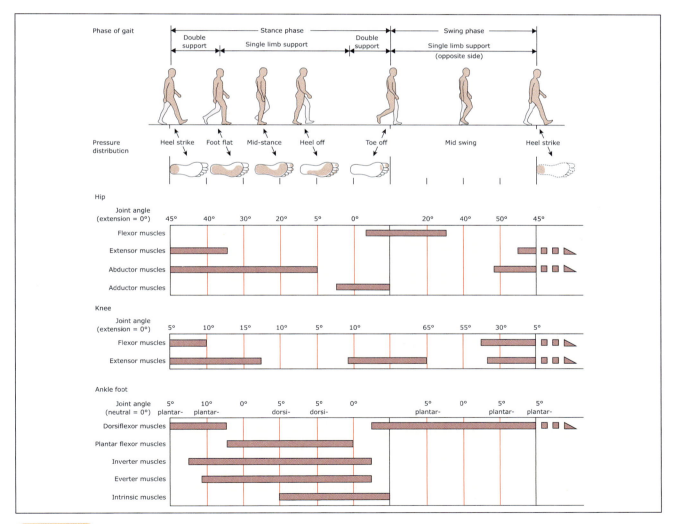

Figure 11-1 Phases of the gait cycle.

Adapted from Susan Standring (Editor-in-Chief). Gray's Anatomy. 39th ed. 2005. Page 1533. Elsevier Churchill Livingstone.

Table 11-1

Muscle Activity During Gait and the Result of Weakness

PORTION OF GAIT	MUSCLE ACTIVITY	RESULT OF WEAKNESS	POSSIBLE COMPENSATION
Heel strike to foot flat	HIP: erector spinae, gluteus maximus, hamstrings KNEE: quadriceps contract initially to hold knee in extension (loading response), then eccentrically to control knee flexion. Gastrocnemius (late in phase) begins contraction. ANKLE & FOOT: pretibial group works eccentrically to control plantar flexion.	Excessive hip flexion and anterior pelvis tilt Quadriceps: excessive knee flexion Gastrocnemius: excessive knee flexion Foot slap	Forceful trunk extension and backward leaning to prevent excessive hip flexion Trunk lurches forward or external rotation of extremity to lock knee into extension Lack of heel strike at initial contact resulting in foot placed flat on floor or toes-first gait
Foot flat through midstance	HIP: gluteus maximus works to oppose hip flexion. KNEE: quadriceps contract in early phase to extend knee, then no activity is required; gastrocnemius and soleus eccentric contraction. Hamstrings: work to prevent genu recurvatum ANKLE & FOOT: gastrocnemius and soleus act eccentrically to control forward advance of tibia	Excessive hip flexion and anterior pelvic tilt Quadriceps: excessive knee flexion Hamstrings: knee hyperextension Excessive dorsiflexion and uncontrolled forward motion of the tibia	Trunk extension initially to prevent excessive hip flexion Plantar flexion at ankle so that foot flat occurs instead of heel strike; eliminates excessive flexion moment of the knee. This occurs early in midstance—no compensation is needed in later part of phase. Ankle may be maintained in plantar flexion to avoid excessive dorsiflexion.
Midstance to heel-off	HIP: extensors in early phase to maintain stability Hip abductors (gluteus medius) work concentrically to control lateral pelvis tilt during swing of opposite limb. KNEE: gastrocnemius and soleus work eccentrically to control advance of the tibia. ANKLE & FOOT: Tibialis posterior isometric	Pelvis drop on swing limb, decreased ability to clear limb Gastrocnemius: excessive dorsiflexion and uncontrolled forward motion of the tibia resulting in knee snapping into extension at late phase Tibialis posterior: controls amount of pronation.	Lateral trunk shift over weak (stance) limb Loss of heel rise at the ankle resulting in dropping of pelvis on this side during pre-swing activities Gastrocnemius: ankle may be maintained in plantar flexion to avoid excessive dorsiflexion; if foot is flat on floor, a steppage gait is produced. Tibialis posterior: excessive pronation of the foot
Heel-off to toe-off	HIP: iliopsoas, adductor magnus, adductor longus for stability of limb position KNEE: quadriceps required to control amount of knee flexion (eccentric contraction) ANKLE & FOOT: gastrocnemius, soleus, peroneus longus/brevis, flexor hallucis longus contract to plantar flex the foot.	Undetermined Quadriceps: excessive heel rise (knee flexion) at initial swing Decreased or no push-off Decreased contralateral step	Undetermined Typically not compensated for Slight lag in forward movement of swing leg; foot is lifted off of floor without push-off.
Acceleration to midswing	HIP: hip flexor activity to initiate swing (iliopsoas, rectus femoris, gracilis, sartorius, tensor fascia lata) KNEE: little or no activity in quadriceps; biceps femoris (short head) gracilis and sartorius act concentrically. ANKLE & FOOT: dorsiflexors contract to bring the ankle into neutral and to prevent toe drag.	Diminished hip flexion causes inability to initiate forward movement of extremity. Biceps femoris: inadequate knee flexion Foot drop and/or toe dragging	Posterior lurch of trunk, circumduction, and/or hip hiking to bring limb forward and clear foot Increased hip flexion, circumduction, or hip hiking to clear foot Increased hip and knee flexion to prevent toe drag, hip hiking, circumduction, or vaulting on opposite limb
Midswing to deceleration	HIP: hip extensors and hamstrings KNEE: hamstrings eccentric contraction ANKLE & FOOT: dorsiflexors contract to maintain dorsiflexion.	Control forward movement of limb, stabilization of hip for stance Control extension movement of knee Foot drop and/or toe dragging	 Knee snaps into extension. Early phase: increased hip and knee flexion to prevent toe drag, hip hiking, circumduction, or vaulting on opposite limb

Muscle activation patterns: gastrocnemius-soleus muscles are active from foot flat through midstance to eccentrically control forward tibial advancement.
3. **Midstance:** the point at which full body weight is taken by the reference or support limb.
Midstance (RLA): the contralateral limb leaves the ground; body weight is taken and advanced over and ahead of the support limb; a period of single limb support.
Muscle activation patterns: hip, knee, and ankle extensors are active throughout stance to oppose antigravity forces and stabilize the limb; hip extensors control forward motion of the trunk; hip abductors stabilize the pelvis during unilateral stance.
4. **Heel-off:** occurs after midstance as the heel of the reference or support limb leaves the ground.
Terminal stance (RLA): the last period of single limb support that begins with heel rise and continues until the contralateral leg contacts the ground.
Muscle activation patterns: peak activity of plantarflexors occurs just after heel-off to push-off and generates forward propulsion of the body.
5. **Toe-off:** the last portion of stance following heel-off, when only the toe of the reference or support limb is in contact with the ground.
Preswing (RLA): the second period of double support from initial contact of the contralateral limb to lift-off of the support limb.
Muscle activation patterns: hip and knee extensors (hamstrings and quadriceps) may contribute to forward propulsion with a brief burst of activity.

Swing Phase

1. **Acceleration:** the first portion of the swing phase from toe-off of the reference limb until midswing.
Initial swing (RLA): the first portion of the swing phase from toe-off of the reference limb until maximum knee flexion of the same extremity.
Muscle activation patterns: forward acceleration of the limb during early swing is achieved through the brief action of quadriceps; by midswing the quadriceps is silent and pendular motion is in effect; hip flexors (iliopsoas) aid in forward limb propulsion.
2. **Midswing:** the midportion of the swing phase when the reference extremity moves directly below the body.
Midswing (RLA): the portion of the swing phase from maximum knee flexion of the reference extremity to a vertical tibial position.
Muscle activation patterns: foot clearance is achieved by contraction of the hip, knee flexors, and ankle dorsiflexors.
3. **Deceleration:** the end portion of the swing phase when the reference extremity is slowing down in preparation for heel strike.
Terminal swing (RLA): the portion of the swing phase from a vertical tibial position of the reference extremity to just prior to initial contact.
Muscle activation patterns: hamstrings act during late swing to decelerate the limb in preparation for heel strike; quadriceps and ankle dorsiflexors become active in late swing to prepare for heel strike.

Pelvic Motion

1. The pelvis rotates in a transverse plane (relative forward and backward motion of each side).
   a. The pelvis on the side of the swing limb moves forward to advance the limb; mean rotation is 4°.
   b. The contralateral side also rotates 4° when it is the swing limb (total of 8°).
2. The pelvis rotates in the frontal plane (lateral pelvic tilt): 5°; controlled by hip abductor muscles.
   a. The side contralateral to the stance limb drops during loading response.
3. The pelvis rotates in the sagittal plane (anterior/posterior tilt). The pelvis is naturally anterior tilted 10–15°, and is pulled anterior as the hip flexors reach the end range of terminal stance.
4. The pelvis moves side to side 4 cm, moving toward the stance limb during loading response.

Cadence

1. The number of steps taken per unit of time.
2. Mean cadence is approximately 110 steps/minute.
3. Increased cadence while maintaining the same speed is the result of shorter step length.
4. Running occurs when the period of double support disappears, typically at a cadence of 180 steps/minute.

Step

1. Step length: the anterior-posterior distance between the heel at initial contact on subsequent steps (ipsi vs. contralateral, in cm or m).
2. Step time: the time (s) between initial contact on the ipsi and contralateral limb.
3. Step width: the distance between feet (e.g., base of support); measured from one heel to the same point on the opposite heel (in cm or m).
   a. Normal step width ranges between 2.54 and 12.7 cm (1 and 5 inches).
   b. Increases as stability demands rise; e.g., wide-based gait in older adults or very small children.

Stride

1. Stride length: the anterior-posterior distance between two consecutive contacts of the same limb (in cm or m).
2. Stride time: the time (s) between initial contact of the same limb on subsequent steps.

Velocity (Walking Speed)
1. The distance traveled divided by the time required (m/sec or miles/hour).
2. Average walking speed is approximately 1.3 m/s (3 miles/hour).
3. Affected by physical characteristics: height, weight, gender.
4. Decreased with age, physical disability, etc.

Acceleration/Deceleration
1. Increase/decrease in walking.
2. Measured as velocity (rate of change/time).

Energy Cost of Walking
1. Commonly measured as normalized rate of consumption (mL/kg/min) or efficiency relative to distance traveled (mL/kg/m).
2. Average oxygen rate for comfortable walking is 12 mL/kg × min.
3. Metabolic cost of walking averages 5.5 kcal/min on level surfaces; energy costs may vary widely depending on speed of walking, stride length, body weight, type of surface, gradient, and activity (e.g., stair climbing).
4. Increased energy costs can occur with age, abnormal gait (e.g., disease, muscle weakness or paralysis, physical disability), or with the use of functional devices (e.g., crutches, orthoses, prostheses).

Common Gait Deviations

Stance Phase or Swing Phase
Muscle weakness, limited range of motion, abnormal tone reflexes, or pain can alter the typical or normal gait pattern. Different deviations will occur depending whether the individual is in the stance or swing phase of gait. See Quick Facts 11-1 for stance phase deviations and Quick Facts 11-2 for swing phase deviations.

QUICK FACTS 11-1 ▶ COMMON GAIT DEVIATIONS: STANCE PHASE

Deviation	Weak Muscle(s) or Joint Limitation	Observations
Trunk and Hip		
Lateral trunk bending	Weak gluteus medius	Lateral trunk bending to the same side as the weakness (a.k.a., Trendelenburg gait) Note: This pattern may also be observed with hip pain.
Backward trunk lean	Weak gluteus maximus	Difficulty going up stairs or ramps
Forward trunk lean	Weak quadriceps	Muscle weakness decreases flexor movement at the knee Note: Hip and knee flexion contractures may cause same observation.
Excessive hip flexion	Weak hip extensors Tight hip and/or knee flexors	Excessive hip flexion during stance
Limited hip extension	Tight or spastic hip flexors	Hip extension will be limited in stance compared to opposite side, gait may appear halted.
Limited hip flexion	Weak hip flexors Tight hip extensors	Hip flexion will be limited in stance compared to uninvolved side.
Abnormal synergistic activity (e.g., stroke)	Muscle tone impaired by synergistic activity	Excessive hip adduction combined with hip and knee extension, plantarflexion Scissoring or adducted gait pattern
Antalgic gait (painful gait)	Decreased ability to tolerate stance on affected limb	Stance time is abbreviated on the painful limb that results in an uneven gait pattern. Uninvolved limb has a shortened step length since it must bear weight sooner than normal.
Knee		
Excessive knee flexion	Weak quadriceps Knee flexor contracture	Knee wobbles or buckles with weight bearing Will also see difficulty going down stairs or ramps Forward trunk bending can compensate for weak quadriceps
Hyperextension	Weak quadriceps Plantar flexion contracture Extensor spasticity (quadriceps, plantar muscles)	Knee hyperextension with weight bearing

(Continued)

QUICK FACTS 11-1 ▶ COMMON GAIT DEVIATIONS: STANCE PHASE (Continued)

Deviation	Weak Muscle(s) or Joint Limitation	Observations
Ankle and Foot		
Toe first	Weak dorsiflexors Spastic or tight plantarflexors Shortened knee (leg length discrepancy) Painful heel Positive support reflex	Initial contact during stance is the toe of the foot rather than the heel
Foot slap	Weak dorsiflexors Hypotonia	The foot makes floor contact with an audible slap at initial contact or immediately following initial contact; compensated for with steppage gait. Foot flat: entire foot contacts ground; the result of weak dorsiflexors, limited range of motion (ROM) Excessive dorsiflexion with uncontrolled forward motion of the tibia (calcaneus gait): the result of weak plantarflexors
Foot flat	Weak dorsiflexors Limited range of motion	Entire foot contacts ground at initial contact Is an immature gait pattern (neonatal)
Excessive plantarflexion (equinus gait)	Spasticity or contracture of the plantar flexors	Heel does not touch the ground; will see poor eccentric contraction and advancement of the tibia
Supination	Spastic invertors Weak evertors Pes varus or genu varum	Excessive lateral contact of foot during stance with varus position of calcaneus May occur at initial contact and correct at foot flat with weight acceptance or remain throughout stance
Pronation	Weak invertors Spasticity Pes valgus or genu valgum	Excessive medial contact of foot during stance with valgus position of calcaneus
Toes claw	Spastic toe flexors May also be a hyperactive plantar grasp reflex	Excessive to clawing (curling) during stance phase
Inadequate push-off	Weak plantar flexors Decreased ROM Pain in the forefoot	Stance phase to initial swing phase will present with limited push-off into swing phase

QUICK FACTS 11-2 ▶ COMMON GAIT DEVIATIONS: SWING PHASE

Deviation	Weak Muscle(S) or Joint Limitation	Observations
Trunk and Hip		
Insufficient forward pelvic rotation (stiff pelvis, pelvic retraction)	Weak abdominal muscles Weak flexor muscles	Decreased pelvic motion (forward) during swing phase (e.g., post stroke)
Insufficient hip and knee flexion	Weak hip and knee flexors	Presents with inability to lift the leg and move it forward during swing phase
Circumduction	Weak hip and knee flexors	The leg swings out to the side (abduction/external rotation followed by adduction/internal rotation)
Hip hiking (quadratus lumborum action)	Weak hip and knee flexors Extensor spasticity	Hip will hike (or lift) during swing phase

(Continued)

QUICK FACTS 11-2 ▶ COMMON GAIT DEVIATIONS: SWING PHASE (Continued)

Deviation	Weak Muscle(S) or Joint Limitation	Observations
Excessive hip and knee flexion (a.k.a., steppage gait)	Weak dorsiflexors (e.g., neuropathy of the fibular nerve)	Is a compensatory response to shorten the leg during swing phase
Abnormal synergistic activity (e.g., stroke)	Muscle tone impaired by synergistic activity	Excessive hip and knee flexion with abduction
Knee		
Insufficient knee flexion	Extensor spasticity; Pain/decreased ROM; Weak hamstrings	Minimal or decreased knee flexion during swing phase, may result in steppage gait pattern, hip circumduction, or toe drag
Excessive knee flexion	Flexor spasticity; Flexor withdrawal reflex	Excessive knee flexion, beyond typical 30–40 degrees, during swing phase
Ankle and Foot		
Foot drop (equinus)	Weak or delayed contraction of the dorsiflexors; Spastic plantarflexors	Diminished dorsiflexion during swing phase, may result in increased hip flexion to assist with foot clearance; potentially circumduction, lateral trunk lean or contralateral vaulting (rising on the ball of the foot, elevated pelvis)
Varus or inverted foot	Spastic or weak invertors (anterior tibialis); Weak peroneals; Abnormal synergistic Pattern (e.g., stroke)	Results in increased internal rotation of the ankle during swing; Spasticity into loading response may interfere with ability to get good heel strike
Equinovarus	Spasticity of the posterior tibialis and/or gastrocnemius-soleus	Results in increased inversion and/or plantarflexed position of the foot and ankle, often due developmental; Abnormality or abnormal tone; If persists into initial contact, can interfere with loading response

Ambulatory Aids

Canes

Indications
1. Widen base of support to improve balance; provide limited stability and unweighting (can unload forces on involved extremity by 30%); can be used to relieve pain, antalgic gait.

Cane Measurement
1. 20–30 degrees of elbow flexion is desirable.
2. Measure from the greater trochanter to a point 6 inches to the side of the toes.

Types
1. Wood or aluminum (adjustable with push pin lock).
2. Standard, single point cane: handle and shaft may be standard (J-shaped) or offset.
3. Quad cane: four contact points with the ground; provides increased stability but slows gait.
   a. Small-based quad cane (SBQC): useful for stairs.
   b. Wide-based quad cane (WBQC): does not fit on stairs.

Gait
1. Cane is held in the hand opposite to the involved extremity; cane and involved extremity are advanced together, followed by the uninvolved extremity.

Gait Sequencing
1. The cane is held in the hand opposite the involved extremity.
2. Beginning gait pattern: cane advanced first, followed by the involved extremity (stepping to or through [past] the cane), then the uninvolved extremity; this results in a slower, more stable gait pattern.

3. Advanced gait pattern: the involved extremity and the cane are advanced simultaneously, followed by the uninvolved extremity.

Crutches

Indications
1. Used to increase the base of support, provide moderate degree of stability, or relieve weight bearing on the lower extremities.

Crutch Measurement
1. 20–30 degrees of elbow flexion is desirable.
2. For standing patients, subtract 16 inches from the patient's height or measure from a point 2 inches below the axilla to a point 6 inches in front and 2 inches lateral to the foot.
3. For supine patients, measure from the axilla to a point 6–8 inches lateral to the heel.
4. Forearm crutches: the cuff should cover the proximal third of the forearm, 1–1½ inches below the elbow.

Types
1. Axillary crutches: wood or aluminum designs; handgrip height and crutch height adjusted by wingnuts; push-button locks with telescoping legs on some aluminum crutches; axillary pads cushion the top of crutch.
   a. Provide increased upper-extremity weight bearing over forearm crutches.
   b. May be difficult to use in small areas.

   RED FLAG: Prolonged leaning on the axillary bar can result in vascular and/or nerve damage (axillary artery/radial nerve).

2. Forearm (Lofstrand) crutches: have a forearm cuff and a hand grip; provide slightly less stability but increased ease of movement; frees hands for use without dropping the crutch (secured by cuff).
3. Forearm platform crutches: allow weight bearing on the forearm; used for patients who are unable to bear weight through their hands; e.g., patients with arthritis; platforms can also be attached to walkers.
4. Crutch tips: rubber ~1.5 inches in diameter; provide suction, minimize slippage.

Walkers

Indications
1. Widen base of support, provide increased lateral and anterior stability, can reduce weight bearing on one or both lower extremities; easy to use; frequently prescribed for patients with debilitating conditions, poor balance, or lower extremity injury when use of crutches is precluded; e.g., elderly patients. Negative features include no reciprocal arm swing and increased flexor posture.

Types of Walkers
1. Standard, rigid walker.
2. Folding (collapsible): facilitate mobility in the community, cars.
3. Rolling (wheeled): available with either two or four wheels (four wheels require hand brake to provide added stability in stopping); facilitates walking as a continuous movement sequence (step-through gait pattern); allows for increased speed.
4. Heavy-duty, extra wide walker: designed for use with patients/clients in the bariatric population; designed to support weights between 400 and 700 pounds.
5. Stair-climbing walker: has two posterior extensions and additional handgrips off the rear legs for use on stairs.
6. Reciprocal walkers: hinged, allow advancement of one side of walker at a time; used with reciprocal gait patterns, reciprocating orthoses.
7. Hemi walker: modified for use with one hand only.
8. Attachments: fold-down seats, carrying baskets.

Measurement
1. Hand grip height should be at the level of the ulnar styloid or wrist crease to allow for 20–30 degrees of elbow flexion.

Additions to Gait Devices

Platforms
1. Allow weight bearing on the forearm; used for patients who are unable to bear weight through their hands (e.g., patients with arthritis, limited wrist extension).
2. Can be added to crutches or walkers.

Crutch/Cane Tips
1. Made of rubber; must be maintained for safety to provide suction and minimize slippage.
2. Ice grippers made of metal or other material provide a non-slip surface.

Bariatric Equipment
1. Heavy-duty equipment specifically designed for increased weight capacity and girth.
2. Heavy-duty mechanical lifts available to assist with transfers.
3. See discussion of obesity in Chapter 6.

Gait Patterns: Use of Assistive Devices

Weight-Bearing Status Determines Gait Pattern
1. Non–weight bearing: no weight bearing is permitted.
   a. Three-point pattern is required (see below).
2. Toe-touch or touch-down weight bearing: toes (also may include foot flat or heel) of affected extremity are allowed to touch the ground and bear very little weight but allow for balance.
   a. Three-point gait pattern is required.
3. Partial weight bearing: plantar surface of involved extremity contacts the floor, a percentage of the patient's weight (e.g., 25%, 50%) is allowed on involved extremity; remaining weight is absorbed through the upper extremities.
   a. Weight can be objectively controlled by means of a limb load monitor.
   b. Typically used with three-point or modified three-point gait pattern (see below).
4. Weight bearing as tolerated: the patient bears as much weight as can be tolerated without discomfort.
5. Full weight bearing: full weight is permitted on the involved extremity.

Two-Point Gait
1. One assistive device (cane or crutches) and opposite extremity move together, followed by the opposite crutch and extremity; requires use of two assistive devices.
2. Allows for natural arm and leg motion during gait, good support and stability from two opposing points of contact.

Three-Point Gait (Non Weight Bearing)
1. Both assistive devices and involved leg advance together—no weight is taken through involved limb and then uninvolved leg is advanced forward; requires use of two assistive devices or a walker.
2. Indicated for use with involvement of one extremity or lower extremity fracture.

Modified Three-Point Gait (Weight Bearing)
1. Both assistive devices and involved leg are advanced together and weight is taken through involved leg; uninvolved leg advances either to (in the instance of poorer balance) or through/past the assistive devices (better balance).
2. Requires use of two assistive devices (crutches, canes) or a walker.
3. Indicated for use with involvement of one extremity or lower extremity fracture.

Four-Point Gait
1. A slow, stable gait in which one assistive device (cane or crutch) is advanced forward and placed on the floor, followed by advancement of the opposite leg; then the remaining crutch is advanced forward followed by the opposite remaining leg.
2. Sequence: left crutch → right leg → right crutch → left leg.
3. Requires use of two assistive devices.
4. Provides maximum stability with three points of support while one limb is moving; used for patients with poor balance.

Swing-to and Swing-Through
1. Are utilized when both lower extremities are involved, such as with paraplegia or spina bifida and when there is trunk instability.
2. Swing-to:
   a. Both crutches (typically Lofstrand) are advanced forward together, and weight is then shifted onto hands for support and both legs are swung (or dragged) forward to meet the crutches.
   b. Requires the use of two crutches or a walker.
3. Swing-through:
   a. Both crutches are advanced forward together; weight is shifted onto the hands for support and both legs are swung forward beyond the point of the crutch placement; requires the use of two crutches.
   b. Not as safe as swing-to pattern.
   c. Requires better balance and strength than swing-to gait pattern.

Stairs
1. Ascent: the stronger (uninvolved) leg steps up first, followed by the assistive device and/then the involved leg.
2. Descent: the assistive device and/then the weaker (involved) leg steps down first, followed by the uninvolved leg.
3. Mnemonic to teach the patient: "The good go up to heaven, the bad go down to hell," "Up with the good, down with the bad."

Gait Patterns with Rigid Walkers
1. Patient instruction.
   a. All four legs of the walker should be picked up and placed down simultaneously (provides maximum stability) or rolled forward (wheeled walker).
   b. Advance walker about an arm's length forward (back legs should be in line with patient's toes).
   c. Avoid: forward trunk flexion, stepping too close to or beyond forward edge of walker and rocking from back to front legs during gait.

2. Full weight bearing.
   a. Advance walker.
   b. Followed by lower extremity (weaker first if applicable).
   c. Followed by remaining lower extremity.
3. Partial weight bearing:
   a. Advance walker.
   b. Then advance involved leg.
   c. Transfer body weight through upper extremities and bear partial weight (as prescribed) on involved leg.
   d. Advance uninvolved leg to (step-to) or past (step-through) involved leg.
4. Non weight bearing:
   a. Advance walker.
   b. Then advance involved leg forward—do not place on ground.
   c. Transfer full weight through upper extremities and move uninvolved leg forward with a small hop.

Guarding

Protocol
1. Indication: protects the patient from falling; requires the use of a gait belt for initial training for most patients.
2. Control: use key points of control for all gait training activities.
   a. as printed
   b. as printed
3. Use of key points of control for all gait training activities.
   a. Shoulder, bilateral or unilateral pelvis, gait belt.
   b. Do not grasp clothing or the patient's extremities.

Stairs
1. Therapist position is always below the patient/client.
   a. Ascent: stand behind and slightly to the involved side.
   b. Descent: stand in front and slightly to the involved side.

Sit-to-Stand Transfers
1. Stand to one side and slightly behind the patient.
2. Increased levels of assistance may require therapist to stand in front of patient.

Locomotor Training

Conventional Over-Ground Training
1. Depends on an observational gait assessment.
2. Manual or verbal cues are used to provide input or guidance.
3. Often starts in parallel bars or other safe setting (e.g., body weight support).
4. Support and cues, in form of augmented and visual (mirror) feedback, are progressively decreased.

Body Weight Supported (BWS) and Treadmill Training (TT)
1. BWS: overhead harness or pressured air chamber are used to support body weight.
   a. Initially, support is high (e.g., 40% of body weight) and is progressively decreased.
   b. BWS is contraindicated if it significantly interferes with gait cycle (e.g., unable to achieve flat foot during stepping).
2. Progressive treadmill training.
   a. Progresses from treadmill walking with slow speeds (e.g., 0.6–0.8 mph) to faster, near-normal walking speeds (e.g., 2.6–2.8 mph).
   b. Progresses from level walking to slight incline walking.
   c. Progresses from treadmill walking to overground walking.
3. Manual assistance.
   a. Level of assistance decreases as training progresses (maxA, to modA, to minA, to no assistance).
   b. Assistance can include hands on pelvis (assisted pelvic motions) and hands on lower extremity (assisted stepping).

Robotic-Assisted Walking
1. An exoskeletal frame with motorized, fitted braces is used with patients with complete SCI; braces support both LEs and part of upper body.
   a. A backpack containing a computer and power supply is worn. Computer program controls hip and knee motions.
   b. Crutches or walker are required.
2. Single robotic leg brace: assists walking in individuals with single limb paralysis (e.g., chronic stroke).
3. Often paired with BWS and TT.
4. Progression is to overground walking.
5. High cost limits availability of devices.

Manual Assistance
1. Level of assistance decreases as training progresses (maxA, to modA, to minA, to no assistance).
2. Assistance can include hands on pelvis (assisted pelvic motions) and hands on lower extremity (assisted stepping).

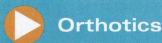
Orthotics

General Concepts

Orthosis: A Rigid or Semi-Rigid Device
1. Used to reduce functional loss due to weak, painful, diseased, or deformed joint.
2. Supports, accommodates, or protects a joint or body segment.
3. Restricts or facilitates motion.
4. Corrects alignment.

Three-Point Pressure Principle
1. Forms the mechanical basis for orthotic correction.
2. A single force is placed at the area of deformity or angulation; two additional counterforces act in the opposing direction.

Splint
1. Colloquial term to describe a temporary device that may serve the same functions.
2. Materials generally not as durable, able to withstand prolonged use.

Device Fitting and Alignment
1. Correct alignment permits effective function.
2. Limb alignment maintained or corrected to prevent further deformity.
3. Restrict or assist motion using rigid blocking or spring-like elements.
4. Transfer load to alternate structures.
5. Reduce pain and/or minimize forces by transferring them away from pressure-sensitive tissues.
6. Proper device alignment minimizes movement between limb and orthoses (e.g., pistoning) and facilitates proper device function.

Lower-Limb Orthoses: Components/Terminology

Shoes
1. The foundation for an orthosis; can substantially influence orthosis function.
2. Often used to provide support or cushioning, including reducing areas of localized high pressure.
3. Traditional leather orthopedic shoes or athletic sneakers can be worn with orthoses; attachments can be external (to the outer part of a leather shoe's sole) or internal (a molded shoe insert).
4. Components include upper, heel counter, midsole, insole, outsole, vamp, toe box.
5. Blucher opening: has vamps (the flaps contain the lace stays) that open wide apart from the anterior margin of the shoe for ease of application.
6. Bal (Balmoral) opening: has stitched down vamps, not suitable for orthotic wear.

Foot Orthosis (FO)
1. May be attached to the interior of the shoe (e.g., an inserted pad) or the exterior of the shoe (e.g., Thomas heel).
2. Soft inserts (i.e., viscoelastic plastic or rubber pads or relief cut-outs) reduce areas of high loading, restrict forces, and protect painful or sensitive areas of the feet.
   a. Metatarsal pad: located posterior to metatarsal heads; moves pressure from the metatarsal heads to the metatarsal shafts; allows more push-off in weak or inflexible feet.
   b. Cushion heel: cushions and absorbs forces at heel contact; used to relieve strain on plantar fascia in plantar fasciitis.
   c. Heel-spur pad.
3. Longitudinal arch supports: prevent depression of the subtalar joint and correct for pes planus (flat foot); flat foot can be flexible or rigid.
   a. UCBL (University of California Biomechanics Laboratory) insert: a semirigid plastic molded insert to correct for flexible pes planus.
   b. Scaphoid pad: used to support the longitudinal arch.
   c. Thomas heel: a heel wedge with an extended anterior medial border used to support the longitudinal arch and correct for flexible pes valgus (pronated foot).
4. Posting.
   a. Rearfoot posting: alters the position of the subtalar joint (STJ), or rearfoot, from heel strike to footflat. Must be dynamic, control but not eliminate STJ motion.
      • Varus post (medial wedge): limits or controls eversion of the calcaneus and internal rotation of the tibia after heelstrike. Reduces calcaneal eversion during running.
      • Valgus post (lateral wedge): controls the calcaneus and subtalar joint that are excessively inverted and supinated at heel strike.
   b. Forefoot posting: supports the forefoot.
      • Medial wedge prescribed for forefoot varus.
      • Lateral wedge prescribed for forefoot valgus.
   c. Contraindicated in the insensitive foot.

5. Heel lifts (or heel platform).
   a. Accommodates for leg length discrepancy; can be placed inside the shoe (up to 3/8 inch) or attached to the outer sole.
   b. Accommodates for limitation in ankle joint dorsiflexion.

> **RED FLAG:** For an insensitive foot, avoid modifications such as heel lifts or rocker bars, which may increase localized forefoot pressure.

6. Rocker bar: located proximal to metatarsal heads; improves weight shift onto metatarsals.
7. Rocker bottom: builds up the sole over the metatarsal heads and improves push-off in weak or inflexible feet. May also be used with insensitive feet.

Ankle-Foot Orthosis (AFO)

1. Typically consists of a foot plate, ankle joint or strut, and a proximal cuff or leg band below the knee.
   a. Can be either custom molded or off the shelf. Can be fabricated using many different materials including leather, thermoplastics, steel, carbon fiber, foamed plastic, or rubber. See Table 11-2.
2. Shoe attachments.
   a. Foot plate: a molded plastic shoe insert; allows application of the brace before insertion into the shoe, ease of changing shoes of same heel height.
   b. Stirrup: a metal attachment riveted to the sole of the shoe; split stirrups allow for shoe interchange; solid stirrups are fixed permanently to the shoe and provide for maximum stability.
3. Ankle controls.
   a. Free motion: provides mediolateral stability that allows free motion in dorsiflexion and plantar flexion.
   b. Solid ankle: allows no movement; indicated with severe pain or instability.
   c. Limited motion: allows motion to be restricted in one or both directions.
      - Bichannel adjustable ankle lock (BiCAAL): an ankle joint with the anterior and posterior channels that can be fit with pins to reduce motion or springs to assist motion.
      - Anterior stop (dorsiflexion stop): determines the limits of ankle dorsiflexion. In an AFO, if the stop is set to allow slight dorsiflexion (~5 degrees), knee flexion results; can be used to control for knee hyperextension; if the stop is set to allow too much dorsiflexion, knee buckling could result.
      - Posterior stop (plantar flexion stop): determines the limits of ankle plantar flexion. In an AFO, if the stop is set to allow slight plantar flexion (~5 degrees), knee extension results; can be used to control for an unstable knee that buckles; if the stop is set to allow too much plantar flexion, recurvatum or knee hyperextension could result.
      - Solid AFO: limits all foot and ankle motion.
   d. Dorsiflexion assistance.
      - Spring assist (Klenzak housing): double upright metal AFO with a single anterior channel for a spring assist to aid dorsiflexion.
      - Posterior leaf spring (PLS): a plastic AFO that inserts into the shoe; widely used to prevent drop foot.
   e. Varus or valgus correction straps (T straps): control for varus or valgus forces at the ankle. Medial strap buckles around the lateral upright and corrects for valgus; lateral strap buckles around the medial upright and corrects for varus.
4. Uprights and attachments (bands or shells).
   a. Conventional AFOs have metal uprights (aluminum, carbon graphite, or steel) and a hinged ankle joint allowing plantarflexion and dorsiflexion. Provides maximum support; if the patient's condition is changing (e.g., peripheral edema), conventional metal AFOs may be easier to alter to accommodate changes than molded AFOs.
      - Double metal uprights extend upward from the ankle on both sides of the leg and attach to a calf band.
      - Conventional AFO, calf band (metal with leather lining or plastic); provides for proximal stabilization on leg; anterior opening and buckle or Velcro closure.
   b. Molded AFOs are made of molded plastic and are lighter in weight and cosmetically more appealing; contraindicated for individuals with changing leg volume.
      - Posterior leaf spring (PLS): has a flexible, narrow posterior shell; functions as dorsiflexion assist; holds foot at 90-degree angle during swing; displaced during stance; provides no medial-lateral stability.
      - Modified AFO: has a wider posterior shell with trimlines just posterior to malleoli; foot plate includes more of medial and lateral borders of foot; provides more medial-lateral stability (control of calcaneal and forefoot inversion and eversion).
      - Static or solid ankle AFO: has widest posterior shell with trimlines extending forward to malleoli; controls (prevents) dorsiflexion, plantarflexion, inversion, and eversion.
      - Spiral AFO: a molded plastic AFO that winds (spirals) around the calf; provides limited control of motion in all planes.
      - Hinged plastic AFOs are available.
   c. Specialized AFOs.
      - Patellar-tendon-bearing brim: allows for weight distribution on the patellar shelf similar to patellar-tendon-bearing prosthetic socket; reduces weight-bearing forces through the foot.

Table 11-2

Ankle Foot Orthoses: Indications, Advantages, and Disadvantages

NAME	INDICATION	DESCRIPTION	ADVANTAGES	DISADVANTAGES
ANKLE FOOT ORTHOSES (AFOS)				
Posterior leaf spring	Dorsiflexion assist	Plastic insert; "off the shelf" or custom fit. Posterior component attached to foot plate, secured in shoe and with calf band	Relatively light compared to metal components. Can easily switch to different shoes	May not provide enough assist in the instance of high plantar flexor tone
ToeOFF® or Ypsilon™	Dorsiflexion assist	Brand name dorsiflexion assist AFOs. Consist of a foot plate secured in shoe, a lateral and lateral-to-medial upright secured with a calf band proximally. Made of carbon material. For use with mild to moderate foot drop	ToeOFF® good for mild to severe foot drop accompanied with mild to moderate ankle instability. Ypsilon™ good for mild to moderate isolated foot drop; provides free ankle movements	Not indicated for use with moderate to severe spasticity. Ypsilon™ not suitable in instance of ankle instability.
Plastic hinged ankle AFO; posterior stop metal upright	Dorsiflexion assist—through plantar flexion resistance	Plastic hinged AFO: hinged ankle joint with a dorsiflexion assist (flexible rubber at ankle joint) and plantar flexion stop (posting at posterior upright). Metal upright joint shape prevents plantar flexion at heel strike. Metal uprights can be made of steel, aluminum, carbon graphite or titanium.	Helps prevent knee from hyperextending at heel strike	May alter gait pattern by forcing knee flexion earlier than normally occurring following heel strike. Plastic AFO contraindicated in instance of fluctuating edema. Newer, lighter metals make for a more expensive AFO.
Solid ankle-foot orthosis	Full ankle control for dorsiflexion and plantar flexion, as well as medial/lateral motion	Plastic AFO that encompasses posterior, medial and lateral calf areas as well as malleoli; may or may not be hinged. Hinged version may have plastic overlap at ankle, plastic rod ankle or metal ankle.	Hinged version increases cadence, step length and velocity. Metal ankle can be adjusted to alter excursion of ankle motion.	Heavier and bulkier than posterior leaf spring or hinged AFO. Contraindicated in instance of fluctuating edema
Spiral AFO	Control of ankle motion in all planes; does not eliminate motion	A single upright spirals up from foot plate medially around leg and stops at calf band. Typically made of polypropylene, nylon or carbon fiber	Minimally conspicuous compared to larger AFOs	Contraindicated in instance of fluctuating edema
Floor reaction orthosis	Knee extension assist	Anterior upright portion attached to foot plate, provides knee extension force during stance phase	Controls knee during stance phase to maintain extension	Pressure on anterior tibia may be difficult to tolerate or cause tissue irritation.
Klenzak joint AFO	Dorsiflexion assist	Solid stirrup and metal uprights attached to sole (heel area) of shoe with spring at ankle	Spring can be adjusted for amount of assistance required	Fixed to pair of shoes, not interchangeable. Heavy and bulky
BiCAAL (bichannel adjustable ankle locks)	Full range of ankle dorsiflexion and plantar flexion control	Metal uprights attached to sole of shoe with hinges. Hinges have ability for motion assist and resistance through use of pins and springs.	Full range of control for ankle motions, resistance and assistance	Bulky and heavier than plastic AFOs. Attached directly to shoe, not interchangeable between shoes. Sole should have a rocker bottom bar to assist with roll over at late stance.
Valgus correction strap	Limits valgus movement of ankle	Typically used with metal upright AFOs. A "T" strap attached to lateral border of shoe and secured around medial upright	Uses three-point pressure system to control valgus movement at ankle	

- Tone-reducing orthosis: molded plastic AFO that applies constant pressure to spastic or hypertonic muscles (plantarflexors and invertors); snug fit is essential to achieve the benefits of reciprocal inhibition.
- Ground reaction AFO (GRAFO): controls forward progression of the tibia, primarily for PF weakness. Can influence the knee by decreasing extensor moment during stance, resisting DF at the ankle.
- Patellar tendon bearing AFO (PTBAFO): unloads the distal limb, primarily for PF weakness. Anterior shell with weight-bearing capabilities, shelf transfers force to the medial tibial flare, patellar tendon bar-like prosthetic socket.
- Charcot restraint orthotic walker (CROW) boot: immobilizes and protects the foot and ankle; includes a rocker bottom and custom molded insert. This serves as an alternative to total contact casting in individuals with diabetes mellitus; eliminates shear forces on the plantar surface.

Knee-Ankle-Foot Orthosis (KAFO)

1. Consists of a shoe attachment, ankle control, uprights, knee control, and bands or shells for the calf and thigh.
2. Knee controls.
   a. Hinge joint: provides mediolateral and hyperextension control while allowing for flexion and extension.
      - Offset: the hinge is placed posterior to the weight-bearing line (trochanter-knee-ankle [TKA] line); assists extension, stabilizes knee during early stance; patients may have difficulty on ramps where knee may flex inadvertently.
   b. Locks.
      - Drop ring lock: ring drops over joint when knee is in full extension to provide maximum stability; a retention button may be added to hold the ring lock up, permit gait training with the knee unlocked.
      - Pawl lock with bail release: the pawl is a spring-loaded posterior projection (lever or ring) that allows the patient to unlock the knee by pulling up or hooking the pawl on the back of a chair and pushing it up; adds bulk and may unlock inadvertently with posterior knee pressure.
   c. Knee stability.
      - Sagittal stability achieved by bands or straps used to provide a posteriorly directed force.
         - Anterior band or strap (knee cap): attaches by four buckles to metal uprights; may restrict sitting, increases difficulty in putting on KAFO.
         - Anterior bands: pretibial or suprapatellar or both.
      - Frontal plane controls: for control of genu varum or genu valgum.
         - Posterior plastic shell.
         - Older braces utilize valgum (medial) or varum (lateral) correction straps, which buckle around the opposite metal upright; less effective as controls than plastic shell.
3. Thigh bands.
   a. Proximal thigh band.
   b. Quadrilateral or ischial weight-bearing brim: reduces weight bearing through the limb.
      - Patten bottom: a distal attachment added to keep the foot off the floor; provides 100% unweighting of the limb; a lift is required on the opposite leg, e.g., used with Legg-Calvé-Perthes disease.
4. Specialized KAFOs.
   a. Craig-Scott KAFO: commonly used appliance for individuals with paraplegia; consists of shoe attachments with reinforced foot plates, BiCAAL ankle joints set in slight dorsiflexion, pretibial band, pawl knee locks with bail release, and single thigh bands.
   b. Oregon orthotic system: a combination of plastic and metal components allows for triplanar control in three planes of motion (sagittal, frontal, and transverse).
   c. Fracture braces: a KAFO device with a calf or thigh shell that encompasses the fracture site and provides support.
   d. Functional electrical stimulation (FES) orthosis: orthotic use and functional ambulation is facilitated by the addition of electrical stimulation to specific muscles; the pattern and sequence of muscle activation by portable stimulators is controlled by an externally worn miniaturized computer pack; requires full passive range of motion (PROM); good functional endurance; in limited use with individuals with paraplegia, drop foot; also scoliosis.
5. Standing frames.
   a. Standing frames: allows for standing without crutch support; may be stationary or attached to a wheeled mobility base (e.g., used with some patients with spinal cord injury).
   b. Parapodium: allows for standing without crutch support; also allows for ease in sitting with the addition of hip and knee joints that can be unlocked (e.g., used with children with myelodysplasia).

Specialized Knee Orthosis (KO)

1. Articulated KO: controls knee motion and provides added stability.
   a. Postsurgery KO protects repaired ligaments from overload.
   b. Functional KO is worn long-term in lieu of surgery or during selected activities (sports competitions).
   c. Examples include Lenox Hill, Pro-AM, Can-Am, Don Joy.

2. Swedish knee cage: provides mild control for excessive hyperextension of the knee.
3. Patellar stabilizing braces.
   a. Improve patellar tracking; maintain alignment.
   b. Lateral buttress (often made of felt) or strap positions patella medially.
   c. A central patellar cutout may help positioning and minimizes compression.
4. Neoprene sleeves.
   a. Nylon-coated rubber material.
   b. Provide compression, protection, and proprioceptive feedback.
   c. Provide little stabilization unless metal or plastic hinges are added.
   d. Retains body heat, which may increase local circulation.
   e. A central cutout minimizes patellar compression.
   f. Can be used in other areas of the body, such as elbow, thigh, and so on.

Hip-Knee-Ankle-Foot Orthosis (HKAFO)
1. Contain a hip joint and pelvic band added to a KAFO.
2. Hip joint: typically a metal hinge joint.
   a. Controls for abduction, adduction, and rotation.
   b. Controls for hip flexion when locked, typically with a drop ring lock; a locked hip restricts gait pattern to either swing-to or swing-through.
3. Pelvic attachments: a leather-covered, metal pelvic band; attaches the HKAFO to the pelvis between the greater trochanter and iliac crest; adds to difficulty in donning and doffing; adds weight and increases overall energy expenditure during ambulation.

Specialized Trunk-Hip-Knee-Ankle-Foot Orthosis (THKAFOs)
1. Contains a trunk band added to a HKAFO.
2. Reciprocating gait orthosis (RGO): utilizes plastic molded solid-ankle orthoses with locked knees, plastic thigh shells, a hip joint with pelvic and trunk bands; the hips are connected by steel cables, which allow for a reciprocal gait pattern (either four-point or two-point); when the patient leans on the supporting hip, it forces it into extension, while the opposite leg is pushed into flexion; allows limb advancement.

Specialized Lower Limb Devices
1. Denis Browne splint: a bar connecting two shoes that can swivel; used for correction of club foot or pes equinovarus in young children.
2. Frejka pillow: keeps hips abducted; used for hip dysplasia or other conditions with tight adductors in young children.
3. Toronto hip abduction orthosis: abducts the hip; used in treatment of Legg-Calvé-Perthes disease.

Spinal (Trunk) Orthoses: Components/Terminology

Corset
1. Provides abdominal compression, increases intra-abdominal pressure.
2. Assists respiration in individuals with spinal cord injury.
3. Relieves pain in low back disorders; sacroiliac support; e.g., pregnancy.

Lumbosacral Orthosis (LSO)
1. Controls or limits lumbosacral motions.
2. Flexible LSO—corset.
   a. Uses abdominal compression to increase intraabdominal pressure.
   b. Provides tactile reminder for postural correction.
   c. Indications: low back pain, compression of abdominal incision, respiratory assist in individual with spinal cord, sacroiliac support for pregnancy, post-operative protection, etc.
3. Rigid LSO—shell (custom or off the shelf).
   a. Uses three-point pressure system, intra-abdominal pressure and total contact to control flexion, extension and lateral flexion of lumbar and sacral spinal segments.
   b. Provides tactile reminder for positioning.
   c. Trimlines/fitting:
      • Anterior: below the xiphoid process to symphysis pubis.
      • Posterior: below the inferior angle of scapula to sacro-coccygeal junction.
   d. Indications: post-op protection, stenosis, low back pain, spondylolisthesis, etc.

Thoracolumbosacral Orthosis (TLSO)
1. Controls or limits thoracic and lumbosacral motions.
2. TLSO shell (custom or OTS).
   a. Uses three-point pressure system, intra-abdominal pressure, and total contact to control flexion, extension, lateral flexion and rotation of the thoracic, lumbar and sacral spinal segments.
   b. Trimlines/fitting:
      • Anterior: distal to the sternal notch to symphysis pubis.
      • Posterior: distal to spine of scapula to sacro-coccygeal junction.
   c. Indications: post-op protection, stable vertebral fracture, scoliosis (with additional thoracic pad to counter spinal curve), spinal cord injury, etc.
3. Anterior control TLSO jewett orthosis or cruciform anterior spinal hyperextension (CASH) orthosis (both available OTS).

a. Uses three-point pressure system and tactile reminders to control primarily flexion of thoracic and lumbar spinal segments.
b. Fitting: sternal pad just distal to sternal notch, pubic pad just proximal to symphysis pubis, posterior pad over the thoracolumbar junction.
c. Indications: thoracolumbar anterior vertebral compression fractures.

Cervical Orthosis (CO)
1. Soft collar.
   a. Provides minimal levels of control of cervical motion.
   b. Provides tactile reminder for postural correction.
   c. Indications: cervical pain, whiplash, cervical weakness, etc.
2. Semirigid (e.g., Miami J or Philadelphia collars):
   a. Uses three-point pressure system and tactile cues to control flexion, extension, lateral flexion, and rotation of cervical spinal segments.
   b. Trimlines/fitting:
      - Anterior: mandible to sternal notch.
      - Posterior: occiput to T1.
   c. Indications: post-op protection, stable cervical vertebral injury, whiplash, etc.
3. Rigid-halo orthosis:
   a. Provides maximal control of all cervical motion with halo attachment to the skull, four uprights connect from the halo to thoracic jacket.
   b. Indications: unstable cervical vertebral fracture, spinal cord injury.
4. Minerva orthosis/cervical thoracic orthosis (CTO).
   a. Has a semi-rigid cervical collar connected to a thoracic jacket via metal uprights.
   b. Provides good control of all cervical motions.
   c. Indications: stable cervical and upper thoracic fractures and fusions.

Specialized Trunk Orthoses
1. Milwaukee orthosis: a cervical, thoracic, lumbosacral orthosis (CTLSO) used to control scoliosis; it has a molded plastic pelvic jacket with one anterior and two posterior uprights extended to a superior neck or chest ring; pads and straps are used to apply pressure to areas of convexity of spinal curves; bulky, less cosmetic; may be used for all kyphotic and scoliotic curves of ≤40 degrees.
2. Boston orthosis (TLSO): a low-profile, molded plastic orthosis for scoliosis; more cosmetic, can be worn under clothing; used for midthoracic or lower scoliosis curves of ≤40 degrees; also used to treat spondylolisthesis and conditions of severe trunk weakness; e.g., muscular dystrophy.

Upper-Limb Orthoses or Splints: Components/Terminology

Goals of Upper Extremity Orthoses/Splints
1. Immobilization
2. Protection/support
3. Correction or prevention of deformities
4. Substitute for weak or absent upper extremity function
5. Serve as a base of attachment for ADL equipment

Wrist Cock-Up Splint
1. An anterior or palmar splint that contains forearm and metacarpals. May include phalanges as well if needed for positioning.
2. Wrist can be held in neutral or in 10°–20° wrist extension.
3. For weak or absent hand strength: orthosis should support the full hand phalanges slightly flexed and with thumb in partial opposition and abduction.
4. For wrist pathologies: trim lines should be at the distal palmar crease and thenar crease to maximize hand function.
5. Used for patients with rheumatoid arthritis, fractures of carpal bones, Colles' fracture, carpal tunnel syndrome, stroke with paralysis, etc.

Thumb Spica Splint
1. A hand-based splint designed to immobilize the first carpometacarpal joint.
2. Thumb positioned in partial opposition and abduction with thumb interphalangeal joint left free for maximal function.
3. Hand-based: used for first CMC arthritis.
4. Forearm-based: used for scaphoid fracture, scaphoid-lunate instability, de Quervain's, etc.

Dorsal Wrist Splint
1. Frees the palm for feeling and grasping through use of grips that curve around over the second and fifth metacarpal heads.
2. Allows attachment of dorsal devices (i.e., rubber bands) to form a dynamic device.
3. Used for flexor tendon repairs.

Airplane Splint
1. Positions the patient's arm out to the side at 90 degrees of abduction, with elbow flexed to 90 degrees.
2. The weight of the outstretched arm is borne on a padded lateral trunk bar and iliac crest band.
3. A strap holds the device across the trunk.
4. Used to immobilize the shoulder following fracture or burn injury to prevent contracture of the axillary region.

Tenodesis Splint
1. Assists patients in use of wrist extensors to approximate the thumb and forefingers (grip) in the absence of active finger flexion.
2. Facilitates tenodesis grasp in patients with quadriplegia.

Finger Splints
1. Mallet Finger: palmar DIP gutter splint to support distal phalange.
2. Boutonniere's Deformity: palmar PIP gutter splint to support middle phalange.
3. Swan Neck Deformity: ring splints over PIP joint to prevent PIP hyperextension.

Dynamic Devices
1. Wrist-driven prehension orthosis (flexor hinge orthosis): assists patients in use of wrist extensors to approximate the thumb and forefingers (grip) in the absence of active finger flexion; e.g., facilitates tenodesis grasp in patients with quadriplegia.
2. Motor-driven flexor hinge orthosis: complex control systems that allow for grasp; not generally in widespread use.

Physical Therapy Intervention

Physical Therapy Team
1. The physical therapist functions as a member of an orthotic clinic team that includes the physician, orthotist, physical therapist, and physical therapist assistant.
2. The physical therapist assistant functions to provide patient education and instruction in the use of the device, performing inspection and orthotic check for fit, and patient training.

Examination
1. Preorthotic assessment and prescription evaluate:
   a. Joint mobility.
   b. Sensation.
   c. Strength and motor function.
   d. Functional level.
   e. Psychological status.
2. Physical therapist orthotic prescription and considerations.
   a. Patient's abilities and needs.
      - Level of impairments, functional limitations, disability.
      - Status: Consider whether the patient's condition is permanent or changing.
   b. Level of function, current lifestyle.
      - Consider whether the patient is going to be a community ambulator versus a household ambulator.
      - Consider recreational and work-related needs.
   c. Overall weight of orthotic devices, energy capabilities of patient. Some individuals abandon their orthoses quickly in favor of wheelchairs because of the high-energy demands of ambulating with orthoses; e.g., patients with high levels of paraplegia.
   d. Manual dexterity, mental capacity of the individual. The donning and use of devices may be too difficult or complicated for some individuals.
   e. Pressure tolerance of the skin and tissues.
   f. Use of a temporary orthosis to assess likelihood of functional independence, reduce costs; e.g., patients with high levels of paraplegia.
3. Orthotic check-out.
   a. The PT and PTA actively participate in the check-out process to ensure proper fit, function, and construction of the orthosis.
   b. Static assessment.
      - Examine alignments for lower limb orthoses: in midstance, foot should be flat on floor.
        ○ Orthotic hip joint: 0.8 cm (0.3 in) anterior and superior to greater trochanter.
        ○ Medial knee joint: ~2 cm (~0.8 in) above joint space, vertically midway between medial joint space and adductor tubercle.
        ○ Ankle joint: at tip of malleolus.
        ○ Plastic shells or metal uprights, thigh and calf bands: conform to contours of limb.
        ○ No undue tissue pressure or restriction of function.
   c. Dynamic assessment.
      - Fit and function during activities of daily living (ADLs), functional mobility skills; e.g., sit-to-stand.
      - Fit and function during gait.

Orthotic Training
1. Instruct the patient in procedures for orthotic maintenance: routine skin inspection and care.

> **RED FLAG:** Check for impaired sensation and areas of excessive pressure. This is important for all patients but critical for patients with impaired neurovascular status (e.g., diabetic neuropathy).

2. Ensure orthotic acceptance.
   a. Patient should clearly understand functions, limitations of an orthosis.
   b. Can use support groups to assist.
3. Teach proper application (donning/doffing) of the orthosis.
4. Teach proper use of the orthosis.
   a. Balance training.
   b. Gait training.
   c. Functional activities training.
5. Reassess fit, function, and construction of the orthosis at periodic intervals; assess habitual use of the orthosis.
6. Teach procedures for routine maintenance of device.

Selected Orthotic Gait Deviations

1. Lateral trunk bending: patient leans toward the orthotic side during stance.
   a. Possible causes: KAFO medial upright too high; insufficient shoe lift; hip pain, weak or tight abductors on the orthotic side; short leg; poor balance.
2. Circumduction: during swing, leg swings out to the side in an arc.
   a. Possible causes: locked knee; excessive plantar flexion (inadequate stop, plantar flexion contractures); weak hip flexors or dorsiflexors. All of these could also cause vaulting (rising up on the sound limb to advance the orthotic limb forward).
3. Anterior trunk bending: patient leans forward during stance.
   a. Possible causes: inadequate knee lock; weak quadriceps; hip or knee flexion contracture.
4. Posterior trunk bending: patient leans backward during stance.
   a. Possible causes: inadequate hip lock; weak gluteus maximus; knee ankylosis.
5. Hyperextended knee: excessive extension during stance.
   a. Possible causes: inadequate plantar flexion stop; inadequate knee lock; poor fit of calf band (too deep); weak quadriceps; loose knee ligaments or extensor spasticity; pes equinus.
6. Knee instability: excessive knee flexion during stance.
   a. Possible causes: inadequate dorsiflexion stop; inadequate knee lock; knee and/or hip flexion contracture; weak quadriceps or insufficient knee lock; knee pain.
7. Foot slap: foot hits the ground during early stance.
   a. Possible causes: inadequate dorsiflexor assist; inadequate plantarflexor stop; weak dorsiflexors.
8. Toes first: on-toes posture during stance.
   a. Possible causes: inadequate dorsiflexor assist; inadequate plantarflexor stop; inadequate heel lift; heel pain, extensor spasticity; pes equinus; short leg.
9. Flat foot: contact with entire foot.
   a. Possible causes: inadequate longitudinal arch support; pes planus.
10. Pronation: excessive medial foot contact during stance, valgus position of calcaneus.
    a. Possible causes: transverse plane malalignment; weak invertors; pes valgus; spasticity; genu valgum.
11. Supination: excessive lateral foot contact during stance, varus position of the calcaneus.
    a. Possible causes: transverse plane malalignment; weak evertors; pes varus; genu varum.
12. Excessive stance width: patient stands or walks with a wide base of support.
    a. Possible causes: KAFO height of medial upright too high; HKAFO hip joint aligned in excessive abduction; knee is locked; abduction contracture; poor balance; sound limb is too short.

Adhesive Taping

General Concepts

Purpose
1. Limit ROM of specific joints.
2. Support injured body segment.
3. Secure protective devices such as felt, foam, gel, or plastic padding, orthoplast or plastazote.
4. Keep dressings and bandages in place and secure.
5. Preventive support for a joint that is at risk.
6. Realign position and reduce pain; e.g., McConnell treatment for patellofemoral pain.
7. May enhance proprioception.
8. Elastic therapeutic tape (e.g., Kinesio tape) is an acrylic, adhesive-backed elastic tape. It is used with athletes and others ostensibly to alleviate pain, enhance performance, relax muscles, support muscles, and reduce inflammation. Research has shown limited evidence of benefit except for reducing pain.

Preparation
1. Part to be taped should be properly positioned and supported.
2. Select appropriate type and width of tape.
3. Body hair should be shaved, skin should be clean. Foam underwrap or stockinet may be used.
4. Lubricated pads should be placed over areas of potential blister formation from friction. e.g.; heel and lace-area pads on the foot.
5. Occlusive dressings should be applied over wounds or skin conditions to be covered by the tape.
6. Skin adherent such as benzoin should be applied to increase adhesion of the tape and to aid in toughening the skin to decrease irritation.

Application
1. If the part has not been previously injured, it should be taped in a neutral position.

2. Injured ligaments should be held in a shortened position.
   a. Lateral or inversion ankle sprains should be taped in an everted position.
   b. Tape should follow body contours and be applied primarily from medial to lateral in the case of an inversion sprain.
3. Tape should be applied with even pressure, and with overlap of previous tape strip by one-half.
4. Circular strapping should be applied very cautiously due to potential circulatory compromise.
5. Avoid creases and folds.
6. If tape is too tight, adjust by removing or modifying strips or reapply.
7. Elastic therapeutic tape is applied in a variety of configurations according to manufacturer's specifications.

Complications

> **RED FLAGS:**
> - Allergic reactions to the tape.
> - Skin irritation.
> - Reduced circulation.
> - If tape is too tight, it might compromise the ability of the patient to perform the skill intended.
> - Tape may lose its effectiveness in an hour or so, and may need to be reapplied.

Prosthetics

General Concepts

Prosthesis
1. A replacement of a body part with an artificial device; an artificial limb.

Levels of Amputation
Amputations occur at different levels. See Quick Facts 11-3 for common lower extremity and upper extremity levels of amputation.

Components
1. All prosthetic devices contain a socket and terminal device with varying components in between.
2. Sockets are custom-molded to the residual limb; total contact is desired, with the load distributed to all tissues; assists in circulation and provides maximal sensory feedback.
   a. Functions to:
      - Contain the residual tissues.
      - Provide a means to suspend the prosthetic limb.
      - Transfer forces from the prosthesis to the residual limb.
   b. Selective loading: pressure-tolerant areas are built up to increase loading (i.e., build-ups for tendon-bearing areas), while pressure-sensitive areas are relieved to decrease loading (i.e., relief for bony prominences, nerves, and tendons).
   c. Liners.
      - Use in every suspension system except anatomical suction.
      - Comprised of silicone or gels to protect the residual limb and minimize the shear forces between the socket and the skin.
   d. Socks.
      - Used in every suspension system except suction.
      - Provide a soft interface between the residual limb and the socket; minimize shear forces between socket and skin.
      - Changing sock thickness or adding more socks can assist in accommodating to changes in volume of residual limb, prevent pistoning.
      - Excessive thickness of socks (>15 ply) can alter fit and weight-bearing ability of the socket.
3. Terminal device (TD).
   a. Provides an interface between the amputee's prosthesis with the external environment.
   b. Lower-limb prosthesis: TD is a foot.
   c. Upper-limb prosthesis: TD is a hook or hand.

Lower-Limb Prosthetics (LLPs)

Partial-Foot Prosthesis
1. Plastic foot replacement: restores foot length, protects amputated stump.
2. Function may be assisted by the addition of a rocker bottom or plastic calf shell.

Transtibial (Below Knee) Prosthesis
1. Foot-ankle assembly.
   a. Functions to:
      - Absorb shock at heel strike.
      - Plantarflex in early stance, permits metatarsophalangeal hyperextension in late stance.
      - Cosmetic replacement of foot.
   b. There are four basic types of foot orthoses. See Quick Facts 11-4.

QUICK FACTS 11-3 ▶ LEVELS OF AMPUTATION

Amputation Level	Location
Lower Extremity Amputations	
Transmetatarsal	Partial foot amputation
Ankle disarticulation (Syme's)	Amputation through the ankle joint; heel pad is preserved and attached to distal end of tibia for weight bearing
Transtibial	Below-knee (BK) amputation; ideally, 20%–50% of the tibial length is spared; short transtibial is <20% of tibial length
Knee disarticulation	Amputation through the knee joint; femur is intact
Transfemoral	Above-knee (AK) amputation; ideally 35%–60% of the femoral length is spared; short transfemoral is <35% of femoral length
Hip disarticulation	Amputation of entire lower limb, pelvis is preserved
Hemipelvectomy	Amputation of entire lower limb, lower half of the pelvis is resected
Hemicorporectomy	Amputation of both lower limbs and pelvis below L4, L5 level
Upper Extremity Amputations	
Transradial	Below-elbow (BE) amputation
Elbow disarticulation	Amputation through the elbow joint
Transhumeral	Above-elbow (AE) amputation
Shoulder disarticulation	Amputation through the shoulder joint

QUICK FACTS 11-4 ▶ TYPES OF FOOT ORTHOSIS

Solid ankle cushion heel (SACH) foot	The most commonly prescribed foot; nonarticulated; contains an energy-absorbing cushion heel and internal wooden keel that limits sagittal plane motion, primarily to plantarflexion Permits a very small amount of mediolateral (frontal plane) and transverse plane motion Assists in hyperextension of knee (knee stability) during stance
Solid ankle flexible endoskeleton (SAFE) foot	Solid ankle flexible endoskeleton (SAFE) foot: a flexible, nonarticulated foot (similar to SACH) Permits more nonsagittal plane motions Prescribed for more active individuals
Flex-foot: a leaf-spring shank (not a foot)	Used with an endoskeletal prosthesis; the long band of carbon fiber originates directly from the shank Stores energy in early stance for later use during push-off Prescribed for more active individuals
Single axis foot	An articulated foot with the lower shank; motion is controlled by anterior and posterior rubber bumpers that limit dorsiflexion and plantarflexion More stable (permits only sagittal plane motion) May be prescribed for individuals with bilateral transfemoral amputations

2. Shank.
   a. Functions to:
      - Provide leg length and shape.
      - Connect and transmit weight from socket to foot.
   b. Exoskeletal: conventional components, usually made of wood with a plastic laminated finish; colored for cosmesis; durable.
   c. Endoskeletal: contains a central metal shank (aluminum, titanium, and other high-strength alloys), covered by soft foam and external stocking; offers improved cosmesis; modular components allows for increased ease of prosthetic adjustment.
3. Socket.
   a. PTB (patellar tendon-bearing) socket: a total contact socket that allows for moderate loading over the area of the patellar tendon.
   b. Pressure-sensitive areas of the transtibial residual limb include:
      - Anterior tibia.
      - Anterior tibial crest.

- Fibular head and neck.
- Fibular nerve.
- Distal cut end of tibia and fibula.
c. Pressure-tolerant areas of the typical transtibial residual limb include:
  - Patellar tendon.
  - Medial tibial plateau.
  - Tibial and fibular shafts.
  - Distal end (rarely, may be sensitive).
  - Gastrocnemius muscles.
d. TSB (total surface bearing) socket: total contact socket with lower profile and rounder shape than PTB socket for more intimate fit.
  - Weight is borne equally throughout the socket on bones and soft tissues.
  - Must use a gel-type liner for suspension and to distribute pressures.
4. Suspension.
  a. Suction: silicone liners rolled over the residual limb for increased suspension and proprioception. Uses either a pin lock or cuff to attach/seal to socket.
  b. Supracondylar (SC) socket suspension: medial and lateral walls of the socket extend up and over the femoral condyles; a removable medial wedge assists in donning and removal; more cosmetic (no buckles or straps); provides increased mediolateral stability.
  c. Supracondylar/suprapatellar (SC/SP) socket suspension: similar to SC but with a high anterior wall; assists in suspension of short residual limbs.
  d. External suspension sleeve: neoprene-type sleeve that covers the proximal socket and distal thigh to suspend the limb.
    - May be used alone or in conjunction with other suspension options.
  e. Thigh corset suspension: a hinged joint with metal uprights attached to a thigh corset; provides larger surface for weight bearing; prescribed for individuals with sensitive skin on the residual limb; the knee joint allows for knee control (locks); pistoning may be a problem.

Transfemoral (Above-Knee) Prosthesis

1. Knee unit (ranked by stability).
  a. Manual locking knee.
    - Lock is engaged for standing and walking; manually unlocked for sitting.
    - Maximal stability for individuals with significant weakness in the lower extremity.
    - Difficulty with clearance of the leg during swing can be controlled by shortening the total prosthetic limb length.
  b. Microprocessor/Computerized knee.
    - Knee stability in stance and ability to flex in swing are controlled electronically.
    - Prevents knee from buckling when weighted.
    - Adapts swing resistance automatically to allow variable gait speeds.
    - Can be used to ascend and descend stairs step over step.
  c. Single axis/weight activated stance control.
    - Permits knee motions to occur around a fixed axis.
    - Weight activated friction braking increases friction at midstance to prevent knee flexion, but permits smooth knee motion through the rest of the gait cycle.
    - Requires extension assist: internal coiled spring that assists in terminal knee extension during late swing.
  d. Polycentric systems (multiple axes): changing axis of motion allows for adjustments to the center of knee rotation
    - Stable in stance phase due to knee center position.
  e. Hydraulic knee units (fluid-controlled) or pneumatic knee units (air-controlled): adjusts resistance dynamically to the individual's walking speed
    - Appropriate for younger, more active individuals
  f. Single axis/constant friction.
    - Continuous resistance is provided by a clamp that acts on the knee mechanism.
    - Least stable knee as friction does not increase in stance phase; must have good hip extensor strength to promote knee extension in midstance.
2. Socket.
  a. Ischial containment socket
    - Triangular shaped socket that holds the femur in an adducted position.
    - Lateral wall of socket extends more proximally to provide lateral stability and to ensure the ischial tuberosity is seated within the socket for a more intimate fit.
  b. Quadrilateral socket:
    - Rectangular shaped socket with a broad horizontal posterior shelf for seating of the ischial tuberosity and gluteals.
    - The medial wall is the same height as the posterior wall, while the anterior and lateral walls are 2½–3 inches higher.
    - A posterior directed force is provided by the anterior and lateral walls to ensure proper seating.
    - Reliefs are provided for the adductor longus tendon, hamstring tendons, sciatic nerve, gluteus maximus, and rectus femoris.
3. Suspension.
  a. Anatomical suction suspension.
    - Suction is employed to maximize contact and suspension; air is pumped out through a one-way air release valve located at the socket's bottom.
    - Good proprioception due to direct skin to socket total contact.

b. Silicone suction suspension.
- Silicone liner with either a locking pin and/or cuff is used to maintain the prosthesis on the limb.
- Reduces shear within the socket and provides pressure relief for the residual limb to increase comfort.

c. TES (Total Elastic Suspension):
- Neoprene belt is applied to prosthesis and wraps around the pelvis to anchor the prosthesis on the residual limb. Can be used alone or in conjunction with other methods.
- Adjustable and readily accommodates to volume changes.
- May cause pistoning of the residual limb in the socket when it is the sole type of suspension.

d. Silesian belt.
- Strap that anchors the prosthesis by reaching around the pelvis (below iliac crest).
- Able to controls rotation in the transverse plane.
- Used as an auxiliary suspension.
- Poor cosmesis.

e. Hinge suspension.
- Hinged hip joint attached to a metal/leather pelvic band, anchored around the pelvis.
- Adds control for medial/lateral stability of hip (rotation, abduction/adduction).
- Reduces Trendelenburg gait deviation, but adds extra weight and bulk.

Knee Disarticulation Prosthesis
1. Functional, allows weight bearing on the distal end of the femur.
2. Problems with cosmesis, added thigh length with the knee joint attached, especially noticeable in sitting.
3. Lower shank is shortened to balance leg length in standing.

Hip Disarticulation Prosthesis
1. Socket is molded to accommodate the pelvis; weight bearing occurs on ischial seat, iliac crests.
2. Endoskeletal components frequently used, decreases weight of prosthesis.
3. Stability achieved with hip extension aid; posterior placement of knee joint with anterior placement of the hip joint to the weight-bearing line.

Immediate Postoperative Prosthesis (Rigid Dressing)
1. Plaster of Paris socket is fabricated in the operating room with the capability to attach a foot and pylon.
2. Advantages.
   a. Allows early, limited weight-bearing ambulation within days of surgery.
   b. Limits postoperative sequelae: edema, postoperative pain.
   c. Enhances wound healing.
   d. Allows for earlier fit of permanent prosthesis.
3. Limitations.
   a. Requires skilled application and close monitoring.
   b. Does not allow for daily wound inspection; contraindicated for older patients with cardiovascular compromise and increased risk for wounds.

Upper-Limb Prosthetics (ULPs)

Below Elbow (BE) Prosthesis
1. Contains terminal device (TD), wrist joint, and forearm socket.

Above Elbow (AE) Prosthesis
1. Contains a terminal device (TD), wrist device, elbow joint, and upper arm socket.

Types of UE Prostheses
1. Conventional/body-powered system.
   a. Power for voluntary opening of the TD (hook or hand) is transmitted by a cable from a figure-of-eight shoulder harness to the TD.
   b. Rubber bands are used for closure and prehensile strength.
   c. Forearm rotation is done by manual prepositioning of the TD through the wrist joint.

Movement Control
1. BE prosthesis: bilateral scapular abduction, depression, or ipsilateral flexion of the humerus is used to pull on the cable and force opening of the hook.
2. AE prosthesis (dual control system): the same motions can be used to flex the elbow in the AE prosthesis; when the elbow is locked out, the forces are then transmitted to operate the TD.

Myoelectric System
1. Utilizes surface electrical activity of various muscles (e.g., wrist flexors/extensors, scapular, and pectoral muscles).
2. Small electric motors (battery-powered) are powered to operate the TD. The intensity of the signal from the muscle allows for different functions and graded power output to the TD.
   a. Benefits: Improves ease of function, prehensile strength and requires no harnessing.
   b. Disadvantages: Adds weight, increased maintenance, cost.

Physical Therapy Intervention

Team
1. In the clinic, the physical therapist functions as a member of the prosthetic clinic team that includes physician, orthotist, physical therapist, and physical therapist assistant.

2. The physical therapist assistant functions to provide patient education and instruction in the use of the prosthetic, performing inspection and check for fit, and patient training.

Preprosthetic Management

1. Preprescription examination.
   a. Skin: inspect incision for healing; scar tissue; other lesions.
   b. Residual limb.
      - Circumference measurements: check for edema.
      - Length: bone, soft tissue length.
      - Shape: should be cylindrical or conical; check for abnormalities (i.e., bulbous end, dog ears, adductor roll).
   c. Vascular status of sound limb, residual limb: examine pulses, color, temperature, trophic changes, pain/intermittent claudication.
   d. AROM and PROM: examine for contractures that might interfere with prosthetic prescription (e.g., hip and knee flexion contractures).
   e. Sensation.
      - Proprioception, visual, vestibular function, contributions to balance; loss of proprioception in the amputated limb will necessitate a compensatory shift to the other senses for balance control.
      - Phantom limb sensation: a feeling of pressure or paresthesia as if coming from the amputated limb. Sensations are normal, not painful; may last for the lifetime of the individual.
      - Phantom pain: an intense burning or cramping pain; disabling, frequently interferes with rehabilitation.
   f. Strength: examine strength of residual limb as tolerated; strength of the sound limb, trunk, and upper extremities needed for function.
   g. Functional status.
      - Functional mobility skills: bed mobility, transfers, wheelchair use.
      - Activities of daily living: basic, instrumental (use of telephone, shopping, etc.).
   h. Cardiopulmonary function, endurance.
      - The shorter the amputation limb, the greater the energy demands; i.e., oxygen consumption is increased 65% over normal walking in the patient with transfemoral amputation; similar to fast walking in those without amputations for the patient with transtibial amputation.
      - Functional capacity further limited by: concomitant diseases (e.g., cardiovascular disease, diabetes), individual fitness level, pain.
   i. Neurologic factors.
      - Cognitive function.
      - Check for neuropathy.
      - Check for neuroma: an abnormal growth of nerve cells that occurs in the residual limb after amputation.
   j. Psychosocial factors: motivation, adjustment and acceptance, availability of support systems.
2. Preprosthetic training: goals and interventions.
   a. Ideally begins preoperatively and continues postoperatively.
   b. Facilitate psychological acceptance.
   c. Postoperative dressings: applied to the residual limb; helps to limit edema, accelerate healing, reduce postoperative pain, and shape the residual limb.
      - Elastic wraps: flexible, soft bandaging, inexpensive; requires frequent reapplication, with pressure greatest distal to proximal; if wraps are allowed to loosen, may have problems with edema control; avoid circular wrapping, which produces a tourniquet effect.
      - Stump shrinkers: flexible, soft, inexpensive, readily available in different sizes.
      - Semirigid dressings: Unna paste dressing (zinc oxide, gelatin, glycerin, and calamine); applied in the operating room.
      - Rigid dressings: plaster of Paris dressing; applied in the operating room; a component of immediate postoperative fitting; allows for edema reduction and early ambulation with a temporary prosthesis (pylon and foot). Good for young patients who are good candidates for a permanent prosthesis.
   d. Desensitizing activities: pressure, rubbing, stroking, bandaging of the residual limb.
   e. Hygiene: inspection and care of the residual limb.

> **RED FLAGS:** Positioning for prevention of contracture; positions to avoid include:
> - Transtibial: prolonged flexion and external rotation at the hip, knee flexion; counteract with use of a posterior board to keep knee straight while in wheelchair; regularly scheduled time in prone-lying.
> - Transfemoral: flexion, abduction, external rotation of hip; counteract with regularly scheduled time in prone-lying.

   f. Flexibility exercises.
      - Full AROM and PROM, active stretching, especially in hip and knee extension.
      - Flexibility of sound limb and trunk.
   g. Strengthening: utilize a general strengthening exercise program with special emphasis on:
      - Hip extensors: especially for the patient with transfemoral amputation.
      - Knee extensors: the patient with transtibial amputation.
      - Hip abductors: for stance phase pelvic stability.

- Dynamic exercises: utilize gravity and body weight to provide resistance during functional mat activities.
  h. Functional mobility training.
     - Sit-to-stand transitions, transfers, standing.
     - Wheelchair independence.
     - Hopping on the sound limb; mobility in the seated position; i.e., scooting for patients with bilateral transfemoral amputation.
     - Early walking with crutches or walker; consider early ambulation with a temporary prosthesis.
  i. Bilateral lower-extremity amputation.
     - Wheelchair training important. Will be primary means of locomotion.
     - Prolonged wheelchair time increases likelihood of hip and knee flexion contractures; prone positioning program is important.
     - Energy expenditure during prosthetic ambulation is increased dramatically; a trial period with temporary prostheses can be used to evaluate ambulation potential with permanent prostheses; especially useful with the elderly.
     - Bilateral transfemoral amputation: ambulation usually requires walker; loss of lower-extremity proprioception increases balance difficulties; loss of knee extensor function will result in significant later difficulties with stair-climbing, curbs, stepping.
     - Bilateral transfemoral amputation: patients can be fitted with shortened prostheses (stubbies) consisting of a socket and foot component (modified rocker feet) with no knee joints; increases ease of use and function; generally poor acceptance due to cosmesis.

Prosthetic Management

1. Prosthetic check-out.
   a. Prosthesis: delivered as ordered, proper functioning; inspect both on and off the patient.
   b. Static assessment.
      - Alignment and comfort in standing, sitting.
      - Leg length discrepancy: pelvis level.
      - Fit and suspension: pistoning when pelvis is lifted.
   c. Dynamic assessment.
      - Sit-to-stand transitions.
      - Gait: smooth, safe gait, absence of gait deviations; gait speeds normally decrease to reduce high levels of energy expenditure.
      - Stairs and inclines.

RED FLAGS: Inspection of the residual limb with the prosthesis off.
- Proper loading: transient redness is to be expected in pressure-tolerant areas after prosthetic use.
- No redness should be seen in pressure-sensitive areas.

2. Prosthetic training: goals and interventions.
   a. Donning and doffing of the prosthesis: training specific to type of socket and type of suspension.
   b. Strengthening, flexibility exercises.
      - Emphasis on hip extension and knee extension (transtibial) with the prosthesis on.
   c. Balance and coordination.
      - Symmetrical stance and weight bearing on prosthetic limb.
      - Weight shifting to limits of stability.
      - Dynamic balance control; e.g., stepping activities.
   d. Gait training.
      - Conventional training: focus on smooth weight transfer from sound limb to prosthetic limb, continuous movement sequence.
      - Biofeedback training: limb load devices to facilitate prosthetic weight acceptance.
      - Training with use of least restrictive assistive device; parallel bars may interfere with learning and independent ambulation in some patients.
   e. Functional activities training: including transfers, stairs, curbs, ramps, down and up from floor, recreational activities, etc.
   f. Regular inspection and maintenance of the prosthesis.
   g. Hygiene: care of stump socks, interior of the socket.
   h. Facilitate prosthetic acceptance.

Selected Prosthetic Gait Deviations

1. Transfemoral amputation. See Table 11-3.
   a. Circumduction: the prosthesis swings out to the side in an arc. Possible causes: a long prosthesis, locked knee, small or loose socket, inadequate suspension, foot plantar flexed, abduction contracture, poor knee control.
   b. Abducted gait: prosthesis is laterally displaced to the side. Possible causes: crotch or medial wall discomfort, long prosthesis, low lateral wall or malalignment, tight hip abductors.
   c. Vaulting: the patient rises up on the sound limb to swing the prosthesis through. Possible causes: prosthesis too long, inadequate suspension, socket too small, prosthetic foot set in too much plantarflexion, too little knee flexion.
   d. Lateral trunk bending during stance: the trunk bends toward the prosthetic side. Possible causes: low lateral wall, short prosthesis, high medial wall; weak abductors, abductor contracture, hip pain, short amputation limb.
   e. Forward flexion during stance: the trunk bends forward. Possible causes: unstable knee unit, short ambulatory aids, hip flexion contracture.
   f. Lumbar lordosis during stance: exaggeration of the lumbar curve. Possible causes: insufficient support from anterior or posterior walls, painful ischial

Table 11-3

Prosthetic Gait Analysis and Deviations

BELOW-KNEE AMPUTATIONS

PORTION OF PHASE	DEVIATION	PROSTHETIC CAUSES	ANATOMIC CAUSES
Initial contact (early stance)	Excessive knee flexion	High shoe heel; insufficient plantar flexion; stiff heel cushion; socket too far anterior; socket excessively flexed; cuff tabs too posterior	Flexion contracture; weak quadriceps
	Insufficient knee flexion	Low shoe heel; excessive plantar flexion; soft heel cushion; socket too far posterior; socket insufficiently flexed	Extensor hyperreflexia; weak quadriceps; anterodistal pain; arthritis
Mid stance	Excessive lateral thrust	Excessive foot inset	
	Excessive medial thrust	Excessive foot outset	
Late stance	Early knee flexion: drop off	High shoe heel; insufficient plantar flexion; keel too short; dorsiflexion stop too soft; socket too anterior; socket excessively flexed; cuff tabs too posterior	Flexion contracture
	Delayed knee flexion: walking up hill	Low shoe heel; excessive plantar flexion; keel too long; dorsiflexion stop too stiff; socket too posterior; socket not flexed enough	Extensor hyperreflexia

ABOVE-KNEE AMPUTATIONS

PHASE	DEVIATION	PROSTHETIC CAUSES	ANATOMIC CAUSES
Stance	Abduction	Long prosthesis; abducted hip joint; inadequate lateral wall adduction; sharp or high medial wall	Abduction contracture; weak abductors; laterodistal pain; instability
Swing	Circumduction	Long prosthesis; locked knee unit; loose friction; inadequate suspension; small socket; loose socket; foot plantar flexed	Abduction contracture; poor knee control
Stance	Lateral bend	Short prosthesis; inadequate lateral wall adduction; sharp or high medial wall	Abduction contracture; weak abductors; hip pain; instability; short amputation limb
Stance	Forward flexion	Unstable knee unit; short walker or crutches	
Stance	Lordosis	Inadequate socket flexion	Hip flexion contracture; weak extensors
Heel off	Medial (lateral) whip	Faulty socket contour; knee bolt externally (internally) rotated; foot malrotated; prosthesis donned in malrotation	With sliding friction unit; fast pace
Heel contact	Foot rotation	Stiff heel cushion; malrotated foot	
Early swing	High heel rise	Inadequate friction; slack extension aid	
Late swing	Terminal impact	Inadequate friction; taut extension aid	Forceful hip flexion
Swing	Vaulting	See above: circumduction	With sliding friction unit; fast pace
Swing	Hip hike	See above: circumduction	Hip flexion contracture
	Uneven step length	Uncomfortable socket; insufficient socket flexion	instability

weight bearing, hip flexion contracture, weak hip extensors or abdominals.

g. **High heel rise:** during early swing, the heel rises excessively. Possible causes: inadequate knee friction, too little tension in the extension aid.

h. **Terminal swing impact:** the prosthesis comes to a sudden stop as the knee extends during late swing. Possible causes: insufficient knee friction or too much tension in the extension aid; patient fears that the knee will buckle; forceful hip flexion.

i. **Swing phase whips:** at toe-off, the heel moves either medially or laterally. Possible causes: socket is rotated, knee bolt is rotated, foot is malaligned.

j. **Foot rotation at heel strike:** as the heel contacts the ground, the foot rotates laterally, sometimes with vibratory motion. Possible causes: foot is malaligned, stiff heel cushion, or plantar flexion bumper.

k. **Foot slap:** excessive plantar flexion at heel strike. Possible cause: heel cushion or plantar flexion bumper is too soft.

1. Uneven step length: patient favors sound limb and limits weight-bearing time on the prosthetic limb. Possible causes: socket discomfort or poor alignment; hip flexion contracture or hip instability.
2. Transtibial amputation.
    a. Excessive knee flexion during stance. Possible causes: socket may be aligned too far forward or tilted anteriorly; plantar flexion bumper is too hard and limits plantar flexion; high heel shoes; knee flexion contracture or weak quadriceps.
    b. Inadequate knee flexion during stance. Possible causes: socket may be aligned too far back or tilted posteriorly; plantar flexion bumper or heel cushion too soft; low heel shoes; anterodistal discomfort, weak quadriceps.
    c. Lateral thrust at midstance. Possible causes: foot is inset too much.
    d. Medial thrust at midstance. Possible causes: foot is outset too much.
    e. Drop off or premature knee flexion in late stance. Possible causes: socket is set too far forward or excessively flexed; dorsiflexion bumper is too soft, resulting in excess dorsiflexion of the foot; prosthetic foot keel too short; knee flexion contracture.
    f. Delayed knee flexion during late stance: patient feels as though walking "uphill." Possible causes: socket is set too far back or lacks sufficient flexion; dorsiflexion bumper is too stiff causing excess plantar flexion; prosthetic foot keel too long.

Wheelchairs

Components

Postural Support System

1. Seating.
    a. Sling seat: standard on wheelchairs. Hips tend to slide forward, thighs tend to adduct and internally rotate. Reinforces poor pelvic position (posterior pelvic tilt).
    b. Insert or contour seat creates a stable, firm sitting surface; made of wood or plastic, padded with foam.
        - Improves pelvic position (neutral pelvic position).
        - Reduces the tendency for the patient to slide forward or sit with a posterior pelvic tilt (sacral sitting).
    c. Seat cushion: distributes weight-bearing pressures. Assists in preventing decubitus ulcers in patients with decreased sensation, prolongs wheelchair sitting times.
        - Pressure-relieving, contoured foam cushion: uses dense, layered foam; accommodates moderate to severe postural deformity. Easy for caregivers to reposition patients, low maintenance. May interfere with slide transfers.
        - Pressure-relieving fluid/gel or combination cushion (fluid/gel plus foam). Can be custom-molded. Accommodates moderate to severe postural deformity. Easy for caregivers to reposition patients. Requires some maintenance, heavier, more expensive.
        - Pressure-relieving air cushion. Accommodates moderate to severe postural deformity. Lightweight, improved pressure distribution. Expensive, base may be unstable for some patients. Requires continuous maintenance.
    d. Adds to measurements to determine back height.

RED FLAG: Pressure relief activities are required, typically every 15–20 minutes (e.g., for the patient with SCI). Examples include wheelchair push-ups, lateral or forward leaning, tilt-in space, or reclining wheelchairs.

2. Back: support to the midscapular region is provided by most standard sling-back wheelchairs.
    a. Lower back height may increase functional mobility, i.e., sports chairs; may also increase back strain.
    b. High back height may be necessary for patients with poor trunk stability or with extensor spasms.
    c. Insert or contour backs: improve trunk extension and overall upright alignment.
    d. Lateral trunk supports: improve trunk alignment for patients with scoliosis, poor stability.
3. Armrests.
    a. Full-length or desk length; desk length facilitates use, proximity to a desk or table.
    b. Fixed-height or adjustable height; adjustable-height arm rests can be raised to facilitate sit-to-stand transfers.
    c. Removable armrests: facilitate transfers.
    d. Wraparound (space saver) armrests: reduce the overall width of the chair by 1½ inches.
    e. Upper extremity support surface (trays or troughs) can be secured to the armrests; provides additional postural assistance for patients with decreased use of upper extremities.

4. Leg rests.
   a. Fixed.
   b. Swing-away, detachable: facilitates ease in transfers, front approach to wheelchair when ambulating.
   c. Elevating: indicated for LE edema control, postural support; contraindicated for patients with knee flexor (hamstring) hypertonicity or tightness.
5. Footrests.
   a. Footplates: provide a resting base for feet, feet are neutral with knees flexed to 90 degrees; footplates can be raised or removed to facilitate transfers.
   b. Heel loops: help maintain foot position, prevent posterior sliding of the foot.
   c. Straps (ankle, calf): can be added to stabilize the feet on the foot plates.

Wheeled Mobility Base

1. Frame.
   a. Fixed or folding.
      - Folding facilitates mobility in the community, ease of storage.
      - Rigid frame facilitates stroke efficiency; increases distance per stroke.
   b. Available in heavy-duty, standard, lightweight, active-duty lightweight, ultra-lightweight construction.
      - In general, the lighter the weight of the frame, the greater the ease of use.
      - Level of expected activity and environment should be taken into account when deciding on frame construction.
2. Wheels, handrims.
   a. Casters: small front wheels, typically 8 inches in diameter; caster locks can be added to facilitate wheelchair stability during transfers.
   b. Drive wheels: large rear wheels used for propulsion; outer rims allow for hand grip and propulsion.
      - Projections may be attached to the rims (vertical, oblique, or horizontal) to facilitate propulsion in patients with poor handgrip, e.g., quadriplegia; horizontal or oblique projections widen the chair and may limit maneuvering in the home.
      - Friction rims/leather gloves: increase handgrip friction, ease of propulsion in patients with poor handgrip.
      - Construction of drive wheels: standard spokes or spokeless wheels.
3. Tires.
   a. Standard hard rubber tires: durable, low maintenance.
   b. Pneumatic (air-filled) tires: provide a smoother ride, increased shock absorption; require more maintenance.
4. Brakes.
   a. Most brakes consist of a lever system with a cam.
   b. Brakes must be engaged for all transfers in and out of chair.
   c. Extensions may be added to increase ease in both locking and unlocking; e.g., for upper extremity weakness, arthritis.
5. Additional attachments.
   a. Seat belts (pelvic positioner): belt should grasp over the pelvis at a 45-degree angle to the seat.
   b. Seat positioners: can add lateral positioners at hip and knee or medial positioner at knee (adductor pommel) to maintain alignment of lower extremities, control for spasticity; seat wedge or tilt-in-space seat can be used for extensor spasms or thrusting.
   c. Seat back positioners: can add lateral trunk positioners to maintain alignment, control for scoliosis.
   d. Antitipping device: a posterior extension attached to the lower horizontal supports, prevents tipping backward in the chair; also limits going up curbs or over door sills.
   e. Hill-holder device: a mechanical brake that allows the chair to go forward, but automatically brakes when the chair goes in reverse; useful for patients who are not able to ascend a long ramp or hill without a rest.

Specialized Wheelchairs

1. Reclining back: indicated for patients who are unable to independently maintain upright sitting position.
   a. Reclining wheelchairs include an extended back and typically elevating leg rests; head and trunk supports may also be added.
   b. Electric reclining back helps to redistribute weight bearing if patient cannot do active push-ups or pressure-relief maneuvers.
2. Tilt-in-space: motorized; entire seat and back may be tipped backward (normal seat to back angle is maintained); indicated for patients with extensor spasms that may throw the patient out of the chair, or for pressure relief.
3. One-arm drive: drive mechanisms are located on one wheel, usually with two outer rims (or by push lever); patient propels the wheelchair by pushing on both rims (or lever with one hand); difficult for some patients to use, e.g., patients with left hemiplegia, cognitive/perceptual impairments.
4. Hemiplegic chair (hemi chair): designed to be low to the ground, allowing propulsion with the noninvolved upper and lower extremities.
5. Amputee chair: wheelchair is modified by placing the drive wheels posterior to the vertical back supports (2 inches backward); increases the length of the base of support and posterior stability; prescribed for patients with bilateral lower-extremity amputations, whose center of gravity is now located more posterior when seated in the wheelchair.
6. Powered wheelchair: utilizes a power source (battery) to propel the wheelchair; prescribed for patients who are not capable of self-propulsion or who have very low endurance.

a. Microprocessors allow the control of the wheelchair to be adapted to various controls; i.e., joystick, head controls.
b. Proportional drives: changes in pressure on the control result in directly corresponding changes in speeds.
c. Microswitching systems: speed is preset; controls turn system on and off; i.e., puff-n-sip tubes for individuals with quadriplegia.
7. Bariatric wheelchair: heavy-duty, extra-wide wheelchair designed to assist mobility in individuals who are obese.
 a. Selection based on patient characteristics, safety, and function.
 b. The bariatric client has a center of body mass that is positioned several inches forward compared to the normal-sized person.
  - In order to ensure wheelchair stability, the rear axle is displaced forward compared to the standard wheelchair.
  - This forward position allows for a more efficient arm push (full-arm stroke with less wrist extension).
 c. Bariatric wheelchair can be ordered with special adaptations:
  - Hard tires versus pneumatic tires for increased durability.
  - Adjustable backrest to accommodate excessive posterior bulk.
  - Specially made seat cushions can be found to accommodate patients up to 650 pounds.
  - Reclining wheelchair to accommodate excessive anterior bulk, cardiorespiratory compromise.
  - Power application attached to a heavy duty wheelchair to accommodate excessive fatigue.
8. Sports wheelchair: variable; generally includes lightweight, solid frame, low seat, low back, seat that accommodates a tucked position, leg straps, slanted drive wheels, small push rims.

Wheelchair Measurements

General Concepts
1. Overall, the size of the wheelchair must be proportional to the size of the patient and take into account the demands of expected use and the environment in which the chair will be used.
2. Assessments should be taken with the patient on a firm surface (seated or supine).

Six Key Measurements
1. Seat width.
 a. Measurement on the patient: width of the hips at the widest part.
 b. Chair measurement: add 2 inches to the patient's measurement.
 c. Potential problems.
  - Excessive width of the wheelchair will result in added difficulties in reaching the drive wheels and propelling the chair.
  - Wheelchair width should accommodate width of doorways; can use a narrowing device; requires coordination to turn the cranking device.
  - A wheelchair that is too narrow will result in pressure/discomfort on the lateral pelvis and thighs; lateral space should allow for changes in the thickness of clothing.
 d. The bariatric client with a pear shape will have increased gluteal femoral weight distribution. Measurement should consider the widest portion of the seated position (e.g., at the forward edge of the seated position). Also consider room for weight-shifting maneuvers for pressure relief, and possible use of lift devices.
2. Seat depth.
 a. Measurement on the patient: posterior buttock to the posterior aspect of the lower leg in the popliteal fossa.
 b. Chair measurement: subtract 2–3 inches from the patient's measurement.
 c. Potential problems.
  - Seat depth that is too short fails to support the thigh adequately.
  - Seat depth that is too long may compromise posterior knee circulation or result in a kyphotic posture, posterior tilting of pelvis and sacral sitting.
3. Leg length/seat to footplate length.
 a. Measurement on the patient: from the bottom of the shoe (customary footwear) to just below the thigh in the popliteal fossa; when a seat cushion is used, the height must be subtracted from the patient's measurement.
 b. Potential problems.
  - Excessive leg length will encourage sacral sitting and sliding forward in the chair.
  - Length that is too short will create uneven weight distribution on thigh and excessive weight on the ischial seat.
4. Seat height.
 a. No patient measurement.
 b. Chair measurement: minimum clearance between the floor and the footplate is 2 inches, measured from the lowest point on the bottom of the footplate.
 c. Add 2 inches to the patient's leg length measurement.
5. Arm rest height (hanging elbow height).
 a. Measurement on the patient: from the seat platform to just below the elbow held at 90 degrees with the shoulder in neutral position.
 b. Chair measurement: add 1 inch to the patient's hanging elbow measurement.

c. Potential problems.
- Armrests that are too high will cause shoulder elevation.
- Armrests that are too low will encourage leaning forward.

6. Back height: height will vary depending upon the amount of support the patient needs.
   a. Measurement on the patient: from the seat platform to the lower angle of the scapula, midscapula, top of shoulder, based on the degree of support desired.
   b. If the patient plans to use a seat cushion, the height of the cushion must be added to the patient's measurement.
   c. Potential problems.
      - Added back height may increase difficulty in getting the chair into a car or van.
      - Added back height may also prevent the patient from hooking onto the push handle for stabilization and weight relief; e.g., the patient with quadriplegia.

Standard Dimensions

1. Custom-made wheelchairs add significantly to the cost of a wheelchair. See Table 11-4.
2. Whenever possible, patients should be matched to standardized chairs.

Wheelchair Training

Basic Instruction

1. Many first-time users require instruction on the use and care of a wheelchair.
2. Instruct in good sitting posture and pressure relief.
   a. Instruct in use of wheelchair cushion: care and maintenance, schedule of use (whenever sitting); limitations of cushion.
   b. Instruct in periodic pressure reliefs: arm push-ups; weight shifts (leaning to one side then other, forward bending).

Table 11-4

Standard Wheelchair Dimensions (In Inches)

CHAIR STYLE	SEAT WIDTH	SEAT DEPTH	SEAT HEIGHT
Adult	18	16	20
Narrow adult	16	16	20
Slim adult	14	16	20
Hemi/low seat			17.5
Junior	16	16	18.5
Child	14	11.5	18.75
Tiny tot	12	11.5	19.5

Wheelchair Propulsion

1. Instruct in manual wheelchair propulsion.
   a. Both arms on drive (push) wheels, one arm on drive wheel/one foot pulls diagonally across floor under chair (e.g., the patient with hemiplegia), or one arm (one-arm drive, both outer rims located on one side).
   b. Propulsion: forward/backward, flat surfaces, uneven surfaces.
   c. Turning: pushing harder with one hand than other; sharp turning: pull one wheel backward while pushing other wheel forward.
   d. Negotiation of obstacles.
2. Power chair training: focus on driving skill and safety; instruct in use of switches (on/off, turns), joystick; maneuverability, safe stopping.

Wheelchair Management

1. Instruct in use of wheel locks (brakes), foot supports (foot plate, leg rest), elevation of leg rests, and arm rests.
2. Instruct in routine maintenance of wheelchair; normal cleaning and maintenance, power chair (battery) maintenance.

Community Mobility

1. Ramps.
   a. Ascending: forward lean of head and trunk, use shorter strokes; move hands quickly for propulsion.
   b. Descending ramps: grip hand rims loosely, control chair's descent; or descend in wheelie position (steep ramp).
2. Wheelies: instruct in how to "pop a wheelie" in order to negotiate curbs; the patient learns how to come up onto and balance on the rear wheels with the front casters off the ground (e.g., the patient with paraplegia).
   a. Practice maintaining balance point in wheelie position (therapist tips chair back into position).
   b. Practice moving into wheelie position: patient places hands well back on hand rims; then pulls (moves) them forward abruptly and forcefully. The head and trunk are moved forward to keep from going over backward. Use lightweight wheelchair to facilitate training.
   c. Balancing in wheelie position: chair tips further back when wheels are pushed forward; chair tips toward upright when wheels are pulled back.
   d. Practice curb ascent: place the front casters up on the curb, the patient then pushes rear wheels up curb; momentum used to assist.
   e. Practice curb descent: descending backward with forward head and trunk lean; descending forward in wheelie position.
3. Practice ascending/descending stairs: in wheelchair, on buttocks.
4. Instruct in how to fall safely, return to wheelchair.
5. Instruct in how to transfer into a car, place wheelchair inside car by pulling wheelchair behind the car seat, or to use a wheelchair lift (van-equipped).

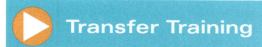
Transfer Training

Dependent Transfers

General Concept
1. Depend transfers require minimal or no active participation by the patient/client

Dependent Lift Transfer ("Quad-Pivot" Transfer)
1. Wheelchair is positioned parallel to surface.
2. Patient is flexed forward at hips in tucked position with hips and knees flexed.
3. Therapist locks patient's tucked knees between legs; places one hand under buttocks and one hand on transfer belt.
4. Patient is rocked forward and lifted using a backward weight shift with therapist in a semisquat position.
5. Therapist then pivots using small steps and gently lowers patient to support surface.

Depend Stand-Pivot Transfer
1. Similar to above except the patient's lower extremities are extended and in contact with floor.

Hydraulic Lift Transfer
1. Positioning and widening of the base of device is critical to stability and safety while using the device.

Assisted Transfers

General Concepts
1. Requires some participation by patient; levels of assistance include stand-by, minimal, moderate, or maximal assistance.
2. Includes verbal cueing or manual assistance for lift, support, or balance control.
3. Transfer belts, trapeze bars, overhead loops can be used to provide additional control.

Assisted Stand-Pivot Transfer
1. Used for patients who are unable to stand independently and can bear some weight on lower extremities (e.g., patients with cerebrovascular accident [CVA], incomplete SCI, hip fracture/replacement).
2. Wheelchair is placed parallel to surface (on the patient's sound or stronger side).
3. Therapist can block out one or both of the patient's knees to provide stability; support can be added by placing both hands on the patient (on both buttocks, both on upper back, or one on buttock/one on upper back).
4. Patient rocks forward and pushes up into standing.
5. Therapist assists patient with forward weight shift and standing, pivoting toward chair, and controlled lowering toward the support surface.
6. Variation: assisted squat-pivot transfer for patients who are unable to stand fully; e.g., with marked weakness in both lower extremities.

Assisted Transfer Using a Sliding Board
1. Used for patients with good sitting balance who can lift most but not all of weight of buttocks; e.g., patients with complete level C5 SCI.
2. Wheelchair is placed parallel to surface.
3. Patient moves forward in chair and board is placed well under buttocks.
4. Patient performs transfer by doing a series of push-ups and lifts along board.
5. Therapist assists in lift (hands on buttocks, on transfer belt, or one on buttock/one on belt).
6. Care must be taken not to pinch fingers under board or drag/traumatize skin.
7. Feet can remain on foot pedals or be positioned on the floor.
8. Patients with complete level C6 SCI can be independent with transfer board on level surfaces.

Sit-Pivot (Squat-Pivot)
1. Used for patients with good sitting balance who can lift buttocks clear of sitting surface; can be a progression in transfer training from using a transfer board.
2. The patient with complete C7 SCI can be independent in transfers without a sliding board.
3. The patient utilizes the head-hips relationship to successfully complete the transfer (movement of head in one direction results in movement of hips in the opposite direction/toward the support surface being transferred to).

Training

Practice
1. In and out of bed.
2. In and out of wheelchair.
   a. Level surfaces.
   b. Unlevel surfaces: to floor.
3. On and off toilet, tub seat.
4. In and out of car.

Instructions
1. Inform patient about the transfer, as well as expectations for the patient.
2. Synchronize actions using commands and counts.
3. Reduce assistance as appropriate.

Bariatric Specific Equipment

Equipment

Beds
1. Mechanized beds for ease of use.
   a. Includes ability to raise/lower entire bed, convert to a chair, move into Trendelenburg's, and reverse Trendelenburg's positions.
   b. Often include a built-in scale to easily weigh patient/client.
2. Mattress may be low-air-loss or air suspension. Contains several segmented bladders or compartments that are individually controlled for air pressure per patient needs (skin condition, mobility level, weight, etc.).
   a. If cardiopulmonary resuscitation becomes necessary, a rigid board must be inserted between the patient and the mattress to ensure a firm surface.
3. Designed to accommodate weights of 300–1000 pounds.
   a. Bariatric beds are heavier than typical hospital beds.

Wheelchairs
1. See wheelchairs section above.

Stretcher Chair
1. Mechanized (typically) chair utilized to position the patient into a sitting position.
2. Typically built to support up to 1000 pounds, is up to 40 inches in width, and comes with adjustable footrests.
3. A supine transfer technique may be used to transfer the patient/client to the stretcher chair.

Treatment Tables
1. Specialized treatment tables provide additional features to assist in the safe handling and management of patients during therapy sessions.
2. Features include: built-in transfer bars, adjustable and motorized back support (including head supports), and seat belts.

Assistive Devices for Transferring

Safety
1. Utilize transfer assist devices to help improve patient and healthcare worker safety.
2. When safe and practical, as with any other functional activity, instruct the patient/client to assist as able.
3. Follow principles of body mechanics for safe, effective transfer techniques.
4. Seek assistance from other healthcare providers to assist with transfers and equipment management.
   a. Follow general rules for multi-person assist transfer by assigning the "lead" person to direct the transfer activities and instruct the patient/client.

Bed Transfer Devices
1. Supine sliding board: used to bridge the gap between surfaces that are relatively similar in height; device helps to decrease tissue pressures on the patient/client.
   a. Note that sitting sliding board transfers are not recommended for this population due to the potential for tissue damage and difficulty maintaining position of the board.
   b. Transfer sheets may be used to accomplish this same transfer; however, they do not bridge the gap between surfaces and pose some risk for tissue damage.
2. Air mattress transfer system: specially designed air mattress is placed under the patient/client for a supine, lateral sliding transfer.
   a. The mattress has many small perforations on the underside that continuously release air when inflated and hooked to an airflow system. This reduces friction between the surface of the air mattress and bedding, thus decreasing effort needed to complete the transfer.
   b. Some may be manufactured to be radiolucent to allow for magnetic resonance imaging (MRI) or x-ray.
3. Bedside sling mechanical lift, floor-based unit: mechanical sling lift used to transfer the patient from bed to/from chair. The sling lift used to transfer the bariatric patient/client should meet these requirements.
   a. Lift capacity sufficient for the patient/client weight.
   b. Base expandable to meet the width of a bariatric chair.
   c. Sufficient clearance under the bariatric bed (typically 6 inches or less).
   d. Single spreader bar of 30 inches; quadrapoint spreader bar of 25 inches point-to-point.
   e. Lift boom to allow sufficient clearance and rotation of the patient.
   f. Two persons should be utilized to rotate the patient/client for the transfer and an additional person to maneuver the lift.

Standing Pole
1. A pole affixed to the floor and ceiling used by the patient/client to hang onto to help pull self into a standing position.

Lift Devices

Standing Lift Device
1. Secures the feet and legs of the patient/client while positioning the upper body weight over the blocked lower extremities.
2. Note the device does not allow for the lower extremity abduction deformity found in some patients/clients in the bariatric population.
3. The device is contraindicated if weight bearing status is limited.

Ceiling Mounted Lift
1. Installed directly into the ceiling and/or building supports.
2. Allows for greater lift capacities and does not pose the risk for tipping over as the bedside mechanical lift does.
3. Disadvantage: they are not portable between patients/clients and can only be used at the location where they are installed.

Overhead A-Frame Lift Device
1. A portable lift device that fits over the bed with its support on the floor.
2. Device is portable from department to department; some models can accommodate patients up to 1000 pounds.
3. Disadvantages: it requires sufficient clearance around the bed.
4. Advantages: lift capacities are virtually unlimited, maintenance is minimal, has the ability to lower the patient below floor height (e.g., lower into a walking pool).

Facility Modifications

Elevators
1. Must be of sufficient load-bearing capacities.
2. Must be of sufficient width to accommodate beds and additional equipment necessary to transport and care for the patient/client.

Toilets
1. Should be floor mounted models versus wall-hung models (wall-hung models are only typically installed to support approximately 300 pounds).

Medical Test Equipment
1. MRI scanners must be of appropriate size.
2. Computed tomographic (CT) scanners or tables, etc., must be of sufficient load-bearing and width to accommodate the bariatric population.

Building
1. Buildings must be built with floor load capacities sufficient to support the patient/client as well as the devices utilized in care.

Environmental Considerations

Environmental Modification

Purpose
1. Assess degree of safety, function, and comfort of the patient in the home, community, and work environments.
2. Provide recommendations to ensure a barrier-free environment, greatest level of functional independence.

Standard Adult Wheelchair Dimensions for Environmental Access
1. Width: 24–26 inches from rim to rim.
2. Length: 42–43 inches.
3. Height (push handles to floor): 36 inches.
4. Height (armrest to floor): 29–30 inches.
5. Footrests may extend for very large people.
6. 360 degrees turning space = 60 inches × 60 inches.
7. 90 degrees turning space = minimum of 36 inches.
8. Minimum clear width for doorways and halls = 32 inches; ideal is 36 inches.
9. High forward reach = maximum of 48 inches from floor; low forward reach = a minimum of 15 inches from the floor.
10. Side reach = maximum of 24 inches.

Home
1. Entrance: accessible; stairs with handrail, ramp, platform to allow for ease of door opening.
2. Floors: nonskid surface, carpeting securely fastened; no scatter rugs.

3. Furniture arrangement: should allow sufficient room to maneuver easily; e.g., with wheelchair, or ambulation with assistive device.
4. Doors: thresholds should be flush or level (no doorsills); standard door width is 32 inches; outside door swing area requires a minimum of 18 inches for walkers and 26 inches for wheelchairs.
5. Stairs: uniform riser heights (7 inches high) with a tread depth (a minimum of 11 inches); handrails, recommended height is 32 inches, ½ to 2 inches in diameter; nonslip surface; well lighted; color code with warm colors (red, orange, yellow) if visual impairments exist.
6. Bedroom: furniture arrangement for easy maneuverability; a minimum of 3 feet on side of bed for wheelchair transfers; firm mattress, stable bed, sufficient height to facilitate sit-to-stand transfers; phone accessibility; appropriate height for wall switches is 36–48 inches; outlets a minimum of 18 inches above the floorboard.
7. Bathroom: optimal toilet seat height is 17–19 inches; tub seat, nonskid tub surface or mat; grab bars securely fastened; optimal height of horizontal grab bars is 33–36 inches.
8. Kitchen: appropriate height of countertops, for wheelchair users no higher than 31 inches; counter depth of at least 24 inches; accessible equipment and storage areas.

Community/Workplace
1. Steps: recommended height is 7–9 inches.
2. Ramps: recommended ratio of slope to rise is 1:12 (for every inch of vertical rise, 12 inches of ramp is required); minimum of 36 inches wide, with nonslip surface; handrail waist high for ambulators (34–38 inches) and should extend 12 inches beyond the top and bottom of runs; ramp should have level landing at top and bottom.
3. Parking (handicapped parking): parking space with adjacent 4-foot aisle for wheelchair maneuverability; accessible within a short distance of buildings; curb cutouts.
4. Building entrance: accessible; accessible elevator.
5. Access to public telephones, drinking fountains, bathrooms.
6. Ergonomic assessment of immediate work area: appropriate lighting, temperature, seating surface, height and size of work counter.
7. Public transportation: accessible.

Acknowledgments: Gerard Dybel

APPENDIX 11A

Ergonomics

THOMAS BIANCO

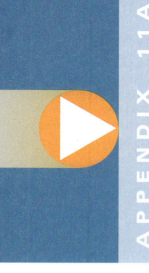

Ergonomics

Definitions
1. Ergonomics is the science of fitting workplace conditions and job demands to the capabilities of the working population.
2. Work demands: determine the physical demands of work tasks including lifting weights, distances, tools used, production levels, and work schedules.
3. Work capacity: objective assessment of worker's current level of ability to perform the physical demands of a specific identified job.

General Concepts
1. Purpose of ergonomics is to assure high productivity, avoid injury and illness risks, and increase satisfaction among workforce.
2. Ergonomics uses scientific and engineering principles to improve the safety, efficiency, and quality of movements involved in work.
3. Ergonomics programs should focus on making the job fit the person.

Hazard Control and Prevention
1. General concepts: common risk factors for musculoskeletal disorders (MSDs) include awkward postures, forceful exertions, repetitive motions, duration, contact stresses, vibration, and workplace conditions (e.g., temperature, machine pace, insufficient breaks).
2. Administrative controls: changes in the way that work is assigned or scheduled to reduce the magnitude, frequency, or duration of exposure to ergonomic risk factors (e.g., job rotation).
3. Engineering controls: reduce the risk of injury by design or modifications of workstations, work methods, and tools to reduce exposure to ergonomic risk factors (e.g., adding lift tables to a workstation).
4. Work style controls: train workers in the recognition of risk factors and instruct in work practices that decrease demands of work tasks.
5. Personal protective equipment (PPE): wrist supports, back belts, or anti-vibration gloves may be effective at reducing risk of injury. Other PPE equipment include respirators, earplugs, safety goggles, hard hats, and safety shoes and are worn to provide a barrier between the worker and the hazard source.
6. Evaluating control effectiveness: follow-up evaluation is needed to ensure that the controls reduced or eliminated the ergonomic risk factors and that no new risk factors were introduced.

Primary Prevention of Occupational Injury
1. Evaluate tasks and workstations to determine biomechanical stresses.
2. Redesign high-risk tasks to ensure that stresses on joints and muscles do not lead to injury.

3. Change workstation layouts to reduce postural stresses.
4. Assess awkward postures to eliminate fatigue and cumulative trauma.
5. Assess highly repetitive manual assembly operations to identify the risk of disorders such as tendinitis, epicondylitis, and carpal tunnel syndrome.
6. Educate workers and managers to increase their awareness of ergonomic prevention.

Role of the Physical Therapist and Physical Therapist Assistant in Occupational Health

Physical Therapist Role: Examination of Employee
1. Work-related injuries and impairments.
2. Functional limitations of employee.
3. Disability (if unable to find reasonable accommodations).
4. Other health-related conditions that prevent individuals from performing work-related tasks.
5. Determine diagnosis, prognosis, and intervention related to work injury and other medical conditions.

Integration of Injury Prevention and General Health and Wellness Programs Into the Consultation, Screening, and Education of Employees

Management of the Acutely Injured Worker
1. Manage lost time and minimize disability.
2. Optimize work capacity while reducing risk of further injury.
3. Assist employee participation in on-site productive light duty program that is appropriate for limitations.
4. Encourage employers to make accommodations to normal duty or provide alternative or transitional duty work.

Management of Work-Related Musculoskeletal Disorders (WMSDs)
1. Diagnose WMSDs and apply interventions to specific tissues affected by injury.
2. Determine safe work activity that will not compromise medical condition.
3. Design safe, progressive rehabilitation program based on worker job demands and within functional and medical limitations of worker.
4. Minimize lost work time with aggressive clinical management and promotion of productive work.

Facilitation of Timely and Appropriate Referrals
1. Monitor signs, symptoms, and medical progress to determine if necessary referrals should be facilitated.
2. Work interdependently with occupational physicians and other health care providers to move worker through employer health care system.

Minimization of Injury/Re-Injury Incident Rate
1. Make ergonomic recommendations for workstation design and worker training regarding specific WMSD.
2. Early intervention for workers with potentially disabling WMSD (e.g., carpal tunnel surgery).
3. Participate in a comprehensive team for the timely dissemination of information including physician, physical therapist, employer representative, safety management, and injured worker.

Phases of Physical Therapy Intervention
1. Admission to a specific phase of care is based on the physical therapy examination, diagnosis, and prognosis of the worker's functional and medical status.
2. Progression from one phase to the next is based on objective, functional tests, and measurements. Duration of treatment is influenced by the level of physical activity required by the job and if a reasonable accommodation is not available.
   a. Acute phase: immediate post-trauma, focuses on control and reduction of localized inflammation, joint or soft tissue restriction, and stabilization of injury.
   b. Post-acute: involve injured worker in functional activities and training to increase ability to perform work-related tasks.
   c. Reconditioning phase: increase intensity of functional activities and exercises and emphasis on work-simulated activities to increase endurance.
   d. Return-to-work phase: if worker is not capable of return to work due to physical, functional, behavioral, or vocational deficits, then complete a functional capacity evaluation before entry into this phase.

Functional Capacity Evaluation (FCE)

Purpose
1. To objectively determine the intensity and duration of work that a patient is capable of safely performing.

Uses
1. Return to work and job placement decisions.
2. Disability evaluation.
3. Determination of work function with non-work-related and work-related injuries.
4. Determination of functional level in nonoccupational settings.
5. Intervention and treatment planning for work conditioning or work hardening.
6. Determination of possible job modifications.
7. Case management and case closure.

Definition
1. A detailed examination and evaluation that objectively measures the worker's current level of function within the context of competitive employment demands.
2. Measurements of the FCE are compared to the physical demands of a job or other functional activity.

FCE Protocols
1. Most common FCEs are 4–6 hours long and objectively measure work demands such as lifting, carrying, walking, bending, overhead work, and hand coordination.
2. FCEs replicate work tasks in order to find realistic values for the return to work statement needed to conclude the rehabilitation process.
3. Work Capacity Evaluations (WCEs) are job-specific tests and measures applied consistently to workers with reference to a specific job.

Definitions of Work Intensity
1. Sedentary: up to 10 lbs. of force occasionally, negligible weight frequently or constantly, 1.5–2.1 METS.
2. Light: up to 20 lbs. occasionally, 10 lbs. frequently, negligible weight constantly, 2.2–3.5 METS.
3. Medium: up to 50 lbs. occasionally, 20 lbs. frequently, 10 lbs. constantly, 3.6–6.3 METS.
4. Heavy: up to 100 lbs. occasionally, 50 lbs. frequently, 20 lbs. constantly, 6.4–7.5 METS.
5. Very heavy: > 100 lbs. occasionally, > 50 lbs. frequently, > 20 lbs. constantly, > 7.5 METS.

Definitions of Work Frequency
1. Never.
2. Occasionally: up to one third of the work day.
3. Frequently: from one third to two thirds of the work day.
4. Constantly: greater than two thirds of the work day.

Work Conditioning and Work Hardening Programs

Definitions
1. Work conditioning programs.
   a. Intensive, work-related, goal-oriented conditioning programs.
   b. Designed specifically to restore systemic neuromusculoskeletal functions, muscle performance, motor function, ROM, and cardiovascular/pulmonary functions.
2. Work hardening programs.
   a. Highly structured, goal-oriented, individualized intervention programs designed to return the patient/client to work.
   b. Multidisciplinary programs that use real and simulated work activities designed to restore physical, behavioral, and vocational functions.

Program Content
1. Work conditioning.
   a. Requires work conditioning examination and evaluation.
   b. Utilizes work conditioning and functional activities related to work.
   c. Provide multihour sessions of up to 4 hours/day, 5 days/week, 8 weeks.
   d. Addresses physical and functional needs provided by one discipline.
2. Work hardening.
   a. Requires work hardening examination and evaluation.
   b. Utilizes real or simulated work activities.
   c. Provided in multihour sessions of up to 8 hours/day, 5 days/week, 8 weeks.
   d. Addresses physical, functional, behavioral, and vocational needs within a multidisciplinary model.

Manual Material Handling and Lifting Limits

Factors Affecting "Safe" Load Lifting
1. Biomechanical factors.
   a. Greatest biomechanical stressors and the largest moments during lifting occur in the lumbar spine, specifically the L5-S1 disc.
   b. Disc compressive forces, shear forces, and torsional forces are believed to be largely responsible for vertebral end-plate fractures, disc herniations, and nerve root irritation.

c. The weight of the load and the distance from the load to the base of the spine are significant contributors to lumbosacral compressive and shear forces when using either a squat or stooped lifting posture.
2. Physiological factors.
   a. The worker's ability to perform dynamic, repetitive lifting is limited by his or her maximal aerobic capacity.
   b. Repetitive lifting tasks could exceed the worker's normal energy capacities, which decrease strength and increase the risk of injury.
   c. Age, gender, and physical conditioning may affect a worker's ability to perform repetitive lifting.
   d. Lifting from floor to knuckle height requires greater whole-body work, although performing lifts above waist height requires greater shoulder and arm muscle work.
3. Psychophysical factors.
   a. The maximal acceptable weight of lift defines what a person can lift repeatedly for an extended period of time without excessive fatigue.
   b. The psychophysical approach provides a means of estimating the combined effects of biomechanical and physiological stressors on manual lifting.

Guidelines for Seated Work

Definition
1. Sitting transfers body weight to supporting areas.
   a. Seat pan through ischial tuberosities.
   b. Backrest through soft tissues.
   c. Armrests through forearms.
   d. Floor.
2. Sitting posture varies with the design of the chair and the task being performed.
   a. Lumbar spine posture during sitting.
   b. Pelvis rotates posteriorly and lumbar spine flattens when moving from standing to unsupported sitting.
   c. Knee and hip angles control spinal posture during sitting, caused by the insertion of various muscles on the pelvis and legs.
3. Lumbar disc pressure during sitting.
   a. Compression forces measured at L3 disc: pressures measured with the subject standing are about 35% lower than the pressure measured when the subject is sitting without support.
   b. Use of a lumbar support decreases lumbar disc pressure.
   c. Backward inclination of the backrest from 90°–110° results in decreased lumbar disc pressure.
   d. Decreased disc pressure when arm rests were used.
4. Chair dimensions for seated work.
   a. Chair height: sufficient to allow the feet to be placed firmly on the floor or a foot support.
   b. Knee flexion angle is 90° with the popliteal fold about 2–3 cm (0.8–1.2 in) above the seat surface. If too low, there is excessive knee flexion, the spine is flexed, and the pelvis is posteriorly rotated. If too high, the feet do not reach the floor and there is excessive pressure on the back of the thighs.
   c. Chair length/depth: the seat pan should provide 10 cm clearance from the popliteal fossa to allow for leg movement and prevent pressure on the back of the knees.
   d. Seat pan slope: a backward slope of 5° is suggested for normal, upright sitting.
   e. Arm rest height: the elbow should be flexed to 90° and the shoulder should be in neutral position.

Review Questions

Functional Training, Equipment, and Devices

1. Identify and describe three different pelvis motions that occur during normal gait.

2. What function does an anterior stop of an ankle foot orthosis (AFO) serve?

3. Describe how applying tape to an injured ligament and joint differs from taping the same uninjured ligament or joint.

4. Contrast the terms *pressure-tolerant* and *pressure-sensitive* areas as they relate to a residual limb. Identify pressure-tolerant and pressure-sensitive areas for transtibial and transfemoral residual limbs.

5. Identify three drawbacks to a sling seat in a wheelchair.

6. What dimensions should a clinician recommend to a family member building a ramp for a front door entrance of a residence that has two 8-inch steps out front?

12
Teaching and Learning

KAREN E. RYAN

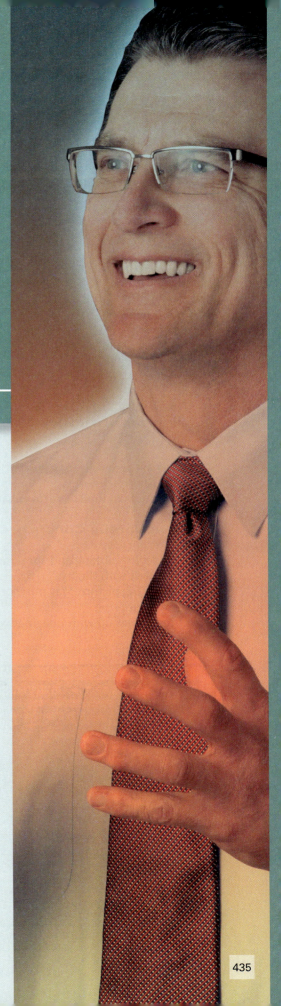

Chapter Outline

- Educational Theories, 436
  - Learning Styles, 436
  - Active vs. Passive Learning, 436
  - Learning Theories, 436
  - Educational Concepts, 437
- Instruction, 437
  - Instructional Process, 437
  - Instructional Activities, 438
  - Instruction Modes, 438
  - Implementation of Instruction, 439
- Motor Learning, 440
  - Description, 440
  - Phases of Motor Learning, 440
  - Implications for Intervention or Instruction, 442
  - Assessment of Performance/Learning, 442
- Communication, 443
  - Verbal, 443
  - Nonverbal, 443
  - Effective Communication Strategies, 444
  - Speech/Language Disorders, 444
  - Treatment Considerations with Aphasia, 445
- Review Questions, 446

Educational Theories

Learning Styles

Description
1. A preferred method (or style) by which an individual attains knowledge and processes it into new meaningful information.

Kinesthetic Learner
1. Learns by doing.
2. Prefers to have "hands-on" experiences.
3. "Touch" helps enhance the learning experience.

Visual Learner
1. Prefers use of the following.
   a. Diagrams.
   b. Maps.
   c. Pictures to enhance the learning experience.
2. Written or spoken words will have less significance without visual aids.

Auditory Learner
1. Prefers to take in information that is heard, versus read.
2. May read text out loud to self to enhance understanding.

Intuitive Versus Concrete Learner
1. Intuitive.
   a. Abstract in thinking and speaking.
   b. Deals well with theory.
   c. Sees the big picture. May miss, or doesn't deal with, the details.
   d. Often comes up with imaginative solutions.
2. Concrete.
   a. Prefers details, specifics, and set patterns.
   b. Does not deal well with theoretical information.
   c. Sees things as black or white, not gray.
   d. Solutions will be less imaginative.

Active vs. Passive Learning

Both active/independent and passive/dependent learning styles are valuable tools for learning. Neither learning style is better than the other, and in fact, a combination of the two may prove best to help the learner retain and apply learned concepts. See Quick Facts 12-1.

Learning Theories

Three Main Theories
Learning theories fall into three broad categories of learning: behaviorism, cognitivism, and constructivism. These learning theories help one to understand how information is learned. These can be used to recognize and support different learning abilities, as well as constructing different learning experiences, for patients, clients, and audiences. See Quick Facts 12-2.

Characteristics of Adult Learners
1. Theorists: Knowles, Kidd.
2. Characteristics of the adult learner.
   a. Highly motivated and self-directed learner.

QUICK FACTS 12-1 ▶ ACTIVE VS. PASSIVE LEARNER COMPARISON

Active/Independent Learning	Passive/Dependent Learning
Actively seeks knowledge: • Participates in discussions • Asks questions • Draws conclusions • Exhibits initiative • Likes to work independently • Thinks for self **Benefits of active/independent learning:** • Increases critical thinking • Allows for feedback of comprehension • Increases attention to subject • Stimulates discussion • May work well for visual learners	**Passively seeks knowledge:** • Learner is responsible for absorbing information presented • Information is delivered by the instructor, learner listens, defines, and describes **Benefits of passive/dependent learning:** • Allows instructor to deliver concrete and organized presentation loaded with information • Allows student to listen to or read information, take notes • May work well for auditory learner

QUICK FACTS 12-2 ▶ LEARNING THEORIES	
Learning Theory	**Characteristics**
Behaviorism (Behaviorists: Skinner, Watson, Magner)	Information is acquired through a series of associations, learning environment is structured to lead learner to correct behaviors. Learning takes place in a series of reinforced steps. Learning is arranged from simple to complex; active practice is important.
Cognitivism (Cognitivists: Piaget, Bruner, Bandura)	Information is learned through internal processing of information; cognitive abilities occur in stages. • Symbolic function, ages 2–8 • Concrete mental operations, ages 8–12 • Conceptual thought, ages 12 and up Learner seeks ways to understand and process information that has been received. Learner gradually assumes greater responsibility for problem solving as information is learned.
Constructivists (Constructivists: Dewey, Montessori)	Learners construct their own meaningful perspective based on context, individual experiences, and internal knowledge. Instructor is responsible to supply correct tools for learning and creates conditions in which learning takes place.

b. Motivated by activities that learner perceives as being directly related to the learner's need for learning (don't like to waste time).
c. Brings an accumulation of life experiences.
  • Can serve as a resource for fellow students.
  • Can also serve as obstacle to overcome.
    ○ May tend to be less flexible than the younger learner.

○ Wants to participate in the decision-making process as it relates to assessment of needs, setting goals, choosing activities.
• May enjoy less structured opportunities to experiment with knowledge.
• May choose ungraded learning opportunities as opposed to graded assignments.
• Tends to be more interested in mastering or attaining knowledge versus simply achieving a grade.
3. Teaching the adult student (patient, family member, colleague, community group member, etc.).
   a. The instructor:
      • Selects activities in which the student can actively participate and in which the learning outcome is clear and meaningful.
      • Involves the student in decision making and goal setting.
      • Incorporates the learner's life experiences into classroom discussions.

Educational Concepts

Clinical Application
1. PTAs need to be able to construct learning environments for patients, clients, peers, and community groups.
2. Learning is impacted by the participant's learning style, preferences, and characteristics.
   a. Learning can also be influenced by language or cultural differences, socioeconomic status, age, gender, gender roles, diseases, or conditions impacting cognitive function.
3. The instructor's ability to recognize and adapt to different learning styles of participants can have significant impact on learning outcomes.
   a. The instructor must also keep in mind the intended goal or outcome of the presentation and employ teaching techniques designed to best influence that (e.g., use demonstration and return demonstration with feedback if the learner is to perform a task).

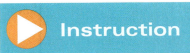 Instruction

Instructional Process

Needs Assessment
1. Identify therapeutic/cognitive needs of the audience (patient, family, peer, etc.).
   a. Identify existing perceptual deficits, visual impairment, communication deficits, confusion, emotional or memory impairment.
   b. Consider psychosocial readiness, support systems.
2. Incorporate active listening, positive verbal and nonverbal interaction, and use of open-ended questions.

3. Assess: past and/or current knowledge and experiences, readiness to learn.

Assess Barriers
1. Determine barriers to learning and design a teaching method that takes these needs into consideration.
2. Recognize that learner motivation, energy level, and emotional condition may vary.

Implementation
1. Determine objectives. Consider priorities, learning environment, and equipment needs.
2. Develop teaching tools to meet learner needs and established objectives.
   a. Presentation, lecture, discussion.
   b. Demonstration.
   c. Visual tools: handouts, video, etc.
3. Engage the learner in setting clear goals and outcomes.
4. Build learning from basic to more complex concepts.
5. Actively involve the audience in the learning process, include trial and error, control the learning environment, and incorporate experiential learning activities to help solidify concepts.

Evaluation
1. Assess audience mastery of concepts, ability to progress to next phase or concept, and build on prior knowledge.
   a. Ask for return teaching: Is audience able to verbalize concepts learned?
   b. Assess audience ability to demonstrate concepts or techniques learned.

Instructional Activities

Patient/Client Instruction
1. Teaching a patient/client the necessary information or exercise for him or her to improve/maintain his or her condition.
2. Takes on many forms.
   a. Discussion.
   b. Demonstration.
   c. Return demonstration.
   d. Illustration of written and video information.
3. Should be designed to provide information to enhance the patient/client understanding of the diagnosis and specific rationale for interventions.
4. Is enhanced through use of applicable:
   a. Models.
   b. Diagrams.
   c. Illustrations.
   d. Hands-on guidance of correct movement patterns.

5. Outcome is often for patient/client to continue independently from treatment session to treatment session and after discharge.
6. The patient/client is empowered to use this information to manage his or her condition, or adapt to the home or work environment.

Care Provider Instruction
1. Specific goal is to instruct care provider in specific techniques to enhance, promote, and produce identified outcomes with the patient/client. Instruction is focused on safety for the provider and patient/client.
2. Instruction can take on many forms, including:
   a. Discussion.
   b. Demonstration.
   c. Return demonstration.
   d. Illustration of written and video information.

In-Service
1. Therapist and/or assistant prepare short educational programs designed to impart specific aspects of knowledge to peers.

Clinical Education
1. Therapist and/or assistant participate in guiding the learning experiences of a student in the clinical environment.
2. Typically occurs prior to the student's graduation from his or her formal educational program in the academic setting.
   a. Takes the form of modeling clinical techniques.
   b. Involves observing learner performance.
   c. Requires structured critique and feedback of the learner's performance.
   d. Experiences and expectations progress from basic to complex, building on previous learning.

Instruction Modes

Presentation/Demonstration
1. Present most important information first.
2. Keep content brief and to the point.
3. Emphasize the most important points.
4. Organize the presentation into subsets of information.
5. Be specific with instructions.
6. Use a variety of methods/ways to present information.
7. Present at a level the learner can comprehend.
8. Provide hands-on demonstration of techniques or ideas when possible.
   a. Use terminology easily understood by the audience.
     - Avoid technical terms for an audience of laypersons.
     - Limit unnecessary extraneous information that will distract the learner from the intended outcome.

Lecture
1. Keep it short.
2. Involve the participants in discussions of key points.
3. Build on information the learner already has processed.
4. Add visual aids to enhance important points or concepts.
    a. Diagrams.
    b. Illustrations.
    c. Models.
        - Provide handouts with important points outlined.
        - Identify these in the presentation.

Written Handout for Exercise
1. Should be specific about:
    a. Repetitions.
    b. Amount of resistance.
    c. Positions for performing.
    d. Number of sets or bouts per day.
2. Include diagrams and identify affected and unaffected limbs as necessary.
3. Include signs/symptoms of intolerance and when to decrease or stop activity.
4. Include contact information for the therapist, PTA, or clinic.

Video
1. Videos can be made to specifically meet the learner's needs.
2. The video should include a review at the start of what the presentation includes.
    a. Identify any equipment the participant will need.
    b. Explain any technical terms used.
    c. Speak clearly.
    d. Focus the camera on critical aspects of the performance.
    e. Limit unnecessary background distractions.

Return Demonstration
1. Allows the presenter to assess how well the learner grasped the concepts presented.
2. Performance activity.
    a. Observe the learner's performance of the task.
        - Critique.
        - Praise.
        - Help refine the learner's performance until consistency is established.
3. Cognitive information.
    a. Ask the learner to explain the information as he or she understands it.
        - Critique.
        - Praise.
        - Help refine the learner's understanding until understanding is demonstrated.

Implementation of Instruction

Patients/Clients
1. Assess the patients'/clients' abilities and learning styles; identify obstacles to learning.
    a. The instructional method will need to adapt to a patient/client who has cognitive deficits or learning disabilities.
    b. If language is a problem, identify resources available or adapt presentation.
    c. Use a variety of teaching methods to involve several learning styles at the same time.
2. Assess the patients'/clients' readiness to learn.
    a. If they are uninterested in learning, your efforts will be unsuccessful.
        - Identify how the learning is relevant to the patients'/clients' needs.
        - Example:
            ○ Learning to roll in the bed will help lead to independence in bed mobility.
3. Develop teaching methods to meet the patients'/clients' learning needs.
    a. If they are visual learners, use handouts and diagrams.
    b. If they are kinesthetic learners, develop a teaching method that allows them hands-on experiences.
    c. Keep instructions simple and to the point.
        - Avoid extra or unnecessary information.
4. Create an environment that the patients/clients feel comfortable in.
    a. Anxiety, pain, and distractions will interfere with learning.
5. Implement the instructional method.
    a. Assess its success.
    b. Adapt it as necessary to meet the patients'/clients' needs.
6. Actively involve patients/clients.
    a. Have them do a return demonstration of a task.
    b. Or have them explain a procedure to you.
7. Review what has been learned and answer any questions.

Families
1. Assess the family members' abilities and learning styles.
    a. Identify obstacles to learning.
    b. The instructional method will need to adapt to the specific needs.
    c. If language is a problem, identify resources available or adapt presentation.
    d. Use a variety of teaching methods to involve several learning styles at the same time.
2. Assess the family members' readiness to learn; if they are uninterested in learning, your efforts will be unsuccessful.

a. Identify how the learning is relevant to their needs and the patient's/client's needs.
     - By learning to transfer the patient/client, they may be able to take their family member home, as opposed to moving the family member to a long-term care facility.
3. Develop teaching methods to meet the family members' learning needs.
4. Create an environment that the family and patient/client feel comfortable in.
   a. Limit distractions, which will interfere with learning.
5. Implement the instructional method.
   a. Assess its success.
   b. Adapt it as necessary to meet the patient's/client's needs.
6. Actively involve the family member.
   a. Have the family do a return demonstration of a task.
   b. Or have them explain a procedure to you.
7. Review what has been learned and answer any questions.

Health Care Providers

1. Assess the needs of the health care provider and identify obstacles to learning.
   a. The instructional method will need to meet their specific needs.
   b. If language is a problem, identify resources available or adapt presentation.
   c. Use a variety of teaching methods to involve several learning styles at the same time.
2. Assess the health care provider's readiness to learn.
   a. If they are uninterested in learning, your efforts will be unsuccessful.
      - Identify how the learning is relevant to their needs and the patient's/client's needs.
      - By learning to transfer the patient/client more therapeutically, they will cause less pain to the patient and will reinforce therapy goals.
      - By learning and using good body mechanics, they can limit their potential for pain or injury.
3. Develop teaching methods to meet their learning needs and capture their interest.
4. Create an environment that the health care provider feels comfortable in; create a fun, relaxed and interactive environment.
   a. Limit distractions, which will interfere with learning.
5. Implement the instructional method.
   a. Assess its success.
   b. Adapt it as necessary to meet the health care provider's needs.
6. Actively involve the health care provider in the learning process.
   a. Have the participants do a return demonstration of a task.
   b. Or have them explain a procedure to you.
7. Review what has been learned and answer any questions.

Motor Learning

Description

Motor Control and Learning
1. Motor control is the ability of a participant to regulate or direct motor actions to accomplish a task.
2. Motor learning considers the process the participant uses to practice and eventually "learn" the skills necessary to accomplish a task.

Phases of Motor Learning (Table 12-1)

Cognitive Stage
1. The learner understands the goal of the tasks.
   a. Develops strategies to perform the task.
   b. Learners need to specifically think about how to perform the task.

Associative Stage
1. Actions are perfected during this phase to produce the most efficient action.
   a. The learner thinks about performing the steps to accomplish the task with greater refinement and precision. This establishes an "internal reference of correctness" of the performance.

Automatic (Autonomous) Stage
1. The learner is able to accomplish the task with very little thinking; it is automatic.
   a. The learner is able to perform the task with a high level of skill in a multitude of environments with a multitude of distracters. The learner is able to perform multiple tasks at the same time.

Table 12-1

Stages of Motor Learning and Training Strategies

COGNITIVE STAGE CHARACTERISTICS	TRAINING STRATEGIES
The learner • develops an understanding of task, *cognitive mapping* • assesses abilities, task demands • identifies stimuli, contacts memory • selects response, performs initial approximations of task • structures motor program • modifies initial responses *"What to do"* decision	Highlight purpose of task in functionally relevant terms. Demonstrate ideal performance of task to establish a *reference of correctness* Have patient verbalize task components and requirements. Point out similarities to other learned tasks Direct attention to critical task elements **Select appropriate feedback** • Emphasize intact sensory systems, intrinsic feedback systems • Carefully pair extrinsic feedback with intrinsic feedback • High dependence on vision: have patient watch movement • Provide **Knowledge of Performance (KP):** focus on errors as they become consistent; do not cue on large number of random errors • Provide **Knowledge of Results (KR):** focus on success of movement outcome Ask learner to evaluate performance, outcomes; identify problems, solutions Use reinforcements (praise) for correct performance and continuing motivation **Organize feedback schedule** • *Feedback* after every trial improves performance during early learning • *Variable feedback* (summed, fading, bandwidth designs) increases depth of cognitive processing, improves retention; may decrease performance initially **Organize initial practice** • Stress controlled movement to minimize errors • Provide adequate rest periods using *distributed practice* if task is complex, long, or energy costly or if learner fatigues easily, has short attention, or has poor concentration • Use manual guidance to assist as appropriate • Break complex tasks down into component parts, teach both parts and integrated whole • Use *bilateral transfer* as appropriate • Use *blocked (repeated)* practice of same task to improve performance • Use *variable practice* (serial or random practice order) of related skills to increase depth of cognitive processing and retention; may decrease performance initially • Use *mental practice* to improve performance and learning, reduce anxiety **Assess, modify arousal levels as appropriate** • High or low arousal impairs performance and learning • Avoid stressors, mental fatigue **Structure environment** • Reduce extraneous environmental stimuli, distractors to ensure attention, concentration • Emphasize closed skills initially gradually progressing to open skills
ASSOCIATED STAGE CHARACTERISTICS	**TRAINING STRATEGIES**
The learner • practices movements • refines motor program • spatial and temporal organization • decreases errors • extraneous movements Dependence on visual feedback decreases, increases for use of proprioceptive feedback; cognitive monitoring decreases *"How to do"* decision	**Select appropriate feedback** • Continue to provide KP; intervene when errors become consistent • Emphasize proprioceptive feedback, "feel of movement" to assist in establishing an internal reference of correctness • Continue to provide KR; stress relevance of functional outcomes • Assist learner to improve self-evaluation, decision-making skills • Facilitation techniques, guided movements are counterproductive during this stage of learning **Organize feedback schedule** • Continue to provide feedback for continuing motivation; encourage patient to self-assess achievements • Avoid excessive augmented feedback • Focus on use of variable feedback (summed, fading, bandwidth) designs to improve retention **Organize practice** • Encourage consistency of performance • Focus on variable practice order (serial or random) of related skills to improve retention **Structure environment** • Progress toward open, changing environment • Prepare the learner for home, community, work environments

(Continued)

Table 12-1

Stages of Motor Learning and Training Strategies (*Continued*)

AUTONOMOUS STAGE CHARACTERISTICS	TRAINING STRATEGIES
The learner • practices movements • continues to refine motor responses • spatial and temporal highly organized • movements are largely error-free • minimal level of cognitive monitoring "How to succeed" decision	Assess need for conscious attention, automaticity of movements **Select appropriate feedback** • Learner demonstrates appropriate self-evaluation, decision-making skills • Provide occasional feedback (KP, KR) when errors evident **Organize practice** • Stress consistency of performance in variable environments, variations of tasks (open skills) • High levels of practice (massed practice) are appropriate **Structure environment** • Vary environments to challenge learner • Ready the learner for home, community, and work environments Focus on competitive aspects of skills as appropriate; e.g., wheelchair sports

From O'Sullivan S, Schmitz T. Physical Rehabilitation. 6th ed, Philadelphia, FA Davis, 2014, pg 397–398, with permission.

Implications for Intervention or Instruction

Learner Readiness
1. Assess.
    a. Motivation.
    b. Fatigue.
    c. Attention to task.
    d. Cognitive abilities of the participant.
2. Take into account that these variables may change from day to day, treatment to treatment. Adjust interventions accordingly.

Identify the Task and Importance
1. Identify the task the learner is to accomplish.
2. Break it into component parts.
3. Identify the importance the task has for the learner's overall function.

Demonstration
1. Demonstrate the task for the participant to gain an appreciation for ideal performance.
2. Break the task into component parts for practice.
3. Provide hands-on facilitation of movements required to accomplish the task.

Progress from Simple to Complex in Treatment Approach
1. Identify components of a task and begin practice with those components.
    a. Introduce multiple components when the learner is ready.
    b. Progress to accomplishing the whole task without breaking it into component parts.
2. Control the environment to assure success.
    a. Decrease distractions.
    b. Ensure level surfaces for transfer or ambulation if appropriate.

Feedback Should Vary with Learner's Ability to Accomplish
1. Begin with greater verbal and tactile cues for successful accomplishment of task.
2. Identify potential problem areas so the participant is aware of them and can plan for them.
3. Eventually decrease the amount of verbal or tactile cues provided to assist the learner to accomplish the task.
4. Allow the learner to make mistakes and correct self while maintaining a safe environment.
5. Progress to environments in which the participant needs to plan the performance around obstacles and problem solve independently.

Assessment of Performance/Learning

As Learning Occurs
1. The level of accuracy in movements to accomplish the tasks will improve.
2. The performance will become more automatic and require less cognitive awareness to accomplish.
3. The speed of accurately performing the task will increase.

As Skill Retention Occurs
1. The learner will be able to perform the skill after a period of not practicing the specific skill.

As Skill Variability Occurs
1. The learner will be able to perform the skill in varied environments, from varied or modified positions.

Measuring Outcomes
1. Identify level of independence in performing task.
2. Identify level of function in performing task.
3. Identify the amount of effort required to accomplish task.

Performance Fatigue
1. Identify causes of performance decline or avoidance.
2. Provide reinforcements relevant to the learner.
3. Identify motivation for performance and consequences for nonperformance.

Communication

Verbal

Messages
1. Verbal messages are conveyed from the sender to the receiver.

Level of Understanding Is Dependent on
1. The perception of the person receiving the message.
2. The clarity of the message sent.
3. The complexity of the message.

Message Direction
1. Communication can take place as one-way or two-way communication. The mode chosen should be based on desired outcome. One-way communication can be quick; however, it limits the options of both the sender and receiver. See Quick Facts 12-3 for traits of each style.

Nonverbal

Description
1. Includes those messages that are conveyed through mediums other than the spoken word.

Body Language
1. Postures and gestures that convey messages from the sender to the receiver and vice versa.
2. Open postures convey a willingness to receive a message.
   a. Open postures.
      - Arms at sides.
      - Legs uncrossed.
      - Erect posture.
      - Face the sender.
      - Position yourself at eye level with the receiver.
3. Closed postures convey an unwillingness to receive a message.
   a. Closed postures.
      - Arms and/or legs crossed.
      - Slumped posture.
      - Turned away from the sender.
4. There are many cultural influences and variations that have a bearing on body language.
   a. Eye contact may or may not be appropriate.
      - A nod of the head does not mean the same thing in all cultures.

Facial Expression/Gestures and Eye Contact
1. Can convey acceptance or rejection of thoughts and ideas presented.
   a. Acceptance.
      - Smile.
      - Direct eye contact.
      - Head nodding.
   b. Rejection.
      - Frown or flat expression.
      - Rolling the eyes.
      - Looking up, down or away from the sender.
      - Head shaking.

QUICK FACTS 12-3 ▶ ONE-WAY VS. TWO-WAY COMMUNICATION

One-Way Communication	Two-Way Communication
• Typically less effective	• Typically more effective
• Does not allow receiver to clarify message	• Allows for both sender and receiver to clarify message
• Does not allow sender to question how message was interpreted	• Helps assure understanding of message intent

Effective Communication Strategies

Active Listening
1. The use of "I statements," to clarify what you think you heard the patient/client tell you.
2. Restate the patient's problem as you heard it stated.
   a. "You mean you don't feel as good today as you did yesterday?"
3. Reflect on what you heard the patient/client tell you, and on the feelings he or she implied in the message.
   a. "You don't feel as good today as you did yesterday and that really concerns you."
4. Clarify or summarize the message you thought you heard the patient/client send you.
   a. Summarize the spoken words you heard your patient/client convey to you to clarify the message, thoughts and frustrations you heard.
      - "When you started therapy you improved rapidly and thought you would continue to feel better each day. Now that you have had some days that you feel the same and the progress has slowed, you are concerned about how long this process will take."

Ensure Understanding of the Patient/Client Goals Right from the Start of Care
1. What problem does the patient/client want help with?
2. Accomplish this by asking questions to clarify what you think you hear the patient/client telling you.
3. Focus on the patient/client, not your next appointment or the phone call you need to return.
4. Develop trust with your patient/client. Follow up with questions, activities or ideas.

Develop Your Ability to Empathize or Sympathize with Your Patient/Client
1. Definition.
   a. Ability to identify with how the patient/client may be feeling.
      - Be empathetic with the patient's condition/situation, yet maintain a professional relationship.
2. Resist pitying patient/client.
   a. This conveys an inequality between you and your patient.
      - Conveys that patient/client is somehow less than you with this situation or condition.
3. Do not offer reassurances. "It can't be all that bad," or "It's only for a short time."
   a. This discounts the patient's feeling or thoughts and conveys an unwillingness to really listen.

Develop Rapport with Your Patient/Client
1. Use open body language when interacting with your patient/client.
2. Be sure facial expressions convey a genuine interest in the patient and his or her needs.
3. Listen actively to determine what the patient's/client's needs are.
   a. Ask open-ended questions to gain a greater perspective.
4. Speak in even, moderate tones using language the patient/client can understand.
   a. Choose words and language sensitive to the patient's/client's level of understanding and cultural background.
5. Respect patient's/client's concerns, questions and ideas.
6. Be honest about what you can do and cannot do for him or her.
   a. Identify what the patient's responsibilities are to help him- or herself.
   b. It is critical that patients/clients understand that part of the healing process lies in their hands as well as yours.

Speech/Language Disorders

Description
1. A language disorder related to brain damage.
   a. The specific type of aphasia is related to the area of the brain that is damaged.

Dysarthria
1. Incoordination of the facial muscles, lips, tongue and jaw that results in apraxic speech production.
   a. Results from damage to the central or peripheral nervous system.
   b. Often the result of a cerebral vascular attack (CVA).
2. Presentation.
   a. The patient/client has difficulty pronouncing words.
   b. Usually retains the ability to comprehend speech.
3. Patient/client instruction.
   a. Will not be able to verbally repeat instructions but can give a return demonstration of techniques learned.

Expressive Aphasia
1. Word-finding difficulty or the inability to speak despite intact oral musculature.
2. Presentation.
   a. May be very frustrated secondary to not being understood.
3. Guard against assuming that there is a problem with the thought process.
   a. May be able to understand, but are unable to vocalize this.

4. Test for accurate yes/no responses.
5. Usually capable of problem solving and learning from demonstration.

Receptive Aphasia
1. Difficulty understanding spoken or written language despite intact auditory ability.
   a. Most patients/clients are able to verbalize ideas accurately.
2. Multilingual patients/clients may lose both their birth (primary) language and/or secondary language skills.
   a. May only lose the secondary language.
      - If the secondary language is lost, instructions should be provided in the primary language.
3. Guard against assuming they understand because they nod in response to questions or are able to speak well.
4. Patient/client instruction.
   a. Will respond better to:
      - Pictures.
      - Diagrams.
      - Physical demonstration.
      - Gestures.

Global Aphasia
1. Characterized by loss of both expressive language and receptive language.
   a. Cannot form clear spoken words or understand spoken or written words.
2. Patient interaction.
   a. Guard against the impression that the patient/client understands:
      - Gestures.
      - Voice tone changes.
      - Facial expression.
   b. May seem to comprehend when patient/client does not understand what is being asked.

Treatment Considerations with Aphasia

Speech and Language Pathologist
1. Seek assistance for patient specific communication strategies as necessary.
2. Throughout treatment session reinforce identified communication strategies and goals.

Influences
1. Patient posture, reflex movements, and respirations can influence the ability to form words clearly.
2. Treatment techniques should be directed at limiting influences that negatively affect the ability to communicate.

Eye Contact
1. Eye contact with the patient/client (as appropriate) can help improve communication efforts.
   a. Be aware of cultural differences in it's importance and appropriateness.

The Assistant Should
1. Be clear.
2. Use concise instructions.
3. Speak slowly.
4. Limit distractions during treatment as much as possible.
5. Involving the family and providing education is important.
6. Consider timing.
   a. Avoid wordiness with instructions.
   b. If yes/no responses are accurate, use closed-ended questions to facilitate communication.

Present Material to Include Multiple Learning Styles
1. Verbal.
2. Kinesthetic.
3. Visual.

Avoid
1. Talking "down" to the patients/clients as if they are children.
2. Increasing voice volume as if the patient/client were hard of hearing.

Use Realistic Testing and Training Situations
1. Carryover from hypothetical or simulated situations may be poor.
2. Therapists will often overestimate the patients'/clients' ability to comprehend.

Aphasia Can Improve Over Time
1. Greatest gains will be seen in the initial rehabilitation phase.
2. Could involve months or years.

Review Questions

Teaching and Learning

1. Identify four steps necessary in preparing a presentation to a community group. These steps are the same steps used when instructing a patient/client.

2. Describe what training strategies are most useful for a patient/client during the cognitive (early) versus the associative (acquiring skills) stage of learning.

3. Identify at least three effective communication strategies.

13

Management, Safety, and Professional Roles

JANE BALDWIN

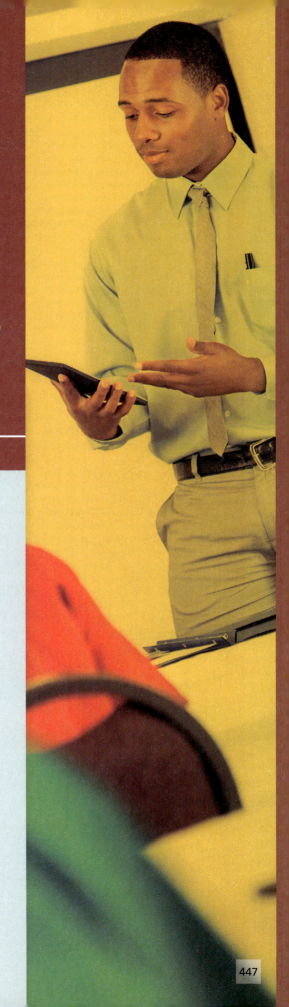

Chapter Outline

- **Facility Department Management, 449**
  - Medical Records Management, 449
  - Risk Management, 451
  - Policy and Procedures, 452
  - Quality Assurance/Continuous Quality Improvement, 452
  - Human Resource Responsibilities, 453
  - Emergency Preparedness, 455
- **Patient Safety and Protection, 455**
  - Fall Risk and Prevention, 455
  - Use of Equipment, 456
  - Use of Restraints, 456
  - Patient/Client Rights, 457
  - First Aid, 458
  - Basic Life Support and CPR, 460

- Illegal Practice and Malpractice, 462
  - Statutory Laws, 462
  - Goals of Statutory Laws Impacting Physical Therapy, 462
  - Nondiscrimination Laws, 462
  - Common Law, 462
- Injury Prevention, 463
  - Overview, 463
- Body Mechanics: General Concepts, 463
  - Principles, 463
  - Inpatient Care, 464
  - Instructions for Patient/Client, 464
  - Other Injury Prevention Information, 464
- Roles and Responsibilities, 464
  - The PT/PTA Team, 464
  - Principles of Collaboration, 465
  - Caregiver Definition and Roles, 465
- American Physical Therapy Association (APTA) Documents
  - Appendix 13A: APTA Guidelines for Documentation of Patient/Client Management, 469
  - Appendix 13B: Standards of Practice for Physical Therapy, 471
  - Appendix 13C: Direction and Supervision of the PTA, 474
  - Appendix 13D: Guide for Conduct of the Physical Therapist Assistant, 476
- Review Questions, 482

Facility Department Management

Medical Records Management

Documentation Format/Problem Oriented Medical Record (POMR)

1. Record system for documentation.
   a. Subjective.
      - Information from the patient or family member.
   b. Objective.
      - Measurable outcomes that a PT or PTA gathers.
      - Measurements can be gathered during the evaluation, treatment sessions, or reevaluations.
      - Document in objective, measurable, functional terms.
   c. Assessment.
      - Analysis of problems, impairments, and functional limitations including short- and long-term goals/outcomes as determined by the PT at evaluation.
      - Ongoing assessment is conducted by the PT or PTA treating the patient on a weekly or daily basis.
      - Document patient's response to treatment session.
      - Frequency of reporting is determined by the insurance or facility requirements.
   d. Plan.
      - Specific treatment plan for the identified problems of the patient.
      - Determined by the PT on the initial evaluation.
2. Documentation is completed for each patient treatment session.

International Classification of Functioning, Disability, and Health Resources (ICF) Model

1. Developed by the World Health Organization (WHO) and endorsed by the American Physical Therapy Association (APTA) and other international organizations.
2. The ICF model identifies dimensions of functioning (body functions and body structures, activities, participation) and dimensions of disability (impairments, activity limitations, participation restrictions). See Box 13-1 for complete definitions.
3. ICF terms serve as a platform for choosing terminology to identify limitations the individual experiences at the level of the body, the environment, or in society.
4. ICF terminology represents a shift from terminology used in the medical model, which focuses on the condition or the disease affecting the individual.

BOX 13-1 Terminology: Functioning, Disability, and Health

Health condition is an umbrella term for disease, disorder, injury, or trauma and may also include other circumstances, such as aging, stress, congenital anomaly, or genetic predisposition. It may also include information about pathogenesis and/or etiology.

Body Functions are physiological functions of body systems (including psychological functions).

Body Structures are anatomical parts of the body such as organs, limbs, and their components.

Impairments are the problems in body function or structure, such as a significant deviation or loss.

Activity is the execution of a task or action by an individual.

Participation is involvement in a life situation.

Activity Limitations are difficulties an individual may have in executing activities.

Participation Restrictions are problems an individual may experience in involvement in life situations.

Contextual Factors represent the entire background of an individual's life and living situation.

- **Environmental Factors** make up the physical, social, and attitudinal environment in which people live and conduct their lives, including social attitudes, architectural characteristics, legal, and social structures.
- **Personal Factors** are the particular background of an individual's life, including gender, age, coping styles, social background, education, profession, past and current experience, overall behavior pattern, character, and other factors that influence how disability is experienced by an individual.

Performance describes what an individual does in his/her current environment.

Capacity describes an individual's ability to execute a task or an action (highest probable level of functioning in a given domain at a given moment).

From *The World Health Organization. International Classification of Functioning, Disability, and Health Resources (ICF).* World Health Organization, Geneva, 2002. http://www.who.int/classifications/en/

Documentation Methods

1. Various methods used for documentation depending on setting, state and federal regulations, and third-party reimbursement requirements.

Reasons for Documenting

1. Record accurate and current status of the patient.
2. Provide history or "story" of the patient's condition and treatments provided by the entire medical team.

3. In physical therapy, is utilized as a system to track and document patient goals, expected outcomes, and determine interventions for achievement of identified goals.
4. Record patient response to interventions and assists in clinical decisions to determine whether interventions are appropriate and effective.
5. Provide legal documentation.
   a. This information can be subpoenaed if necessary.
6. Utilized as a communication tool between PT and PTA, as well as other health care professionals, to facilitate the decision making process.

Guidelines for Documentation (Appendix A)
1. All documentation must comply with jurisdictional and regulatory requirements.
2. Compliance with all insurance and Medicare guidelines is required to ensure reimbursement.
3. The patient's right to privacy must always be respected and protected.
4. Release of any medical information must be authorized by the patient in writing.
   a. The PTA always refers the person who is asking for medical information to the supervising PT.
5. Records must be kept in a safe and secure place for a certain number of years, usually 7 years.

Basic Principles of Documentation
1. Documentation must be consistent with the APTA's Standards of Practice (Appendix B).
2. All documents must be legible.
3. Medically approved abbreviations or symbols can be used. Many facilities have specific approved lists.
4. All documentation should be written in blue or black ink.
5. Mistakes should be crossed out with a single line through the error.
   a. Should be initialed and dated by the assistant.
   b. The mistake must be legible to anyone reviewing the chart.
6. Obtaining formal informed consent for treatment prior to treatment is the responsibility of the physical therapist.
   a. Must be signed by a competent adult.
   b. Minor child or adult deemed incompetent: parent or appointed guardian must sign.
7. Every treatment has to be documented.
   a. Specifics of documentation vary greatly depending on setting, insurance guidelines, and state and federal regulations.
8. The patient's name, medical ID number, and date of birth should be on each page.
9. Date each entry and document the length of each visit.
10. Sign each of your entries with first and last name as it reads on your PTA license and your professional designation (PTA).
11. Record all communications with any of the team members.
    a. Team members could include: physical therapists, nurses, physicians and/or social workers, etc.

Progress Notes
1. Document specific treatment, equipment provided. Include signature of therapist or assistant providing care.
2. Document patient response to treatment, functional progress, goals achieved, revision of goals, and suggestions for treatment plan modification.
3. Interim progress notes can be written by:
   a. Physical therapist (PT).
   b. Physical therapist assistant (PTA).
   c. Student (PT, PTA) notes must be cosigned by supervising therapist.

Reevaluation/Reassessment
1. Completed as indicated by the supervising PT (minimally every 30 days for Medicare patients). Includes.
   a. Restatement of initial problems.
   b. Length of time patient has been treated.
   c. Progress or regression since last assessment or initial evaluation (whichever occurred last).
   d. Rationale for continued care.
   e. Revision of goals and outcomes.
      • Discussed with PTA.
      • Patient is in agreement.
   f. Revision of plan of care.
      • Discussed with PTA.
      • Patient is in agreement.
2. Must be written by the supervising PT.
3. Frequency of reevaluations/reassessments varies according to setting, insurance guidelines, and state and federal regulations.

Discharge Summary
1. Must be written by the supervising PT.
2. The PTA can and should provide objective tests and measures to the PT.
3. Includes: progress toward goals and outcome achievements.

Discharge Plan
1. Must be written by supervising PT.
2. The PTA can and should provide input into discharge plan and participate in setting up follow-up and home services.

Common Reasons for Payment Denials

1. Insufficient/incomplete documentation. Missing data and insufficient detail and descriptions may cause a denial of payment.
2. Incorrect documentation. Wrong date of service, incorrect billing units, mismatched billing date with date in documentation. May result in denial of payment.
3. Medically unnecessary. Poor documentation that does not fully explain medical reason for interventions may result in denial of payment. If documentation reflects maintenance level of care and no continued progress, this may result in denial of payment.
4. Incorrect coding. Failure to document the proper CPT, ICD-9, or other codes may result in denial of payment.
5. Pay for performance. As pay for performance programs grow, poor documentation that does not reflect best practice may result in reduced payments for services.

Successful Documentation Practices

1. Demonstrate progress toward goals in specific and functional terms.
2. Document medical necessity and reasons for skilled care.
3. If progress not being made, state confounding factors such as medical setbacks, exacerbations of condition, etc.
4. Documentation should stand up in court. Avoid jargon, obscure abbreviations.
   a. Document in full words and avoid abbreviations if in doubt.
   b. Write legibly.
   c. Be factual and objective.
   d. Sign and date all entries.

Risk Management

Physical Therapist Assistant Role

1. PTAs will be responsible to understand and follow specific risk management practices utilized at the facility where they work.
2. PTAs may be placed in roles of responsibility to monitor, enforce, and review risk management practices.

Risk Management Program

1. Designed to identify, evaluate, and take corrective action against risk(s) to staff, visitors, and/or patients/clients.
2. Identifies potential property loss or damage:
   a. Financial loss.
   b. Legal liability.

Incident and Occurrence Reports

1. Staff is required to report unusual occurrences.
   a. Report in objective manner what happened and the result of the occurrence/incident.
   b. Do not include opinions or judgments.
   c. Report is submitted to supervisor and risk management team.
2. Reports are not used for punitive or corrective action.
3. Reports are used in the quality improvement process to change policy, procedures, and attitudes.

Risk Management in Physical Therapy Practice

1. Equipment maintenance.
   a. Yearly check and documentation of electrical equipment.
   b. Procedure for identifying, marking, and reporting malfunctioning equipment.
2. Ongoing staff education.
   a. Safety training for all staff in the use of equipment.
   b. Basic life support certification.
   c. Infection control.
3. Daily check of emergency cart.

Occurrence/Incident and Sentinel Event Reporting

1. Occurrence/incident report is used to document events that involve patients and/or staff which result in harm and/or potential for harm to patient and/or staff.
   a. Are not part of the medical record, nor should they be mentioned in the medical record.
   b. Used to document additional information, circumstances, contributing factors that would not be appropriate to include in the medical record.
   c. Only facts are documented in an occurrence/incident report. No subjective data is given. Statements of what people said should be in quotes. Document factors leading up to the event, what occurred during the event, and actions taken after the event.
   d. Used as part of an internal quality improvement program. May be used to evaluate systems and processes that may have contributed to the event in order to evaluate and improve underlying causes or contributing factors.
   e. May be used as part of an individual employee performance appraisal.
2. A sentinel event is a specific patient-related occurrence in which an unexpected finding or outcome can be analyzed to improve processes, systems, or therapist/assistant performance to reduce the likelihood of reoccurrence.
   a. Sentinel events signal the need for immediate investigation and response.

b. A sentinel event is an unexpected occurrence involving death or serious physical or psychological injury or the risk thereof.
c. Includes any process variation for which a recurrence would carry a significant chance of a serious adverse outcome.
d. Is part of a comprehensive quality assurance and improvement program to analyze and improve processes, systems, or therapist performance to reduce the likelihood of reoccurrence.
e. Many regulatory and accrediting agencies require sentinel event reporting and analysis be done, particularly on specific types of events.

Assuring Patient Safety and Reducing Risk in the Healthcare Environment

1. Efforts taken to decrease risk in physical therapy.
   a. Equipment maintenance, e.g., biannual check of electrical equipment.
   b. Staff education, e.g., safety training for new equipment.
   c. Proper procedure for identifying and notification of malfunctioning equipment.
   d. Regular check of essential safety equipment.
   e. Policies to clean equipment and reduce potential for spreading infections.
2. Patient and staff safety: review all occurrence/incident reports.
3. Identify risk factors in patient care or therapist safety; e.g., if there are greater than three staff back injuries, implement an in-service on proper body mechanics.
4. Proper and timely reporting of adverse patient reactions or occurrences (sentinel event) as required by federal and/or state statute. May include:
   a. Adverse drug reaction.
   b. Abuse or neglect of patient.
   c. Outbreak of disease which may affect public safety, e.g., influenza.
   d. Violence against patient and/or staff.
5. Annual certification/recertification of staff in cardiopulmonary resuscitation (CPR).

Policy and Procedures

Policy and Procedure Manual

1. Provides extensive information on what is to be accomplished and how it is to be accomplished in an organization, physical therapy department, and/or specific units or clinics.
2. Policy and procedure manuals are required by:
   a. The Joint Commission of Accreditation of Healthcare Organizations (JCAHO).
   b. Commission on Accreditation of Rehabilitation Facilities (CARF).

Policies are Broad Statements Used as a Guide in Decision-Making

1. Operational policies.
   a. Billing policies.
   b. Medical record management.
   c. Quality assurance and improvement activities.
2. Human resources policies.
   a. Vacation/time off.
   b. Probationary period as a new employee.
   c. Leave of absence/maternity leave.
   d. Dress code.
3. Policies vary greatly depending on facility and its organizational structure.

Procedures

1. Procedures are specific guides to job behaviors for all personnel such as:
   a. Safety and emergency procedures.
   b. Equipment management.
   c. Hand washing.
   d. Hazardous waste management.
   e. Disciplinary action.
   f. Reporting of abuse.
2. Policies outline specific procedures that all employees need to follow.
3. Disregard for policies and procedures can lead to disciplinary action and possible termination.

Quality Assurance/Continuous Quality Improvement

Quality Assurance (QA)

1. Monitor quality.
2. Monitor appropriateness of care.
3. Resolve identified problems/inconsistencies.

Continuous Quality Improvement (CQI)

1. Can also be known as continuous performance improvement (CPI).
2. Systematic process that involves ongoing, deliberate, and continuous monitoring of systems and processes affecting patient care to attain the best quality outcomes possible.

Utilization Review (UR)

1. Monitors quality of services delivered and appropriateness of care.
2. Resolves identified problems with the quality of service and care delivered.

3. Can be done in a variety of ways.
   a. Peer review.
      - A system in which quality, appropriateness, and effectiveness of work/treatments are reviewed by peers.
      - Results are educational, not punitive.
      - The goal is to improve the quality of care.
      - Focuses on how well services are performed in the delivery of care under review.
      - Determines if the patient's needs have been met.
   b. Concurrent review.
      - Review of documentation of ongoing treatment.
      - Determine if services rendered are necessary, appropriate, and comprehensive in relation to the patient's needs.
   c. Retrospective reviews.
      - Conducted after services have been rendered.
      - Method to ensure appropriate care was given.
      - Time-consuming and expensive method for third-party payers.
   d. Professional review organization (PRO).
      - A group of reviewers who evaluate the appropriateness of services and quality of care under reimbursement and/or state licensure requirements.
      - Reviews services provided to Medicare and Medicaid beneficiaries and some managed care plans.
      - Determines the appropriateness of services delivered to patients.

Prospective Review
1. Evaluation of proposed treatment plan, including specifics of how care will be provided.
2. Used by third-party payers to approve physical therapy services.

Program Evaluation
1. Assessment of the management of patients with a specific diagnosis.
2. Objectives are established for patients and program, e.g., total hip replacement (THR) rehab.
3. Outcomes are evaluated in terms of range of motion (ROM), strength, gait, function, etc.
4. Comparisons made between therapists, facilities, units, etc.
5. Programs modified and improved according to findings.

CQI Projects
1. Once an area of concern or deficit is identified, a plan or process to correct the situation is developed.
2. Projects are not only identified for direct patient care but can be related to operational procedures.
3. The process of developing this plan.
   a. Prioritize the outcomes that need to change or be achieved.
   b. Conduct a more thorough review of the care/procedures.
   c. Identify problems or areas of concern.
   d. Develop a plan to change patient care or procedures.
   e. Implement the plan.
   f. Monitor plan and changes in behavior.
   g. Assess if changes result in desired outcome.

Human Resource Responsibilities

Interview
1. Performed by director, supervisor, and possible representative from human resources.
2. Purpose is to meet prospective employees/employers.
   a. Exchange questions and answers for both the employer and candidate to make an informed decision.
   b. Questions asked are informational for both the employee and candidate requiring details and not just "yes" or "no": e.g., "Give me an example of how you handled the last stressful situation you experienced with a coworker."
   c. No questions can be asked about age, race, religion, sexual orientation, marital status, number of children, political views, etc.
   d. May ask about academic record, educational program, past performance, but must obtain permission from candidate.
3. Many employers require criminal background checks, which require candidate's permission.
4. Employers look for the following.
   a. Decision-making skills.
   b. Communication skills.
   c. Interpersonal skills (body language, tact, ability to work with others).
   d. Leadership.
   e. Employment record.
   f. Personal goals/direction.
5. Interviewer should provide.
   a. Organizational structure.
   b. Benefits (e.g., health insurance, vacation time, sick time, tuition reimbursement).
   c. Career ladder.
   d. Salary.
   e. Job description.
6. Documents reviewed for employment.
   a. Application.
   b. Previous experience.
   c. Transcript from educational program.
   d. Resume.
   e. References.

Job Descriptions

1. General summary of responsibilities.
   a. Includes overview of position, supervisory structure, both administrative and clinical.
2. Specific job responsibilities.
   a. Task-specific responsibilities.
   b. Performance standards established.
   c. Outlines skilled and nonskilled duties.
   d. Outlines supervisory relationships.
      - Position title.
      - Department division.
      - Supervisor's title (administrative).
      - Supervisor's title (clinical).
3. Job specifications.
   a. Educational requirements.
   b. Licensure requirements.
   c. Essential job functions (physical and cognitive).
      - Lifting requirements.
      - Transferring requirements.
      - Positioning/ambulatory requirements.
      - Reading/writing/comprehension requirements.
      - Communication requirements.
4. Expectations regarding ability to organize and plan time; overall work habits.
5. Required problem-solving skills.

Performance Review/Appraisal

1. Assesses an employee's performance in relation to objective performance criteria.
2. Written report, discussed with employee in person.
   a. Usually have probationary period of 90 days at start of employment.
   b. Reviews are often performed annually.
3. Reviews correlate to job description as well as organizational goals.
4. Feedback should be objective and specific.
5. Outcome of performance review may be used for promotion and raises.
6. Performance reviews may identify areas needing improvement.

Continuing Education

1. Ongoing educational activities to foster life-long learning.
   a. Enhances clinical knowledge.
   b. Exposes, instructs, and teaches therapists/assistants new techniques and technologies.
2. Educational programs can be delivered a variety of ways.
   a. On-site programs.
      - In-services.
      - Journal clubs.
      - Case presentations.
   b. Off-site programs.
      - Continuing education programs.
      - National and state physical therapy meetings.
      - Special interest group–sponsored courses.
3. Frequency can vary according to time and resources.
4. Employers should support and may subsidize staff member's attendance. Should promote professionalism, educational development, and continued competence.
5. Each state has its own requirements and expectations for licensee continuing education.

OSHA (Occupational Safety and Health Administration)

1. Federal agency whose role is to assure safe and healthful working conditions for working men and women.
2. Provides funds for research, information, education, and training in the field of occupational safety and health.
3. Any workplace needs to comply with OSHA standards pertaining to such things as blood-borne pathogens, needle sticks, and construction safety.
4. Respond to worker's complaints of unsafe work conditions.
5. Performs inspections of workplaces.
   a. Inspects physical aspect of work environment.
   b. Meets with and interviews workers.
   c. Reviews policies and procedures addressing worker safety.
   d. Philosophy of continuous quality improvement. Policies are constantly reviewed to assure optimal safety for workers in the workplace.
   e. Areas specific to physical therapy that OSHA addresses.
      - Bloodborne pathogens.
      - Ergonomics.
      - Slips/falls.
      - Hazardous chemicals.
      - Equipment hazards.

Sexual Harassment

1. All employees are protected through both state and federal laws through the EEOC (Equal Employment Opportunity Commission).
2. Sexual advances, requests for sexual favors, and verbal or physical conduct of a sexual nature.
   a. Submission to or rejection of such advances is made (explicitly or implicitly) a term or condition of employment and/or may affect promotions or other things such as vacations, etc.
   b. Such advances have the purpose or effect of unreasonably interfering with an individual's work performance by creating an intimidating, hostile, humiliating, or sexually offensive work environment.
3. Either sex may be the harasser.

4. Sexual harassment may occur regardless of the intentions of the harasser.
5. Harasser can be the victim's supervisor, a supervisor in another area, a coworker, or a nonemployee.
6. Harasser's conduct must be unwelcome.
7. Examples of sexual harassment.
   a. Sexual jokes.
   b. Leering, whistling, and brushing against the body.
   c. Display of sexually graphic art, cartoons, objects.
   d. Request for sexual favors in exchange for job benefits.
8. Employee education and prevention is the best tool against sexual harassment.
9. Individual can file a complaint through the human resources department.
10. Unlawful to retaliate against an individual for filing a complaint.

Emergency Preparedness

Emergency Plan
1. All workplaces must have emergency plans that address emergencies within the facility as well as how to respond to emergencies outside the facility.

Workplaces Must Have Written Emergency Plans
1. Available for employees to review at any time.
2. Procedures for reporting fire or other emergency.
3. Procedures for emergency evacuation, including type of evacuation and exit route assignments.
4. Procedures to account for all patients and employees after evacuation.
5. Procedures to be followed by employees performing rescue or medical duties.

Alarm System
1. Workplaces must also have an alarm system that has a distinctive signal for each purpose (e.g., fire, evacuation, tornado).
2. Some examples include responses to fire, evacuation, tornado, and hurricane.

Employee Training
1. An employer must designate and train employees to assist in a safe and orderly evacuation of patients and other employees.
2. Employers must review the emergency action plan with employees on a yearly basis or when the following occurs.
3. Training also occurs when:
   a. Changes are made to the plan.
   b. When the plan is developed or the employee is assigned initially to a job.
   c. When the employee's responsibilities under the plan change.

External Emergencies
1. Facilities also have emergency plans to respond to external emergencies.
2. Local disasters (train wreck, multiple car wreck on major highway, chemical spill).
3. Natural disasters (floods, earthquakes, forest fires).
4. Terrorist attacks.

Practice
1. Drills to cover both internal and external disasters occur on a regular basis.
2. Employees are to follow facility specific procedures when drills occur and in case of a true disaster.

Patient Safety and Protection

Fall Risk and Prevention

Role of PTs and PTAs
1. Reducing falls and identifying those who are at risk for falls are initiatives of many organizations/facilities.
2. Developing programs for individuals who are at risk for falling that follow best practices for fall prevention.

Risk Factors in Different Environments
1. Identifying risk factors in the facility environment.
   a. Call light, TV control, phone, etc., are within reach of patient.
   b. Spills are cleaned up quickly.
   c. Room is well lit.
   d. IVs, catheters, etc., are secure and out of way.
   e. Patient is frequently checked.

2. Identifying risk factors in the home environment.
   a. Scatter rugs removed.
   b. All stairs have sturdy handrails.
   c. Rooms are well lit and night lights are used.
   d. Bathroom has needed adaptations, e.g., raised toilet seat, grab bars.
   e. Area rugs are secured down with tape and/or non-skid treads.
   f. Phone is within easy reach.
   g. All clutter is removed from hallways and stairs.
   h. Phone and electrical cords are tucked away.
   i. Chairs are sturdy, have arms, and are easy to get in and out.
   j. Frequently used items in kitchens and closets are stored at waist level.

Characteristics
1. Common characteristics for individuals at risk for falls include the following.
   a. Visual deficit.
   b. Lower extremity weakness.
   c. Balance deficit.
   d. History of falls.
   e. Over 80 years of age.
   f. Use of assistive device.
   g. Depression and/or cognitive impairment.
   h. Decreased sensation in lower extremities.
   i. Multiple prescription medications.

Standardized Balance Testing
1. Use to identify the level or risk for falls. These tests can include:
   a. Berg Balance Scale.
   b. Timed Up and Go (TUG).
   c. Functional Reach.
   d. Dynamic Gait Index.
   e. Tinetti Assessment Tool.

Program Development and Implementation
1. Identify need and develop a program to identify/monitor fall risks as well as individuals at risk for falls as indicated.
2. Perform baseline assessments.
   a. Assess environmental factors.
   b. Assess individuals using a standardized balance test appropriate to the individual.
3. Implement program.
   a. Modify environment based on assessment.
   b. Administer balance and falls prevention and/or rehabilitation program specific to identified needs and deficits.
4. Evaluation of program effectiveness.
5. Modify as indicated.

Use of Equipment

Minimal/No Lift Guidelines
1. Many states/jurisdictions now have minimal lift guidelines in place; various jurisdictions have different laws and guidelines.
2. Facility-specific guidelines may also be in place.

Intent of Guidelines
1. To minimize injuries to the worker; e.g., injuries to the back, neck, or shoulder, etc.
2. To minimize injuries to patients/clients.
3. To promote an environment where the usage of assistive equipment is encouraged and expected.

Indications for Use
1. Equipment should be utilized when a patient/client exceeds minimal assistance for transfer activities.
2. Increase safety and efficiency of worker; at the same time, increase confidence of the patient.

Various Types of Equipment Can Assist with Lifting/Transfers
1. Slide boards.
2. Total mechanical lift.
3. Hoyer lift.
4. Sit-stand mechanical lift (SARA lift).
5. Transfer/gait belt.

Training
1. Proper training in the use of equipment as well as training in proper body mechanics is indicated and appropriate.

Use of Restraints

Regulation
1. JCAHO and other regulators determined facilities should be as "restraint-free" as possible.
2. Guiding principle is to create a physical, social, and cultural safe environment that preserves patient rights yet protects patients from injury.

Decision to Use Restraints
1. The decision to use a restraint is based on a comprehensive review of the patient/resident with concern for safety.
2. A restraint will be used when it is deemed that there is greater risk to the patient/resident if no restraint is used.
   a. Use of restraints can be reduced if environmental or alternative strategies are implemented instead.
   b. Examples include bed alarms and sitters.

3. If restraints are needed, less restrictive method is used.
4. Use of restraints is evaluated regularly and restraint is discontinued at earliest possible time.

Patient/Client Rights

Health Insurance Portability and Accountability Act (HIPAA)

1. Federal law established in 1996 applies to health information created or maintained by healthcare providers.
2. Assures privacy of all healthcare information, especially information that is electronic.
   a. Gives individuals rights over their health information.
   b. Sets rules and limits of who can look at and receive health information.
3. All the following must abide by law:
   a. All healthcare providers: physicians, nurses, physical therapists/assistants, pharmacists, etc.
   b. Health insurance companies, Health Maintenance Organizations (HMOs), employer group health plans.
   c. Medicare and Medicaid.
4. Information that is protected:
   a. Information entered in the medical record.
   b. Conversations among caregivers and between patient and caregivers.
   c. Billing information.
5. Information can be shared in order to:
   a. Provide appropriate care and coordination of care.
   b. Pay physicians, facilities, and other individuals who provided care.
   c. Protect public (i.e., report cases of flu or whooping cough).
   d. Complete required reports to authorities (i.e., gunshot wounds to police).
6. Information cannot be shared in order to:
   a. Give information to the employer.
   b. Develop marketing or advertising campaigns.
   c. Share notes about mental health or psychiatric counseling.
7. Providers who must comply with this law:
   a. Take reasonable steps to keep health information secure.
   b. Instruct and train staff as to how information may and may not be used and shared.

Americans with Disabilities Act (ADA)

1. Signed into law in July 1990, the ADA is wide-ranging legislation intended to make society more accessible to people with disabilities.
2. The ADA's protection applies primarily to "disabled" individuals.
3. An individual is considered disabled if he/she meets at least one of the criteria:
   a. Has a physical or mental impairment that substantially limits one or more of his/her major life activities.
   b. Has a record of such an impairment.
   c. Is regarded as having such impairment.
4. Other individuals protected by the ADA:
   a. Parents of an individual with a disability.
   b. Those that are coerced or subjected to retaliation for assisting people with disabilities in asserting their rights under the ADA.
5. The ADA is divided into four titles.
   a. Employment: business must provide reasonable accommodations such as restructuring jobs, altering the layout of work-stations, or modifying equipment.
   b. Public services: state and local government, commuter authorities cannot deny to people with disabilities services, programs, or activities that are available to people without disabilities. Public transportation must be accessible to individuals with disabilities.
   c. Public accommodations: all new construction and modifications must be accessible to individuals with disabilities. Public accommodations include facilities such as restaurants, hotels, grocery stores, retail stores, etc.
   d. Telecommunications: companies offering telephone service to the general public must have telephone relay service to individuals who use telecommunication devices for the deaf, Text Telephone (TTYs) or similar devices.
6. Employment rules apply to those who employ 15 or more employees.
7. Public accommodations rules apply to all, no matter the size, including all governmental offices.

Individuals with Disabilities Education Act (IDEA)

1. Originally enacted in 1975, allowing children with disabilities from birth through age 21 to receive a free, appropriate education in the least restrictive environment.
2. Federal funding is given to individual school systems to help cover the cost of educating students with special needs.
3. IDEA mandates that students receive related services (e.g., PT, occupational therapist [OT], speech therapist) to meet their educational needs.
4. Related services must be provided by qualified personnel.

5. Students who qualify for services must be evaluated every three years and an Individual Educational Plan (IEP) must be devised.
   a. Parent/guardian must approve and sign off on the IEP.
   b. Team meeting including the parent and student (when appropriate) must take place to discuss plan and outcomes.
6. Related services such as PT are provided to the student to meet their educational needs and to allow the student to access their school environment.

Abuse and Neglect

1. PTs and PTAs are mandated reporters of neglect and/or abuse of children, elders, and the disabled in all 50 states.
2. Each state may have specific reporting systems and requirements.
3. All 50 states have a hotline to report abuse/neglect.
4. Facilities will have specific protocols to report such findings.
5. States have varying levels of knowledge that trigger a report.
   a. Some states may require only a "reasonable suspicion."
   b. Other states may require a higher threshold of "know or suspect."
6. All states have legislation that provides for immunity from prosecution arising out of the reporting abuse/neglect.
7. In most states a person who reports suspected child abuse in "good faith" is immune from criminal and civil liability.
8. Victims are not likely to report abuse, as they are often dependent on the abuser.
9. Elder abuse/neglect.
   a. Individuals 50 years of age or older.
   b. Any action that constitutes the willful infliction of injury, unreasonable confinement, intimidation, or cruel punishment with resulting physical harm, pain or mental anguish.
   c. Denial of goods or services (e.g., food, medical care) to an elder with the intent to cause physical harm, mental anguish, or mental illness.
   d. Abuse/neglect can be physical, emotional, medical, financial, and/or sexual.
   e. Signs of abuse/neglect.
      - Unexplained physical injuries.
      - Withdrawal.
      - Increased agitation.
      - Increased depression.
      - Malnutrition.
      - Substandard care or poor physical hygiene.

Sexual Harassment/Advances

1. It is unlawful and unethical for a PT or PTA to have a sexual relationship with a patient/client.
2. Sexual harassment can be in the form of:
   a. Sexual jokes.
   b. Leering, whistling, rude, and unwanted sexual comments.
   c. Display of sexually graphic art, cartoons, objects.
   d. Request for sexual favors in exchange for treatment.
   e. Inappropriate touching or physical exam given diagnosis.
3. Even if contact is consensual, it is still unethical.
4. If patient/client makes advances to the PT/PTA, the practitioner has to be clear that those actions are inappropriate.
   a. Caution should be taken; work with those patients in an open area with others in the area.
      - If situation continues, care should be transferred to another therapist.
5. PTs and PTAs are obligated to report any caregivers who engage in sexual activity with their patients/clients.

First Aid

External Bleeding

1. Minor bleeding.
   a. Usually clots within 10 minutes.
   b. If patient/client taking aspirin or non-steroidal anti-inflammatory drugs (NSAIDs), clotting time may be longer.
2. Severe bleeding characteristics.
   a. Blood spurting from a wound.
   b. Blood fails to clot even after measures to control bleeding have been taken.
   c. Arterial bleed: high pressure, spurting, red blood.
   d. Venous bleed: low pressure, steady flow, dark red or maroon blood.
   e. Capillary bleed: low pressure, oozing, dark red blood.
3. Controlling external bleeding.
   a. Use standard precautions such as wearing gloves.
   b. Apply gauze pads using firm pressure. If no gauze available, use a clean cloth, towel, a gloved hand, or patient's own hand. If blood soaks through, do not remove any gauze; add additional layers.
   c. Elevate the part if possible unless it is deformed or it causes significant pain when elevated.
   d. Apply a pressure bandage, such as roller gauze, over the gauze pads.
   e. If necessary, apply pressure with the heel of your hand over pressure points. The femoral artery in the

groin and the brachial artery in the medial aspect of the upper arm are two such points.
f. Monitor A, B, Cs, and overall status of the patient. Administer supplemental oxygen if nearby. Seek more advanced care as necessary.

Internal Bleeding

1. Could be the result of a fall, blunt force, trauma, or a fracture rupturing a blood vessel or organ.
2. Severe internal bleeding may be life threatening.
3. Characteristics.
   a. Ecchymosis (black and blue) in the injured area.
   b. Body part, especially the abdomen, may be swollen, tender, and firm.
   c. Skin may appear blue, gray, or pale and may be cool or moist.
   d. Respiratory rate is increased.
   e. Pulse rate is increased and weak.
   f. Blood pressure is decreased.
   g. Patient may be nauseated or vomit.
   h. Patient may exhibit restlessness or anxiety.
   i. Level of consciousness may decline.
4. Management of internal bleeding.
   a. If minor, follow RICE procedure: rest, ice, compression, elevation.
   b. Major internal bleeding.
      - Summon advanced medical personnel.
      - Monitor A, B, Cs, and vital signs.
      - Keep the patient comfortable and quiet. Prevent either overheating or getting chilled.
      - Reassure patient or victim.
      - Administer supplemental oxygen if available and nearby.

Shock (Hypoperfusion)

1. Failure of the circulatory system to perfuse vital organs.
2. At first, blood is shunted from the periphery to compensate.
   a. Victim may lose consciousness as the brain is affected.
   b. Heart rate increases resulting in increased oxygen demand.
   c. Organs ultimately fail when deprived of oxygen.
   d. Heart rhythm is affected, ultimately leading to cardiac arrest and death.
3. Types and causes of shock.
   a. Hemorrhagic: severe internal or external bleeding.
   b. Psychogenic: emotional stress causes blood to pool in body away from the brain.
   c. Metabolic: loss of body fluids from heat or severe vomiting or diarrhea.
   d. Anaphylactic: allergic reaction from drugs, food, or insect stings.
   e. Cardiogenic: MI or cardiac arrest results in pump failure.
   f. Respiratory: respiratory illness or arrest results in insufficient oxygenation of the blood.
   g. Septic: severe infections cause blood vessels to dilate.
   h. Neurogenic: traumatic brain injury (TBI), spinal cord injury (SCI), or other neural trauma causes disruption of autonomic nervous system, resulting in disruption of blood vessel dilation/constriction.
4. Signs and symptoms.
   a. Pale gray or blue, cool skin.
   b. Increased weak pulse.
   c. Increased respiratory rate.
   d. Decreased blood pressure.
   e. Irritability or restlessness.
   f. Diminishing level of consciousness.
   g. Nausea or vomiting.
5. Care for shock.
   a. Obtain a history if possible.
   b. Examine the victim for airway, breathing, circulation, and bleeding.
   c. Assess level of consciousness.
   d. Determine skin characteristics and perform capillary refill test of finger tips.
      - Capillary refill: squeeze fingernail for 2 seconds. In healthy individuals, the nail will blanch and turn pink when pressure is released. If nail bed does not refill and turn pink within 2 seconds, the cause could be that blood is being shunted away from the periphery to vital organs or to maintain core temperature.
   e. Treat any specific condition if possible: control bleeding, splint a fracture, Epi-Pen for anaphylaxis, and so on.
   f. Keep the victim from getting chilled or overheated.
   g. Elevate the legs 12 inches unless there is suspected spinal injury or painful deformities of the lower extremities.
   h. Reassure the victim and continue to monitor A, B, Cs.
   i. Administer supplemental oxygen if nearby.
   j. Do not give any food or drink.
   k. Summon more advanced medical care.

Basic Life Support and CPR (Box 13-2)

BOX 13-2 ▷ Basic Life Support (BLS) and Cardiopulmonary Resuscitation (CPR)

Most adult victims of sudden cardiac arrest (SCA) experience ventricular fibrillation (VF), requiring resuscitation and defibrillation performed within the first 5 minutes after collapse. Asphyxial cardiac arrest is more common in infants and children. CPR is critical both before and after defibrillation. The sequence of CAB (Compressions-Airway-Breathing) is standard practice to minimize the time to chest compression in order to circulate the blood. Current CPR guidelines for healthcare (HC) providers include the following:

1. For sudden collapse in victims of all ages, HC providers should call for help (911 or if in hospital a "code" and get an automated external defibrillator [AED] [when readily available]), return to the victim and begin CPR and use the AED.
2. For unresponsive victims of all ages (e.g., asphyxial arrest), the HC provider should deliver about five cycles of CPR (about 2 minutes) before calling for help and getting the AED. Upon return, begin CPR and use the AED.
3. Initial Breathing: the HC provider should open the airway (use head-tilt/chin-lift maneuver) and deliver two rescue breaths. If trauma is suspected, use jaw thrust to open airway; do not tilt head.
   - Pinch nose shut and seal lips around the victim's mouth or mouth and nose if an infant.
   - Mouth-to-Mouth Rescue Breathing: deliver two rescue breaths at 1-second/breath that make the chest rise.
   - Mouth-to-Barrier Device Breathing: place pocket face mask over victim's mouth and nose. Continue to tilt head and lift chin, give two slow rescue breaths into opening of pocket mask.
   - For individuals with respiratory arrest and a perfusing rhythm (pulses), provide rescue breaths without chest compressions at 10–12 breaths per minute for the adult and 12–20 breaths per minute for the infant (less than 1 year) and child (1–8 years). Recheck pulse every 2 minutes.
4. After two rescue breaths, the HC provider should feel for a pulse (carotid pulse). If no pulse within 10 seconds, the provider should begin cycles of chest compressions and ventilations.
   - Overall compression rate is at least 100/minute for adults, infants, and children.
   - Compression-ventilation ratio is 30:2 for all adults (one or two rescuers); 30:2 for single rescuer (child); 15:2 for infant and child (two rescuers). Allow for complete chest recoil between compressions.
   - Victim must be supported on a hard surface.
   - Compression landmarks: place heel of one hand on the lower half of the sternum between the nipples; the other hand is placed on top of first hand. For the infant, use two fingers to compress the chest just below the nipple line.
   - Push hard and fast and release completely; compression depth should be at least 2 inches for adults; at least 1/3 the anterior-posterior (about 2 inches for children, about 1½ inches for infants) depth of the chest for an infant and child. Minimize interruptions in compressions.
   - Reevaluate patient's pulse after 1 minute and every 1–3 minutes thereafter. If pulse returns but not breathing, continue with rescue breathing only.
   - Continue with CPR until advanced life support (ALS) providers take over, or victim starts to move.

   Lay rescuers should immediately begin cycles of chest compressions and ventilations after delivering two rescue breaths for an unresponsive victim. Lay rescuers are not taught to assess for pulse or signs of circulation for an unresponsive victim. Lay rescuers are not taught to provide rescue breathing without chest compressions.

BOX 13-2 ▸ Basic Life Support (BLS) and Cardiopulmonary Resuscitation (CPR) (Continued)

Summary of Key Basic Life Support (BLS) Components

COMPONENT	ADULTS	CHILDREN	INFANTS
When to intervene	Unresponsive, no breathing, not breathing normally (e.g., only gasping)	Same as for adults	Same as for adults
CPR sequence	CAB	CAB	CAB
Hand placement	Two hands on the lower half of the sternum, avoiding the xiphoid process	One hand on the lower half of the sternum, avoiding the xiphoid process	Two fingers used placed just below the intermammary line
Compression rate	At least 100/minute	Same as for adults	Same as for adults
Compression depth	At least 2 inches	At least 1/3 AP depth, about 2 inches	At least 1/3 AP depth, about 1½ inches
Compression to ventilation ratio	30:2 (1 or 2 rescuer)	30:2 single rescuer 15:2 2 HCP rescuer	30:2 single rescuer 15:2 2 HCP rescuer
Airway	Head tilt-chin lift (if HCP suspects trauma: jaw thrust)	Same as for adults	Same as for adults

From *2017 American Heart Association Guidelines for CPR and ECG*. https://eccguidelines.heart.org/index.php/circulation/cpr-ecc-guidelines-2/

5. Defibrillation AED.
   - All basic life support providers should be trained to use AED/defibrillator.

     Whenever defibrillation is attempted, rescuers must coordinate good CPR with defibrillation to minimize interruptions in chest compressions and to ensure immediate resumption of chest compressions after shock delivery.
   - When any rescuer witnesses an out-of-hospital arrest and an AED is immediately available on-site, the rescuer should use the AED as soon as possible. HC providers who treat cardiac arrest in hospitals and other facilities with AEDs on-site should provide immediate CPR and should use the AED/defibrillator as soon as it is available.
   - When an out-of-hospital cardiac arrest is not witnessed by EMS personnel, they may give about five cycles of CPR before checking the ECG rhythm and attempting defibrillation.
   - If not shockable, resume CPR immediately for five cycles. Check rhythm every five cycles.
   - For children (1–8 years old), use pediatric AED system if available. Defibrillation not recommended for infants <1 year of age.
   - Continue until ALS providers take over or victim starts to move.

6. Foreign-Body Airway Obstruction (choking).
   - Examine for signs of airway obstruction by a foreign body. "Are you choking?" "Can you speak?"
   - Universal distress signal: victim clutches his or her neck with the thumb and index finger.
   - Difficulty speaking, high-pitched sounds while inhaling.
   - Poor, ineffective coughs.
   - Bluish skin color (cyanosis).
   - Procedure for obstructed airway.
   - If victim is conscious and standing, use Heimlich's maneuver. Make a fist with one hand, place thumb side of fist on victim's abdomen, below breast bone and above navel. Grasp around victim with other hand and provide quick upward thrusts into the victim's abdomen. Repeat until object is expelled.
   - For child, use back slaps and chest thrusts.

From: *2005 American Heart Association Guidelines for Cardiopulmonary Resuscitation and Emergency Cardiovascular Care*. Circulation 112:IV–12–IV–17, 2005.

Illegal Practice and Malpractice

Statutory Laws

Legislative
1. Passed by the legislature and impacting physical therapy.
   a. Licensure laws.
   b. Workers' Compensation Acts.
   c. Medicare/Medicaid.
   d. Americans with Disabilities Acts (ADA).

Goals of Statutory Laws Impacting Physical Therapy

Jurisdiction or State Laws
1. Professional licensing laws are enacted by all states.
2. Protect the consumer against practitioners who are incompetent.
3. Determine the minimal standards of educational preparation and the scope of practice.
   a. Graduation from an accredited program or its equivalent in physical therapy.
   b. Successful completion of a national licensing examination.
   c. Ethical and legal standards relating to continuing practice of physical therapy.
   d. Each state determines criteria to practice and issues a license.

Nondiscrimination Laws

Employment
1. Prevent a facility from discrimination against employees.
2. Title VII of the Civil Rights Act of 1964 prohibits employment discrimination based on:
   a. Race.
   b. Color.
   c. Sex.
   d. Religion.
   e. National origin.

The Age Discrimination and Employment Act of 1967
1. Prohibits employers from discriminating against persons from 40–70 years of age in any area of employment.

1973 Rehabilitation Act
1. Prohibits employment discrimination based on disability in:
   a. Federal executive agencies.
   b. All institutions receiving Medicare, Medicaid, and other federal support.

The Americans with Disability Act (ADA), 1990
1. Prevents discrimination against people with disabilities.
2. Ensures their integration into mainstream life.
3. The definition "disabilities" encompasses a wide range of physical and mental conditions.
4. Requires businesses of 15 or more employees to reasonably accommodate the needs of persons with disabilities to facilitate their economic independence in both the public and private sector.
5. Equal Employment Opportunity Commission (EEOC) oversees issues and interprets regulations.
6. Reasonable accommodations in the workplace by removing barriers must be made unless it would cause "undue hardship."
   a. Installing an elevator so the individual could access the upper floors may be considered an undue hardship.

Common Law

Has Evolved from Legal Decisions and Impacts in Physical Therapy in Several Areas

Malpractice
1. Physical therapists and physical therapist assistants are personally responsible for negligence and other acts that may result in harm to a patient through professional/patient relationships.
2. Negligence.
   a. Failure to do what a reasonably competent practitioner would have done under similar circumstances.
   b. To find a practitioner negligent, harm must have occurred to the patient.
   c. Every individual is liable for his/her own negligence.

3. Supervisors or superiors may also be found "vicariously" negligent because of the actions of their workers, if they provided faulty supervision or inappropriate delegation of responsibilities.
4. Patients may contribute to their own negligence if they do not follow directions from the assistant or therapist.
5. The institution usually is found "vicariously" negligent if a patient was harmed as a result of an environmental problem.
   a. Slippery floor.
   b. Fall in a poorly lit hall.
6. The institution is also liable if an employee was incompetent or not properly licensed.
7. Statute of limitations is a legal time limit in which an injured party can make a claim of medical malpractice.
   a. Time limitation is from 1–4 years after the injury occurred.
8. A physical therapist assistant may be asked to be an expert witness or testify in a malpractice case for:
   a. The plaintiff (victim).
   b. The defendant (accused).

Injury Prevention

Overview

Injuries
1. Back injuries are one of the leading causes of lost work days among healthcare workers.
2. Patient lifts and transfers were found to be the most common causes of reported back injury among healthcare workers.

Prevention
1. Injuries can be prevented through the use of proper body mechanics as well as effective use of appropriate assistive equipment.
2. Ongoing training and effective policy are necessary.

Common Back Musculoskeletal Injuries
1. Strained ligaments.
2. Strained muscles.
3. Injury to muscle or ligaments from repetitive motions.

Common Causes of Injury
1. Single high-load incident.
2. Awkward postures for lifting or for sustained periods of time.
3. Fatigue; not taking breaks when tired.
4. Repetitive and sustained activities in one direction.
5. Stressful situations with increased workload demand.

Prepare
1. Assessment of the situation prior to lift or transfer is key in preventing injuries.
2. Determine level of assistance patient requires.
3. Assess the environment.
   a. Transfer/patient area should be free of clutter.
   b. Transfer/patient area should allow easy access to patients and visitors.
   c. Adjustments in technique may be needed in small areas such as bathrooms.
   d. Bed or wheelchair should be moved to allow access from both sides.
   e. Proper footwear is needed for both patient and healthcare worker.
   f. If floor too slippery due to high polish or wet (e.g., floor of tub/shower), cover with nonslip material.

Body Mechanics: General Concepts

Principles
1. Back should be held in a neutral position to maintain the spine's natural curves
   a. This position protects the back and tolerates larger compressive forces.

Avoid Twisting
1. Discs are weaker and more vulnerable when flexing is combined with twisting.
2. Move feet to maintain alignment of the hips and shoulders.

Keep Weight Close to the Body (Center of Gravity, Lower Abdominal Area)
1. Supporting weight at increased distances from the center of gravity increases stresses placed on the spine.

Utilize Slow Planned Movements
1. Jerking movements limit the ability of the body to recruit all the muscles necessary for a safe lift.

Bend at the Hips and Lift with the Legs
1. The large muscles of the legs have greater strength and power than the back muscles to do the lifting.
2. Tighten the lower abdominal muscles to provide more support to the lower back.

Maintain a Wide Base of Support for Improved Balance

Push Rather Than Pull or Carry Heavy Loads

Inpatient Care

Prior to the Lift
1. Consider use of a mechanical lift given the patient's size and the amount of assistance he or she is able to offer.
2. Ask for help from another healthcare worker when in doubt or when necessary.
3. Keep in mind all of the body mechanic principles when lifting/transferring a patient.
4. Assess and set up the environment prior to the transfer.

During the Lift
1. Explain procedure to patient/client and assure comprehension.
2. Instruct the patient to do as much as they can themselves.
3. If needed, lift in stages; use slide board to assist and give a surface to rest on.
4. If a patient or object slips, lower gently to the floor.

Instructions for Patient/Client

Safe Handling
1. Patient and caregiver instructions for safe handling should cover the following.
   a. Correct and safe use of transfer equipment, e.g., wheelchairs, sliding boards, gait belt.
   b. Correct positioning of equipment, patient/client, helper.
   c. Body mechanics guidelines for the helper.
   d. Mechanical principles to assist in transfer and bed mobility activities, e.g., "nose over the toes" to assist in standing, weight shift away from direction of scoot on sliding board.

Other Injury Prevention Information

Furniture and Equipment
1. Purchase furniture and equipment with patient handling and patient use in mind.
2. Furniture and equipment should have removal arm rests and leg rest to assist with ease of transfers.
3. Beds should always be lowered or raised in order to make transfers easy.
4. Bathrooms, toilets, and showers should be designed and set up so pushing and pulling of shower chairs is as easy as possible.

Staff Management
1. On a regular basis, ensure staff is properly trained in use of equipment and body mechanics.
2. Employee conditioning, such as cardiovascular conditioning, strengthening, and flexibility exercises, can help prevent work-related injury.

Roles and Responsibilities

The PT/PTA Team

Guidelines
1. The PT is the only individual who can clinically direct and supervise a PTA; the PTA must practice under the direction of a PT.
2. Each jurisdiction has specific guidelines/rules as to what type of supervision a PTA requires and how often that supervision needs to occur.
3. Various practice environments and facilities will have different policies as to the required supervision of the PTA.

4. The PTA must follow the plan of care established by the PT.
   a. If the PTA identifies a possible need for change or update to the plan of care, the PTA discusses this with the PT.
5. In working as a team member, the PTA works closely with other healthcare professionals (see below).
6. In working with and discussing patient care with other professionals, the PTA must convey the prognosis, plan of care, goals, and outcomes established by the PT.

Principles of Collaboration

Definition
1. A team is a group of equally important individuals with a common interest, collaborating to develop shared goals, building trusting relationships to achieve these shared goals.

Members of the Healthcare Team
1. The patient/client/consumer.
2. Patient family members.
3. Significant others.
4. Caregivers.
5. Healthcare professionals.
6. Insurance company or assigned liaison.
7. Professional members on the team will vary with practice setting.

The Caregiver as a Team Member
1. The consumer, family member, significant other, and/or caregiver role on the team have become increasingly important as the focus on healthcare has changed.
2. Collaboration with these individuals is mandated by law.

Factors That Influence and Increase the Effectiveness of a Functioning Team
1. Identifying member's skills and knowledge level.
2. Team members' commitment to the patient's goals.
3. Team members must be effective communicators to all other team members.
4. Membership composition must address all of the patient's medical needs.
5. Members must share a common language.
6. Members have to be effective leaders.

Caregiver Definition and Roles

Physical Therapy Director
1. Oversees the function of the department.
2. Ensures policies and procedures are carried out effectively.
3. Acts as a liaison with the facility administration.
4. Sets goals and strategic plans for the department.

Physical Therapy Supervisor
1. Qualified experienced clinician with a variety of skills.
   a. Good clinical knowledge of tasks performed.
   b. Ability to motivate subordinates and communicate effectively with supervisors.
   c. Ability to evaluate staff and give oral and written feedback effectively.
   d. Ability to delegate tasks to appropriate staff.

Physical Therapist (PT)
1. A skilled healthcare professional who is licensed by the state jurisdiction.
2. Every PT is licensed by each state or jurisdiction following successful performance on the national physical therapy examination.
3. Role of the PT:
   a. Examines patients.
   b. Evaluates data.
   c. Establishes diagnosis.
   d. Establishes prognosis.
   e. Establishes plan of care.
   f. Executes interventions.
   g. Supervises treatment.
4. PTs can delegate portions of treatments to PTAs.
5. PTs have the authority to supervise and direct supportive personnel (PTA and PT aides or techs) in designated tasks.
6. Reevaluates and adjusts the patient's plan of care as indicated.
7. Performs and documents initial/reevaluation/final evaluation, establishes discharge and follow-up plans.

Physical Therapist Assistant (PTA)
1. A PTA is a technically educated healthcare provider who assists the PT in the provision of physical therapy.
2. The PTA is a graduate of a PTA associate degree program accredited by the Commission on Accreditation in Physical Therapy Education (CAPTE).
3. Required to pass a national examination in most jurisdictions.
4. Utilization of the physical therapist assistant:
   a. The PT is directly responsible for the actions of the PTA related to patient/client management (Appendices II and III).

b. The PTA may perform selected physical therapy interventions under the direction and at least general (the PT is not required to be on-site during patient care) supervision of the PT.
- Some state bylaws require direct or on-site supervision (refer to individual state bylaws for clarification).
- The ability of the PTA to perform the selected interventions as directed shall be assessed on an ongoing basis by the supervising PT.
- The PTA may modify an intervention in accordance with changes in patient/client status within the scope of the established plan of care.

5. In all practice settings, the performance of selected interventions by the PTA must be consistent with safe and legal PT practice and shall be predicated on the following factors:
   a. The complexity and acuity of the patient's/client's needs.
   b. The proximity and accessibility to the PT.
   c. The supervision available in the event of an emergency or during critical events.
   d. The type of setting in which the service is provided.
6. The PTA is also expected to work within outlined ethical guidelines. These are outlined in APTA documents and may also be found in individual state documents (Appendix C).
7. Supervision of the PTA in off-site settings: The following requirements must be observed (Appendix C).
   a. A PT must be accessible by telecommunications to the PTA at all times while the PTA is treating patients/clients.
   b. There must be regularly scheduled and documented conferences with the PTA regarding the patient/client.
      - The frequency is determined by the needs of the patient/client and the needs of the PTA.
   c. When the PTA is involved in the care of a patient/client, supervisory visits by the PT will be made:
      - Upon the PTA's request for a reexamination.
      - When a change in the treatment plan of care is needed.
      - Before any planned discharge.
      - In response to a change to the patient's/client's medical status.
   d. Supervisory visits should occur at least once a month.
      - A higher frequency may be established by the PT, in accordance with the needs of the patient.
   e. Supervisory visits should include.
      - An on-site reexamination of the patient/client by the physical therapist.
      - On-site review of the plan of care with appropriate revision or termination.

Physical Therapy Aide
1. Is a nonlicensed worker.
   a. Specifically trained under the direction of a PT or PTA.
      - When permissible by the individual state practice act, PTAs can supervise physical therapy aides.
2. Functions only with continuous on-site supervision of a PT or PTA.
3. Performs designated routine tasks related to the operation of the physical therapy service.
4. Job responsibilities.
   a. Patient transportation.
   b. Equipment maintenance.
   c. Secretarial or housekeeping duties.
      - May set up patients for treatments where permissible by state law (e.g., assist in application of heat, cold, or participate in basic whirlpool treatments).
5. Medicare and some insurance companies do not reimburse for the services provided by the physical therapy aide.

PT and PTA Students
1. Performs duties commensurate with level of education.
2. PT or PTA clinical instructor (CI) is responsible for all actions and duties of the affiliating student and must provide on-site supervision at all times.
3. All student documentation must be cosigned by clinical instructor.
4. Patients must be informed that they will be treated by a student and have the right to refuse treatment.

Home Health Aide (HHA)
1. A nonlicensed worker.
   a. Provide personal care and home management services.
      - Assist patients to remain in the home setting.
2. Responsibilities.
   a. Bathing.
   b. Grooming.
   c. Light housework.
   d. Shopping.
   e. Cooking.
   f. Provide supervision/assistance to the patient to perform a home exercise program (HEP) after receiving instruction/supervision from the PT and/or PTA.
3. Home health aides are supervised directly by nursing or the physical therapist.

Occupational Therapist (OTR/L)
1. A skilled healthcare professional who is licensed by the state jurisdiction.
2. Required to pass a national examination.

3. Responsibilities.
   a. Provides education and training in activities of daily living.
   b. Development and fabrication of orthoses (splints).
   c. Provides training, recommendations, and selecting of adaptive equipment.
   d. Provides therapeutic activities.
      - Functional performance.
      - Cognitive/perceptual function.

Occupational Therapist Assistant (COTA)
1. A skilled technician holding an associate's degree who is licensed by the state jurisdiction.
2. Required to pass a national examination.
3. Works under the supervision of the occupational therapist in carrying out established treatment plans. COTA relationship follows similar guidelines to the PT/PTA.

Speech-Language Pathologist (Speech Therapist)
1. A skilled healthcare professional licensed in the state jurisdiction.
   a. Has completed 1 year of supervised field experience.
2. Required to pass a national examination.
3. Develops and conducts treatments to restore or improve communication of patients with language and speech impairments:
   a. Physiological deficits.
   b. Neurological disturbances.
   c. Defective articulation.
4. Works closely with occupational therapy to correct swallowing problems and cognitive processing deficits.

Certified Orthotist
1. Designs, fabricates, and fits orthoses prescribed by physicians.
   a. Braces.
   b. Splints.
   c. Cervical collars.
   d. Corsets.
   e. Orthotics/shoe inserts.
2. Successfully completed the examination by the American Orthotist and Prosthetist Association.

Certified Prosthetist
1. Designs, fabricates, and fits prostheses for patients with partial or total absence of a limb.
2. Successful passage on the examination by the American Orthotist and Prosthetist Association.

Certified Respiratory Therapy Technician (CRRT) (Respiratory Therapist)
1. Technically trained with an associate's degree from an accredited program.
2. Administers treatment as prescribed and supervised by a physician.
   a. Pulmonary function tests.
   b. Treatments: nebulizers, aerosols, oxygen therapy.
   c. Maintains all respiratory equipment and assists patient with its use (e.g., ventilators, continuous positive airway pressure [CPAP]).

Registered Nurse (RN)
1. Skilled healthcare professional who is a graduate of an accredited program and who has successfully passed a licensure exam.
2. Primary liaison between patient and physician.
3. Supervises other levels of nursing care (e.g., licensed practical nurse (LPN), certified nursing assistants, home health aides).
4. Makes referrals under the direction of the physician.
5. Dispenses medication but cannot change drug dosages.

Social Worker
1. Skilled healthcare professional who is a graduate of an accredited program and after 1 year of practical field work is licensed or registered by the state.
2. Can serve as a family and patient counselor.
3. Can serve as a case manager coordinating patient's care and transition from one setting to another.
   a. Assist family/patient with applications for financial assistance.
   b. Assist family/patient with search of nursing home or other facilities for transfer of care.
   c. Assures all discharge plans and referrals are in place.
   d. Advocate for patient in family and dealing with outside agencies and procuring continued services (e.g., insurance companies, home health agencies).
   e. Mediates between family/patient and team surrounding discharge plans and ongoing care.

Rehabilitation Counselor (Vocational Counselor)
1. Technically educated healthcare worker.
2. Counsels individuals with physical and/or cognitive disabilities.
3. Administers vocational testing which can assist in determining optimal occupational choices for an individual.
4. Will assist individuals with job placement and may arrange job-specific training.

Audiologist
1. Skilled healthcare professional who is a graduate of an accredited program and has successfully passed a licensure exam.
2. Specialist in hearing disorders:
   a. Uses audiometric tests to assess sensitivity of sense of hearing and of hearing loss.
   b. Uses speech audiometric tests to assess the ability to understand the spoken word.

Physiatrist
1. A physician specializing in physical medicine and rehabilitation.
2. Completes board certification as a specialist.
3. Primary focus is maximal restoration of physical, psychological, social, vocational function and to alleviate pain.
4. Often serves as the attending physician on inpatient rehab units.

Primary Care Physician (PCP)
1. Serves to manage routine healthcare needs.
2. Can be an internist, family medicine physician, or general practitioner.
3. Can serve as "gate keepers" of medical care.
   a. Many times, individuals need a referral from their PCP prior to seeing any specialist, including physical therapist.

Physician Assistant (PA, PA-C) or Nurse Practitioner (NP)
1. Skilled healthcare professional who is a graduate of an accredited program and who has successfully passed a licensure exam.
2. Considered a "physician extender."
3. Under supervision of the physician, can perform routine diagnostic, preventive, therapeutic interventions.
4. Can practice in a variety of settings.
5. Able to provide physical therapy referral and prescribe certain medications.
6. Nurse practitioner must complete RN training and pass licensure board prior to training as a nurse practitioner.

Athletic Trainer
1. Skilled healthcare professional who is a graduate of an accredited program and who has successfully passed a national certification exam.
2. Integral provider of care to athletes.
   a. Works with athletes to prevent injuries.
   b. Works with athletes after an injury for rehabilitation and return to sport.
3. Setting for delivery of care: public schools, colleges and universities, professional athletic teams, and private or hospital-based clinics.
   a. If working in private or hospital-based clinics, various jurisdictions have various rules and regulations of how an athletic trainer can be used in the clinic.

APPENDIX 13A: APTA Guidelines for Documentation of Patient/Client Management

Documentation Authority for Physical Therapy Services—May 2007

Physical therapy examination, evaluation, diagnosis, prognosis, and plan of care (including interventions) shall be documented, dated, and authenticated by the physical therapist who performs the service. Interventions provided by the physical therapist or selected interventions provided by the physical therapist assistant under the direction and supervision of the physical therapist are documented, dated, and authenticated by the physical therapist or, when permissible by law, the physical therapist assistant.

Other notations or flow charts are considered a component of the documented record but do not meet the requirements of documentation in or of themselves.

Students in physical therapist or physical therapist assistant programs may document when the record is additionally authenticated by the physical therapist or, when permissible by law, documentation by physical therapist assistant students may be authenticated by a physical therapist assistant.

Guidelines: Physical Therapy Documentation of Patient/Client Management

General Guidelines

- Documentation is required for every visit/encounter.
- All documentation must comply with the applicable jurisdictional/regulatory requirements.
- All handwritten entries shall be made in ink and will include original signatures. Electronic entries are made with appropriate security and confidentiality provisions.
- Charting errors should be corrected by drawing a single line through the error and initialing and dating the chart or through the appropriate mechanism for electronic documentation that clearly indicates that a change was made without deletion of the original record.
- All documentation must include adequate identification of the patient/client and the physical therapist or physical therapist assistant.
- The patient's/client's full name and identification number, if applicable, must be included on all official documents.

- All entries must be dated and authenticated with the provider's full name and appropriate designation:
- Documentation of examination, evaluation, diagnosis, prognosis, plan of care, and discharge summary must be authenticated by the physical therapist who provided the service.
- Documentation of intervention in visit/encounter notes must be authenticated by the physical therapist or physical therapist assistant who provided the service.
- Documentation by physical therapist or physical therapist assistant graduates or other physical therapists and physical therapist assistants pending receipt of an unrestricted license shall be authenticated by a licensed physical therapist, or, when permissible by law, documentation by physical therapist assistant graduates may be authenticated by a physical therapist assistant.
- Documentation by students (SPT/SPTA) in physical therapist or physical therapist assistant programs must be additionally authenticated by the physical therapist or, when permissible by law, documentation by physical therapist assistant students may be authenticated by a physical therapist assistant.
- Documentation should include the referral mechanism by which physical therapy services are initiated:
  - Self-referral/direct access.
  - Request for consultation from another practitioner.
- Documentation should include indication of no-shows and cancellations.

Visit/Encounter

- Documentation of each visit/encounter shall include the following elements:
  - Patient/client self-report (as appropriate).
  - Identification of specific interventions provided, including frequency, intensity and duration as appropriate. Examples include:
    - Knee extension, three sets, 10 repetitions, 10# weight.
    - Transfer training bed to chair with sliding board.
    - Equipment provided.
  - Changes in patient/client impairment, functional limitation, and disability status as they relate to the plan of care.
  - Response to interventions, including adverse reactions, if any.
  - Factors that modify frequency or intensity of intervention and progression goals, including patient/client adherence to patient/client-related instructions.
  - Communication/consultation with providers/patient/client/family/significant other.
  - Documentation to plan for ongoing provision of services for the next visit(s), which is suggested to include, but not be limited to:
    - The interventions with objectives.
    - Progression parameters.
    - Precautions, if indicated.

Excerpts from the American Physical Therapy Association's Board of Directors Guidelines for Documentation. Last updated December 2008.

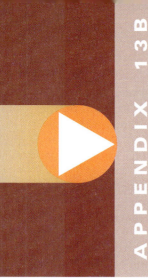

Standards of Practice for Physical Therapy

Standards of Practice for Physical Therapy October 2013 Preamble

The physical therapy profession's commitment to society is to promote optimal health and function in individuals by pursuing excellence in practice. The American Physical Therapy Association attests to this commitment by adopting and promoting the following *Standards of Practice for Physical Therapy*. These Standards are the profession's statement of conditions and performances that are essential for provision of high quality professional service to society and provide a foundation for assessment of physical therapist practice.

Ethical/Legal Considerations

1. Ethical Considerations.
   The physical therapist practices according to the *Code of Ethics* of the American Physical Therapy Association.
   The physical therapist assistant complies with the *Standards of Ethical Conduct for the Physical Therapist Assistant* of the American Physical Therapy Association.

2. Legal Considerations.
   The physical therapist complies with all the legal requirements of jurisdictions regulating the practice of physical therapy.
   The physical therapist assistant complies with all the legal requirements of jurisdictions regulating the work of the assistant.

Administration of the Physical Therapy Service

1. Statement of Mission, Purposes and Goals.
   The physical therapy service has a statement of mission, purposes and goals that reflects the needs and interests of the patients/clients served, the physical therapy personnel affiliated with the service and the community.

2. Organizational Plan.
   The physical therapy service has a written organizational plan.

3. Policies and Procedures.
   The physical therapy service has written policies and procedures that reflect the operation, mission, purposes, and goals of the service and are consistent

with the Association's standards, policies, positions, guidelines, and *Code of Ethics*.
4. Administration.
   A physical therapist is responsible for the direction of the physical therapy service.
5. Fiscal Management.
   The director of the physical therapy service, in consultation with physical therapy staff and appropriate administrative personnel, participates in the planning for and allocation of resources. Fiscal planning and management of the service is based on sound accounting principles.
6. Improvement of Quality of Care and Performance.
   The physical therapy service has a written plan for continuous improvement of quality of care and performance of services.
7. Staffing.
   The physical therapy personnel affiliated with the physical therapy service have demonstrated competence and are sufficient to achieve the mission, purposes, and goals of the service.
8. Staff Development.
   The physical therapy service has a written plan that provides for appropriate and ongoing staff development.
9. Physical Setting.
   The physical setting is designed to provide a safe and accessible environment that facilitates fulfillment of the mission, purposes and goals of the physical therapy service. The equipment is safe and sufficient to achieve the purposes, and goals of physical therapy.
10. Collaboration.
    The physical therapy service collaborates with all disciplines as appropriate.

Patient Client Management

1. Physical Therapist of Record.
   The physical therapist of record is the therapist who assumes responsibility for patient/client management and is accountable for the coordination, continuation, and progression of the plan of care.
2. Patient/Client Collaboration.
   Within the patient/client management process, the physical therapist and the patient/client establish and maintain an ongoing collaborative process of decision-making that exists throughout the provision of services.
3. Initial Examination/Evaluation/Diagnosis/Prognosis.
   The physical therapist performs an initial examination and evaluation to establish a diagnosis and prognosis prior to intervention. Wellness and prevention visits/encounters may occur without the presence of disease, illness, impairments, activity limitations, or participation restrictions.
4. Plan of Care.
   The physical therapist establishes a plan of care and manages the needs of the patient/client based on the examination, evaluation, diagnosis, prognosis, goals, and outcomes of the planned interventions for identified impairments, activity limitations, and participation restrictions.
   The physical therapist involves the patient/client and appropriate others in the planning, implementation, and assessment of the plan of care.
5. Intervention.
   The physical therapist provides or directs and supervises the physical therapy intervention consistent with the results of the examination, evaluation, diagnosis, prognosis and plan of care. The physical therapy intervention may be provided in an episode of care, or in a single visit/encounter such as for a wellness and prevention visit/encounter or a specialty consultation or for a follow-up visit/encounter after episodes of care, or may be provided intermittently over longer periods of time in cases of managing chronic conditions.
   An episode of care is the managed care provided for a specific problem or condition during a set time period and can be given either for a short period or on a continuous basis, or it may consist of a series of intervals marked by one or more brief separations from care.
6. Reexamination.
   The physical therapist reexamines the patient/client as necessary during an episode of care, during follow-up visits/encounters after an episode of care, or periodically in the case of chronic care management, to evaluate progress or change in patient/client status. The physical therapist modifies the plan of care accordingly or concludes the episode of care.
7. Conclusion of Episode of Care.
   The physical therapist concludes an episode of care when the anticipated goals or expected outcomes for the patient/client have been achieved, when the patient/client is unable to continue to progress toward goals, or when the physical therapist determines that the patient/client will no longer benefit from physical therapy.
8. Communication/Coordination/Documentation.
   The physical therapist communicates, coordinates and documents all aspects of patient/client management including the results of the initial examination and evaluation, diagnosis, prognosis, plan of care, interventions, response to interventions, changes in patient/client status relative to the intervention, reexamination, and episode of care summary. The physical therapist of record is responsible for "hand off" communication.

Education

The physical therapist is responsible for individual professional development. The physical therapist assistant is responsible for individual career development.

The physical therapist and the physical therapist assistant, under the direction and supervision of he physical therapist, participate in the education of students.

The physical therapist educates and provides consultation to consumers and the general public regarding the purposes and benefits of physical therapy.

The physical therapist educates and provides consultation to consumers and the general public regarding the roles of the physical therapist and the physical therapist assistant.

Research

The physical therapist applies research findings to practice, and encourages, participates in and promotes activities that establish the outcomes of patient/client management provided by the physical therapist.

Community Responsibility

The physical therapist demonstrates community responsibility by participating in community and community agency activities, educating the public, formulating public policy or providing pro bono physical therapy services.

APPENDIX 13C

Direction and Supervision of the PTA

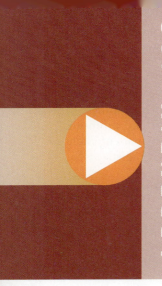

Direction and Supervision of the Physical Therapist Assistant—June 2005

Physical therapists have a responsibility to deliver services in ways that protect the public safety and maximize the availability of their services. They do this through direct delivery of services in conjunction with responsible utilization of physical therapist assistants who assist with selected components of intervention. The physical therapist assistant is the only individual permitted to assist a physical therapist in selected interventions under the direction and supervision of a physical therapist.

Direction and supervision are essential in the provision of quality physical therapy services. The degree of direction and supervision necessary for assuring quality physical therapy services is dependent upon many factors, including the education, experiences, and responsibilities of the parties involved, as well as the organizational structure in which the physical therapy services are provided.

Regardless of the setting in which the physical therapy service is provided, the following responsibilities must be borne solely by the physical therapist:

1. Interpretation of referrals when available.
2. Initial examination, evaluation, diagnosis, and prognosis.
3. Development or modification of a plan of care which is based on the initial examination or reexamination and which includes the physical therapy goals and outcomes.
4. Determination of when the expertise and decision-making capability of the physical therapist requires the physical therapist to personally render physical therapy interventions and when it may be appropriate to utilize the physical therapist assistant. A physical therapist shall determine the most appropriate utilization of the physical therapist assistant that provides for the delivery of service that is safe, effective and efficient.
5. Reexamination of the patient/client in light of their goals and revision of the plan of care when indicated.
6. Establishment of the discharge plan and documentation of discharge summary/status.
7. Oversight of all documentation for services rendered to each patient/client.

The physical therapist remains responsible for the physical therapy services provided when the physical therapist's plan of care involves the physical therapist assistant to assist with selected interventions. Regardless of the setting in which the service is provided, the determination to utilize physical therapist assistants for selected interventions requires the education, expertise and professional judgment of a physical therapist as described by the *Standards of Practice, Guide to Professional Conduct and Code of Ethics.*

In determining the appropriate extent of assistance from the physical therapist assistant (PTA), the physical therapist considers:

- The PTA's education, training, experience, and skill level.
- Patient client criticality, acuity, stability, and complexity.
- The predictability of the consequences.
- The setting in which the care is being delivered.
- Federal and state statutes.
- Liability and risk management concerns.
- The mission of physical therapy services for the setting.
- The needed frequency of reexamination.

Physical Therapist Assistant

Definition The physical therapist assistant is a technically educated healthcare provider who assists the physical therapist in the provision of physical therapy. The physical therapist assistant is a graduate of a physical therapist assistant associate degree program accredited by the Commission on Accreditation in Physical Therapy Education (CAPTE).

Utilization The physical therapist is directly responsible for the actions of the physical therapist assistant related to patient/client management. The physical therapist assistant may perform selected physical therapy interventions under the direction and at least general supervision of the physical therapist. In general supervision, the physical therapist is not required to be on-site for direction and supervision, but must be available at least by telecommunications. The ability of the physical therapist assistant to perform the selected interventions as directed shall be assessed on an ongoing basis by the supervising physical therapist. The physical therapist assistant makes modifications to selected interventions either to progress the patient/client as directed by the physical therapist or to ensure patient/client safety and comfort.

The physical therapist assistant must work under the direction and at least general supervision of the physical therapist. In all practice settings, the performance of selected interventions by the physical therapist assistant must be consistent with safe and legal physical therapist practice and shall be predicated on the following factors: complexity and acuity of the patient's/client's needs; proximity and accessibility to the physical therapist; supervision available in the event of emergencies or critical events; and type of setting in which the service is provided.

When supervising the physical therapist assistant in any off-site setting, the following requirements must be observed:

1. A physical therapist must be accessible by telecommunications to the physical therapist assistant at all times while the physical therapist assistant is treating patients/clients.
2. There must be regularly scheduled and documented conferences with the physical therapist assistant regarding patients/clients, the frequency of which is determined by the needs of the patient/client and the needs of the physical therapist assistant.
3. In those situations in which a physical therapist assistant is involved in the care of a patient/client, a supervisory visit by the physical therapist will be made:
   a. Upon the physical therapist assistant's request for reexamination, when a change in the plan of care is needed, prior to any planned discharge and in response to a change in the patient's/client's medical status.
   b. At least once a month, or at a higher frequency when established by the physical therapist, in accordance with the needs of the patient/client.
   c. A supervisory visit should include:
      i   An on-site reexamination of the patient/client.
      ii. On-site review of the plan of care with appropriate revision or termination.
      iii. Evaluation of need and recommendation for utilization of outside resources.

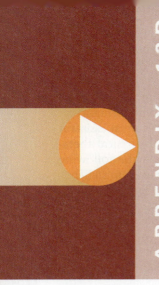

Guide for Conduct of the Physical Therapist Assistant

Purpose

This Guide for Conduct of the Physical Therapist Assistant (Guide) is intended to serve physical therapist assistants in interpreting the Standards of Ethical Conduct for the Physical Therapist Assistant (Standards) of the American Physical Therapy Association (APTA). The APTA House of Delegates in June of 2009 adopted the revised Standards, which became effective on July 1, 2010.

The Guide provides a framework by which physical therapist assistants may determine the propriety of their conduct. It is also intended to guide the development of physical therapist assistant students. The Standards and the Guide apply to all physical therapist assistants. These guidelines are subject to change as the dynamics of the profession change and as new patterns of health care delivery are developed and accepted by the professional community and the public.

Interpreting Ethical Standards

The interpretations expressed in this Guide reflect the opinions, decisions, and advice of the Ethics and Judicial Committee (EJC). The interpretations are set forth according to topic. These interpretations are intended to assist a physical therapist assistant in applying general ethical standards to specific situations. They address some but not all topics addressed in the Standards and should not be considered inclusive of all situations that could evolve.

This Guide is subject to change, and the Ethics and Judicial Committee will monitor and timely revise the Guide to address additional topics and Standards when necessary and as needed.

Preamble to the Standards

The Preamble states as follows:

The Standards of Ethical Conduct for the Physical Therapist Assistant (Standards of Ethical Conduct) delineate the ethical obligations of all physical therapist assistants as determined by the House of Delegates of the American Physical Therapy Association (APTA). The Standards of Ethical Conduct provide a foundation for conduct to which all physical therapist assistants shall adhere. Fundamental to the Standards of Ethical Conduct is the special obligation of physical therapist assistants to enable patients/clients to achieve greater independence, health and wellness, and enhanced quality of life.

No document that delineates ethical standards can address every situation. Physical therapist assistants are encouraged to seek additional advice or consultation in instances where the guidance of the Standards of Ethical Conduct may not be definitive.

Interpretation

Upon the Standards of Ethical Conduct for the Physical Therapist Assistant being amended effective July 1, 2010, all the lettered standards contain the word "shall" and are mandatory ethical obligations. The language contained in the Standards is intended to better explain and further clarify existing ethical obligations. These ethical obligations predate the revised Standards. Although various words have changed, many of the obligations are the same. Consequently, the addition of the word "shall" serves to reinforce and clarify existing ethical obligations. A significant reason that the Standards were revised was to provide physical therapist assistants with a document that was clear enough such that they can read it standing alone without the need to seek extensive additional interpretation.

The Preamble states that "[n]o document that delineates ethical standards can address every situation." The Preamble also states that physical therapist assistants "are encouraged to seek additional advice or consultation in instances where the guidance of the Standards of Ethical Conduct may not be definitive." Potential sources for advice or counsel include third parties and the myriad resources available on the APTA Web site. Inherent in a physical therapist assistant's ethical decision-making process is the examination of his or her unique set of facts relative to the Standards.

Standards

Respect

Standard 1A states as follows:

1A. Physical therapist assistants shall act in a respectful manner toward each person regardless of age, gender, race, nationality, religion, ethnicity, social or economic status, sexual orientation, health condition, or disability.

Interpretation

Standard 1A addresses the display of respect toward others. Unfortunately, there is no universal consensus about what respect looks like in every situation. For example, direct eye contact is viewed as respectful and courteous in some cultures and inappropriate in others. It is up to the individual to assess the appropriateness of behavior in various situations.

Altruism

Standard 2A states as follows:

2A. Physical therapist assistants shall act in the best interests of patients/clients over the interests of the physical therapist assistant.

Interpretation

Standard 2A addresses acting in the best interest of patients/clients over the interests of the physical therapist assistant. Often this is done without thought, but sometimes, especially at the end of the day when the clinician is fatigued and ready to go home, it is a conscious decision. For example, the physical therapist assistant may need to make a decision between leaving on time and staying at work longer to see a patient who was 15 minutes late for an appointment.

Sound Decisions

Standard 3C states as follows:

3C. Physical therapist assistants shall make decisions based upon their level of competence and consistent with patient/client values.

Interpretation

To fulfill 3C, the physical therapist assistant must be knowledgeable about his or her legal scope of work as well as level of competence. As a physical therapist assistant gains experience and additional knowledge, there may be areas of physical therapy interventions in which he or she displays advanced skills. At the same time, other previously gained knowledge and skill may be lost due to lack of use. To make sound decisions, the physical therapist assistant must be able to self-reflect on his or her current level of competence.

Supervision

Standard 3E states as follows:

3E. Physical therapist assistants shall provide physical therapy services under the direction and supervision of a physical therapist and shall communicate with the physical therapist when patient/client status requires modifications to the established plan of care.

Interpretation

Standard 3E goes beyond simply stating that the physical therapist assistant operates under the supervision of the physical therapist. Although a physical therapist retains responsibility for the patient/client throughout the episode of care, this standard requires the physical therapist assistant to take action by communicating with the supervising physical therapist when changes in the patient/client status indicate that modifications to the plan of care may be needed. Further information on supervision via APTA policies and resources is available on the APTA Web site.

Integrity in Relationships

Standard 4 states as follows:

4: Physical therapist assistants shall demonstrate integrity in their relationships with patients/clients, families, colleagues, students, other health care providers, employers, payers, and the public.

Interpretation

Standard 4 addresses the need for integrity in relationships. This is not limited to relationships with patients/clients, but includes everyone physical therapist assistants come into contact with in the normal provision of physical therapy services. For example, demonstrating integrity could encompass working collaboratively with the health care team and taking responsibility for one's role as a member of that team.

Reporting

Standard 4C states as follows:

4C. Physical therapist assistants shall discourage misconduct by health care professionals and report illegal or unethical acts to the relevant authority, when appropriate.

Interpretation

When considering the application of "when appropriate" under Standard 4C, keep in mind that not all allegedly illegal or unethical acts should be reported immediately to an agency/authority. The determination of when to do so depends upon each situation's unique set of facts, applicable laws, regulations, and policies.

Depending upon those facts, it might be appropriate to communicate with the individuals involved. Consider whether the action has been corrected, and in that case, not reporting may be the most appropriate action. Note, however, that when an agency/authority does examine a potential ethical issue, fact finding will be its first step. The determination of ethicality requires an understanding of all of the relevant facts, but may still be subject to interpretation.

The EJC Opinion titled: Topic: Preserving Confidences; Physical Therapist's Reporting Obligation With Respect to Unethical, Incompetent, or Illegal Acts provides further information on the complexities of reporting.

Exploitation

Standard 4E states as follows:

4E. Physical therapist assistants shall not engage in any sexual relationship with any of their patients/clients, supervisees, or students.

Interpretation

The statement is fairly clear—sexual relationships with their patients/clients, supervisees or students are prohibited. This component of Standard 4 is consistent with Standard 4B, which states:

4B. Physical therapist assistants shall not exploit persons over whom they have supervisory, evaluative or other authority (eg, patients/clients, students, supervisees, research participants, or employees).

Next, consider this excerpt from the EJC Opinion titled Topic: Sexual Relationships With Patients/Former Patients (modified for physical therapist assistants):

A physical therapist [assistant] stands in a relationship of trust to each patient and has an ethical obligation to act in the patient's best interest and to avoid any exploitation or abuse of the patient. Thus, if a physical therapist [assistant] has natural feelings of attraction toward a patient, he/she must sublimate those feelings in order to avoid sexual exploitation of the patient.

One's ethical decision making process should focus on whether the patient/client, supervisee or student is being exploited. In this context, questions have been asked about whether one can have a sexual relationship once the patient/client relationship ends. To this question, the EJC has opined as follows:

The Committee does not believe it feasible to establish any bright-line rule for when, if ever, initiation of a romantic/sexual relationship with a former patient would be ethically permissible.

……

The Committee imagines that in some cases a romantic/sexual relationship would not offend ... if initiated with a former patient soon after the termination of treatment, while in others such a relationship might never be appropriate.

Colleague Impairment

Standard 5D and 5E state as follows:

5D. Physical therapist assistants shall encourage colleagues with physical, psychological, or substance-related impairments that may adversely impact their professional responsibilities to seek assistance or counsel.

5E. Physical therapist assistants who have knowledge that a colleague is unable to perform their professional responsibilities with reasonable skill and safety shall report this information to the appropriate authority.

Interpretation

The central tenet of Standard 5D and 5E is that inaction is not an option for a physical therapist assistant when faced with the circumstances described. Standard 5D states that a physical therapist assistant shall encourage colleagues to seek assistance or counsel while Standard 5E addresses reporting information to the appropriate authority.

5D and 5E both require a factual determination on the physical therapist assistant's part. This may be challenging in the sense that you might not know or it might be difficult for you to determine whether someone in fact has a physical, psychological, or substance-related impairment. In addition, it might be difficult to determine whether such impairment may be adversely affecting someone's work responsibilities.

Moreover, once you do make these determinations, the obligation under 5D centers not on reporting, but on encouraging the colleague to seek assistance. However, the obligation under 5E does focus on reporting. But note that 5E discusses reporting when a colleague is unable to perform, whereas 5D discusses encouraging colleagues to seek assistance when the impairment may adversely affect his or her professional responsibilities. So, 5D discusses something that may be affecting performance, whereas 5E addresses a situation in which someone is clearly unable to perform. The 2 situations are distinct. In addition, it is important to note that 5E does not mandate to whom you report; it gives you discretion to determine the appropriate authority.

The EJC Opinion titled Topic: Preserving Confidences; Physical Therapist's Reporting Obligation With Respect to Unethical, Incompetent, or Illegal Acts provides further information on the complexities of reporting.

Clinical Competence

Standard 6A states as follows:

6A. Physical therapist assistants shall achieve and maintain clinical competence.

Interpretation

6A should cause physical therapist assistants to reflect on their current level of clinical competence, to identify and address gaps in clinical competence, and to commit to the maintenance of clinical competence throughout their career. The supervising physical therapist can be a valuable partner in identifying areas of knowledge and skill that the physical therapist assistant needs for clinical competence and to meet the needs of the individual physical therapist, which may vary according to areas of interest and expertise. Further, the physical therapist assistant may request that the physical therapist serve as a mentor to assist him or her in acquiring the needed knowledge and skills. Additional resources on Continuing Competence are available on the APTA Web site.

Lifelong Learning

Standard 6C states as follows:

6C. Physical therapist assistants shall support practice environments that support career development and lifelong learning.

Interpretation

6C points out the physical therapist assistant's obligation to support an environment conducive to career development and learning. The essential idea here is that the physical therapist assistant encourage and contribute to the career development and lifelong learning of himself or herself and others, whether or not the employer provides support.

Organizational and Business Practices

Standard 7 states as follows:

7. Physical therapist assistants shall support organizational behaviors and business practices that benefit patients/clients and society.

Interpretation

Standard 7 reflects a shift in the Standards. One criticism of the former version was that it addressed primarily face-to-face clinical practice settings. Accordingly, Standard 7 addresses ethical obligations in organizational and business practices on a patient/client and societal level.

Documenting Interventions

Standard 7D states as follows:

7D. Physical therapist assistants shall ensure that documentation for their interventions accurately reflects the nature and extent of the services provided.

Interpretation

7D addresses the need for physical therapist assistants to make sure that they thoroughly and accurately document the interventions they provide to patients/clients and document related data collected from the patient/client. The focus of this Standard is on ensuring documentation of the services rendered, including the nature and extent of such services.

Support—Health Needs

Standard 8A states as follows:

8A. Physical therapist assistants shall support organizations that meet the health needs of people who are economically disadvantaged, uninsured, and underinsured.

Interpretation

8A addresses the issue of support for those least likely to be able to afford physical therapy services. The Standard does not specify the type of support that is required. Physical therapist assistants may express support through volunteerism, financial contributions, advocacy, education, or simply promoting their work in conversations with colleagues. When providing such services, including pro bono services, physical therapist assistants must comply with applicable laws, and as such work under the direction and supervision of a physical therapist. Additional resources on pro bono physical therapy services are available on the APTA Web site.

Issued by the Ethics and Judicial Committee
American Physical Therapy Association
October 1981
Last Amended November 2010

Standards of Ethical Conduct for the Physical Therapist Assistant

HOD S06-09-20-18 [Amended HOD S06-00-13-24; HOD 06-91-06-07; Initial HOD 06-82-04-08] [Standard]

Preamble

The Standards of Ethical Conduct for the Physical Therapist Assistant (Standards of Ethical Conduct) delineate the ethical obligations of all physical therapist assistants as determined by the House of Delegates of the American Physical Therapy Association (APTA). The Standards of Ethical Conduct provide a foundation for conduct to which all physical therapist assistants shall adhere. Fundamental to the Standards of Ethical Conduct is the special obligation of physical therapist assistants to enable patients/clients to achieve greater independence, health and wellness, and enhanced quality of life.

No document that delineates ethical standards can address every situation. Physical therapist assistants are encouraged to seek additional advice or consultation in instances where the guidance of the Standards of Ethical Conduct may not be definitive.

Standards

Standard #1: Physical therapist assistants shall respect the inherent dignity, and rights, of all individuals.

1A. Physical therapist assistants shall act in a respectful manner toward each person regardless of age, gender, race, nationality, religion, ethnicity, social or economic status, sexual orientation, health condition, or disability.

1B. Physical therapist assistants shall recognize their personal biases and shall not discriminate against others in the provision of physical therapy services.

Standard #2: Physical therapist assistants shall be trustworthy and compassionate in addressing the rights and needs of patients/clients.

2A. Physical therapist assistants shall act in the best interests of patients/clients over the interests of the physical therapist assistant.

2B. Physical therapist assistants shall provide physical therapy interventions with compassionate and caring behaviors that incorporate the individual and cultural differences of patients/clients.

2C. Physical therapist assistants shall provide patients/clients with information regarding the interventions they provide.

2D. Physical therapist assistants shall protect confidential patient/client information and, in collaboration with the physical therapist, may disclose confidential information to appropriate authorities only when allowed or as required by law.

Standard #3: Physical therapist assistants shall make sound decisions in collaboration with the physical therapist and within the boundaries established by laws and regulations.

3A. Physical therapist assistants shall make objective decisions in the patient's/client's best interest in all practice settings.

3B. Physical therapist assistants shall be guided by information about best practice regarding physical therapy interventions.

3C. Physical therapist assistants shall make decisions based upon their level of competence and consistent with patient/client values.

3D. Physical therapist assistants shall not engage in conflicts of interest that interfere with making sound decisions.

3E. Physical therapist assistants shall provide physical therapy services under the direction and supervision of a physical therapist and shall communicate with the physical therapist when patient/client status requires modifications to the established plan of care.

Standard #4: Physical therapist assistants shall demonstrate integrity in their relationships with patients/clients, families, colleagues, students, other health care providers, employers, payers, and the public.

4A. Physical therapist assistants shall provide truthful, accurate, and relevant information and shall not make misleading representations.

4B. Physical therapist assistants shall not exploit persons over whom they have supervisory, evaluative or other authority (eg, patients/clients, students, supervisees, research participants, or employees).

4C. Physical therapist assistants shall discourage misconduct by health care professionals and report illegal or unethical acts to the relevant authority, when appropriate.

4D. Physical therapist assistants shall report suspected cases of abuse involving children or vulnerable adults to the supervising physical therapist and the appropriate authority, subject to law.

4E. Physical therapist assistants shall not engage in any sexual relationship with any of their patients/clients, supervisees, or students.

4F. Physical therapist assistants shall not harass anyone verbally, physically, emotionally, or sexually.

Standard #5: **Physical therapist assistants shall fulfill their legal and ethical obligations.**

5A. Physical therapist assistants shall comply with applicable local, state, and federal laws and regulations.

5B. Physical therapist assistants shall support the supervisory role of the physical therapist to ensure quality care and promote patient/client safety.

5C. Physical therapist assistants involved in research shall abide by accepted standards governing protection of research participants.

5D. Physical therapist assistants shall encourage colleagues with physical, psychological, or substance-related impairments that may adversely impact their professional responsibilities to seek assistance or counsel.

5E. Physical therapist assistants who have knowledge that a colleague is unable to perform their professional responsibilities with reasonable skill and safety shall report this information to the appropriate authority.

Standard #6: **Physical therapist assistants shall enhance their competence through the lifelong acquisition and refinement of knowledge, skills, and abilities.**

6A. Physical therapist assistants shall achieve and maintain clinical competence.

6B. Physical therapist assistants shall engage in lifelong learning consistent with changes in their roles and responsibilities and advances in the practice of physical therapy.

6C. Physical therapist assistants shall support practice environments that support career development and lifelong learning.

Standard #7: **Physical therapist assistants shall support organizational behaviors and business practices that benefit patients/clients and society.**

7A. Physical therapist assistants shall promote work environments that support ethical and accountable decision-making.

7B. Physical therapist assistants shall not accept gifts or other considerations that influence or give an appearance of influencing their decisions.

7C. Physical therapist assistants shall fully disclose any financial interest they have in products or services that they recommend to patients/clients.

7D. Physical therapist assistants shall ensure that documentation for their interventions accurately reflects the nature and extent of the services provided.

7E. Physical therapist assistants shall refrain from employment arrangements, or other arrangements, that prevent physical therapist assistants from fulfilling ethical obligations to patients/clients

Standard #8: **Physical therapist assistants shall participate in efforts to meet the health needs of people locally, nationally, or globally.**

8A. Physical therapist assistants shall support organizations that meet the health needs of people who are economically disadvantaged, uninsured, and underinsured.

8B. Physical therapist assistants shall advocate for people with impairments, activity limitations, participation restrictions, and disabilities in order to promote their participation in community and society.

8C. Physical therapist assistants shall be responsible stewards of health care resources by collaborating with physical therapists in order to avoid overutilization or underutilization of physical therapy services.

8D. Physical therapist assistants shall educate members of the public about the benefits of physical therapy.

Review Questions

Management, Safety, and Professional Roles

1. Identify four common reasons for denial of payment by an insurance company for physical therapy services.

2. What services does the Individuals with Disabilities and Education Act (IDEA) provide?

3. Identify four specific criteria that must be considered when restraints are used with patients/residents.

4. Differentiate between a policy and a procedure an employee will find in a policy and procedure manual.

14

Research and Evidence-Based Practice

SUSAN B. O'SULLIVAN

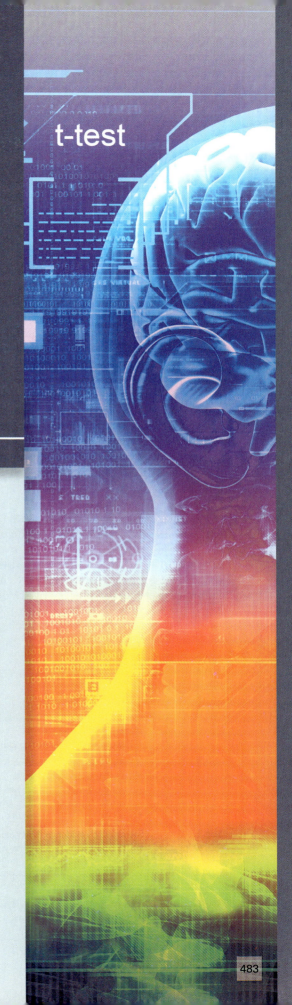

Chapter Outline

- Roles and Responsibilities, 484
  - PTs and PTAs Use Evidence-Based Practice (EBP), 484
  - Clinical Prediction Rule (CPR), 484
- Research Design, 485
  - Methods, 485
  - Variables, 485
  - Hypothesis, 486
  - Levels of Measurement, 486
  - Sampling, 486
  - Instrumentation, 487
  - Informed Consent, 487
  - Determining the Quality of Research, 487
- Evaluating the Evidence: Levels of Evidence and Grades of Recommendation, 489
  - Definitions, 489
  - Levels of Evidence, 489
- Review Questions, 491

Roles and Responsibilities

PTs and PTAs Use Evidence-Based Practice (EBP)

Definition of EBP
1. The "conscientious, explicit and judicious use of current best evidence in making decisions about the care of individual patients" (Sackett et al, 2000).

Clinical Decisions Are Based on
1. Systematic review of research evidence: studies included are rigorous and clinically relevant, "best available external clinical evidence" (e.g., randomized trials and meta-analysis).
2. Clinical expertise of the therapist; proficiency and judgment acquired through clinical practice, acquisition of clinical skills, and continued educational development. For example, the clinician accurately identifies the patient's health status and needs, the risks and benefits of possible interventions.
3. Patient values: values and unique qualities (preferences, concerns, expectations) are identified and integrated into clinical decisions.

EPB Is a Four-Step Process
See Table 14-1 for a description of the process.

Electronic Medical Databases
See Table 14-2 for a list of relevant electronic medical databases useful to the practice of physical therapy.

Clinical Practice Guidelines (CPGs)
1. Systematically developed statements to assist the clinician and patient in decisions about appropriate courses of action.
2. CPGs are developed through a combination of current best scientific evidence (e.g., systematic research and meta-analysis), expert judgment, and analysis of patient preferences combined with outcome-based guidelines.
3. Guidelines issued by professional groups and governmental agencies are developed by expert consensus.
   a. APTA currently has a program to assist CPG development, resources, and a submission/acceptance process.

Clinical Prediction Rule (CPR)
1. A combination of clinical findings that have statistically demonstrated meaningful predictability in guiding clinical decision making.
2. A mathematical, evidence-based tool that can be used to assist clinicians in determining a diagnosis (diagnostic CPRs), prognosis (prognostic CPRs), or intervention (prescriptive CPRs).
3. Combined with clinical expertise and patient preference to improve overall quality of care.

Table 14-1

Steps in Evidence-Based Practice	
Step 1	A clinical problem is identified and an answerable research question is formulated. • The question is clearly defined and related to a clinical decision (e.g., whether to use a therapeutic, preventive, or diagnostic intervention). • The question is focused to clarify the target of the literature search.
Step 2	A systematic literature review is conducted and best evidence is collected. • Sources of evidence include books, journals, clinical protocols, colleagues. • Stronger sources of evidence include a systematic review using an electronic search of the medical literature; see Electronic Medical Databases (Table 14-2). • Articles are selected that are most likely to provide valid results (e.g., randomized controlled trials [RCTs]).
Step 3	The research evidence is summarized and critically analyzed. • The type (design) of the study is identified. • Study methods are identified (e.g., Were all patients who entered the trial properly accounted for and attributed at the conclusion of the study? Were appropriate samples of patients used? What are the inclusion and exclusion criteria?) • Statistical methods and analysis are identified (e.g., Are results presented clearly? Statistically significant?)
Step 4	The research evidence is synthesized and applied to clinical practice. • Best evidence is available and applied to clinical practice using clinical decision analysis.

Table 14-2

Electronic Medical Databases

- PubMed—U.S. National Library of Medicine's search service to Medline and Pre-Medline (database of medical and biomedical research) http://www.ncbi.nlm.nih.gov/pubmed/
- APTA PTNow, www.ptnow.org (formerly Open Door at APTA.org) provides APTA members easy access to journals and other resources relevant to clinical practice at ArticleSearch@apta.org
- Cochrane Database of Systemic Reviews (Cochrane Reviews) (database of systematic reviews of RCTs; primary source for clinical effectiveness information) http://www.cochrane.org/reviews
- CINAHL (database of nursing and allied health research) http://www.cinahl.com
- Physiotherapy Evidence Database (PEDro) (database of physical therapy RCTs, systematic reviews, and evidence-based clinical practice guidelines) http://www.pedro.fhs.usyd.edu.au/index.html
- The Sheffield Evidence for Effectiveness and Knowledge http://www.shef.ac.uk/seek/infosearch.htm#guide
- The Centre for Health Evidence http://www.cche.net/
- ERIC (database of education research) http://www.eric.ed.gov/
- Ovid (database of health and lifescience research) http://www.ovid.com
- DARE (database of abstracts of reviews of evidence from medical journals) http://www.ovid.com/site/products/ovidguide/daredb.htm
- RehabDATA (database of disability and rehabilitation research) http://www.naric.com/research
- Center for International Rehabilitation Research Information and Exchange (database of rehabilitation research) http://www.cirrie.buffalo.edu

Physical Therapy Outcomes Registry (APTA)

1. An organized system for collecting data to evaluate patient function.
2. Includes clinically relevant measures for the population of patients receiving physical therapy services.
3. Use of standardized outcome measures improves practice (patient outcomes, patient satisfaction, PT/PTA clinical decision-making), informs payment for physical therapy services, and promotes research.

Research Is in Clinical and Academic Settings

1. The research question/proposal is developed and submitted for ethical approval and funding (Institutional Review Board).
2. The research study is conducted.
3. The research data is analyzed and reported (i.e., presentation and written publication).

Research Evidence Is Incorporated into Clinical Practice

1. Steps: See Table 14-1.
2. Sources: evidence is presented in publications, websites (Table 14-2), discussion groups, presentations.
3. Changes in clinical practice are based on consultation with the patient, to arrive at a determination of which option best suits the patient (a client-centered approach).
4. PTs and PTAs must exercise good clinical-judgment in determining applicability of the research results to the specific patient (i.e., similarity to the research group).
    a. PTAs should discuss research outcomes, CPGs, and CPRs prior to application to patient populations to ensure alignment for application to interventions with patient populations.

Research Design

Methods

Common Denominators
1. Research includes:
    a. Statement of the problem.
    b. Formation of a research question.
    c. Collection and analysis of data.
    d. Conclusions.

Variables

General Concepts
1. Independent variable: a variable that stands alone and isn't changed by any other variables being measured, e.g., age and time; in an experiment, the variable that is being manipulated.

2. Dependent variable: the variable that is being studied and measured; in an experiment, it changes when the independent variable is manipulated, e.g., how tall you are at different ages.

Hypothesis

General Concepts
1. Hypothesis is a tenative and testable explanation of the relationship between variables; the results of an experiment determine whether the hypothesis is accepted or rejected.
2. Directional hypothesis (research hypothesis): a generalization that predicts an expected relationship between variables.
3. Null hypothesis: states that no relationship exists between variables, a statistical hypothesis; any relationship found is the result of chance or sampling error.
   a. The null hypothesis is rejected; meaning that a significant difference was observed between groups or treatments.
   b. The null hypothesis is accepted; meaning that no significant difference was observed between groups or treatments.

Levels of Measurement

Data Types (See Table 14-3)
1. Nominal scale: classifies variables or scores into two or more mutually exclusive categories based on a common set of characteristics; the lowest level of measurement; e.g., subjects are classified as male or female, tall or short, etc.
2. Ordinal scale: classifies and ranks variables or scores in terms of the degree to which they possess a common characteristic.
   a. Intervals between ranks are NOT equal; e.g., subjects are ranked in a graduating class according to grade point average; manual muscle test grades (normal, good, fair, poor, trace, zero) are ranked as an ordinal scale.
3. Interval scale: classifies and ranks variables or scores based on predetermined equal intervals.
   a. Does not have a true zero point; e.g., an IQ test with scores ranging from 0–200; temperature scales (fahrenheit or celsius).
4. Ratio scale: classifies and ranks variables or scores based on equal intervals and a true zero point.
   a. The highest, most precise level of measurement; e.g., goniometry, scales for height, weight, or force allow the use of precise physical measures (ratio data) for research.

Sampling

Selection of Sample
1. The selection of individuals for a study from a population. The sample represents the larger group from which they were selected.
2. Random: all individuals in a population have an equal chance of being chosen for a study.

Table 14-3

Examples of Statistical Analyses According to the Study's Purpose and the Data's Level of Measurement

PURPOSES	LEVELS OF MEASUREMENT	STATISTICS
Describe the Variable	Nominal	Frequency, Percentage
	Ordinal	Median, Mode, Range
	Interval	Mean, Median, Mode, Range, Standard Deviation, Skew of the Distribution
Relationship	Nominal	Chi Square
	Ordinal	Spearman's Rank Order or Kendall's Tau Correlations
	Interval	Pearson's Product Moment Correlation, Partial Correlation, Multiple Correlation, Multiple Regression
Difference	Nominal	One group: Chi Square Two groups: Independent: Chi Square; Paired: McNemar Test More than two groups: Independent: Chi Square; Paired: Cochran's Q
	Ordinal	Two groups: Independent: Mann-Whitney U; Paired: Wilcoxon Signed Rank More than two groups: Independent: Kruskal-Wallis; Paired: Friedman ANOVA
	Interval	Two groups: Independent: t-test; Paired: Paired t-test; Statistical Control: ANCOVA More than two groups: Independent: ANOVA; Across time: Repeated ANOVA; Statistical Control: ANCOVA

Nominal: characteristics into categories
Ordinal: rank ordering, no specific intervals between ranks
Interval: values rank ordered on a scale that has equal distances (intervals) between points on that scale
Prepared by Nina Coppens, PhD, RN, University of Massachusetts, Lowell.

3. Systematic: individuals are selected from a population list by taking individuals at specified intervals; e.g., every 10th name.
4. Stratified: individuals are selected from a population from identified subgroups based on some predetermined characteristic; e.g., by height, weight, or gender.
5. Double-blind study: an experiment in which the subject and the investigator are not aware of group assignment.
6. Effect size: the size (quantity, magnitude) of the differences between sample means; allows a statistical test to find a difference when one really does exist.
7. Generalizability: the degree to which a study's findings based on a sample apply to an entire population.

Instrumentation

Selection
1. Instruments are chosen with established validity and reliability.
2. Gold standard: an instrument with established validity can be used as a standard for assessing other instruments.

Informed Consent

General Concepts
1. A document that includes consent of an individual prior to participation in a study with full disclosure of risks and benefits; ethical disclosure.
2. Components.
   a. Information about the general nature of what is to take place.
   b. Any risks to the individual and what will be done to minimize the risks.
   c. Possible benefits.
   d. An ethical disclosure.

Determining the Quality of Research

Control
1. The researcher attempts to remove the influence of any variable other than the independent variable in order to evaluate its effect on the dependent variable.
   a. Control group: the group in a research study that resembles the experimental group but which does not receive the new or different treatment (e.g., treated as usual); provides a baseline for interpretation of results.
   b. Experimental group: the group in a research study that receives a new or novel treatment that is under investigation.
   c. Intervening variable: a variable that alters the relationship (intervenes) between the independent and dependent variable; may not be directly observable or easy to control (e.g., anxiety).

Validity
1. The degree to which a test, instrument, or procedure accurately measures what it is supposed to or intended to measure.
2. Types.
   a. Internal validity: the degree to which the observed differences on the dependent variable are the direct result of manipulation of the independent variable and not some other variable.
   b. External validity: the degree to which the results are generalizable to individuals (general population) or environmental settings outside of the experimental study.
   c. Face validity: the assumption of validity based on the appearance of an instrument as a reasonable measure of a variable; may be used for initial screening of a test instrument but psychometrically unsound.
   d. Content validity: the degree to which an instrument measures an intended content area.
      - Determined by expert judgment.
      - Requires both item validity and sampling validity.
   e. Concurrent validity: the degree to which the scores on one test are related to the scores on another criterion test with both tests being given at relatively similar times; usually involves comparison to the gold standard.
   f. Predictive validity: the degree to which a test is able to predict future performance.
   g. Construct validity: the degree to which a test measures an intended hypothetical abstract concept (nonobservable behaviors or ideas).

Threats to Validity
1. Sampling bias (selection bias): the researcher introduces systematic sampling error; e.g., a sample of convenience (the use of volunteers or available groups) instead of random selection of subjects.
2. Failure to exert rigid control over subjects and conditions: intervening variables interact with the dependent variable; e.g., in a longitudinal pediatric study, the outcome is due to the maturation of the child rather than the treatment intervention.

3. The administration of the pretest influences scores on the posttest; e.g., a learning effect occurs as a result of taking a test.
4. The measurement instrument is not accurate, the test does not measure the characteristic it purports to measure; e.g., muscle strength, not motor control.
5. Pretest-treatment interaction: subjects respond differently to the treatment because of the pretest.
6. Multiple treatment interference: more than one treatment is being given to the subjects at the same time; or carry-over effects from an earlier treatment influence the results of a later treatment, e.g., effects of ultrasound following application of a hot pack.
7. Experimenter bias: expectations of the researcher about the expected outcomes of the study influence the results of a study.
8. Hawthorne effect: the subject's knowledge of participation in an experiment influences the results of a study.
9. Placebo effect: subjects respond to a sham treatment with positive effects; e.g., taking a sugar pill instead of an experimental drug results in a change.

Reliability
1. The degree to which an instrument measures a phenomenon accurately, dependably, time after time, and without variation.
   a. Interrater (intertester) reliability: the degree to which two or more independent raters can obtain the same rating for a given variable; the consistency of multiple raters.
   b. Intrarater (intratester) reliability: the degree to which one rater can obtain the same rating for a given variable on multiple measurement trials; an individual's consistency of rating.
   c. Test-retest reliability: the degree to which the scores on a test are stable or consistent over time; a measure of instrument stability.
   d. Split-half reliability: the degree of agreement when a test is split in half and the reliability of first half is compared to the second half; a measure of internal consistency of an instrument.

Threats to Reliability
1. Errors of measurement: random errors or systematic errors; e.g., repeat measurements of blood pressure may vary as a result of physiological changes (fear, anxiety).

Objectivity
1. Agreement among expert judges on what is observed or what is done; e.g., scoring of a perceptible sign or symptom is the same, regardless of who is observing the phenomena (e.g., licensure exam).

Subjectivity
1. Refers to a testing format that may differ depending upon the person grading the test (e.g., figure skating judging).

Sensitivity and Specificity
1. Sensitivity: a test's ability to correctly identify the proportion of individuals who truly have a disease or condition (a true positive).
2. Specificity: a test's ability to correctly identify the proportion of individuals who do not have a disease or condition (a true negative).
3. Predictive value: a test's ability to estimate the likelihood that a person will test positive (or negative) for a target condition.
4. True positive: individuals are correctly identified as having the target condition.
5. True negative: individuals are correctly identified as not having the target condition.
6. False positive: individuals are identified as having the target condition when they do not.
7. False negative: individuals are identified as not having the target condition when they do.
8. Both sensitivity and specificity are expressed as values between 0 and 1. Values very close to 1 are ideal.
9. Sensitivity and specificity values may be combined to obtain a likelihood ratio, used to determine how much the test influences identification of a condition or limitation in function.

Responsiveness
1. Used to determine if a measure is sufficiently sensitive to reflect meaningful change in status.
2. Minimal detectable change (MDC): the smallest amount of change in a measurement that exceeds the measurement error of the instrument; reflects a true change in status.
3. Minimally important clinical difference (MCID): is the smallest difference in a measured variable that signifies a clinically important change in status.

Evaluating the Evidence: Levels of Evidence and Grades of Recommendation

Definitions

Systematic Review (SR)
1. SR is a type of literature review in which the primary studies are summarized, critically appraised, and statistically combined.
2. Usually quantitative in nature (RCTs) with specific inclusion/exclusion criteria.
3. Meta-analysis is a statistical analysis that combines the results of multiple conceptually similiar scientific studies; results in a higher statistical power and more robust findings.

Random zed Controlled Trial (RCT)
1. RCT is an experimental study in which participants are randomly assigned to either an experimental or control group to receive different interventions or a placebo.

Cohort Study
1. A cohort study is a prospective (forward-in-time) study; a group of participants (cohort) with a similar condition is followed for a defined period of time.
2. Comparison is made to a matched group that does not have the condition.

Homogeneity/Heterogeneity
1. Homogeneity: a SR free of variations in the directions and degree of results between individual studies.
2. Heterogeneity: a SR with variations.

Case-Control Study
1. A retrospective (backward-in-time) study.
2. A group of individuals with a similar condition (disease) is compared with a group that does not have the condition to determine factors that may have played a role in the condition.

Case Report Study
1. A type of descriptive research in which only one individual is studied in depth, often retrospectively.

Levels of Evidence

Grades (See Table 14-4)
1. Includes criteria to determine the level of evidence and the accompanying grade of recommendation.
2. Level I is based on the highest level of evidence and Level V is the lowest level of evidence.
3. Grades are used when evaluating interventions and supporting action statements for best practice (CPGs).
4. Synopses of CPGs are presented in individual chapters.

Table 14-4

Levels of Evidence and Grades of Recommendation

LEVEL	DESCRIPTION
I	Evidence is based on SR of high-quality RCTs (or meta-analyses) with adequate size to ensure low risk of bias, substantial agreement of size and direction of treatment effects; or individual RCT with narrow confidence level, treatment effects precisely defined, and low risk of bias; prospective studies.
II	Evidence is based on SR lesser-quality RCT, e.g., too small to provide Level I evidence; weaker diagnostic criteria and reference standards, improper randomization; < than 80% follow-up of subjects enrolled in study or SR of cohort studies with homogeneity; prospective studies.
III	Evidence is based on SR of nonrandomized, controlled cohort studies or individual case-control study; retrospective studies.
IV	Evidence is based on case series studies and poor-quality cohort or case-control studies (comparison groups not adequately defined, exposures and outcomes not measured objectively, lack of control for confounders, insufficient follow up—cohort studies only).
V	Evidence is based on expert opinion without critical appraisal, or based on physiology, bench research.

GRADES OF RECOMMENDATION BASED ON	STRENGTH OF EVIDENCE
A—Strong evidence	A preponderance of Level I and/or Level II studies support the recommendation. This must include at least one Level I study.
B—Moderate evidence	A single, high-quality RCT or a preponderance of Level II studies support the recommendation.
C—Weak evidence	A single Level II study or a preponderance of Level III and IV studies, including statements of consensus by content experts support the recommendation.
D—Conflicting evidence	Higher-quality studies conducted on this topic that disagree on conclusions. The recommendation is based on these conflicting studies.
E—Theoretical/foundational evidence	A preponderance of evidence from animal or cadaver studies, from conceptual models/principles, or from basic sciences/bench research support this conclusion.
F—Expert opinion	Best practice based on the clinical experience of the guidelines development team.

RCT = randomized controlled trials; SR = systematic review

Grades of recommendation adapted from Knee Pain and Mobility Impairments: Meniscal and Articular Cartilage Lesions. Clinical Practice Guidelines linked to the International Classification of Functioning, Disability, and Health from the Orthopedic Section of the American Physical Therapy Association, Summary of Recommendations. JOSPT 6(40): A30, 2010.

Review Questions

Research and Evidence-Based Practice

1. Explain the difference between independent and dependent variables.

2. Rank and briefly explain the following levels of evidence. Which of these provides a better level of evidence from which to base treatment decisions?
    – Case-control study
    – Randomized controlled trial (RCT)
    – Cohort study

3. Differentiate the terms *sensitivity* versus *specificity*.

4. Describe what a clinical prediction rule (CPR) is and how it can be used in practice.

15 Chapter Review Questions and Answers

- Therapeutic Exercise Foundations, 494
- Musculoskeletal Physical Therapy, 496
- Neuromuscular Physical Therapy, 498
- Cardiac, Vascular, and Lymphatic Physical Therapy, 500
- Pulmonary Physical Therapy, 502
- Other Systems, 504
- Integumentary Physical Therapy, 506
- Geriatric Physical Therapy, 508
- Pediatric Physical Therapy, 510
- Therapeutic Modalities, 512
- Functional Training, Equipment, and Devices, 514
- Teaching and Learning, 515
- Management, Safety, and Professional Roles, 516
- Research and Evidence-Based Practice, 517

Chapter 1 Review Questions

Therapeutic Exercise Foundations

1. Describe these three specific principles as they relate to developing muscle strength:
   Overload
   Specificity
   Reversibility

   - Overload principle: to increase strength in a muscle it must be challenged, or overloaded, beyond its current force capability in order to develop (hypertrophy of muscle fibers).
   - Specificity: training effects are specific to the overload imposed; therefore, the mode of strengthening must be specific to the desired training effects.
   - Reversibility: hypertrophy and training effects are not maintained without continuous challenge; detraining effects include muscle fiber atrophy and decreased muscle recruitment.

2. Identify the benefits and precautions/contraindications of the following types of resistance exercise.

Type of Exercise	Benefit	Precaution/Contraindication
Isometric	Strengthens muscle at specific point in ROM.	Can cause an increase in blood pressure; monitor for Valsalva's maneuver.
Isotonic	Strengthens muscle at the weakest point in range of motion. Variable resistance strengthens the muscle throughout the range of motion.	Incorrect use of machines or free weights can lead to injury.
Isokinetic	Provides maximum resistance at all points of the range of motion.	Same as isotonic and isometric.
Eccentric	Requires less energy than concentric contraction. Useful for functional training and injured muscles. Useful to prepare muscles for functional activities.	More apt to cause DOMS (delayed-onset muscle soreness) when working with maximal contractions.

3. Differentiate between dynamic, static, and ballistic stretching techniques. Include how to perform the technique and what it is best used for. Identify any precautions or contraindications to each.

   - Dynamic: slowly to moderately moving a joint through available range of motion following a general (whole-body, light jog) easy warmup (40% max HR). Perform active or passive controlled and repeated movements, beneficial to mimic those required for activity (e.g., high stepping or marching for a hurdler or soldier, straight-leg raises with opposite arm reach for a sprinter). Indicated for warmup for sport as it does not diminish the torque-producing ability of muscle; precaution should be used without prior warmup and in tissues that are recovering from injury.
   - Static: a prolonged stretch applied to a muscle (active or passive) at its end range of motion for purpose of lengthening short tissues. Effective stretch is held for 30–60 seconds; research is highly variable, it is generally accepted that less than 30 seconds does not result in long-term ROM gains. Indicated for decreased ROM. Contraindicated prior to sport activity because it has been shown to diminish torque-producing ability of muscle. Precaution and diminished intensity should be implemented in tissues recovering from injury.

- Ballistic: a high-velocity, high-frequency, short-duration "bouncing"-type stretch performed by contracting the opposite muscle group and/or using body weight and momentum to stretch; can be performed actively or passively. It is performed beyond the available ROM of the muscle and facilitates the stretch reflex within the muscle which actually increases tension in the muscle being stretched. Velocity rates in research are highly variable, inconclusive as to what frequency results in better outcomes. Indication—best used following warmup for individuals preparing to participate in ballistic-type sports (e.g., basketball, tennis). Contraindicated in injured and rehabilitating muscles; should be avoided in weakened or injured tissues.

4. Discuss conditions or situations when precaution must be exercised when implementing a strengthening program that includes mechanical resistance. Describe a technique to reduce post-exercise muscle soreness.

- Fatigue: both general and local muscle fatigue diminish the muscles' ability to develop peak torque forces and places the individual at greater risk for injury secondary to diminished energy stores, e.g., glycogen, lowers blood sugar, potassium depletion.
- Persons with medical conditions can fatigue more quickly and suffer longer-term residual effects (includes those who are significantly overweight, have cardiac disease, multiple sclerosis, or lower motor neuron diseases such as postpolio syndrome, for example).
- Osteoporosis is a precaution for resistance strengthening exercises; clinicians should pay particular attention to avoid dangerous positions that may place the client at risk for fracture. For example, avoid the traditional sit-up position or flexion activities for an individual with thoracic fractures.
- Muscle soreness develops during, or immediately after, exercise that has been performed to point of fatigue. It is the result of a temporary buildup of lactic acid and potassium. Post-exercise and delayed-onset muscle soreness (DOMS) can be limited by participating in a cool-down period of low-intensity exercise (20%–30% max HR, lower or no resistance) following strenuous exercise. This facilitates return of oxygen to the muscle.

5. Describe the body's response to exercise in hot weather. Identify appropriate precautions a physical therapy clinician should implement.

- In an effort to cool the core (brain, heart), the body shunts blood to the periphery of the system; while appropriate, this mechanism can deprive muscles of oxygen.
- As core temperature increases, perspiration also increases to create a cooling effect as evaporation of the perspiration occurs. This can lead to loss of fluid levels as well as diminished or altered electrolyte balance, typically occurring in extreme humidity or heat. Recognize that exercise in conditions in which the relative humidity is 60% or greater diminishes the effect of evaporation of sweat, making it an ineffective mechanism to cool the individual. Individuals who are obese may be at risk for overheating more quickly than others in similar circumstances; excess adipose tissue can slow the conduction of heat to the periphery.
- Appropriate precautions: maintaining blood/fluid levels by encouraging intake of fluid throughout or following the activity is typically sufficient; colder fluid empties from the stomach more rapidly than room temperature fluid. Remind individuals to remove jackets as they warm up.
- Clinicians should note that in cases of extreme physical exertion fluid should be replaced with glucose-polymer drinks—specifically manufactured to provide electrolytes and carbohydrates. For the recreational athlete, water is typically appropriate.

  Recognize signs and symptoms of heat exhaustion or stroke.

6. Outline the progression of developing controlled mobility for an individual with ataxia.

- Develop a stable core in the stationary position, progressing to include weight shifting and movement as skill develops.

  Begin with large-range controlled movements → to small-range controlled movement → to holding steady.

Chapter 2 Review Questions

Musculoskeletal Physical Therapy

1. What joint accessory motion is used when performing mobilization techniques to increase joint range of motion? Identify and describe it.
   - Glide/slide—it is a translatory motion of one surface gliding on another, e.g., when a braked wheel skids.

2. In what circumstance might a physician order a plain film radiograph (x-ray) versus a CT scan?
   - An x-ray is used to demonstrate the integrity of bony tissues.
   - A CT scan (a computer-enhanced x-ray–type image) is better for examining complex fractures, facet dysfunction and disc disease, stenosis of the spinal canal or intervertebral foramen.

3. Compare and contrast the symptoms a patient or client might describe for facet joint dysfunction versus spinal stenosis.

Facet Joint Dysfunction	Spinal Stenosis
– Stiffness upon rising; pain eases within an hour.	– Pain that is related to position.
– Loss of motion accompanied by pain.	– Flexed postures decrease pain; extended postures increase pain.
– Pain that is sharp with certain movements.	– Feelings of numbness, tightness, or cramping.
– Movement in pain-free range usually reduces symptoms.	– Walking brings on symptoms.
– Stationary positions increase symptoms.	– Pain may persist for hours after assuming a resting position.

4. Compare and contrast physical therapy treatment strategies and goals for patients and clients with arthritic, soft tissue, and bony tissue conditions.

Similarities among All	Condition Specific
– Maintain/improve joint mechanics and connective tissue functions.	Arthritic and bony tissue conditions:
– Implement aerobic capacity/endurance conditioning or reconditioning as needed.	– Provide joint protection strategies.
– Implement graded strengthening program as appropriate for activity.	– Implement flexibility exercises to maintain/improve normal joint motion and length of muscles.
– Application of appropriate therapeutic modalities to reduce pain and inflammation.	– Implement manual therapy for maintenance of normal joint mechanics, for joint biomechanics and soft tissues.

5. Describe the rehabilitation process for an individual rehabilitating from surgical repair of an anterior-inferior dislocation of the shoulder.

- Most shoulder dislocations occur when the abducted shoulder is forcefully externally rotated; this causes tearing of the inferior glenohumeral ligament, anterior capsule, and possibly the glenoid labrum.
- Avoid the apprehension position –90° flexion, 90° abduction, and 80° external rotation until repaired tissues are healing and able to withstand tension.
- Initiate passive motion, therapeutic modalities, and positioning to assist with pain control and resist tissue adhesions during healing. Joint motion should be performed by the patient/client and clinician; grade I and II joint mobilization, Codman's exercises and PROM for pain reduction, tissue mobility, and joint nutrition.
- Introduce active, non-resisted and minimal discomfort motion as tissue healing occurs. Refer to Table 2-1, Tissue Healing Times, in this chapter.
- Continue joint mobilization techniques, increasing intensity if required to achieve joint capsule ROM and normal biomechanics.
- Build muscle endurance and normal joint biomechanics of associated musculature as well as adjacent musculature (scapular control and mobility are critical, assess acromioclavicular and sternoclavicular joint mechanics as well).
- Build strength and progress to sport- or function-specific activities necessary for ADLs, work, and recreation.

Chapter 3 Review Questions

Neuromuscular Physical Therapy

1. Describe two to three predictable deficits a clinician can expect to observe when each of the following areas of the brain is damaged: (1) frontal lobe, (2) temporal lobe, and (3) cerebellum.

Lobe	Predictable Deficit
Frontal lobe	Contralateral weakness
	Personality changes/antisocial behavior
	Ataxia
	Broca's aphasia
	Delayed or poor initiation
Temporal lobe	Hearing impairments (dominant)
	Memory and learning deficits
	Wernicke's aphasia
	Antisocial behaviors
Cerebellum	Ataxia
	Lack of trunk and extremity coordination
	Intention tremor
	Balance deficits
	Dysdiadochokinesia
	Dysmetria

2. Identify what an exteroceptor is as it relates to sensory responses. Now identify two proprioceptive facilitation techniques and two proprioceptive exteroceptive inhibition techniques that can be used with patients/clients with neurological deficits.

    - Exteroceptors are sensory nerve endings that are responsible for receiving superficial sensations from the environment. Sensations include light touch, pressure, pain, and temperature.
    - Exteroceptive inhibition techniques include maintained pressure or touch, slow continuous stroking, prolonged icing, and neutral warmth.
    - Proprioceptive facilitation techniques include quick stretching or tapping of a muscle belly or tendon, resistance to movement, joint approximation, and joint traction.
    - See Table 3-22 for additional Proprioceptive Techniques.

3. A PTA is working with a patient who has a spinal cord injury (SCI). The PT has ordered a manual wheelchair with projection rims. What level of SCI is the highest-level injury a PTA should expect to be able to use this type of wheelchair?

    A patient with a C6 SCI. An individual with this level injury will be unable to produce an effective grip for a typical hand rim. An individual with a C5 injury will not have the ability to utilize a manual wheelchair. An individual with a C7 injury is likely able to produce sufficient grip to manage a manual wheelchair without projections.

4. Differentiate equilibrium and nonequilibrium coordination tests. Describe two equilibrium and two nonequilibrium coordination tests.

- Equilibrium coordination tests: those tests that incorporate both static and dynamic components of balance and posture when in an upright position.
- Nonequilibrium coordination tests: those tests that identify both static and mobile components of gross and fine motor activities when in a seated position.
- See Table 3-15 for Nonequilibrium Coordination Tests.
- See Table 3-16 for Equilibrium Coordination Tests and Intervention to Improve.

5. A PTA is working with an individual who has neurological balance deficits. The patient is able to perform static and dynamic sitting activities with little to no difficulties. Identify three ideas for progression of balance activities at this point.

- Increase the number of body segments the patient has to control by:
  1) Attempting sitting on a movable base, e.g., exercise ball or balance disc.
  2) Attempting quadruped.
  3) Attempting standing.
- See Table 3-19 for additional mechanisms to increase or decrease the difficulty level of exercises or activities.

Chapter 4 Review Questions

Cardiac, Vascular, and Lymphatic Physical Therapy

1. List three non-modifiable and three modifiable risk factors for coronary artery disease.
   - Non-modifiable risk factors: (1) age, (2) sex, and (3) race
   - Three modifiable risk factors include: (1) cigarette smoking, (2) high blood pressure, and (3) elevated cholesterol levels and LDL levels. Also included in the list of risk factors are elevated blood homocystine, obesity, sedentary lifestyle, stress, and family history.

2. Describe the signs and symptoms of left-sided congestive heart failure (CHF) versus right-sided CHF.
   - Left-sided CHF signs and symptoms include dyspnea, fatigue and muscle weakness, increasing kidney dysfunction, pulmonary edema.
   - Right-sided CHF signs and symptoms include jugular venous distension, cyanosis in nail beds, peripheral edema, nausea, weight gain, ascites.

3. Differentiate these signs and symptoms of cardiovascular disease.
   Chest pain
   Dyspnea
   Claudication
   - Chest Pain: can be described as tightness or pressure and may radiate to the neck, jaw, shoulder, upper trapezius area, upper back, and arms. Could be indicative of a myocardial infarction. How is this chest pain different from gastroesophogeal reflux disease (GERD)? With GERD, the patient's chest pain often subsides with a change in position.
   - Dyspnea (shortness of breath): may occur at rest or with exertion, termed dyspnea on exertion (DOE). DOE can be caused by left ventricular impairment. Dyspnea can be a result of cardiac or pulmonary conditions.
   - Claudication: patient may complain of pain or cramping in the lower extremities, and this symptom is often secondary to peripheral vascular disease (arterial or venous; know the difference), and claudication can significantly limit the tolerance of standing or walking.

4. Discuss the clinical significance of cardiovascular laboratory tests and values—SaO_2 and hematocrit percentages. Identify normal and abnormal values. Identify modifications a PTA should make during a patient treatment session when values are abnormal.
   - Laboratory values and tests allow the PTA to review and continue to monitor patient status before, during, and after physical therapy intervention.
   - Tables 4-2 and 6-3 indicate normal and abnormal values, as well as modifications and signs and symptoms the PTA should be aware of.

   Arterial Blood Gases:
   - SaO_2: normal is greater than or equal to 95%, below 90% often requires supplemental oxygen; during treatment if saturation drops below 90%, the patient should stop the exercise he or she is doing, sit down, and take deep breaths. PTA should monitor the saturation levels, indicate what activity the patient was doing when the drop occurred, how long recovery took, get assistance if recovery above 90% is not occurring.
   - Hematocrit (Hct): normal for males is 42%–52% and for females is 37%–47%. If the Hct is greater than 25% but less than normal, the patient can do light exercise only; if the Hct is less than 25%, then exercise is contraindicated. A high Hct percentage could be due to dehydration or shock, and a low Hct percentage could be from an acute hemorrhage or severe anemia.

5. What effect does taking a beta-blocker have on a patient who is exercising?
    - A beta-blocker decreases the force of the cardiac contraction and therefore decreases the heart rate which creates a decrease demand on the heart and also decreases blood pressure. When a patient is exercising while using a beta blocker, the heart rate will stay consistent. Thus, monitoring the heart rate with exercise will not provide accurate feedback about exercise work load.
    - For this patient, it is most appropriate to use the rate of perceived exertion scale (RPE) for monitoring physiological response.

      It is also important to monitor for bradycardia and signs of orthostatic hypotension.

6. Compare and contrast Phase 1 to Phase 2 management for individuals with edema secondary to lymphatic dysfunction.
    - During Phase 1 treatment compression bandaging/garments are worn 24 hours per day and strenuous activities, jogging, ballistic movements, and rotational motions are contraindicated. During Phase 2 treatment compression garments and bandaging may be modified to be worn at night. Exercise can be initiated, combined with compression garments. Low pressure sequential pumps may be used.
    - Patient education regarding skin care and positioning remains constant throughout phases of rehabilitation for lymphedema management.

Chapter 5 Review Questions

Pulmonary Physical Therapy

1. Identify normal pH levels, at normal room air. What pH value indicates a state of respiratory acidosis and alveolar hypoventilation? What signs and symptoms might a patient exhibit in the state of respiratory acidosis?

   - pH at normal room air = 7.35–7.45.
   - Respiratory acidosis (alveolar hypoventilation) = pH <7.35.
     Signs and symptoms = early: anxiety, restlessness, dyspnea, headache; late: confusion, sleepy/drowsy, coma.

2. Define inspiratory reserve volume (IRV), expiratory reserve volume (ERV), and vital capacity.

   - IRV: volume of gas that can be inhaled beyond a normal resting tidal inhalation; it is a measure of lung volume.
   - ERV: volume of gas that can be exhaled beyond normal resting tidal exhalation; it is a measure of lung volume.
   - Vital capacity: the amount of air that is under volitional control; it is a measure of lung capacity.

3. Describe the active cycle of breathing technique. Describe how a clinician should instruct a patient/client to perform the technique.

   - Describe/define: active cycle of breathing technique (ACBT) is an independent program used to assist in the removal of the more peripheral secretions that coughing alone may not clear. It is performed in three phases that are repeated in cycles—breathing control, thoracic expansion, forced expiratory technique (FIT).
   - Instructing the patient/client: the patient/client may sit or position himself or herself into the appropriate postural drainage position.
   - The patient:
     (1) Breathes in a controlled diaphragmatic fashion.
     (2) Performs thoracic expansion exercises by taking a deep breath (with or without percussion and shaking) with a hold at the top if possible. A sniff or hold at end of inspiration helps facilitate distribution of air into collapsed segments of lungs. Expiration is passive. The patient may place a hand over the area of the lungs being treated to encourage chest wall movement in that area.
     (3) Forced expiration phase: the patient performs a series of huffing techniques (see huffing in previous section) and breathing control after one to two huffs. Repeat cycles as necessary.

4. Differentiate between the adventitious breath sounds—crackles, wheezes, and rhonchi. Which portion of the stethoscope should be used for each?

Crackles (rales, crepitations)	Wheezes	Rhonchi
– Low pitch; sounds like rubbing hairs between fingers. – Discontinuous sound during inspiration. – Indicates condition in peripheral airways, or pathology (atelectasis, fibrosis, pulmonary edema). – Bell portion of stethoscope may be more beneficial.	– High-pitch, musical. – Heard during expiration; with severe airway constriction (croup) may be heard at inspiration. – Caused by airway obstruction. – Diaphragm portion of stethoscope may be more beneficial.	– Low-pitched; sounds like a snore. – Continuous sound heard on both inspiration and expiration. – Indicates obstructive process in larger, more central airways. – Bell portion of stethoscope may be more beneficial.

5. Describe the palpation method used to assess chest wall excursion of the apical segments of the right upper lobe and the right middle lobe of the lung. When assessing chest wall excursion, should palpation be performed unilaterally or bilaterally? What type of pathological condition might cause a unilateral restriction in chest wall expansion?

The therapist assistant stands or sits facing the patient and places his or her hands gently on the patient to assess rib motion as the patient inhales and exhales.

(1) Upper lobe motion: place hands so that heel of the hand is at approximately the fourth rib, fingers rest across the upper trapezius area and thumbs rest horizontally meeting at the sternum. Ask patient to inhale and assess for symmetry and extent of movement.

(2) Anterolateral and middle lobe motion: place hands so that the palms lie on the anterolateral rib area with web space between thumb and first finger resting below nipple line, thumbs rest horizontally meeting at the sternum. Ask patient to inhale and assess for symmetry and extent of movement.

When assessing chest wall excursion, it is most effective to palpate bilaterally; comparisons are then made between the two lungs.

Unilateral restrictions in lung excursion are more typical in conditions affecting individual lobes such as lobar pneumonia; conditions such as COPD are more likely to restrict excursion bilaterally.

6. What is a central venous catheter? Describe where it might be located on a patient and what type of patient may have a central venous catheter. What activity restrictions and precautions apply to physical therapy intervention?

- A central venous catheter, also known as a central venous access device (CVAD) or vascular access device, is a catheter inserted into larger, more proximal veins in the patient. It is likely to be used when repeated injections or blood draws are necessary; it is also used for long-term IV therapy delivery. This method might also be used when the medication administered (e.g., chemotherapy drugs) may cause irritation to the smaller vessels.

- Locations: directly into the internal or external jugular vein; may also be tunneled just under the skin below the clavicle and inserted into the cephalic, internal or external jugular vein. The internal tip ends in the superior vena cava. There are also implanted central venous access ports or infusion ports that, when used, are placed subcutaneously in the upper chest just below the clavicle and have an access port that extends through the skin.

- There are no activity or positioning restrictions associated with a central venous catheter. Caution should be observed to avoid entangling the external catheter during activity. Use caution to avoid tugging on the catheter or displacing the end cap on the injection port.

Chapter 6 Review Questions

Other Systems

1. Name the primary immune and helper cells the body deploys in reaction to infectious agents. How are these affected when an individual has an immune deficient disease?

   - Lymphocytes—T and B.
   - Macrophages—accessory cells that process and present antigens to the lymphocytes.
   - CD molecules (CD4 helper cells) serve as master regulators of the immune response by influencing the function of all other immune cells.
   - Immunodeficiency—these cells are depressed or absent and unable to effectively respond to threats.
     - Primary immunodeficient disorders result from a defect in T and B lymphocytes or lymphoid tissues (lymph system and lymph nodes, spleen).
     - Secondary immunodeficiency disorders are caused by underlying pathology or treatment that suppress the immune system. Diseases include: leukemia, bone marrow tumor, chronic diabetes, renal failure, cirrhosis, cancer treatments such as chemotherapy and radiation.

2. Identify secondary infections or complications that may be a result of the compromised immune system of a patient who has acquired immunodeficiency syndrome.

   - Opportunistic infections—most commonly pneumocystis carinii pneumonia, oral and esophageal candidiasis (fungal infection—thrush), cytomegalovirus infection, chronic herpes simplex, toxoplasmosis, mycobacterium tuberculosis.
   - Malignancies—most commonly Kaposi's sarcoma, which is a malignant blood vessel and skin condition, and non-Hodgkin's lymphoma.

   Neurological disease—focal encephalitis (CNS toxoplasmosis), cryptococcal meningitis, AIDS dementia complex, herpes zoster.

3. Describe the clinical presentation/characteristics of a patient with chronic fatigue versus fibromyalgia syndrome. Describe physical therapy intervention for each.

   - Common symptoms: generalized or persistent fatigue, sleep disturbances, irritable bowel and GI disturbances, anxiety, or depression.
   - Chronic fatigue syndrome (CFS): significantly lower level of tolerance for activity—does not resolve with sleep, general flu-like symptoms, tender lymph nodes (neck, armpit), mental fog, dizziness or fainting (difficulty with upright position), visual disturbances—light sensitivity, blurring, eye pain.
   - Fibromyalgia syndrome (FMS): general myalgia and aching, fatigue may be mental as well as physical, morning stiffness, restless legs, atypical patterns of numbness and tingling.
   - PT intervention is very similar for both syndromes—it is important to remember that regular, smaller bouts and non-maximal exercise and activity are encouraged for both syndromes.
   - It is important to note that regular exercise has been proven beneficial in diminishing the signs, symptoms, and disability associated with each syndrome.

4. Compare the mode of transmission and protective measures for norovirus, hepatitis A, and measles.

   - Norovirus is transmitted by infected droplet—via the cough or sneeze of an infected individual, suctioning of endotracheal fluid may produce droplets; capable of traveling fairly short distances, ≤ 3 feet. Protective measures include use of a masks, standard and contact precautions.
   - Measles can be spread through airborne transmission, microorganisms are transmitted on droplet nuclei carried on air currents; capable of traveling long distances. Protective measures include use of specifically designed masks and specially designed ventilation systems.

   Note: Standard precautions and infection control procedures are summarized in Box 6-1.

5. Describe physical therapy management for the conditions of sacroiliac dysfunction, varicose veins, and post-cesarean childbirth.
   - Sacroiliac dysfunction: instruction in core stabilization exercises and strengthening of hip abductors, external stabilization devices, patient instruction to avoid single-limb weight-bearing activities.
   - Varicose veins: patient instruction in avoiding crossing of legs, elevation of extremities, wearing compression stockings when up.
   - Post-cesarean childbirth: post-operative TENS for pain at incision site, instruction in diaphragmatic breathing and cough to prevent pulmonary complications; inclusion of gentle, supported abdominal exercises, pelvic floor exercises, instruction to avoid heavy lifting and proper lifting techniques.

6. What is the difference between stress, urge, and functional incontinence? Describe different methods of management of incontinence.

Stress	Urge	Functional
Is the sudden, unintended, release of urine. Due to increases in intra-abdominal pressure, e.g., coughing, laughing, exercise. Due to weakness and laxity of pelvic floor musculature, sphincter weakness, e.g., postpartum incontinence, menopause, damage to pudendal nerve.	Bladder begins contracting and urine is leaked after sensation of bladder fullness is perceived; an inability to delay voiding until the toilet is reached. Due to detrusor muscle instability or hyperreflexia, e.g., following stroke; or sensory instability—hypersensitive bladder.	Leakage associated with inability or unwillingness to toilet, may be due to: impaired cognition (dementia), impaired physical function (stroke), environmental barriers.

   - Dietary management: control/limit foods that aggravate the bladder or incontinence—citrus fruit or juices, caffeine, chocolate; control fluid intake and fluid intake times.
   - Medical management: medications for urge, stress and overflow incontinence—estrogen with phenylpropanolamine; control of medications that may aggravate incontinence—diuretics, anticholinergic or psychotropic drugs. Catheterization for overflow incontinence. Surgery for bladder neck suspension, removal of prostate obstructions, suprapubic cystostomy.
   - Other management:
     - Prompted voiding–toileting schedule—using the bathroom at regular intervals (may be part of an integrated program for a patient/resident in an in-patient, rehabilitation, or long-term care environment).
     - Physical therapy management for strengthening—teach pelvic floor muscle exercises, functional electrical stimulation for retraining, biofeedback, progressive weighted vaginal cones or pelvic floor exerciser, teach incorporation of Kegel's exercise into ADLs, activity and exercise; behavioral training—voiding diary, discussion and education of condition.
     - Physical therapy management for environmental conditions—environmental modification, e.g., install handrails or raised toilet seat for safe toilet transfers; provide protection—underpads or adult diapers.
     - Psychological support—can be socially isolating.

Chapter 7 Review Questions

Integumentary Physical Therapy

1. Name four different assessments performed during inspection of a wound.
   - Location—describe in relationship to anatomical landmarks.
   - Size—length, width, depth, tunneling, undermining.
   - Exudate—type (serous, purulent, sanguineous), amount (may be dry), odor, consistency.
   - Temperature—of wound and of surrounding tissues.
   - Periwound area—halo of erythema, warmth, edema (cellulitis present?), maceration, coloring (cyanotic), trophic changes.
   - Sensory integrity—limb and surrounding area.
   - Signs of infection—edema, erythema, red streaks, foul discharge.

2. What viral infection produces pain and tingling along a spinal or cranial nerve dermatome? It often appears as raised red papules and vesicles that follow along a nerve path. What causes this condition and is it contagious? Identify the following: (a) describe associated signs and symptoms, (b) describe management of the condition.
   - The infection described is a viral infection called Herpes zoster or shingles. IT IS A CONTAGIOUS INFECTION caused by the varicella-zoster virus—better known as chickenpox. It is a reaction of the virus lying dormant in cerebral ganglia or ganglia of posterior nerve roots.
   - Associated signs and symptoms: in addition to the red papules and vesicles occurring along the dermatome, the infected individual experiences pain—often significant pain; is it often accompanied by fever, chills, malaise and potentially gastrointestinal disturbances. It should be noted that postherpetic neuralgia pain can last constantly or intermittently for weeks or months following initial onset.
   - Management: there is no curative agent; significant doses of antiviral medications slow the progress, especially when started immediately at onset of the condition. Symptomatic treatment for itching may consist of corticosteroids. Symptomatic treatment of pain may include oral or cream-based analgesics. Patients should not be treated in open areas, and the infected area should not be touched or exposed to surfaces used by other individuals.

3. Differentiate between these two immune disorders of the skin—systemic lupus erythematosus (SLE) and scleroderma. Describe the condition, symptoms, management, and precautions for each.

Condition	Systemic lupus erythematosus	Scleroderma
Description	Chronic, systemic inflammatory disorder affecting multiple organ systems, including skin, joints, kidneys, heart, nervous system and mucous membranes; it can be fatal. Commonly affects young women.	Chronic, diffuse disease of connective tissues—causes fibrosis of skin, joints, blood vessels and internal organs (GI tract, lungs, heart, kidneys). Usually accompanied by Raynaud's phenomenon.
Symptoms	Fever, malaise, characteristic butterfly rash across bridge of nose, skin lesions, chronic fatigue, arthralgia, arthritis, skin rashes, photosensitivity, anemia, hair loss, Raynaud's phenomenon	Taut, firm, edematous skin that is firmly bound to subcutaneous tissues. <u>Limited disease</u>: symmetrical skin involvement of distal extremities and face; slow progression, late involvement of viscera. <u>Diffuse disease</u>: skin thickening symmetrical, widespread skin involvement of distal and proximal extremities, face and trunk; rapid progression of skin changes and early involvement of viscera.

Condition	Systemic lupus erythematosus	Scleroderma
Management	No cure. Topical corticosteroid treatment of skin lesions, salicylates or indomethacin when fever and pain are present; immunosuppressive agents with life-threatening disease.	No specific treatment. Supportive therapy can include corticosteroids, vasodilators, analgesics, and immunosuppressive agents. Physical therapy can slow development of contracture and deformity.
Precautions	Observe for side effects of corticosteroids: edema, weight gain, acne, hypertension, bruising, purplish stretch marks. Long-term use: associated with increased risk of infection, osteoporosis, myopathy, tendon rupture, diabetes, gastric irritation, low potassium.	Use caution with sclerosed skin, sensitive to pressure. Acute hypertension may occur and regular blood pressure checks must be done.

4. What type of wound may appear as a partial-thickness wound with shaggy edges and present with good blood flow, granulation tissue, and a yellow fibrous covering on it?

- A venous wound.
- For additional review, create a table differentiating the clinical signs/symptoms of, as well as treatment for, different wounds.

5. Compare and contrast between a foam and a hydrocolloid wound dressing.

Foam	Hydrocolloid
• Semipermeable membrane that varies in thickness, absorptive capacity and adhesive properties. • Indicated for partial and full-thickness wounds with minimal to moderate exudate; can be used as secondary dressing for wound with packing to provide additional absorption. • Advantages: insulates, provides padding, most are non-adherent, comfortable, newer products are designed for deep cavities. • Disadvantages: may require secondary dressing or tape to hold in place, poor conformability for deep wounds, may need to protect surrounding intact tissues to prevent maceration.	• Adhesive wafer containing hydroactive/absorptive particles that interact with wound fluid to form a gelatinous mass over wound bed; may be occlusive or semi-occlusive. Also available in paste form that can be used as wound filler for shallow cavity wound. • Indicated for protection of partial-thickness wounds; allows for autolytic debridement of necrosis or slough and absorbs mild exudate. • Advantages: waterproof barrier that maintains moist wound environment and supports autolytic debridement, non-adhesive to healing tissue, impermeable to external bacteria and contaminants, thin forms can diminish friction. • Disadvantages: may soften and change shape with heat or friction, odor and yellow drainage when dressing removed, dressing edges may curl; is not recommended for deep wounds, wounds with heavy exudate, sinus tracts, or infections.

Chapter 8 Review Questions

Geriatric Physical Therapy

1. Summarize changes in the following systems as a result of aging:
   Muscular System
   Skeletal System
   Vestibular System

   - Muscular system: some loss of muscle strength and mass is a part of the aging process; however, strength can be increased and maintained with regular exercise. Muscles will fatigue more readily (decreased oxidative capacity and blood flow) and power will diminish. Girth measurements are not valid to determine strength gain.
   - Skeletal system: decreased levels of activated vitamin D_3 (for calcium absorption); decreased hormone levels, both estrogen and progesterone. Other factors contributing to bone loss can include hyperthyroidism and steroid therapy. Postural changes may lead to forward head, increased kyphosis, and flattened lumbar spine.
   - Vestibular system: the vestibular ocular reflex (VOR) diminishes with aging, resulting in delayed reaction times and longer response times; may lead to some blurred vision as VOR function diminishes and retinal image stability is affected. May become more dependent upon somatosensory system as other senses diminish.

2. Identify what a normal T-score is and what a lower T-score indicates. Identify medical management of an individual who has low T-scores.

   - A T-score is the measurement of bone density. A normal T-score is −1 to +4 SD from the young normal mean reference population.
   - Osteopenia is represented as a T-score of −1 to 2.5 SD below the normal mean reference population; Osteoporosis is diagnosed with a T-score ≤ 2.5 SD below the normal mean reference.
   - Medical management for low T-scores can include medications as well as increased calcium intake.
     - Calcium absorption is largely dependent on vitamin D intake and often medical management includes taking calcium supplements in conjunction with increased vitamin D intake.
     - Daily calcium intake for individuals 50 or older is recommended at 1200 mg/day, and vitamin D is recommended at 800–1000 IU/day.
     - Table 8-2 identifies medications that may be prescribed for individuals with low bone density.

3. Identify three physical therapy interventions each for osteoarthritis and rheumatoid arthritis that have good evidence supporting their use in treatment programs.

   - Osteoarthritis: aerobic conditioning, strengthening exercises, and joint mobilizations.
   - Rheumatoid arthritis: supervised exercise programs for strength and aerobic conditioning for individuals who are medically controlled, adherence to joint protection principles.

4. Differentiate modifiable and non-modifiable risk factors for stroke/cerebrovascular accident.

   - Modifiable: high blood pressure, healthy diet, regular exercise.
   - Non-modifiable: age, ethnicity, gender.

5. Which balance assessment test is more appropriately used for a community-dwelling older adult—the Dynamic Gait Index (DGI) or the Performance Oriented Mobility Assessment (POMA) test? Compare and contrast these two balance assessments.

- The Dynamic Gait Index (DGI) has been demonstrated reliable in testing function in community-dwelling older adults and is highly predictive of identifying those at greater risk for incidence of disability.

DGI	POMA
– The test presents external demands to balance responses by including changes in gait speed, head turns, pivot turns, obstacles, and stairs. A score of 19 or less is indicative of increased fall risk. – Most sensitive in community-dwelling older adults; also useful for individuals with vestibular dysfunction. – Has good test-retest and inter/intrarater reliability. Is valid and predictive of risk.	– The test includes both a balance and a gait subset of activities to perform. A score of <19 indicates a high risk for falls. – Balance and mobility test effective for use in the elderly population in residential care. – Demonstrates 68% sensitivity and 75% specificity.

We suggest you take this opportunity to review standardized balance assessment tests so that you are familiar with which tests are best used for different populations and are able to identify scoring. Table 3-17 summarizes this information.

Chapter 9 Review Questions

Pediatric Physical Therapy

1. What does the IDEA (Public Law 108-446) require?

   - It is a federal program overseen by the states and implemented at the district level in each state.
   - Part C provides services for children from birth to 3 years of age and their families. Those services include activities to identify children at risk and in need of services, services are delivered in "natural environments" and an Individualized Family Service Plan (IFSP) is developed for the child and family by the provider.
   - Part B provides for services for individuals between 3 and 21 years of age. Those services include what is needed to support the child's individual educational needs—NOT for medical needs. An Individualized Educational Plan (IEP) is devised for each child. Transition plans must be in place within the IEP for individuals by the time the individual is 16 years of age.

2. What impairments are expected in a child with Duchenne muscular dystrophy? Identify three physical therapy interventions/goals for a child with Duchenne muscular dystrophy.

   - Progressive weakness, typically beginning proximally and progressing distally. Onset is between 3 and 4 years of age, life expectancy is young adulthood or early 20s.
   - Contractures and deformity likely to develop due to muscular imbalances, especially heel cords, tensor fascia latae. Pseudohypertrophic muscles appear as muscle is replaced by fat and connective tissue, commonly in calves, deltoids, quadriceps, and tongue.
   - Progressive cardiopulmonary limitations.
   - Spinal deformities: decreasing lumbar lordosis, kyphoscoliosis.
   - Physical therapy interventions/goals:
     - Maintain range of motion by positioning, splinting, and stretching.
     - Maintain ambulation and standing skills; utilize assistive devices as needed—crutches, braces, standing frame, dynamic stander.
     - Maintain functional skills: mobility (motorized wheelchair), alternative communication devices.
     - Maintain cardiorespiratory function: avoid traditional strengthening exercises to preserve muscle tissue. Aquatic therapy is a good alternative; it can help build strength and endurance while not increasing the rate of tissue breakdown.

3. In what position should a splint for an infant with congenital hip dysplasia position the hips?

   The hips should be placed in a flexed and abducted position, the closed packed position. This allows for development of the hip socket and stability within the joint.

4. What characteristic impairments should a PTA working with a child who has a Pervasive Developmental Disorder (PDD) expect the child to present with?

   Children with PDD, e.g., autism, typically have impairments in social, behavioral and communication skills. Motor skills can certainly be affected in any population; however, this is not a common occurrence resulting from the PDD diagnosis.

5. A PTA is working with a teenager with spina bifida at S1 level to address increased lower extremity weakness that is limiting walking. During treatment, the PTA notes the teenager appears fatigued. The teenager reports a headache, recent sleep disturbances, and recent problems with bowel and bladder control. What should the PTA suspect is the problem and report immediately to the supervising physical therapist?

> The signs and symptoms reported are similar to those experienced with cord tethering. Cord tethering is a concern for children with spina bifida, especially during a growth spurt; a growth spurt would be expected during the teenage years.

Chapter 10 Review Questions

Therapeutic Modalities

1. When is a patient/client who is receiving a hot pack treatment at greatest risk for burn? What is the correct temperature range for a hydrocollator unit containing hot packs?

   - A patient/client is at greatest risk during the first 5 minutes of treatment. Tissue inspection should be performed within this time frame to minimize the chances of a burn.
   - Hydrocollator temperature range is 165°–170°.

2. Describe how to best manage tissue heating when using a capacitor heating unit with a short-wave diathermy device. What type of tissue responds best to short-wave diathermy?

   - Capacitor plates that are placed closer together will produce higher tissue temperatures; tissues at the center of the electrical field receive greater current density.
   - The sensation of heat is proportionate to the electrode distance from the skin. Plates that are placed closer to the skin produce greater superficial heating.
   - Tissues that are most resistant to current flow develop the most heat. For example, muscle, blood, and fat. Clinicians using capacitor heating plates must be cautious when treating individuals with greater fat content.

3. How would the application of cervical traction change when used to treat a patient/client who has a degenerative joint condition versus a protruding disc in the cervical spine at the C5–C6 level?

   - Degenerative joint conditions: Spine positioned in 25°–30° of cervical flexion. Treatment times for degenerative joint conditions and muscle spasm are typically between 10 and 30 minutes using an intermittent duty cycle.
   - Cervical disc dysfunction: best treated in the neutral spine position, approximately 20° of flexion. Treatment times for disc dysfunction are typically between 5 and 10 minutes using a static duty cycle.

4. What type of nerve and motor tissue response will an electrical current that is 0.5 msec in duration and applied at 80 pulses per second achieve?

   - A pulse duration that is >0.06 and <1 msec is most likely to produce a response from a motor nerve that is innervated. Denervated muscle requires pulse durations >1 msec.
   - Pulse frequencies between 1 and 10 pulses/second will produce brief, or twitch muscle contractions with each stimulus. Pulse frequencies that are generally >10 pulses/second will produce tetanic muscle contractions.

5. Zinc oxide may be used to treat dermal ulcers. What lead should be attached to the active electrode to drive ions of zinc oxide into the tissues?

   - Zinc is the positive medicinal ion; the active electrode should be attached to the positive lead.

6. Name five contraindications to the use of electrical stimulation with a patient/client.

   Contraindications:
   - Anywhere in the body for patients with demand-type pacemakers, unstable arrhythmias, suspected epilepsy or seizure disorder.
   - Over or in the areas of the carotid sinus, thrombosis or thrombophlebitis, eyes, thoracic region, phrenic nerve, urinary bladder stimulators, and abdomen or low back during pregnancy.
   - Transcerebrally or transthoracically.
   - In the presence of active bleeding or infection.
   - Superficial metal implants.
   - Pharyngeal or laryngeal muscles.
   - Motor-level stimulation should not be applied in conditions that prohibit/restrict motion.

   Precautions:
   - Candidates should also review precautions and understand the differences between precautions and contraindications. Review these in Chapter 10.

Chapter 11 Review Questions

Functional Training, Equipment, and Devices

1. Identify and describe three different pelvis motions that occur during normal gait.
   - Transverse motion: pelvis moves forward/backward during gait, forward on the unsupported (swing) limb, backward on the weight-bearing limb; total pelvic motion is approximately 8°.
   - Lateral pelvic motion: pelvis moves up and down approximately 5°, motion is controlled by hip abductors; high point occurs during midstance and low point occurs during double support.
   - Side-to-side motion: follows stance limb, approximately 5° of motion.

2. What function does an anterior stop of an ankle foot orthosis (AFO) serve?
   - It controls dorsiflexion of the ankle.
     When set for slight dorsiflexed position, it can help control knee hyperextension; if set at too great of an angle, it can cause the knee to buckle.

3. Describe how applying tape to an injured ligament and joint differs from taping the same uninjured ligament or joint.
   - Injured ligament or joint: should be taped in a shortened and protected position.
   - Uninjured ligament or joint: should be taped in a neutral position.

4. Contrast the terms *pressure tolerant* and *pressure sensitive* areas as they relate to a residual limb. Identify pressure tolerant and pressure sensitive areas for transtibial and transfemoral residual limbs.

Residual limb	Pressure tolerant	Pressure sensitive
Transfemoral residual limb	Ischial tuberosity Gluteals Lateral sides of the residual limb (over the muscle belly)	Distolateral end of femur Pubic symphysis Perineal area
Transtibial residual limb	Patellar tendon Medial tibial plateau Tibia and fibula shafts Distal end	Anterior and distal end of tibia Anterior tibial crest Fibular neck and head Fibular nerve

5. Identify three drawbacks to a sling seat in a wheelchair.
   - Hips tend to slide forward.
   - Thighs and hips tend toward internal rotation.
   - Reinforces posterior pelvic tilt sitting position.

6. What dimensions should a clinician recommend to a family member building a ramp for a front door entrance of a residence that has two 8-inch steps out front?
   - Slope to rise of a ramp is 12 inches of slope for every 1 inch of rise; this ramp should be 192 inches in length.
   - Ramp should be 36 inches in width.
   - Handrail should extend 12 inches beyond the top and bottom of the run of the ramp.

Chapter 12 Review Questions

Teaching and Learning

1. Identify four steps necessary in preparing a presentation to a community group. These steps are the same steps used when instructing a patient/client.
   - Identify the needs of the audience.
   - Set educational objectives and goals.
   - Select educational methods and design the presentation.
   - Implement and carry out the educational process.
   - Evaluate and revise the presentation.

2. Describe what training strategies are most useful for a patient/client during the cognitive (early) versus the associative (acquiring skills) stage of learning.

Cognitive	Associative
– During this phase, the learner for the most part consciously controls movements and tasks.	– During this phase, the learner is beginning to incorporate some automatic, subconscious tasks without previous cognitive planning.
– Training strategies include facilitating success of tasks, providing physical and/or verbal guidance, providing praise and continuing motivation, providing feedback and guidance, using blocked/repeated practice trials, beginning to use variable practice patterns.	– Training strategies include encourage self-assessment, vary feedback to learner (e.g., provide fading amounts), encourage consistency of performance, progress to changing environments.

3. Identify at least three effective communication strategies.
   - Use active listening skills, "I statements."
   - Establish patient desired goals and work toward those; establish trust.
   - Empathize with the patient/client.
   - Develop rapport with patient/client.

Chapter 13 Review Questions

Management, Safety, and Professional Roles

1. Identify four common reasons for denial of payment by an insurance company for physical therapy services.
    - Incomplete/insufficient documentation.
    - Medically unnecessary services.
    - Incorrect coding.
    - Insufficient functional outcomes.

2. What services does the Individuals with Disabilities and Education Act (IDEA) provide?
    - Ensures children with disabilities receive appropriate, free public education.
    - Provides statutes and guidelines for states and school districts regulating the provision of special education and related services.
    - Establishes early intervention programs including PT, OT, and ST as well as other services needed.

3. Identify four specific criteria that must be considered when restraints are used with patients/residents.
    - Restraints must be used for a specific reason, e.g., patient safety.
    - Restraints are considered temporary and may not be used for infinite amounts of time.
    - A patient/resident in restraints must be checked on at least every 30 minutes.
    - Restraints are NOT intended to be used for punishment and are not a substitute for proper staff supervision.

4. Differentiate between a policy and a procedure an employee will find in a policy and procedure manual.
    - Policy: broad statements that are used as a guide in decision making; for example, for medical records management, the policy would identify that records are maintained for a minimum of 7 years after the last date of service.
    - Procedure: a specific guideline for job behaviors for all personnel; for example, hand washing must be performed for 30–45 seconds using warm soapy water between patient/client visit.

Chapter 14 Review Questions

Research and Evidence-Based Practice

1. Explain the difference between independent and dependent variables.
   - An independent variable is the factor that is believed to bring about the change in the dependent variable; the cause or treatment.
   - A dependent variable is the change or difference in behavior that is the result of the intervention (independent variable); the outcome that is being evaluated.

2. Rank and briefly explain the following levels of evidence. Which of these provides a better level of evidence from which to base treatment decisions?
   – Case-control study.
   – Randomized controlled trial (RCT).
   – Cohort study.
   - A randomized controlled trial provides the best level of evidence from this list. A systematic review of multiple, homogenous RCTs provides even better evidence than one RCT. A RCT is an experimental study in which participants are randomly assigned to either an experimental or control group to receive different interventions or a placebo.
   - A cohort study is a prospective (forward-in-time) study; a group of participants (cohort) with a similar condition is followed for a defined period of time. A comparison is then made to a matched group that does not have the condition.
   - A case-control study is the lowest level of evidence included in this list; a case report provides a lower level of evidence than a case-controlled study. A case-controlled study is a retrospective (backward-in-time) study in which a group of individuals with a similar condition (disease) is compared with a group that does not have the condition. It is used to determine factors that may have played a role in the condition.

3. Differentiate the terms *sensitivity* versus *specificity*.
   - Sensitivity is a measure of the test's ability to correctly identify the proportion of those that truly have the condition, impairment, or disease being measured. It is a measure of true positive.
   - Specificity is a measure of the test's ability to correctly identify the proportion of those who do NOT have the condition, impairment, or disease being measured. It is a measure of true negative.

4. Describe what a clinical prediction rule (CPR) is and how it can be used to practice.
   - A CPR is a combination of clinical findings that have statistically demonstrated meaningful predictability in guiding clinical decision making. It can be used to assist the clinician in determining a diagnosis, a prognosis, or an intervention.
   - When these CPRs are used with clinical expertise and patient preference they can help to improve the overall quality of care.

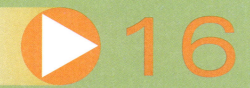

Online Examinations

With this book you also receive access to the TherapyEd Online Learning Portal containing three complete practice exams. The Access Code to the learning portal can be found either in this text or was sent to you in a confirmation email. In the learning portal you may take an entire practice exam, or you can choose to take smaller mini-tests focused on specific areas of practice, which are drawn from the full exams. After you complete the mini-tests or full exams, your performance will be analyzed across the six domains and five categories of the NPTE content outline. You can then refer to the following section to review the questions, the correct and incorrect choices, and understand the content and reasoning rationales for each item.

Questions with Answers and Rationales

Domains

- Cardiovascular, Pulmonary, and Lymphatic
- Musculoskeletal
- Neuromuscular and Nervous
- Integumentary
- Other Systems: Metabolic and Endocrine, Gastrointestinal, Genitourinary, System Interactions
- Nonsystem

Categories

- Diseases and Conditions Impacting Intervention
- Data Collection
- Interventions
- Equipment, Devices, and Therapeutic Modalities
- Safety and Protection, Professional Responsibilities, Research, and Evidence-Based Practice

Diagnostic Level Question

 Inductive Reasoning   Inference   Analysis

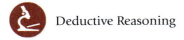 Deductive Reasoning   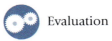 Evaluation

Examination A

A1

Musculoskeletal | Interventions

A patient sustained a fracture to the left proximal humerus, which is now healed. The left scapula now protracts, elevates early, and moves excessively with shoulder flexion. Which of the following physical therapy interventions should be emphasized?

Choices:
1. Stretching of scapular stabilizers and strengthening of the pectoralis major and minor muscles.
2. Scapulothoracic mobilization and strengthening of the pectoralis major and minor muscles.
3. Glenohumeral mobilization and strengthening of scapular stabilizer muscles.
4. Glenohumeral mobilization, and strengthening of the rotator cuff muscles.

Teaching Points

Correct Answer: 3

Compensation for glenohumeral restrictions is often exhibited as excessive scapular movement. Therefore, mobilization of the glenohumeral joint and strengthening of scapular stabilizers is needed to regain normal scapulohumeral motion.

Incorrect Choices:
Strengthening of the scapula, not mobilization or stretching, is needed to prevent scapula protracting. Although glenohumeral mobilization is needed, strengthening of the scapular musculature rather than the rotator cuff is appropriate.

Type of Reasoning: Inductive
One must determine the best therapeutic approach for a patient with excessive scapular movement. This requires knowledge of the diagnosis and therapeutic approaches for it, which is an inductive reasoning skill. For this case, the assistant should emphasize glenohumeral mobilization and strengthening the scapular stabilizers. If answered incorrectly, review intervention approaches for excessive scapular movement.

A2

Cardiac | Interventions

A physical therapist assistant is supervising the exercise of a cardiac rehabilitation outpatient class on a very hot day, with temperatures expected to be above 90°F. The class is scheduled for 2 p.m. and the facility is not air conditioned. What is the **BEST** strategy?

Choices:
1. Decrease the exercise intensity by slowing the pace of exercise.
2. Increase the warm-up period to equal the total aerobic interval in time.
3. Continue with planned intensity for exercise class and encourage participants to drink more water.
4. Shift to intermittent exercise but decrease the rest time.

Teaching Points

Correct Answer: 1

Clinical decisions should focus on reducing the environmental costs of exercising (change the time of day of the exercise class to reduce the heat stress) or reducing the overall metabolic costs of the activity (decrease the pace of exercise, add more rest periods).

Incorrect Choices:

Altering the warm-up period, or increasing water intake do not lower the overall cost of the aerobic exercise. While shifting to intermittent exercise is appropriate, a clinician would want to increase rest time, not decrease rest time, in order to reduce the cost of exercising.

Type of Reasoning: Evaluative

One must determine a best course of action for a group of clients exercising in hot temperatures. The test taker must weigh the potential courses of action and outcomes to arrive at a correct conclusion, which is an evaluative reasoning skill. For this case, the best strategy is to decrease the exercise intensity by slowing the pace of exercise. If answered incorrectly, review cardiac rehabilitation guidelines, including exercise in warmer temperatures.

A3

Nonsystem | Equipment and Devices

A patient with a transtibial amputation has recently been fitted with a patellar tendon-bearing (PTB) socket. Following gait training, the patient removes the prosthesis. If the prosthesis is fitted correctly, which area should the physical therapist assistant NOT expect to find skin redness?

Choices:
1. Anterior tibia and tibial crest.
2. Patellar tendon and tibial tuberosity.
3. Medial tibial and fibular plateaus.
4. Medial and lateral distal ends of the residual limb.

Teaching Points

Correct Answer: 1

In a PTB socket, reliefs are provided for pressure-sensitive areas: the anterior tibia and tibial crest, fibular head and peroneal nerve.

Incorrect Choices:

All the other choices, with the exception of the tibial tuberosity, are considered pressure-tolerant areas and will likely have redness present even with a properly fitting prosthesis.

Type of Reasoning: Inferential

One must infer or draw a reasonable conclusion about gait training with a PTB socket and areas that are not likely to show redness after walking. This requires one to determine what may not occur with the patient, necessitating an inferential reasoning skill. For this situation, one should not expect to find redness on the anterior tibia and tibial crest. If answered incorrectly, review properties of a PTB socket and pressure relief.

A4

NonSystem | Therapeutic Modalities

The plan of care indicates ultrasound treatment for a muscle spasm of the piriformis. The piriformis is compressing the sciatic nerve and producing pain in the posterior hip region. The pain has been worsening over the past 3 months. What is the **MOST** beneficial ultrasound setting for this case?

Choices:
1. 3 MHz continuous at 1.0 w/cm.2
2. 3 MHz pulsed at 1.0 w/cm.2
3. 1 MHz pulsed at 1.0 w/cm.2
4. 1 MHz continuous at 1.0 w/cm.2

Teaching Points

Correct Answer: 4

One MHz of continuous ultrasound provides deep heating to a depth of 3–5 cm. At this frequency, attenuation (absorption) is less in superficial tissues. This allows more energy to be absorbed; thus, more heat is produced in deeper tissue layers. Continuous ultrasound is applied to achieve thermal effects (e.g., for chronic pain), and pulsed ultrasound is used when nonthermal effects are desired (e.g., for acute soft-tissue injuries).

Incorrect Choices:
The 3 MHz would only heat superficially and the piriformis is a deep muscle. 1 MHz continuous US is the only choice that offers deep thermal effects. 3 MHz offers a superficial heating effect, and pulsed US offers mechanical effects.

Type of Reasoning: Inductive
This question requires one to determine the most beneficial ultrasound setting for a patient with a muscle spasm of the piriformis. This requires clinical judgment to arrive at a correct conclusion, necessitating inductive reasoning skill. For this scenario, it is most beneficial to administer ultrasound at 1 MHz continuously at 1.0 w/cm^2 to achieve desired deep-heating thermal effects. If answered incorrectly, review ultrasound guidelines for patients with chronic pain.

A5

Neuromuscular | Diseases and Conditions Impacting Intervention

A patient is recovering from a complete spinal cord injury, at the level of L2. What is the expected outcome in this case?

Choices:
1. A spastic or reflex bladder.
2. Some recovery of function.
3. Loss of motor function, pain, and temperature sensation below the level of lesion.
4. Greater loss of upper-extremity function than of lower-extremity function.

Teaching Points

Correct Answer: 2

A spinal cord lesion below L1 is a cauda equina lesion, thus a lower motor neuron injury to peripheral roots and nerves. Because some regeneration is possible, some recovery in function can be expected.

Incorrect Choices:

A spastic or reflex bladder is associated with upper motor neuron injury. Other choices describe the deficits associated with anterior cord syndrome or central cord syndrome.

Type of Reasoning: Inferential

One must determine the most likely outcome for a patient with a complete spinal cord injury to arrive at a correct conclusion. Questions that require the test taker to project what may occur in the future often require inferential reasoning skill. For this case, the patient would most likely demonstrate some recovery of function because damage is to peripheral nerve roots. If answered incorrectly, review outcomes for cauda equina spinal cord injuries.

A6

Nonsystem | Professional Roles

The physical therapist assistant (PTA) is scheduled to perform gait training with a patient recently fitted with an ankle-foot orthosis but is running behind schedule. The PTA asks the physical therapist assistant student, on day 2 of his first affiliation, to work with this patient although the student has never performed tissue inspection of an ankle foot orthosis. Which of the following procedures is the **MOST** appropriate for the patient's skin inspection?

Choices:
1. Direct the student to perform.
2. Request the supervising physical therapist to perform.
3. Request another PTA working in the area to perform.
4. Send the patient to their room and request the nurse perform.

Teaching Points

Correct Answer: 2

In this case, the physical therapist is the most appropriate practitioner to perform the examination as he or she is familiar with the patient and knows the patient's baseline skin condition.

Incorrect Choices:

Physical therapy students should not perform advanced tasks for the first time without any instruction or direct supervision. This might be unsafe for the patient. The task of tissue inspection is most appropriately performed by an experienced physical therapist assistant or physical therapist. The skin inspection cannot wait and should not be delayed in case there is an issue with the skin.

Type of Reasoning: Evaluative

This question requires one to determine a best course of action when staffing issues are present in a busy clinic and a student is present. This requires one to weigh the courses of action and determine an appropriate response, which requires evaluative reasoning skill. For this case, because the student has not performed the task before, the task of tissue inspection should be given to the physical therapist in charge of the case. If answered incorrectly, review student supervisory guidelines.

A7

Musculoskeletal | Interventions

A patient has been diagnosed with acute synovitis of the temporomandibular joint. Which intervention is **MOST BENEFICIAL** to help resolve early stage acute inflammation?

Choices:
1. Application of an intraoral appliance and phonophoresis.
2. Joint mobilization and postural awareness.
3. Instruction to eat a soft-food diet and phonophoresis.
4. Temporalis stretching and joint mobilization.

Teaching Points

Correct Answer: 3
Phonophoresis and education regarding consumption of only soft food could help resolve the acute inflammatory process in the temporomandibular joint. Phonophoresis will help to reduce inflammation, and eating soft foods will decrease the stress/demand on the TMJ thereby helping to reduce inflammation.

Incorrect Choices:
Application of an intraoral appliance occurs only when the acute inflammation is not resolved or bruxism continues. Joint mobilization should not be attempted with an acute inflammation.

Type of Reasoning: Inductive
One must utilize knowledge of intervention approaches for the temporomandibular joint to arrive at a correct conclusion. This necessitates clinical judgment, which is an inductive reasoning skill. For this situation, the most beneficial intervention approach is instruction to eat a soft-food diet and phonophoresis. If answered incorrectly, review intervention approaches for patients with acute synovitis of the temporomandibular joint.

A8

Neuromuscular | Data Collection

Which behavior represents a fine motor skill that should be established by 9 months of age?

Choices:
1. Picking up a raisin with a fine pincer grasp.
2. Building a tower of four blocks.
3. Holding a cup by the handle while drinking.
4. Transferring objects from one hand to the other.

Teaching Points

Correct Answer: 4
Transferring objects from one hand to the other is a task developmentally appropriate for an 8- or 9-month-old.

Incorrect Choices:
Using a fine pincer grasp and building a tower of four blocks are skills that develop in the 12–15 month range. Holding a cup by the handle while drinking usually occurs by 12 months of age.

Type of Reasoning: Deductive
For this question, the test taker must recall developmental guidelines of infants in fine motor skills to arrive at a correct conclusion. This requires recall of factual information, which is a deductive reasoning skill. For this case, a 9-month-old infant should demonstrate transfer of objects from one hand to another. Review developmental milestones of infants, especially fine motor skills, if answered incorrectly.

A9

Nonsystem | Professional Roles

A patient who is scheduled to undergo surgery for a chronic shoulder dislocation asks the physical therapist assistant to explain the rehabilitation following the scheduled surgical reconstructive procedure. Which is the **BEST** response?

Choices:
1. Explain the surgical procedure in detail for the patient.
2. Suggest the patient ask the surgeon for information about the procedure and appropriate rehabilitation.
3. Explain how patients typically respond to the surgery and outline the progression of exercises.
4. Refer the patient to a physical therapy clinical specialist who is an expert on shoulder reconstructive rehabilitation.

Teaching Points

Correct Answer: 3

The physical therapist assistant should assess the needs of the patient and provide appropriate information based on the expected rehabilitation process. Physical therapist assistants should be knowledgeable about rehabilitation following orthopedic surgeries. The postop course of treatment should be familiar to the PTA and would not necessarily need the expertise of a clinical specialist. Do not "pass the buck" unless the information is outside the assistant's scope of work.

Incorrect Choices:

Information about the surgical procedure is in the realm of the surgeon. Rehabilitation is the physical therapy domain.

Type of Reasoning: Evaluative

One must determine the best course of action when explaining the rehabilitation process to a patient about to undergo surgery. One must evaluate the courses of action provided and determine the one that effectively addresses the patient's needs. This is an evaluative reasoning skill. For this scenario, the assistant should explain how patients typically respond to the surgery and outline the progression of exercises. If answered incorrectly, review scope of practice guidelines for the physical therapist assistant.

A10

Musculoskeletal | Data Collection

Which of the following processes will **MOST** accurately measure the circumference of a patient's lower leg following a knee arthroplasty?

Choices:
1. Begin at the area of the greatest edema, then every 2 inches proximal and 2 inches distal.
2. Begin at the inferior angle of the greater trochanter of that extremity and continue distally until the inferior angle of the lateral malleolus.
3. Begin at the inferior angle of the lateral malleolus, and in 2–4-inch increments proximally, stopping proximal to the edematous area.
4. Begin at the bend of the knee and proceeding distally every 2 cm, stopping distal to the edematous area.

Teaching Points

Correct Answer: 3

Circumferential measurement must be based from a bony landmark that is reproducible for future measurements. The measurements should include areas immediately proximal and distal to the edematous area. Circumferential measurements are best taken with an anthropometric measuring tape that has a pressure gauge on one end to ensure consistent pressure on the tape during measurement.

Incorrect Choices:

The option including the greater trochanter does begin with a bony landmark; however, it includes the entire thigh and would not likely be necessary for edema in the calf. Soft tissues change with changes in edema and are not a reproducible landmark from which to base measurements, the area of greatest edema may change from day to day. The bend of the knee is not a bony landmark.

Type of Reasoning: Deductive

This question requires the test taker to recall the procedures for circumferential measurement of a patient's calf following a total knee arthroplasty. This necessitates the recall of guidelines and procedures, which is a deductive reasoning skill. For this case, the assistant should measure beginning at the inferior angle of the lateral malleolus, and in 4-inch increments proximally, stopping proximal to the edematous area. If answered incorrectly, review the circumferential measurement procedures for the lower extremity.

A11

Neuromuscular | Interventions

A patient with T10 paraplegia has recently been fitted with bilateral knee-ankle-foot orthoses and is receiving initial ambulation training with axillary crutches. The patient is unable to ambulate with a reciprocal gait pattern. Which of the following gait patterns is the **BEST INITIAL** choice to teach the patient?

Choices:
1. 4-point.
2. Swing-to.
3. 2-point.
4. Swing-through.

Teaching Points

Correct Answer: 2

A swing-to gait pattern is indicated for individuals with limited use of both lower extremities and trunk instability. It is slower and more stable than a swing-through gait pattern (a gait pattern this patient can be progressed to after initial training).

Incorrect Choices:

This patient is unable to perform a reciprocal gait, and therefore, 4-point or 2-point gait patterns are not feasible.

Type of Reasoning: Inductive

This question requires the test taker to determine the best initial gait pattern for a patient with T10 paraplegia. This requires knowledge of the diagnosis and typical gait patterns to arrive at a correct conclusion. This necessitates inductive reasoning skill. For this case, the assistant should teach a swing-to gait pattern. Review gait patterns and gait training for patients with T10 paraplegia if answered incorrectly.

A12

Nonsystem | Professional Roles

After mastectomy, a patient receiving home care cannot accept the loss of her breast. She reports being weepy all the time with loss of sleep. She is constantly tired and has no energy to do anything. Which of the following represents the **BEST** course of action for the physical therapist assistant treating this individual?

Choices
1. Contact the supervising physical therapist and suggest a psychological consult.
2. Report observations to the nurse case manager to monitor the patient closely.
3. Tell her depression is common at first but will resolve with time.
4. Request that her spouse observe her closely for possible suicidal tendencies.

Teaching Points

Correct Answer: 1
The patient is experiencing grief over her loss. Significant persistent symptoms are an indication for referral to a qualified professional (psychologist) to help her deal with her loss. Given that this depression is out of the scope of physical therapy practice, a referral to an appropriate health professional is needed. The physical therapist needs to make that referral request to the physician.

Incorrect Choices:
Depression does not necessarily resolve with time and is not an expected consequence of mastectomy. The nurse case manager does not necessarily treat the client or see them on a regular basis, thus unlikely able to regularly monitor the patient's behavior. The question does not identify the patient has expressed suicidal tendencies.

Type of Reasoning: Evaluative
For this question, the test taker must determine a best course of action for a patient experiencing grief over the loss of her breast. This requires evaluative reasoning skill, as the test taker must weigh the courses of action to determine the best approach for the patient. For this case, the assistant should contact the supervising physical therapist and suggest a psychological consult. If answered incorrectly, review approaches for assisting patients dealing with grief and loss.

A13

Metabolic and Endocrine | Diseases and Conditions Impacting Intervention

An individual with a body mass index (BMI) of 33 kg/m^2 is referred to an outpatient exercise program. Which of the following risk factors should the physical therapist assistant recognize this patient is susceptible to?

Choices:
1. Hyperthermia during exercise.
2. Hypothermia during exercise.
3. Rapid weight loss during the initial weeks.
4. Increased anxiety and depression.

Teaching Points

Correct Answer: 1
A patient with a BMI of 33 kg/m^2 is obese (BMI >30 kg/m^2) and is at increased risk for heat intolerance or hyperthermia during exercise (as well as orthopedic injury).

Incorrect Choices:
Hypothermia is cold intolerance and not related to increased BMI. Weight loss is the result of complex interplay between diet and exercise and not the result of exercise alone. A balanced program of exercise and diet will produce effects over time, not just in the initial weeks. An appropriately prescribed exercise program should decrease anxiety and depression.

Type of Reasoning: Deductive
One must recall the risk factors for patients with obesity and engagement in exercise to arrive at a correct conclusion. This is factual information, necessitating deductive reasoning skill. For this scenario, patients with obesity are at an increased risk for hyperthermia during exercise. Review exercise guidelines for patients with obesity and risk factors if answered incorrectly.

A14

Nonsystem | Evidence-Based Practice

In a research study resulting in a skewed distribution that includes extreme scores on a balance measure that deviate from the total group performance, which of the following measures **MOST** accurately represents the central tendency?

Choices:
1. Mean.
2. Mode.
3. Median.
4. Standard deviation.

Teaching Points

Correct Answer: 3
The median is the middle score of all the scores. The most accurate measure of performance in skewed distribution with extreme scores is the median.

Incorrect Choices:
The mean is a measure of central tendency that is calculated by adding up all the scores and dividing the total by the number of scores. Standard deviation is not a measure of central tendency. The mode is the most frequently occurring score.

Type of Reasoning: Deductive
One must recall research guidelines including measures of central tendency to arrive at a correct conclusion. This is factual information and recall of a research definition, which is a deductive reasoning skill. For this case, the most accurate representation of central tendency is median. If answered incorrectly, review research terminology, especially median scores.

A15

Nonsystem | Equipment and Devices

A patient is recovering from a right cerebrovascular accident (CVA) resulting in severe left hemiplegia and visuospatial deficits. Additionally, there is a large diabetic ulcer on the left foot with pitting edema. What is the **MOST** appropriate wheelchair prescription for this patient?

Choices:
1. Hemiplegic chair with elevating leg rest on the left.
2. Powered wheelchair with joystick and elevating leg rests.
3. Lightweight active duty wheelchair with elevating leg rests.
4. One-arm drive chair with elevating leg rest on the left.

Teaching Points

Correct Answer: 1
A hemiplegic chair has a lower seat height (17 ½ inches compared with the standard height of 19 ½ inches) and is the best choice for this patient; the patient can propel the wheelchair by using both the sound upper and lower extremities.

Incorrect Choices:
The elevating leg rest on the left will assist in managing the wound and edema in the left lower extremity; however an electric wheelchair is not indicated. A one-arm drive wheelchair has both drive mechanisms located on one wheel to enable the patient to propel the wheelchair by using one hand. It is contraindicated in patients with cognitive or perceptual deficits which often accompany a patient with a right CVA, making it inappropriate in this case. Additionally, to be the most successful in using a powered chair one should have good visuospatial awareness which may be affected in this case scenario.

Type of Reasoning: Inductive
This question requires one to utilize clinical judgment to determine the most appropriate wheelchair prescription for a patient with a CVA and hemiplegia. This requires knowledge of wheelchair prescription guidelines and clinical judgment, which is an inductive reasoning skill. For this case, the most appropriate wheelchair is a hemiplegic chair with elevating leg rest on the left. If answered incorrectly, review wheelchair prescription guidelines for patients with CVA and hemiplegia.

A16

Nonsystem | Therapeutic Modalities

A patient fractured the right mid-tibia in a skiing accident 3 months ago. After cast removal, a severe foot drop was noted. The plan of care includes electrical stimulation orthotic substitution. During which phase of gait should the physical therapist assistant set up the functional electrical stimulation to contract the appropriate muscles?

Choices:
1. Heel-off (terminal stance).
2. Midswing (midswing).
3. Foot flat (loading response).
4. Toe-off (preswing).

Teaching Points

Correct Answer: 2
Foot drop is a swing phase deficit. Stimulation of the dorsiflexor muscles during the swing phase places the foot in a more neutral position and prevents the toes from contacting the ground and interfering with the gait pattern.

Incorrect Choices:
Heel-off and toe-off are when the gastrocsoleus is activated, not the dorsiflexors. Foot flat again is activation of the gastrocsoleus but eccentrically.

Type of Reasoning: Analytical
One must analyze the deficits of the patient to determine the appropriate use of functional electrical stimulation during gait training. This requires analytical reasoning skill. For this situation, the functional electrical stimulation should be set up to contract the muscles during the swing phase. If answered incorrectly, review functional electrical stimulation guidelines for use with patients with foot drop.

A17

Nonsystem | Safety

A physical therapist assistant has weeping dermatitis on the back of the hand and is scheduled to treat a patient with HIV for management of a wound. Which represents the **BEST** course of action for the physical therapist assistant?

Choices:
1. Double glove and treat as scheduled.
2. Use sterile precautions with mask and gloves.
3. Continue with treatment as scheduled but wash hands thoroughly before and after.
4. Refrain from patient care but arrange for treatment by another practitioner.

Teaching Points

Correct Answer: 4
Blood and Body Fluid Precautionary Guidelines from the Centers for Disease Control and Prevention (CDC) state that a health care worker with exudative lesions or weeping dermatitis should refrain from all direct patient care and from handling patient-care equipment until the condition resolves.

Incorrect Choices:
Other responses all include the PTA working with patient/client which is contraindicated when the clinician has open lesions.

Type of Reasoning: Evaluative
One must utilize judgment to determine a best course of action when the assistant has weeping dermatitis and is scheduled to treat a patient with human immunodeficiency virus. This requires the test taker to weigh the courses of action to arrive at a correct conclusion. This necessitates evaluative reasoning skill. For this case, the assistant should refrain from treating the patient but arrange for treatment by another practitioner. If answered incorrectly, review CDC guidelines for treating patients with human immunodeficiency virus when one has weeping dermatitis.

A18

Neuromuscular and Nervous | Diseases and Conditions Impacting Intervention

The initial evaluation for a patient with a right cerebrovascular accident (CVA) identifies that the patient has a profound deficit of homonymous hemianopsia. Which of the following represents the **BEST INITIAL** strategy to assist the patient in compensating for this deficit?

Choices:
1. Teach the patient to turn the head to the affected left side.
2. Provide constant reminders, printed notes on the left side, telling the patient to look to the left.
3. Place items, eating utensils on the patient's left side.
4. Rearrange the room so while the patient is in bed the left side is facing the doorway.

Teaching Points

Correct Answer: 1
A patient with homonymous hemianopsia needs to be made aware of his or her deficit and instructed to turn the head to the affected left side (a compensatory training strategy).

Incorrect Choices:
The question asks for initial strategies. Initial strategies include placing items on the right (unaffected side) not the left or positioning the patient so that the doorway is on the right (unaffected side) not the left so that the patient can successfully interact with the environment. Later, as there is ability to compensate, items can be moved to midline and finally to the affected left side. Placing items on the left (affected side) initially is too advanced for an initial strategy.

Type of Reasoning: Inductive
This question requires one to determine a best initial strategy for patient with a CVA and homonymous hemianopsia to arrive at a correct conclusion. This requires inductive reasoning skill. For this patient the assistant's best initial strategy is to teach the patient to turn the head to the affected left side. If answered incorrectly, review compensatory training strategies for patients with homonymous hemianopsia.

A19

Neuromuscular | Diseases and Conditions Impacting Intervention

A patient with multiple sclerosis exhibits moderate fatigue during a 30-minute exercise session. When the patient returns for the next regularly scheduled session 2 days later, the patient reports going home after the last session and immediately going to bed. The patient was exhausted and unable to get out of bed until the late afternoon of the next day. Which of the following strategies is **BEST** for further treatment?

Choices:
1. Treat the patient in a warm, relaxing environment.
2. Utilize a massed practice schedule.
3. Utilize a distributed practice schedule.
4. Switch the patient to a pool therapy program.

Teaching Points

Correct Answer: 3
Common problems in multiple sclerosis include fatigue and heat intolerance. Exercise intensity should be reduced and a distributed practice schedule used in which rest times equal or exceed exercise times.

Incorrect Choices:
A massed practice schedule in which the exercise time exceeds the rest time is contraindicated. A cool environment (e.g., cooling suit) can reduce heat intolerance and fatigue that commonly accompany exercise. A warm environment or pool therapy in a warm pool is contraindicated as both can increase fatigue.

Type of Reasoning: Inductive
One must utilize clinical judgment to determine a best strategy for a patient with multiple sclerosis. This requires inductive reasoning skill. For this case, given the patient's experience with the previous treatment session, the best strategy is to utilize a distributed practice schedule. Review treatment scheduling for patients with multiple sclerosis to prevent fatigue if answered incorrectly.

A20

Integumentary | Interventions

A patient with a venous stasis ulcer near the left medial malleolus is referred to physical therapy. Stasis dermatitis is evident in the lower extremity. Which nonoperative physical therapy intervention is the **MOST** beneficial for venous stasis ulcers?

Choices:
1. Daily walking for 30–60 minutes.
2. Elastic wraps and daily exercises.
3. Daily warm water baths and exercise.
4. Compression therapy with exercise.

Teaching Points

Correct Answer: 4

Compression therapy is the mainstay of nonoperative treatment of venous stasis ulcers and works with exercise to facilitate movement of excess fluid from the lower extremity. Dressings are applied before compression bandages. Pliable, nonstretchable dressing wraps (e.g., Unna boot) or custom-fitted graduated compression stockings can be used to assist in venous circulation.

Incorrect Choices:

Elastic wraps are easy to apply but provide only light support and do little to assist circulation. Prolonged hydrotherapy is contraindicated for venous ulcers due to risk of infection as well as having the limb in a dependent position for extended periods of time. Daily walks for 30 to 60 minutes would not be appropriate due to the dilated greater saphenous vein and the chance for edema having the limb in a dependent position. Skin changes associated with venous disease include pigmentation, venous eczema and lipodermatosclerosis.

Type of Reasoning: Inductive

One must recall the treatment guidelines for patients with venous stasis ulcers to arrive at a correct conclusion. This necessitates clinical judgment, which is an inductive reasoning skill. For this situation, the most important nonoperative intervention is compression therapy with exercise. If answered incorrectly, review treatment guidelines for patients with venous stasis ulcers, including nonoperative approaches.

A21

Neuromuscular | Diseases and Conditions Impacting Intervention

A patient recovering from stroke is having difficulty bearing weight on the left lower extremity. The patient is unable to advance the tibia forward and abbreviates the end of the stance phase on the left going directly into swing phase. Which factor following stroke is **MOST** likely to result in failure to advance the lower extremity when walking?

Choices:
1. Weakness or contracture of hip extensors.
2. Spasticity or contracture of the plantar flexors.
3. Spasticity of the anterior tibialis muscle.
4. Weakness or contracture of the dorsiflexors.

Teaching Points

Correct Answer: 2
Forward advancement of the tibia from midstance to heel-off is controlled by eccentric contraction of the plantar flexors; from heel-off to toe-off the plantar flexors contract concentrically. Either spasticity or contracture of the plantar flexors would limit this forward progression by limiting the amount of dorsiflexion the ankle can move in to. Patients compensate by moving right into swing, typically with a circumducted gait or with increased hip and knee flexion because there is no push-off. This is commonly seen in the patient with stroke.

Incorrect Choices:
Excessive spasticity of the anterior tibialis would limit the plantarflexion and would prevent the patient from achieving foot flat. Weakness or contracture of the hip extensors would affect the swing phase of gait.

Type of Reasoning: Inferential
One must infer or draw a reasonable conclusion about the most likely reason for failure to advance the lower extremity when walking after stroke. A test taker must determine what may be true of this situation, necessitating inferential reasoning skill. For this scenario, the likely reason for this failure is spasticity or contracture of the plantar flexors. If answered incorrectly, review gait patterns for patients with stroke, especially failure to advance the affected leg.

A22

Neuromuscular | Data Collection

Which of the following functional activities would a physical therapist assistant **NOT** expect a 4 ½-year-old child to perform?

Choices:
1. Skilled tandem walking.
2. Jumping down off a step.
3. Toe-walking.
4. Jumping from two feet.

Teaching Points

Correct Answer: 1
The ability to perform tandem walking typically develops at 5+ years of age; one would not expect a 4 ½ -year-old child to be able to perform this skill.

Incorrect Choices:
The ability to perform jumping from two feet and jumping down off a step typically develop between the ages of 3 and 4 years. A physical therapist assistant performing an intervention with this child could expect the child to be able to perform the jumping tasks. Toe-walking is usually seen when the child first begins to walk and would resolve well before the child is 4 ½ years old.

Type of Reasoning: Inferential
This question requires the test taker to infer or draw a reasonable conclusion about the functional activities of a child and abilities not likely to be seen for a child this age. This requires inferential reasoning skill. For this case, one should not expect to see skilled tandem walking at 4 ½ years of age. If answered incorrectly, review developmental milestones of young children, including motor skills of 4-year-olds.

A23

Nonsystem | Teaching and Learning

Which of the following represents the MOST appropriate feedback strategy for a physical therapist assistant to utilize when providing gait training for a patient who has been receiving gait training for 3 weeks?

Choices:
1. Immediate feedback given after each practice trial.
2. Intermittent feedback given at scheduled intervals, every other practice trial.
3. Continuous feedback with ongoing verbal cuing during gait.
4. Occasional feedback given when consistent errors appear.

Teaching Points

Correct Answer: 4

In learning a psychomotor skill, the patient needs to be able to actively process information and self-correct responses. Occasional feedback provides the best means of allowing for introspection and is appropriate for later practice (associated and autonomous phases of motor learning).

Incorrect Choices:
Continuous feedback and immediate feedback are used when first training and when in the cognitive phase of motor learning. Intermittent feedback is best used during the associated stage of motor learning.

Type of Reasoning: Inductive
This question requires the test taker to determine a best approach when one is providing feedback for a patient during gait training. This requires clinical judgment, which is an inductive reasoning skill. For this situation, after 3 weeks of gait training, the assistant should provide occasional feedback when consistent errors appear. Review gait training guidelines and the use of feedback to improve performance if answered incorrectly.

A24

Cardiac | Diseases and Conditions Impacting Intervention

A patient who is prescribed digitalis (digoxin) will demonstrate understanding of the adverse side effects of this medication by recognizing the importance of informing the physical therapist assistant of which of the following symptoms during exercise?

Choices:
1. Confusion and memory loss.
2. Slowed heart rate.
3. Involuntary movements and shaking.
4. Weakness and palpitations.

Teaching Points

Correct Answer: 4

Class III heart disease is characterized by marked limitation of physical activity; the patient is comfortable at rest, but less than ordinary physical activity causes fatigue, palpitations, dyspnea, or anginal pain. Digitalis (digoxin) is frequently used to treat congestive heart failure (it slows heart rate and increases force of myocardial contraction). Adverse side effects of digitalis can include muscle weakness and supraventricular or ventricular arrhythmias, including ventricular fibrillation, without premonitory signs.

Incorrect Choices:
The other symptoms are not side effects of digitalis, as well as all the other symptoms can be observed by the therapist and would not need to be reported.

Type of Reasoning: Inferential
One must infer the response by the patient that indicates that the patient understands the adverse side effects of digitalis medication. This requires the test taker to determine what may be true of a situation, which is an inferential reasoning skill. For this case, the patient understands the adverse side effects of the medication if the patient knows to report symptoms of weakness and palpitations. If answered incorrectly, review side effects of digitalis medication.

A25

Nonsystem | Safety and Protection

A physical therapist assistant is working with a patient with active hepatitis B infection. How can the PTA **MOST** effectively minimize transmission of the disease?

Choices:
1. Wash hands before and after treatment.
2. Wear gloves during any direct contact with blood or body fluids.
3. Wear a gown and mask during treatment.
4. Have the patient wear gloves to prevent direct contact with the therapist.

Teaching Points

Correct Answer: 2
Standard precautions specify that health care workers wear gloves when they come into direct contact with blood or body fluids. Health care workers should wear moisture-resistant gowns and masks for protection from the splashing of blood, other body fluids, or respiratory droplets.

Incorrect Choices:
Although hand washing is important, it is not as important as wearing gloves when direct contact is made with blood or body fluids. Hepatitis B is a blood-borne pathogen that is transmitted via contact with blood; therefore, the therapist needs to prevent coming into contact with blood. The other options do not prevent the therapist from being in contact with blood.

Type of Reasoning: Inferential
One must determine the most effective means of minimizing exposure to the hepatitis B virus to arrive at a correct conclusion. This requires recall of guidelines regarding standard precautions first and then determining the most effective approach according to these guidelines, which is an inferential reasoning skill. For this situation, the most effective means of minimizing risk is to wear gloves during any direct contact with blood or body fluids. Review standard precautions for the hepatitis B virus if answered incorrectly.

A26

Nonsystem | Therapeutic Modalities

A patient reports pain (7/10) and limited range of motion of the right shoulder as a result of chronic overuse. The therapist has identified procaine hydrochloride iontophoresis as part of a physical therapy intervention. Which of the following treatments would be correct?

Choices:
1. Continuous biphasic current with the medication under the anode.
2. Continuous monophasic current with the medication under the anode.
3. Continuous monophasic current with the medication under the cathode.
4. Interrupted biphasic current with the medication under the cathode.

Teaching Points

Correct Answer: 2
Because like charges are repelled, the positively charged medication would be forced into the skin under the positive electrode (anode). A continuous, unidirectional current flow is very effective in repelling ions into the skin.

Incorrect Choices:
A pulsed or bidirectional current generates less propulsive force owing to the discontinuous nature of the current. Procaine is a positive medicinal ion and will be repelled from the anode (positive pole).

Type of Reasoning: Deductive
One must recall the guidelines for use of iontophoresis to arrive at a correct conclusion. This is factual information, which necessitates deductive reasoning skill. For this case, it is best to administer the substance with continuous monophasic current with the medication under the anode. If answered incorrectly, review iontophoresis guidelines and the use of medication for treatment of pain.

A27

Cardiac | Diseases and Conditions Impacting Intervention

Prior to initiating joint mobilization as directed in the plan of care, which of the following situations should necessitate the physical therapist assistant consulting with the physical therapist?

Choices:
1. Reflex muscle guarding.
2. Long-term corticosteroid therapy.
3. Concurrent inhalation therapy.
4. Functional chest wall immobility.

Teaching Points

Correct Answer: 2
Although chest wall immobility is present with COPD, this is not a contraindication for joint mobilization. Very often patients with chronic pulmonary disease have been managed with corticosteroid therapy, and long-term steroid use affects ligamentous integrity which often produces joint hypermobility.

Incorrect Choices:
Inhalation therapy is a common treatment for COPD but again has no contraindications for joint mobilization. Muscle guarding may be a response to joint mobilization; however it is not a contraindication.

Type of Reasoning: Deductive
One must recall the contraindications for joint mobilization in patients with chronic pulmonary disease to arrive at a correct conclusion. This necessitates the recall of factual guidelines, which is a deductive reasoning skill. For this situation, a contraindication to joint mobilization for a patient with chronic pulmonary disease is long-term corticosteroid therapy. If answered incorrectly, review contraindications for joint mobilization treatment, especially for patients with chronic pulmonary disease.

A28

Nonsystem | Professional Roles

A physical therapist assistant is responsible to oversee departmental equipment safety. Which task is beyond the scope of the assistant's responsibilities?

Choices:
1. Training all staff to do "simple" repairs on all electrical equipment if a breakdown should occur.
2. Supervising new staff and students in the use of all newly purchased equipment.
3. Documenting all preventive maintenance and keeping this information on file.
4. Conducting educational sessions for staff regarding the indications and contraindications for all equipment.

Teaching Points

Correct Answer: 1
Electrical equipment is repaired by the manufacturer or local vendor, or in some cases, the maintenance department—not by physical therapy staff. It is not in the scope of physical therapy practice to fix electrical equipment.

Incorrect Choices:
Supervising new staff in the use of new equipment, documenting preventative maintenance, and conducting educational sessions may all be appropriately assigned to the physical therapist assistant per procedures and policies of the institution.

Type of Reasoning: Evaluative
This question requires the test taker to use knowledge of the physical therapy scope of practice to determine a best course of action when managing equipment safety. This requires evaluative reasoning skill. For this case, it is NOT within the scope of practice for the assistant to train all staff to do simple repairs on all electrical equipment if a breakdown should occur. If answered incorrectly, review scope of practice guidelines.

A29

Integumentary | Data Collection

An elderly and frail resident of an extended-care facility presents with hot, red, and edematous skin over the shins of both lower extremities. The patient also has a mild fever. These are signs and symptoms of which condition?

Choices:
1. Dermatitis.
2. Cellulitis.
3. Herpes simplex infection.
4. Scleroderma.

Teaching Points

Correct Answer: 2
Cellulitis is an inflammation of the cellular or connective tissue in or close to the skin. It is characterized by skin that is hot, red, and edematous. Fever is a common finding.

Incorrect Choices:
Dermatitis produces red, weeping, crusted skin lesions but is not commonly accompanied by fever. Location on shins makes herpes an unlikely choice, and there are no skin eruptions or vesicles. Scleroderma is a collagen disease producing tight, drawn thickened skin.

Type of Reasoning: Analytical

This question provides symptoms, and the test taker must determine the most likely problem. Questions of this nature often require analysis of the symptoms, which is an analytical reasoning skill. For this scenario, the symptoms are indicative of cellulitis and should be reported to the physical therapist by the assistant. If answered incorrectly, review signs and symptoms of cellulitis.

A30

Nonsystem | Therapeutic Modalities

A 12-year-old child presents with pain (4/10) and limited knee range of motion (5°–95°) following surgical repair of the medial collateral and anterior cruciate ligaments. Which modality should be used with caution in this case?

Choices:
1. Premodulated interferential current.
2. Continuous short-wave diathermy.
3. High-rate transcutaneous electrical stimulation.
4. Low-dose ultrasound.

Teaching Points

Correct Answer: 4

Because the epiphyseal plates do not close until the end of puberty, ultrasound energy should be applied with caution around the epiphyseal area because of the potential for causing bone growth disturbances. However, there is no documented evidence that ultrasound creates any direct untoward effects on the growth plates, especially if applied at low dosage.

Incorrect Choices:

Electrical stimulation or deep thermotherapy would have no deleterious effects on the epiphyseal plates because no mechanical effects on hard tissue are associated with their use.

Type of Reasoning: Inductive

This question requires one to utilize clinical judgment to determine the treatment modality that can be used with precaution on a 12-year-old. This necessitates inductive reasoning skill. For this case, low-dose ultrasound can be used with caution around the epiphyseal area. If answered incorrectly, review use of ultrasound in children and precautions.

A31

Musculoskeletal | Interventions

A weight lifter exhibits marked hypertrophy after embarking on a strength training regime. At what point in training can hypertrophy of major muscle groups be expected to occur?

Choices:
1. 2–4 weeks of training.
2. 4–6 weeks of training.
3. 6–8 weeks of training.
4. 8–10 weeks of training.

Teaching Points

Correct Answer: 3
Hypertrophy is the increase in muscle size as a result of resistance training and can be observed following at least 6–8 weeks of training. Individual muscle fibers are enlarged, contain more actin and myosin, and have more, larger myofibrils.

Incorrect Choices:
Prior to 6–8 weeks of training muscle fibers will gain in endurance and strength before significant hypertrophy develops.

Type of Reasoning: Inferential
One must infer or draw a reasonable conclusion about the likely expectation of hypertrophy with strength training. This requires one to determine what may be true of a situation, necessitating inferential reasoning skill. For this situation, one can expect hypertrophy after 6–8 weeks of training. If answered incorrectly, review outcomes of strength training and hypertrophy.

A32

Musculoskeletal | Diseases and Conditions Impacting Intervention

A diagnosis of bicipital tendonitis has been made following an evaluation of a patient with shoulder pain. Which shoulder position will **BEST** expose the tendon of the long head of the biceps for application of phonophoresis?

Choices:
1. Lateral (external) rotation and extension.
2. Medial (internal) rotation and abduction.
3. Horizontal adduction.
4. Abduction.

Teaching Points

Correct Answer: 1
The long head of the biceps is best exposed in shoulder lateral (external) rotation and extension owing to its attachment at the supraglenoid tubercle of the scapula, which is at the medial aspect of the shoulder joint.

Incorrect Choices:
Medial (internal) rotation and abduction place the long head of the biceps deep to the anterior deltoid and pectoralis major muscles. The anterior surface of the shoulder, including the long head of the biceps, loses exposure with horizontal adduction.

Type of Reasoning: Inductive
This question requires the test taker to utilize clinical judgment to determine the best shoulder position for application of phonophoresis to the long head of the biceps. This is an inductive reasoning skill. For this scenario, the long head of the biceps is best exposed in shoulder lateral rotation and extension. Review anatomy of the shoulder and treatment guidelines for bicipital tendonitis and use of phonophoresis if answered incorrectly.

A33

Musculoskeletal | Data Collection

The initial evaluation indicates that a patient has a weak gluteus maximus. What gait deviation should the physical therapist assistant expect to see with this patient during stance phase?

Choices:
1. Lateral bending of the trunk to the same side.
2. Lateral bending of the trunk to the opposite side.
3. Backward trunk lean.
4. Forward trunk lean.

Teaching Points

Correct Answer: 3

A backward trunk lean is the substitution pattern most commonly used by a person with a weak gluteus maximus. This position helps to maintain hip extension by relying on the tension of the hip joint capsule and ligaments.

Incorrect Choices:
A lateral trunk lean to the same side is a common gait deviation demonstrated by a patient with a weak gluteus medius. A lateral trunk lean to the opposite side may be demonstrated by the presence of a weak hip flexor. A forward trunk lean may be a function of a weak quadriceps or a hip or knee flexion contracture.

Type of Reasoning: Inferential
This question requires the test taker to draw a reasonable conclusion about the likely gait deviation expected for a patient with a weak gluteus maximus. This necessitates inferential reasoning skill as the test taker is determining what may be true for a patient. In this case, one should expect a backward trunk lean during the stance phase. If answered incorrectly, review substitution patterns for patients with a weak gluteus maximus.

A34

Integumentary | Diseases and Conditions Impacting Intervention

A patient is transferred to a burn clinic with partial-thickness burns over 30% of the body. What type of healing will this type of wound be characterized by?

Choices:
1. Blisters and minimal edema with spontaneous healing.
2. Depressed skin area that heals with grafting and scarring.
3. Moderate edema with spontaneous healing and minimal grafting.
4. Marked edema with slow healing and extensive hypertrophic scarring.

Teaching Points

Correct Answer: 4

Deep partial-thickness burns involve destruction of the epidermis with damage of the dermis down into the reticular area. Appearance is mixed red/white color with sluggish capillary refill. Superficial sensation is decreased while sense of deep pressure is retained. The burn will heal spontaneously in 3–5 weeks if no infection develops (infection can convert the burn to full-thickness). There is most likely marked edema with excessive scarring (hypertrophic).

Incorrect Choices:
Superficial burns heal with minimal edema, whereas superficial partial-thickness burns heal spontaneously with moderate edema and minimal scarring; they do not require grafting. Full-thickness burns require skin grafting; appearance is depressed with significant scarring.

Type of Reasoning: Inferential
This question provides a diagnosis, and the test taker must infer the likely presentation of symptoms. Questions of this nature often require inferential reasoning skill. For this situation, healing of this burn is characterized by marked edema with slow healing and extensive hypertrophic scarring. Review burn healing guidelines for patients with deep partial-thickness burns if answered incorrectly.

A35

Nonsystem | Equipment and Devices

A patient with a complete spinal cord injury at the T6 level is being discharged home after 2 months of rehabilitation. In preparation for discharge, the rehabilitation team visits the home and finds three standard-height steps going into the home. What length ramp will need to be constructed for wheelchair access into this home?

Choices:
1. 60 inches (5 feet).
2. 192 inches (16 feet).
3. 120 inches (10 feet).
4. 252 inches (21 feet).

Teaching Points

Correct Answer: 4
The architectural standard for rise of a step is 7 inches (steps may vary from 7–9 inches). The recommended ratio of slope to rise is 1:12 (an 8% grade). For every inch of vertical rise, 12 inches of ramp will be required. A straight ramp will have to be 252 inches or 21 feet long.

Incorrect Choices:
A ramp less than 252 inches (21 feet) long will not meet identified standard ratio for slope to rise—for every inch of vertical rise, 12 inches of ramp is required.

Type of Reasoning: Deductive
This question requires one to recall guidelines for the construction of a wheelchair ramp to arrive at a correct conclusion. Questions of this nature, where factual information is used to make decisions, often require deductive reasoning skill. For this case, guidelines indicate that the ramp should be 252 inches or 21 feet long. If answered incorrectly, review Americans with Disabilities Act guidelines for wheelchair ramp construction.

A36

Cardiac | Data Collection

What symptoms should the physical therapist assistant recognize as symptoms of left-sided, class II, heart failure?

Choices:
1. Uncomfortable chest pain that increases with any physical activity.
2. Weight gain with dependent edema.
3. Anorexia and nausea with abdominal pain and distention.
4. Dyspnea with fatigue and muscular weakness.

Teaching Points

Correct Answer: 4

Left-sided heart failure is the result of the left ventricle failing to pump enough blood through the arterial system to meet the body's demands. It produces pulmonary edema and disturbed respiratory control mechanisms. Patients can be expected to demonstrate progressive dyspnea (exertional at first, then paroxysmal nocturnal dyspnea), fatigue and muscular weakness, pulmonary edema, cerebral hypoxia, and renal changes.

Incorrect Choices:

Severe chest pain and shortness of breath are symptoms of impending myocardial infarction. Weight gain and dependent edema as well as anorexia, nausea with abdominal pain and distention are all symptoms associated with right-sided ventricular failure.

Type of Reasoning: Inferential

This question provides a diagnosis, and the test taker must infer the likely symptoms. Questions of this nature often require inferential reasoning skill as one is determining what may be true for a patient. For this situation, the patient can be expected to demonstrate dyspnea with fatigue and muscular weakness. If answered incorrectly, review signs and symptoms of left-sided heart failure.

A37

Musculoskeletal | Interventions

A physical therapist assistant is instructing a physical therapist assistant student in proper positioning to prevent the typical contractures in a patient with a transfemoral amputation. What position should the assistant stress?

Choices:
1. Prone-lying with the residual limb in neutral rotation.
2. A wheelchair with a gel cushion and adductor roll.
3. Supine-lying with the residual limb resting on a small pillow.
4. Side-lying on the residual limb.

Teaching Points

Correct Answer: 1

The typical contractures with a transfemoral amputation are hip flexion, typically from too much sitting in a wheelchair. The residual limb also rolls out into abduction and lateral (external) rotation. When the patient is in bed, hip extension should be emphasized (e.g., prone-lying). Time in extension (prone, supine or standing) should counterbalance time sitting in a wheelchair.

Incorrect Choices:

When the patient is sitting in the wheelchair, neutral hip rotation should be emphasized (e.g., using an abductor roll). The hip flexors need to be stretched and side lying and sitting are not going to do that. Some hip flexor lengthening may occur with the patient in supine if the patient is positioned flat, but not when the limb is resting on a pillow.

Type of Reasoning: Inductive

One must utilize clinical judgment to determine positioning guidelines for a patient with transfemoral amputation. This requires inductive reasoning skill. For this situation, it is important to position the patient in the prone-lying position with the residual limb in neutral rotation to prevent contractures. If answered incorrectly, review positioning guidelines for patients with transfemoral amputations and prevention of contractures.

A38

Metabolic and Endocrine | Diseases and Conditions Impacting Intervention

A physical therapist assistant is following the plan of care to provide gait training for a patient who is insulin dependent. In a review of the patient's medical record, the assistant notices that the blood glucose level for that day is 310 mg/dL. What is the assistant's **BEST** course of action?

Choices:
1. Refrain from ambulating the patient, reschedule for tomorrow before other therapies.
2. Ambulate the patient as planned but monitor closely for signs of exertional intolerance.
3. Postpone therapy and consult with the nurse as soon as possible.
4. Talk to the nurse about walking the patient later that day after lunch.

Teaching Points

Correct Answer: 3

Normal fasting plasma glucose is less than 115 mg/dL, whereas a fasting plasma glucose level greater than 126 mg/dL on more than one occasion is indicative of diabetes. This patient is hyperglycemic with high glucose levels (equal to or greater than 250 mg/dL). Clinical signs that may accompany this condition include ketoacidosis (acetone breath) with dehydration, weak and rapid pulse, nausea/vomiting, deep and rapid respirations (Kussmaul's respirations), weakness, diminished reflexes and paresthesias. The patient may be lethargic and confused and may progress to diabetic coma and death if not treated promptly with insulin. Coordination with the nurse is crucial so that the patient's blood glucose levels drop to a point that is safe for ambulation.

Incorrect Choices:
Refraining from treating the patient, or scheduling intervention for later in the day, does not address the condition of hyperglycemia identified. Ambulating the patient is not safe management of this patient/client. Physical therapy intervention is contraindicated; exercise can lead to further impaired glucose uptake.

Type of Reasoning: Evaluative
This question requires one to evaluate the courses of action presented to determine the best course of action to effectively address the patient's symptoms. This requires evaluative reasoning skill. For this scenario the assistant's best course of action is to postpone therapy and consult with the nurse as soon as possible. If answered incorrectly, review intervention approaches for patients with hyperglycemia.

A39

Musculoskeletal | Interventions

An infant was referred to physical therapy for right torticollis. In order to **MOST** effectively stretch the muscle, the head and neck should be positioned into which position?

Choices:
1. Flexion, left side-bending, and left rotation.
2. Extension, right side-bending, and left rotation.
3. Flexion, right side-bending, and left rotation.
4. Extension, left side-bending, and right rotation.

Teaching Points

Correct Answer: 4
Right torticollis involves tightness and spasm of the sternocleidomastoid muscle. The right sternocleidomastoid produces left lateral (external) rotation and right lateral flexion of the cervical spine as well as flexion of the spine. The right sternocleidomastoid is in lengthened position with the head turned to the right, laterally flexed to the left and the cervical spine extended.

Incorrect Choices:
Other choices do not include all of the appropriate positions to effectively stretch the sternocleidomastoid muscle; the positions are incomplete to render an effective treatment.

Type of Reasoning: Inductive
One must use knowledge of intervention approaches for torticollis to arrive at a correct conclusion. This necessitates clinical judgment, which is an inductive reasoning skill. For this situation, the most effective method to stretch the muscle is by positioning the head and neck into extension, left side-bending, and right rotation. If answered incorrectly, review intervention approaches for torticollis.

A40

Neuromuscular | Interventions

A patient is recovering from a stroke and demonstrates good recovery in the lower extremity (out-of-synergy movement control). Timing deficits are apparent during gait. What can isokinetic training be used to help improve?

Choices:
1. Rate control at slow movement speeds.
2. Rate control at varying movement speeds.
3. Both reaction and movement times.
4. Initiation of movement.

Teaching Points

Correct Answer: 2
Patients during the later stages of recovery from stroke frequently exhibit problems with rate control. They are able to move at slow speeds, but as speed of movement increases, control decreases. An isokinetic device can be an effective training modality to remediate this problem.

Incorrect Choices:
Typically patients are able to control movement at slow speeds and would not need to utilize isokinetic equipment to enhance. Isokinetic equipment is not likely to assist with initiation of movement or reaction times.

Type of Reasoning: Inferential
One must determine the intervention approach that will be most beneficial for a patient with a stroke and timing deficits during gait to arrive at a correct conclusion. This requires inferential reasoning skill. For this situation, isokinetic training can be used to improve rate control at varying movement speeds. If answered incorrectly, review gait training guidelines for patients with stroke, especially for those with rate control problems.

A41

Musculoskeletal | Interventions

An older adult patient with a transfemoral amputation is having difficulty wrapping the residual limb. Which of the following strategies should the physical therapist assistant utilize to assist a patient with a transfemoral amputation who is having difficulty wrapping the residual limb?

Choices:
1. Suggest the use of a shrinker.
2. Redouble efforts to teach proper Ace bandage wrapping.
3. Apply a temporary prosthesis immediately.
4. Consult with the vascular surgeon about the application of an Unna's paste dressing.

Teaching Points

Correct Answer: 1

A shrinker is a suitable alternative to elastic wraps. It is important to select the right size shrinker to limit edema and accelerate healing. It is important to have some sort of pressure wrap on the residual limb in order to shape and shrink the limb.

Incorrect Choices:

An Unna's paste dressing is applied at the time of initial surgery and is used to help heal open wounds. Use of a temporary prosthesis should be a prosthetic team decision and is based on additional factors such as age, balance, strength, cognition, and so forth. Continued attempts at teaching are not appropriate and may delay necessary compression to the residual limb which ultimately can lead to an ill-formed residual limb and make prosthetic fitting difficult.

Type of Reasoning: Inductive

This question necessitates clinical judgment to determine the best course of action for a patient who is having difficulty with residual limb wrapping. This is an inductive reasoning skill. For this case, the assistant should suggest the use of a shrinker rather than elastic wraps. If answered incorrectly, review care for the residual limb, especially the use of shrinkers.

A42

Pulmonary | Interventions

A physical therapist assistant is assisting a patient who has a segment of a lobe of the lung removed. Which of the following patient instructions is **BEST** to facilitate chest expansion exercises?

Choices:
1. Breathe in through the nose and raise the shoulders with inhalation.
2. Round the shoulders forward with inhalation.
3. Lean forward and rest the forearms on the thighs or on a countertop with inhalation.
4. Breathe in through the nose and push the ribs out against hands placed on the lower ribs.

Teaching Points

Correct Answer: 4

Breathing patterns to encourage chest expansion include the patient performing lateral costal breathing, or expanding the ribs with inhalation. This cue encourages use of the intercostal muscles and facilitates as much thoracic expansion as possible.

Incorrect Choices:

Although patients should be encouraged to breathe in through their nose, they should be discouraged from raising their shoulders with inhalation as this encourages use of accessory musculature. Forward bending and supporting the forearms on the thigh or on a countertop helps to facilitate relaxation for persons with obstructive or restrictive breathing conditions. This position is often used by patients to decrease dyspnea. The forward rounded shoulder position should be discouraged.

Type of Reasoning: Inductive

One must utilize clinical judgment to determine the best approach for facilitating chest expansion during exercise. This requires knowledge of therapeutic procedures for chest expansion exercises, which is an inductive reasoning skill. For this case, the assistant should instruct the patient to breathe in through the nose and push the ribs out against hands placed on the lower ribs. Review chest expansion exercises if answered incorrectly.

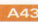

Neuromuscular | Data Collection

The physical therapist evaluation identifies that a patient has scored low on the Berg Balance Scale. What functional activities should the physical therapist assistant recognize have been assessed?

Choices:
1. Hold a single-limb standing position without losing balance.
2. Perform multiple daily activities including turning, stepping up or down, and reaching.
3. Reach forward without losing balance.
4. Rise from a chair, walk and return to a chair and sit back down.

Teaching Points

Correct Answer: 2

The Berg Balance Scale assessment identifies the patient's ability to maintain posture and control during a variety of daily activities, such as stepping onto and off a step, turning and looking over a shoulder, and stooping to pick something off the floor.

Incorrect Choices:

The Timed Up and Go test (#4) assesses the patient's ability to rise from a chair, walk 3 m and return to and sit back down in a chair. Single limb stance (#1) and the Forward Reach test (#3) specific measures of balance control that assess the patient's ability to perform those specific tasks.

Type of Reasoning: Deductive

One must recall the parameters of the Berg Balance Scale to arrive at a correct conclusion. This necessitates the recall of factual information, which is a deductive reasoning skill. For this situation, the Berg Balance Scale identifies the patient's ability to perform multiple daily activities including turning, stepping up or down and reaching. If answered incorrectly, review the Berg Balance Scale and assessment parameters.

A44

Cardiac | Interventions

A patient had a myocardial infarction 4 weeks ago. Which **BEST** represents restrictions that should be followed for resistive training using weights to improve muscular strength and endurance?

Choices:
1. Ensure exercise intensities are kept below 85% maximal voluntary contraction.
2. Exercise tolerance is greater than 5 METs with no anginal symptoms or ST segment depression.
3. Initiate program at 4–6 weeks as long as judicious monitoring of heart rate is used.
4. Wait until post–acute phase III cardiac rehabilitation.

Teaching Points

Correct Answer: 2
Resistance training is typically initiated after patients have completed 4–6 weeks of supervised cardiorespiratory endurance exercise. Lower intensities are prescribed. Careful monitoring of blood pressure is necessary as blood pressure will be higher and heart rate lower than for aerobic exercise. Contraindications to resistance training include unstable angina, uncontrolled arrhythmias, recent history of congestive heart failure, left ventricular outflow obstruction, severe valvular disease, and uncontrolled hypertension. Patients should demonstrate an exercise capacity greater than 5 METs without anginal symptoms or ST segment depression (Source: American College of Sports Medicine: Guidelines for Exercise Testing and Prescription, Ed 6).

Incorrect Choices:
Up to 85% max would be too intense for 4 weeks s/p MI. Phase III cardiac rehab is postacute and is more than 4 weeks post-MI. Exercises can be more intense with higher METs at that point.

Type of Reasoning: Inductive
One must have knowledge of cardiac rehabilitation guidelines for patients with myocardial infarction to arrive at a correct conclusion. This knowledge is coupled with clinical judgment, which necessitates inductive reasoning skill. For this situation, resistive training using weights to improve muscular strength and endurance is appropriate if the exercise capacity is greater than 5 METs with no anginal symptoms or ST segment depression. If answered incorrectly, review cardiac rehabilitation guidelines and use of resistive training.

A45

Nonsystem | Equipment and Devices

A patient diagnosed with lumbar spinal root impingement caused by narrowing of the intervertebral foramen has been referred to physical therapy. The physical therapist has indicated use of mechanical traction in the plan of care. What is the lowest percentage of body weight that should be considered for the **INITIAL** traction force?

Choices:
1. 25%.
2. 15%.
3. 55%.
4. 85%.

Teaching Points

Correct Answer: 1

To overcome the coefficient of friction of the body moving horizontally over the surface of a table, the traction force should be at least 25% of the body weight when one is using a split table or 50% when one is using a non-split table. The minimum 25% for initial treatment would provide sufficient joint distraction by stretching the ligamentous tissue and widening the intervertebral foramen.

Incorrect Choices:

Traction forces set to 55% and 85% are too high for an initial trial of traction. A traction force of 15% is not enough to provide an effective treatment.

Type of Reasoning: Deductive

This question requires the test taker to recall the guidelines for the use of mechanical traction. This necessitates the recall of factual guidelines, which is a deductive reasoning skill. For this case, the lowest percentage of body weight that should be considered for the initial traction force is 25%. If answered incorrectly, review mechanical traction guidelines and configuration of traction force.

A46

Neuromuscular | Interventions

Which of the following physical therapy interventions is **MOST** appropriate to use at school during class for a child with decreased sitting balance and normal tone?

Choices:
1. Sitting on a therapy ball while performing desktop activities.
2. Sitting in an adaptive wheelchair with lateral supports and lap tray.
3. Standing on a static prone-stander with lap tray.
4. Sitting in an appropriate height chair with lateral postural supports.

Teaching Points

Correct Answer: 2

The goal of school physical therapy is to directly facilitate the educational process—for example, interacting in class, viewing the blackboard, etc. The adaptive wheelchair is the best choice for this child because it allows the child to move around in the classroom while maintaining a stable position.

Incorrect Choices:

Sitting on a therapy ball is too advanced for a child with decreased sitting balance. The prone-stander is restrictive and does not promote sitting, and a chair with lateral supports would assist with sitting but would not assist with overall mobility of the student.

Type of Reasoning: Inductive

One must utilize clinical judgment to determine the most beneficial intervention approach for a child with decreased sitting balance. This necessitates inductive reasoning skill. For this case, the most appropriate approach is sitting in an adaptive wheelchair with the lateral supports and lap tray. If answered incorrectly, review school-based intervention approaches for children with decreased sitting balance.

A47

Neuromuscular | Diseases and Conditions Impacting Intervention

A patient with Parkinson's disease demonstrates a gait pattern typical of this diagnosis. Which activity could present a danger if used by the physical therapist assistant?

Choices:
1. Standing, using body weight support from a harness.
2. Sidestepping and cross-stepping using light touch-down support of hands.
3. Gait training using a rolling walker.
4. Rhythmic stepping using a motorized treadmill.

Teaching Points

Correct Answer: 3
The patient with Parkinson's disease typically presents with postural deficits of forward head and trunk with hip and knee flexion contractures. Gait is narrow-based and shuffling. A festinating gait typically results from persistent forward posturing of the body near the forward limits of stability. A rolling walker is contraindicated because it has the potential to increase forward postural deformities and festinating gait.

Incorrect Choices:
All other choices are appropriate training activities to improve upright standing balance and gait for an individual who has Parkinson's disease.

Type of Reasoning: Inferential
This question requires one to determine what may present a danger to a patient with Parkinson's disease to arrive at a correct conclusion. This requires inferential reasoning skill. For this situation, gait training with the use of a rolling walker could present a danger as this can increase forward postural deformities and festinating gait. If answered incorrectly, review contraindications for assistive device use with patients with Parkinson's disease.

A48

Neuromuscular | Diseases and Conditions Impacting Intervention

A physical therapist assistant is working with a patient recovering from a stroke. In which of these conditions would it be **MOST** important for the assistant to implement additional safety precautions during treatment?

Choices:
1. Anosognosia.
2. Ideational apraxia.
3. Unilateral neglect.
4. Ideomotor apraxia.

Teaching Points

Correct Answer: 1
Anosognosia is a more severe form of neglect with lack of awareness and denial of the severity of one's paralysis.

Incorrect Choices:
With ideomotor apraxia, a patient cannot perform a task upon command but can do the task when on his or her own. With ideational apraxia, a patient cannot perform a requested task at all. Unilateral neglect might lead the patient to ignore something positioned on the involved side.

Type of Reasoning: Inferential
One must infer or draw a reasonable conclusion about the level of safety precautions required for a patient with a stroke. This requires inferential reasoning skill. For this case, a patient with anosognosia would require additional safety measures during treatment to address the severity of the patient's neglect and denial of severity of paralysis. If answered incorrectly, review safety guidelines for patients with stroke, including patients with anosognosia.

A49

Nonsystem | Equipment and Devices

A patient with a transfemoral amputation has been fitted with a prosthesis that utilizes a quadrilateral socket. Following gait training, where should the physical therapist assistant expect to observe evidence of weight bearing on the residual limb?

Choices:
1. Ischial tuberosity and lateral sides of residual limb.
2. Adductor magnus and medial side of residual limb.
3. Distolateral end of femur and ischial seat.
4. Perineal area and medial side of the residual limb.

Teaching Points

Correct Answer: 1
A quadrilateral socket in a transfemoral amputation is designed to selectively load tissues that are pressure tolerant. The ischial tuberosity, gluteals, and lateral sides of the residual limb are pressure-tolerant areas.

Incorrect Choices:
All the other areas identified are inappropriate areas for weight bearing, and evidence of weight bearing in these areas indicates an ill-fitting prosthesis and must be corrected prior to any additional gait training.

Type of Reasoning: Deductive
This question requires the test taker to recall the pressure-tolerant areas of the quadrilateral socket to arrive at a correct conclusion. This necessitates the recall of factual information, which is a deductive reasoning skill. For this scenario, the pressure-tolerant areas include the ischial tuberosity and lateral sides of the residual limb. If answered incorrectly, review pressure tolerance areas for a quadrilateral socket.

A50

Musculoskeletal | Interventions

A patient has been confined to bed for a period of 2 months and now demonstrates limited range of motion in both lower extremities. Range in hip flexion is 5°–115° and knee flexion is 10°–120°. The physical therapist has indicated that flexibility activities should be implemented to improve the range of motion in preparation of standing activities. Which represents the **MOST** appropriate intervention to improve flexibility and ready this patient for standing?

Choices:
1. Manual passive stretching, 10 repetitions each joint, two times a day.
2. Tilt table standing, 20 minutes daily.
3. Mechanical stretching using traction and 5-lb weights, 2 hours, twice daily.
4. Hold–relax techniques followed by passive range of motion, 10 repetitions, two times a day.

Teaching Points

Correct Answer: 3

Prolonged mechanical stretching involves a low-intensity force (generally 5–15 lb) applied over a prolonged period (30 minutes to several hours). It is generally the most effective way to manage long-standing flexion contractures.

Incorrect Choices:

Manual passive stretching and tilt table standing are shorter duration stretches that are not likely to be effective in this case. Hold–relax techniques can be used to improve flexibility in the presence of shortening of muscular elements but are not likely to be effective in this case because of the short duration and long-standing contracture affecting connective tissue elements.

Type of Reasoning: Inductive

This question requires the test taker to have knowledge of muscle stretching guidelines for patients with prolonged periods of immobility to arrive at a correct conclusion. This necessitates clinical judgment, which is an inductive reasoning skill. For this situation, the most appropriate intervention is mechanical stretching using traction and 5 lb weights, twice per day. If answered incorrectly, review muscle stretching procedures for patients with prolonged immobility.

A51

Nonsystem | Professional Roles

A physical therapist assistant has recently attended a professional conference on myofascial release. The physical therapist assistant has been asked to share this information with colleagues during an in-service. Which represents the assistant's **BEST INITIAL** activity?

Choices:
1. Ask colleagues to select a suitable time and place for the in-service.
2. Provide a comprehensive packet of handouts in advance of the in-service.
3. Organize a PowerPoint presentation and prepare a handout.
4. Survey colleagues about their current level of knowledge by using a brief questionnaire.

Teaching Points

Correct Answer: 4
Prior to any teaching it is best to assess the baseline knowledge of the learner. To better share the information, the assistant needs to determine what information and skills colleagues currently have. A brief questionnaire is an effective means to achieve this goal.

Incorrect Choices:
The other choices demonstrate planning of the learning experience WITHOUT benefit of a needs assessment. This can lead to an in-service that is ineffective and does not meet audience needs.

Type of Reasoning: Inductive
One must utilize clinical judgment to determine the best initial approach to providing an in-service to colleagues to arrive at a correct conclusion. This necessitates inductive reasoning skill. For this situation, the assistant should survey colleagues about their current level of knowledge before providing the in-service. If answered incorrectly, review guidelines for planning in-services.

A52

Musculoskeletal | Interventions

When preparing a patient who has incomplete T12 paraplegia for ambulation, which muscle groups should strengthening be focused on?

Choices:
1. Upper trapezius, rhomboids, and levator scapulae.
2. Deltoid, triceps, and wrist flexors.
3. Middle trapezius, latissimus dorsi, and triceps.
4. Lower trapezius, latissimus dorsi, and triceps.

Teaching Points

Correct Answer: 4
The upper-quadrant muscles that are most important to strengthen for crutch gaits include the lower trapezius, latissimus dorsi, and triceps. Shoulder depression and elbow extension strength are crucial for successful crutch gait.

Incorrect Choices:
The other muscles listed do not help in actions needed to depress shoulder and extend elbow in order for the UEs to take on the body weight to allow for movement of the LEs.

Type of Reasoning: Inductive
This question requires the test taker to determine the most important muscles to strengthen in the upper quadrant for a patient with T12 paraplegia. This requires clinical judgment, which is an inductive reasoning skill. For this case, the assistant should strengthen the lower trapezius, latissimus dorsi, and triceps in preparation for crutch use. If answered incorrectly, review gait training approaches for patients with T12 injury, especially crutch use and musculature needed.

A53

System Interactions | Interventions

A physical therapist assistant is discussing an aerobic exercise program with a pregnant woman. Which represents accurate information for the patient?

Choices:
1. She should discontinue aerobic exercise until after she gives birth.
2. She must limit participation in aerobic exercise to the first and second trimesters and then discontinue.
3. She may notice that she reaches her maximum or preferred work level more quickly than she did prior to pregnancy.
4. She should limit her aerobic exercise choices to bicycling or swimming.

Teaching Points

Correct Answer: 3

A woman who has an established aerobic exercise program will likely continue to tolerate her exercise program during pregnancy; she may, however, notice that she reaches her desired workout level or maximum exercise capacity more quickly than she did prior to pregnancy.

Incorrect Choices:

A woman does not have to discontinue her aerobic exercise program during pregnancy, nor does she have to limit participation to the first and second trimesters or to just bicycling or swimming. Women who do not participate in a regular aerobic program prior to pregnancy may tolerate swimming, walking, or biking more easily than running, however exercise options are not limited to these options.

Type of Reasoning: Deductive

This question requires one to recall the guidelines for exercise with pregnancy to arrive at a correct conclusion. This necessitates the recall of factual information, which is a deductive reasoning skill. For this situation, the assistant should inform the woman that she may notice that she reaches her maximum work level more quickly than she did prior to pregnancy. If answered incorrectly, review exercise guidelines during pregnancy.

A54

Musculoskeletal | Diseases and Conditions Impacting Intervention

Following major surgery of the right hip, a patient walks with a Trendelenburg gait. The initial evaluation reveals right hip abductor weakness and range-of-motion limitations in flexion and lateral (external) rotation. Which application describes the **BEST** placement for functional electrical stimulation?

Choices:
1. Stimulation applied to the right abductors during swing on the right.
2. Stimulation applied to the right abductors during stance on the right.
3. Stimulation applied to the left abductors during stance on the right.
4. Stimulation applied to the left abductors during swing on the right.

Teaching Points

Correct Answer: 2

During the stance phase of gait, the hip abductors of the weight-bearing limb are activated to maintain the pelvis in a relative horizontal position. This allows the opposite foot to clear the floor during swing. If there is weakness of the weight-bearing limb the pelvis will drop, which is called a Trendelenburg. The right hip abductors need to be stimulated during stance in order to prevent the pelvis from dropping.

Incorrect Choices:

Stimulation of the right abductors throughout swing or the left hip abductors during swing or stance would not compensate for the weakness of the right hip abductors during the support period.

Type of Reasoning: Inductive

This question requires one to determine the best placement for functional electrical stimulation to improve gait pattern. This requires knowledge of functional electrical stimulation protocols as well as clinical judgment, which is an inductive reasoning skill. For this case, the assistant should focus on the right abductors during stance on the right to improve the Trendelenburg gait. If answered incorrectly, review functional electrical stimulation guidelines to improve Trendelenburg gait.

A55

Musculoskeletal | Diseases and Conditions Impacting Intervention

A physical therapist assistant is working with a patient who has a diagnosis of supraspinatus impingement with possible tear. The patient has been receiving physical therapy care for 4 weeks. What physical therapy intervention should be included in this early subacute rehabilitation stage of recovery?

Choices:
1. Active assistive pulley exercises.
2. Modalities to reduce pain and inflammation.
3. Small-amplitude oscillations performed to the limit of tissue resistance to the glenohumeral joint.
4. Resistance exercises for the affected muscles.

Teaching Points

Correct Answer: 1

During the early subacute phase, active assistive pulley exercises are indicated to promote healing of the supraspinatus muscle and maintain active range of motion of the glenohumeral joint.

Incorrect Choices:

Acute physical therapy intervention would focus on reduction of pain and inflammation. Oscillations to the limit of tissue resistance (joint mobilization) and resistance exercises are too vigorous at this stage.

Type of Reasoning: Inductive

One must determine the best approach for treating a supraspinatus impingement to arrive at a correct conclusion. This requires clinical judgment and knowledge of therapeutic approaches, which is an inductive reasoning skill. For this case, the assistant should progress to active assistive pulley exercises. If answered incorrectly, review treatment approaches for supraspinatus impingement, especially for the subacute phase.

A56

Nonsystem | Evidence-Based Practice

Two therapists are asked to perform a test on the same group of patients by using the Functional Independence Measure (FIM). The results of both sets of measurements reveal differences in therapists' scores but **NOT** in the repeat measurements. What type of measurement problem are these results indicative of?

Choices:
1. Concurrent validity.
2. Intrarater reliability.
3. Interrater reliability.
4. Construct validity.

Teaching Points

Correct Answer: 3

Interrater reliability is the degree to which two or more independent raters can obtain the same rating for a given variable. In this case, two therapists obtained different FIM scores for the same group of patients, indicating a problem in interrater reliability.

Incorrect Choices:

Intrarater reliability is the consistency of an examiner on repeat tests. Issues of validity (Does the test measure what it says it measures?) are not relevant.

Type of Reasoning: Deductive

This question requires the test taker to recall the parameters of interrater reliability to arrive at a correct conclusion. This is factual information, which requires deductive reasoning skill. For this case, the description of the differences in the therapists' scores indicates a problem with interrater reliability. If answered incorrectly, review research guidelines, including interrater reliability.

A57

Neuromuscular | Interventions

A patient is recovering from a complete spinal cord injury with C5 tetraplegia. The physical therapist assistant is performing passive range of motion exercises on the mat when the patient complains of a sudden pounding headache and double vision. The physical therapist assistant notices that the patient is sweating excessively, and measures the patient's blood pressure at 240/95 mm Hg. What is the **BEST** course of action in response to these findings?

Choices:
1. Lie the patient down immediately, elevate the patient's lower extremities and then call for a nurse.
2. Place the patient in a supported sitting position and continue to monitor blood pressure, then call for a nurse.
3. Sit the patient up, check/empty catheter bag and then call for emergency medical assistance.
4. Lie the patient down, open the patient's shirt and monitor the respiratory rate closely.

Teaching Points

Correct Answer: 3

The patient is exhibiting autonomic dysreflexia (an emergency situation). The assistant should first sit the patient up and check for irritating or precipitating stimuli (e.g., a blocked catheter, tight clothing). The next step is to call for emergency medical assistance.

Incorrect Choices:

Placing the patient supine can aggravate the situation by not assisting the bladder to drain and possibly increasing the blood pressure (#1 and #4). It is an emergency situation so action needs to be taken and monitoring is not enough (#2 and #4).

Type of Reasoning: Evaluative

This question requires one to determine a best course of action to effectively address the patient's symptoms from the choices provided. This requires one to have an understanding of the significance of the problem. This requires evaluative reasoning skill. For this scenario, the assistant should sit the patient up, check and empty the catheter bag, and then call for emergency medical assistance. If answered incorrectly, review signs and symptoms of autonomic dysreflexia and intervention approaches.

A58

Nonsystem | Equipment and Devices

Which represents an external shoe modification that shifts weight bearing from the metatarsal joints to the metatarsal shafts?

Choices:
1. Thomas heel.
2. Scaphoid pad.
3. Metatarsal pad.
4. Metatarsal bar.

Teaching Points

Correct Answer: 4

A metatarsal bar is an external modification indicated to take pressure off the metatarsal heads and improve push off.

Incorrect Choices:

The metatarsal pad is an internal shoe modification that does the same thing. Scaphoid pads and Thomas heels help to manage flexible flat foot.

Type of Reasoning: Deductive

This question requires one to recall the device that shifts weight bearing from the metatarsal joints to the metatarsal shafts to arrive at a correct conclusion. This is factual recall of information, which is a deductive reasoning skill. For this case, the device described is a metatarsal bar. If answered incorrectly, review shoe modifications, especially external and internal shoe modifications.

A59

Integumentary | Interventions

A child with full-thickness burns to both upper extremities is developing hypertrophic scars. What is the **BEST** intervention to manage these scars?

Choices:
1. Primary excision followed by autografts.
2. Application of custom-made pressure garments.
3. Application of compression wraps.
4. Application of occlusive dressings.

Teaching Points

Correct Answer: 2
Following burns, edema and hypertrophic scarring can be effectively controlled with pressure garments. Custom garments are the best choice. Pressure should be maintained 23 hours per day, often for 6–12 months.

Incorrect Choices:
Surgery is the option of last choice. Compression wraps (elastic bandages) and occlusive dressings have no impact on hypertrophic scarring.

Type of Reasoning: Inductive
One must use knowledge of hypertrophic scarring management guidelines to arrive at a correct conclusion. This requires clinical judgment, which is an inductive reasoning skill. For this situation, the best intervention to manage the scars is application of custom-made pressure garments. If answered incorrectly, review burn treatment guidelines, including management of hypertrophic scarring.

A60

Pulmonary | Data Collection

A patient with chronic obstructive pulmonary disease has developed respiratory acidosis. What should the patient be monitored closely for?

Choices:
1. Disorientation.
2. Tingling or numbness of the extremities.
3. Dizziness or lightheadedness.
4. Hyperreflexia.

Teaching Points

Correct Answer: 1
A patient with respiratory acidosis may present with many symptoms of increased carbon dioxide levels in the arterial blood. Significant acidosis may lead to disorientation, stupor or coma.

Incorrect Choices:
The other choices are signs and symptoms of respiratory alkalosis or a decrease of carbon dioxide in the arterial blood.

Type of Reasoning: Deductive
One must recall the risk factors for patients with chronic obstructive pulmonary disease and respiratory acidosis to arrive at a correct conclusion. This is factual information, which necessitates deductive reasoning skill. For this situation, the patient is at risk for disorientation, and the patient should be monitored closely for this symptom. If answered incorrectly, review risk factors for respiratory acidosis in patients with chronic obstructive pulmonary disease.

A61

System Interactions | Interventions

Which of the following is an appropriate exercise modification for a woman who is 15 weeks into her pregnancy?

Choices:
1. Encouraging unilateral exercise of the lower extremities.
2. Standing rather than supine lower-extremity resistive band exercises.
3. Avoiding quadruped exercise activities.
4. Placing a small wedge under right hip during supine exercise.

Teaching Points

Correct Answer: 4
After the first trimester a pregnant women should avoid supine positioning for greater than 5 minutes at a time. When performing supine exercises, placement of a wedge under the right hip helps to decrease the effects of uterine compression on abdominal vessels and improves cardiac output.

Incorrect Choices:
Asymmetrical stretching or strengthening activities of the lower extremities can contribute to joint instability, especially of the lower back and sacroiliac joint area. Quadruped positioning is an appropriate modification for prone activities; however, note that hip extension activities should be limited to midline, and hip extension beyond midline should be avoided as this position can place asymmetrical forces through the sacroiliac joint and lower back area.

Type of Reasoning: Inductive
One must utilize clinical judgment to determine the best exercise modification for a patient who is 15 weeks pregnant. This requires knowledge of exercise guidelines during pregnancy, which is an inductive reasoning skill. For this case, the assistant should recommend placing a small wedge under the right hip during supine exercise. If answered incorrectly, review exercise modifications during pregnancy.

A62

Nonsystem | Equipment and Devices

When working with a patient who is obese, what equipment would a physical therapist assistant use to assist in transferring the patient from sit to stand?

Choices:
1. Sliding board.
2. Gait belt.
3. Standing pole.
4. Bariatric wheelchair.

Teaching Points

Correct Answer: 3

A standing pole provides the patient something to grip and pull on allowing them to assist the physical therapist assistant in transferring from sit to stand.

Incorrect Choices:

A sliding board assists in transferring from one surface to another but does nothing to assist in standing. The use of a sliding board transfer is not recommended for individuals who are obese. A gait belt is used for all transfers and may not be safe for use by the bariatric patient given the patient's weight and the stress it would place on the guarding belt. A bariatric wheelchair, although appropriate for position and mobility, will not assist in getting from a sitting to a standing position.

Type of Reasoning: Inferential

This question requires one to determine what may be true for a patient who is obese and needs assistance during a transfer. This requires knowledge of adaptive devices for patients who are obese to arrive at a correct conclusion. For this situation, the likely equipment to be used for the transfer is a standing pole. If answered incorrectly, review assistive devices for transfer skills with bariatric patients.

A63

Neuromuscular | Diseases and Conditions Impacting Intervention

What muscle groups and technique should a physical therapist assistant instruct a patient with complete C6 tetraplegia to use while learning to transfer using a sliding board?

Choices:
1. Shoulder depressors and triceps, keeping the hands flexed to protect tenodesis grasp.
2. Pectoral muscles to stabilize elbows in extension and scapular depressors to lift the trunk.
3. Shoulder extensors, lateral (external) rotators, and anterior deltoid to position and lock the elbow.
4. Serratus anterior to elevate the trunk with elbow extensors stabilizing.

Teaching Points

Correct Answer: 3

The patient with complete C6 quadriplegia will lack triceps and should be taught to lock the elbow for push-up transfers by using shoulder lateral (external) rotators and extensors to position the upper extremity; the anterior deltoid locks the elbow by reverse actions (all of these muscles are functional).

Incorrect Choices:

Triceps and elbow extensors are not active due to the level of injury (#1 and #4) and the pectoral muscles do not stabilize the elbow in to extension.

Type of Reasoning: Inductive

One must utilize knowledge of sliding board transfer skills for patients with tetraplegia to arrive at a correct conclusion. This requires inductive reasoning skill. For this case, the patient should be instructed to use shoulder extensors, lateral (external) rotators, and anterior deltoid to position and lock the elbow during the transfer. If answered incorrectly, review transfer techniques for patients with tetraplegia, especially C6 injuries.

A64

Nonsystem | Professional Roles

A physical therapist assistant volunteered to teach a stroke education class on positioning techniques for family members and caregivers. At the conclusion of the class, caregivers will be expected to utilize the skills taught. Which represents the **BEST** choice of teaching method?

Choices:
1. Assistant demonstration, caregiver practice, and follow-up individual discussion.
2. Assistant demonstration with caregiver role-playing patient.
3. Multimedia (PowerPoint and handouts) that accompany an oral presentation.
4. Question and answer addressing the specific individual concerns of the caregivers.

Teaching Points

Correct Answer: 1

A variety of teaching methods including demonstration, practice, and discussion has the best chance of reinforcing learning in a diverse group. Using only one type of teaching methodology is not likely to be as successful in meeting the needs of all the group members. Psychomotor skills are best learned by practice, not lecture or just question and answer. Feedback is essential for learning and should include both knowledge of performance and knowledge of results.

Incorrect Choices:

Without return demonstration by the learner there is no way to assess if he or she has learned the psychomotor skill. Numbers 2, 3, and 4 have no component of return demonstration.

Type of Reasoning: Inductive

One must determine the best approach for teaching caregivers positioning techniques to arrive at a correct conclusion. This requires clinical judgment, which is an inductive reasoning skill. For this case, the assistant should demonstrate the skills, facilitate caregiver practice and follow-up with individual discussion. If answered incorrectly, review training techniques and guidelines for caregivers.

A65

Nonsystem | Safety

A patient with active tuberculosis is referred for physical therapy. Which of the following is an appropriate precaution?

Choices:
1. The patient must wear a tight-fitting mask while being treated in his or her room.
2. The assistant must wash hands only upon leaving the patient's room.
3. The assistant must wear a tight-fitting mask, gown, and gloves while treating the patient.
4. The patient must be in a private, negative-pressurized room.

Teaching Points

Correct Answer: 4

The assistant should wash hands upon entering and leaving every patient's room. This is not unique to TB. When the patient is suspected of having tuberculosis, the patient should be in a private, negative-pressurized room. The room is considered a potentially infective environment, and the assistant should don a tight-fitting mask prior to entering the room.

Incorrect Choices:
Gown and gloves are not always necessary because TB is airborne and not contact. The patient only needs to wear a mask if there is a need to leave the room (for a medical test, etc.).

Type of Reasoning: Deductive
One must recall the guidelines for standard precautions when working with patients who have active tuberculosis. This is factual information and recall of guidelines, which is a deductive reasoning skill. For this case, the assistant should realize that the patient should be in a private, negative-pressurized room. If answered incorrectly, review transmission-based guidelines for patients with tuberculosis in this textbook.

A66

Musculoskeletal | Interventions

The plan of care for a patient following acute whiplash of the cervical spine calls for initiating cervical stabilization exercises. The patient is tolerating cervical nodding exercises and has a pain rating of 5 out of 10 (10 being the worst pain). As the patient maintains the cervical nod, how should the physical therapist assistant progress the cervical nodding exercise?

Choices:
1. Perform active shoulder flexion to 90° while sitting on a ball.
2. Perform active shoulder flexion to 180° while supine.
3. Perform active shoulder flexion to 90° while supine.
4. Perform active shoulder flexion to 180° while standing.

Teaching Points

Correct Answer: 3

Because the patient is only tolerating a cervical nod and has a pain rate of 5, the exercises should be progressed slowly. The correct progression from maintaining a cervical nod is to initiate partial shoulder range of motion with the head and trunk in a supported position.

Incorrect Choices
Once the patient can do this successfully without significant increase in pain, then further progressions will include full range motion of the shoulders in a supported position (#2). Once able to do full range with body supported, body support will be taken away (#4) and then challenged (#1) with decreasing trunk support as the patient tolerates.

Type of Reasoning: Inductive
This question requires the test taker to utilize knowledge of intervention approaches for whiplash injury to arrive at a correct conclusion. This necessitates inductive reasoning skill, as clinical judgment is paramount to choosing a correct solution. For this case, the assistant should begin by performing active shoulder flexion to 90° while supine. If answered incorrectly, review intervention approaches for whiplash injuries.

A67

Musculoskeletal | Interventions

A patient has undergone surgery and subsequent immobilization to stabilize the olecranon process. The patient now exhibits an elbow flexion contracture. What is an absolute **CONTRAINDICATION** for joint mobilization in this situation?

Choices:
1. Soft end-feel.
2. Springy end-feel.
3. Empty end-feel.
4. Firm end-feel.

Teaching Points

Correct Answer: 3
An empty end-feel (no real end-feel) may be indicative of severe pain and muscle guarding associated with pathological conditions.

Incorrect Choices:
Springy and firm end-feels may be expected after elbow surgery. Soft end-feel is an indication of range limited because of tissue compression (e.g., in knee flexion there is contact between the posterior lower extremity and the posterior thigh).

Type of Reasoning: Deductive
This question requires the test taker to recall the contraindications for joint mobilization to arrive at a correct conclusion. This necessitates the recall of factual guidelines, which is a deductive reasoning skill. For this situation, the contraindication for joint mobilization is an empty end-feel. If answered incorrectly, review joint mobilization guidelines and contraindications.

A68

Nonsystem | Interventions

A physical therapist assistant is providing early stage gait training for a patient after a left total hip arthroplasty. The patient is using crutches and is practicing on a level surface. What represents the **BEST** position for the physical therapist assistant to guard the patient?

Choices:
1. Stand slightly behind the patient on the intact side, one hand on the gait belt.
2. Stand in front of the patient, walking backward, with one hand on the gait belt and one hand on the shoulder.
3. Stand behind and to the left side of the patient, one hand on the gait belt.
4. Stand behind the patient with both hands on the gait belt.

Teaching Points

Correct Answer: 3

The correct guarding technique to protect a patient from falling is to stand slightly behind and to one side (the involved or left side). One hand should be on the gait belt and the other hand should be at the shoulder or trunk depending on how much assistance the patient requires.

Incorrect Choices:

It is not appropriate to stand in front of a patient when guarding on levels (#2). It is appropriate to stand on the involved side NOT the intact side (#1). Both hands should not be on the gait belt (#4)—one hand needs to be free to guard at the trunk or shoulders.

Type of Reasoning: Inductive

One must recall the guidelines for guarding techniques during gait training to arrive at a correct conclusion. This necessitates clinical judgment, which is an inductive reasoning skill. For this scenario, the assistant should stand behind and to the left side with one hand on the gait belt. If answered incorrectly, review gait training guidelines for patients with total hip arthroplasties, especially with the use of crutches.

A69

Musculoskeletal | Interventions

A patient has lumbar spinal stenosis encroaching on the spinal cord. What activity should the physical therapist assistant instruct the patient to **AVOID**?

Choices:
1. Bicycling on hills.
2. Use of a rowing machine.
3. Tai Chi activities.
4. Swimming using a crawl stroke.

Teaching Points

Correct Answer: 4

Continuous positioning in spinal extension increases symptoms in patients with spinal stenosis. Activities such as swimming using a crawl stroke place the spine in extension which needs to be avoided.

Incorrect Choices:
All other activities (numbers 1, 2, and 3) described do not require the patient to maintain a continuous extended spinal position and do not need to be avoided.

Type of Reasoning: Analytical
One must analyze the activities presented to determine the activity that will increase symptoms for a patient with spinal stenosis because of continuous positioning in spinal extension. This requires analytical reasoning skill. For this case, swimming using a crawl stroke should be avoided to prevent an increase in symptoms. If answered incorrectly, review contraindications for functional activities in patients with spinal stenosis.

A70
Nonsystem | Equipment and Devices

A patient with postpolio syndrome is being treated in outpatient physical therapy with symptoms of myalgia and increasing fatigue. The patient has been using a knee–ankle–foot orthosis for 10 years. During gait training the physical therapist assistant observes the patient rise up on the sound extremity to advance the extremity with the orthosis forward. What muscle weakness is **MOST** likely the cause of this gait deviation?

Choices:
1. Quadriceps on the affected extremity.
2. Iliopsoas on the affected extremity.
3. Gluteus medius on sound extremity.
4. Gastrocsoleus on the sound extremity.

Teaching Points

Correct Answer: 2
This patient is vaulting (rising up on the sound extremity to advance the orthosis extremity forward). This is most likely because of weakness of the iliopsoas (hip flexors) on the affected extremity. This gait deficit increases the energy demands of gait and is most likely contributing to fatigue. The myalgia and fatigue are also direct impairments of postpolio syndrome.

Incorrect Choices:
The quadriceps muscle may assist with hip flexion; however, weakness of it is more likely to result in a steppage-type gait deviation. In addition, because the patient is in an knee–ankle–foot orthosis, the knee extensors are eliminated as the knee is locked in extension. Weakness of the gluteus medius on the sound extremity would likely result in lateral trunk bending to the sound side. The gastrocsoleus on the sound extremity is most likely overdeveloped secondary to the current gait deviation.

Type of Reasoning: Inferential
This question requires one to infer or draw a reasonable conclusion about the likely muscle that is weak and causing vaulting during ambulation. Therefore, one must determine what may be true for a patient, which is an inferential reasoning skill. For this case, the iliopsoas muscle on the affected extremity is most likely weakened. If answered incorrectly, review causes of vaulting during walking.

A71

Nonsystem | Therapeutic Modalities

An athlete presents with pain (5/10) and muscle spasm of the left upper trapezius as the result of a strain that occurred 2 weeks previously. The plan of care indicates the use of a combination of ultrasound and electrical stimulation. What **BEST** represents appropriate treatment parameters for this client?

Choices:
1. Continuous ultrasound with intense motor-level electrical stimulation.
2. Continuous ultrasound and comfortable sensory-level electrical stimulation.
3. Pulsed ultrasound with motor-level electrical stimulation.
4. Pulsed ultrasound at 50% duty cycle with comfortable motor-level electrical stimulation.

Teaching Points

Correct Answer: 2

Continuous ultrasound is indicated to create increased temperatures in the tissues; sensory level stimulation will help contribute to decreasing muscle spasm.

Incorrect Choices:
Pulsed ultrasound is not indicated as this is not an acute injury. Motor-level stimulation at this subacute phase may be irritating to the tissues that are still in the healing phase and is better indicated to reduce long-standing muscle spasm.

Type of Reasoning: Deductive
One must recall the guidelines for the use of ultrasound and electrical stimulation for the treatment of pain and muscle spasm to arrive at a correct conclusion. This requires the recall of protocols and guidelines, which is a deductive reasoning skill. For this situation, the most appropriate treatment parameters are continuous ultrasound and comfortable sensory-level electrical stimulation. If answered incorrectly, review protocols for electrical stimulation and ultrasound for pain and muscle spasm.

A72

Nonsystem | Evidence-Based Practice

A researcher states that he expects that there will be a significant difference between 20- and 30-year-olds after a 12-week exercise training program using exercise heart rates and myocardial oxygen consumption as measures of performance. What kind of hypothesis is being used in this study?

Choices:
1. Quasi-experimental hypothesis.
2. Research hypothesis.
3. Null hypothesis.
4. Nondirectional hypothesis.

Teaching Points

Correct Answer: 2

A research hypothesis is a generalization that predicts an expected relationship between variables.

Incorrect Choices:

The null hypothesis is a statistical hypothesis that states that there is no relationship (or difference) between variables. Any relationship found will be a chance relationship, not a true one. A research hypothesis predicts an expected relationship between variables (e.g., 20-year-olds will demonstrate improved measures of performance compared with 30-year-olds). Quasi-experimental means that the subjects cannot be randomly assigned to groups. Nondirectional means that a direction of change cannot be predicted.

Type of Reasoning: Deductive

One must recall the definition of a research hypothesis to arrive at a correct conclusion. This necessitates the recall of factual information, which is a deductive reasoning skill. For this case, the prediction for this study presented is that of a research hypothesis. If answered incorrectly, review research terminology, especially research hypotheses.

A73

Neuromuscular | Interventions

A patient has a 3-year history of multiple sclerosis. One of the disabling symptoms is persistent and severe diplopia, which leaves the patient frequently nauseated and immobile. Which represents an appropriate intervention strategy to assist the patient to successfully participate in rehabilitation?

Choices:
1. Provide the patient with special glasses that magnify images.
2. Instruct the patient to close both eyes and practice movements without visual guidance.
3. Provide the patient with a soft neck collar to limit head and neck movements.
4. Patch one eye.

Teaching Points

Correct Answer: 4

Double vision (diplopia) can be managed by patching one eye. Patients are typically on an eye-patching schedule that alternates the eye that is patched. Loss of depth perception can be expected with eye-patching but is not as disabling as diplopia.

Incorrect Choices:

It is not beneficial for this patient to wear magnification glasses. Closing eyes to perform movements without visual guidance will not help diminish or eliminate diplopia. A soft collar to limit neck movements will not diminish or eliminate diplopia.

Type of Reasoning: Inferential

One must determine an intervention approach that will effectively address the patient's deficits. This requires one to determine what will be most beneficial for a patient, which is an inferential reasoning skill. For this scenario, the most effective intervention strategy for the patient's diplopia is to patch one eye. If answered incorrectly, review intervention approaches for diplopia for patients with multiple sclerosis.

A74

Neuromuscular | Interventions

Which of the following represents the **MOST** appropriate positioning strategy for a patient recovering from acute stroke who is in bed and presents with a flaccid upper extremity?

Choices:
1. Supine with the affected upper extremity flexed with hand resting on stomach.
2. Side-lying on the sound side with the affected shoulder protracted, and upper extremity extended resting on a pillow.
3. Supine with the affected elbow extended and upper extremity positioned close to the side of the trunk.
4. Side-lying on the sound side with the affected upper extremity flexed overhead.

Teaching Points

Correct Answer: 2
Most patients with stroke recover from the flaccid stage and develop spasticity. Positioning for the patient with early stroke promotes two principles: (1) protection against ligamentous strain and the development of a painful subluxed shoulder and (2) positions counter to the typical spastic posture of flexion and adduction with pronation. Side-lying with the affected upper extremity supported on a pillow with the shoulder protracted and elbow extended accomplishes both of these goals.

Incorrect Choices:
The other choices identified in the question do not account for appropriate joint protection and positioning.

Type of Reasoning: Inductive
One must utilize clinical judgment to determine the most appropriate positioning strategy for a patient with acute stroke. This is an inductive reasoning skill. For this case, the most appropriate positioning strategy is side-lying on the sound side with the affected shoulder protracted and upper extremity extended resting on a pillow. If answered incorrectly, review positioning strategies for a patient with stroke.

A75

Gastrointestinal | Diseases and Conditions Impacting Intervention

A physical therapist assistant is gait training an older adult in the home setting who has had a recent total hip arthroplasty. The patient is complaining of new tenderness in the groin, anterior hip, and thigh area. What additional diagnosis could tenderness in these areas be an indication of?

Choices:
1. Constipation.
2. Diarrhea.
3. Inflammatory bowel disease.
4. Gastritis.

Teaching Points

Correct Answer: 1
Constipation can cause abdominal pain and tenderness in the anterior hip, groin, or thigh area. The assistant working with a patient who is homebound should recognize that a decreased activity level and the addition of pain medications can both lead to constipation.

Incorrect Choices:
The identified tenderness is not a likely symptom of diarrhea, inflammatory bowel disease, or gastritis. Inflammatory bowel disease and gastritis do not refer pain to the hip/groin, pain is persistent in the stomach and gut.

Type of Reasoning: Analytical

This question provides a group of symptoms, and the test taker must determine the most likely cause for these symptoms. This requires one to analyze the various symptoms to draw a correct conclusion, which is an analytical reasoning skill. For this case, the symptoms are indicative of constipation. If answered incorrectly, review signs and symptoms of constipation.

A76

Integumentary | Data Collection

A patient presents with a large plantar ulcer that will be debrided. The foot is cold, pale, and painless. Which of the following conditions **BEST** meets the described clinical presentation?

Choices:
1. Chronic arterial insufficiency.
2. Chronic venous insufficiency.
3. Acute arterial insufficiency.
4. Deep venous thrombosis.

Teaching Points

Correct Answer: 2

Venous ulcers are often painless, or present with minimal pain compared with arterial ulcers, which are painful (claudication and rest pain). Chronic venous insufficiency is also characterized by thickening, coarsening, and brownish pigmentation of the skin around the ankles. The skin is usually thin, shiny, and cyanotic.

Incorrect Choices:
Deep venous thrombosis may be asymptomatic initially. When symptoms occur, patients typically report a dull ache, tightness, or pain in the calf. Both acute or chronic arterial insufficiency are painful conditions.

Type of Reasoning: Analytical

This question provides symptoms for a patient with a plantar ulcer and one must determine the most likely cause for such symptoms. This requires analytical reasoning skill, as symptoms are analyzed to reach a conclusion. For this situation, the symptoms indicate chronic venous insufficiency. If answered incorrectly, review signs and symptoms of chronic venous insufficiency.

A77

Nonsystem | Therapeutic Modalities

A patient has been referred for physical therapy following a fracture of the femur 6 months ago. The cast was removed, but the patient was unable to volitionally contract the quadriceps. To address this problem the physical therapist indicates utilization of electrical stimulation to the quadriceps muscle in the plan of care. Which of the following **BEST** describes the appropriate electrode size and placement for this patient?

Choices:
1. Large electrodes, closely spaced.
2. Small electrodes, closely spaced.
3. Large electrodes, widely spaced.
4. Small electrodes, widely spaced.

Teaching Points

Correct Answer: 3
Large electrodes are used on large muscles to disperse the current (minimize current density under the electrode) enabling a more comfortable delivery of current.

Incorrect Choices:
Widely spaced electrodes permit the current to travel deeper into the muscle to stimulate a greater number of deeper muscle fibers. Small electrodes will increase density of stimulus and will likely not be tolerated by the client.

Type of Reasoning: Deductive
One must recall the guidelines for electrode size and placement for electrical stimulation to arrive at a correct conclusion. This necessitates the recall of factual protocols and guidelines, which is a deductive reasoning skill. For this case, the therapist should select large electrodes, widely spaced. If answered incorrectly, review electrical stimulation guidelines for stimulation of the quadriceps, especially electrode size and placement.

A78

Neuromuscular | Diseases and Conditions Impacting Intervention

A patient suffered a severe traumatic brain injury and multiple fractures following a motor vehicle accident. The patient is recovering in the intensive care unit. The physical therapy referral requests passive range of motion and positioning. On day one, the patient is semi-alert and drifts in and out during treatment. On day two, the patient is less alert and the status is changing. Which of the following signs and symptoms require immediate consultation with the patient's nurse and physician?

Choices:
1. Developing irritability and disorientation.
2. Decreasing function of eye movements.
3. Rigidity in the neck muscles.
4. Decreasing consciousness with slowing of pulse.

Teaching Points

Correct Answer: 4
Signs of increased intracranial pressure secondary to cerebral edema and brain herniation include decreasing consciousness with slowing of pulse.

Incorrect Choices:
The other choices are signs and symptoms associated with traumatic brain injury. All of the problems listed are serious. Developing irritability and rigidity in many cases are frequent symptoms seen in TBI but are not life threatening. The correct choice is life threatening.

Type of Reasoning: Inferential
One must infer or draw a reasonable conclusion about the symptoms that would indicate a life-threatening emergency and need for emergency consultation to arrive at a correct conclusion. This requires inferential reasoning skill. For this situation, symptoms of decreasing consciousness with slowing of pulse are indicative of an emergency and need for consultation, as they are signs of increased intracranial pressure. If answered incorrectly, review signs and symptoms of intracranial pressure and emergency procedures for patients with traumatic brain injuries.

A79

Neuromuscular | Diseases and Conditions Impacting Intervention

A physical therapist assistant is working with a patient who has neurapraxia involving the ulnar nerve secondary to an elbow fracture. Which of the following statements represents the typical progression of this condition?

Choices:
1. Nerve dysfunction is likely to reverse in 4–6 months.
2. Nerve dysfunction is likely to reverse in 4–6 weeks.
3. Regeneration is likely after 1–1½ years.
4. Regeneration is unlikely because surgical approximation of the nerve ends was not performed.

Teaching Points

Correct Answer: 2

Neurapraxia is a mild peripheral nerve injury (conduction block ischemia) that causes transient loss of function. Nerve dysfunction is rapidly reversed, generally within 4–6 weeks. An example is a compression injury to the radial nerve from falling asleep with the upper extremity over the back of a chair (Saturday night palsy).

Incorrect Choices:
Regeneration of compression type injuries should occur prior to 6 months. Surgical approximation is not necessary in a compression type injury.

Type of Reasoning: Inferential
This question provides a diagnosis and one must infer the likely progression of recovery to arrive at a correct conclusion. This requires one to determine what may be true for a patient, which is an inferential reasoning skill. For this case, one should expect that nerve dysfunction will be rapidly reversed, generally in 4–6 weeks. If answered incorrectly, review ulnar nerve neurapraxia and progression of recovery.

A80

System Interactions | Diseases and Conditions Impacting Intervention

A home health physical therapist assistant is working with an older adult patient who has a history of hypertension and hyperlipidemia. On this day the patient is confused with shortness of breath and generalized weakness. What information should the physical therapist assistant immediately report to the supervising physical therapist?

Choices:
1. Mental changes are indicative of early Alzheimer's disease.
2. The patient may be experiencing unstable angina.
3. The patient forgot to take his or her hypertension medication.
4. The patient may be presenting with early signs of myocardial infarction.

Teaching Points

Correct Answer: 4

An elderly patient with a cardiac history may present with initial symptoms of mental confusion, the result of oxygen deprivation to the brain during developing myocardial infarction. The shortness of breath and generalized weakness may also be attributable to generalized circulatory insufficiencies coexisting with the developing myocardial infarction.

Incorrect Choices:

Alzheimer's disease would not present with shortness of breath. An individual with unstable angina would complain of pain. Forgetting hypertension medications would most likely present itself as increased blood pressure.

Type of Reasoning: Analytical

This question provides a group of symptoms and the test taker must determine the most likely cause for them. This requires analytical reasoning skill. For this case, the patient's symptoms are most indicative of early signs of myocardial infarction, given the history of hypertension and hyperlipidemia. If answered incorrectly, review early signs and symptoms of myocardial infarction.

A81

Musculoskeletal | Diseases and Conditions Impacting Intervention

A baseball pitcher is being seen following surgical repair of a glenoid labrum lesion of the pitching upper extremity. In follow-up care, the physical therapist assistant needs to pay attention to the pitching motion. What phase of throwing motion places the glenohumeral labrum and shoulder joint capsule at greatest stress?

Choices:
1. Wind-up.
2. Cocking.
3. Acceleration.
4. Deceleration.

Teaching Points

Correct Answer: 2

During the cocking phase, the upper extremity is taken into the end range of humeral lateral (external) rotation. At that point, the anterior aspects of the capsule and labrum are acting as constraints to prevent excessive anterior glide of the humerus.

Incorrect Choices:

Acceleration, deceleration, and wind-up are most affected by muscle performance and are not at the end range.

Type of Reasoning: Analytical

One must analyze the conditions presented when pitching and utilize knowledge of stress factors for the labrum and capsule during pitching to arrive at a correct conclusion. This requires analytical reasoning skill. For this case, the greatest stress during pitching occurs during the cocking phase. If answered incorrectly, review effects of pitching on glenoid labrum and capsule stress.

A82

Integumentary | Interventions

A frail older adult is confined to bed in a nursing facility and has developed a small superficial wound over the sacral area. Because only small amounts of necrotic tissue are present, the physical therapist has decided to use autolytic wound débridement. How will this intervention **BEST** be achieved?

Choices:
1. Wound irrigation using a syringe.
2. Transparent film dressing.
3. Wet-to-dry gauze dressing with antimicrobial ointment.
4. Sharp débridement.

Teaching Points

Correct Answer: 2

Autolytic wound débridement allows the body's natural enzymes to promote healing by trapping them under a synthetic, occlusive dressing. Moisture-retentive dressings are applied for short durations (less than 2 weeks). Choices include transparent film dressings, hydrocolloid, or hydrogel dressings.

Incorrect Choices:

The other choices are wound management techniques; however, they are not autolytic.

Type of Reasoning: Analytical

One must recall the parameters for autolytic wound débridement and effective approaches to arrive at a correct conclusion. This requires one to analyze the approaches presented to determine the approach that will be most effective for wound healing. For this situation, transparent film dressing is best. If answered incorrectly, review wound healing guidelines for superficial wounds, especially autolytic wound débridement and dressings.

A83

Musculoskeletal | Diseases and Conditions Impacting Intervention

The plan of care includes strengthening for a patient who reports subpatellar pain after participation in an aerobic exercise program for two weeks. The physical therapist's examination shows a large Q angle, pain with palpation at the inferior pole of the patella, and mild swelling at both knees. Which intervention will **BEST** meet the dysfunctions identified by the physical therapist examination?

Choices:
1. Vastus medialis muscle strengthening.
2. Lateral patellar tracking.
3. Vastus lateralis strengthening.
4. Hamstring strengthening.

Teaching Points

Correct Answer: 1

Q angles greater than 15° could be indicative of abnormal lateral patellar tracking. Vastus medialis muscle strengthening can reduce the tendency for the patella to track laterally.

Incorrect Choices:

Vastus lateralis strengthening can promote greater lateral patellar tracking and further irritation of the patellofemoral joint. Vastus lateralis strengthening may promote an outward pull or dislocation of the patella. Hamstring strengthening does not directly affect tracking of the patella. In the closed chain, problems at the hip or foot can also contribute to patellofemoral pain syndrome.

Type of Reasoning: Inductive

One must utilize clinical judgment to determine a best course of action for a patient with subpatellar pain and a large Q angle. This requires inductive reasoning skill. For this case, the assistant should focus intervention efforts on vastus medialis strengthening. If answered incorrectly, review intervention approaches for subpatellar pain and large Q angle.

A84

Neuromuscular | Interventions

A physical therapist assistant is working with a patient in the patient's home. The patient is being seen for right hemiparesis. The physical therapy evaluation indicates that the patient demonstrates good recovery; both involved extremities are categorized as out-of-synergy. The patient is ambulatory with a small-based quad cane. Which activity is **MOST** appropriate for a patient at this stage of recovery?

Choices:
1. Supine, bending the hip and knee up to the chest with some hip abduction.
2. Sitting, marching in place (alternate hip flexion movements).
3. Standing, picking the foot up behind and slowly lowering it.
4. Standing, small-range knee extension movements to gain quadriceps control.

Teaching Points

Correct Answer: 3

This stage of recovery is characterized by some movement combinations that do not follow paths of either flexion or extension obligatory synergies. Knee flexion in standing is an out-of-synergy movement.

Incorrect Choices:

All other choices represent synergistic movements: the supine and sitting options are flexion synergy movements whereas the other standing option focuses on knee extensor movement within an extended position.

Type of Reasoning: Inductive

One must determine the most appropriate activity for a patient with hemiparesis and decline in spasticity. This requires knowledge of rehabilitation guidelines for patients with spasticity to arrive at a correct conclusion. This requires inductive reasoning skill. For this case, the most appropriate activity for a patient is standing, picking the foot up behind and slowly lowering it. If answered incorrectly, review rehabilitation guidelines for patients with spasticity.

A85

Neuromuscular | Data Collection

A clinician has moved a patient's joint through its available range of motion and stops to hold the joint near end range, then asks the patient to identify the position of the joint. What sense is the clinician testing?

Choices:
1. Tactile localization.
2. Kinesthesia.
3. Proprioception.
4. Pressure perception.

Teaching Points

Correct Answer: 3

Proprioception tests are performed by positioning a patient's affected joint into a position, following an instructional trial, and asking the patient to verbally (or visually using the uninvolved extremity) report which position the joint is in.

Incorrect Choices:
Kinesthesia awareness is tested by moving the patient's affected joint through a portion of its range of motion and asking the patient to identify or replicate the range of movement performed. Tactile localization is assessing the patient's ability to identify the location of a touch stimulus provided by the clinician, e.g., radial condyle, web space of hand. Pressure perception is tested by applying pressure to a specific location using a fingertip or cotton swab and asking the patient to respond "yes" or "no" when they feel pressure.

Type of Reasoning: Deductive
One must recall the testing procedures for proprioception to arrive at a correct conclusion. This necessitates the recall of factual procedures and guidelines, which is a deductive reasoning skill. For this situation, the test procedure described is that of proprioception. If answered incorrectly, review proprioception testing procedures.

A86

Pulmonary | Diseases and Conditions Impacting Intervention

What is a preferred treatment position when one is providing strengthening exercises for a patient who is diagnosed with pulmonary edema?

Choices:
1. Supine with the lower extremities elevated.
2. Sitting with the lower extremities dangling.
3. Side-lying.
4. Prone with the head down.

Teaching Points

Correct Answer: 2
The sitting position helps decrease the work of breathing and reduces venous return.

Incorrect Choices:
Supine lying is a more difficult position for breathing. The side-lying or prone positions do not alleviate the difficulty with breathing.

Type of Reasoning: Inductive
This question requires one to determine the best position for strengthening exercises for a patient with pulmonary edema. This necessitates clinical judgment, which is an inductive reasoning skill. For this situation, the assistant should position the patient in sitting with the lower extremities dangling. If answered incorrectly, review positioning techniques for patients with pulmonary edema.

A87

Nonsystem | Equipment and Devices

A patient with bilateral short transfemoral amputations will require a wheelchair for functional mobility in the home and community. What is an important feature to include in a wheelchair prescription for this patient?

Choices:
1. Placement of the drive wheels 2 inches anterior to the vertical back supports.
2. Lowering the seat height by 3 inches.
3. Increasing the seat depth by 2 inches to accommodate the length of the residual extremities.
4. Placement of the drive wheels 2 inches posterior to the vertical back supports.

Teaching Points

Correct Answer: 4
Placement of the drive wheels 2 inches posterior to the vertical back supports is an appropriate modification for a patient with bilateral transfemoral amputations. This increases the length of the base of support and provides increased posterior stability. This is needed to offset the change in mass given the anterior mass is much less with the loss of the lower extremities.

Incorrect Choices:
Lowering the seat height by 3 inches is an appropriate modification for a patient following a cerebralvascular accident, who will use his or her sound extremities for wheelchair propulsion. Increasing the seat depth is not appropriate as that is not the method of accommodating the residual limb.

Type of Reasoning: Inductive
One must utilize knowledge of wheelchair prescription guidelines to arrive at a correct conclusion. This requires inductive reasoning skill. For this case, it is important for a patient with bilateral transfemoral amputations to have a wheelchair with placement of the drive wheels 2 inches posterior to the vertical back supports. If answered incorrectly, review wheelchair prescription guidelines for patients with bilateral transfemoral amputations.

Musculoskeletal | Interventions

In treating a patient with a diagnosis of right shoulder impingement syndrome, the plan of care is focused on regaining normal scapular–humeral rhythm. What is the **FIRST** priority of treatment for this patient?

Choices:
1. Implement a stretching program for the shoulder girdle musculature.
2. Instruct the patient in proper postural alignment.
3. Achieve complete active range of motion in all shoulder motions.
4. Modulate all pain.

Teaching Points

Correct Answer: 2
Without regaining normal postural alignment and scapular–humeral rhythm, the patient will continue to impinge the supraspinatus and/or biceps tendon at the acromion and never regain normal function of the shoulder.

Incorrect Choices:
It is unlikely that all pain would be controlled. Appropriate active range of motion exercises and/or stretching could be the focus after posture has been corrected.

Type of Reasoning: Inductive
This question requires the test taker to determine a first priority in treatment of a patient with shoulder impingement syndrome. This requires knowledge of the diagnosis and appropriate intervention approaches, which is an inductive reasoning skill. For this situation, the priority should be to instruct the patient in proper postural alignment. If answered incorrectly, review intervention approaches for patients with shoulder impingement syndrome.

A89

Neuromuscular | Data Collection

Which of the following is the **MOST** likely cause of a drooping of the shoulder, winging of the same scapula, and an inability to shrug the shoulder?

Choices:
1. Muscle imbalance.
2. A lesion of the long thoracic nerve.
3. A lesion of the spinal accessory nerve.
4. Strain of the serratus anterior.

Teaching Points

Correct Answer: 3

Although this winging of the scapula could be found with all of the above answers, the shoulder drooping and inability to shrug the shoulder is secondary to a lesion of the spinal accessory nerve (cranial nerve XI), which innervates the trapezius muscle.

Incorrect Choices:

Muscle imbalance is unlikely to create the postural deviations identified. A lesion of the long thoracic nerve could cause scapular winging; however, since the spinal accessory nerve and dorsal scapular nerves are not involved the middle trapezius and rhomboids will likely control scapular winging. A strain of the serratus anterior is unlikely to result in an inability to shrug the shoulder (upper trapezius) or drooping of the shoulder.

Type of Reasoning: Analytical

This question provides a group of symptoms and one must determine the most likely cause for them. This requires analysis of the symptoms to reach a correct conclusion, which is an analytical reasoning skill. For this case, the symptoms indicate a lesion of the spinal accessory nerve. If answered incorrectly, review signs and symptoms of spinal accessory nerve lesion.

A90

Neuromuscular | Data Collection

An elderly and frail patient is being seen for balance instability and frequent falls. The patient arrives for a therapy session complaining of pain and tingling in the forehead, cheek and jaw on the left side of the face. An inspection of the face and trunk reveals the eruption of vesicles in the distribution of the T2 dermatome. What is the physical therapist assistant's **BEST** course of action?

Choices:
1. Discuss this with the physical therapist with potential referral to the primary physician.
2. Utilize a hot pack to help relieve the pain and continue with balance training.
3. Advise the patient to take a pain reliever and contact the physician if the pain worsens.
4. Instruct the patient in cervical stretches to help relax the muscles on the left side of the neck.

Teaching Points

Correct Answer: 1

This patient is exhibiting signs of a herpes zoster infection (varicella zoster virus [VZV]). This is also known as shingles; the same virus causes chickenpox in children. Varicella zoster virus affects the sensory ganglia of the spinal cord or cranial nerves (commonly the trigeminal nerve, cranial nerve V [CNV], and thoracic dermatomes). Early inflammation produces pain and tingling; late symptoms include postherpetic neuralgia (severe aching or burning pain) that can persist for months or years. The physical therapist assistant should recognize these early symptoms and immediately notify the physical therapist who will likely recommend an immediate physician visit. The physician will likely order antiviral medications (e.g., acyclovir) to control the virus; this may also help with pain. Oral medications can be used to control pain; however, recommending this is not within the scope of the assistant.

Incorrect Choices:

Other interventions listed can be used to relieve pain but may be contraindicated without a full diagnostic workup and referral.

Type of Reasoning: Evaluative

This question provides symptoms and the test taker must determine an appropriate course of action based on these symptoms. One must weigh the merits of the potential courses of action to arrive at a correct conclusion, which is an evaluative reasoning skill. For this situation, the assistant should discuss the symptoms with the physical therapist with potential referral to the primary physician, as the symptoms indicate VZV infection. Review signs and symptoms of VZV infection if answered incorrectly.

Nonsystem | Therapeutic Modalities

A patient with spastic hemiplegia is referred to physical therapy. The physical therapy evaluation indicates that the patient is having difficulty in rising to a standing position as a result of co-contraction of the hamstrings and quadriceps. The plan of care calls for the use of biofeedback as an adjunct to help break up this pattern. What should the biofeedback protocol consist of to facilitate knee extension?

Choices:
1. High-detection sensitivity with electrodes placed close together.
2. Low-detection sensitivity with electrodes placed far apart.
3. High-detection sensitivity with electrodes placed far apart.
4. Low-detection sensitivity with electrodes placed close together.

Teaching Points

Correct Answer: 4

When the electrodes are close together, the likelihood of detecting undesired motor unit activity from adjacent muscles (crosstalk) decreases. By setting the sensitivity (gain) low, the amplitude of signals generated by the hypertonic muscles would decrease and keep the electromyograph output from exceeding a visual or auditory range.

Incorrect Choices:

If the setting was set at high detection or if the electrodes were placed far apart, there would be a considerable amount of "extra noise" because of hypertonicity; therefore to receive feedback that is useful the pads must be close together and on low detection.

Type of Reasoning: Deductive

This question requires the test taker to recall the guidelines for use of biofeedback for patients with abnormal co-contraction to arrive at a correct conclusion. This is factual information, which is a deductive reasoning skill. For this case, the biofeedback protocol should consist of low-detection sensitivity with electrodes placed close together. If answered incorrectly, review biofeedback guidelines and electrode placement.

A92

System Interactions | Diseases and Conditions Impacting Intervention

A patient sustained a T10 spinal cord injury 4 years ago and is now referred for an episode of outpatient physical therapy. In the initial examination the physical therapist documented redness over the ischial seat that persisted for 10 minutes when the patient was not sitting. The plan of care includes strengthening and instruction in functional activities. Which of the following activities should the physical therapist assistant include in the therapy session to meet the plan of care?

Choices:
1. Supine chest press with 20-pound barbell.
2. Half-standing transfers between surfaces.
3. Bilateral upper-extremity dips in the parallel bars.
4. Seated, gravity-resisted triceps curls with 10 pounds.

Teaching Points

Correct Answer: 3
Bilateral upper-extremity dips in the parallel bars will best strengthen the musculature needed to assist the patient to improve the ability to perform wheelchair push-ups to relieve pressure on the ischial tuberosities. Excessive ischial pressure and redness from prolonged sitting require an aggressive approach.

Incorrect Choices:
Supine chest presses and gravity-resisted triceps curls only incorporate the triceps muscles and do not incorporate the latissimus; therefore, they are not as comprehensive in muscle recruitment as the parallel bar dips are. Performing the half-standing transfers for the patient is not functional training.

Type of Reasoning: Inductive
This question requires the test taker to determine a best therapeutic approach for a patient with ischial redness. This requires clinical judgment, which is an inductive reasoning skill. For this case, the assistant should include bilateral upper-extremity dips in the parallel bars to strengthen the muscles needed to perform wheelchair push-ups. If answered incorrectly, review pressure relief techniques and exercises for patients with ischial redness.

A93

Nonsystem | Safety and Protection

A physical therapist assistant working in a long-term care facility witnesses a resident's family member collapse to the floor. What should the physical therapist assistant do immediately after calling for help and activating the EMS system?

Choices:
1. Perform a blind finger sweep followed by two rescue breaths.
2. Get an automated external defibrillator (AED) and begin cardiopulmonary resuscitation (CPR) and use of AED.
3. Roll the victim over and deliver two quick abdominal thrusts.
4. Deliver 5 cycles (2 minutes) of CPR before calling for help.

Teaching Points

Correct Answer: 2

When a sudden collapse is witnessed, for victims of all ages, healthcare providers should call for help (emergency response system outside of a care facility, or call for a code [or as directed in policy and procedure manual] in a care facility) and get an AED when readily available. In this instance the assistant is working in a long-term care facility; most likely an AED is immediately available.

Incorrect Choices:

A blind finger sweep is an inappropriate in this instance. When an unresponsive victim is found, a healthcare provider should assess ABCs (airway, breathing, and consciousness) and initiate CPR if appropriate after calling for help and getting an AED. The emergency response system should be initiated prior to delivering 2 minutes of CPR in this setting. Abdominal thrusts are only delivered if it is determined that the victim has choked on something.

Type of Reasoning: Evaluative

This question requires one to weigh the courses of action presented and then make a determination of the action that will best address the person's immediate needs. This requires evaluative reasoning skill. For this situation, the assistant should get an AED and begin CPR and use of AED after calling for help. If answered incorrectly, review CPR and first responder guidelines.

A94

Neuromuscular | Data Collection

During treatment in an outpatient rehabilitation center for an 18-month-old child with developmental delay and an atrioventricular shunt for hydrocephalus, the mother tells the assistant that the child vomited several times this morning, was irritable, and is now lethargic. What is the physical therapist assistant's **BEST** course of action?

Choices:
1. Call for emergency transportation and notify the physical therapist immediately.
2. Apply cold washcloths to try to rouse the child.
3. Place the child in a side-lying position and monitor vital signs.
4. Have the mother give the child clear liquids to avoid dehydration secondary to vomiting.

Teaching Points

Correct Answer: 1

These signs could be the result of increased cerebral edema because of a clogged or infected shunt. Medical attention should be obtained immediately to avoid damage to the brain. This is an emergency situation and needs immediate medical attention.

Incorrect Choices:

Other choices are inappropriate responses to potential problems associated with an atrioventricular shunt.

Type of Reasoning: Evaluative

This question requires one to weigh the symptoms presented and then determine the best course of action that effectively addresses the issue at hand. This requires evaluative reasoning skill. For this case, the assistant should call for emergency transportation and notify the physical therapist immediately, as the symptoms indicate possible cerebral edema. Review signs and symptoms of cerebral edema, as well as first aid guidelines, if answered incorrectly.

A95

Musculoskeletal | Diseases and Conditions Impacting Intervention

A woman recently delivered twins. After delivery she developed a 4-cm diastasis recti abdominis. What is the **BEST** initial intervention for this condition?

Choices:
1. Pelvic tilts and bilateral straight leg raising.
2. Pelvic floor exercises and sit-ups.
3. Gentle stretching of hamstrings and hip flexors.
4. Protection and splinting of the abdominal musculature.

Teaching Points

Correct Answer: 4

Diastasis recti abdominis is a condition in which there is a lateral separation or split of the rectus abdominis. It is important to **FIRST** teach protection (splinting) of the abdominal musculature. The key is INITIAL; once the patient is able to splint and protect the musculature, then it is appropriate to address muscle performance.

Incorrect Choices:

Patients should be instructed to avoid full sit-ups or bilateral straight leg raising. Pelvic floor exercises are done but are not remediation for diastasis recti. Gentle stretching of the hamstring and hip flexors does not apply.

Type of Reasoning: Inductive

One must utilize clinical judgment to determine the best initial intervention for a patient with diastasis recti abdominis. Questions of this nature often require inductive reasoning skill. For this situation, the best initial intervention is teaching protection and splinting of the abdominal musculature. If answered incorrectly, review intervention guidelines for diastasis recti abdominis.

A96

Neuromuscular | Diseases and Conditions Impacting Intervention

A patient has a 2 year history of amyotrophic lateral sclerosis and exhibits moderate functional deficits. The patient is still ambulatory with bilateral canes but is limited in endurance. When implementing treatment, what does the physical therapist assistant need to be careful to prevent?

Choices:
1. Radicular pain and paresthesias.
2. Overwork and damage in weakened, denervated muscle.
3. Further ataxia.
4. Further functional loss as a result of myalgia.

Teaching Points

Correct Answer: 2

Amyotrophic lateral sclerosis is a progressive degenerative disease that affects both upper and lower motor neurons. An important early goal of physical therapy is to maintain the patient's level of conditioning while preventing overwork damage in denervated muscle (lower motor neuron injury).

Incorrect Choices:

Myalgia is common in lower motor neuron lesions; it can be ameliorated but not prevented. Ataxia and radicular pain are not associated with amyotrophic lateral sclerosis.

Type of Reasoning: Inductive

One must utilize clinical judgment to determine therapeutic approaches that the assistant should prevent. This requires knowledge of the diagnosis to arrive at a correct conclusion, which is an inductive reasoning skill. For this situation, the assistant should prevent overworking and damaging the weakened, denervated muscle. If answered incorrectly, review therapeutic approaches for patients with amyotrophic lateral sclerosis and precautions for exercise.

A97

Nonsystem | Equipment and Devices

A patient has extensive full-thickness burns to the dorsum of the right hand and forearm and is being fitted with a resting splint to support the wrists and hands in a functional position. What position should this splint place the wrist and hand in?

Choices:
1. Neutral wrist position with slight finger flexion and thumb flexion.
2. Slight wrist extension with fingers supported and thumb in partial opposition and abduction.
3. Slight wrist flexion with interphalangeal joint extension and thumb opposition.
4. Neutral wrist position with interphalangeal joint extension and thumb flexion.

Teaching Points

Correct Answer: 2

A resting splint that positions the wrist and hand in a functional position includes 10°–20° of wrist extension, fingers supported, and thumb in partial opposition and abduction.

Incorrect Choices:
The neutral and flexed wrist positions are contraindicated for this condition.

Type of Reasoning: Deductive

This question requires one to recall the guidelines for hand splinting after burns. This is factual information, requiring deductive reasoning skill. For this case, the functional hand splinting position includes slight wrist extension with fingers supported, and thumb in partial opposition and abduction. Review splinting guidelines for patients with hand burns if answered incorrectly.

A98

Neuromuscular | Interventions

A young child with Down syndrome and moderate developmental delay is being treated at an early intervention program. What daily training activities should be considered for this patient?

Choices:
1. Stimulation to postural extensors in sitting using rhythmic stabilization.
2. Locomotor training using body weight support and a motorized treadmill.
3. Holding and weight shifting in sitting and standing using tactile and verbal cueing.
4. Rolling activities, initiating movement with stretch and tracking resistance.

Teaching Points

Correct Answer: 3

Children with Down syndrome typically present with generalized hypotonicity. The low tone is best managed by weight-bearing activities in antigravity postures. Typical responses include widened base-of-support and co-contraction to gain stability. Proprioceptors are not in a high state of readiness and the child may be slow to respond to proprioceptive facilitation techniques (i.e., stretch, resistance, rhythmic stabilization). Verbal cueing for redirection is generally the best form of feedback to use along with visually guided postural control.

Incorrect Choices:

With developmental delay this child is not ready for intensive locomotor training. Rhythmic stabilization and initiation are indicated for individuals with low tone, individuals with moderate developmental delay.

Type of Reasoning: Inductive

One must have knowledge of therapeutic activities for children with Down syndrome to arrive at a correct conclusion. This requires clinical judgment, which is an inductive reasoning skill. For this case, the assistant should focus on holding and weight shifting in sitting and standing using tactile and verbal cueing. Review treatment activities for children with Down syndrome if answered incorrectly.

A99

Neuromuscular | Data Collection

A patient with multiple sclerosis demonstrates strong bilateral lower-extremity extensor spasticity in the typical distribution of antigravity muscles. What position should the clinician expect the patient to present with?

Choices:
1. Sitting with the pelvis laterally tilted with increased weight bearing on ischial tuberosities.
2. Sacral sitting with increased extension and adduction of lower extremities.
3. Sitting with both legs abducted and laterally (externally) rotated.
4. Skin breakdown on the ischial tuberosities and lateral malleoli.

Teaching Points

Correct Answer: 2

Spasticity is typically strong in antigravity muscles. In the lower extremities this is usually the hip and knee extensors, adductors, and plantar flexors. Strong extensor tone results in sacral sitting with the pelvis tilted posteriorly.

Incorrect Choices:

Clinicians may see the other sitting postures but the question is related to the lower extremity spasticity pattern which is hip extension, adduction and plantarflexion.

Type of Reasoning: Inferential

One must determine what may be true for a patient with multiple sclerosis to arrive at a correct conclusion. This requires inferential reasoning skill. For this situation, the patient is likely to present with sacral sitting with increased extension and adduction of lower extremities. If answered incorrectly, review signs and symptoms of multiple sclerosis, especially effects of spasticity on functional positioning.

A100

Neuromuscular | Diseases and Conditions Impacting Intervention

A patient with multiple sclerosis (MS) has been on prednisolone for the past 4 weeks. The medication is now being tapered off. This is the third time this year that the patient has received this treatment for an MS exacerbation. What are possible adverse effects of this mediation?

Choices:
1. Weight gain and hyperkinetic behaviors.
2. Hypoglycemia and nausea or vomiting.
3. Muscle wasting, weakness, and osteoporosis.
4. Spontaneous fractures with prolonged healing or mal-union.

Teaching Points

Correct Answer: 3

This patient is receiving systemic corticosteroids to suppress inflammation and the normal immune system response during an MS attack. Chronic treatment leads to adrenal suppression. There are numerous adverse reactions and side effects that can occur. Those affecting the patient's capacity to exercise include muscle wasting and pain, weakness, and osteoporosis. Weight loss is common (anorexia) with nausea and vomiting.

Incorrect Choices:
Adrenal suppression produces hyperglycemia, not hypoglycemia. Hyperkinetic behaviors or spontaneous fractures are not typical or expected adverse effects of prednisolone.

Type of Reasoning: Deductive
One must recall the potential adverse effects of prednisolone to arrive at a correct conclusion. This requires recall of factual guidelines, which is a deductive reasoning skill. For this case, one should expect the potential adverse effects to include muscle wasting, weakness, and osteoporosis. If answered incorrectly, review adverse effects of prednisolone.

A101

Neuromuscular | Data Collection

A patient suffered carbon monoxide poisoning from a work-related factory accident and is left with permanent damage to the basal ganglia. What impairments should the clinician expect the patient to present with?

Choices:
1. Motor paralysis with the use of free weights to increase strength.
2. Muscular spasms and hyperreflexia with the use of ice wraps.
3. Impaired sensory organization of balance with the use of standing balance platform training.
4. Motor planning with the use of guided and cued movement.

Teaching Points

Correct Answer: 4
The basal ganglia functions to convert general motor activity into specific, goal-directed action plans. Dysfunction results in problems with motor planning and scaling of movements and postures (e.g., bradykinesia). Patients benefit from initial guided movement and task-specific training. Proprioceptive, tactile, and verbal cues can also be used prior to and during a task to enhance movement.

Incorrect Choices:
The other listed deficits (choices) are not typically seen with basal ganglia disorders.

Type of Reasoning: Inferential
This question requires the test taker to determine what symptoms are likely to be present and best intervention approaches for a patient with basal ganglia damage. This requires inferential reasoning skill. For this case, one should expect impairments in motor planning and should choose guided and cued movement. If answered incorrectly, review signs and symptoms of basal ganglia damage, as well as intervention approaches for this diagnosis.

A102

Neuromuscular | Data Collection

While assessing the gait of a patient with right hemiplegia, the physical therapist assistant notes foot drop during midswing on the right. What is the **MOST** likely cause of this deviation?

Choices:
1. Inadequate contraction of the ankle dorsiflexors.
2. Excessive extensor synergy.
3. Decreased proprioception of foot and ankle muscles.
4. Excessive flexor synergy.

Teaching Points

Correct Answer: 1
Weakness or delayed contraction of the ankle dorsiflexors or spasticity in the ankle plantar flexors may cause foot drop during midswing.

Incorrect Choices:
Excessive extensor synergy would cause plantar flexion during stance. Decreased proprioception of the foot and ankle muscles would cause difficulties with foot placement and balance during stance. A strong flexor synergy can cause dorsiflexion with hip and knee flexion during swing.

Type of Reasoning: Analytical
This question requires the test taker to analyze the symptoms for a patient with right hemiplegia and foot drop during midswing and determine a likely cause for the deviation. Questions of this nature often require analytical reasoning skill. For this situation, the most likely cause is inadequate contraction of the ankle dorsiflexors. Review causes of foot drop in patients with hemiplegia if answered incorrectly.

A103

Nonsystem | Therapeutic Modalities

Which of the following conditions would allow the clinician to continue with orders to implement ultrasound?

Choices:
1. Plastic implants.
2. Infected tissue.
3. Metal implants.
4. Neoplastic lesions.

Teaching Points

Correct Answer: 3
Several studies have shown the safe use of ultrasound over metal implants. The acoustical energy is dispersed throughout the metal and is absorbed into the surrounding tissue. There is no significant heating within the implant.

Incorrect Choices:
The other choices identified are contraindications for the use of ultrasound.

Type of Reasoning: Deductive
One must recall the guidelines for the use of ultrasound under certain conditions. This requires the recall of guidelines, which is a deductive reasoning skill. For this scenario, it is permissible to use ultrasound over metal implants. If answered incorrectly, review guidelines for safe use of ultrasound.

Neuromuscular | Diseases and Conditions Impacting Intervention

A physical therapist assistant observes genu recurvatum while gait training a patient with hemiplegia. The patient has been using a posterior leaf spring orthosis since discharge from subacute rehabilitation 4 weeks ago. The patient has strong synergies in the lower extremity and **NO** out-of-synergy movement. What is the **MOST** likely cause of this deviation?

Choices:
1. Extensor spasticity.
2. Hip flexor weakness.
3. Dorsiflexor spasticity.
4. Hamstring weakness.

Teaching Points

Correct Answer: 1
A hyperextended knee can be caused by extensor spasticity, quadriceps weakness (a compensatory locking of the knee), or by plantar flexion contractures or deformity. The most likely cause in this case is extensor spasticity, which is consistent with strong obligatory synergies.

Incorrect Choices:
Hip flexor weakness would likely result in difficulty with initiation of swing or use of hip hike to progress the limb forward; hamstring weakness would likely result in lack of knee flexion during swing, and dorsiflexion spasticity would result in excessive dorsiflexion with potential buckling of the knee.

Type of Reasoning: Analytical
This question reveals deficits and the test taker must analyze the symptoms to determine a likely cause for them. Questions of this nature require analytical reasoning skill. For this situation, the most likely cause is extensor spasticity. Review causes of extensor spasticity in patients with hemiplegia if answered incorrectly.

A105

Pulmonary | Data Collection

During a home visit a physical therapist assistant is providing postural drainage in the Trendelenburg position to an adolescent with cystic fibrosis. The patient experiences right-sided chest pain and shortness of breath. Auscultation reveals there are no breath sounds on the right. What should the physical therapist assistant do now?

Choices:
1. Continue treating to dislodge possible mucous plug.
2. Reposition patient with the head of the bed flat.
3. Place the right lung in a gravity-dependent position.
4. Call emergency medical services.

Teaching Points

Correct Answer: 4

The combined signs and symptoms of ABSENT breath sounds, sudden onset of chest pain and shortness of breath indicate a pneumothorax, especially in a adolescent (growth spurt) with pathological changes of lung tissue. This is an emergency situation that requires immediate medical attention.

Incorrect Choices

An individual experiencing a mucous plug is not likely to present with no breath sounds. Repositioning the patient is an ineffective response to a pneumothorax.

Type of Reasoning: Evaluative

This question requires one to weigh the courses of action presented to determine the action that will effectively address the patient's symptoms. This requires evaluative reasoning skill. For this situation, the assistant should call emergency medical services as it may be a pneumothorax. Review first aid approaches for patients with pneumothorax if answered incorrectly.

A106

Neuromuscular | Interventions

A patient with an 8 year history of Parkinson's disease is referred for physical therapy. The initial evaluation identifies the patient as having significant rigidity, decreased passive range of motion in both upper extremities in the typical distribution and frequent episodes of akinesia. What is the BEST exercise intervention to address these identified problems?

Choices:
1. Quadruped position, upper-extremity proprioceptive neuromuscular facilitation (PNF) D2 flexion and extension.
2. Resistance training, free weights for shoulder flexors at 80% of one repetition maximum.
3. Modified plantigrade, isometric holding, stressing upper-extremity shoulder flexion.
4. PNF bilateral symmetrical upper extremity D2 flexion patterns, rhythmic initiation.

Teaching Points

Correct Answer: 4

The patient with Parkinson's disease typically develops elbow flexion and shoulder adduction contractures of the upper extremities along with a flexed, stooped posture. Bilateral symmetrical upper-extremity PNF D2F patterns encourage shoulder flexion and abduction with elbow extension, and upper-trunk extension (all needed motions).

Incorrect Choices:

Both quadruped and modified plantigrade positions encourage postural flexion. Treatment should emphasize initiation of movement due to akinesia not strengthening.

Type of Reasoning: Inductive

One must utilize clinical judgment to determine the best intervention approach for a patient with Parkinson's disease. This is an inductive reasoning skill. For this case, the assistant should use PNF bilateral symmetrical upper-extremity D2 flexion patterns and rhythmic initiation to address the patient's deficits. If answered incorrectly, review intervention approaches for patients with Parkinson's disease, especially PNF approaches.

A107

Neuromuscular | Data Collection

A patient is referred for rehabilitation following a middle cerebral artery stroke. What signs and symptoms should the physical therapist assistant expect the patient to present with?

Choices:
1. Contralateral hemiplegia with thalamic sensory syndrome and involuntary movements.
2. Contralateral hemiparesis and sensory deficits, with the upper extremity more involved than the lower extremity.
3. Decreased pain and temperature to the face and ipsilateral ataxia with contralateral pain and thermal loss of the body.
4. Contralateral hemiparesis and sensory deficits, with the lower extremity more involved than the upper extremity.

Teaching Points

Correct Answer: 2

A cerebrovascular accident (CVA) affecting the middle cerebral artery will result in symptoms of contralateral hemiparesis and hemisensory deficits with greater involvement of the upper extremity than the lower extremity.

Incorrect Choices:

Contralateral hemiplegia with thalamic sensory syndrome and involuntary movements are characteristic of a CVA affecting the posterior cerebral artery syndrome (central territory). Decreased pain and temperature to the face and ipsilateral ataxia, with contralateral pain and thermal loss of the body are characteristic of a CVA affecting the vertebral artery, posterior inferior cerebellar artery (lateral medullary syndrome). Contralateral hemiparesis and sensory deficits, with the lower extremity more involved than the upper extremity, are characteristic of a CVA affecting the anterior cerebral artery.

Type of Reasoning: Deductive

This question requires the test taker to recall the symptoms of middle cerebral artery stroke to arrive at a correct conclusion. This necessitates recall of factual information, which is a deductive reasoning skill. For this diagnosis, the assistant should expect contralateral hemiparesis and sensory deficits, with the upper extremity more involved than the lower extremity. If answered incorrectly, review signs and symptoms of middle cerebral artery stroke.

A108

Cardiac | Data Collection

The cardiac rehabilitation team is conducting education classes for a group of patients. The focus is on risk factor reduction and successful lifestyle modification. A participant asks the physical therapist assistant to explain these cholesterol findings: Total cholesterol is 220 mg/dL, high-density lipoprotein (HDL) cholesterol is 24 mg/dL, and low-density lipoprotein (LDL) cholesterol is 160 mg/dL. What should the physical therapist assistant explain that these readings indicate?

Choices:
1. That the levels of HDL, LDL, and total cholesterol are all abnormally high.
2. That LDL and HDL cholesterol levels are within normal limits and total cholesterol should be below 200 mg/dL.
3. That the levels of HDL, LDL, and total cholesterol are all abnormally low.
4. The levels of LDL and total cholesterol are abnormally high and the level of HDL cholesterol is abnormally low.

Teaching Points

Correct Answer: 4

Increased total blood cholesterol levels (>200 mg/dL) and levels of LDLs (>130 mg/dL) increase the risk of coronary artery disease (CAD); conversely, low concentrations of HDLs (<40 mg/dL for men and <50 mg/dL for women) are also harmful. The link between CAD and triglycerides is not as clear.

Incorrect Choices:
HDL levels are low and LDL levels represented are high.

Type of Reasoning: Analytical
One must analyze the information presented to determine the significance of this information. This requires analytical reasoning skills, as pieces of information are assessed to draw a conclusion. For this situation, the findings indicate that the levels of LDL and total cholesterol are abnormally high and the HDL level is abnormally low. If answered incorrectly, review normal and abnormal blood cholesterol parameters.

A109

Nonsystem | Therapeutic Modalities

When working with a patient in a pool who is submerged to chest level, which clinical effect will be produced?

Choices:
1. The patient will be able to better regulate body temperature in the water.
2. Exercises will be more easily performed with the body part submerged more deeply in the water.
3. The patient's center of gravity (buoyancy in the water) moves higher, closer to the area of the sternum.
4. The more quickly the patient moves the easier the exercises will be.

Teaching Points

Correct Answer: 3

When the patient is submerged in the pool, the patient's center of gravity moves to the area of the sternum. Buoyancy devices will alter this center of gravity, e.g., a buoyancy device placed posteriorly will cause the patient to lean forward.

Incorrect Choices:

Temperature regulation is more challenging while submerged as less skin is exposed to allow heat dissipation through evaporation. Once the body part has overcome the surface tension and has been submerged in the water it will need to overcome the effects of buoyancy and viscosity; being submerged more deeply does not necessarily mean the exercise is harder to perform. Performing an exercise more quickly increases the water turbulence and drag thus making the exercise more difficult.

Type of Reasoning: Inductive

One must utilize clinical judgment to make a determination of the effects of submersion in water to chest level. This requires inductive reasoning skill. For this case, the effects include the center of gravity moving higher and closer to the area of the sternum. If answered incorrectly, review effects of submersion in water on buoyancy and center of gravity.

A110

Lymphatic | Interventions

A patient is being treated for secondary lymphedema of the right upper extremity as a result of a radical mastectomy and radiation therapy. What is the **BEST** physical therapy method to help reverse pitting edema?

Choices:
1. Isokinetics, extremity positioning in elevation, and massage.
2. Active range of motion and extremity positioning in a functional upper extremity/hand position.
3. Isometric exercises, extremity positioning in elevation, and compression bandaging.
4. Intermittent pneumatic compression, extremity elevation, and massage.

Teaching Points

Correct Answer: 4

Lymphedema following surgery and radiation is classified as secondary lymphedema. Stage 1 means that there is pitting edema that is reversible with elevation. The arm may be normal size first thing in the morning with edema developing as the day goes on. It can be effectively managed by external compression and extremity elevation. Manual lymph drainage (massage and passive range of motion) are also appropriate interventions.

Incorrect Choices:

Exercise and positioning alone would not provide the needed lymph drainage; isometric exercise is contraindicated.

Type of Reasoning: Inductive

One must utilize knowledge of lymphedema intervention approaches to arrive at a correct conclusion. This requires clinical judgment, which is an inductive reasoning skill. For this situation, the best method to reverse the pitting edema is intermittent pneumatic compression, extremity elevation, and massage. If answered incorrectly, review intervention approaches for lymphedema, especially reversible pitting edema.

A111

Pulmonary | Interventions

A postsurgical patient is receiving a regimen of postural drainage three times a day. At what point is it appropriate to suggest reducing the frequency of treatments?

Choices:
1. If the consistency of the sputum changes.
2. If the patient becomes febrile.
3. If the patient experiences decreased postoperative pain.
4. If the amount of productive secretions decreases.

Teaching Points

Correct Answer: 4

The purpose of postural drainage is to help remove secretions. If the amount diminishes, this might be an indicator that the treatment has been successful and that the frequency of treatment can be reduced.

Incorrect Choices:

The other choices of fever, sputum consistency, and pain do not provide a rationale to decrease treatment frequency.

Type of Reasoning: Inductive

This question requires the test taker to utilize knowledge of postural drainage guidelines and treatment approaches to arrive at a correct conclusion. This necessitates clinical judgment, which is an inductive reasoning skill. For this case, the assistant should suggest reducing the frequency of treatment if the amount of productive secretions decreases. Review postural drainage treatment approaches and frequency of treatment if answered incorrectly.

A112

Cardiac | Interventions

A patient with coronary artery disease received inpatient cardiac rehabilitation following a mild myocardial infarction. The patient is now enrolled in an outpatient exercise class that utilizes intermittent training. What is the **MOST** appropriate initial spacing of exercise and rest intervals when safely stressing the aerobic system?

Choices:
1. 1:1.
2. 5:1.
3. 2:1.
4. 10:1.

Teaching Points

Correct Answer: 3

Presuming that the exercise goals for inpatient cardiac rehabilitation are met, an exercise-to-rest ratio of 2:1 can be used with this patient to begin exercise in an outpatient setting in a safe manner.

Incorrect Choices:

An exercise-to-rest ratio of 1:1 is appropriate for an initial prescription for inpatient rehabilitation programs with a goal of achieving a 2:1 ratio. Ratios of 5:1 or 10:1 are too stressful to begin outpatient rehabilitation. A 5:1 ratio may be a goal for later exercise programming.

Type of Reasoning: Inductive

One must utilize clinical judgment and knowledge of cardiac rehabilitation guidelines to arrive at a correct conclusion. This requires inductive reasoning skill. For this case, the most appropriate initial spacing of exercise and rest intervals is 2:1. Review cardiac rehabilitation guidelines for patients with mild myocardial infarctions in outpatient settings if answered incorrectly.

A113

Musculoskeletal | Interventions

What is the **BEST** intervention to improve functional mobility in an individual with a stable humeral neck fracture?

Choices:
1. Active resistive range of motion.
2. Isometrics for all shoulder musculature.
3. Pendulum exercises.
4. Modalities to decrease pain.

Teaching Points

Correct Answer: 3

This individual will typically be immobilized with a sling for a period of 6 weeks. After 1 week the sling should be removed to have the patient perform pendulum exercises to prevent shoulder stiffness and to begin mobilization of the joint.

Incorrect Choices:

Resistive exercises are not indicated during this early period and address muscle performance not mobility. Isometrics may be used early in treatment but address muscle performance/strength not mobility. Modalities may be effective in reducing pain but do not improve mobility.

Type of Reasoning: Inductive

This question requires the test taker to determine a best initial intervention approach for a patient with a stable humeral neck fracture. This requires clinical judgment, which is an inductive reasoning skill. For this scenario, the assistant should perform pendulum exercises for the initial intervention approach. Review intervention approaches for patients with stable humeral neck fractures if answered incorrectly.

A114

Musculoskeletal | Diseases and Conditions Impacting Intervention

A dancer with unilateral spondylolysis at L4 is referred for physical therapy. The patient reports generalized low back pain when standing longer than 1 hour. What strengthening exercises should be included in the subacute phase of healing?

Choices:
1. Abdominals working from neutral to full flexion.
2. Multifidi working from neutral to full extension.
3. Abdominals working from full extension to full flexion.
4. Multifidi working from full flexion back to neutral.

Teaching Points

Correct Answer: 4
Performing strengthening exercises to the multifidi from flexion to neutral will not stress the pars defect which is imperative with spondylolysis.

Incorrect Choices:
Abdominal strengthening will not provide the segmental stability needed with this condition. Lumbar extension beyond neutral and rotation will tend to aggravate the condition in the early stages of rehabilitation.

Type of Reasoning: Inductive
For this question, the test taker must utilize knowledge of spondylolysis and intervention approaches to arrive at a correct conclusion. This requires inductive reasoning skill. For this situation, the assistant should include strengthening exercises for the multifidi working from full flexion back to neutral. Review intervention approaches in the subacute phase of rehabilitation for patients with spondylolysis if answered incorrectly.

A115

Musculoskeletal | Diseases and Conditions Impacting Intervention

A patient has fixed forefoot varus malalignment. What compensatory motion(s) or posture(s) might a clinician expect to see in this patient?

Choices:
1. Genu recurvatum.
2. Excessive subtalar pronation.
3. Ipsilateral pelvic lateral (external) rotation.
4. Hallux varus.

Teaching Points

Correct Answer: 2
Possible compensatory motions or postures for forefoot varus malalignment include plantar flexed first ray; hallux valgus; excessive midtarsal or subtalar pronation or prolonged pronation; excessive tibial, tibial and femoral, or femoral and pelvic medial (internal) rotation; and/or all with contralateral lumbar spine rotation.

Incorrect Choices:
Genu recurvatum is seen to compensate for limited dorsiflexion. Hallux valgus is not expected with a forefoot varus deformity. Contralateral and medial rotation deviations are more likely.

Type of Reasoning: Inferential
This question requires the test taker to infer or draw a reasonable conclusion about the likely compensatory motions for a patient with fixed forefoot varus malalignment. This requires inferential reasoning skill. For this situation, the patient is likely to demonstrate excessive subtalar pronation. Review compensatory motions for fixed forefoot varus malalignment if answered incorrectly.

A116

Nonsystem | Safety and Protection

A patient comes into outpatient physical therapy following rotator cuff surgery. The physical therapist assistant initiates resistance band resistive exercise at the beginning of the session then proceeds with soft tissue mobilization and stretching to increase range of motion. Near the end of the therapy session the patient reports having watery eyes and an itchy feeling in the hands. Upon inspection the assistant notes a skin rash on the patient's palms and slight facial swelling. What is the **MOST** likely cause of this response?

Choices:
1. Atopic dermatitis.
2. Rosacea.
3. Latex allergy.
4. Stasis dermatitis.

Teaching Points

Correct Answer: 3

The patient is likely experiencing an immediate hypersensitivity to latex (type I hypersensitivity). Symptoms typically include contact dermatitis and, if severe, swelling and respiratory changes. The assistant should identify this as a latex sensitivity to the patient and have the patient follow up with the physician. The assistant should provide the patient with a latex-free resistance band.

Incorrect Choices:

Atopic dermatitis is a chronic inflammatory skin disease. Rosacea is a chronic form of acne with a vascular component (erythema, telangiectasis) usually of the face in a butterfly pattern around the eyes and nose. In stasis dermatitis, skin is dry and thin with shallow ulcers that develop on the lower legs as a result of venous insufficiency.

Type of Reasoning: Analytical

This question provides a group of symptoms and the test taker must determine the most likely cause. Questions of this nature often require analytical reasoning skill. For this case, the symptoms the patient experienced after exercise are consistent with a latex allergy. If answered incorrectly, review signs and symptoms of latex allergies.

A117

Cardiac, Vascular | Data Collection

A patient has an episode of syncope in the physical therapy clinic. The physical therapist asks the physical therapist assistant to check to see whether the patient is experiencing orthostatic hypotension. How should the physical therapist assistant complete this assessment?

Choices:
1. Check the heart rate (HR) and blood pressure (BP) in supine position after 5 minutes rest, then repeating in semi-Fowler position.
2. Palpate the carotid arteries and taking HR; using the supine position for BP measurements.
3. Check the HR and BP at rest, and after 3 and 5 minutes of cycle ergometry exercise.
4. Check the resting BP and HR in sitting, then repeating measurements after standing for 1 minute.

Teaching Points

Correct Answer: 4

Orthostatic hypotension is a fall in BP with elevation of position, i.e., from supine to sitting or sitting to standing. A small increase or no increase in heart rate upon standing may suggest baroreflex impairment. An exaggerated increase in HR upon standing may indicate volume depletion. A drop in blood pressure with change in position may indicate orthostatic hypotension.

Incorrect Choices:

Orthostatic hypotension is identified by first measuring blood pressure in the seated or reclined position—then progressing to standing; not in consistent reclining positions. Supine measurements must be compared to standing measurements; there is no need to measure the carotid pulse. Checking after 3–5 minutes of activity will provide inaccurate information as the patient's heart rate and blood pressure will be elevated during this ability.

Type of Reasoning: Deductive

This question requires one to recall the procedures for testing orthostatic hypotension. This is a factual procedure, which is a deductive reasoning skill. For this situation, the assistant should check resting BP and HR in sitting, then repeat measurements after standing for 1 minute. If answered incorrectly, review testing procedures for orthostatic hypotension.

A118

Integumentary | Data Collection

An inpatient with a grade 3 diabetic foot ulcer is referred for physical therapy. Panafil is being applied to the necrotic tissue twice a day. The wound has no foul smell; however, the physical therapist assistant notes a green tinge on the dressing. What should the physical therapist assistant do in this case?

Choices:
1. Document the finding and contact the therapist immediately.
2. Begin a trial of acetic acid to the wound.
3. Document the finding and continue with treatment.
4. Fit the patient with a total contact cast.

Teaching Points

Correct Answer: 3

A greenish tinge to the dressing is expected with the use of Panafil. Panafil is a keratolytic enzyme used for selective débridement. A greenish or yellowish exudate can be expected.

Incorrect Choices:

If the exudate were green and had a foul smell, *Pseudomonas aeruginosa* should be suspected and acetic acid would be the topical agent of choice. Beginning acetic acid treatment does not relate to the identification of a green-tinged discharge. A total contact cast can be used only after the wound is free of necrotic tissue.

Type of Reasoning: Evaluative

This question requires the test taker to determine a best course of action for and significance of a wound dressing with a green tinge on it. This requires one to weigh the merits of the courses of action, which is an evaluative reasoning skill. For this case, because a greenish tinge is expected with the use of Panafil, the assistant should document the finding and continue with treatment.

A119

Nonsystem | Safety and Protection

A physical therapist assistant is performing a home assessment to examine the fall risk of an older adult patient who lives alone and has had two recent falls. Which of the following activities represents the **MOST** common risk factor associated with falls in older adults?

Choices:
1. Climbing on a stepstool to reach overhead objects.
2. Walking with a roller walker with hand brakes.
3. Dressing while sitting on the edge of the bed.
4. Turning around and sitting down in a chair.

Teaching Points

Correct Answer: 4

Most falls occur during normal daily activity. Getting up or down from a bed or chair, turning, bending, walking and climbing or descending stairs all are high-risk activities.

Incorrect Choices:

Only a small percentage of individuals fall during clearly hazardous activities (e.g., climbing the stepstool). Proper use of an assistive device reduces the risk of falls.

Type of Reasoning: Inferential

This question necessitates one to infer or draw a reasonable conclusion about the most likely risk factor for falls in the elderly. This requires inferential reasoning skill, as one must determine what is likely to be true for a population. For this scenario, the most common risk factor is turning around and sitting down in a chair. If answered incorrectly, review risk factors for falls in the elderly.

A120

Musculoskeletal | Interventions

During surgery to remove an apical lung tumor, the long thoracic nerve was injured. Muscle weakness is 3+/5. The plan of care indicates strengthening exercises for the weak muscles. Which of the following **BEST** represents initial exercises for this patient?

Choices:
1. Standing, upper-extremity overhead lifts using hand weights.
2. Supine, upper-extremity overhead lifts using weights.
3. Sitting, upper-extremity overhead lifts using a pulley.
4. Standing, wall push-ups.

Teaching Points

Correct Answer: 4

The long thoracic nerve supplies the serratus anterior muscle. With a muscle grade of fair plus (3+/5), the patient can begin functional strengthening by using standing wall push-ups, with resistance provided by the patient's own body.

Incorrect Choices:

The other exercises identified are not optimal exercises for strengthening the serratus anterior with fair plus strength.

Type of Reasoning: Inductive

This question requires clinical judgment to determine the best initial exercise approach for a patient with long thoracic nerve injury. This necessitates knowledge of muscles innervated by the long thoracic nerve and effective exercise approaches, which is an inductive reasoning skill. For this case, the therapist should instruct the patient in wall push-ups in standing. If answered incorrectly, review exercises for the serratus anterior and long thoracic nerve injury.

A121

Musculoskeletal | Interventions

A college soccer player sustained a hyperextension knee injury when kicking the ball with the opposite lower extremity. The physician in the emergency room discharged the patient with a diagnosis of "knee sprain." The patient was sent to physical therapy the **NEXT** day for rehabilitation. The therapist's initial evaluation identifies a positive Lachman's test for anterior cruciate ligament (ACL) integrity. What type of exercise is indicated in the acute phase of treatment?

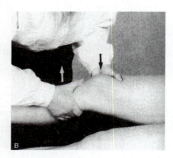

Magee D (2002). Orthopedic Physical Assessment, 4th ed. Philadelphia, W. B. Saunders, Figure 12-27B, page 700, with permission.

Choices:
1. Agility exercises.
2. Closed-chain terminal knee extension exercises.
3. Open-chain terminal knee extension exercises.
4. Plyometric functional exercises.

Teaching Points

Correct Answer: 2

The test that was conducted was a Lachman's test to determine integrity of the ACL. A positive test suggests laxity of the anterior cruciate ligament.

Incorrect Choices:

Quick cutting or lateral movements that occur in agility training and heavy joint loading that occurs with plyometric exercise should be avoided until the muscular restraints that reduce excessive anterior translation of the affected tibiofemoral joint are strengthened. Open-chain knee extension may place excessive load on the ACL. Closed-chain terminal knee extension exercises are safe and effective secondary to the dynamic stability inherent with this type of exercise.

Type of Reasoning: Analytical

One must analyze the symptoms presented to determine the appropriate approach for the acute phase of treatment. This requires analytical reasoning skill. For this case, the exercise approach that is indicated is closed-chain terminal knee extension exercises. If answered incorrectly, review treatment approaches for laxity of the ACL.

A122

Musculoskeletal | Data Collection

A patient with a transtibial amputation is learning to walk with a patellar tendon–bearing prosthesis and is having difficulty maintaining prosthetic stability from heel-strike (initial contact) to foot-flat (loading response). What muscles are **MOST** likely weak during stance phase?

Choices:
1. Knee extensors.
2. Back extensors.
3. Hip flexors.
4. Knee flexors.

Teaching Points

Correct Answer: 1
The quadriceps is maximally active at heel strike (initial contact) to stabilize the knee and counteract the flexion moment. Weakness may result in buckling of the knee.

Incorrect Choices:
Weak back extensors may present as excessive forward flexion of the trunk. Weak hip flexors may present as difficulty in initiation of swing or hip hike to initiate swing. Weak knee flexors may present as decreased knee flexion in swing.

Type of Reasoning: Inferential
One must infer or draw a reasonable conclusion about the likely muscles that are weakened when a patient is demonstrating difficulty maintaining prosthetic stability from heel-strike to foot-flat. This requires inferential reasoning skill. For this situation, the most likely weak muscles are the knee extensors. Review gait deviations with the use of a patellar tendon–bearing prosthesis if answered incorrectly.

A123

Nonsystem | Therapeutic Modalities

A physical therapist assistant is applying high-volt pulsed current to the vastus medialis to improve patellar tracking during knee extension. The patient reports that the current is uncomfortable. To make the current more tolerable to the patient, yet maintain a good therapeutic effect, what parameter should the assistant consider adjusting?

Choices:
1. Pulse rate.
2. Current intensity.
3. Pulse duration.
4. Current polarity.

Teaching Points

Correct Answer: 3
Decreasing the pulse duration reduces the electrical charge of each pulse, making the current more comfortable by decreasing the total current applied while maintaining the full therapeutic effect.

Incorrect Choices:
Pulse rate will not affect the comfort of the current. Lowering the intensity of the intensity can result in the inability to achieve a muscle contraction and thus diminish effectiveness. Current polarity does not affect current tolerance.

Type of Reasoning: Deductive
This question requires one to recall the guidelines for use of high-volt pulsed current and adjustments made to provide comfort for the patient. This is factual information, which is a deductive reasoning skill. For this scenario, the assistant should adjust the pulse duration to make the current more comfortable for the patient. If answered incorrectly, review high-volt pulsed current treatment guidelines.

A124

Neuromuscular | Diseases and Conditions Impacting Intervention

An older adult who is a wheelchair-dependent resident of a community nursing home has a diagnosis of organic brain syndrome, Alzheimer's disease type, stage 2. During an afternoon treatment session, the patient demonstrated limited interaction and mild agitation, and tried to wheel the chair down the hall. As it was late in the day, the assistant decided to resume the treatment the next morning. What is this patient exhibiting?

Choices:
1. Frustration because of an inability to communicate.
2. Disorientation to time and date.
3. Sundowning behavior.
4. Inattention as a result of short-term memory loss.

Teaching Points

Correct Answer: 3
A patient with stage 2 Alzheimer's disease can be expected to exhibit impaired cognition and abstract thinking, sundowning (defined as extreme restlessness, agitation, and wandering that typically occur in the late afternoon), inability to carry out activities of daily living, impaired judgment, inappropriate social behavior, lack of insight, repetitive behavior, and a voracious appetite. Given the treatment was late in the day also indicates the likelihood of sundowning.

Incorrect Choices:
Inability to communicate is characteristic of stage 3. Short-term memory loss and disorientation to time and date are early signs of the disease (stage 1).

Type of Reasoning: Analytical
This question provides a group of symptoms and the test taker must determine the most likely cause for them. This requires analysis of the symptoms, which is an analytical reasoning skill. For this situation, the symptoms exhibited are most consistent with sundowning behavior. Review signs and symptoms of sundowning behavior in patients with Alzheimer's disease if answered incorrectly.

A125

System Interactions | Diseases and Conditions Impacting Intervention

An older, frail adult is receiving physical therapy in the home environment to improve general strength and mobility. The patient has a 4-year history of taking NSAIDs (aspirin) for joint pain and recently began taking a calcium-channel blocker. What adverse side effects should the physical therapist assistant be aware of?

Choices:
1. Increased sweating, fatigue, chest pain.
2. Stomach pain, hypertension, confusion.
3. Weight increase, hyperglycemia, hypotension.
4. Paresthesias, incoordination, bradycardia.

Teaching Points

Correct Answer: 2
With advanced age, the capacity of the individual to break down and convert drugs diminishes secondary to decreased liver and kidney function, reduced hepatic and renal blood flow, etc. Some drugs additionally slow metabolism (e.g., calcium-channel blockers). NSAIDs are associated with potential gastrointestinal (GI) effects (stomach pain, peptic ulcers, GI hemorrhage), peripheral edema, and easy bruising and bleeding. NSAIDs can also lessen the effects of antihypertensive drugs. Central nervous system effects can include headache, dizziness, lightheadedness, insomnia, tinnitus, confusion, and depression.

Incorrect Choices:
The other choices are not expected adverse effects of NSAID or calcium-channel blocker usage.

Type of Reasoning: Deductive
This question requires one to recall the adverse side effects of taking both NSAIDs and calcium-channel blockers to arrive at a correct conclusion. This necessitates the recall of factual information, which is a deductive reasoning skill. For this case, the adverse side effects could include stomach pain, hypertension, and confusion. Review adverse effects of NSAIDs and calcium-channel blockers if answered incorrectly.

A126

Neuromuscular | Data Collection

A patient presents with pain, joint swelling, subcutaneous olecranon nodules, and increased erythrocyte sedimentation rate. What condition are these findings characteristic of?

Choices:
1. Rheumatoid arthritis.
2. Fibromyalgia.
3. Systemic lupus erythematosus.
4. Osteoarthritis.

Teaching Points

Correct Answer: 1
Rheumatoid arthritis (RA) is characterized by morning stiffness, pain, and relatively symmetric joint involvement. Laboratory abnormalities in RA include positive serum rheumatoid factor and elevated erythrocyte sedimentation rate. Articular and extraarticular manifestations include weight loss, malaise, nodulosis, and vasculitis. Synovial fluid analysis reveals elevated white blood cell count and protein count.

Incorrect Choices:

Osteoarthritis, or degenerative joint pain, and fibromyalgia both produce pain but do not produce the laboratory findings reported above or nodulosis. Systemic lupus erythematosus (SLE) is an immunologic disorder characterized by inflammatory lesions in multiple organ systems. It is diagnosed by client history (multiple organ involvement, especially of skin, joints, serous membranes), systemic symptoms (e.g., fever, malaise, fatigability) and appearance of skin rash (erythema). Erythrocyte sedimentation rate is elevated in patients with SLE; however, nodulosis and joint malformations are not expected.

Type of Reasoning: Analytical

This question requires the test taker to analyze a group of symptoms to make a determination of the characteristics and likely problem. This requires analytical reasoning skill. For this situation, the symptoms are characteristic of rheumatoid arthritis. If answered incorrectly, review signs and symptoms of rheumatoid arthritis.

A127

System Interaction | Interventions

A patient is exercising in a phase III outpatient cardiac rehabilitation program that utilizes circuit training. One of the stations utilizes weights. The patient lifts a 5-lb weight, holds it for 20 seconds and then lowers it slowly. The physical therapist assistant corrects the activity and tells the patient to reduce the length of the static hold. What can this static exercise expect to produce?

Choices:
1. Abnormal oxygen uptake.
2. Lower heart rate and arterial blood pressure.
3. Higher heart rate and arterial blood pressure.
4. Reduced normal venous return to the heart and elevated blood pressure.

Teaching Points

Correct Answer: 3

Dynamic exercise facilitates circulation whereas isometric (static) exercise hinders blood flow, producing higher heart rates and arterial blood pressures.

Incorrect Choices:

Abnormal oxygen uptake is more likely indicative of a pulmonary issue and lower HR and arterial blood pressure is an abnormal response to exercise that may have a variety of causes.

Type of Reasoning: Inferential

One must infer the likely effects of static exercise for a patient in a cardiac rehabilitation program to arrive at a correct conclusion. This requires inferential reasoning skill, as one must determine what is likely to be true for a patient. For this case, the static exercise can produce a higher heart rate and arterial blood pressure. If answered incorrectly, review effects of static exercise on patients in cardiac rehabilitation programs.

A128

Other Systems | Diseases and Conditions Impacting Intervention

A teenaged child with a 4 year history of type 2 diabetes is insulin dependent and wants to participate in cross-country running. The physical therapist assistant who has previously worked with the athlete in the clinic advises the athlete to measure plasma glucose concentrations before and after running. What other advice should the physical therapist assistant provide the patient?

Choices:
1. Consume a carbohydrate after practice to avoid hyperglycemia.
2. Increase insulin dosage immediately before running.
3. Consume a carbohydrate before or during practice to avoid hypoglycemia.
4. Avoid carbohydrate-rich snacks within 12 hours of a race.

Teaching Points

Correct Answer: 3

During exercise of increasing intensity and duration, plasma concentrations of insulin progressively decrease. Exercise-induced hypoglycemia is the likely result. Hypoglycemia can also occur up to 4–6 hours after exercise. To counteract these effects, the individual may need to reduce insulin dosage or increase carbohydrate intake before or after running. Consuming a carbohydrate product before or during the race will have a preventive modulating effect on hypoglycemia.

Incorrect Choices:

Consuming carbohydrates after practice or avoiding carbohydrate-rich snacks within 12 hours of activity will not appropriately control blood sugar levels. Consuming a carbohydrate after practice helps avoid hypoglycemia not hyperglycemia.

Type of Reasoning: Evaluative

For this question, the test taker must weigh the information provided in the form of advice given to a patient and determine which advice is best aligned with the patient's diagnosis and current needs. This requires evaluative reasoning skill. For this case, the assistant should advise the patient to consume a carbohydrate before or during practice to avoid hypoglycemia. Review exercise guidelines for patients with type 2 diabetes and intervention approaches for exercise-induced hypoglycemia.

A129

Nonsystem | Therapeutic Modalities

An athlete presents with pain and muscle spasm of the upper back (C7–T8) extending to the lateral border of the scapula. This encompasses a 5 cm by 10 cm area on each side of the spine. The ultrasound unit has a 5 cm² sound head. How should the physical therapist assistant administer the ultrasound?

Choices:
1. Covering the entire area in 5 minutes.
2. Covering the entire area in 10 minutes.
3. Along each side allotting 2.5 minutes for each area.
4. Along each side allotting 10 minutes for each area.

Teaching Points

Correct Answer: 4

The total treatment area is too large for the 5 cm² sound head to produce adequate tissue heating. Moving the transducer too fast to cover both sides adequately in the allotted time does not allow sufficient time for the acoustic energy to produce heat because the head is not in a given area long enough. Sonating each side independently, for 10 minutes on each area, will allow enough time to produce sufficient heating within the tissues to help decrease muscle spasm and pain.

Incorrect Choices:

Just increasing the treatment time will not affect the rate of heat production. Two and a half minutes is too brief to produce sufficient therapeutic tissue heating.

Type of Reasoning: Inductive

This question requires one to utilize clinical judgment to determine a best course of action when one is providing ultrasound treatment over a large surface area. This requires knowledge of ultrasound guidelines and judgment about a best approach, which is an inductive reasoning skill. For this case, the assistant should treat each side allotting 5 minutes for each session. Review ultrasound treatment guidelines for the upper back, especially larger surface areas, if answered incorrectly.

A130

Nonsystem | Therapeutic Modalities

A patient with chronic cervical pain is referred to an outpatient physical therapy clinic. Past medical history reveals appendectomy 12 years ago, chronic heart disease, demand-type pacemaker implanted 8 years ago, and whiplash injury 2 years ago. Presently the patient reports pain and muscle spasm in the cervical region. What modality is contraindicated in this case?

Choices:
1. Mechanical traction.
2. Infrared lamp.
3. Hot pack.
4. Transcutaneous electrical stimulation.

Teaching Points

Correct Answer: 4

All electrical stimulation devices are contraindicated when a patient has a demand-type pacemaker. The electrical signals could interfere with the rhythmic signals of the pacemaker.

Incorrect Choices:

The other modalities are not contraindicated in this case.

Type of Reasoning: Deductive

This question requires one to recall the contraindications for treatment modalities with a patient who has a demand-type pacemaker. This necessitates the recall of factual guidelines, which is a deductive reasoning skill. For this situation, the modality that is contraindicated is transcutaneous electrical stimulation, as the signals can interfere with the pacemaker signals. If answered incorrectly, review use of modalities with patients who have demand-type pacemakers.

A131

Cardiac | Diseases and Conditions Impacting Intervention

A patient in a cardiac exercise class develops muscle weakness and fatigue. The physical therapist's examination reveals lower-extremity cramps and hyporeflexia. The patient also experiences frequent episodes of postural hypotension and dizziness. There are some abnormalities on the electrocardiogram. What do these findings suggest?

Choices:
1. Hyperkalemia.
2. Hypocalcemia.
3. Hyponatremia.
4. Hypokalemia.

Teaching Points

Correct Answer: 4

Hypokalemia, decreased potassium in the blood, is characterized by the above signs and symptoms. Other possible symptoms include respiratory distress, irritability, confusion or depression, and gastrointestinal disturbances. Electrocardiogram abnormalities would include flat T wave, prolonged QT interval, and depressed ST segment.

Incorrect Choices:

Hyperkalemia is excess potassium in the blood and may present with widened PR interval and QRS and tachycardia. Hyponatremia is decreased sodium in the blood which presents with hypotension and tachycardia, and hypocalcemia is decreased calcium in the blood which presents with arrhythmias and hypotension.

Type of Reasoning: Analytical

This question provides a group of symptoms and the test taker must analyze the symptoms to make a determination of the likely diagnosis. This requires analytical reasoning skill. For this situation, the symptoms are characteristic of hypokalemia or low blood potassium. If answered incorrectly, review signs and symptoms of hypokalemia.

A132

Other Systems | Diseases and Conditions Impacting Intervention

A patient has a 5 year history of acquired immunodeficiency syndrome (AIDS). The case worker reports that the patient has had a gradual increase in difficulty with walking. The patient rarely goes out anymore. A referral to physical therapy is initiated. The physical therapist assistant has been directed to provide functional training including bed mobility and transfer training. The physical therapist assistant would expect which of the following neuromuscular symptoms with this patient?

Choices:
1. Paraplegia or tetraplegia.
2. Widespread sensory loss resulting in sensory ataxia.
3. Motor ataxia and paresis with pronounced gait disturbances.
4. Progressive rigidity and akinesia with severe balance disturbances.

Teaching Points

Correct Answer: 3
Alterations in memory, confusion and disorientation are characteristic of AIDS dementia complex, a common central nervous system manifestation of HIV infection. Motor deficits may include ataxia, paresis with gait disturbances, and loss of fine motor coordination. Patients may also develop peripheral neuropathy with distal pain and sensory loss.

Incorrect Choices:
Paraparesis (not paraplegia) might be a finding. The sensory loss is not widespread but is in similar distribution of peripheral neuropathies. Rigidity and akinesia are not associated with AIDS.

Type of Reasoning: Inferential
This question requires the test taker to infer the likely neuromuscular symptoms for a patient with AIDS. This requires inferential reasoning skill, as one must determine what is likely to be true. For this case, the assistant should expect motor ataxia and paresis with pronounced gait disturbances. If answered incorrectly, review neuromuscular symptoms associated with AIDS.

A133

Neuromuscular | Data Collection

A physical therapist assistant is working with a postal worker who reports numbness and tingling in the right hand. Symptoms are reported on the palm, the palmar surface of the first two fingers, and the pad of the thumb. Which nerve should the physical therapist assistant report that the patient was demonstrating diminished sensation in?

Choices:
1. Radial nerve.
2. Ulnar nerve.
3. Median nerve.
4. Accessory nerve.

Teaching Points

Correct Answer: 3
The symptoms best typify median nerve distribution.

Incorrect Choices:
Sensory distribution of the radial nerve covers the dorsum of the thumb and dorsal surface of the thumb and first two fingers. The ulnar nerve covers the thenar eminence, little finger, and medial border of the ring finger.

Type of Reasoning: Deductive
One must recall the symptoms of median nerve dysfunction to arrive at a correct conclusion. This requires the recall of factual symptoms and guidelines, which is a deductive reasoning skill. For this case, the symptoms typify median nerve dysfunction, which should be reviewed if answered incorrectly.

A134

Musculoskeletal | Diseases and Conditions Impacting Intervention

Four weeks following a cesarean section a patient tells the physical therapist assistant she is anxious to return to her pre-pregnancy physical activity level of running 5 miles and 3 times per week weight lifting classes. What is the **BEST** recommendation the physical therapist assistant should provide the patient?

Choices:
1. Begin running and weight lifting at this time.
2. Gentle pelvic floor exercise may begin at 6–8 weeks post surgery.
3. Core and abdominal strengthening can begin at 4–6 weeks post surgery.
4. Begin a walking program now, progress to running in 2 weeks.

Teaching Points

Correct Answer: 2

It is too soon to begin strengthening exercises or running. Pelvic floor exercises can begin at post-op weeks 6–8.

Incorrect Choices:

Weight lifting, advanced core exercises, abdominal strengthening, and running should be avoided for a minimum of 6–8 weeks and may not be well tolerated yet at that point.

Type of Reasoning: Evaluative

One must weigh the merits of the courses of action presented and determine which response best addresses the patient's needs and desires. This requires evaluative reasoning skill. For this case, the assistant should tell the patient to complete pelvic floor and gentle abdominal exercises for the first 4–6 weeks. If answered incorrectly, review post-cesarean exercises and restrictions.

A135

Neuromuscular | Diseases and Conditions Impacting Intervention

What is reasonable to expect for a young child with Down Syndrome?

Choices:
1. Learn to walk by age 6 or 7 years.
2. Learn to walk by age 2 or 3 years.
3. Be unable to walk independently.
4. Keep up with typically developing peers in walking skills.

Teaching Points

Correct Answer: 2

Research shows that most children with Down syndrome learn to walk by the time they are 2–3 years of age. Initially they are delayed in their gross motor skill development compared with their typically developing peers.

Incorrect Choices:

Children with Down syndrome typically can walk independently, and are able to do so by age 3. Children with Down syndrome do achieve their gross motor milestones, but most often these milestones are delayed.

Type of Reasoning: Inferential
This question requires one to determine what may be true for a child with Down syndrome. Questions of this nature often require inferential reasoning skill. For this situation, one can expect a child with Down syndrome to learn to walk by age 2. If answered incorrectly, review developmental milestones and expectations for children with Down syndrome, especially motor skills such as walking.

A136

Musculoskeletal | Interventions

During treatment for chronic shoulder pain in a recreational swimmer, the assistant observes excessive medial (internal) rotation of the shoulders and winging of the scapula during overhead motion. The physical therapist diagnosis is chronic shoulder impingement. What should the physical therapist assistant focus on to restore balance between the anterior chest muscles and posterior trunk muscles?

Choices:
1. Strengthening of pectoral muscles and stretching of upper trapezius.
2. Strengthening of upper trapezius and stretching of pectoral muscles.
3. Strengthening middle and lower trapezius and stretching of pectoral muscles.
4. Strengthening of rhomboids and stretching of upper trapezius.

Teaching Points

Correct Answer: 3
Abnormal posture that produces excessive medial (internal) rotation of the shoulders may result in chronic shoulder impingement syndrome attributable to a loss of scapular stability with overhead motion. Shoulder pain is likely to continue until a balance between anterior and posterior trunk musculature is achieved.

Incorrect Choices:
The anterior chest muscles (pectorals) are shortened and need stretching and posterior trunk muscles (middle and lower trapezius) are stretched and need strengthening.

Type of Reasoning: Inductive
This question requires clinical judgment to determine a best course of action for a patient with chronic shoulder impingement. This requires inductive reasoning skill. For this case, the assistant should focus on strengthening middle and lower trapezius and stretching of pectoral muscles. If answered incorrectly, review treatment approaches for chronic shoulder impingement and loss of scapular stability.

A137

Musculoskeletal | Data Collection

The diagram shown is **MOST** consistent with what condition?

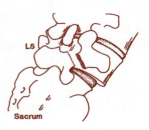

Twomey L, Taylor J (2000) Physical Therapy of the Low Back, 3rd ed. Philadelphia, Churchill Livingstone, Figure 7-1, page 204, with permission.

Choices:
1. Herniated disc.
2. Degenerative joint disease.
3. Stenosis.
4. Spondylolisthesis.

Teaching Points

Correct Answer: 4

The diagram indicates an anterior slippage of one vertebra on the vertebra below, the definition of spondylolisthesis.

Incorrect Choices:

Stenosis is the narrowing of the vertebral canal, which is not visible in the diagram. Neither degenerative joint disease nor a herniated disc are visible on the diagram.

Type of Reasoning: Analytical

This question requires one to analyze the information presented in a diagram to determine the most likely condition the diagram depicts. Questions that require one to analyze information in the form of pictures, charts, and diagrams often necessitate analytical reasoning skill. For this case, the diagram depicts spondylolisthesis. Review signs and symptoms of spondylolisthesis if answered incorrectly.

A138

Musculoskeletal | Diseases and Conditions Impacting Intervention

A physical therapist assistant is working with an office worker, who is a long-term smoker who now has emphysema. The physical therapist diagnosis and treatment plan includes intervention and patient education for thoracic outlet syndrome. The patient reports increased pain and tingling in bilateral hands after sitting at a desk for longer than 1 hour. What should the physical therapist assistant focus treatment on?

Choices:
1. Stretching the pectoralis major and rhomboid muscles.
2. Stretching of the scalenes and pectoralis minor muscles.
3. Stretching the wrist and finger flexors.
4. Stretching of the biceps brachii and brachialis.

Teaching Points

Correct Answer: 2

Patients with emphysema typically present with hypertrophy of the accessory breathing muscles that include the scalenes, which can compress the neurovascular structures of the thoracic outlet; the pectoralis minor can also compress these structures.

Incorrect Choices:

Stretching of the biceps, brachialis, or wrist and finger flexors will not address the cause of the symptoms due to thoracic outlet syndrome. The rhomboids are posterior and not involved in the thoracic outlet.

Type of Reasoning: Inductive

This question requires clinical judgment to determine a best course of action for a patient with emphysema and thoracic outlet syndrome. This requires knowledge of the diagnosis and therapeutic approaches, which is an inductive reasoning skill. For this case, the assistant should focus on stretching of the scalenes and pectoralis minor muscles. If answered incorrectly, review treatment approaches for emphysema and thoracic outlet syndrome.

A139

Other Systems | Diseases and Conditions Impacting Intervention

A physical therapist assistant is working with an individual with a diagnosis of low back pain, degenerative disc disease, and gastroesophageal reflux disease. The patient reports that at night upon going to bed the exercises have resulted in upset stomach and inability to sleep very well. The assistant should instruct the patient to:

Choices:
1. Avoid doing the exercises.
2. Drink plenty of water throughout the day.
3. Sleep in the supine position.
4. Avoid eating large meals later in the day.

Teaching Points

Correct Answer: 4
Patients who suffer from gastroesophageal reflux disease (GERD) should eat smaller meals; avoiding meals close to bed or exercise time can help as well. Sleeping with the head of their bed elevated can help decrease the symptoms.

Incorrect Choices:
The supine position should be avoided. Exercising with the upper trunk supported in the elevated position is also recommended. Avoiding exercise will not necessarily help the low back pain. Drinking plenty of water can help decrease the chances of constipation but does not affect reflux.

Type of Reasoning: Inductive
This question requires one to first determine the cause for the patient's symptoms and then to choose an appropriate course of action. This necessitates clinical judgment, which is an inductive reasoning skill. For this case, the assistant should recommend that the patient avoid eating large meals to alleviate symptoms. Review signs and symptoms of GERD, as well as approaches to alleviating symptoms, if answered incorrectly.

A140

Other Systems | Diseases and Conditions Impacting Intervention

An obese individual who has diabetes is coming to physical therapy to participate in a conditioning program. What should the physical therapist assistant instruct the participant to do?

Choices:
1. Eat a carbohydrate-balanced snack at least 2 hours prior to participating in the conditioning program.
2. Avoid eating foods for several hours prior to participating in the conditioning program.
3. Inject insulin into the large muscle groups such as the quadriceps prior to participating in the conditioning program.
4. Participate in the conditioning program when blood glucose levels are greater than 300 mg/dL.

Teaching Points

Correct Answer: 1
Eating a carbohydrate-balanced snack at least 2 hours prior to participating in the conditioning program will help to ensure regulation of blood sugars.

Incorrect Choices:
Insulin injections should be given in muscles that are not going to be used heavily during exercises; an abdominal injection is recommended, not the quadriceps as those will be used during exercise. Participation in exercise programs is contraindicated with fasting blood glucose levels greater than 300 mg/dL, or less than 70 mg/dL.

Type of Reasoning: Evaluative
One must weigh the merits of the courses of action presented and then determine the response that will most effectively address the patient's needs. This requires evaluative reasoning skill. For this situation, the assistant should recommend that the patient eat a carbohydrate-balanced snack at least 2 hours prior to participating in the conditioning program. Review guidelines for conditioning programs for patients with diabetes and obesity, as well as regulation of blood sugars with exercise, if answered incorrectly.

A141

Musculoskeletal | Diseases and Conditions Impacting Intervention

During the first 8 weeks following a central zone repair of the lateral meniscus, what activity is contraindicated?

Choices:
1. Full active knee extension.
2. Muscle setting exercises.
3. Partial weight bearing at 25%.
4. Knee flexion greater than 60°–70°.

Teaching Points

Correct Answer: 4
Central zone repairs of the meniscus are progressed more conservatively than peripheral zone repairs. Flexion beyond 60°–70° places posterior translation forces on the repaired meniscus, thus increasing the risk of displacement. Muscle setting and A-AAROM exercises begin the day after surgery.

Incorrect Choices:
Restriction of full active knee extension exercises are part of the protocol following anterior cruciate ligament repair, not following meniscus repair. Muscle setting exercises and weight bearing limited to 25% do not present a contraindication following meniscus injury.

Type of Reasoning: Deductive
One must recall the contraindications for activity after a central zone repair of the lateral meniscus. This requires the recall of factual guidelines, which is a deductive reasoning skill. For this scenario, the patient should avoid knee flexion greater than 60°–70°. If answered incorrectly, review contraindications and activity limitations for patients with central zone repair of the lateral meniscus.

A142

Other Systems | Diseases and Conditions Impacting Intervention

A physical therapist assistant is providing home care for an older adult patient. Upon arrival, the assistant notices that the patient is confused. The patient's skin color is pale and the turgor is poor. The patient reports an intestinal upset for the past few days with frequent vomiting and diarrhea. What is the physical therapist assistant's **BEST** course of action?

Choices:
1. Monitor vital signs; if heart rate is not elevated, get the patient up and walking.
2. Notify the family, and insist that the patient not be alone until the illness is over.
3. Cancel therapy for today, carefully document the findings and notify the physician.
4. Give the patient water and notify the physician and physical therapist immediately.

Teaching Points

Correct Answer: 4

The patient is exhibiting signs of dehydration. Confusion is a red flag and requires immediate action: administer fluids and notify the physician and therapist immediately.

Incorrect Choices:

Getting the patient up and walking or warning the family to stay with the patient will not address the dehydration. This situation can develop into a medical emergency and needs immediate medical attention.

Type of Reasoning: Evaluative

One must first analyze the symptoms and then weigh the courses of action to determine the best approach that effectively meets the patient's needs. This requires evaluative reasoning skill. For this case, the patient's symptoms are those of dehydration and the assistant should give the patient water and notify the physician and physical therapist immediately. If answered incorrectly, review signs and symptoms of dehydration as well as first aid approaches for this diagnosis.

A143

Neuromuscular | Data Collection

How should a physical therapist assistant assess a patient's ability to perceive light touch?

Choices:
1. Lightly brush a cotton ball across the area being tested.
2. Lightly touch the tip of a pin on the area being tested.
3. Lightly touch the blunt end of a paper clip on the area being tested.
4. Lightly apply pressure through the tip of a cotton swab on the area being tested.

Teaching Points

Correct Answer: 1

Light touch sensations are tested by brushing the tip of a cotton swab or camel hair brush across the area being tested. The clinician asks the patient to identify by a "yes" or "no" response after the stimulus has been provided.

Incorrect Choices:

The sharp end of a pin or the tip of a straightened paper clip test the patient's ability to perceive pain, the blunt ends of the pin or paper clip are used to assess dull sensation. Pressure applied through the tip of a cotton swab tests pressure sensation. All of these tests assess superficial-level sensations.

Type of Reasoning: Deductive

One must recall the procedures for testing light touch to arrive at a correct conclusion. This necessitates the recall of procedures and guidelines, which is a deductive reasoning skill. For this case, the assistant should brush a cotton ball across the area being tested. If answered incorrectly, review light touch testing procedures.

A144

Musculoskeletal | Interventions

A patient with a traumatic injury to the right hand had a flexor tendon repair to the fingers. When should physical therapy intervention begin?

Choices:
1. After the splint is removed 2–3 weeks to allow full active range of motion of all affected joints.
2. After the splint is removed 4–6 weeks to allow ample healing time for the repaired tendon.
3. Within a few days following surgery to preserve tendon gliding.
4. Within a few days following surgery to allow for early initiation of strengthening exercises.

Teaching Points

Correct Answer: 3

Early passive and active assistive exercises promote collagen remodeling to allow free tendon gliding. When rehabilitation is delayed by several weeks, adhesions form, which restrict free tendon gliding.

Incorrect Choices:

Early initiation of strengthening is not indicated. Waiting two weeks or more to remove the splint and initiate movement is very likely to result in adhesions and restriction of tendon gliding motions.

Type of Reasoning: Inferential

One must infer or draw a reasonable conclusion about the likely intervention approach for a patient with a flexor tendon repair to the fingers. This requires one to determine what may be true of a situation, which is an inferential reasoning skill. For this situation, one should expect interventions to begin within a few days following surgery to preserve tendon gliding. Review intervention approaches for patients with flexor tendon repair if answered incorrectly.

A145

Pulmonary | Data Collection

A physical therapist assistant is gait training a patient who has obstructive pulmonary disease. When assessing the patient's respiratory status what should the physical therapist assistant expect to find?

Choices:
1. The thorax size decreased.
2. Decreased rib excursion with respirations.
3. An uneven rise between the two sides of the thorax.
4. A decreased respiratory rate.

Teaching Points

Correct Answer: 2

Persons with obstructive lung diseases will typically present with decreased rib excursion during respirations and an enlarged thorax, especially in the advanced stages. This occurs secondary to the loss of elastic recoil of the lung tissues.

Incorrect Choices:

One would expect an uneven rise in the thorax if a lung or portion of a lung were collapsed, filled with fluid, or compromised, not in a person with obstructive lung disease. Persons with chronic obstructive pulmonary disease will present with increased and more shallow respirations.

Type of Reasoning: Inferential

This question requires the test taker to determine what is likely to be true for a patient with obstructive pulmonary disease. This requires inferential reasoning skill. For this scenario, the assistant should find decreased rib excursion with respirations. If answered incorrectly, review signs and symptoms associated with obstructive lung disease.

A146

Neuromuscular | Data Collection

A patient is recovering from a left transtibial amputation and reports numbness and tingling of the left great toe and on the dorsum of the left foot. The patient knows the extremity is gone and cannot understand why this is happening. The physical therapist assistant informs the physical therapist of the patient's newly reported symptom. The therapist suspects the source of discomfort is MOST likely pressure from residual limb wrapping and asks the assistant to check to make sure there is NO pressure on the peripheral nerve. The physical therapist assistant should check for pressure on which peripheral nerve?

Choices:
1. Sural nerve.
2. Medial calcaneal nerve.
3. Tibial nerve.
4. Common peroneal (fibular) nerve.

Teaching Points

Correct Answer: 4

The common peroneal nerve supplies sensation to the dorsal foot and big toe. Phantom limb sensation (sensation of an extremity that is no longer there) usually occurs in the immediate postoperative phase and can be stimulated by external pressure (residual limb wrapping or rigid dressing). It typically dissipates over time though some patients may experience the sensation for the rest of their lives. This is a common finding and should not interfere with prosthetic rehabilitation.

Incorrect Choices:

Sensation to the dorsum of the foot and big toe is supplied by the superficial peroneal (fibular) nerve, a branch off the common peroneal (fibular) nerve. The sural nerve is a distal branch of the tibial nerve that supplies the back of the lower extremity and the lateral side of the foot and little toe. The medial calcaneal nerve is also a branch of the tibial nerve that supplies the heel and medial sole of the foot.

Type of Reasoning: Analytical

This question requires the test taker to analyze the symptoms to determine the likely nerve that is affected. This requires analytical reasoning skill. For this situation, the assistant should test the common peroneal (fibular) nerve for pressure, as symptoms indicate dysfunction of this nerve. If answered incorrectly, review signs and symptoms of dysfunction of the common peroneal nerve.

A147

Neuromuscular | Interventions

A patient who sustained a complete spinal cord injury at the level of T10 is ready to begin community wheelchair training. The plan of care includes instructions in wheelchair skills to manage curbs. What is the **BEST** strategy to provide the patient?

Choices:
1. Throw their head and trunk backward to rise up on the large wheels.
2. Place hand on the top of the handrims to steady the chair while throwing the head and trunk forward.
3. Lean backward while moving the hands slowly backward on the rims.
4. Grasp the handrims posteriorly and pull them forward abruptly and forcefully.

Teaching Points

Correct Answer: 4
In order for a wheelchair user to manage curbs the patient needs to learn to "pop a wheelie." A wheelie can be assumed by having the patient place the hands posterior on the handrims and pulling them abruptly and sharply forward. If the patient is unable to lift the casters in this manner, he or she can throw the head back forcefully when pulling the handrims. An alternate technique is to grasp the handrims anteriorly, pull backward, then abruptly and forcefully reverse the direction of pull. The therapist can assist by steadying the chair at the patient's balance point until he or she learns to adjust the position through the use of handrim movements forward and backward.

Incorrect Choices:
In order to perform a wheelie more than just leaning or throwing the body back is needed. The rims need to be forcefully and abruptly moved.

Type of Reasoning: Inductive
One must recall guidelines for curb management using a wheelchair and then utilize clinical judgment to determine the best course of action for teaching a patient with T10 paraplegia to manage curbs. This requires inductive reasoning skill. For this case, the assistant should instruct the patient to grasp the handrims posteriorly and pull them forward abruptly and forcefully. If answered incorrectly, review curb management techniques with wheelchairs.

A148

Nonsystem | Therapeutic Modalities

A patient presents with multiple fractures of both hands and wrists as a result of a mountain bike accident. Now, 5 weeks later, the patient has limited wrist and finger motion, and dry scaly skin over the previously casted areas. What physical agent is **MOST** appropriate to aid in increasing range of motion?

Choices:
1. Paraffin.
2. Hot packs.
3. Functional electrical stimulation.
4. Contact ultrasound.

Teaching Points

Correct Answer: 1
Paraffin bath will provide circumferential heating of the hands and fingers and will aid in softening the skin.

Incorrect Choices:
Active exercise, including functional electrical stimulation, would be more effective after the application of paraffin as tissue extensibility and pliability would be increased. Hot packs or ultrasound using direct contact would not completely cover the area to be treated.

Type of Reasoning: Inductive
This question requires clinical judgment to determine a best course of action to address the patient's symptoms. This is an inductive reasoning skill. For this situation, the most appropriate modality choice to increase range of motion is paraffin. If answered incorrectly, review indications for use of paraffin, especially for increasing range of motion.

A149

Musculoskeletal | Interventions

A male child who plays catcher on his baseball team complains of bilateral knee pain that is exacerbated with forceful quadriceps contraction. The physical therapist examination noted pain and swelling at the distal attachment of the patellar tendon. The therapist has instructed the physical therapist assistant to begin treatment that addresses the pain and swelling. What should **EARLY** management focus on?

Choices:
1. Isometric exercises to decrease inflammation.
2. Active range of motion exercises to prevent contracture.
3. Decreased loading of the knee by the quadriceps femoris muscle.
4. Casting followed by decreased loading of the knee.

Teaching Points

Correct Answer: 3
Baseball catchers must make forceful contractions of the quadriceps muscles each time they stand up to throw the ball to the pitcher. This may precipitate Osgood–Schlatter disease in the adolescent boy. Early intervention of this condition focuses on reduction of the loading by the quadriceps but still retaining normal lower-extremity function.

Incorrect Choices:
Isometric exercises and active range will still "stress" the patella tendon/tibial tubercle causing continued irritation and pain. Casting is not indicated as you do not want to immobilize the limb.

Type of Reasoning: Inductive
This question requires the test taker to determine a best course of action for a child with bilateral knee pain and swelling. This requires clinical judgment, which is an inductive reasoning skill. For this case, the assistant should focus on decreased loading of the knee by the quadriceps femoris muscle. If answered incorrectly, review intervention approaches for knee pain associated with forceful contractions of the quadriceps.

A150

System Interactions | Diseases and Conditions Impacting Intervention

A patient who is 70 pounds overweight is recovering from a myocardial infarction, which occurred 6 weeks ago. The plan of care includes exercise class in conjunction with dietary program to promote weight reduction. Which exercise protocol is **MOST** appropriate for this patient?

Choices:
1. Jogging, for 10 minutes at 4 miles per hour.
2. Walking, intensity set at 50% target heart rate.
3. Walking, intensity set at 75% of heart rate reserve.
4. Swimming, intensity set at 75% age-adjusted heart rate.

Teaching Points

Correct Answer: 2
Obese individuals are typically more sedentary with lower initial levels of physical conditioning. The initial exercise prescription should focus on a lower intensity exercise progressing to longer durations.

Incorrect Choices:
Higher intensity exercise (75% or 85% of heart rate maximum) should be avoided initially. Jogging is also too intense and may yield additional orthopedic problems. Swimming at 75% age-adjusted heart rate is too intense for this individual.

Type of Reasoning: Inductive
One must have knowledge of exercise and reconditioning approaches for patients with obesity to arrive at a correct conclusion. This requires inductive reasoning skill, as clinical judgment is paramount to arriving at a correct conclusion. For this situation, the most appropriate protocol for exercise should include walking with the intensity set at 50% target heart rate. Review exercise guidelines for patients with obesity if answered incorrectly.

Examination B

B1

Musculoskeletal | Interventions

The physical therapist's evaluation of a patient's gait identifies the patient as having a positive Trendelenburg sign on the right. The plan of care includes functional activities for strengthening the affected musculature. Which of the following treatments **BEST** addresses the weakness?

Choices:
1. Bridging.
2. Lateral step-ups bilaterally.
3. Quadruped leg extension.
4. Supine hip abduction.

Teaching Points

Correct Answer: 2

A Trendelenburg gait pattern is the result of weak hip abductors, specifically the gluteus medius. Lateral step-ups bilaterally will increase the strength of the gluteus medius muscle, both on the weight-bearing limb and the lower extremity performing the step-up.

Incorrect Choices:
Supine hip abduction would not likely strengthen the gluteus medius enough to improve the patient's gait as gravity is not a factor. Bridging increases hip extensor strength. Quadruped leg extension increases strength of both the gluteus maximus and the hamstrings.

Type of Reasoning: Inductive
One must determine the best exercise for a patient, given the diagnosis provided. This is an inductive reasoning skill, where clinical judgment is utilized to draw conclusions. For this patient with a Trendelenburg gait pattern, the best intervention approach to address the weakness is lateral step-ups bilaterally. If answered incorrectly, review signs and symptoms of Trendelenburg gait pattern as well as exercises for this diagnosis.

B2

Neuromuscular | Interventions

A patient has muscle weakness in elbow flexion pronation and supination; strength of the forearm is normal. Which of the following muscles **MOST** likely requires strengthening?

Choices:
1. Brachialis.
2. Biceps brachii.
3. Brachioradialis.
4. Coracobrachialis.

Teaching Points

Correct Answer: 1

The brachialis is the only muscle listed that solely performs elbow flexion.

Incorrect Choices:

Because the actions of pronation and supination are normal the muscles that perform that motion, biceps brachii (supination) and brachioradialis (pronation), are not implicated. The coracobrachialis performs shoulder flexion and adduction.

Type of Reasoning: Analytical

One must analyze the symptoms presented and then draw a conclusion about what these symptoms represent. This requires analytical reasoning skill, where various pieces of information are analyzed to draw a correct conclusion. In this case, the pattern of weakness indicates that the brachialis muscle is weak and requires strengthening. Review symptoms of brachialis weakness if answered incorrectly.

B3

Neuromuscular | Interventions

A child with cerebral palsy has persistence of the symmetrical tonic neck reflex. What should the physical therapist assistant do to facilitate the child's ability to maintain stability in the quadruped position during treatment?

Choices:
1. Turn the head to the non-dominant side.
2. Tap on the paraspinal musculature.
3. Apply approximation to both shoulders.
4. Keep the chin elevated.

Teaching Points

Correct Answer: 4

If the symmetrical tonic neck reflex persists, elevating the chin will cause the upper extremities to extend and the lower extremities to flex, thus helping to maintain the quadruped position.

Incorrect Choices:

Turning the head toward the non-dominant side will increase awareness of the non-dominant side. Tapping on the paraspinal musculature is appropriate if the goal is to increase trunk extension. Applying approximation through the shoulder joint can stimulate increased firing of the shoulder joint musculature but will not assist with hip control.

Type of Reasoning: Inductive

One must determine the position that will maintain stability in the quadruped position in a child with cerebral palsy. This requires inductive reasoning skill, a skill that requires clinical judgment to determine a best course of action. In this case, a child with symmetrical tonic neck reflex in the quadruped position should keep the chin elevated to maintain stability in this position. If answered incorrectly, review symmetrical tonic neck reflex, especially head positioning for quadruped stability.

B4

Nonsystem | Therapeutic Modalities

As part of a home program, a patient is using a mechanical cervical traction unit. When the physical therapist assistant arrives, the patient indicates that the cervical condition is improving; however, there is now discomfort in the area of the occiput. Which of the following is the MOST appropriate response?

Choices:
1. Have the patient demonstrate the procedure used, and check to see if the setup is correct.
2. Instruct the patient to place a soft pad between the teeth during traction.
3. Have the patient discontinue the traction.
4. Have the patient decrease the amount of weight used during traction.

Teaching Points

Correct Answer: 1
In this situation, the most likely cause of the discomfort is inappropriate application of the traction. The physical therapist assistant should assess whether the patient is setting up the traction machine correctly.

Incorrect Choices:
There should be no traction force applied through the mandible, and soft pads between the teeth are inappropriate in any situation while using cervical traction. The decision to discontinue is inappropriate if setup has not been assessed. Decreasing the weight may make the traction ineffective and does not address the cause of the discomfort.

Type of Reasoning: Inductive
This question requires one to utilize clinical judgment to determine a best course of action for a patient with discomfort after using mechanical cervical traction. This necessitates inductive reasoning skill. For this case, the assistant should have the patient demonstrate the procedure used and check to see if the setup is correct. Review guidelines for mechanical cervical traction and setup if answered incorrectly.

B5

Musculoskeletal | Interventions

The plan of care calls for manual stretch of a patient's piriformis muscle. Which patient position will BEST accomplish this stretch?

Choices:
1. Supine with the hip flexed to 70° and the knee extended.
2. Side-lying with hip extended and medially (internally) rotated.
3. Side-lying with the hip abducted and laterally (externally) rotated.
4. Supine with the hip flexed to 70° and adducted.

Teaching Points

Correct Answer: 4
Because of its attachments, the piriformis is best elongated and stretched with the hip in a flexed and adducted position.

Incorrect Choices:

The position of 70° hip flexion with knee extension will provide a stretch to the hamstrings. Hip extension and medial (internal) rotation places the piriformis on slack. Hip abduction and lateral rotation will stretch the adductor group.

Type of Reasoning: Deductive

One must recall the guidelines for manual stretch of the piriformis muscle to arrive at a correct conclusion. This is factual information, which requires deductive reasoning skill. For this case, the therapist should position the patient in supine with the hip flexed and laterally (externally) rotated. Review hip-stretching exercises, especially for the piriformis muscle, if answered incorrectly.

B6

Cardiac I Interventions

Four weeks after a myocardial infarction, a patient enters an outpatient physical therapy cardiac rehabilitation program. Now that the patient is in phase 2, what should be the predominant focus of the exercise sessions?

Choices:
1. Low-level weight training using a starting weight at one repetition maximum.
2. Circuit training using various upper-extremity resistance devices.
3. Continuous aerobic activities using large muscle groups.
4. Recreational activities such as running and basketball.

Teaching Points

Correct Answer: 3

Functional work capacity during phase 2 of cardiac rehabilitation is typically determined by metabolic equivalents (METs). When beginning phase 2, activities of 4 to 5 METs are typically used with an exit to phase 3 when the patient can complete activities of 9 METs. Additionally, the goal is to improve the patient's cardiovascular fitness, which is best completed with continuous aerobic activities taxing large muscle groups.

Incorrect Choices:

Completing activities at the patient's one repetition max is inappropriate and does not classify as low level. At the beginning of phase 2 and only 4 weeks after a myocardial infarction, resistive upper-extremity activities are contraindicated. Running and basketball are 8 to 9 METs and are therefore inappropriate at the beginning of phase 2.

Type of Reasoning: Deductive

One must recall factual guidelines of outpatient cardiac rehabilitation to arrive at a correct conclusion. Recall of factual guidelines requires deductive reasoning skill. For this question, the focus for exercise in phase 2 rehabilitation should be continuous aerobic activities using large muscle groups. If answered incorrectly, review cardiac rehabilitation guidelines, especially for phase 2.

B7

Nonsystem | Professional Responsibilities

A physical therapist assistant has just completed instructing a family member in how to transfer a patient from bed to wheelchair and back to bed. The physical therapist assistant needs to document in the **SOAP** note the family member's ability to complete the transfer. What section of the **SOAP** note should this be documented in?

Choices:
1. Subjective.
2. Objective.
3. Assessment.
4. Plan.

Teaching Points

Correct Answer: 3

The Assessment section is the appropriate location for an assistant's interpretation of the treatment session. In this situation, the assistant is utilizing multiple pieces of data to interpret the family member's ability to perform the transfer.

Incorrect Choices:

Subjective information is information provided by the patient or the family member. The Objective portion of the note includes a description of the technique taught to the family member. The Plan section should identify if further training of the family member is planned or indicated.

Type of Reasoning: Deductive

This question requires a test taker to recall the factual guidelines for **SOAP** note documentation. Factual guidelines often necessitate deductive reasoning skill. For this situation, the family member's ability to complete the transfer should be documented in the Assessment section of the **SOAP** note. If answered incorrectly, review **SOAP** note documentation guidelines, including information to be placed in the Assessment section.

B8

Cardiac | Diseases and Conditions Impacting Intervention

A physical therapist assistant treating a patient with congestive heart failure should be alert for signs of digitalis toxicity. Which of the following systems will **MOST** likely be affected?

Choices:
1. Gastrointestinal and central nervous systems.
2. Genitourinary and endocrine systems.
3. Pulmonary and genitourinary systems.
4. Gastrointestinal and integumentary systems.

Teaching Points

Correct Answer: 1

Digitalis toxicity is a somewhat common and potentially fatal adverse reaction. The central nervous system is often impacted with drowsiness, confusion, headache, and visual disturbances. The gastrointestinal system reactions can be in the form of vomiting, diarrhea, and nausea.

Incorrect Choices:
Adverse reactions to digitalis do not affect the genitourinary, integumentary, endocrine, and pulmonary systems.

Type of Reasoning: Deductive
One must recall the signs of digitalis medication toxicity to arrive at a correct conclusion. This is factual information, which is a deductive reasoning skill. For this scenario, the assistant should monitor the patient for adverse reactions affecting the gastrointestinal and central nervous systems, which are symptoms indicating toxicity. If answered incorrectly, review side effects of taking digitalis medication and signs of toxicity.

B9

Nonsystem | Safety & Protection

In an acute care center, a physical therapist assistant is gait training an adult patient who falls to the floor and is unresponsive. The assistant calls a nurse standing nearby and activates the emergency system in the hospital. The assistant assesses the airway, breathing, and circulation and finds a weak, thready pulse and no respirations. What should the assistant do next?

Choices:
1. Respirations at one breath every 15 seconds.
2. Chest compressions at 15 per minute.
3. Respirations at one breath every 5 seconds.
4. Chest compressions at 60–80 per minute.

Teaching Points

Correct Answer: 3
Following the assessment, the physical therapist assistant has identified the patient is not breathing but the heart is still beating. The physical therapist assistant should begin rescue breathing, providing respirations at one breath every 5 seconds.

Incorrect Choices:
Chest compressions are inappropriate at this time as the patient has a pulse, even if it is weak and thready. Respirations at one breath every 15 seconds will not allow for enough oxygen to be introduced to the body.

Type of Reasoning: Deductive
This question requires a test taker to recall the factual guidelines for the administration of cardiopulmonary resuscitation (CPR). Factual guidelines often necessitate deductive reasoning skill. For this situation, after assessing the airway, breathing, and circulation, the assistant should begin respirations at one breath every 5 seconds. If answered incorrectly, review CPR guidelines.

B10

Musculoskeletal | Diseases and Conditions Impacting Intervention

The physical therapist has established a plan of care for a patient with rheumatoid arthritis affecting the hands. Which of the following conditions is **MOST** likely present?

Choices:
1. Stiffness of the fingers of short duration.
2. Osteophytes.
3. Radial drift of the metacarpophalangeal joints.
4. Bilateral symmetrical deformities.

Teaching Points

Correct Answer: 4
Bilateral symmetrical deformities are characteristic of rheumatoid arthritis.

Incorrect Choices:
Short-duration stiffness and bone spurs are characteristic of osteoarthritis. The metacarpophalangeal joints often have ulnar drift, not radial drift.

Type of Reasoning: Inferential
This question provides a diagnosis in which the test taker must determine the most likely symptoms. Questions of this nature often require inferential reasoning skill, which requires one to determine what is most likely to be true of a situation. For this situation, the symptom most consistent with rheumatoid arthritis of the hands is bilateral symmetrical deformities. If answered incorrectly, review symptoms of rheumatoid arthritis, especially those affecting the hands.

B11

Cardiovascular | Diseases and Conditions Impacting Intervention

A physical therapist assistant is working with a patient who is receiving treatment for a venous thrombosis and notes several areas of ecchymosis on both upper extremities. Which of the following medications is **MOST** likely the cause?

Choices:
1. Heparin.
2. Hydrocortisone.
3. Dilantin.
4. Digoxin.

Teaching Points

Correct Answer: 1
Heparin is a blood thinner. Patients receiving heparin need to be cautious, as they will tend to bleed and bruise more easily if injured.

Incorrect Choices:
Hydrocortisone is used to decrease the effects of psoriasis and other skin disorders. Dilantin is used to decrease seizures, especially in patients with epilepsy. Digoxin is used to increase cardiac muscle contractility and decreases heart rate.

Type of Reasoning: Analytical
One must analyze the symptoms presented to determine the medication that is secondary to these symptoms. This requires analytical reasoning skill, where pieces of information are analyzed to draw a conclusion. For this case, the symptoms are secondary to the medication heparin. Review side effects of taking blood thinner medication, especially heparin, if answered incorrectly.

B12

Neuromuscular | Interventions

A child with spastic quadriplegia demonstrates a strong extensor thrust pattern while seated. Which of the adjustments identified will **BEST** help decrease the extensor thrusting response when this patient is sitting in the wheelchair?

Choices:
1. Just the forefoot should touch the foot plates.
2. Both the seat and seat back should be reclined backward approximately 15°.
3. The leg rests should be kept elevated at 80°.
4. The wheelchair should be equipped with an electric reclining back.

Teaching Points

Correct Answer: 2
When both the seat and the seat back are tilted backward, the patient's center of gravity will be displaced posteriorly. This will assist with combating extensor thrusting response and decreases the likelihood of the patient sliding out of the wheelchair.

Incorrect Choices:
Placing just the forefoot on the foot rest is likely to place undue stress on the metatarsal heads and may stimulate a clonus response in the gastrocnemius and soleus musculature. Elevating the leg rests will not decrease overall tone. Using only a reclining back may place the patient at risk for scooting forward in the seat of the wheelchair when the extensor thrusting pattern is initiated. This would place the patient at risk for sliding out the front of the chair.

Type of Reasoning: Inductive
This question requires the test taker to determine the most appropriate position for a patient with a strong extensor thrust while seated in a wheelchair. This requires clinical judgment, which is an inductive reasoning skill. For this case, the wheelchair seat and back should be reclined backward 15° to reduce the extensor thrust. If answered incorrectly, review wheelchair seating and positioning guidelines for children with spastic quadriplegia.

B13

Neuromuscular | Interventions

A patient presents with a flexion synergy pattern and spastic hemiparesis on the left. To **BEST** decrease the tone in the upper-extremity, which treatment activity should be utilized?

Choices:
1. Slow passive range-of-motion exercises of the left upper-extremity in diagonal patterns.
2. Right upper-extremity active exercise with the left upper-extremity placed in a weight-bearing position.
3. Functional activities and right upper-extremity exercise with the left upper extremity supported in a hemi-sling.
4. Slow stretch of the left shoulder extensors, elbow extensors and wrist extensors.

Teaching Points

Correct Answer: 2
Performing weight-bearing activities with the extremity placed out of the synergy pattern is the best mechanism identified in this question to decrease the flexion synergy pattern. Additionally, performing active exercise with the contralateral extremity promotes functional skill performance.

Incorrect Choices:
Performing slow passive range-of-motion exercises will help decrease triggering a spastic response within the movements performed. A hemi-sling is used to protect the extremity but does not help promote normal movement patterns or decrease tone. A slow stretch applied to the antagonists it is not likely to decrease the tone pattern in the agonist muscles.

Type of Reasoning: Inductive
One must determine the best approach to decreasing tone in the upper extremity of a patient with flexor synergy pattern and spastic hemiparesis. This is an inductive reasoning skill, where clinical judgment is utilized to draw conclusions. For this patient, it is best to perform right-extremity active exercise with the left upper extremity placed in a weight-bearing position with the shoulder laterally rotated and wrist extended. If answered incorrectly, review exercise guidelines to decrease tone for patients with flexor synergy.

B14

Neuromuscular | Diseases and Conditions Impacting Intervention

A physical therapist assistant is working with a patient who has Parkinson's Disease and is taking levadopa (Sinemet). Which of the following does this medication affect?

Choices:
1. Alpha motor neuron excitability.
2. Transmission of impulses within the spinal cord.
3. Synaptic transmission at the neuromuscular synapse.
4. Neurochemical imbalances in the basal ganglia.

Teaching Points

Correct Answer: 4
Levodopa (Sinemet) is an anti-Parkinsonism medication. Levodopa replaces dopamine that is normally produced by the basal ganglia but is deficient or absent in patients with Parkinson's disease.

Incorrect Choices:
Valium (diazepam) is a muscle relaxant that affects alpha motor neuron excitability. Baclofen is an antispasticity drug that affects transmission of impulses within the spinal cord. Botulinum toxin is a muscle relaxant that affects synaptic transmission.

Type of Reasoning: Deductive
This question requires the test taker to recall the properties of anti-Parkinsonism medications to arrive at a correct conclusion. This is factual information, which is a deductive reasoning skill. For this situation, the medications will affect neurochemical imbalances in the basal ganglia. If answered incorrectly, review anti-Parkinsonism medication, especially levodopa and Sinemet.

B15

Neuromuscular | Safety and Protection

A patient with a traumatic brain injury has a convulsive seizure during treatment. The patient loses consciousness and presents with tonic-clonic convulsions of all extremities. What is the physical therapist assistant's **BEST** response?

Choices:
1. Position the patient in side-lying and immediately call for emergency assistance.
2. Initiate cardiopulmonary resuscitation (CPR) immediately and call for help to restrain the patient.
3. Position in supine with head supported with a pillow and wait out the seizure.
4. Use straps and blankets to secure the limbs so the patient cannot be harmed.

Teaching Points

Correct Answer: 1
This is an emergency situation and emergency assistance should be called for immediately. To prevent aspiration if the patient is vomiting, the PTA should turn the head to the side or position the patient in side-lying.

Incorrect Choices:
CPR is not indicated at this time as the patient's circulation has not been assessed and a heart rate is likely present. Placing a pillow under the patient's head will narrow the airway and a supine position may result in aspiration if the patient begins to vomit. It is never appropriate to restrain a patient who is having a seizure; the area around the patient, however, should be cleared to prevent injury.

Type of Reasoning: Evaluative
This question requires the test taker to determine the best response for a patient who is experiencing a convulsive seizure during treatment. Questions that require one to weigh the implications of an action or response often require evaluative reasoning skill. For this situation, the best response is to position the patient in side-lying, then check to see if the airway is open and immediately call for emergency assistance. If answered incorrectly, review emergency first aid and CPR guidelines, especially for patients having seizures.

B16

Neuromuscular | Data Collection

A patient has damage to the lower branches of the femoral nerve. The patient is **MOST** likely to have difficulty with which of the following activities?

Choices:
1. Ascending stairs.
2. Walking on level surfaces.
3. Descending stairs.
4. Bridging exercises.

Teaching Points

Correct Answer: 3
The quadriceps muscle group is innervated by the femoral nerve. Eccentric control of the quadriceps is needed to descend the stairs.

Incorrect Choices:

While the quadriceps may be active with ascending stairs and walking on level surfaces, strong hip extensors can compensate for this weakness by creating knee hyperextension. The gluteus maximus and hamstrings muscle group are the primary muscles involved in bridging exercises.

Type of Reasoning: Inferential

Questions that provide a diagnosis and ask the test taker to determine the likely functional difficulties associated with that diagnosis often require inferential reasoning skill. For this question, damage to the lower branches of the femoral nerve will likely produce difficulty with descending stairs. If answered incorrectly, review signs and symptoms of femoral nerve damage, especially engagement in functional activities with damage.

B17

System Interactions | Diseases and Conditions Impacting Intervention

A physical therapist assistant is recovering from a head cold. Which of the following patients should the physical therapist assistant avoid treating?

Choices:
1. Patients who are in the acute stage of rheumatoid arthritis.
2. Patients who are undergoing chemotherapy.
3. Patients who have had a recent cerebrovascular accident.
4. Patients who have recently had a spinal tap.

Teaching Points

Correct Answer: 2

Patients undergoing chemotherapy treatments have a compromised immune system. Precautions should be taken when a treating PTA is experiencing a cold or other infection.

Incorrect Choices:

Patients who have rheumatoid arthritis or experienced a recent cerebrovascular accident or have had a spinal tap will not be as susceptible to the effects of exposure to a person with a head cold.

Type of Reasoning: Inductive

This question requires one to utilize clinical judgment to determine a best course of action. For this case, an assistant with a cold should limit contact with patients who are undergoing chemotherapy because of the patients' compromised immune system. If answered incorrectly, review precautions for working with patients who are immunocompromised, especially patients undergoing chemotherapy.

B18

System Interactions | Diseases and Conditions Impacting Intervention

A patient has been discharged to home following a recent **ORIF** for a pathological fracture of the tibia. The patient also has metastatic carcinoma of the lung. During treatment the patient reports sharp pain in the right hip that frequently causes a loss of sleep. What should the physical therapist assistant do with this information?

Choices:
1. Continue with treatment as tolerated and attribute the pain to increased use during treatment.
2. Suggest the use of heat and monitor the patient's response at the next visit.
3. Modify the treatment to avoid walking and report the hip pain to the physician.
4. Recommend that the patient see the physician as soon as possible and document the report in the patient's chart.

Teaching Points

Correct Answer: 4

New pain, especially at night, is a red flag for possible metastasis to a new site. In addition to suggesting a visit to the physician, the physical therapist assistant should notify the physical therapist and document the findings.

Incorrect Choices:

The other choices minimize stress to the area but do not address the primary concern of possible metastasis.

Type of Reasoning: Evaluative

For this question, the test taker must determine an appropriate course of action for a patient reporting sharp pain in the right hip. This requires one to weigh the significance of all the information presented to arrive at a correct conclusion, which is an evaluative reasoning skill. For this scenario, the assistant should recommend that the patient see the physician as soon as possible, especially in light of the patient's history of metastatic cancer. If answered incorrectly, review signs and symptoms of metastatic cancer.

B19

Lymphatic | Diseases and Conditions Impacting Intervention

Following radiation treatments for prostate cancer, a patient is developing edema in the right lower extremity. What secondary effect of the radiation treatment is likely the cause of this edema?

Choices:
1. Lymphatic obstruction.
2. Disuse atrophy.
3. Orthostatic hypotension.
4. Onset of congestive heart failure.

Teaching Points

Correct Answer: 1

A patient who has completed radiation treatments for prostate cancer may be a candidate for developing lymphatic disease secondary to damage to the lymphatic system from the radiation.

Incorrect Choices:

Disuse atrophy will result in tissue wasting, not edema. Orthostatic hypotension can result from immobility, blood volume depletion, side effects of medication and other causes; however, it is not a secondary effect of radiation therapy or a cause of edema. Although congestive heart failure (CHF) can result in peripheral edema, it is not likely to be unilateral and nothing in the scenario described indicates that the patient is at risk for CHF.

Type of Reasoning: Inferential

One must determine the secondary effects of radiation treatment causing edema in the lower extremity. This requires one to infer what may be true, which is an inferential reasoning skill. For this case, the secondary effects of radiation causing lower-extremity edema can be attributable to lymphatic obstruction. If answered incorrectly, review radiation treatment guidelines for patients with cancer, especially edema associated with radiation treatment.

B20

Nonsystem | Professional Responsibilities

A physical therapist assistant working in an early intervention program arrives at a home to treat a 2-year-old child. Upon arrival the physical therapist assistant is greeted at the door by the 8-year-old sibling. The sibling tells the assistant to come in as the parent has gone to the store. The assistant determines that the two children are at home alone. What should the physical therapist assistant do?

Choices:
1. Call the parent's cell phone.
2. Enter the home as invited and treat the child.
3. Call the Department of Social Services to report the situation.
4. Take the children to the local police station.

Teaching Points

Correct Answer: 3

A physical therapist assistant working in the home care setting is considered to be a mandatory reporter. Mandatory reporters are required to report cases of suspected child abuse or maltreatment.

Incorrect Choices:

It is inappropriate for a mandatory reporter to attempt to contact the parent on the cell phone since the children were found at home alone and unattended. The PTA should not enter the home or take the children away as Social Services will appropriately handle the situation.

Type of Reasoning: Evaluative

One must determine an appropriate course of action for children who have been left home alone. This requires weighing the choices presented to determine the course of action that best resolves the issue. This is an evaluative reasoning skill. For this case, the assistant should call the Department of Social Services to report the issue. If answered incorrectly, review child abuse and maltreatment guidelines, including mandatory reporting guidelines.

B21

Nonsystem | Professional Responsibilities

A physical therapist and physical therapist assistant team are treating a patient whose plan of care includes "therapeutic exercise to strengthen knee stabilizers." The physical therapist assistant documented progressing the exercise program to include single knee extension in supine. Which of the following is the **MOST** accurate observation of the physical therapist assistant's intervention?

Choices:
1. The physical therapist assistant is working within their scope of practice.
2. The physical therapist assistant should have checked with the physical therapist prior to starting the new exercise.
3. The physical therapist assistant should not have progressed the exercise in this situation.
4. The physical therapist assistant is working outside their scope of practice in this situation.

Teaching Points

Correct Answer: 1

It is within the scope of practice for a physical therapist assistant to progress a patient through an exercise program if it is included in the plan of care.

Incorrect Choices:

If the plan of care identifies specific exercises, modalities, or therapeutic activities, the assistant would need to get verbal or written consent from the physical therapist to modify it. The physical therapist assistant is not working beyond the scope of practice in this scenario.

Type of Reasoning: Deductive

This question requires one to recall factual guidelines about physical therapy scope of practice. This is a deductive reasoning skill where factual guidelines are often utilized to make decisions. For this situation, the assistant is working within the scope of practice. If answered incorrectly, review physical therapy scope of practice guidelines.

B22

System Interactions | Diseases and Conditions Impacting Intervention

A patient is referred to physical therapy following 3 weeks of bed rest. The patient has multiple problems including an acute flare-up of rheumatoid arthritis in both hands, a recent surgical repair of an intertrochanteric fracture of the hip, bilateral knee flexion contractures, and an abnormal electrocardiogram (EKG). The patient is now permitted to walk with partial weight bearing on the operated side. The plan of care includes increasing range of motion and improving endurance. Which of the following interventions **BEST** meets the patient's needs?

Choices:
1. Walk as tolerated with a standard walker and perform passive stretch to bilateral hamstrings.
2. Use a recumbent bike and perform contract/relax to bilateral hamstrings.
3. Participate in contract/relax exercises to stretch bilateral hamstrings and walk on a treadmill.
4. Use an upper-extremity ergometer set at moderate resistance and prone-lying passive stretch of the hamstrings.

Teaching Points

Correct Answer: 2

Recumbent bike riding is a safe mechanism to maintain partial weight bearing on the hip while still increasing endurance, and contract/relax is an effective means of stretching the hamstrings.

Incorrect Choices:

The upper-extremity ergometer may not be safe considering the recent abnormal EKG and is not a good choice for a patient with a flare-up of rheumatoid arthritis in the joints of the hands. The treadmill should be avoided as the weight-bearing status would be exceeded. Ambulation as tolerated with the standard walker may increase endurance; however, a passive stretch is not as effective as contract/relax mechanisms to increase range of motion.

Type of Reasoning: Inductive

One must determine the best therapeutic exercise for a patient with a hip fracture, rheumatoid arthritis, and an abnormal EKG. Clinical judgment is utilized with questions of this nature, which require inductive reasoning skill. For this situation, the assistant should use a recumbent bike and perform contract/relax to bilateral hamstrings to best meet the plan of care. If answered incorrectly, review therapeutic exercises for patients with hip fracture, rheumatoid arthritis and abnormal EKGs.

B23

Musculoskeletal | Diseases and Conditions Impacting Intervention

A patient has rheumatoid arthritis in bilateral elbows and is having difficulty tolerating the long hours required at a desk job. Initially, which of the following physical therapy treatments is **MOST** appropriate?

Choices:
1. Use of cold and avoidance of active elbow flexion.
2. Application of topical analgesics and light resistance strengthening.
3. Splinting in 90° of flexion and isometric exercise at 80% effort.
4. Use of heat modalities and joint protection.

Teaching Points

Correct Answer: 4
Initially, the patient should be treated with modalities while avoiding activities that increase tissue irritation. Heat and joint protection will be the most effective.

Incorrect Choices:
Use of cold in a patient with rheumatoid arthritis can be problematic because of the increased likelihood of cold intolerance or Raynaud's phenomenon. At this stage, strengthening is not appropriate. Splinting should be avoided as inactivity often increases the pain in individuals who have rheumatoid arthritis.

Type of Reasoning: Inductive
One must determine the best intervention approach for a patient with rheumatoid arthritis in both elbows. This requires clinical judgment, which is an inductive reasoning skill. For this case, initial intervention should include the use of heat modalities and joint protection to decrease symptoms. If answered incorrectly, review treatment approaches for rheumatoid arthritis.

B24

Neuromuscular | Diseases and Conditions Impacting Intervention

A physical therapist has been asked to consult with a physical education teacher regarding exercises to incorporate with a child who has Down syndrome. Which of the following activities should be avoided?

Choices:
1. Jumping jacks during strength and conditioning training.
2. Batting during softball.
3. Long-distance running on the track.
4. Forward rolls during gymnastics.

Teaching Points

Correct Answer: 4
One complication of Down syndrome is atlanto-axial instability because of ligamentous laxity between the C1 and C2 vertebrae. If this joint is unstable, the pressure exerted through the area with a forward roll could put the patient at risk for spinal cord injury.

Incorrect Choices:
Although not all children will be able to perform the other activities because of personal limitations, they are not contraindicated in this situation.

Type of Reasoning: Evaluative

One must determine the activity to avoid for a child with Down syndrome. This requires the test taker to weigh the information and its significance to reach a correct conclusion. This is an evaluative reasoning skill. For this situation, the child should not participate in exercise that places stress on the atlanto-axial joint, such as forward rolls. If answered incorrectly, review precautions and contraindications for exercise in children with Down syndrome.

B25

Cardiac | Interventions

A physical therapist assistant is gait training a patient with cardiac disease. During the activity the patient becomes hypotensive. What is the physical therapist assistant's **MOST** appropriate response?

Choices:
1. Immediately contact the supervising physical therapist.
2. Terminate the activity, sit the patient down, and elevate the lower extremities.
3. Offer the patient a drink of orange juice.
4. Decrease the speed of walking.

Teaching Points

Correct Answer: 2

If a patient with a history of cardiac disease experiences hypotension with activity, the activity should be stopped; this is an indication the heart cannot keep up with the physical demands of the activity.

Incorrect Choices:
While the PTA should notify the supervising PT of the incident, this should not occur until the patient has terminated the exercise. Orange juice would be appropriate for a patient with diabetes mellitus who was showing signs of hypoglycemia. Decreasing the walking speed will not sufficiently decrease the workload on the heart.

Type of Reasoning: Evaluative
For this question, the test taker must determine an appropriate response for a patient who has become hypotensive during gait training. This requires one to weigh the courses of action and determine the action that effectively addresses the patient's needs. This is an evaluative reasoning skill. For this situation, the assistant should terminate the activity, sit the patient down, and elevate the lower extremities. If answered incorrectly, review guidelines for addressing hypotensive episodes.

B26

Musculoskeletal | Interventions

Which of the following activities should be included in the plan of care for a patient immediately following a cesarean delivery?

Choices:
1. Progressive cardiovascular training.
2. Partial curl-ups.
3. Pelvic floor exercises.
4. Practice lifting techniques.

Teaching Points

Correct Answer: 3

Following a pregnancy and a cesarean delivery, the patient will likely present with decreased tone in the pelvic floor muscles. Pelvic floor exercises should be included to help rebuild muscle strength and control.

Incorrect Choices:

Cardiovascular training and lifting techniques do not address the diagnosis identified and are too intense at this time. Partial curl-ups are contraindicated immediately following cesarean delivery; time must be allowed for appropriate healing of the abdominal muscles and tissues.

Type of Reasoning: Inductive

One must determine the best exercises to include for a patient postcesarean delivery. This requires inductive reasoning skill, a skill that requires clinical judgment to determine a best course of action. In this case, the plan of care should include pelvic floor exercises to help rebuild muscle strength and control. If answered incorrectly, review exercises for patient's postcesarean delivery.

B27

Neuromuscular | Data Collection

Which of the following **BEST** describes the characteristics of a patient who was recently admitted to the hospital with a diagnosis of Guillain-Barré syndrome?

Choices:
1. Symmetrical distribution of extremity weakness with possible involvement of the lower cranial nerves.
2. Asymmetrical weakness with hyperreflexia.
3. Unilateral facial paralysis; affected eye does not close.
4. Sensory loss (stocking and glove distribution) with minor loss of motor function.

Teaching Points

Correct Answer: 1

Guillain-Barré syndrome is an acute polyneuritis characterized by rapid development of progressive muscle weakness that is symmetrical and ascends the body (starting first in the lower extremities, progressing to trunk, upper extremities, and, finally, cranial nerves).

Incorrect Choices:

Asymmetrical weakness is not common in Guillain-Barré syndrome nor is hyperreflexia. Unilateral facial paralysis is indicative of Bell's palsy. Stocking and glove sensory loss could be found but not with minor loss of motor function.

Type of Reasoning: Inferential

This question provides a diagnosis and the test taker must determine the likely symptoms of this diagnosis. Questions of this nature often require inferential reasoning skill. For this case, one should expect the patient to present with symmetrical distribution of extremity weakness with possible involvement of the lower cranial nerves. If answered incorrectly, review signs and symptoms of Guillain-Barré syndrome.

B28

Musculoskeletal | Data Collection

The stationary arm of a goniometer is placed in line with the lateral midline of the trunk, the fulcrum is placed at the greater trochanter, and the movable arm is aligned with lateral femoral condyle. Which of the following actions is **MOST** likely being measured?

Choices:
1. Hip abduction.
2. Trunk lateral flexion.
3. Hip flexion.
4. Trunk extension.

Teaching Points

Correct Answer: 3

This is the correct goniometer placement when measuring hip flexion.

Incorrect Choices:

Hip abduction is measured with the fulcrum on the anterior hip, the stationary arm parallel to the anterior superior iliac spine of the ilium, and the movable arm along the anterior thigh aligned with the patella. Trunk range of motion is more accurately measured with an inclinometer.

Type of Reasoning: Deductive

This question requires one to recall the procedures for measuring hip flexion with a goniometer. This is factual recall of information, which is a deductive reasoning skill. For this situation, the measurement being taken is that of hip flexion.

B29

Nonsystem | Equipment and Devices

What is the **MOST** appropriate wheelchair modification for a patient with bilateral transfemoral amputations?

Choices:
1. Placement of the drive wheels 2 inches anterior to the vertical back supports.
2. Lowering the seat height by 3 inches.
3. Increasing the seat depth by 3 inches to accommodate the length of the residual extremity.
4. Placement of the drive wheels 2 inches posterior to the vertical back supports.

Teaching Points

Correct Answer: 4

Placement of the drive wheels 2 inches posterior to the vertical back supports is an appropriate modification to increase posterior stability in relationship to the patient's altered center of mass.

Incorrect Choices:

Moving the wheels anteriorly will displace the center of mass too far posteriorly and likely cause the chair to tip over backward. Lowering the seat height is an appropriate modification for a patient following a stroke who will use the sound extremity for wheelchair propulsion. Increasing the seat depth does not address the concern of wheelchair stability.

Type of Reasoning: Inductive

This question requires one to utilize clinical judgment to determine the best wheelchair modification for a patient with bilateral transfemoral amputations. This is an inductive reasoning skill. For this case, an appropriate modification is placement of the drive wheels 2 inches posterior to the vertical back supports to increase posterior stability. If answered incorrectly, review wheelchair modification guidelines, including modifications for patients with bilateral lower-extremity amputations.

B30

Musculoskeletal | Data Collection

In sitting, a patient is able to flex the hip through 75% of the available range of motion without manual resistance. In side-lying, the patient is able to flex the hip through the full available range of motion. What should the physical therapist assistant record as the patient's hip flexor muscle grade?

Choices:
1. Fair minus (3–/5).
2. Good (4/5).
3. Fair (3/5).
4. Poor (2/5).

Teaching Points

Correct Answer: 1

A grade of 3–/5 (fair minus) is given when movement against gravity can be achieved through at least half of the available range.

Incorrect Choices:

A grade of 4/5 (good) is given for full movement against gravity with moderate manual resistance applied. When a person can move an extremity through the available range of motion against gravity without manual resistance, the muscle grade is 3/5 (fair). A grade of 2/5 (poor) describes full range of motion in a gravity-eliminated position.

Type of Reasoning: Deductive

One must recall the procedures for manual muscle testing to arrive at a correct conclusion. This is factual recall of guidelines, which is a deductive reasoning skill. For this case, the description of the patient's movement should receive a grade of fair minus for the hip flexor muscle. If answered incorrectly, review manual muscle testing guidelines, especially for the hip.

B31

Neuromuscular | Interventions

A physical therapist assistant is positioning a patient in bed who has spastic left hemiparesis. How should the affected upper extremity be positioned?

Choices:
1. Scapula retracted with the shoulder adducted and medially (internally) rotated.
2. Scapula protracted with the shoulder abducted and laterally (externally) rotated.
3. Scapula retracted with the shoulder abducted and laterally (externally) rotated.
4. Scapula protracted with the shoulder adducted and medially (internally) rotated.

Teaching Points

Correct Answer: 2

This position places the extremity out of tone-dependent and reflex-dependent postures.

Incorrect Choices:

The other three positions described encourage increased tone and synergistic movement in patients with spastic hemiparesis.

Type of Reasoning: Deductive

One must recall the guidelines for positioning a patient with spastic hemiparesis in bed. This is factual information, which necessitates deductive reasoning skill. For this case, the assistant should position the upper extremities so that the scapula is protracted with the shoulder abducted and laterally rotated. If answered incorrectly, review bed positioning for patients with spasticity.

B32

Integumentary | Interventions

A patient with a deep partial thickness burn to the anterior neck is being treated in physical therapy for positioning. Which of the following is the **MOST** appropriate position for this patient?

Choices:
1. Chin tucked.
2. Chin forward.
3. Neck hyperextension.
4. Neck flexion.

Teaching Points

Correct Answer: 3

When a patient has suffered a deep partial thickness burn to the anterior neck, it is best to position the neck in hyperextension to avoid contracture formation in a non-functional position of neck flexion.

Incorrect Choices:

Scar tissue is less flexible than undamaged tissue and can limit range of motion. Placing the neck in flexion or with the chin tucked or forward will create a shortened scar and not allow for functional movement in the neck.

Type of Reasoning: Deductive

This question requires the test taker to recall the guidelines for splinting the neck after burns. This is factual information, which is a deductive reasoning skill. For this situation, the neck should be splinted after a deep partial thickness burn to the anterior neck in hyperextension to prevent contractures. If answered incorrectly, review splinting guidelines for patients with burns, especially burns to the neck region.

B33

Nonsystem | Therapeutic Modalities

Which of the following conditions will require extreme caution when utilizing a cryo cuff?

Choices:
1. Acute inflammatory process.
2. Very fair complexion.
3. Obesity.
4. Raynaud's disease.

Teaching Points

Correct Answer: 4

Extreme caution should be taken when applying cryotherapy to a patient with Raynaud's disease because of the increased sensitivity to cold. Cryotherapy, in many cases, is contraindicated for someone with Raynaud's disease.

Incorrect Choices:

Cryotherapy is the first choice of treatment for an acute inflammatory process. A patient with a very fair complexion may be at risk with the use of radiant heat. Cryotherapy or thermotherapy may not be effective on a person who is obese, but they do not increase concern.

Type of Reasoning: Deductive

One must recall the contraindications and precautions for the use of cryotherapy to arrive at a correct conclusion. This requires the recall of factual information, necessitating deductive reasoning skill. For this scenario, when one is using a cryo-cuff, caution must be taken with patients who have Raynaud's disease. If answered incorrectly, review symptoms of Raynaud's disease and the use of modalities, especially cryotherapy.

B34

Neuromuscular | Data Collection

When assessing a child with myelomeningocele, which complication would **LEAST** likely be observed?

Choices:
1. Increased tone in the lower extremities.
2. Inadequate bladder emptying.
3. Sensory impairment in the lower extremities.
4. Disturbances of bone growth and development.

Teaching Points

Correct Answer: 1

Spina bifida typically results in decreased tone in the lower extremities.

Incorrect Choices:

It is common for a child with myelomeningocele to have inadequate bladder emptying and lower-extremity sensory impairments due to lumbar nerve root damage. Disturbances in bone growth and development are common due to the lack of movement and poor weight bearing since birth.

Type of Reasoning: Inferential

This question provides a diagnosis and the test taker must determine the symptoms not consistent with this diagnosis. This requires one to determine what is not likely to be true, which is an inferential reasoning skill. For this situation, the child with spina bifida is not likely to demonstrate increased tone in the lower extremities. If answered incorrectly, review signs and symptoms of spina bifida.

B35

Nonsystem | Equipment and Devices

A patient status post a cerebrovascular accident uses a wheelchair and is independent with standing pivot transfers. The patient currently ambulates limited distances. What is the **MOST** important feature to consider for this patient's wheelchair?

Choices:
1. A swing-away detachable leg rest.
2. A one-arm drive.
3. Standard non-removable desk arms.
4. Removable desk arms.

Teaching Points

Correct Answer: 1

Because the patient is ambulatory and performing stand-pivot transfers independently, it will be important to remove obstacles that may cause the patient to trip to ensure patient safety. Therefore, a swing-away removable leg rest is the most important feature of a wheelchair for this patient.

Incorrect Choices:

A patient who has hemiplegia may require a one-arm drive, but hemiplegia was not mentioned in this case. Non-removable desk arms do not provide any benefit for this patient. Removable desk arms are important for a patient who transfers by using a sliding board or squat pivot technique.

Type of Reasoning: Inductive

One must utilize clinical judgment to determine the most important feature for a patient's wheelchair. This requires inductive reasoning skill. For this case, the patient with cerebrovascular accident would benefit most from a swing-away detachable leg rest on the wheelchair. If answered incorrectly, review wheelchair prescription guidelines for patients with cerebrovascular accident.

B36

Neuromuscular | Interventions

What is the best strategy to use when working with a patient with Alzheimer's disease who becomes frustrated in mastering a skill during treatment?

Choices:
1. Move the patient to a quiet treatment area to minimize any distractions and enhance concentration.
2. End the treatment session and try the skill later in the day when the patient may be less agitated.
3. Redirect the patient to a less challenging skill.
4. Increase the time and number of demonstrations of the skill before the patient tries it again.

Teaching Points

Correct Answer: 3
When treating a patient with Alzheimer's disease, it is best to keep tasks simple to minimize frustration.

Incorrect Choices:
Although moving the patient to a quiet treatment area may help, the task may still be too difficult and the frustration would continue. The session should not be ended with a negative or frustrating task. If the task is too difficult for the patient's skill level, the patient will not be successful regardless of the amount of repetition or demonstration given.

Type of Reasoning: Inductive
One must determine the best strategy to assist a patient with Alzheimer's disease who is demonstrating frustration during a task. This requires clinical judgment, which is an inductive reasoning skill. For this situation, it is best to redirect the patient to a less challenging skill. If answered incorrectly, review treatment guidelines for patients with Alzheimer's disease.

B37

Neuromuscular | Data Collection

When assessing the development of an 11-month-old child, which of the following should the child be expected to perform?

Choices:
1. Run independently.
2. Stand alone for several seconds.
3. Walk up stairs with assistance.
4. Walk up stairs one step at a time without assistance.

Teaching Points

Correct Answer: 2
Standing alone for several seconds occurs for most children between 10 and 11 months.

Incorrect Choices:
The other developmental milestones listed—run independently (24 months), walk up stairs with assistance (18 months), and walk up stairs one step at a time without assistance (24 months)—are reached at later stages.

Type of Reasoning: Deductive
This question requires the test taker to recall developmental milestones of infants. This is factual information, which is a deductive reasoning skill. For this case, an 11-month-old child can be expected to stand alone for several seconds. Review developmental milestones of infants, especially motor skills of 11-month-old infants, if answered incorrectly.

B38

Musculoskeletal | Data Collection

During a gait assessment, the physical therapist assistant notes the patient's affected hip laterally (externally) rotates during the swing phase of gait. This gait pattern is **MOST** likely compensating for weakness in which muscle?

Choices:
1. Tensor fascia latae.
2. Gluteus medius.
3. Rectus femoris.
4. Iliopsoas.

Teaching Points

Correct Answer: 4

Lateral (external) hip rotation is most likely occurring due to hip flexor weakness. The iliopsoas is the strongest hip flexor and is likely weak in this scenario.

Incorrect Choices:

The tensor fascia latae assists with hip flexion and is causing the increased hip lateral (external) rotation to compensate for the weak iliopsoas muscle. Weakness of the gluteus medius would result in a Trendelenburg gait pattern. The rectus femoris also assists with hip flexion, but would not contribute to the lateral (external) rotation.

Type of Reasoning: Inferential

This question requires one to infer or draw a reasonable conclusion about the likely muscle that is weak with a patient who demonstrates lateral rotation of the hip during the swing phase of gait. This requires inferential reasoning skill. For this situation, the iliopsoas muscle is most likely weak causing the lateral rotation. If answered incorrectly, review gait patterns for patients with weak hip musculature.

B39

Musculoskeletal | Interventions

A physical therapist assistant is initiating gait training per the physical therapist's plan of care for a patient with a transfemoral amputation. Which of the following gait patterns is **MOST** appropriate for this patient?

Choices:
1. 2-point gait.
2. Swing-through gait.
3. 4-point gait.
4. 3-point gait.

Teaching Points

Correct Answer: 3

When first teaching a patient to walk with a prosthesis, the 4-point gait pattern will allow for the most stable gait pattern.

Incorrect Choices:

The other gait patterns listed are not as stable as a 4-point gait pattern and, therefore, not as safe.

640　Examination B

Type of Reasoning: Inductive

One must determine the safest gait pattern to teach a patient with transfemoral amputation to arrive at a correct conclusion. This requires clinical judgment, which is an inductive reasoning skill. For this case, when using a prosthesis for the first time, the patient should be instructed in the use of a 4-point gait pattern. Review gait-training guidelines for patients with lower-extremity amputations if answered incorrectly.

B40

Musculoskeletal | Diseases and Conditions Impacting Intervention

A physical therapist assistant is working with a patient status post a grade 3 rotator cuff tendon repair. Surgery was completed two days ago. Which of the following interventions should the physical therapist assistant **AVOID** performing?

Choices:
1. Pendulum exercises.
2. Submaximal isometric exercise.
3. Passive range of motion.
4. Cryotherapy techniques.

Teaching Points

Correct Answer: 2

The patient is in the acute stage of healing and strengthening exercises are not appropriate during this stage, as the repair could be easily weakened or disrupted. A grade 3 tendon repair includes suturing of a tear in the tissues, and resistance 2 days following suturing of a tear would put the tissue at risk for tearing of the sutures.

Incorrect Choices:
Pendulum exercises, passive range of motion, and cryotherapy are all indicated to promote healing, tissue movement, and decreased inflammation during the acute stage of healing.

Type of Reasoning: Evaluative

One must weigh all of the potential approaches presented to determine the approach that is inappropriate for a patient with grade 3 rotator cuff tendon injury. This is an evaluative reasoning skill. For this situation, it is inappropriate to incorporate submaximal isometric exercise because of the risk for tearing of the sutures. If answered incorrectly, review intervention approaches for patients with rotator cuff repairs, especially grade 3 tendon injuries.

B41

Musculoskeletal | Interventions

A patient has just undergone a total knee arthroplasty secondary to severe degenerative joint disease. Which of the following is a benefit of using a continuous passive movement (CPM) machine with this patient?

Choices:
1. Decreased range of motion.
2. Increased edema.
3. Increased risk of a deep vein thrombosis.
4. Decreased postoperative pain.

Teaching Points

Correct Answer: 4

The continuous passive motion (CPM) machine decreases postoperative pain by keeping the lower-extremity moving, thus preventing the extremity from "stiffening up."

Incorrect Choices:

The CPM will help to increase range of motion, and may actually decrease edema and decrease the risk for deep vein thrombosis by keeping the joint moving.

Type of Reasoning: Deductive

This question requires one to recall the purposes of the CPM machine for patients with a status of post–total knee arthroplasty. This is factual information, which necessitates deductive reasoning skill. For this scenario, the purpose of CPM placement after surgery is to decrease postoperative pain. Review indications for CPM machines after joint arthroplasty if answered incorrectly.

B42

Neuromuscular | Diseases and Conditions Impacting Interventions

Which of the following gait abnormalities **MOST** accurately describes the typical gait pattern of a patient with spastic diplegia and flexor hypertonicity?

Choices:
1. Excessive hip and knee flexion with decreased stride length.
2. Increased double limb support with decreased stride width.
3. Pillar-like rigidity on weight bearing with ankle varus.
4. Excessive hip flexion with increased stride width.

Teaching Points

Correct Answer: 1

The typical position of the lower extremities for a patient with spastic diplegia and flexor hypertonicity is excessive hip and knee flexion, with adduction and medial (internal) rotation of the hips. Having the lower extremities both adducted and medially (internally) rotated will decrease the stride length.

Incorrect Choices:

Double limb support is not typically affected. Ankle valgus and decreased stride width are more commonly seen.

Type of Reasoning: Inferential

One must infer or draw a reasonable conclusion about the likely features of a gait pattern for a patient with spastic diplegia. This requires one to determine what may be true, which is an inferential reasoning skill. For this case, one should expect the patient to most likely demonstrate excessive hip and knee flexion with decreased stride length. Review gait patterns for patients with spastic diplegia if answered incorrectly.

B43

Nonsystem | Equipment and Devices

A patient with post-polio syndrome exhibits foot slap at initial contact. Which of the following components will be **MOST** appropriate in an ankle-foot orthosis for this patient?

Choices:
1. Medial T strap.
2. Lateral T strap.
3. Posterior stop.
4. Anterior stop.

Teaching Points

Correct Answer: 3

Foot slap is a result of eccentric weakness of the dorsiflexors. A posterior stop will limit the amount of plantar flexion allowed thus limiting foot slap.

Incorrect Choices:

An anterior stop is used if a patient exhibits increased dorsiflexion. Medial and lateral T straps are used to decrease excessive abduction or adduction of the foot or to decrease excessive supination.

Type of Reasoning: Inductive

One must utilize clinical judgment to determine the appropriate ankle-foot orthosis for a patient with postpolio syndrome and a foot slap. This is an inductive reasoning skill. For this situation, the ankle-foot orthosis should include a posterior stop to address the foot slap. Review orthoses for patients with weak dorsiflexors if answered incorrectly.

B44

Neuromuscular | Data Collection

A physical therapist assistant is providing moderate perturbation forces that displace the patient anteriorly. What muscle group should be activated to maintain balance in a patient who is demonstrating appropriate balance responses?

Choices:
1. Hip extensors.
2. Hip flexors.
3. Trunk extensors.
4. Dorsiflexors.

Teaching Points

Correct Answer: 1

To preserve the center of gravity with a moderate perturbation force, the patient will most likely contract the hip extensors to reestablish the trunk position.

Incorrect Choices:

The hip flexors and dorsiflexors would be utilized in the event of a posterior displacement. The trunk extensors are not typically utilized unless a large disturbance is provided or the patient's balance responses are poor.

Type of Reasoning: Inferential

One must determine what may be true for a patient with balance deficits whose balance is displaced forward during balance testing to arrive at a correct conclusion. This requires inferential reasoning skill. For this scenario, the muscle group that is likely to contract strongly to reestablish the trunk position is the hip extensors. If answered incorrectly, review standing balance guidelines and the role of muscles in maintaining balance during balance disturbances.

B45

Musculoskeletal | Interventions

The physical therapist assistant is teaching a group of workers to lift heavy objects off the floor. Which of the following concepts of lifting should be taught to the group?

Choices:
1. Keep the lumbar spine flexed during the lift.
2. Stoop down to the object before trying to lift it.
3. Increase the lordotic posture to increase stability when lifting.
4. Keep objects as far away from the center of gravity as possible.

Teaching Points

Correct Answer: 2

When instructing workers to lift heavy objects, the PTA must emphasize proper body mechanics. One of the main principles of body mechanics is to stoop down (squat) to the object first, allowing the patient the ability to "lift with the legs."

Incorrect Choices:
The spine should be held in a "neutral position," neither flexed or in increased lordosis. The workers should also be instructed to keep objects close to the body.

Type of Reasoning: Deductive
One must recall body mechanics guidelines to arrive at a correct conclusion for this question. This is factual information, which is a deductive reasoning skill. For this scenario, the assistant should instruct the workers to stoop down to the object before trying to lift it. If answered incorrectly, review proper body mechanics for lifting heavy objects from the floor.

B46

Integumentary | Interventions

A patient presents with a 20 degree plantarflexion contracture 6 months status post a deep partial thickness burn of the distal lower extremity. Prior to stretching the ankle joint, what massage technique is **MOST** appropriate to help release soft tissue adhesions?

Choices:
1. Kneading.
2. Effleurage.
3. Percussion.
4. Friction.

Teaching Points

Correct Answer: 4

The patient who has deep partial thickness burns is at an increased risk for developing hypertrophic scarring, scarring and shortening of the tissue caused the contracture; the scar needs to become more supple to increase range of motion and stretch the area. Friction massage is the technique used to "break up" scar tissue, and should be used prior to stretching the area.

Incorrect Choices:

Kneading and effleurage are massage techniques used for relaxation and to address muscle tightness. Percussion is used primarily as a chest physical therapy technique.

Type of Reasoning: Inductive

This question requires the test taker to use knowledge of massage techniques to arrive at a correct conclusion. This necessitates clinical judgment, which is an inductive reasoning skill. For this case, the most appropriate massage technique for a patient with a plantar flexion contracture after deep partial thickness burns is friction massage. Review massage techniques for hypertrophic scarring after burns if answered incorrectly.

B47

Neuromuscular | Interventions

To encourage functional reintegration of the affected side, how should a patient with hemiplegia be encouraged to roll from a supine position to sitting up over the edge of the bed?

Choices:
1. Rotate the upper trunk toward the unaffected side to encourage use of the hemiplegic extremities when pushing to sitting.
2. Grab the bed rail with the unaffected upper extremity first to help roll to the side of hemiplegia.
3. Flex and rotate the upper trunk diagonally toward the side of hemiplegia to achieve a side-lying position on-elbow posture first.
4. Flex the upper trunk by extending both shoulders to achieve a bilateral on-elbows position before rolling onto the unaffected side.

Teaching Points

Correct Answer: 3

Having the patient roll to a side-lying position on-elbow posture on the affected side facilitates weight bearing through the affected extremity and initial functional use of the extremity by pushing through the extremity. This will best help to functionally reintegrate the affected side.

Incorrect Choices:

Rotating the upper trunk toward the unaffected side would not likely allow completion of the skill as the weakness in the affected upper extremity would not allow pushing to a sitting position without the assistance of the lower extremities and/or a position between supine and full sitting on the edge of the bed. A patient with hemiplegia will have great difficulty in rolling toward the unaffected side because the affected side must initiate the movement.

Type of Reasoning: Inductive

One must utilize clinical judgment to determine the best approach for encouraging bed mobility for a patient with hemiplegia. This is an inductive reasoning skill. For this situation, the patient should be encouraged to roll and sit up over the edge of the bed from a supine position by flexing and rotating the upper trunk diagonally toward the hemiplegic side to achieve a side-lying on-elbow posture. Review bed mobility guidelines for patients with hemiplegia if answered incorrectly.

B48

Nonsystem | Equipment and Devices

A physical therapist assistant is using ultrasound to assist in the healing and flexibility of a first degree strain to the musculotendinous junction 23 days after injury. What is the **MOST** effective application of ultrasound?

Choices:
1. Stretching of the tissues followed by continuous ultrasound then resting in a support device for protection.
2. Ultrasound at a continuous setting followed immediately by gentle stretching and active assistive use of the muscle in the newly acquired range.
3. Active exercising of the muscle followed by a gentle static stretch to end range with pulsed ultrasound.
4. Continuous ultrasound to the tissues followed by active exercise within the available range of motion.

Teaching Points

Correct Answer: 2
Ultrasound is effective in the subacute phase of healing if applied at mild thermal ranges. Tissue extensibility will be the greatest following ultrasound treatment. It has been demonstrated that tissues will best remain at the lengthened state when used in that newly gained range of motion while warm.

Incorrect Choices:
The incorrect choices include splinting the area, stretching to end range (not beyond), and exercising within the available range; none will effectively address increasing range of motion. Non-thermal ultrasound (pulsed) is utilized in the acute phase, not the subacute phase.

Type of Reasoning: Inductive
This question requires the test taker to determine the most effective application of ultrasound for a patient with an injury to the musculotendinous junction. This requires knowledge of ultrasound guidelines and clinical judgment, which is an inductive reasoning skill. For this situation, the most effective application of ultrasound should include a continuous setting followed immediately by gentle stretching and active assistive use of the muscle in the newly acquired range. Review ultrasound guidelines for patients with musculotendinous junction injury if answered incorrectly.

B49

Musculoskeletal | Data Collection

During observation of a patient's gait in the sagittal view, the physical therapist assistant observes the patient fully extend the knee and hip at midstance and hyperextend the trunk in the stance phase. Weakness of which muscle results in knee, hip, and trunk extension during stance phase?

Choices:
1. Rectus femoris.
2. Gluteus medius.
3. Gluteus maximus.
4. Gastrocnemius.

Teaching Points

Correct Answer: 3
To compensate for a weak gluteus maximus, the patient fully extends the knee and hip while extending the trunk to "lock" the kinetic chain and assist with maintaining hip extension during stance.

Incorrect Choices:
Weakness of the rectus femoris would result in knee flexion during stance phase. Weakness of the gluteus medius would result in a Trendelenburg gait pattern with an observable hip drop during stance phase. Weakness of the gastrocnemius would result in excessive dorsiflexion and diminished toe off.

Type of Reasoning: Analytical
One must assess the patient's gait deviation features to determine the muscle that is likely weak and contributing to the deviation. This requires analytical reasoning skill. For this case, the knee, hip, and trunk extension during the stance phase indicates weakness of the gluteus maximus. Review common gait deviations and their cause if answered incorrectly.

B50

Neuromuscular | Data Collection

A patient with a supracondylar fracture of the humerus has radial nerve involvement. Which of the following problems would the physical therapist assistant expect this patient to demonstrate?

Choices:
1. Inability to flex the fingers.
2. Impaired sensation to the volar surface of the hand.
3. Inability to flex the metacarpophalangeal joints.
4. Deviation of the wrist to the ulnar side.

Teaching Points

Correct Answer: 4
The radial nerve innervates the extensor carpi radialis as well as the abductor pollicis, both of which are responsible for radial deviation. Because these muscles are inactive, the wrist will exhibit ulnar deviation.

Incorrect Choices:
Inability to flex the fingers is a result of damage to the ulnar and median nerves, as is impaired sensation to the volar aspect. Inability to flex the metacarpophalangeal joints is the result of damage to the ulnar nerve.

Type of Reasoning: Inferential
This question provides a diagnosis and the test taker must determine the likely symptoms, which is an inferential reasoning skill. For this patient with a supracondylar fracture and radial nerve involvement, one should expect to see deviation of the wrist to the ulnar side. If answered incorrectly, review signs and symptoms of radial nerve damage.

B51

Musculoskeletal | Interventions

What is the **MOST** likely rationale for the application of large and small amplitude oscillatory joint mobilization techniques at the beginning of range of motion?

Choices:
1. Decrease pain.
2. Increase range of motion.
3. Increase pain.
4. Decrease range of motion.

Teaching Points

Correct Answer: 1

Large and small amplitude oscillatory techniques are used to decrease pain by enhancing synovial fluid movement and stimulating mechanorecptors, including A beta fibers.

Incorrect Choices:

Increasing pain or decreasing range of motion is not a plausible outcome. Increasing range of motion will occur with joint glides III and IV.

Type of Reasoning: Inductive

One must utilize clinical judgment to determine the most appropriate condition for utilizing large- and small-amplitude oscillation joint mobilization techniques and myofascial techniques. This requires inductive reasoning skill. For this situation, the condition appropriate for these treatment techniques is locked facet joints of the lumbar vertebra. Review indications for joint mobilization techniques, as well as myofascial techniques, if answered incorrectly.

B52

Musculoskeletal | Diseases and Conditions Impacting Interventions

A patient with spinal stenosis wants to return to recreational swimming. Which of the following swimming strokes is the **MOST** appropriate for the patient?

Choices:
1. Back stroke.
2. Breast stroke.
3. Butter fly.
4. Front crawl.

Teaching Points

Correct Answer: 1

When swimming the back stroke the lower back is in a flexed position. This relieves stress on the joints in the lower back.

Incorrect Choices:

The breast stroke, butter fly stroke, and the front crawl all place the lower back in a more hyperextended position, which can place increased pressure on the joints of the spine. This can cause increased pain and irritation in the joints of the spine and should be avoided.

Type of Reasoning: Inductive

For this question, the test taker must determine the appropriate water exercise for a patient with spinal stenosis. This requires knowledge of the diagnosis and precautions, which is an inductive reasoning skill. For this case, the assistant should instruct the patient to perform the backstroke in place of the crawl swim to avoid an extended spine during activities. If answered incorrectly, review water-based exercises for patients with spinal stenosis.

B53

Musculoskeletal | Interventions

A patient presents with neck pain and spasm of the left sternocleidomastoid muscle. To apply myofascial techniques and a gentle stretch, what motions should the physical therapist assistant perform with the cervical spine?

Choices:
1. Lateral flexion to the right with flexion.
2. Lateral flexion to the right and rotation to the left with extension.
3. Lateral flexion and rotation to the right with extension.
4. Lateral flexion to the left and rotation to the right with flexion.

Teaching Points

Correct Answer: 2
To apply a stretch, the physical therapist assistant must move the muscle in the opposite direction. The left sternocleidomastoid laterally flexes the neck to the left, rotates the neck to the right, and flexes the neck. Stretching the muscle should then incorporate lateral flexion to the right, rotation to the left, and extension of the neck.

Incorrect Choices:
A stretch of the sternocleidomastoid muscle must include lateral flexion, flexion, and rotation; failing to incorporate all of the degrees of motion of the muscle will not fully elongate the muscle. Placing the muscle into the motions it performs will not provide a stretch.

Type of Reasoning: Inductive
One must utilize clinical judgment to determine the appropriate cervical motions for a patient with sternocleidomastoid spasm and neck pain. This is an inductive reasoning skill. For this scenario, the assistant should perform lateral neck flexion to the right and rotation to the left to stretch the muscle. If answered incorrectly, review myofascial techniques, especially for the cervical region.

B54

Musculoskeletal | Interventions

Where is the trigger point for the levator scapula most likely palpated?

Choices:
1. Immediately medial to the superior portion of the acromion process.
2. Immediately medial to the inferior angle of the vertebral border of the scapula.
3. Just superior to the superior angle of the vertebral border of the scapula.
4. Just inferior to the mastoid process.

Teaching Points

Correct Answer: 3
The trigger points for the levator scapula are just superior to its attachment on the superior angle of the scapula and immediately inferior to its attachment on the occiput.

Incorrect Choices:
The trapezius has trigger points just medial to the acromion process on the superior portion as well as at the midway point of the vertebral border of the scapula. The sternocleidomastoid muscle has a trigger point just inferior to the mastoid process.

Type of Reasoning: Deductive

This question requires the test taker to recall factual information regarding a trigger point for the levator scapula muscle. This is a deductive reasoning skill, as guidelines are utilized to reach a reasonable conclusion. For this case, the trigger point is located just superior to the superior angle of the vertebral border of the scapula. If answered incorrectly, review trigger points for the cervical muscles.

B55

Nonsystem | Therapeutic Modalities

A physical therapist assistant reads a stated goal in the plan of care to stimulate a denervated anterior tibialis muscle. Which of the following types of current is the **MOST** appropriate type of current to use?

Choices:
1. Interrupted alternating current (biphasic current).
2. Continuous direct current (monophasic current).
3. Transcutaneous electrical neural stimulation (monophasic or biphasic current).
4. Interrupted direct current (monophasic current).

Teaching Points

Correct Answer: 4

Interrupted direct current (monophasic current) is used to stimulate denervated muscles by producing residual charges in the tissues under the cathode and anode.

Incorrect Choices:

Use of a biphasic current stimulates neural tissue to produce an action potential; a denervated muscle cannot be stimulated in this manner, as there is no nerve innervation remaining. Continuous direct current is primarily used for applying iontophoresis. Transcutaneous electrical neural stimulation is used to treat pain.

Type of Reasoning: Deductive

One must recall the guidelines for use of electrical stimulation to stimulate denervated muscles. This is factual information, which necessitates deductive reasoning skill. For this situation, to stimulate a denervated anterior tibialis muscle, the assistant should use interrupted direct current (monophasic current). If answered incorrectly, review electrical stimulation guidelines for denervated muscles.

B56

Musculoskeletal | Diseases and Conditions Impacting Interventions

A physical therapist assistant is working with a patient presenting with alkylosing of the subtalar joints bilaterally. Which of the following conditions would the patient **MOST** likely have difficulty with when ambulating?

Choices:
1. Uneven terrain.
2. Up ramps.
3. Level surfaces.
4. Down stairs.

Teaching Points

Correct Answer: 1

An ankylosed joint has limited motion and may, in fact, be fused. The subtalar joint allows for medial and lateral movements that enable the foot to adjust to uneven surfaces. Therefore, the patient who has ankylosis of both subtalar joints will have difficulty walking on uneven terrain.

Incorrect Choices:

The other walking activities listed require sufficient dorsiflexion and plantar flexion motions, both of which occur at the talocrural joint.

Type of Reasoning: Inferential

One must infer or draw a reasonable conclusion about the likely difficulty a patient with ankylosis of both subtalar joints will have while walking. This requires one to determine what may be true, which is an inferential reasoning skill. For this case, the patient will have the most difficulty walking on uneven terrain. Review ankylosis of the subtalar joints if answered incorrectly, especially challenges in walking.

B57

System Interaction | Interventions

A patient with congestive heart failure (CHF) is to undergo postural drainage of the posterior basal segment of the left lower lobe. Which of the following is the **MOST** appropriate strategy to modify the patient's position to prevent additional complications from the heart failure?

Choices:
1. Side-lying on the right with the bed flat.
2. Side-lying on the right with the foot of the bed elevated 18 inches.
3. Prone with the foot of the bed elevated 18 inches.
4. Prone with the bed flat.

Teaching Points

Correct Answer: 4

A patient with CHF will not tolerate the Trendelenburg position (foot of the bed elevated 18 inches). An appropriate modification involves placing the patient prone but maintaining the bed flat, allowing gravity to assist in draining the posterior segments of the lung.

Incorrect Choices:

Although the ideal method to drain the basal segment of the lung is with a Trendelenburg position, it is contraindicated for a patient with CHF. Side-lying on the right with the bed flat would be an appropriate modification for draining the anterior basal segments of the lower lobe in a patient with CHF.

Type of Reasoning: Inductive

One must determine the best modified position for postural drainage for a patient with congestive heart failure. This requires clinical judgment and knowledge of the diagnosis to arrive at a correct conclusion, which is an inductive reasoning skill. For this situation, the position should be modified to prone with the bed flat. If answered incorrectly, review postural drainage techniques and positioning for patients with CHF.

B58

Neuromuscular | Interventions

A patient has a lesion at T10, resulting in paraplegia. Which of the following mat activities promotes weight bearing through the hips in order to facilitate initial control of the lower trunk and hips?

Choices:
1. Supine on elbows.
2. Quadruped.
3. Long sitting.
4. Prone on elbows.

Teaching Points

Correct Answer: 2

Having the patient in the quadruped position on the mat allows for weight bearing through the femur into the hip joint. In this position, the lower trunk musculature must work to keep the hips aligned and to prevent lateral sway and/or anterior/posterior sway.

Incorrect Choices:

The remaining positions do not allow weight bearing through the hips, nor do they facilitate use of the lower trunk musculature.

Type of Reasoning: Analytical

One must analyze the activities presented to determine the activity that facilitates weight bearing to the hips and initial control of the lower trunk and hips. This requires analytical reasoning skill. For this situation, the first position in the mat activity sequence for this patient should be quadruped. Review mat activity for patients with thoracic spinal cord injury, especially lower thoracic injuries, if answered incorrectly.

B59

Nonsystem | Safety and Protection

During gait training at home, an adult patient falls and strikes his/her head. The physical therapist assistant determines that the patient is unconscious, has no pulse and is no longer breathing. The assistant is the only person present. What is the **NEXT** thing the physical therapist assistant should do?

Choices:
1. Assess the wound to the patient's head.
2. Begin rescue breathing.
3. Activate the emergency response system.
4. Initiate on-person cardiopulmonary resuscitation (CPR).

Teaching Points

Correct Answer: 3

When the physical therapist assistant is alone with an adult patient and help is not readily available, after determining the patient is unresponsive and is in need of emergency assistance, the PTA should activate the emergency medical (EMS) system.

Incorrect Choices:
While there may be a lesion/wound to the head that needs to be assessed, in order of priority, this is not a top priority. Rescue breathing is not a correct response when an individual has no pulse. CPR is an appropriate response after the emergency medical services system has been contacted.

Type of Reasoning: Evaluative
This question requires the test taker to weigh the courses of action and determine the action that best addresses the patient's immediate concerns. This is an evaluative reasoning skill. For this scenario, the next thing the assistant should do is call the emergency response system before administering care. If answered incorrectly, review emergency first aid and CPR guidelines.

B60

Musculoskeletal | Diseases and Conditions Impacting Intervention

A patient who has just undergone surgical repair for a chronic anterior shoulder dislocation is participating in an exercise program. Early rehabilitation should **AVOID** which of the following glenohumeral motions?

Choices:
1. Lateral (external) rotation.
2. Abduction.
3. Medial (internal) rotation.
4. Flexion.

Teaching Points

Correct Answer: 1
Lateral (external) rotation will move the humeral head forward and place the repair in a position of stress, increasing the likelihood of anterior dislocation.

Incorrect Choices:
Abduction primarily moves the humeral head inferiorly. Medial (internal) rotation causes the head of the humerus to move posteriorly. Flexion results in posterior movement of the humeral head.

Type of Reasoning: Inductive
One must utilize clinical judgment and knowledge of chronic anterior shoulder dislocation to arrive at a correct conclusion. This necessitates inductive reasoning skill. For this situation, early rehabilitation should avoid glenohumeral lateral rotation to avoid anterior dislocation. If answered incorrectly, review chronic anterior shoulder dislocation guidelines and intervention approaches.

B61

Musculoskeletal | Interventions

The supervising physical therapist has asked the physical therapist assistant to provide stretching exercises to a patient with traumatic brain injury (TBI). The patient has hip flexor tightness and decreased knee extension bilaterally. What is one optimal position in which to place the patient to achieve maximum efficiency for stretching?

Choices:
1. Sitting.
2. Prone.
3. Supine.
4. Side-lying.

Teaching Points

Correct Answer: 4

If the patient is in side-lying, the physical therapist assistant is able to stretch both the hips and knees into extension. This is especially important for the patient who has suffered a TBI as side-lying is a supportive and relaxed position.

Incorrect Choices:

The sitting position will make it difficult to stretch the patient into hip extension. While the assistant will be able to stretch the patient in a prone position, the patient may exhibit an increase in flexion and flexor tone if the tonic labyrinthine reflex is present, which is common in patients following a TBI. The supine position also limits the ability to get the hip into an extended position.

Type of Reasoning: Inductive

This question requires the test taker to use knowledge of muscle-stretching guidelines and TBI to reach a correct conclusion. This requires clinical judgment, which is an inductive reasoning skill. For this case, the optimal position to place the patient in to achieve maximal range of motion is side-lying. If answered incorrectly, review muscle-stretching guidelines for the lower extremity in patients with TBI.

B62

Pulmonary | Data Collection

While reviewing the patient's medical record prior to gait training, the physical therapist assistant notes that the patient is experiencing increased shortness of breath and the physician has just written an order for a ventilation perfusion scan. What is the **MOST** appropriate response now for the physical therapist assistant?

Choices:
1. Withhold treatment and contact the supervising therapist.
2. Proceed with the treatments as usual because there is no definitive change in the patient's status.
3. Modify treatment plan to focus on breathing exercises.
4. Proceed with the treatments while monitoring the patient's respiration rate and vital signs very carefully.

Teaching Points

Correct Answer: 1

A ventilation perfusion scan is performed to identify the presence of a pulmonary embolus (PE). If there is a possibility of a PE, the safest thing to do is to delay the treatment (remember, safety first). The physical therapist assistant should contact the supervising physical therapist for him/her to determine whether the patient is appropriate for treatment.

Incorrect Choices:

Number 2 and 4 are incorrect options as they involve therapeutic intervention. Physical therapy is contraindicated if there is a possibility of a PE. The physical therapist assistant should also not change the treatment plan without consulting the supervising physical therapist (option 3).

Type of Reasoning: Evaluative

One must weigh the value of the approaches provided to determine the approach that is most appropriate for the patient and the potential diagnosis of PE. For this situation, having knowledge of the reasons for a physician ordering a ventilation perfusion scan, the assistant should withhold treatment and contact the supervising therapist. If answered incorrectly, review ventilation perfusion scan information.

B63

Integumentary | Diseases and Conditions Impacting Interventions

A patient who is receiving home physical therapy reports experiencing increased aching in the left lower extremity, which is only alleviated when the lower extremity is elevated. The physical therapist assistant inspects the feet and lower extremities and notes some mild edema, a darker pigmentation to the tissues, and a dermatitis-type condition on the medial distal lower extremity. These symptoms are consistent with what type of ulcer?

Choices:
1. Diabetic ulcers.
2. Venous ulcers.
3. Arterial ulcers.
4. Pressure ulcers.

Teaching Points

Correct Answer: 2

The presented characteristics are all consistent with a venous ulcer, primarily resulting from a collection of deoxygenated blood in the affected extremity.

Incorrect Choices:
Arterial ulcers likely result in pain with leg elevation, trophic changes, and a pale, ischemic appearance. Diabetic ulcers are typically not painful though paresthesias may be present; they typically have a more round or "punched-out" appearance. Pressure ulcers typically appear over bony landmarks in weight-bearing areas.

Type of Reasoning: Analytical
This question provides symptoms and the test taker must determine the possible diagnosis of the patient. This requires one to analyze the symptoms presented to draw a conclusion, which is an analytical reasoning skill. For this case, the symptoms are consistent with venous ulcers. Review signs and symptoms of venous ulcers if answered incorrectly.

B64

Musculoskeletal | Data Collection

If a physical therapist assistant measures the patient's ankle range of motion to be 25° to –7°, what is the **BEST** interpretation?

Choices:
1. The patient has 25° of dorsiflexion and –7° of plantar flexion.
2. The patient has 25° of dorsiflexion and 7° of plantar flexion.
3. The patient has 25° of plantar flexion and 7° of dorsiflexion.
4. The patient has 25° of plantar flexion and –7° of dorsiflexion.

Teaching Points

Correct Answer: 4

Normal range of motion of the ankle is typically reported as 50° to 0° to 20°, indicating 50° of plantar flexion, the ability to return to neutral ankle position, and 20° of dorsiflexion. This patient's range of motion for ankle dorsiflexion is –7°, indicating the inability to achieve the neutral ankle position of zero.

Incorrect Choices:

A negative number reported for ROM signifies a movement that does not obtain the neutral position for the joint. For the ankle, this signifies a lack of dorsiflexion. While this patient has 25° of plantar flexion, the ankle is 7° short of the neutral position.

Type of Reasoning: Analytical

One must analyze the range-of-motion numbers presented for the ankle and determine their significance to arrive at a correct conclusion. This requires analytical reasoning skill, as pieces of information are analyzed to determine significance. For this situation, the range-of-motion numbers indicate 7° of ankle dorsiflexion. If answered incorrectly, review range-of-motion measurement guidelines for the ankle.

B65

System Interactions | Safety and Protection

An adult runner collapses after being brought to the first aid station. Ambient temperature is 92°F (33°C) and body temperature is measured at 101°F (38°C). The runner presents with a rapid pulse, rapid respirations, and skin that is warm and dry to touch. When questioned, the runner is confused. What type of shock are these symptoms are consistent with?

Choices:
1. Hypovolemic shock.
2. Hypervolemic shock.
3. Anaphylactic shock.
4. Septic shock.

Teaching Points

Correct Answer: 1

This runner is demonstrating signs and symptoms of dehydration, which leads to hypovolemic shock.

Incorrect Choices:

While the signs noted are common to many types of stroke, it is the cause that distinguishes what type of shock occurs. Anaphylactic shock is an allergic reaction to drugs, food or insect stings. Septic shock results from a severe infection in the blood. Hypervolemia, an excess in blood volume, does not typically result in shock.

Type of Reasoning: Analytical

This question provides a group of symptoms and the test taker must determine a possible cause. This requires analysis of pieces of information to draw a correct conclusion, which is an analytical reasoning skill. For this scenario, the findings seem consistent with hypovolemic shock. If answered incorrectly, review symptoms of hypovolemic shock.

B66

Cardiac | Data Collection

A home health physical therapist assistant is treating an older adult patient. On this day the patient is confused and presents with shortness of breath and generalized weakness. What does the physical therapist assistant suspect is occurring?

Choices:
1. Mental changes indicative of early Alzheimer's disease.
2. Unstable angina.
3. Early signs of myocardial infarction.
4. Forgetting to take prescribed hypertension medication.

Teaching Points

Correct Answer: 3

An elderly patient with a cardiac history may present initially with mental confusion when experiencing early myocardial infarction as a result of oxygen deprivation to the brain. The shortness of breath and generalized weakness may also be caused by generalized circulatory insufficiencies coexisting with the developing myocardial infarction.

Incorrect Choices:
Mental changes associated with Alzheimer's disease would not develop as rapidly as this patient's symptoms, nor would it be accompanied by shortness of breath and generalized weakness. Unstable angina would likely present with the additional sign of chest and/or referred pain to the jaw, left upper extremity or back. Failure to take the prescribed hypertension medications would not likely result in mental confusion, but signs such as headache, vision changes and diaphoresis.

Type of Reasoning: Analytical
This question requires the test taker to determine a cause for the patient's symptoms. Questions that require one to determine a diagnosis based on a group of symptoms often require analytical reasoning skill. For this situation, the assistant could conclude that the patient's symptoms indicate early signs of myocardial infarction. If answered incorrectly, review signs and symptoms of myocardial infarction, especially in older adults.

B67

Neuromuscular | Interventions

A patient with musculoskeletal pain and spasm of the upper back and neck secondary to emotional stress at work is being taught a relaxation protocol. Which of the following choices is **LEAST** likely a part of this program?

Choices:
1. Active strengthening exercises to the affected musculature.
2. Progressive tensing, holding and releasing of the affected muscle groups.
3. Hot packs to the neck and back for 20 minutes.
4. Controlled, diaphragmatic breathing.

Teaching Points

Correct Answer: 1
Active strengthening exercises are not considered a relaxation technique.

Incorrect Choices:
Progressive tensing and release as well as controlled breathing are key concepts of a relaxation protocol. Although hot packs are a modality, heat is typically used in conjunction with relaxation techniques and would therefore be an appropriate component of the relaxation protocol.

Type of Reasoning: Deductive

One must recall the relaxation protocol for patients with pain and spasm to arrive at a correct conclusion. This requires the recall of factual information, which is a deductive reasoning skill. For this case, the only approach that is not part of a relaxation protocol is active strengthening exercises to the affected musculature. If answered incorrectly, review relaxation guidelines for patients with musculoskeletal pain and spasm.

B68

Neuromuscular | Interventions

As a result of a traumatic brain injury, a patient is demonstrating significant static standing balance deficits. Which of the following is the **BEST** intervention strategy for this patient?

Choices:
1. Use of a standing equilibrium board.
2. Rhythmic stabilization in standing.
3. Weight shifting to pick up objects from the floor.
4. Performing reaching tasks outside the base of support.

Teaching Points

Correct Answer: 2

Rhythmic stabilization applied in the standing position will help to increase the patient's static standing balance.

Incorrect Choices:
The incorrect answers involve activities that address the patient's dynamic standing balance.

Type of Reasoning: Inductive

This question requires one to determine the best intervention strategy for a patient with static standing balance deficits. This requires knowledge of the intervention approaches to arrive at a correct conclusion, which is an inductive reasoning skill. For this situation, the best intervention strategy is rhythmic stabilization in standing. Review static standing balance approaches for patients with traumatic brain injury, especially static standing activities, if answered incorrectly.

B69

Nonsystem | Therapeutic Modalities

An athlete with no other medical conditions incurred blunt trauma to the right thigh. An ice pack was applied for 20 minutes. What **INITIAL** skin changes should the physical therapist assistant expect after removing the ice pack?

Choices:
1. Erythema followed by blanching at about 30 minutes.
2. Blanching followed by decreased blood pressure and increased pulse rate.
3. Reflex vasodilation followed by increased blood pressure and decreased pulse rate.
4. Blanching followed by erythema at about 10 minutes.

Teaching Points

Correct Answer: 4
Blanching, caused by vasoconstriction of the superficial blood vessels, is the initial response to cold. With extended exposure, the body's response is to move relatively warmer blood to the affected area, which results in erythema.

Incorrect Choices:
Changes in blood pressure or heart rate are not expected responses of a local cold application to a healthy individual. If blanching develops after extended exposure, the tissues are demonstrating intolerance for cold and may be frostbitten.

Type of Reasoning: Inferential
One must infer the likely initial response of the skin to blunt trauma and cryotherapy to arrive at a correct conclusion. This requires inferential reasoning skill. For this scenario, the assistant should expect the skin to initially exhibit blanching followed by erythema at about 10 minutes. If answered incorrectly, review skin responses to cryotherapy after injury.

B70

Neuromuscular | Interventions

When a physical therapist assistant is writing a home program to be administered by family members for a child with cerebral palsy, what is the primary consideration?

Choices:
1. Educational level of the family members.
2. Gender of the child.
3. Religion or beliefs of the family.
4. Nationality of the family.

Teaching Points

Correct Answer: 1
The physical therapist assistant should not develop a program written higher than the family members' level of understanding in order to facilitate completion of the home program.

Incorrect Choices:
The gender of the child, the religious beliefs of the family, and their nationality are not primary considerations of the home program.

Type of Reasoning: Inductive
One must determine the primary consideration when providing a home program for family members. This requires one to determine the outcomes of each of the choices presented to assess the primary benefit of these choices. This is an inductive reasoning skill. For this situation, primary consideration should be the educational level of the family members to ensure understanding of the program and follow-through. If answered incorrectly, review development of home programs for family members.

B71

Integumentary | Diseases and Conditions Impacting Interventions

A physical therapist assistant is asked to perform gait training with a patient who has a venous insufficiency ulcer on the medial side of the left ankle. After gait training, the assistant should specifically ensure which of the following considerations?

Choices:
1. The lower extremity is elevated and a support garment or elastic bandage is in place.
2. The dressing is changed and an antiseptic ointment is applied to the wound.
3. The patient returns to bed and that the head of the bed is moderately elevated.
4. There are no signs of deep venous thrombosis.

Teaching Points

Correct Answer: 1

For a patient with a venous insufficiency ulcer, the lower extremity should not be left in a dependent position, as this will contribute to the development of further edema and decreased ulcer healing. Application of a support garment or elastic bandage is also beneficial to decrease edema.

Incorrect Choices:
Dressing changes are not part of gait training and, therefore, would fall outside the plan of care. Elevating the head of the bed would worsen the patient's lower-extremity edema. The patient should be assessed for signs of a deep venous thrombosis prior to, not following, gait training.

Type of Reasoning: Inductive
This question requires one to have knowledge of venous insufficiency ulcers to arrive at a correct conclusion. This requires inductive reasoning skill. For this situation, after gait training, the assistant should ensure that the affected lower extremity is elevated and a support garment or elastic bandage is in place. If answered incorrectly, review treatment guidelines for patients with venous insufficiency ulcers.

B72

Nonsystem | Therapeutic Modalities

A patient is receiving iontophoresis using hydrocortisone for chronic overuse tendonitis. The hydrocortisone is used for which of the following therapeutic effects?

Choices:
1. Analgesic.
2. Antispasmodic.
3. Anti-inflammatory.
4. Antifungal.

Teaching Points

Correct Answer: 3
Hydrocortisone and dexamethasone are the anti-inflammatory agents delivered via iontophoresis.

Incorrect Choices:
Lidocaine or xylocaine are used to decrease pain, calcium or magnesium are used to decrease muscle spasm, and copper may be used to treat fungal infections.

Type of Reasoning: Deductive

One must recall the benefits for using hydrocortisone in iontophoresis. This is factual information and recall of guidelines, which is a deductive reasoning skill. For this scenario, the hydrocortisone is used as an anti-inflammatory agent. If answered incorrectly, review iontophoresis guidelines, including indications for the use of hydrocortisone.

B73

Musculoskeletal | Interventions

The physical therapist assistant is instructed to provide gait training for an older adult patient who has a grade 2 left ankle sprain and impaired balance. If the patient is instructed to maintain partial weight bearing during gait which of the following is the MOST appropriate gait-training strategy?

Choices:
1. Wheeled walker using a reciprocal gait.
2. Standard walker, advancing the left lower extremity, then the right.
3. Axillary crutches using a 3-point partial-weight-bearing gait.
4. Bilateral small-base quad canes using a 3-point gait pattern.

Teaching Points

Correct Answer: 2

A standard walker with the involved lower extremity advancing followed by the unaffected lower extremity will allow for maintaining partial weight bearing as indicated.

Incorrect Choices:

Axillary crutches and quad canes are less stable than the walker, which would pose a safety risk to a patient with impaired balance. A reciprocal gait pattern with a wheeled walker will not allow for partial weight bearing.

Type of Reasoning: Inductive

One must determine the most appropriate gait-training method for an older adult with grade 2 ankle sprain and fair balance to arrive at a correct conclusion. This requires clinical judgment, which is an inductive reasoning skill. For this case, gait training should include use of a standard walker, advancing the left lower extremity, then the right. Review gait-training guidelines for patients with ankle sprain and balance deficits if answered incorrectly.

B74

Neuromuscular | Diseases and Conditions Impacting Intervention

When working with a group of patients who have multiple sclerosis, which of the following is the MOST appropriate course of action?

Choices:
1. Use a therapeutic pool.
2. Avoid resistance exercises.
3. Implement exercise sets with specific repetitions for each.
4. Schedule morning treatment sessions.

Teaching Points

Correct Answer: 4

Patients who have multiple sclerosis (MS) can fatigue easily and will likely respond best to treatment scheduled in the morning to avoid the afternoon fatigue.

Incorrect Choices:

A therapeutic pool will likely be kept at a temperature that is too high for a patient with MS and can contribute to fatigue. Group exercise sessions should allow for patients with varying levels of ability, strength, and endurance; therefore, a variety of resistance strengths and exercise repetitions would be appropriate.

Type of Reasoning: Evaluative

This question requires the test taker to evaluate the courses of action and determine the one that is most beneficial for a group of patients with MS. This requires evaluative reasoning skill. For this scenario, it is most important to schedule morning treatment sessions to avoid afternoon fatigue. If answered incorrectly, review signs and symptoms of MS and intervention approaches.

Musculoskeletal | Interventions

Which of the following positions is the **BEST** choice to stretch the pectoralis major muscle?

Choices:
1. Sitting on heels, forward trunk flexion, with upper extremities in 180° of shoulder flexion.
2. Supine with the shoulder abducted to 45° and medially (internally) rotated.
3. Supine with the shoulder flexed and abducted to 145°.
4. With hands clasped together behind the low back and extended.

Teaching Points

Correct Answer: 3

To stretch the pectoral muscles, the shoulders must be abducted and laterally (externally) rotated. This is best accomplished in supine with the shoulder flexed and abducted to 145° with the weight of gravity providing a stretching force.

Incorrect Choices:

The incorrect options listed do not place the pectoralis on a stretch. Sitting on heels and performing forward trunk flexion with arms outstretched affects the low back flexors and latissimus. Lying supine with the shoulder abducted to 45° and medially rotated is ineffective in stretching the pectoralis major. Hands clasped behind the back and extended is effective for stretching the anterior chest if scapular retraction is performed simultaneously.

Type of Reasoning: Deductive

One must recall the guidelines for stretching the pectoralis major muscle to arrive at a correct conclusion. This is factual information, which is a deductive reasoning skill. For this case, the pectoralis major muscle should be stretched in supine with the shoulder flexed and abducted 145°. If answered incorrectly, review muscle-stretching techniques for the pectoralis major.

B76

Nonsystem | Safety and Protection

A physical therapist assistant observes a patient suddenly fall to the ground while walking into the clinic. When the assistant arrives at the patient's side, the patient is unresponsive. What is the assistant's **MOST** appropriate response?

Choices:
1. Call out for someone to activate the emergency response, open the airway and assess breathing.
2. Contact the physical therapist, determine heart rate, and, if absent, begin chest compressions.
3. Call for emergency help, take vital signs, and begin chest compressions as needed.
4. Call a code, stay with the patient, monitor vital signs, and wait for the emergency team.

Teaching Points

Correct Answer: 1

This is an emergency situation and immediate action is appropriate. Because the physical therapist assistant is in the clinic, calling out for help is an appropriate first step, followed immediately by opening the airway and assessing the individuals ABCs (airway, breathing, circulation).

Incorrect Choices:

Calling the physical therapist or waiting for the emergency team to arrive may cost the individual their life. Initiation of chest compressions is inappropriate until assessment of a lack of pulse is completed and no pulse is detected.

Type of Reasoning: Evaluative

One must evaluate the courses of action presented and then determine the action that will effectively address the patient's needs. This requires evaluative reasoning skill. For this situation, the assistant should call out for someone to activate a code, open airway, and assess breathing. If answered incorrectly, review emergency first aid and CPR guidelines. Information about CPR and rescue breathing guidelines is found in the Management, Safety and Professional Roles chapter.

B77

Musculoskeletal | Interventions

Which of the following is true regarding the use of isokinetic exercises?

Choices:
1. Speed of exercise should be preset and resistance will vary depending upon the patient's ability.
2. Resistance should be preset and the speed of exercise will vary depending upon the patient's ability.
3. Resistance should be increased if the patient can achieve a preset 10-repetition maximum.
4. Speed of exercise should be increased for the patient to generate greater torque.

Teaching Points

Correct Answer: 1

In isokinetic exercise, the speed is preset and the resistance changes. As the patient "works" harder, the machine responds by increasing the resistance while keeping the speed constant.

Incorrect Choices:

The speed of exercise is constant during isokinetic exercise while the resistance varies based on the effort exerted by the patient. When the speed of exercise is increased, the torque produced will be decreased.

Type of Reasoning: Inductive

This question requires one to recall the benefits of isokinetic exercises to arrive at a correct conclusion. This requires knowledge of isokinetic exercise guidelines, which necessitates inductive reasoning skill. For this case, in carrying out this form of exercise, the speed of exercise should be preset and resistance will vary depending upon the patient's ability. If answered incorrectly, review isokinetic exercise guidelines.

B78

Other Systems | Diseases and Conditions Impacting Intervention

What does current research support about the use of exercise when treating a patient who has a diagnosis of HIV in stage I?

Choices:
1. Exercise will further suppress the immune system.
2. Exercise will help increase the helper CD4 T cells.
3. Exercise training should be performed at 50%–60% of maximum heart rate.
4. Exercise is contraindicated.

Teaching Points

Correct Answer: 2

Current research demonstrates that exercise is important and effective in enhancing the helper CD4 T cells as well as the overall health of the person with HIV, especially in the earlier stages.

Incorrect Choices:

Exercise training, which should be done at 70%–80% of maximum heart rate to achieve the best results. Exercise does not suppress the immune system but rather enhances it. Exercise is not contraindicated in early stages of HIV unless there are extenuating circumstances; none were identified in the question.

Type of Reasoning: Inferential

This question requires one to draw a reasonable conclusion about current research regarding exercise for patients with AIDS. This requires inferential reasoning skill. For this scenario, current research demonstrates that exercise will help increase the helper CD4 T cells, thereby enhancing overall health. If answered incorrectly, review current research regarding benefits of exercise for patients with AIDS. Information about the use of exercise with patients who have HIV or AIDS is found in the Other Systems and Conditions chapter.

B79

Neuromuscular | Data Collection

A physical therapist assistant working with a patient who has a lower motor neuron injury should expect the patient to present with which of the following elements?

Choices:
1. Positive Babinski sign.
2. Clonus.
3. Extensor muscle spasms.
4. Flaccidity.

Teaching Points

Correct Answer: 4

Symptoms of a lower motor neuron injury include decreased reflexes, muscle fasciculations and severe muscle wasting.

Incorrect Choices:

Positive Babinski sign, clonus, and extensor muscle spasm are all signs of upper motor neuron lesions.

Type of Reasoning: Inferential

One must infer or draw a reasonable conclusion about the likely presentation of a patient with lower motor neuron injury. This requires one to determine what may be true of a patient, which is an inferential reasoning skill. For this situation, one should expect the patient to present with flaccidity. If answered incorrectly, review signs and symptoms of lower motor neuron injury. Information about the signs and symptoms of upper versus lower motor neuron lesions is found in Chapter 2.

B80

Musculoskeletal | Interventions

During a gait observation, the physical therapist assistant notes that the patient has decreased hip extension during stance phase. Which of the following deficits is likely to result in this gait deviation?

Choices:
1. Decreased range of motion of the biceps femoris.
2. Decreased range of motion of the iliopsoas.
3. Weakness of the hip flexors.
4. Weakness of the hip extensors.

Teaching Points

Correct Answer: 2

Decreased hip extension in stance phase most likely illustrates decreased range of motion of the hip flexors, the biggest of which is the iliopsoas.

Incorrect Choices:

Decreased range of motion of the biceps femoris will likely result in decreased knee extension and will affect both the stance and swing phases. Weakness of the hip flexors affects the amount of hip flexion achieved during swing phase. Weakness of the hip extensors will result in lateral or backward bending of the trunk during stance phase.

Type of Reasoning: Inferential

This question provides a deficit and the test taker must determine the most likely cause for it. This requires one to infer the reason for the deficit, which is an inferential reasoning skill. For this situation, the most likely reason for the deficit is decreased range of motion of the iliopsoas muscle. If answered incorrectly, review gait abnormalities, including decreased hip extension during stance phase. Information about the causes of common gait deviations is found in the Gait, Functional Training, Equipment, and Devices chapter.

B81

Cardiac | Data Collection

While assisting a physical therapist in treating a critically ill patient in the intensive care unit, the therapist asks the physical therapist assistant to quickly find out the most recent PO_2 and PCO_2 results for the patient. Where in the medical record can these values be located?

Choices:
1. Pulmonary function test results.
2. Hematocrit results.
3. Arterial blood gases.
4. Vital signs.

Teaching Points

Correct Answer: 3

PO_2 and PCO_2 values, which indicate the levels of oxygen and carbon dioxide in the blood, are called arterial blood gases or ABGs.

Incorrect Choices:

Pulmonary function test results include such information as tidal volume, vital capacity, and total lung capacity. Hematocrit results will be found in the complete blood count (CBC). Vital signs will primarily be located in the nursing notes.

Type of Reasoning: Deductive

This question requires one to recall the abbreviations indicating arterial blood gas values to arrive at a correct conclusion. This is factual information, necessitating deductive reasoning skill. For this situation, PO_2 and PCO_2 can be found in the medical record by looking for arterial blood gas values. If answered incorrectly, review lab values for patients in the intensive care unit, including arterial blood gases. Information about laboratory tests and values, including ABGs, is found in the Cardiac, Vascular, and Lymphatic chapter.

B82

Nonsystem | Equipment and Devices

Posting on a lower extremity orthosis is typically used to help correct which of the following conditions?

Choices:
1. Pes planus (flat foot).
2. Weak dorsiflexors.
3. A lower-extremity length discrepancy.
4. Rearfoot varus.

Teaching Points

Correct Answer: 4

Posting is a wedge that is placed on the forefoot or rearfoot portion of an orthosis to correct for a varus or valgus deformity.

Incorrect Choices:

A longitudinal arch support will help prevent pes planus and help control the subtalar joint. Weak dorsiflexors are best managed with an ankle-foot orthosis with a dorsiflexion assist or plantar flexion stop. A lower-extremity length discrepancy will likely be managed with a heel lift.

Type of Reasoning: Deductive

One must recall the purpose of posting on a lower-extremity orthosis to arrive at a correct conclusion. This is factual recall of guidelines, which is a deductive reasoning skill. For this case, posting on the orthosis will help correct for rearfoot varus. If answered incorrectly, review lower-extremity orthotics, especially orthotics for correction of rearfoot varus.

B83

Musculoskeletal | Equipment and Devices

A patient who has rheumatoid arthritis is **MOST** likely to use which of the following devices?

Choices:
1. Airplane splint.
2. Cock-up splint.
3. Dynamic wrist extension splint.
4. Milwaukee brace.

Teaching Points

Correct Answer: 2

A cock-up or resting splint will likely be used to protect and rest the wrist; the smaller joints of the wrist and hand are often affected when a person has rheumatoid arthritis.

Incorrect Choices:

An airplane splint is used to position the shoulder at 90° of abduction, and 90° of elbow flexion following a fracture or surgery when the neutral position is not desirable. A dynamic wrist extension splint will facilitate the tenodesis grasp in a patient with quadriplegia. A Milwaukee brace is a specialized trunk orthosis used to control scoliosis.

Type of Reasoning: Inferential

This question requires one to determine the likely device that would be used by a patient who has rheumatoid arthritis. The test taker must infer the likely conclusion, which is an inferential reasoning skill. For this case, the patient is likely to wear a cock-up splint, as these splints are often worn to protect and rest the wrists. If answered incorrectly, review splinting guidelines for patients with rheumatoid arthritis.

B84

Integumentary | Interventions

When discussing the care of a patient in the home environment, a physical therapist assistant should explain to the family that pressure ulcers primarily develop in what location for a patient who is wheelchair bound?

Choices:
1. Ischial tuberosity.
2. Greater trochanter.
3. Lateral malleolus.
4. Sacrum.

Teaching Points

Correct Answer: 1

In a sitting position, the greatest amount of weight is supported by the ischial tuberosities, thus making them most susceptible to pressure ulcers.

Incorrect Choices:

The greater trochanter and lateral malleolus would be most susceptible to breakdown in side-lying while the sacrum would have the most pressure when the patient is positioned in supine.

Type of Reasoning: Deductive

One must recall the causes of pressure ulcers to arrive at a correct conclusion. This necessitates the recall of factual information, which is a deductive reasoning skill. For this situation, the primary cause of decubitus ulcers is excess pressure. If answered incorrectly, review decubitus ulcer guidelines and common causes.

B85

Neuromuscular | Therapeutic Modalities

An athlete received a contusion to the left thigh nearly a week ago. The plan of care includes superficial heat prior to exercise. What is the **MOST** likely rationale for this intervention?

Choices:
1. Anesthetize the area.
2. Decrease muscle spasm.
3. Decrease tissue extensibility.
4. Decrease the extensibility of collagen tissue.

Teaching Points

Correct Answer: 2

Application of superficial heat will increase the extensibility of collagen tissue resulting in the reduction of muscle spasms.

Incorrect Choices:

Anesthetizing the area, decreasing tissue extensibility, and decreasing extensibility of collagen tissue are all results of the application of cryotherapy.

Type of Reasoning: Inferential

One must determine the likely reason for use of a hot pack on a site of contusion prior to exercise to arrive at a correct conclusion. This requires one to determine what may be true of a situation, which is an inferential reasoning skill. For this scenario, it is most likely that the hot pack is being used to decrease muscle spasm prior to exercise. If answered incorrectly, review benefits and indications for use of heat prior to exercise. Information about the indications and contraindications for superficial heat is found in the Therapeutic Modalities chapter.

B86

Musculoskeletal | Data Collection

Gait observation reveals a patient ambulating with a steppage gait pattern. What is the MOST likely cause of this compensatory gait pattern?

Choices:
1. Weakness of the gastrocnemius and soleus muscles.
2. Spasticity of the tibialis anterior muscle.
3. Weakness of the extensor digitorum longus and tibialis anterior muscles.
4. Extensor spasticity of both the quadriceps and gastrocnemius soleus muscles.

Teaching Points

Correct Answer: 3

In order to compensate for weakness of the extensor digitorum longus and tibialis anterior, the patient will demonstrate exaggerated hip and knee flexion during swing phase, termed a steppage gait.

Incorrect Choices:

Weakness of the gastrocnemius and soleus muscles will affect knee stability at midstance, and, most significantly, limit push-off into swing phase. Spasticity of the tibialis anterior muscle will result in a varus or inverted foot. Extensor spasticity of the quadriceps and gastrocnemius soleus muscles would result in hip hiking or eqinovarus.

Type of Reasoning: Inferential

One must infer or draw a reasonable conclusion about the most likely cause for a patient ambulating with a steppage gait pattern. This requires inferential reasoning skill. For this case, the most likely cause is weakness of the extensor digitorum longus and tibialis anterior muscles. If answered incorrectly, review gait pattern deviations, including steppage gait pattern.

B87

Integumentary | Data Collection

A patient presents with a partial thickness burn wound to the palmar surface of the right hand. Which of the following wound bed appearances should the physical therapist assistant expect to observe?

Choices:
1. Red with slight edema, no blisters and some tenderness.
2. Black or charred, and dry; edema is present with little pain.
3. Blistered and inflamed with no pain.
4. Reddened or white, with edema and/or blistering, with severe pain.

Teaching Points

Correct Answer: 4

A partial thickness burn involves the epidermis and dermis and will appear red or white with edema and/or blistering. Due to injury to the nerve endings, the patient will have severe pain.

Incorrect Choices:

Superficial burns appear red, with slight edema and no blistering. A full thickness burn will appear black or charred, have a dry surface with a scab, and present with little pain as the nerve endings have been destroyed. Pain is a hallmark of partial thickness burns and will be present.

Type of Reasoning: Deductive

One must recall the features of a partial thickness burn to arrive at a correct conclusion. This is factual recall of information, which is a deductive reasoning skill. For this situation, one should expect the wound bed to appear reddened or white, with edema and/or blistering, and with severe pain. Review characteristics of partial thickness burns if answered incorrectly.

B88

Neuromuscular | Interventions

A newborn has a brachial plexus injury that is a result of a breech birth presentation. Nerve roots C8 and T1 have been affected. The infant will **MOST** likely present with which of the following manifestations?

Choices:
1. Paralysis of the intrinsic muscles and wrist flexors.
2. A shoulder that is adducted and medially (internally) rotated shoulder.
3. A waiter's tip deformity.
4. Winging of the scapula.

Teaching Points

Correct Answer: 1

The nerve roots of C8 and T1 and the peripheral nerves that come from these roots innervate the muscles of the wrist flexors and the intrinsic muscles of the hand.

Incorrect Choices:

Damage to the C5–C7 nerve roots would result in Erb's palsy, characterized by a waiter's tip deformity, adducted and medially rotated shoulder, and winging of the scapula.

Type of Reasoning: Inferential

This question provides a diagnosis and the test taker must determine the most likely symptoms of this diagnosis. This requires inferential reasoning skill. For this case, an incident with C8 and T1 nerve root damage will most likely present with paralysis of the intrinsic muscles and wrist flexors. If answered incorrectly, review brachial plexus injuries in infants, including Klumpke's paralysis.

B89

System Interactions | Diseases and Conditions Impacting Intervention

Following an organ transplant, a patient has been on a long-term regimen of corticosteroids. What are the possible side effects of this course of treatment?

Choices:
1. Dyspnea, increased blood pressure, and weight loss.
2. Osteoporosis, slowness of wound healing, and weight gain.
3. Low blood sugar levels, increased heart rate, and weight gain.
4. Osteoporosis, increased healing, and weight loss.

Teaching Points

Correct Answer: 2

There are many side effects from using steroids, including weight gain, decreased healing, and osteoporosis.

Incorrect Choices:

All of the options listed are a result of steroid use except weight loss and low blood sugar levels.

Type of Reasoning: Deductive
One must recall the side effects of long-term corticosteroid use to arrive at a correct conclusion. This is factual recall of information, which is a deductive reasoning skill. For this scenario, possible side effects of corticosteroids include osteoporosis, slowness of wound healing, and weight gain. If answered incorrectly, review side effects of corticosteroid use.

B90

Neuromuscular | Interventions

A physical therapist assistant is working with a patient who has a C6-level spinal cord injury. The physical therapist assistant should expect the patient to be able to demonstrate which of the following functional levels?

Choices:
1. Dependent for all self-care activities.
2. Independent with wheelchair push-ups for pressure relief.
3. Independent performing a sliding board transfer on level surfaces.
4. Grasping objects by contracting the finger flexors to form a tight grip.

Teaching Points

Correct Answer: 3
A patient with a C6 spinal cord injury should be able to perform sliding board transfers on level surfaces.

Incorrect Choices:
While a patient with a C8–T1 injury would be independent with self-care, a patient with a C6 injury would be able to perform some self-care activities. Independent performance of wheelchair push-ups for pressure relief is more likely to occur in a patient with innervated triceps (C7 injury). Grasping object with a strong grip using the finger flexors will also be more appropriate for a patient with a C7 injury.

Type of Reasoning: Inferential
This question requires one to determine what may be true for a patient with C6 spinal cord injury. Questions of this nature often require inferential reasoning skill. For this situation, one should expect that the patient is able to perform a sliding board transfer on level surfaces. If answered incorrectly, review functional abilities for patients with C6 spinal cord injury, especially transfer abilities.

B91

Nonsystem | Professional Responsibilities

Which of the following hospital engineering controls should be employed to decrease the potential for an employee to be exposed to a blood-borne pathogen?

Choices:
1. Color-coded red or labeled containers.
2. Gloves.
3. Face shield.
4. Eye irrigation station.

Teaching Points

Correct Answer: 1

The Occupational Safety and Health Administration (OSHA) regulates work environments and has identified engineering controls that isolate or remove the biohazard from employees, namely the use of puncture-resistant and leak-proof containers that are color-coded red or labeled.

Incorrect Choices:

Work practice requirements cover the use of personal protective equipment (gloves, face shield, etc.) and the mechanism for eye irrigation in the event of an exposure.

Type of Reasoning: Deductive

One must recall engineering control guidelines to arrive at a correct conclusion. This is factual information, which is a deductive reasoning skill. For this scenario, an example of an engineering control to reduce the risk of exposure to bloodborne pathogens is color-coded red or labeled containers. If answered incorrectly, review OSHA guidelines for engineering controls to reduce exposure to bloodborne pathogens.

B92

Integumentary | Interventions

Scar tissue mobilization is safe to initiate during which stage of healing?

Choices:
1. First, or inflammatory phase.
2. Third, or fibroblastic phase.
3. Second, or granulation phase.
4. Fourth, or maturation phase.

Teaching Points

Correct Answer: 2

During the fibroblastic phase, collagen fibers are laid down with weaker hydrostatic bonds that make tissue elongation easier and safe.

Incorrect Choices:

During the first and second phases of healing, granulation tissue is being laid down. Granulation tissue is fragile and care must be taken not to damage it. While scar mobilization can occur during the maturation phase, it should not be initiated this late in the healing process, as it is significantly more difficult to remodel tissues.

Type of Reasoning: Deductive

Knowledge of scar tissue mobilization guidelines is paramount to arriving at a correct conclusion for this question. This requires the recall of factual information, which is a deductive reasoning skill. For this situation, it is safe to initiate scar tissue mobilization during the third or fibroblastic phase of healing. Review scar tissue mobilization guidelines if answered incorrectly.

B93

Pulmonary | Data Collection

Which of the following chronic pulmonary changes is expected following a left pneumonectomy?

Choices:
1. Decreased tidal volume.
2. Increased tidal volume.
3. Decreased breath sounds on the right.
4. Decreased residual volume.

Teaching Points

Correct Answer: 4
Residual volume will decrease as there is less air housed in the lung at the end of exhalation since there is only one lung present.

Incorrect Choices:
Tidal volume (the amount of air inhaled and exhaled during rest) will not change, i.e., it will not increase or decrease. Decreased breath sounds would be expected on the side of the pneumonectomy.

Type of Reasoning: Inferential
One must infer or draw a reasonable conclusion about the likely chronic pulmonary changes following a pneumonectomy. Questions of this nature require one to determine what may be true, which is an inferential reasoning skill. For this case, chronic pulmonary changes should include decreased residual volume. If answered incorrectly, review pulmonary changes following pneumonectomy.

B94

Nonsystem | Therapeutic Modalities

In providing ultrasound treatment for a patient with acute medial epicondylitis, which of the following settings is appropriate for the physical therapist assistant to utilize?

Choices:
1. 3.3 w/cm^2.
2. 1.0 MHz.
3. 1.0 w/cm^2.
4. 3.3 MHz.

Teaching Points

Correct Answer: 4
The superficial tissues over the epicondyle require 3.3 MHz ultrasound.

Incorrect Choices:
A 1.0 MHz ultrasound would penetrate too deeply into the tissues and may cause periosteal pain. Watts per centimeter squared (w/cm^2) is a measurement of intensity. An intensity of 3.3 w/cm^2 is too high and could burn the patient; 1.0 w/cm^2 may be an appropriate intensity; however, there is no mention of how long the treatment is delivered which makes the answer inappropriate.

Type of Reasoning: Deductive
One must recall the guidelines for ultrasound treatment for patients with acute medial epicondylitis. This requires recall of factual guidelines, which is a deductive reasoning skill. For this situation, the assistant should administer ultrasound at 3.0 MHz to treat the superficial tissues over the epicondyle. If answered incorrectly, review ultrasound treatment guidelines for medial epicondylitis.

B95

Cardiac | Data Collection

A physical therapist assistant determines the resting heart rate of an infant is 115 beats per minute. How should this be documented?

Choices:
1. Tachycardia.
2. A normal heart rate.
3. Tachypnea.
4. Bradycardia.

Teaching Points

Correct Answer: 2

The normal heart rate of an infant is a range of 70–170 beats per minute.

Incorrect Choices:

Tachycardia (rapid heart rate) and bradycardia (slow heart rate) are not appropriate descriptors. Tachypnea refers to a rapid respiratory rate.

Type of Reasoning: Deductive

One must recall the normal resting heart rate of an infant to arrive at a correct conclusion. This is factual recall of guidelines, which is a deductive reasoning skill. For this case, the resting heart rate of 115 beats per minute indicates a normal heart rate. If answered incorrectly, review resting heart rates of infants.

B96

Neuromuscular | Interventions

A physical therapist assistant is working with a patient who has been diagnosed with a brain injury. The patient displays agitation while in therapy sessions. What is the **BEST** way to decrease this behavior?

Choices:
1. Treat the patient in a calm, non-stimulating environment.
2. Ignore the agitation as it is to be expected.
3. Reward good behavior if the patient controls the agitation.
4. Discontinue treatment when the agitation occurs.

Teaching Points

Correct Answer: 1

Moving the patient to a calm, non-stimulating environment will potentially decrease his or her agitation and help him or her to attend to therapy sessions.

Incorrect Choices:

Agitation often occurs in response to overstimulation, therefore discontinuing treatment is not necessary and simple modification of the environment is appropriate. The other strategies are not appropriate in managing agitation but are utilized when addressing inappropriate behaviors.

Type of Reasoning: Inductive

This question requires clinical judgment to determine a best course of action for a patient displaying agitation while in therapy. Questions of this nature often require inductive reasoning skill. For this situation, it is best to treat the patient in a calm, non-stimulating environment. If answered incorrectly, review intervention techniques for patients with brain injury, including behavioral intervention guidelines.

B97

Musculoskeletal | Diseases and Conditions Impacting Intervention

A patient has unilateral weakness of the gastrocnemius/soleus and shortening of the tibialis anterior on the same side. Which of the following activities will this patient have the **MOST** difficulty performing?

Choices:
1. Walking up an incline.
2. Ascending stairs.
3. Walking down an incline.
4. Descending stairs.

Teaching Points

Correct Answer: 3

Shortening of the tibialis anterior will limit plantar flexion. In addition, weakness of the gastrocnemius and soleus muscles will result in weak plantar flexion. When a person descends an incline, plantar flexion range is necessary for the foot to be flat on surface, and the plantar flexors must act in reverse action to hold back the tibia.

Incorrect Choices:
Walking up an incline requires sufficient dorsiflexion range of motion and anterior tibialis strength. Ascending and descending stairs relies more on appropriate motion and strength of the hip and knee.

Type of Reasoning: Inductive
One must have knowledge of the impact of weakness of the gastrocnemius/soleus with shortening of the tibialis anterior to arrive at a correct conclusion. This requires clinical judgment, which is an inductive reasoning skill. For this case, it would be most difficult for this patient to walk down an incline because of the limited and weak plantar flexion. If answered incorrectly, review functional limitations from lower-extremity weakness, especially gastrocnemius/soleus weakness and tibialis anterior shortening.

B98

Nonsystem | Therapeutic Modalities

A physical therapist assistant is preparing to perform electrical stimulation on a patient for pain management following the principles of the Gate Control Theory. Which of the following parameters is appropriate for the physical therapist assistant to utilize?

Choices:
1. A rate of 15 pps.
2. A rate of 100–130 pps.
3. A pulse width of 150 μsec.
4. A treatment duration of 5 minutes.

Teaching Points

Correct Answer: 2

Electrical stimulation following the Gate Control Theory utilizes a pulse rate between 100–150 pulses per second (pps).

Incorrect Choices:

A pulse rate lower than 10 pps is used to apply the endorphin release theory. A pulse width of 150 μsec is high enough to get a muscle contraction, which is not appropriate when using this theory. A treatment duration of 20–60 minutes is recommended for pain relief following the principles of the Gate Control Theory.

Type of Reasoning: Deductive

One must recall the guidelines for performing electrical stimulation for pain management following principles of the Gate Control Theory. This is factual recall of guidelines, which is a deductive reasoning skill. For this situation, the assistant should select a rate of 80–100 pps. If answered incorrectly, review electrical stimulation guidelines for pain management and the Gate Control Theory.

B99

Nonsystem | Therapeutic Modalities

What is the **BEST** form of cryotherapy to both reduce muscle spasm and facilitate the stretching of a tight muscle group?

Choices:
1. Cold pack.
2. Ice massage.
3. Contrast bath.
4. Vapocoolant spray.

Teaching Points

Correct Answer: 4

Vapocoolant spray will cool the area and serves as an analgesic to decrease the pain. By interrupting the pain cycle and "blocking" some of the pain the physical therapist assistant will be able to stretch the muscle more effectively. "Numbing" the area and decreasing or eliminating the pain input can disrupt the pain/spasm cycle.

Incorrect Choices:

The analgesic effects of vapocoolant spray are longer lasting than those of cold packs or ice massage. Contrast baths are better used to stimulate circulation and not appropriate to decrease the pain response to allow tissue stretching.

Type of Reasoning: Inductive

One must have knowledge of cryotherapy techniques for muscle spasm and stretching to arrive at a correct conclusion. This requires clinical judgment, which is an inductive reasoning skill. For this scenario, the best form of cryotherapy to reduce muscle spasm and facilitate stretching of tight muscles is vapocoolant spray. If answered incorrectly, review cryotherapy guidelines, including uses of vapocoolant spray.

B100

Nonsystem | Professional Responsibilities

The physical therapist has modified a patient's plan of care to include lateral costal expansion. In the medical record, which section of the **SOAP** note will this information be located?

Choices:
1. Subjective.
2. Objective.
3. Assessment.
4. Plan.

Teaching Points

Correct Answer: 4

This information will be in the Plan section of the note as it outlines the interventions to be used for treatment and any changes to be made for future treatments.

Incorrect Choices:

The Subjective section of the note is what the patient says or reports. The Objective section is the measurable data obtained through observation, tests, and measures. The Assessment section is for the professional opinion of what the outcome may be and how the patient may respond to treatment.

Type of Reasoning: Deductive

This question requires a test taker to recall the factual guidelines for **SOAP** note documentation. Factual guidelines often necessitate deductive reasoning skill. For this situation, the plan to include lateral costal expansion should be documented in the Plan section of the **SOAP** note. If answered incorrectly, review **SOAP** note documentation guidelines, including information to be placed in the Plan section.

B101

Musculoskeletal | Interventions

A patient presents with hip drop of the swing limb at midstance during gait training. The physical therapist assistant should provide facilitation of what muscle to correct this gait deviation?

Choices:
1. Gluteus medius on the swing limb.
2. Iliopsoas on the stance limb.
3. Quadratus lumborum on the swing limb.
4. Hamstrings on the swing limb.

Teaching Points

Correct Answer: 3

A "hip drop" on the swing limb can be caused by a weak quadratus lumborum on that side or a weak gluteus medius on the stance limb; facilitation of either will help to decrease the gait deviation.

Incorrect Choices:

Facilitation of the iliopsoas will improve hip flexion during initial swing. Facilitation of the hamstrings will assist with knee flexion during swing or control knee "snap" at terminal swing if facilitated at the appropriate time.

Type of Reasoning: Inductive

One must determine the best therapeutic approach for a patient with a hip drop. This requires knowledge of the diagnosis and appropriate courses of action, which is an inductive reasoning skill. For this case, the assistant should provide facilitation to the quadratus lumborum on the swing limb to decrease the gait deviation. If answered incorrectly, review intervention approaches for hip drop.

B102

Neuromuscular | Interventions

What is the benefit of performing graded oscillation techniques at the limit of available motion?

Choices:
1. Improve free movement of the joint surfaces.
2. Improve joint nutrition.
3. Decrease pain.
4. Decrease accessory motions of the joints.

Teaching Points

Correct Answer: 1

Grades III and IV oscillation techniques are used to improve joint capsule range of motion (accessory motion) and joint motion at the end ranges of motion.

Incorrect Choices:

Grades I and II oscillation techniques are used at the beginning of the joint range of motion and are used to decrease pain and promote joint nutrition through stimulation of the synovium. Decreased accessory motion of the joint is a reason for performing graded oscillation but is not a benefit of the technique.

Type of Reasoning: Deductive

This question requires one to recall the indications for use of graded oscillation techniques performed at the limit of available motion to arrive at a correct conclusion. This is factual recall of information, which is a deductive reasoning skill. For this scenario, grades III and IV oscillation techniques are used to improve free movement of the joint surfaces. Review joint mobilization techniques if answered incorrectly, especially indications for grade III and IV techniques.

B103

Nonsystem | Professional Responsibilities

A physical therapist assistant is treating a patient who immigrated from Asia. What is the **FIRST** consideration to be employed when treating the patient?

Choices:
1. Teach the patients what is to be expected and acceptable regarding health care delivery in the United States.
2. Find a translator who is not a family member to objectively determine the patient's state of health.
3. Try to understand the patient's attitudes and beliefs regarding health care.
4. Ensure that the plan of care is tailored to meet the needs of the patient.

Teaching Points

Correct Answer: 3

The physical therapist assistant will need to first understand the attitudes and beliefs of the patient. Attitudes, expectations, and beliefs will greatly affect treatment, outcomes, and what interventions will be appropriate for this patient.

Incorrect Choices:
Although teaching the patient what is expected of the health care system in the United States is important, the assistant must first assess whether the patient understands the delivery of health care. Finding a translator and objectively determining the patient's state of health is important; however, that is not the first action to take. Tailoring the plan of care for each individual is appropriate for all patients, and is not specific to this situation.

Type of Reasoning: Evaluative
One must evaluate the potential courses of action presented and determine the action that is most effective in addressing the immediate needs of the patients. This requires one to weigh the merits of the actions, which is an evaluative reasoning skill. For this situation, it is important to first try to understand each patient's attitudes and beliefs regarding health care. If answered incorrectly, review guidelines for working with culturally diverse patients.

B104

Musculoskeletal | Data Collection

The physical therapist assistant is assessing the joint range of motion for ankle dorsiflexion and plantarflexion. Which of the following statements is the correct goniometric alignment for the measurement?

Choices:
1. Stationary arm parallel to the midline of the fibula; moving arm parallel to the fifth metatarsal with the knee stabilized and fully extended.
2. Stationary arm parallel to the midline of the tibia; moving arm parallel to the first metatarsal with a towel roll under the knee.
3. Stationary arm parallel with the tibia; moving arm parallel to the first metatarsal with the knee stabilized and fully extended.
4. Stationary arm parallel to the fibula; moving arm parallel to the fifth metatarsal with a towel roll under the knee.

Teaching Points

Correct Answer: 4
When measuring ankle dorsiflexion and plantar flexion, the goniometer is aligned on the lateral aspect of the lower extremity. The stationary arm is aligned along midline of the fibula and the moving arm is parallel to the fifth metatarsal. The knee should be slightly flexed to put slack on the long head of the gastrocnemius so ankle dorsiflexion is not limited by this muscle.

Incorrect Choices:
The tibia and first metatarsal are on the medial side of the lower leg; therefore, these are incorrect bony landmarks to use when measuring ankle dorsiflexion and plantarflexion. As previously noted, the knee must be somewhat flexed to prevent the gastrocnemius from limiting accurate measurement of dorsiflexion range of motion.

Type of Reasoning: Deductive
This question requires the test taker to recall procedural guidelines for range-of-motion measurement of the ankle. This necessitates the recall of factual information, which is a deductive reasoning skill. For this case, the ankle should be measured by aligning the stationary arm of the goniometer parallel to the midline of the fibula and the movable arm parallel to the fifth metatarsal, keeping the patient's knee somewhat flexed. If answered incorrectly, review range-of-motion measurement procedures, especially for the ankle.

B105

Nonsystem | Equipment and Devices

Which of the following patients would **MOST** benefit from the use of rim projections, friction rims, and leather gloves?

Choices:
1. Patients whose grip strength is 4–/5.
2. Patients whose grip strength is 3–/5.
3. Patients with quadriplegia at the C4 neurological level.
4. Patients who race in wheelchairs at relatively high speeds.

Teaching Points

Correct Answer: 2

Rim projections, friction rims, and leather gloves will help compensate for weak or decreased grip strength; a patient with a 3–/5 strength has less strength than a patient with 4–/5 strength.

Incorrect Choices:

Patients with quadriplegia at the C4 level have no hand function; therefore, a manually propelled wheelchair is inappropriate. Those who race wheelchairs must use leather gloves to adequately grip the rim and to prevent abrasions or blisters on their hands and fingers; however, they would not need rim projections.

Type of Reasoning: Analytical

This question requires one to analyze the adaptive devices presented and determine the type of patient who would be most appropriate to utilize such devices. This requires analytical reasoning skill as the evaluation of the devices is utilized to arrive at a correct conclusion. For this situation, the use of rim projections, friction rims, or leather gloves for wheelchair mobility is most appropriate for patients whose grip strength is 3–/5. If answered incorrectly, review indications for use of rim projections, friction rims and leather gloves for wheelchair mobility.

B106

Cardiac | Diseases and Conditions Impacting Intervention

A patient with a complete spinal cord lesion at the C6 level exhibits signs of orthostatic hypotension. What is the appropriate course of action?

Choices:
1. Reacclimate the patient to the upright position.
2. Walk the patient in the parallel bars using an abdominal binder and elastic wraps on the limbs to prevent venous pooling.
3. Immediately check the catheter for blockage.
4. Have the patient concentrate on diaphragmatic breathing and lateral costal expansion.

Teaching Points

Correct Answer: 1

To prevent orthostatic hypotension, the physical therapist assistant should gradually bring the patient upright to reacclimate the patient to a standing position, helping to decrease the sudden drop in blood pressure that is occurring.

Incorrect Choices:
Ambulation is not an option because a patient with a lesion at the C6 level will not be ambulatory. Immediately checking the catheter for blockage is the first course of action if autonomic dysreflexia (also known as autonomic hyperreflexia) is suspected. Diaphragmatic breathing and lateral costal expansion will help with aeration of the lungs, but will not help to prevent a drop in blood pressure.

Type of Reasoning: Evaluative
This question requires one to determine a best course of action for a patient with orthostatic hypotension. One must weigh the benefits of the courses of action presented to determine the action that will have the most beneficial outcome, which is an evaluative reasoning skill. For this case, the best course of action is to reacclimate the patient to an upright position. Review guidelines for intervention with patients with spinal cord injury who experienced orthostatic hypotension if answered incorrectly.

B107

Other Systems | Diseases and Conditions Impacting Intervention

Which of the following signs is **NOT** typically seen in the medical record of a patient with early stage cystic fibrosis?

Choices:
1. Excessive appetite and weight gain.
2. Increased pulmonary secretions with airway obstruction.
3. Frequent recurrent respiratory infections.
4. Salty skin and sweat.

Teaching Points

Correct Answer: 1
Cystic fibrosis (CF) affects the exocrine glands of the hepatic, digestive, and respiratory systems. Excessive weight gain is rarely a finding in a patient with CF.

Incorrect Choices:
Early clinical manifestations of CF include excessive secretion of purulent sputum, an inability to gain weight despite excessive appetite and adequate caloric intake, and a positive "sweat test," indicating chloride excretion.

Type of Reasoning: Inferential
One must infer or draw a reasonable conclusion about the potential symptoms of a patient with CF to determine the symptoms the assistant would be unlikely to document in the medical record. This requires knowledge of the diagnosis and determining what may be true of a situation, which is an inferential reasoning skill. For this case, it would be unusual to document weight gain for this disease. If answered incorrectly, review signs and symptoms of CF.

B108

Other Systems | Diseases and Conditions Impacting Intervention

A patient with human immunodeficiency virus is hospitalized with a viral infection and has a history of four infectious episodes within the past year. The physical therapist assistant should recognize that ongoing systemic effects for this patient are likely to include which of the following complications?

Choices:
1. Low-grade fever, malaise, anemia, and fatigue.
2. Decreased erythrocyte sedimentation rate.
3. Redness, warmth, swelling, and pain.
4. Fever, tachycardia, and hypermetabolic state.

Teaching Points

Correct Answer: 1

Repeat infections produce a chronic inflammatory state with systemic effects that include low-grade fever, weight loss, malaise, anemia, fatigue, leukocytosis, and lymphocytosis.

Incorrect Choices:

Inflammatory activity produces an elevated erythrocyte sedimentation rate. Redness, warmth, swelling, and pain are signs of the systemic effects of an acute inflammation. Fever, tachycardia, and hypermetabolic state are associated with an acute infection.

Type of Reasoning: Inferential

One must utilize knowledge of the diagnosis and likely symptoms to arrive at a correct conclusion. This determination of likely symptoms necessitates inferential reasoning skill. For this case, ongoing systemic effects are likely to include low-grade fever, malaise, anemia, and fatigue. If answered incorrectly, review signs and symptoms of human immunodeficiency virus, including ongoing systemic effects of the condition.

B109

Nonsystem | Therapeutic Modalities

A patient was instructed to apply high rate transcutaneous electrical nerve stimulation to the low back to modulate a chronic pain condition. The patient now states that the transcutaneous nerve stimulation unit is no longer effective in reducing the pain in spite of increasing the intensity to maximum. How should the settings be altered secondary to the patient's subjective complaints?

Choices:
1. Switch to low-rate.
2. Increase the treatment frequency.
3. Switch to modulation mode.
4. Decrease the pulse duration.

Teaching Points

Correct Answer: 3

With long-term continuous use of TENS, the sensory receptors are likely to accommodate to the continuous current and respond with less intensity to the same level of stimuli. Neural receptors are less likely to accommodate to a modulated current (wave length, frequency, amplitude).

Incorrect Choices:
Low-rate TENS is indicated for acute pain conditions. Increasing the treatment frequency would increase the likelihood of continued accommodation. Decreasing the pulse duration would not provide for accurate stimulation of the target tissues. Additionally, all of these changes should be made by the PT, as they are significantly altering the treatment provided.

Type of Reasoning: Inductive
This question requires one to utilize clinical judgment to determine a best course of action. This requires knowledge of the application of TENS to arrive at a correct conclusion, which is an inductive reasoning skill. For this scenario, the patient should be switched to modulation mode TENS. If answered incorrectly, review treatment parameters for TENS for patients with chronic pain.

B110

Musculoskeletal | Interventions

A physical therapist assistant is working with a patient who delivered her first child 2 weeks ago. The physical therapist diagnosis is a 4 cm diastasis recti. What is the **MOST** appropriate initial intervention to teach this patient?

Choices:
1. Pelvic tilts and bilateral straight leg raising.
2. Pelvic floor exercises and sit-ups.
3. Gentle stretching of hamstrings and hip flexors.
4. Protection and splinting of the abdominal musculature.

Teaching Points

Correct Answer: 4
With the presence of a lateral separation or split of the rectus abdominis muscle, it is important to initially teach protection (splinting) of the abdominal musculature.

Incorrect Choices:
Pelvic floor exercises are appropriate for a postpartum patient but are not remediation for diastasis recti. Patients should be instructed to avoid full sit-ups or bilateral straight leg raising. Stretching of the hamstrings and hip flexors will not remediate the diastasis recti.

Type of Reasoning: Inductive
One must utilize clinical judgment to determine the best initial intervention for a patient with diastasis recti abdominis. Questions of this nature often require inductive reasoning skill. For this situation, the best initial intervention is teaching protection and splinting of the abdominal musculature. If answered incorrectly, review intervention guidelines for diastasis recti abdominis.

B111

Neuromuscular | Interventions

To facilitate functional capabilities in children with considerable developmental delay and persistence of the tonic labyrinthine reflex, what is the **BEST** position to place the child when reaching for objects?

Choices:
1. Supine.
2. Prone.
3. Long-sitting.
4. Side-lying.

Teaching Points

Correct Answer: 4
The tonic labyrinthine reflex presents itself when the child is placed in a supine or prone position. To limit the effect of this reflex, the side-lying position should be utilized.

Incorrect Choices:
Placing the child in supine results in increased extensor tone while placing the child in prone results in increased flexor tone. Placing a child in long-sitting would likely be too difficult for the child to maintain while also reaching for objects.

Type of Reasoning: Inductive
This question requires the test taker to use clinical judgment to determine a best course of action. This necessitates inductive reasoning skill. For this scenario, the best position for the child with tonic labyrinthine reflex is in side-lying while practicing reaching for objects. If answered incorrectly, review the tonic labyrinthine reflex and the influence of positioning on tone.

B112

Neuromuscular | Interventions

Following a cerebrovascular accident, a patient with right hemiplegia is beginning ambulation using a large-base quad cane after completing gait training in the parallel bars. The patient is having difficulty advancing the right lower extremity. What is the **MOST** appropriate initial feedback that the physical therapist assistant should provide for this patient?

Choices:
1. Verbally cue to shift the weight to the left.
2. Physically assist the patient to shift the weight to the left.
3. Verbally instruct the patient to lift the right lower extremity.
4. Physically assist the patient to advance the right lower extremity.

Teaching Points

Correct Answer: 1
To advance the right lower extremity the patient must first shift the weight toward the left—the stance limb. The most appropriate use of feedback is to verbally cue the patient, because the technique was previously mastered in the parallel bars.

Incorrect Choices:
If the patient is unable to complete the task with verbal cues, it would be appropriate to physically assist the patient to perform the weight shift. Cueing the patient to lift the right lower extremity should not be performed until a weight shift has occurred.

Type of Reasoning: Inductive
For this question, one must have knowledge of gait-training guidelines for patients with stroke to arrive at a correct conclusion. This necessitates clinical judgment, which is an inductive reasoning skill. For this case, the patient with difficulty advancing the right lower extremity during ambulation should be given a verbal cue to shift weight to the left. If answered incorrectly, review gait-training guidelines for patients with stroke, especially difficulty advancing a leg during ambulation.

B113

Nonsystem | Equipment and Devices

What is the **BEST** choice when selecting a device to control medial ankle joint motion in a patient who has spasticity?

Choices:
1. Floor reaction orthosis.
2. Valgus correction strap.
3. Solid, molded plastic ankle-foot orthosis (AFO).
4. Patellar tendon-bearing brim.

Teaching Points

Correct Answer: 3

Using a molded plastic ankle-foot orthosis is the best mechanism to control medial-lateral motion.

Incorrect Choices:

A floor reaction orthosis is typically used to resist knee flexion. A valgus correction strap will control medial ankle joint motion but is not as effective as the solid AFO. A patellar tendon-bearing brim is used to decrease weight through the foot.

Type of Reasoning: Inductive

One must determine the best choice to control medial ankle joint motion in a patient with spasticity to arrive at a correct conclusion. This requires knowledge of orthotic devices and therapeutic benefits, which is an inductive reasoning skill. For this situation, the best choice is a solid, molded plastic AFO. If answered incorrectly, review orthotic devices to control ankle motion in patients with spasticity.

B114

Pulmonary | Interventions

Which of the following positions is **MOST** effective for a patient with advancing chronic lung disease to catch one's breath?

Choices:
1. Supine in the recumbent position.
2. Sitting and leaning forward on the hands or forearms.
3. Side-lying opposite the symptomatic side.
4. Prone over a pillow.

Teaching Points

Correct Answer: 2

Sitting and leaning forward on the forearms or hands assists the patient with chronic lung disease to utilize the pectoralis and serratus anterior as accessory motions for ventilation.

Incorrect Choices:

The other positions will likely increase the amount of energy required to breathe and should be avoided.

Type of Reasoning: Inductive

This question requires the test taker to have knowledge of advancing chronic lung disease and strategies for catching one's breath to arrive at a correct conclusion. This requires inductive reasoning skill. For this situation, it is most effective to catch one's breath by assuming a "tripod posture" or sitting and leaning forward on the hands or forearms. If answered incorrectly, review breathing strategies and postures for chronic lung disease.

B115

Nonsystem | Safety and Protection

A physical therapist assistant is visiting a patient at home. There is no air conditioning and the day is hot and humid. The patient reports having a headache, being dizzy, and experiencing nausea. The patient refuses to take part in therapy. What is the **MOST** appropriate intervention to be performed by the physical therapist assistant?

Choices:
1. Call the emergency response system, report a case of heat stroke and remain with the patient until help arrives.
2. Move the patient to a cool place and administer salt tablets if available.
3. Elevate the patient's lower extremities and begin stroking massage to improve circulation.
4. Give the patient cold water and elevate the lower extremities.

Teaching Points

Correct Answer: 4

The patient's symptoms indicate the early signs of dehydration. Elevating the lower extremities (to prevent distal edema), giving the patient cold water, and attempting to decrease the patient's body temperature are the most appropriate ways to address the situation.

Incorrect Choices:

The situation described is not a medical emergency and the emergency response system should not be activated. Moving the patient to a cool place is a good option, but administering salt tablets is not within the scope of care for a physical therapist assistant. There is no indication of a problem with the patient's circulation; therefore, massage is not indicated.

Type of Reasoning: Evaluative

This question requires one to determine the best course of action for a patient with symptoms of dehydration. One must weigh the courses of action and determine the one that best addresses the patient's symptoms, which is an evaluative reasoning skill. For this scenario, the assistant should give the patient cold water and elevate the lower extremities. If answered incorrectly, review first aid approaches for dehydration.

B116

Pulmonary | Interventions

A physical therapist assistant is preparing to perform postural drainage on a patient. Which of the following is a precaution for postural drainage with the patient in the Trendelenburg position?

Choices:
1. Humeral fracture.
2. Claustrophobia.
3. Rib fractures.
4. Congestive heart failure.

Teaching Points

Correct Answer: 4
Congestive heart failure is a precaution for postural drainage in the Trendelenburg position as this potentially increases the workload on an already damaged heart by returning excess fluids from the lower extremities to the heart.

Incorrect Choices:
A humeral fracture is a contraindication for positioning in side-lying on the side of the fracture. For rib fractures, prone positioning would be concerning. The Trendelenburg position should not bother a person who is claustrophobic.

Type of Reasoning: Deductive
One must recall the precautions for postural drainage to arrive at a correct conclusion. This necessitates the recall of factual information, which is a deductive reasoning skill. For this situation, a precaution for postural drainage in the Trendelenburg position is congestive heart failure. If answered incorrectly, review precautions for postural drainage techniques, especially the Trendelenburg position.

B117

Nonsystem | Professional Responsibilities

A patient is uncooperative and frequently expresses displeasure about what is being done during treatment sessions. What should the physical therapist assistant do **FIRST**?

Choices:
1. Ask the supervisor to discharge this patient from the assistant's patient load as there is no therapeutic relationship.
2. Accept the patient's criticism as a phase of anger related to the disability.
3. Tell the patient that the negative attitude could retard rehabilitation.
4. Ask the patient to be more specific about why there is so much dissatisfaction with treatment.

Teaching Points

Correct Answer: 4
When a patient frequently expresses displeasure regarding a treatment session, the physical therapist assistant should ask the patient to be more specific about why he or she is dissatisfied to more accurately address the problem(s).

Incorrect Choices:
Neither switching assistants nor accepting the patient's criticism as a phase of anger will address the dissatisfaction. Indicating that a negative attitude could retard rehabilitation will most likely only increase the patient's anger.

Type of Reasoning: Evaluative
This question requires the test taker to weigh the merits of the courses of action presented and then determine the response that will most effectively resolve the patient's concerns. This requires evaluative reasoning skill. For this scenario, the assistant should first ask the patient to be more specific about the dissatisfaction with treatment to accurately address the problem. If answered incorrectly, review patient interaction skill guidelines and conflict resolution procedures.

B118

Nonsystem | Therapeutic Modalities

A patient is using a portable functional electrical stimulator at home to regain functional wrist extension. The PTA should instruct the patient to increase the amplitude until which response is achieved?

Choices:
1. A muscle contraction to achieve full wrist extension.
2. A very strong muscle stimulus is felt.
3. A visualized twitch contraction of the wrist extensor muscles.
4. A visualized contraction to begin to raise the hand off of the treatment surface.

Teaching Points

Correct Answer: 1
The amplitude of electrical stimulation for functional strength gains must create a strong, tetanic, muscle contraction; a maximal contraction meets that criteria.

Incorrect Choices:
When a patient feels a very strong stimulus, the goal is most likely pain control. A twitch contraction will not create appreciable gains in strength of a muscle for functional use. A contraction to raise the hand off the treatment surface may not be strong enough to increase the strength of the muscle.

Type of Reasoning: Inductive
One must utilize knowledge of functional electrical stimulation to arrive at a correct conclusion for this question. This necessitates clinical judgment, which is an inductive reasoning skill. For this scenario, the assistant should instruct the patient to increase the amplitude until the patient obtains a maximal wrist extension contraction. If answered incorrectly, review guidelines for selecting functional electrical stimulation parameters.

B119

Musculoskeletal | Data Collection

A physical therapist assistant inspects the sneakers of an active child who reports experiencing foot pain. The sneakers have a flimsy, non-supportive heel counter and minimal medial arch support. This type of inadequate foot support will **MOST** likely lead to what type of foot positioning?

Choices:
1. Depressed metatarsal heads.
2. Excessive pronation.
3. Excessive supination.
4. Pes cavus (claw foot).

Teaching Points

Correct Answer: 2
Excessive pronation results in the medial aspect of the foot touching the ground during weight-bearing. This can occur because of inadequate support of the medial arch and/or a flimsy heel counter.

Incorrect Choices:
Depressed metatarsal heads are usually a result of wearing high heels. Excessive supination and pes cavus are caused by anatomical malalignment or neurological deficits rather than inadequate footwear.

Type of Reasoning: Inferential

One must infer the most likely condition that can result from inadequate foot support when a child is wearing non-supportive shoes. This requires one to determine what may be true of a situation, which is an inferential reasoning skill. For this case, inadequate foot support will most likely lead to excessive pronation. If answered incorrectly, review guidelines for appropriate footwear and support for children.

B120

Musculoskeletal | Interventions

A patient has limited wrist extension following removal of a cast for a fracture of the distal third of the radius. How should the physical therapist assistant position the patient's forearm for wrist extension with gentle stretching?

Choices:
1. Supinating the forearm and extending the wrist and fingers.
2. Pronating the forearm and extending the wrist while allowing the fingers to flex.
3. Supinating the forearm and extending the wrist while allowing the fingers to flex.
4. Pronating the forearm and extending the wrist and fingers.

Teaching Points

Correct Answer: 2

Gently stretching to improve wrist extension would involve extending the wrist and allowing the fingers to flex. This allows the two joint muscles (long finger flexors) to stretch over only one joint. Keeping the forearm pronated allows the wrist and finger flexors to be slack.

Incorrect Choices:

Beginning in supination places the wrist flexors in an already lengthened position. Extending both the wrist and fingers would be appropriate in the later stages of rehabilitation but not right after cast removal.

Type of Reasoning: Inductive

One must determine a best approach for gentle stretching after a distal radius fracture to arrive at a correct conclusion. This requires clinical judgment, which is an inductive reasoning skill. For this situation, gentle stretching can be initiated by pronating the forearm and extending the wrist while allowing the fingers to flex. If answered incorrectly, review stretching guidelines for the upper extremity after cast removal, especially the wrist.

B121

Other Systems | Diseases and Conditions Impacting Intervention

A patient with uncontrolled diabetes mellitus is being seen in physical therapy for a prosthetic checkout. The patient appears very lethargic and begins to experience vomiting and abdominal pain. The physical therapist assistant notes weakness and some confusion. What condition should the physical therapist assistant recognize these symptoms of?

Choices:
1. Ketoacidosis.
2. Respiratory acidosis.
3. Ketoalkalosis.
4. Lactic acidosis.

Teaching Points

Correct Answer: 1

A patient with uncontrolled diabetes mellitus is at risk of developing diabetic ketoacidosis. All of the listed signs and symptoms are consistent with this complication.

Incorrect Choices:

The other complications are not typically seen in a patient with uncontrolled diabetes mellitus.

Type of Reasoning: Analytical

This question provides symptoms from a patient in which the test taker must determine the likely problem that necessitates informing the therapist immediately. This requires analyzing the symptoms to draw a reasonable conclusion, which is an analytical reasoning skill. For this case, the patient's symptoms indicate ketoacidosis. If answered incorrectly, review signs and symptoms of ketoacidosis.

B122

Other Systems | Diseases and Conditions Impacting Intervention

Which of the following are likely to occur in a patient with hyperthyroidism?

Choices:
1. Trigger points and bradycardia.
2. Rheumatoid-like symptoms and muscle stiffness.
3. Muscular and joint edema, and poor peripheral circulation.
4. Proximal muscle weakness and potential dysrhythmia.

Teaching Points

Correct Answer: 4

A patient with hyperthyroidism will commonly present with muscle weakness and fatigue, muscle atrophy, and chronic periarthritis symptoms as well as increased pulse rate, cardiac output and blood volume.

Incorrect Choices:

The other symptoms listed all are manifestations of hypothyroidism.

Type of Reasoning: Inferential

This question provides a diagnosis and the test taker must infer the likely symptoms of this diagnosis. This requires one to determine what may be true for a patient's diagnosis, which is an inferential reasoning skill. For this scenario, one should expect to see proximal muscle weakness and potential dysrhythmia. If answered incorrectly, review signs and symptoms of hyperthyroidism.

B123

Cardiac | Diseases and Conditions Impacting Intervention

A patient with the diagnosis of left-sided heart failure, class II, is being seen in physical therapy. Which of the following should the physical therapist assistant expect the patient to demonstrate during exercise?

Choices:
1. Dyspnea with fatigue and muscular weakness.
2. Uncomfortable chest pain with shortness of breath.
3. Weight gain with dependent edema.
4. Anorexia, nausea with abdominal pain and distention.

Teaching Points

Correct Answer: 1
Left-sided heart failure produces pulmonary edema and symptoms associated with lack of oxygen to the body. Patients can be expected to demonstrate progressive dyspnea (exertional at first, then paroxysmal nocturnal dyspnea), fatigue and muscular weakness, pulmonary edema, cerebral hypoxia, and renal changes.

Incorrect Choices:
Severe chest pain and shortness of breath are symptoms of impending myocardial infarction. The other choices describe symptoms associated with right-sided ventricular failure.

Type of Reasoning: Inferential
One must infer or draw a reasonable conclusion about the likely symptoms of a patient who has left-sided heart failure. This requires inferential reasoning skill, as one must determine what may be true of a diagnosis. For this situation, one can expect the patient to demonstrate dyspnea with fatigue and muscular weakness. If answered incorrectly, review signs and symptoms of left-sided heart failure.

B124

Neuromuscular | Data Collection

Which test should a physical therapist assistant employ to assess fine motor activity?

Choices:
1. Bilateral, symmetrical foot tapping.
2. Rapid, alternating forearm pronation/supination.
3. Bilateral finger-to-thumb opposition.
4. Unilateral finger-to-nose activity.

Teaching Points

Correct Answer: 3
Finger-to-thumb opposition is fine motor activity.

Incorrect Choices:
The remaining activities would be used to assess gross motor functioning.

Type of Reasoning: Inductive
One must utilize clinical judgment to determine the best test to employ to assess fine motor activity. This requires inductive reasoning skill. For this case, the only test that assesses fine motor activity is bilateral finger-to-thumb opposition. If answered incorrectly, review assessment guidelines for fine motor skills.

B125

Neuromuscular | Interventions

Following surgery, a patient has effusion of the right knee joint and is unable to initiate quadriceps-setting exercises. What is the **BEST** facilitation method to implement in this situation?

Choices:
1. Transcutaneous nerve stimulation to the thigh.
2. Quick icing to the quadriceps muscle.
3. Prolonged stretch of the quadriceps muscle.
4. Firm pressure on the patellar tendon.

Teaching Points

Correct Answer: 2
Quick icing is the most appropriate method to facilitate a muscle contraction. The icing may also have a secondary effect of decreasing the joint effusion.

Incorrect Choices:
Transcutaneous nerve stimulation will facilitate quadriceps activity; however, it could be quite uncomfortable and is not the easiest or most efficient method for doing so. Prolonged stretch and firm pressure on the patellar tendon would be used to inhibit the quadriceps.

Type of Reasoning: Inductive
This question requires the test taker to utilize knowledge of modalities to facilitate quadriceps activity to arrive at a correct conclusion. This requires clinical judgment, which is an inductive reasoning skill. For this case, the best facilitation method is quick icing to the quadriceps muscle. Review muscle facilitation methods, especially quadriceps facilitation, if answered incorrectly.

Nonsystem | Evidence-Based Practice

Researchers performed a meta-analysis to examine the benefits of strength training on functional performance in older adults. What type of study review is this?

Choices:
1. Pooling of data from multiple randomized controlled studies to yield a larger sample.
2. A mechanism to critically evaluate case reports.
3. Data analysis performed by the Cochrane Collaboration.
4. The retrospective study of individuals with similar conditions.

Teaching Points

Correct Answer: 1
Meta-analysis refers to pooling of data of randomized controlled trials (RCTs) to yield a larger sample.

Incorrect Choices:
Meta-analysis utilizes only RCTs and, therefore, does not include case reports. The Cochrane Collaboration is one source of meta-analysis reviews. A retrospective review of a group of individuals with similar conditions is an example of a case-control study.

Type of Reasoning: Deductive
This question requires one to recall the guidelines for a meta-analysis to arrive at a correct conclusion. This is factual information, necessitating deductive reasoning skill. For this scenario, meta-analysis refers to the pooling of data of randomized controlled studies to yield a larger sample. If answered incorrectly, review meta-analysis study guidelines.

B127

Integumentary | Interventions

A patient has a deep wound on the thigh secondary to the incision from a saphenous vein harvest site failing to heal. There are moderate to large amounts of exudate, tunneling, and fragile wound edges. Which of the following dressing categories is the **BEST** selection for this patient?

Choices:
1. A hydrocolloid dressing.
2. A transparent film cut 2 inches larger than the wound edges.
3. A rope-shaped alginate covered with a thick gauze pad.
4. Hydrophilic foam.

Teaching Points

Correct Answer: 3

Alginate absorbs significant amounts of wound exudates. A rope-shaped alginate is an effective treatment to fill up dead space in the wound tunnel. The thick gauze pad would allow additional absorption of the exudate.

Incorrect Choices:
A hydrocolloid dressing is best used for wounds with less drainage and is not recommended for fragile tissues. A transparent film is non-absorptive and not recommended for fragile wound edges. Although foams can absorb moderate amounts of exudates, they do not conform well to wound beds.

Type of Reasoning: Inductive
One must utilize knowledge of wound-dressing techniques to arrive at a correct conclusion for this question. The use of clinical judgment to determine a best course of action often necessitates inductive reasoning skill. For this case, the best dressing selection for this patient is a rope-shaped alginate covered with a thick gauze pad. If answered incorrectly, review wound dressing techniques, especially for wounds with tunneling and significant amounts of exudate.

B128

Cardiac | Interventions

A patient who has recently and successfully completed a 2-week program of phase III cardiac rehabilitation will **MOST** likely demonstrate a decrease in which of the following?

Choices:
1. Heart rate at a given level of submaximal work.
2. CO_2 elimination in maximal work.
3. Cardiac output in maximal work.
4. Stroke volume at a given level of submaximal work.

Teaching Points

Correct Answer: 1

Successful cardiac rehabilitation will result in decreased heart rate at a given level of submaximal work as conditioning of the heart musculature will result in more effective pumping with decreased contractions.

Incorrect Choices:
The other choices are indications of a cardiac system that is not efficient and are not expected outcomes of phase III cardiac rehabilitation.

Type of Reasoning: Inferential

One must infer or draw a reasonable conclusion about the most likely characteristics of a patient in a cardiac rehabilitation program. This requires one to determine what may be true, which is an inferential reasoning skill. For this situation, the patient will most likely demonstrate a decrease in heart rate at a given level of submaximal work. If answered incorrectly, review cardiac rehabilitation guidelines, especially patient characteristics, after phase III program completion.

B129

Neuromuscular | Interventions

The plan of care for a patient who recently returned home with right hemiparesis indicates the patient demonstrates good recovery. Spasticity is in decline, there is no indication of synergistic movement, and the patient is ambulatory with a small-based quad cane. What is the **MOST** appropriate activity for a patient at this stage of recovery?

Choices:
1. Standing, picking the foot up behind, and slowly lowering it.
2. Supine, bending the hip and knee up to the chest with some hip abduction.
3. Sitting, marching in place (alternate hip flexion movement).
4. Standing, small-range knee extension movement to gain quadriceps control.

Teaching Points

Correct Answer: 1

This phase of recovery is characterized by movement combinations that do not follow the paths of either flexion or extension obligatory synergies. Knee flexion in standing is an out-of-synergy movement.

Incorrect Choices:

All other choices represent synergistic movements: the supine and sitting options are flexion synergy movements and the other standing option focuses on knee extensor movement within an extended position.

Type of Reasoning: Inductive

One must determine the most appropriate activity for a patient with hemiparesis and decline in spasticity. This requires knowledge of rehabilitation guidelines for patients with spasticity to arrive at a correct conclusion. This requires inductive reasoning skill. For this case, the most appropriate activity for a patient is standing, picking the foot up behind, and slowly lowering it. If answered incorrectly, review rehabilitation guidelines for patients with spasticity.

B130

System Interactions | Diseases and Conditions Impacting Intervention

Following a deep contusion to the lower back, a patient has been advised to take ibuprofen. The patient asks what the medication does. What should the physical therapist assistant explain to the patient about ibuprofen?

Choices:
1. It is a corticosteroid that will help to inhibit inflammatory reactions.
2. It is a muscle relaxant that relieves serious muscle spasms associated with painful conditions.
3. It is a nonsteroidal anti-inflammatory drug that is useful in treating mild to moderate pain and inflammation.
4. It is an analgesic generally used to provide symptomatic relief from pain.

Teaching Points

Correct Answer: 3

Ibuprofen is a nonsteroidal anti-inflammatory drug (NSAID). NSAIDs are used to treat mild to moderate inflammation and pain.

Incorrect Choices:
Ibuprofen does not fall into the categories of corticosteroid, muscle relaxant, or analgesic.

Type of Reasoning: Deductive
This question requires the test taker to recall the properties of ibuprofen to arrive at a correct conclusion. This is factual recall of guidelines, which is a deductive reasoning skill. For this case, ibuprofen is a nonsteroidal anti-inflammatory drug that is used to treat mild to moderate pain and inflammation. If answered incorrectly, review indications for use of ibuprofen.

B131

Pulmonary | Interventions

When trying to improve the breathing pattern of a patient with a diagnosis of chronic emphysema, what technique should the physical therapist assistant emphasize?

Choices:
1. Having the patient supine with a pillow under the knees.
2. Pursed-lip expiration.
3. Forceful inspiration.
4. Maximal use of accessory muscles during the breathing pattern.

Teaching Points

Correct Answer: 2

The primary problem for patients with emphysema is air trapping, resulting in overly inflated lungs. A pursed-lip breathing pattern facilitates the goal of emptying the lungs.

Incorrect Choices:
A seated rather than supine position is best. Expiration, not inspiration, should be emphasized.
Use of accessory muscles will only increase the trapping of the air and continue the over-inflation of the lungs.

Type of Reasoning: Deductive
Knowledge of breathing techniques for patients with chronic emphysema is paramount for arriving at a correct conclusion for this question. One must recall breathing technique guidelines, which is a deductive reasoning skill. For this situation, the assistant should emphasize pursed-lip breathing strategies to facilitate emptying the lungs. If answered incorrectly, review breathing strategies and techniques for patients with chronic emphysema.

B132

Nonsystem | Equipment and Devices

What procedure should the physical therapist assistant instruct the patient who is descending a curb with a cane to use?

Choices:
1. Side of weakness, with the weaker extremity and cane descending first.
2. Side of weakness, with the stronger extremity descending first.
3. Strong side, with the stronger extremity descending first.
4. Strong side, with the weaker extremity and cane descending first.

Teaching Points

Correct Answer: 4
When using a one-handed device, the device is used opposite the weaker lower extremity. When descending a step, the patient should lead with the weaker lower extremity to allow the stronger lower extremity to eccentrically lower the body to the next step.

Incorrect Choices:
The cane should not be held on the strong side as this places increased force on the weak hip abductor muscles and decreases the base of support when the patient is bearing weight on the weaker extremity. Descending with the stronger extremity will require the patient to perform the majority of the lowering with the weaker extremity and could result in the patient falling.

Type of Reasoning: Deductive
One must recall the proper procedures for descending a curb utilizing a cane to arrive at a correct conclusion. This necessitates the factual recall of guidelines and procedures, which is a deductive reasoning skill. For this case, the patient should hold the cane on the side opposite the weaker extremity, with the weaker extremity and cane leading when descending, followed by the stronger extremity. If answered incorrectly, review gait-training guidelines, including procedures for descending a curb with an assistive device.

B133

System Interactions | Diseases and Conditions Impacting Intervention

A patient who is 3 months post–cerebrovascular accident is being treated in physical therapy for adhesive capsulitis of the right shoulder. Today, the patient reports new symptoms including burning pain in the right upper extremity that is increased by the dependent position along with lowered pain threshold and heightened sensitivity to light touch. The right hand is mildly edematous and the skin is dry and warm to touch. Which of the following interventions should be **AVOIDED** by the physical therapist assistant?

Choices:
1. Stress-loading activities with weight-bearing on the affected extremity.
2. Passive manipulation of the shoulder.
3. Positional elevation, compression and gentle massage.
4. Active assistive range of motion exercises of the shoulder.

Teaching Points

Correct Answer: 2

This patient is demonstrating early signs of complex regional pain syndrome (CRPS), type I (also known as reflex sympathetic dystrophy). Stage I (early) changes include those described in the question and typically begin up to 10 days following injury. Passive manipulation should be avoided as it may aggravate sympathetically maintained pain.

Incorrect Choices:

All of the other treatments listed are appropriate for managing a patient in the early stages of CRPS.

Type of Reasoning: Analytical

This question provides symptoms and the test taker must first determine the likely diagnosis and the intervention approach to be avoided. This requires analytical reasoning skill. For this case, the intervention to be avoided is passive manipulation of the shoulder, as the symptoms indicate complex regional pain syndrome. If answered incorrectly, review intervention guidelines for complex regional pain syndrome.

B134

Cardiac | Interventions

A physical therapist assistant is working with a patient who had a myocardial infarction 4 weeks ago. When is it appropriate to utilize resistive training to improve muscular strength and endurance?

Choices:
1. If exercise intensities are kept below 85% maximal voluntary contraction.
2. If exercise capacity is greater than 5 METs with no anginal symptoms or ST segment depression.
3. During all phases of rehabilitation if judicious monitoring of heart rate is used.
4. Only during post–acute phase III cardiac rehabilitation.

Teaching Points

Correct Answer: 2

Resistance training is typically initiated after patients have completed 4–6 weeks of supervised cardiorespiratory endurance exercise. Patients should demonstrate an exercise capacity greater than 5 METs without anginal symptoms or ST segment depression before beginning resistive training.

Incorrect Choices:

Lower intensities are used early in cardiac rehabilitation; therefore, 85% maximal voluntary contraction would be too intense. Resistive training should not be implemented in the earliest stages and, when utilized, require careful monitoring of blood pressure. It is not necessary to wait until phase III cardiac rehabilitation to begin resistive training.

Type of Reasoning: Inductive

One must have knowledge of cardiac rehabilitation guidelines for patients with myocardial infarction to arrive at a correct conclusion. This knowledge is coupled with clinical judgment, which necessitates inductive reasoning skill. For this situation, resistive training using weights to improve muscular strength and endurance is appropriate if the exercise capacity is greater than 5 METs with no anginal symptoms or ST segment depression. If answered incorrectly, review cardiac rehabilitation guidelines and use of resistive training.

B135

Musculoskeletal | Interventions

To perform assisted hamstring stretching in the pool, a patient should submerge to the waist, place a buoyant ankle weight around the ankle and perform which of the following?

Choices:
1. Walk forward and backward, taking very large steps and not allow the foot to raise toward the top of the water.
2. Stand facing the wall and allow knee flexion to occur.
3. Stand with the back against the pool wall, allowing hip flexion to occur.
4. Lie supine in the water and perform large, slow flutter kicks.

Teaching Points

Correct Answer: 3
Standing with the back against the pool wall and allowing the buoyant ankle weight to float will assist with hamstring range of motion by creating a flexion movement at the hip.

Incorrect Choices:
Both walking with large steps and performing flutter kicks will increase the work of the lower-extremity musculature and strengthen, not stretch, the muscles. Standing and facing the wall while allowing the knee to flex will stretch the quadriceps.

Type of Reasoning: Inductive
This question requires clinical judgment to determine a best course of action for a patient performing hamstring stretches in a pool. This requires knowledge of therapeutic muscle-stretching guidelines, which is an inductive reasoning skill. For this case, the patient should stand with the back against the pool wall, allowing hip flexion to occur. If answered incorrectly, review water-based stretching exercises, especially hamstring stretches.

B136

Pulmonary | Diseases and Conditions Impacting Intervention

A patient with chronic obstructive pulmonary disease has developed respiratory acidosis. The physical therapist assistant should monitor the patient carefully for which of the following?

Choices:
1. Disorientation.
2. Tingling or numbness of the extremities.
3. Dizziness or lightheadedness.
4. Hyperreflexia.

Teaching Points

Correct Answer: 1
A patient with respiratory acidosis may present with many symptoms of increased carbon dioxide levels in the arterial blood, including disorientation, stupor or coma.

Incorrect Choices:
The other choices are signs and symptoms of respiratory alkalosis or a decrease of carbon dioxide in the arterial blood.

Type of Reasoning: Deductive

This question requires one to recall the common symptoms of respiratory acidosis to arrive at a correct conclusion. This is factual information, which is a deductive reasoning skill. For this case, one should monitor the patient closely for disorientation, a common symptom of respiratory acidosis. If answered incorrectly, review signs and symptoms of respiratory acidosis.

B137

Nonsystem | Safety and Protection

A physical therapist assistant is working in a single-story, long-term care facility. The emergency call for a tornado warning has been announced over the speaker system. How should the physical therapist assistant respond?

Choices:
1. Evacuate the residents from the building to the designated gathering location outside the building.
2. Remove the residents from rooms, closing doors, and placing residents in hallways.
3. Remove the residents from the location of the building most affected and closing safety doors at the entrance to that hallway.
4. Immediately discontinue treatment in the gym area and return residents to their rooms.

Teaching Points

Correct Answer: 2
In a tornado situation the general rule is to remove residents from the exterior of the building near windows, shutting room doors and keeping residents and personnel on the interior of the building away from glass and flying debris.

Incorrect Choices:
Evacuating residents from a building or removing them from an area and isolating that area is the response in the case of a fire. Residents should not be returned to their rooms, as it is easier to protect all of the residents when they are in the same vicinity.

Type of Reasoning: Evaluative
One must determine the best course of action by weighing the merits of the actions presented to determine a correct conclusion. This requires evaluative reasoning skill, where one evaluates actions and determines their benefits. For this case, the assistant should remove residents from rooms, closing doors, and placing residents in hallways. Review tornado response guidelines in health care facilities if answered incorrectly.

B138

Neuromuscular | Interventions

What is the **MOST** appropriate position for a patient recovering from acute stroke who is in bed and demonstrates a flaccid upper extremity?

Choices:
1. Side-lying on the sound side with the affected shoulder protracted, and arm extended resting on a pillow.
2. Supine with the affected arm flexed with hand resting on stomach, pillow placed under knees.
3. Supine with the affected elbow extended and arm positioned close to the side of the trunk.
4. Side-lying on the sound side with the affected upper extremity flexed overhead.

Teaching Points

Correct Answer: 1
Positioning for the patient with early stroke involves protecting against ligamentous strain and in a position counter to the typical spastic posture that can develop after the flaccid stage. Side-lying with the affected upper extremity supported on a pillow with the shoulder protracted and elbow extended accomplishes both of these goals.

Incorrect Choices:
Supine with the arm flexed and hand resting on the stomach will place stress on the shoulder ligaments. Supine with the elbow extended and shoulder adducted will position the patient toward a typical extension spasticity pattern. Flexing the upper extremity over the head when in side-lying will place a significant amount of stress on the shoulder.

Type of Reasoning: Deductive
One must recall the guidelines for positioning patients with stroke and a flaccid upper extremity in bed to arrive at a correct conclusion. This is factual information, necessitating deductive reasoning skill. For this situation, the patient should be positioned side-lying on the sound side with the affected shoulder protracted, and arm extended resting on a pillow. If answered incorrectly, review bed positioning guidelines for patients with stroke.

B139

Nonsystem | Therapeutic Modalities

Which of the following will **NOT** occur by placing a hot pack around the ankle?

Choices:
1. Increased subcutaneous tissue temperature.
2. Hyperemia.
3. Increased sympathetic response.
4. Increased collagen tissue extensibility.

Teaching Points

Correct Answer: 3
A sympathetic response does not occur when peripheral/superficial heat is applied to an area.

Incorrect Choices:
All of the other options will occur directly as a result of application of superficial heat.

Type of Reasoning: Inferential
This question requires one to determine what will not occur when one is using a hot pack. This requires one to infer a potential outcome, which is an inferential reasoning skill. For this case, increased sympathetic response will not occur by placing a hot pack around the ankle. If answered incorrectly, review outcomes of using superficial heat on joints.

B140

Other Systems | Data Collection

Which of the following is appropriate for a patient who has a blood glucose level of 68 mg/dL after 15 minutes of exercise?

Choices:
1. Consume a carbohydrate snack and continue to exercise unless further symptoms occur.
2. Request the physical therapist assistant call for immediate emergency assistance and prepare to initiate life-saving measures.
3. Continue to exercise as usual.
4. Consume a carbohydrate snack and retest in 15 minutes prior to proceeding.

Teaching Points

Correct Answer: 4
Blood glucose levels below 70 mg/dL warrant consumption of a carbohydrate snack. After waiting 15 minutes, the blood glucose level should be retested to ensure appropriate levels prior to beginning activity.

Incorrect Choices:
It is not appropriate to continue with exercise when the patient's blood glucose is at or below 70 mg/dL, regardless of the presence or absence of other symptoms. This is not an emergency situation as the patient is still conscious and can consume a carbohydrate snack in an effort to raise the blood glucose reading.

Type of Reasoning: Evaluative
This question requires one to determine the benefits of the courses of action presented to determine the one that will effectively resolve the patient's issue. This is an evaluative reasoning skill. For this scenario, the assistant should administer a carbohydrate snack and retest in 15 minutes prior to proceeding. If answered incorrectly, review intervention approaches for patients with low blood glucose.

B141

Musculoskeletal | Data Collection

During gait training the physical therapist assistant observes a patient exhibit an anterior trunk lean from heel strike through midstance. Which of the following is likely the cause of this gait deviation?

Choices:
1. Weak hip extensors.
2. Weak knee extensors.
3. Weak hip flexors.
4. Tight hip extensors.

Teaching Points

Correct Answer: 2
Leaning forward from heel strike through midstance will biomechanically lock the knee to compensate for the weakened quadriceps muscles.

Incorrect Choices:
A patient with weak hip extensors would demonstrate a backward trunk lean during stance. Weak hip flexors would result in a circumduction or vaulting gait pattern. Tight hip extensors would result in a shortened step length.

Type of Reasoning: Inferential

One must determine the likely reason for an anterior trunk lean from heel strike through midstance to arrive at a correct conclusion. This requires one to determine what may be true of a situation, which is an inferential reasoning skill. For this case, the likely reason for this gait deviation is weak knee extensors. If answered incorrectly, review gait deviation patterns, including patterns resulting from week knee extensors.

B142

Cardiac | Interventions

Three days following a myocardial infarction, which of the following activities is contraindicated?

Choices:
1. Upper-extremity exercise using 5-pound weights.
2. Exercise that increases the heart rate 10–15 beats per minute over the resting level.
3. Exercises in the 2–3 MET range.
4. Short-duration exercise sessions.

Teaching Points

Correct Answer: 1

Upper-extremity resistive exercise is contraindicated immediately following a myocardial infarction.

Incorrect Choices:

The other options are all appropriate for a patient immediately following a myocardial infarction provided the patient has been stable for at least 24 hours.

Type of Reasoning: Deductive

This question requires the test taker to recall the contraindications for exercise for patients with myocardial infarction to arrive at a correct conclusion. This is factual recall of guidelines, which is a deductive reasoning skill. For this situation, it is contraindicated to include upper-extremity exercise using 5-pound weights. If answered incorrectly, review cardiac rehabilitation guidelines for patients with myocardial infarction.

B143

Pulmonary | Interventions

Which of the following is appropriate when instructing a patient in diaphragmatic breathing?

Choices:
1. Ensure that the upper chest, not the abdomen, rises on inspiration.
2. Place the hands at the lateral costal margins.
3. Place the hands on the rectus abdominis just below the anterior costal margin.
4. Have the patient shrug the shoulders on inspiration to facilitate diaphragmatic movement.

Teaching Points

Correct Answer: 3

Diaphragmatic breathing is taught with the hands over the abdomen and anterior ribs.

Incorrect Choices:
The upper chest may rise along with the abdomen, but it should not rise in place of the abdomen. Lateral costal expansion is not desirable when emphasizing diaphragmatic breathing. The shoulders should not be shrugged as this facilitates accessory muscle use and is not desired when teaching diaphragmatic breathing.

Type of Reasoning: Deductive
One must recall the diaphragmatic breathing guidelines to arrive at a correct conclusion. This necessitates the recollection of factual information, which is a deductive reasoning skill. For this case, the assistant should place the hands on the rectus abdominis just below the anterior costal margin. If answered incorrectly, review diaphragmatic breathing guidelines.

B144

Nonsystem | Evidence-Based Practice

A researcher expects to find **NO** significant difference between 20- and 30-year-olds after a 12-week exercise-training program using exercise heart rates and myocardial oxygen consumption as measures of performance. What kind of hypothesis is this an example of?

Choices:
1. Experimental hypothesis.
2. Research hypothesis.
3. Null hypothesis.
4. Directional hypothesis.

Teaching Points

Correct Answer: 3
The null hypothesis states that there is no relationship (or difference) between variables.

Incorrect Choices:
A directional or research (experimental) hypothesis predicts an expected relationship between variables.

Type of Reasoning: Analytical
This question provides a research definition and the test taker must determine the term associated with this principle. This requires one to analyze the information provided to determine the appropriate definition, necessitating analytical reasoning skill. For this scenario, the definition is an example of a null hypothesis. If answered incorrectly, review research guidelines, especially hypothesis definitions.

B145

Integumentary | Interventions

Following a dorsal hand burn, an upper-extremity orthosis designed to provide functional positioning should place the wrist and hand in what position?

Choices:
1. Slight wrist extension, MCP extension, and IP extension.
2. Slight wrist flexion, MCP flexion, and IP flexion.
3. Slight wrist extension, MCP flexion, and IP extension.
4. Slight wrist flexion, MCP extension, and IP flexion.

Teaching Points

Correct Answer: 3

The functional position of the hand is slight wrist extension, metacarpophalangeal (MCP) flexion, and interphalangeal (IP) extension.

Incorrect Choices:

Splinting the MCP joints in extension may lead to contractures limiting hand closure. Wrist flexion positioning may lead to contractures that prevent the patient's ability to produce a power grip with hand closure.

Type of Reasoning: Deductive

This question requires one to recall the guidelines for hand splinting after burns. This is factual information, requiring deductive reasoning skill. For this case, the functional hand splinting position includes slight wrist extension, MCP flexion and IP extension. Review splinting guidelines for patients with hand burns if answered incorrectly.

B146

Neuromuscular | Interventions

The first step in a motor-relearning program includes observation and analysis of the functional activity. What is the **NEXT** step?

Choices:
1. Practicing the activity in the realistic environment.
2. Practicing components of the activity in a controlled environment.
3. Practicing the activity in a controlled environment.
4. Practicing components of the activity in an open environment.

Teaching Points

Correct Answer: 2

Components of the functional activity are practiced before the entire activity to focus on the patient relearning correct movement patterns.

Incorrect Choices:

As components of tasks are mastered, the entire activity itself may then be practiced. A controlled environment is utilized early; transfer to new, open environments is the final step of motor learning.

Type of Reasoning: Deductive

One must recall the steps in a motor-relearning program to arrive at a correct conclusion. This necessitates the recall of a therapeutic procedure, which is factual information and a deductive reasoning skill. For this situation, the next step is to practice components of the activity in a controlled environment. If answered incorrectly, review motor-relearning program procedures.

B147

Nonsystem | Safety and Professional Roles

A patient with diabetes reports feeling weak, dizzy, and somewhat nauseous during exercise. The physical therapist assistant notices that the patient is sweating profusely and is unsteady when standing. What is the physical therapist assistant's **FIRST** course of action?

Choices:
1. Administer orange juice for developing hypoglycemia.
2. Call emergency services for an insulin reaction.
3. Have a nurse administer an insulin injection for developing hyperglycemia.
4. Insist the patient sit down until the orthostatic hypotension resolves.

Teaching Points

Correct Answer: 1

The patient, who is diabetic, is showing signs and symptoms of hypoglycemia and should be given an oral sugar (e.g., orange juice).

Incorrect Choices:

Emergency services should not be contacted as the patient is capable of ingesting an oral sugar to raise the blood glucose level. The signs and symptoms are not consistent with hyperglycemia. Profuse sweating does not usually accompany orthostatic hypotension.

Type of Reasoning: Evaluative

For this question, the test taker must determine an appropriate course of action among the choices provided to determine the action that will effectively resolve the patient's symptoms. This requires evaluative reasoning skill. For this case, the assistant's first course of action should be to administer orange juice for developing hypoglycemia. If answered incorrectly, review first aid procedures for patients with hypoglycemia.

B148

Other Systems | Data Collection

A physical therapist assistant is reviewing the plan of care of a patient prior to initiating balance-training activities. The initial evaluation revealed that upon admission the patient had a positive fecal blood test. Which lab value is **MOST** important for the assistant to check prior to administering balance-retraining activities today?

Choices:
1. Hematocrit.
2. Leukocytes.
3. Platelet count.
4. Erythrocyte sedimentation rate.

Teaching Points

Correct Answer: 1

If the hematocrit (HCT) value is within the normal range for both males and females it indicates that the fecal blood loss is not significant at treatment time and should not affect the patient's ability to tolerate activity. Low HCT levels can lead to decreased exercise tolerance, decreased endurance, and orthostatic intolerance.

Incorrect Choices:
Leukocytes, platelets, and erythrocyte sedimentation rate can be low but will not impact balance.

Type of Reasoning: Inductive
One must utilize clinical judgment to determine the most important lab value to check prior to administering balance retraining activities for patients with a positive fecal blood test. This is an inductive reasoning skill. For this scenario, it is most important to check the hematocrit prior to administering balance retraining, as it can provide an indication of fecal blood loss. If answered incorrectly, review lab values for patients with blood loss.

B149

Other Systems | Diseases and Conditions Impacting Intervention

Patients with diabetes are at risk for developing plantar ulcers and should be reminded to avoid which of the following?

Choices:
1. Pressure from footwear and walking barefoot.
2. Soaking the feet daily in tepid water.
3. Applying mineral oil or lotion to the feet daily.
4. Wearing well-fitting jogging shoes instead of leather shoes for use as primary footwear

Teaching Points

Correct Answer: 1
Pressure from footwear can lead to pressure ulcers and walking barefoot can result in lesions to the foot that may not be felt, both of which may not heal well due to the patient's circulation and sensory impairments.

Incorrect Choices:
The remaining options will assist the patient in maintaining the integrity of the skin on the plantar surface of the foot and are appropriate foot care for patients with diabetes.

Type of Reasoning: Inductive
One must utilize knowledge of diabetic foot care guidelines to arrive at a correct conclusion. This requires inductive reasoning skill, as clinical judgment is paramount to arriving at a correct conclusion. For this case, the patient should be instructed to avoid pressure from footwear and walking barefoot to avoid pressure ulcers. If answered incorrectly, review diabetic foot care guidelines and appropriate footwear.

B150

Neuromuscular | Data Collection

A physical therapist assistant working with a patient who had an injury to the median nerve following a Colles' fracture should expect to see a strength deficit of which muscle?

Choices:
1. Pronator teres.
2. Extensor indicis.
3. Flexor digiti minimi.
4. Flexor digitorum superficialis.

Teaching Points

Correct Answer: 4

The flexor digitorum superficialis (FDS) is innervated by the median nerve distally and is commonly injured following a Colles' fracture.

Incorrect Choices:

The pronator teres is innervated by the median nerve but would most likely be damaged with a proximal radial/ulnar fracture. The extensor indicis is innervated by the radial nerve, and the flexor digiti minimi is innervated by the ulnar nerve.

Type of Reasoning: Inferential

One must infer or draw a reasonable conclusion about the likely muscle that will be weakened after a Colles' fracture. This requires the test taker to determine what may be true for a diagnosis, which is an inferential reasoning skill. For this scenario, one should expect to see a strength deficit of the flexor digitorum superficialis. If answered incorrectly, review muscle strength deficits following a Colles' fracture.

Examination C

C1

Musculoskeletal | Interventions

A physical therapist has directed a physical therapist assistant to provide strengthening exercises for a patient with a painful arc of motion resulting from a chronically inflamed biceps brachii muscle. What is the **MOST** efficient type of exercise to utilize with this patient?

Choices:
1. Isometric exercises at the end of range of movement.
2. Active concentric contractions through partial range of motion.
3. Active eccentric contractions in the pain-free range.
4. Isokinetic exercises through the full range of motion.

Teaching Points

Correct Answer: 3

For a muscle that is chronically inflamed, focus should be placed on eccentric contractions because there is less effort and stress placed on the contractile units compared with concentric contractions at the same level of work.

Incorrect Choice:
Isokinetic, isometric, and isotonic exercises do not allow for pain-free muscle contractions and can cause further inflammation of the muscle.

Type of Reasoning: Inductive
This question requires one to assess the benefits of each of the intervention approaches presented and then to determine the approach that will minimize pain and improve function. This requires inductive reasoning skill, which is often utilized when one is making judgments about a best therapeutic approach. In this situation, the assistant should choose active eccentric contractions in the pain-free range. If answered incorrectly, review therapeutic exercises for chronically inflamed muscles.

C2

Nonsystem | Professional Responsibilities

A patient who is terminally ill with cancer begins to cry during the physical therapy session. What is the assistant's **MOST** appropriate response?

Choices:
1. Ask the patient questions while continuing to administer therapy.
2. Ignore the tears and focus on therapy in a compassionate manner.
3. Take time to allow the patient to express any feelings.
4. Encourage denial to enable the patient to better cope with the challenges that lie ahead.

Teaching Points

Correct Answer: 3

It is important to allow a patient who is confronting death to verbalize feelings and frustrations. This will help the patient develop a level of trust with the PTA and facilitate engagement in therapy.

Incorrect Choice:

At this point, therapeutic intervention will not likely be beneficial until the patient is able to progress through the stages of death and dying. Ignoring the patient's feelings and encouraging denial are not acceptable methods of helping a patient cope with the dying process.

Type of Reasoning: Evaluative

This question requires one to determine the best approach for a patient who is confronting death. Questions of this nature that ask one to evaluate the statements made to others and their effectiveness require evaluative reasoning skill. In this situation, it is best to take time to allow the patient to express any feelings. If answered incorrectly, review strategies for helping patients cope with illness experiences.

C3

System Interactions | Data Collection

A patient with a right transtibial amputation secondary to complications of diabetes has just completed ambulating 100 feet with a walker. The patient reports dizziness, shaking, fatigue and weakness. Upon questioning, the patient also reports not having eaten breakfast because of lack of appetite. What is the **MOST** appropriate action for the physical therapist assistant?

Choices:
1. Have the patient take insulin.
2. Give the patient orange juice.
3. Give the patient a glass of water.
4. Have the patient rest, and then continue therapy.

Teaching Points

Correct Answer: 2

The patient is exhibiting signs of hypoglycemia and needs a quick intake of glucose, which orange juice contains.

Incorrect Choice:

Continuing therapy, water intake, and insulin will decrease the blood sugar level and be more detrimental to the patient.

Type of Reasoning: Analytic

This question requires the test taker to analyze the symptoms presented and then determine the cause for these symptoms. Once this determination is made, one must then decide the best course of action. This necessitates analytical reasoning skill. For this case, the patient's symptoms are caused by hypoglycemia and the best course of action is to give the patient orange juice. If answered incorrectly, review symptoms of and remedies for hypoglycemia.

C4

Cardiac | Data Collection

A physical therapist assistant is working with a patient who has pulmonary disease and is being monitored continuously with a pulse oximeter. The patient's saturation levels are approximately 92%–94%. The physical therapist assistant should stop treatment and notify the physical therapist when the oximeter reading initially drops below what level?

Choices:
1. 78%.
2. 82%.
3. 86%.
4. 90%.

Teaching Points

Correct Answer: 4

Normal oxygen saturation levels are between 96% and 100% and systems are being deprived of oxygen if the oxygen saturation point is below 90%.

Incorrect Choice:

Although the other options are concerning as well, they are not the initial point at which concern should be noted.

Type of Reasoning: Inductive

One must determine the pulse oximetry reading that indicates the need to stop treatment. This requires inductive reasoning skill, a skill that requires clinical judgment to determine a best course of action. In this case, when the initial reading drops below 88%, the treatment should stop. If answered incorrectly, review pulse oximetry monitoring guidelines, especially when to stop activity during monitoring.

C5

Nonsystem | Data Collection

A physical therapist assistant checks the vital signs of a patient who has a history of cardiac disease. The heart rate is steady at 60 beats per minute; respiratory rate is eight breaths per minute; blood pressure is 120/70 mm Hg and the oral temperature is 98.6°F. Which vital sign presents the greatest concern at this time?

Choices:
1. Respiratory rate.
2. Heart rate.
3. Blood pressure.
4. Temperature.

Teaching Points

Correct Answer: 1

The normal adult respiratory rate should be 12–18 breaths per minute. A rate of eight breaths per minute will cause changes in other vital signs over time.

Incorrect Choice:

Although the heart rate is on the low end of normal, it is not a cause for concern at this time. The blood pressure and temperature are within normal limits for an adult.

Type of Reasoning: Deductive

One must review all of the vital signs presented and then determine the vital sign that is of greatest concern, based on one's understanding of factual guidelines. This is a deductive reasoning skill, where factual guidelines are utilized to determine normal versus abnormal parameters. In this case, the only vital sign that is not within normal parameters is the patient's respiratory rate. If answered incorrectly, review vital signs guidelines, especially normal respiratory rate.

C6

Nonsystem | Equipment and Devices

The physical therapist has identified that a patient needs a spiral ankle–foot orthosis. What is the primary purpose of this type of orthosis?

Choices:
1. Limiting dorsiflexion.
2. Limiting plantar flexion.
3. Medial or lateral instability of the ankle.
4. Increasing plantar flexion.

Teaching Points

Correct Answer: 3

A spiral ankle–foot orthosis can correct either medial or lateral ankle instability.

Incorrect Choice:
A spiral ankle–foot orthosis would not limit or increase dorsiflexion or plantar flexion as it does not provide anterior or posterior control.

Type of Reasoning: Inferential
One must infer or draw a reasonable conclusion about the purpose of a spiral ankle–foot orthosis. This necessitates inferential reasoning skill, which often requires one to determine what may be true of a therapeutic process or procedure. In this case, the spiral ankle–foot orthosis is utilized primarily for medial or lateral instability of the ankle. Review lower-extremity orthotics, especially spiral ankle–foot orthosis, if answered incorrectly.

C7

Integumentary | Data Collection

Prior to beginning prosthetic training with a patient, the physical therapist assistant notices an area of redness and a slight blister on the distal aspect of the residual limb. How should this be documented?

Choices:
1. Stage I pressure ulcer.
2. Stage II pressure ulcer.
3. Stage III pressure ulcer.
4. Normal tissue response to weight bearing in the new prosthesis.

Teaching Points

Correct Answer: 2
A stage II pressure ulcer presents clinically as an abrasion, blister or shallow crater.

Incorrect Choice:
A stage I pressure ulcer presents clinically as non-blanchable erythema of intact skin. Stage III pressure ulcers would involve a crater that extends through the epidermis and dermis. This is not a pressure tolerant area for weight bearing and, therefore, is not a normal tissue response.

Type of Reasoning: Analytical
One must analyze the symptoms presented and then draw a conclusion about what these symptoms represent. This requires analytical reasoning skill, where various pieces of information are analyzed (such as symptoms) to draw a conclusion. In this case, the symptoms indicate a stage II pressure ulcer. Review symptoms and features of pressure ulcers if answered incorrectly.

C8

Neuromuscular | Diseases and Conditions Impacting Intervention

A physical therapist assistant working with a patient 4 weeks following a right-sided cerebrovascular accident (CVA) should expect the patient to exhibit which of the following?

Choices:
1. Poor judgment and decreased safety awareness.
2. Negative disposition, self-deprecating comments, and depression.
3. Slow, cautious behaviors.
4. Hesitancy, requiring more feedback and support.

Teaching Points

Correct Answer: 1
A patient who has suffered a right-sided CVA will typically demonstrate poor judgment with numerous safety issues.

Incorrect Choice:
A patient will demonstrate cautious, slow behaviors and require more positive feedback and support following a left-sided CVA. Negative disposition and depression are more associated with a left-sided CVA.

Type of Reasoning: Inferential
Questions that ask one to determine the likely presentation or deficits of a patient often necessitate inferential reasoning skill. Inferential reasoning skill asks one to determine what is likely to be true in a situation, though one cannot always be absolutely certain. In this case, the patient with a right-sided CVA will most likely exhibit poor judgment and decreased safety awareness. If answered incorrectly, review differences between right- versus left-sided CVA symptomatology, especially symptoms of right-sided CVA.

C9

Neuromuscular | Diseases and Conditions Impacting Intervention

A physical therapist assistant is treating a patient with Parkinson's disease. Which of the following should the assistant expect to see during ambulation?

Choices:
1. Shuffling gait pattern and weakness on one side.
2. Decreased trunk rotation and decreased arm swing.
3. Decreased step length bilaterally and unilaterally decreased weight bearing.
4. Forward stooped posture and internally rotated hips bilaterally.

Teaching Points

Correct Answer: 2

Decreased trunk rotation, decreased arm swing, decreased step length, shuffling gait, and stooped posture are characteristic gait changes in a patient with Parkinson's disease.

Incorrect Choice:

Each of the incorrect options contains a deviation that is more commonly seen in a diagnosis other than Parkinson's disease. Unilateral weakness would be expected in a person who has suffered a stroke. A patient would demonstrate decreased unilateral weight bearing following a hip arthroplasty. Spastic cerebral palsy would be more likely to result in bilateral internally rotated hips.

Type of Reasoning: Inferential

One must determine the most likely ambulation pattern of a patient who has Parkinson's disease. This requires one to infer the likely features, which is an inferential reasoning skill. For this situation, the assistant should expect to see decreased trunk rotation and decreased arm swing. Review symptoms of Parkinson's disease if answered incorrectly, especially ambulation patterns.

C10

Musculoskeletal | Interventions

A physical therapist has directed a physical therapist assistant to provide therapeutic exercises to a patient in the early stages of care for a musculoskeletal injury to the shoulder. Which of the following exercises should be implemented?

Choices:
1. Pendulum exercise.
2. Active range-of-motion exercises focused on abduction and lateral (external) rotation.
3. Strengthening of the rhomboids and lower trapezius.
4. Strengthening of the rotator cuff muscles.

Teaching Points

Correct Answer: 1

During the initial phase of rehabilitation the damaged structures should be protected to allow healing. Pendulum exercises do not stress the damaged tissues and provide movement of the joint surfaces to maintain movement and nutrition within the joint.

Incorrect Choice:

Active range-of-motion exercises into abduction and lateral (external) rotation would place too much stress on the tissues. Immediately following a muscular or soft tissue injury, resistance should be avoided to protect the structures.

Type of Reasoning: Inductive

One must determine the best exercises to implement for a patient, considering the diagnosis provided. This is an inductive reasoning skill, where clinical judgment is utilized to draw conclusions. For this patient with musculoskeletal injury to the shoulder, it is best to initiate intervention with pendulum exercises. If answered incorrectly, review indications for use of pendulum exercises and interventions for musculoskeletal shoulder injuries.

C11

Neuromuscular | Data Collection

The physical therapist has directed the physical therapist assistant to monitor a patient's equilibrium reactions during functional activity training. Which of the following activities is appropriate to meet this direction?

Choices:
1. Have the patient reach forward while sitting unsupported and observe the patient's recovery.
2. Have the patient bring his or her knee to the chest in sitting while the assistant applies manual resistance.
3. Have the patient alternate touching his or her finger from the nose to the assistant's finger.
4. Have the patient tap his or her toe as fast as possible.

Teaching Points

Correct Answer: 1
To test a patient's equilibrium reactions a physical therapist assistant can observe whether a patient has adequate recovery when reaching outside the base of support.

Incorrect Choice:
Knee to chest with overpressure is used for testing strength of the hip flexors. Finger to nose and toe tapping test the patient's coordination.

Type of Reasoning: Inferential
This question requires one to determine the best way to assess a patient's equilibrium reactions. This necessitates inferential reasoning skill, where the test taker infers a best course of action. In this scenario, the assistant should perform this test by having the patient sit unsupported while reaching forward and observing the patient's recovery. If answered incorrectly, review equilibrium reaction testing guidelines.

C12

Neuromuscular | Data Collection

Which of the following accurately lists the development of the grasp reflex in an infant?

Choices:
1. Voluntary release first, then transfers from hand to hand, followed by reflexive grasp, and finally voluntary grasp.
2. Voluntary grasp first, then reflexive grasp, followed by voluntary release, and finally transfers from hand to hand.
3. Reflexive grasp first, then voluntary release, followed by voluntary grasp, and finally transfers from hand to hand.
4. Reflexive grasp first, then voluntary grasp, followed by voluntary release, and finally transfers from hand to hand.

Teaching Points

Correct Answer: 4
Grasping skills progress from a reflexive grasp to a voluntary grasp. Only after the child can grasp voluntarily do release skills develop. Transferring skills need both voluntary grasp and release.

Incorrect Choice:
Choices 1 and 2 incorrectly place voluntary grasp before reflexive grasp. Choice 3 incorrectly places voluntary release before grasp.

Type of Reasoning: Deductive

One must recall factual guidelines of infant motor development to arrive at a correct conclusion. Recall of factual guidelines requires deductive reasoning skills. For this question, the grasp reflex in an infant develops with reflexive grasp first, then voluntary grasp, followed by voluntary release, and transfers from hand to hand. If answered incorrectly, review infant motor development guidelines, especially the grasp reflex.

C13

Nonsystem | Safety and Protection

A patient with hepatitis B receives a bleeding skin tear on the right calf during a treatment session. To prevent transmission of the disease while cleaning up, what should the physical therapist assistant do?

Choices:
1. Wash both hands before and after cleaning up.
2. Wipe up the blood with gauze and dispose of it in a trash container.
3. Wear disposable gloves.
4. Wear a mask with a splash guard.

Teaching Points

Correct Answer: 3

Hepatitis B is a bloodborne pathogen that is transmitted only via body fluids to non-infected people. Universal (standard) precautions should be followed, including wearing gloves.

Incorrect Choice:

Washing hands prior to patient contact does nothing to prevent transmission of the pathogen. The blood should be wiped up but must be disposed of in a biohazard container. This situation is unlikely to cause blood or body fluid spray and a mask with a splash guard is not necessary.

Type of Reasoning: Deductive

One must recall the guidelines for universal (standard) precautions to arrive at a correct conclusion. This is a factual guideline that requires deductive reasoning skill. For this case the therapist should wear disposable gloves to prevent transmission of the hepatitis B virus. Review universal (standard) precautions if answered incorrectly.

C14

Neuromuscular | Diseases and Conditions Impacting Intervention

Which of the following symptoms is present in an individual with cystic fibrosis?

Choices:
1. Rapid respirations with a prolonged exhalation phase.
2. Persistent cough, shortness of breath, thick greasy stools.
3. Persistent cough and thickening of the lining of the bronchial passages.
4. Cough, fever and chest pain with deep breathing.

Teaching Points

Correct Answer: 2

Cystic fibrosis is an obstructive disorder that results in the production of thickened mucus in the lungs and other organs of the body. This results in a persistent cough, shortness of breath, and thick, greasy stools.

Incorrect Choice:
Emphysema often results in rapid respirations with a prolonged exhalation phase. Chronic bronchitis produces thickening of the lining of the bronchial passages. A cough associated with fever and chills is symptomatic of pneumonia.

Type of Reasoning: Inferential
This question provides a diagnosis and the test taker must determine the symptoms that are associated with cystic fibrosis. Questions of this nature often require inferential reasoning skill, which requires one to infer what is most likely to be true of a situation. For this situation, the symptoms most consistent with cystic fibrosis are persistent cough, shortness of breath, and thick, greasy stools. If answered incorrectly, review symptoms of cystic fibrosis.

C15

Cardiac | Interventions

A physical therapist assistant is treating a patient on the tilt table secondary to orthostatic hypotension. The patient has been gradually raised from supine to 60° when the blood pressure begins to suddenly decrease. What is the **MOST** appropriate manner for the assistant to lower the tilt table?

Choices:
1. Immediately lower the table to 0° and call the physical therapist for assistance.
2. Lower the patient in 5°–10° increments until the blood pressure stabilizes.
3. Return the table to 45° and stay at this level for the remainder of the session.
4. Immediately lower the table to 0° and call a medical emergency.

Teaching Points

Correct Answer: 2
The drop in blood pressure indicates the heart's inability to adapt to the increased demand of being upright. The table should be lowered slowly until the blood pressure stabilizes.

Incorrect Choice:
Immediately lowering the table to 0° can cause an unsafe rush of blood to the brain and place the patient at risk of intracranial pressure increasing too rapidly or a CVA. While returning the table to 45° may occur, it is not necessary to remain at this level as elevation can resume once the patient's blood pressure stabilizes.

Type of Reasoning: Inductive
This question requires one to utilize clinical judgment to determine a best course of action for a patient with orthostatic hypotension. This necessitates inductive reasoning skill. For this case, the physical therapist assistant should lower the tilt table down in 5°–10° increments until the blood pressure stabilizes. Review guidelines for the use of a tilt table for orthostatic hypotension if answered incorrectly.

C16

Musculoskeletal | Interventions

A physical therapist assistant is treating a patient who has a diagnosis of right shoulder adhesive capsulitis with accessory motion dysfunction and loss of proper scapulohumeral rhythm. Which of the following interventions is **MOST** likely to help achieve proper scapulohumeral rhythm of the shoulder complex?

Choices:
1. Strengthening exercises for the parascapular muscles and stretching the glenohumeral structures.
2. Immobilization to protect joint biomechanics.
3. Strengthening exercises for the glenohumeral joint at end range.
4. Manual stretch to achieve normal internal and external rotation at the glenohumeral joint.

Teaching Points

Correct Answer: 1
Stretching the glenohumeral structures will promote normal joint biomechanics and strengthening the scapular stabilizers will help maintain the appropriate biomechanical relationship of scapulohumeral rhythm.

Incorrect Choice:
Immobilization will not restore the effective balance of length and strength for the shoulder girdle muscles. The glenohumeral structures need to be stretched, not strengthened. Scapulohumeral rhythm has greater impact for flexion and abduction than medial (internal) and lateral (external) rotation.

Type of Reasoning: Inferential
This question requires the test taker to determine an intervention approach that will most likely result in functional improvement. Questions that ask one to determine what may be most beneficial in a therapeutic approach often require inferential reasoning skill. For this scenario, the assistant should initiate strengthening exercises for the parascapular muscles and stretch the glenohumeral structures to achieve the most benefit. If answered incorrectly, review intervention guidelines for adhesive capsulitis.

C17

Integumentary | Diseases and Conditions Impacting Intervention

The physical therapy team members should be **MOST** concerned about the development of keloid scarring with what patient population?

Choices:
1. Persons of Asian descent.
2. Infants and children.
3. The elderly.
4. Persons of African American descent.

Teaching Points

Correct Answer: 4
The development of keloid scarring is a concern with persons of African or African American descent.

Incorrect Choice:
Persons of Asian descent do not typically develop keloid scarring. While age is not a factor in the development of keloid scarring, it may contribute to slower healing times.

Type of Reasoning: Inductive
One must utilize clinical judgment to determine the patient population that would present the most concern with the development of keloid scarring. Questions that require clinical judgment often necessitate inductive reasoning skill. For this scenario, team members should be most concerned about keloid scarring in persons of African American descent. If answered incorrectly, review information related to keloid scar development.

C18

Nonsystem | Safety and Protection

A physical therapist assistant comes upon an unresponsive adult on the floor of the hospital room. After properly positioning the patient, the physical therapist assistant opens the airway and attempts two slow breaths but the air does not go in. What should the physical therapist assistant do next?

Choices:
1. Perform the Heimlich maneuver.
2. Have someone else perform chest compressions.
3. Reposition the head and attempt two more breaths.
4. Do nothing as the person has expired.

Teaching Points

Correct Answer: 3

If the initial two rescue breaths are unsuccessful, the patient's head may not have been properly positioned the first time or the tongue may have fallen into the back of the throat and is blocking it. The PTA should re-tilt the head and give two breaths before assuming it is an airway obstruction.

Incorrect Choice:

After the re-tilt of the head and a second attempt to get air into the lungs is unsuccessful, the Heimlich maneuver should be performed. Cardiac compressions are not utilized unless the patient has no pulse. Only the medical professionals at a hospital can pronounce a patient as expired.

Type of Reasoning: Deductive

This question requires a test taker to recall the factual guidelines for the administration of cardiopulmonary resuscitation (CPR). Factual guidelines often necessitate deductive reasoning skill. For this situation, after one has tried to administer two slow breaths and the air does not go in, the head should be repositioned and two more breaths should be attempted. If answered incorrectly, review CPR guidelines.

C19

Integumentary | Data Collection

What should the physical therapist assistant expect when providing intervention to the lower extremity of a patient with a diagnosis of venous insufficiency?

Choices:
1. Abnormal nail growth, hair loss, dry skin, and increased pain.
2. Hemosiderin staining, wounds at the proximal medial malleolus, and area warm to touch.
3. Tissues that appear whitish in color and are very painful.
4. Mild pain, edema in one extremity, numbness, and tingling.

Teaching Points

Correct Answer: 2

Venous insufficiency results in hemosiderin staining (brown pigmentation) and increased tissue temperatures with wounds at the proximal, medial malleolus.

Incorrect Choice:

Arterial insufficiency is painful and produces trophic changes such as abnormal nail growth, hair loss, and dry skin. Raynaud's disease typically produces whitish skin and severe pain. Lymphedema presents as edema of the affected extremity with resultant numbness and tingling.

Type of Reasoning: Inferential

One must infer or draw a reasonable conclusion about the likely signs and symptoms of venous insufficiency. Determining what may be true of a situation often requires inferential reasoning skill. For this situation, one would expect hemosiderin staining, wounds at the proximal medial malleolus, and increased tissue temperatures. If answered incorrectly, review signs and symptoms of venous insufficiency.

C20

Cardiac | Interventions

A physical therapist assistant working in an outpatient clinic has been assigned a group exercise program with patients in phase III of their cardiac rehabilitation program. For this phase of rehabilitation, which of the following interventions is **MOST** appropriate?

Choices:
1. Resistance exercises using less than 15 pounds when in a sitting position.
2. Slowly performing active range-of-motion activities of the upper and lower extremities.
3. Walking on a treadmill at 2 mph.
4. Running on a treadmill at 5 mph.

Teaching Points

Correct Answer: 1

Patients in phase III of a cardiac rehabilitation program should have returned to their previous functional levels and be able to safely perform resistance exercises in a sitting position using less than 15 pounds.

Incorrect Choice:

Slowly performing active range-of-motion activities will not increase the heart rate enough for cardiac rehabilitation in phase III. Walking on a treadmill at 2 mph is included in phase II of the cardiac rehabilitation program. Running on a treadmill at 5 mph exceeds the MET level appropriate for many of the patients in this patient population and may be unsafe.

Type of Reasoning: Inductive

One must determine the most appropriate therapeutic exercise for patients in phase III of a cardiac rehabilitation program. This requires clinical judgment, which is an inductive reasoning skill. For this case the most appropriate therapeutic exercise is resistance exercise using less than 15 pounds, in a sitting position. If answered incorrectly, review cardiac rehabilitation guidelines, especially phase III cardiac rehabilitation and exercises.

C21

Musculoskeletal | Interventions

The plan of care for a patient in the third trimester of pregnancy includes strengthening exercises for the abdominal muscles. Which of the following exercises represents the **MOST** conservative modification for abdominal exercise with this patient?

Choices:
1. Supine "short-arc bicycle" exercises.
2. Supine single-leg heel slides.
3. Curl-ups and curl-downs while hands approximate the rectus muscle.
4. Head lift with pelvic tilt while hands approximate the rectus muscle.

Teaching Points

Correct Answer: 2
Strengthening of the abdominal muscles should be performed with caution to avoid causing or progressing the separation of the fibers of the rectus abdominis muscle. Supine single-leg heel slide exercise does not require the woman to overcome gravity, thus making it the most conservative and least strenuous for the woman to perform.

Incorrect Choice:
All exercises listed are appropriate modifications to protect the rectus muscle during pregnancy. The incorrect options, however, require the woman to overcome gravity to perform the exercise and, therefore, are more strenuous.

Type of Reasoning: Inductive
This question requires the test taker to determine the most conservative modification for abdominal exercise during pregnancy. Clinical judgment is utilized to arrive at a correct conclusion, which necessitates inductive reasoning skill. For this situation, the most conservative modification for abdominal exercise during pregnancy is supine single heel sliding. Review abdominal exercises during pregnancy if answered incorrectly.

C22

Vascular | Diseases and Conditions Impacting Intervention

After reading a patient's medical history, the physical therapist assistant notes that the patient has arterial insufficiency. Which of the following conditions is **MOST** likely to limit the patient's participation in therapy?

Choices:
1. Signs of intermittent claudication.
2. Increased pedal pulses.
3. Peripheral neuropathy.
4. Cool skin.

Teaching Points

Correct Answer: 1
Arterial insufficiency results in ischemia to the exercising muscle causing intermittent claudication, which is a precaution for therapy. The patient experiences cramping in the calf area with increased use such as walking. Relief of pain is accomplished by resting the extremity.

Incorrect Choice:
Pedal pulses actually diminish with arterial insufficiency. Caution in daily living activities is needed for peripheral neuropathy and cool skin.

Type of Reasoning: Inferential
One must infer or draw a reasonable conclusion about the likely limitations for participation in therapy by a patient who has arterial insufficiency. Inferential reasoning is utilized whenever one must determine what may be true in a therapeutic circumstance. For this case, participation in therapy is likely to be limited by intermittent claudication. If answered incorrectly, review arterial insufficiency signs and symptoms as well as intermittent claudication.

C23

Musculoskeletal | Equipment and Devices

To decrease the progression of a scoliosis curvature, a child has been fitted with a wheelchair seating system with a three-point support. What are the three points of support used to stabilize?

Choices:
1. Both sides of the pelvis and the upper trunk on the convex side of the curve.
2. The pelvis and the upper rib cage on the concave side of the curve, and the apex of the curve on the convex side.
3. The head, pelvis, and rib cage.
4. The shoulder, pelvis, and knee, all on the convex side of the curve.

Teaching Points

Correct Answer: 2
To minimize the progression of a spinal curve, the apex of the curve needs to be supported as well as the stabilizing counterpoints on the pelvis and upper ribcage on the opposite side of the body.

Incorrect Choice:
When both sides of the pelvis are supported, there is no counterforce to pressure on the upper trunk on the convex side. The head, shoulder, and knee are not involved in stabilizing the spine.

Type of Reasoning: Deductive
One must recall the features of a wheelchair seating system with three-point support. This is factual information, which requires deductive reasoning skill. For this situation, a three-point support system stabilizes the pelvis and the upper rib cage on the concave side and the apex of the curve on the convex side. If answered incorrectly, review wheelchair seating systems, especially three-point supports.

C24

Musculoskeletal | Diseases and Conditions Impacting Intervention

Passive stretching exercises are not recommended for a child with which of the following diagnoses?

Choices:
1. Cerebral palsy.
2. Osteogenesis imperfecta.
3. Duchenne's muscular dystrophy.
4. Spina bifida.

Teaching Points

Correct Answer: 2
Children with osteogenesis imperfecta have very fragile bones and hypermobile joints that can be easily damaged with passive stretching.

Incorrect Choice:
Passive stretching is recommended for children with cerebral palsy, Duchenne's muscular dystrophy, and spina bifida.

Type of Reasoning: Inductive

This question requires one to use clinical judgment to determine the diagnosis that is inappropriate for passive stretching. Questions requiring reasoning through clinical situations often necessitate inductive reasoning skill. For this scenario, passive stretching is not recommended for a child with osteogenesis imperfecta. If answered incorrectly, review exercises for children with osteogenesis imperfecta as well as contraindicated exercises.

C25

Musculoskeletal | Interventions

A patient returns for therapy 2 days after receiving cervical traction for the first time and reports increased pain. The established plan of care calls for traction, therapeutic exercise, education regarding proper body mechanics, and modalities to decrease pain. Consultation with the supervising physical therapist will most likely identify the focus of today's therapy session as which component of the plan of care?

Choices:
1. Modalities to decrease the pain.
2. Cervical traction, but with decreased tension or pull.
3. Therapeutic exercises to strengthen the cervical musculature.
4. Educating the patient about correct body mechanics with all activities of daily living.

Teaching Points

Correct Answer: 1

The patient has increased pain after the initial traction treatment, and the best intervention at this time is to decrease the patient's pain.

Incorrect Choice:

The traction should not be performed again as it appears to have aggravated the cervical condition. Strengthening the cervical musculature and education about proper body mechanics will not be fully beneficial until the pain has decreased.

Type of Reasoning: Inductive

One must determine a best course of action for a patient with increased pain after traction. This requires clinical judgment, which is an inductive reasoning skill. For this case, the therapy session should focus on modalities to decrease the pain. If answered incorrectly, review cervical traction guidelines, especially interventions for pain after traction.

C26

Nonsystem | Equipment and Devices

A physical therapist has directed a physical therapist assistant to measure a patient for a manual wheelchair. The patient's measurements are 22 inches from hip to hip and 16 inches from buttocks to the back of the knees. What is the **MOST** appropriate size wheelchair for this patient?

Choices:
1. Standard adult.
2. Narrow adult.
3. Extra-wide adult.
4. Standard child.

Teaching Points

Correct Answer: 3

Because a standard adult chair measures 18 inches in width, this patient requires an extra-wide wheelchair.

Incorrect Choice:

A standard adult chair is 18″ in width. A narrow adult chair is 16″ in width. A standard child chair is 10″–14″ in width.

Type of Reasoning: Deductive

One must recall the factual guidelines for wheelchair measurement to arrive at a correct conclusion. The recall of facts often requires deductive reasoning skill. For this case, the patient's measurements indicate that an extra-wide adult wheelchair is most appropriate. If answered incorrectly, review wheelchair prescription guidelines, especially wheelchair measurements.

C27

Musculoskeletal | Interventions

A patient is attending outpatient physical therapy for a right rotator cuff strain that occurred 2 weeks ago. The plan of care indicates beginning with isometric exercises for the rotator cuff muscles. What is the advantage of isometric exercises in this case?

Choices:
1. Limiting the joint position of the exercise.
2. Facilitation of greater work by the rotator cuff muscles.
3. Increased muscle action to increase swelling and decrease circulation.
4. A low risk of joint irritation.

Teaching Points

Correct Answer: 4

The fixed range of motion of isometric exercises promotes a low risk of joint irritation.

Incorrect Choice:

While the joint position is limited during the exercise, this is not considered an advantage. There is no movement with isometric exercises so no work is performed by the rotator cuff muscles. Isometrics decrease swelling and increase circulation, not vice versa as stated.

Type of Reasoning: Inferential

One must determine the advantages of isometric exercises to arrive at a correct conclusion. This requires one to infer the benefits of such an approach, which is an inferential reasoning skill. For this situation the advantage of isometric exercises is a low risk of joint irritation. Review benefits of isometric exercise guidelines if answered incorrectly.

C28

Nonsystem | Therapeutic Modalities

The physical therapy plan of care for a patient with a diagnosis of acute biceps tendonitis includes modalities to decrease inflammation. What is the **MOST** appropriate modality for this patient?

Choices:
1. Iontophoresis using lidocaine at 40 mAmp minutes.
2. Iontophoresis using dexamethasone at 40 mAmp minutes.
3. Phonophoresis using a 50% duty cycle for 5 minutes.
4. Phonophoresis using a 100% duty cycle for 8 minutes.

Teaching Points

Correct Answer: 2
This patient's diagnosis calls for modalities that decrease inflammation. Dexamethasone is appropriately used to decrease inflammation.

Incorrect Choice:
Lidocaine is used to decrease pain. Phonophoresis used with a duty cycle greater than 20% will introduce heat into the area, which can increase inflammation.

Type of Reasoning: Inductive
This question requires the test taker to determine the most appropriate modality for a patient with acute biceps tendonitis. This requires clinical judgment, which is an inductive reasoning skill. In this case, the therapy plan of care should include iontophoresis using dexamethasone at 40 mAmp minutes. If answered incorrectly, review treatment modalities for acute biceps tendonitis, especially iontophoresis.

C29

Musculoskeletal | Data Collection

The physical therapist assistant is working with a patient who has lymphedema of the lower extremity following radiation treatment for cancer of the prostate. What is the **MOST** appropriate method to measure girth of the limb?

Choices:
1. Centimeters, every 10 centimeters proximally from the metatarsal heads to the groin.
2. Inches, at 5-inch increments proximally to the groin.
3. Centimeters, at 3-centimeter increments proximally to the superior patellar angle.
4. Inches, at 1-inch increments proximally to an area just proximal to the area of edema.

Teaching Points

Correct Answer: 1
Circumference is best measured in centimeters as it is more sensitive than inches. Measurements along the length of the limb should begin at a bony landmark and be conducted in increments sufficient (about every 1–2 inches) to identify the extent of the edema.

Incorrect Choice:
Because the condition affects the entire lower extremity, ending at the superior patellar angle is not sufficient.

Type of Reasoning: Deductive
This question requires one to recall the guidelines for lower-extremity measurement of lymphedema. Deductive reasoning skills are utilized whenever one must recall factual guidelines or protocols. For this scenario, the limb should be measured in centimeters, every 10 cm proximally from the metatarsal heads to the groin. If answered incorrectly, review lymphedema measurement guidelines of the lower extremity.

C30

Integumentary | Interventions

A patient is recovering from a full-thickness burn to the shoulder, anterior chest, and axillary area. Range-of-motion activities should focus on what shoulder motions?

Choices:
1. Abduction, medial (internal) rotation, and flexion.
2. Extension, lateral (external), and medial (internal) rotation.
3. Flexion, abduction, and lateral (external) rotation.
4. Adduction, extension, and medial (internal) rotation.

Teaching Points

Correct Answer: 3

Range of motion should focus on preventing the common contractures of flexion, abduction, and lateral (external) rotation.

Incorrect Choice:

While the other shoulder motions are important, they do not include the specific area of concern for preventing contracture and deformity.

Type of Reasoning: Inductive

This question requires the use of clinical judgment to determine a best course of action. Questions requiring clinical judgment often necessitate inductive reasoning skill. For this question, one must recall the common deformity for burns to the shoulder and axillary area to determine the best range-of-motion activities. In this case, range-of-motion activities should focus on shoulder flexion, abduction, and lateral rotation. If answered incorrectly, review range-of-motion exercises for patients with burns to the upper body.

C31

Nonsystem | Safety and Protection

A physical therapist assistant is monitoring a patient in a work conditioning program. When the patient squats to lift a box, the physical therapist assistant observes that the client lifts with a posteriorly rounded lower back. What is the **MOST** appropriate instruction in order to utilize proper lifting technique?

Choices:
1. Perform a slight anterior pelvic tilt.
2. Keep the back in a neutral position.
3. Exaggerate the posterior rounded low back.
4. Maintain the extension of the knees and increase hip flexion.

Teaching Points

Correct Answer: 2

The back should be maintained in the patient's neutral position.

Incorrect Choice:

Increased flexion (posterior rounded low back) or extension (anterior pelvic tilt) puts the spine in a position of weakness and the patient at greater risk of injury during the lift. The hips and knees should be in a flexed position.

Type of Reasoning: Deductive
One must recall the guidelines for proper lifting techniques to arrive at a correct conclusion. This is factual information, which is a deductive reasoning skill. For this case, the assistant's instructions should include keeping the back in a neutral position. If answered incorrectly, review proper lifting techniques, especially biomechanical alignment.

C32

Neuromuscular | Diseases and Conditions Impacting Intervention

A child with cerebral palsy has a strong asymmetrical tonic neck reflex (ATNR) when the head is turned to the right side. What activity will the child have the **MOST** difficulty performing?

Choices:
1. Brushing the teeth while sitting in a wheelchair.
2. Bringing a spoon to the mouth with the right hand when the head is facing forward.
3. Activating a head switch placed on the right side of the wheelchair head support using neck rotation and extension.
4. Extending both arms into a T-shirt that is being held to the right side.

Teaching Points

Correct Answer: 4
The stimulus for the ATNR is turning the head to the side. The response is flexion of the extremities on the scalp side, and extension of the extremities on the face side. Extending both arms while the head is turned to the side is impossible for the child because of this reflex.

Incorrect Choice:
Brushing teeth and bringing a spoon to the mouth are accomplished by keeping the head facing forward and, therefore, would not stimulate the ATNR reflex. Activating a switch by the head would likely be a reproducible movement as the effect of her reflex on the extremities will not interfere with task performance.

Type of Reasoning: Inferential
This question requires the test taker to infer the most challenging activity to complete with the presence of the ATNR reflex. Questions that require one to determine what may be true of this situation often require inferential reasoning skill. For this case, the child will have the most difficulty with extending both arms into a T-shirt that is being held to the right side. Review ATNR reflex, especially functional activities with the presence of this reflex, if answered incorrectly.

C33

System Interactions | Diseases and Conditions Impacting Intervention

A physical therapist assistant providing cardiac rehabilitation to a patient who has Graves' disease should avoid which of the following situations?

Choices:
1. Bradycardia.
2. Cool exercise environment.
3. Overheating the patient.
4. Decreased blood pressure.

Teaching Points

Correct Answer: 3

Persons with hyperthyroid diseases (e.g., Graves' disease) are more susceptible to heat intolerance, and precautions must be taken during exercise to avoid overheating.

Incorrect Choice:
Bradycardia and decreased blood pressure as well as exercising in a cool environment are more likely associated with hypothyroidism.

Type of Reasoning: Deductive
This question requires the recall of precautions and contraindications when one is working with a patient who has Graves' disease. This is factual recall of information, which is a deductive reasoning skill. For this scenario, the assistant should be cautious to avoid overheating the patient because of the susceptibility of heat intolerance associated with the disease. If answered incorrectly, review Graves' disease, especially precautions for rehabilitation.

C34

Neuromuscular | Data Collection

During observation of a young patient attempting bed mobility activities, the physical therapist assistant notes the child exhibits increased extension of the extremities while supine and increased flexion of the extremities and neck while prone. The child is displaying which reflex?

Choices:
1. Asymmetrical tonic neck reflex.
2. Symmetrical tonic neck reflex.
3. Righting response.
4. Tonic labyrinthine reflex.

Teaching Points

Correct Answer: 4

The tonic labyrinthine reflex is influenced by position. If the patient is supine, both the upper and lower extremities will go into extension. If the patient is prone, both the upper and lower extremities will flex.

Incorrect Choice:
The other reflexes listed are affected by head movements or position, not body position.

Type of Reasoning: Analytical
One must analyze the information presented to determine the most likely reflex present during this functional activity. Whenever pieces of information are analyzed to determine a diagnosis or deficit, analytical reasoning skills are utilized. For this case, the description is consistent with tonic labyrinthine reflex. If answered incorrectly, review childhood reflexes, especially tonic labyrinthine reflex.

C35

Neuromuscular | Diseases and Conditions Impacting Intervention

The physical therapist assistant is preparing to treat a patient diagnosed with Guillain-Barré syndrome. In the early rehabilitation phase, which of the following characteristics should the physical therapist assistant expect the patient to demonstrate?

Choices:
1. Asymmetrical weakness of the upper extremities with hyperreflexia.
2. Symmetrical distribution of weakness, progressing from lower extremities to upper extremities.
3. Decreased muscle tone of one side of the face, with drooping mouth and an exaggerated open eye.
4. Asymmetrical distribution of weakness and tingling, progressing from the upper extremities to the lower extremities.

Teaching Points

Correct Answer: 2
Guillain-Barré syndrome is an acute polyneuritis characterized by rapid development of progressive muscle weakness. It is typically symmetrical and begins in the distal lower extremities, progressing to the upper extremities.

Incorrect Choice:
Asymmetrical distribution is not typical. Loss of muscle tone on one side of the face, with drooping mouth and exaggerated open eye are symptoms of Bell's palsy. Bell's palsy results in the decreased muscle tone of the facial muscles and typically presents on one side.

Type of Reasoning: Inferential
One must determine the likely presentation of symptoms of a patient with Guillain-Barré syndrome. This necessitates inferential reasoning skill, which is often utilized when one is determining the likely symptoms or deficits of the patient. In this case, one should expect the patient to present with symmetrical distribution of weakness, progressing from the lower extremities to the upper extremities. If answered incorrectly, review signs and symptoms of Guillain-Barré syndrome.

C36

Neuromuscular | Diseases and Conditions Impacting Intervention

Which of the following is expected in a child diagnosed with myelomeningocele with an L3–4 lesion?

Choices:
1. Intact lower extremity sensation.
2. Intact bowel and bladder control.
3. Active hip flexion.
4. Complete inability to hip hike.

Teaching Points

Correct Answer: 3
Children with myelomeningocele at the L3–4 level will be able to perform active hip flexion.

Incorrect Choice:
Children with an L3–4 lesion would not have intact lower extremity sensation (L1-S3) or bowel and bladder control (S2-S4). Hip hiking is produced by the quadratus lumborum which is innervated from the mostly intact/functional T12–L3 levels.

Type of Reasoning: Inferential

This question requires the test taker to infer the likely symptoms of a child with spina bifida, which requires inferential reasoning skill. For this particular situation, a child with spina bifida at the L3–4 level would most likely demonstrate active hip flexion. If answered incorrectly review signs and symptoms of different types of spina bifida, especially effects on the lumbar region.

C37

System Interactions | Diseases and Conditions Impacting Intervention

An elderly patient is being treated for depression following the death of a spouse and is currently taking a tricyclic antidepressant medication. Which of the following symptoms should the physical therapist assistant monitor the patient for?

Choices:
1. Hyperalertness.
2. Cardiac arrhythmias.
3. Dyspnea.
4. Postural hypotension.

Teaching Points

Correct Answer: 4

Tricyclic antidepressants (e.g., Elavil) can be effective in relieving depression but may cause postural hypotension, fainting, or confusion, thus increasing fall risk.

Incorrect Choice:
Hyperalertness, cardiac arrhythmias, or dyspnea are not typical side effects of tricyclic antidepressants.

Type of Reasoning: Deductive

One must recall the common side effects of taking tricyclic antidepressants to arrive at a correct conclusion. This is factual information, which is a deductive reasoning skill. For this scenario, the assistant should monitor the patient for signs of postural hypotension, a common side effect of taking this medication. If answered incorrectly, review side effects of tricyclic antidepressants.

C38

Neuromuscular | Interventions

For a patient with Down syndrome, the plan of care includes promoting increased muscle tone. Which intervention should the physical therapist assistant perform to meet this goal?

Choices:
1. Perform slow, rhythmic movements.
2. Lightly bounce the child on his or her lap.
3. Assist the child to perform facilitated somersaults.
4. Perform gentle passive range of motion.

Teaching Points

Correct Answer: 2
Most children with Down syndrome have low tone. Bouncing and vigorous movement help stimulate muscle activity and, therefore, increase tone.

Incorrect Choice:
Slow, rhythmic, and passive movements tend to relax a child. Somersaults are never appropriate with a child with Down syndrome because of the risk of atlantoaxial dislocation.

Type of Reasoning: Inductive
One must determine the best therapeutic activity for a child with Down syndrome. Clinical judgment is utilized with questions of this nature, which require inductive reasoning skill. For this situation, the child should be lightly bounced on the assistant's lap to stimulate muscle activity and increased tone. If answered incorrectly, review therapeutic activities for Down syndrome, especially activities to stimulate muscle activity and improve hypotonicity.

C39

Neuromuscular | Data Collection

Protective extension backwards will **MOST** likely be exhibited by an infant at what age?

Choices:
1. 3–4 months old.
2. 5–6 months old.
3. 7–8 months old.
4. 9–10 months old.

Teaching Points

Correct Answer: 4
Protective extension backwards usually develops by 9–10 months of age.

Incorrect Choice:
Children 5–6 months of age may be able to protect themselves from falling forward, while children ages 7–8 months can protect themselves from falling laterally.

Type of Reasoning: Deductive
One must recall the guidelines for the development of the protective extension reflex to arrive at a correct conclusion. This is factual recall of information, which necessitates deductive reasoning skill. In this case, protective extension backwards usually develops by 9–10 months of age. If answered incorrectly, review the protective extension and similar protective reflexes and age of development.

C40

Musculoskeletal | Diseases and Conditions Impacting Intervention

A physical therapist assistant is working with a young, active patient who had a transtibial amputation two weeks ago whose condition is complicated by a wound at the incision site. The patient is anxious to begin weight bearing and would like to be measured and fit for a prosthesis immediately. What is the assistant's **MOST** appropriate response?

Choices:
1. Inform the patient that he or she cannot be measured or fit for prostheses until 3 months after the amputation.
2. Inform the patient that his or her arms are not strong enough to assist with sit to stand this soon after the surgery.
3. Inform the patient that the wound on the residual limb needs to heal and swelling needs to minimize before the prosthesis can be measured.
4. Inform the patient that the physician will address that concern at the next visit.

Teaching Points

Correct Answer: 3

It is within the physical therapist assistant's scope to address the patient's concerns, providing him/her with accurate information about when he can expect to be fit for the prosthesis.

Incorrect Choice:

Determination for when the patient will be measured and fit for a prosthesis is not based on time since the surgery. The patient is young and strong and could certainly bear weight on crutches to support his weight. Asking the patient to wait until he/she sees the physician does not show respect for the patient's concerns or needs and is not necessary.

Type of Reasoning: Evaluative

This question requires the test taker to determine the best response for a patient who is requesting to be fit for a prosthesis and who has a wound at the incision site. Questions that require one to weigh the implications of an action or response often require evaluative reasoning skill. For this situation, the most appropriate response is to explain that the wound on the residual limb needs to heal and swelling needs to minimize before fitting for a prosthesis. If answered incorrectly, review prosthetic fitting guidelines, especially for wounds on the residual limb. Additional information on guidelines for prosthetic fitting is located in the Gait, Functional Training, Equipment and Devices chapter.

C41

Neuromuscular | Diseases and Conditions Impacting Intervention

A patient has been diagnosed with a stroke of the middle cerebral artery. Which of the following conditions should the physical therapist assistant expect to see?

Choices:
1. Contralateral sensory loss and hemiparesis with the leg more involved than the arm.
2. Unilateral neglect, homonymous hemianopsia, and aphasia.
3. Contralateral sensory loss, thalamic sensory syndrome, and cortical blindness.
4. Decreased level of consciousness, dysarthria, tetraplegia, and diplopia.

Teaching Points

Correct Answer: 2

Symptoms describing a middle cerebral artery occlusion include unilateral neglect, homonymous hemianopsia, and aphasia.

Incorrect Choice:

Occlusion of the anterior cerebral artery results in contralateral sensory loss and hemiparesis with the leg more involved than the arm. A posterior cerebral artery occlusion usually results in contralateral sensory loss, thalamic sensory syndrome, cortical blindness, prosopagnosia (inability to recognize faces, even one's own), and visual agnosia. Vertebrobasilar syndrome can result in decreased level of consciousness, dysarthria, tetraplegia, and diplopia.

Type of Reasoning: Inferential

Questions that provide a diagnosis and ask the test taker to determine the likely symptoms of that diagnosis often require inferential reasoning skill. For this question, a stroke of the middle cerebral artery will likely produce unilateral neglect, memory and behavioral impairments, and aphasia. If answered incorrectly, review signs and symptoms of stroke, especially of the middle cerebral artery.

C42

Nonsystem | Professional Responsibilities

An adolescent is in a high school class for those with severe disabilities. The physical therapist evaluated the student's physical therapy needs and set up a positioning, standing, and strengthening program that the teacher and classroom staff are to carry out. The Individualized Education Plan states that the student is to get consult services from physical therapy. What is the appropriate role for the physical therapist assistant when providing services for this child?

Choices:
1. Reassess the student's strength and functional skills on a weekly basis.
2. Be available to the teacher and classroom aides to help implement appropriate activities.
3. Recommend discharge from physical therapy as the student has no needs.
4. Provide therapeutic intervention as the physical therapist has indicated in the plan of care.

Teaching Points

Correct Answer: 2

Being available to consult with the physical therapist assistant regularly should meet this child's needs for physical therapy between evaluations by the physical therapist.

Incorrect Choice:

The plan of care does not require weekly data collection or therapeutic intervention. Recommending discharge is outside the scope of care for the physical therapist assistant.

Type of Reasoning: Inductive

This question requires one to determine the appropriate role for the physical therapist assistant in a high-school setting providing consult services. This requires clinical judgment and knowledge of school-based therapy guidelines, which necessitates inductive reasoning skill. For this situation, the assistant should be available to the teacher and classroom aides to help implement appropriate activities, which best provides consultation services. If answered incorrectly, review school-based consult services for physical therapy.

C43

Integumentary | Diseases and Conditions Impacting Intervention

A physical therapist assistant is assigned to perform a paraffin treatment for a patient with thick, scaly plaques on the skin that have a silvery appearance. What is the skin disorder **MOST** likely being described?

Choices:
1. Polymyositis.
2. Scleroderma.
3. Eczema.
4. Psoriasis.

Teaching Points

Correct Answer: 4

Psoriasis is an immune skin disorder that presents with scaly, silvery skin caused by rapid skin cell reproduction. Heat, paraffin baths, and splinting can be effective in reducing symptoms and helping to improve range of motion.

Incorrect Choice:

The clinical presentation of polymyositis, scleroderma, and eczema is not thick, scaly plaques on the skin. Additionally, these conditions require more intense medical management than whirlpool treatments.

Type of Reasoning: Analytical

This question provides a group of symptoms and the test taker must determine the most likely diagnosis. Questions of this nature require analytical reasoning skill as pieces of information are evaluated to determine a diagnosis. For this case, the symptoms are indicative of psoriasis. If answered incorrectly, review signs and symptoms of psoriasis. Additional information on skin disorders is located in the Integumentary Physical Therapy chapter.

C44

Neuromuscular | Interventions

A physical therapist assistant is working with a patient following a traumatic brain injury. The patient has developed a flexion synergy pattern in the right upper extremity. To inhibit this pattern during functional activities, how should the physical therapist assistant position the right upper extremity?

Choices:
1. Scapular retraction, shoulder abduction, and elbow extension.
2. Scapular protraction, shoulder lateral (external) rotation, and elbow flexion.
3. Shoulder medial (internal) rotation, elbow extension, and forearm pronation.
4. Elbow extension, forearm supination, and wrist flexion.

Teaching Points

Correct Answer: 3

To inhibit a synergy pattern during functional activities, the extremity should be positioned out of the pattern of influence. For a flexion synergy the patient should be positioned in shoulder medial (internal) rotation, elbow extension, and forearm pronation.

Incorrect Choice:

Placing the patient in scapular retraction, shoulder abduction, shoulder lateral (external) rotation, elbow flexion, forearm supination, and/or wrist flexion would not be out of the flexion synergy pattern.

Type of Reasoning: Inductive

One must utilize clinical judgment to determine the best position to inhibit a flexor synergy pattern. Inductive reasoning skills are utilized whenever one must determine a best therapeutic technique for optimal outcomes. For this situation, the assistant should position the right shoulder into internal rotation, elbow extension, and forearm pronation. If answered incorrectly, review flexor synergy patterns of the upper extremity, especially after traumatic brain injury.

C45

Nonsystem | Safety and Protection

A physical therapist assistant finishing gait training with a patient who is on contact precautions secondary to a MRSA infection is preparing to leave the patient's private room. What is the order of how the physical therapist assistant should proceed?

Choices:
1. Store the gait belt in the patient's room, remove the gloves and protective gown, and wash the hands before leaving the patient's room.
2. Remove the protective gown and gloves, place the gait belt in the lab coat pocket, and wash the hands before leaving the patient's room.
3. Place the gait belt in a biohazard laundry bag and transport it to the designated laundry area down the hall, wash the hands immediately after disposing of contaminated laundry.
4. Remove the mask and dispose of it in the biohazard trash, store the gait belt in the patient's room, remove the protective gown and gloves, wash the hands, place the gown in the biohazard laundry bag, and transport it to the contaminated laundry area.

Teaching Points

Correct Answer: 1

MRSA requires contact precautions that call for a private room with dedicated patient care equipment, wearing of gloves and gown when in contact with the patient, and hands washed with antiseptic soap immediately upon leaving the room.

Incorrect Choice:

It is inappropriate to use the gait belt with other patients or to remove it from the room. It is also inappropriate to remove the biohazard bag without washing the hands after disposing of it.

Type of Reasoning: Deductive

This question requires a test taker to recall the sequential procedures for contact precautions. This is a factual guideline, which necessitates deductive reasoning skill. For this scenario, the assistant should first store the gait belt in the patient room, then remove gloves and protective gown and finally wash hands before leaving the patient's room. If answered incorrectly, review contact precautions procedures, especially for MRSA.

C46

Musculoskeletal | Interventions

A patient presents with limited shoulder abduction secondary to adhesive capsulitis. The supervising physical therapist determines that grade 2 and 3 joint mobilization techniques will assist in promoting the return of normal joint accessory motion and shoulder abduction. What is the correct direction for applying the mobilization?

Choices:
1. Superior glide of the humerus on the scapula.
2. Inferior glide of the humerus on the scapula.
3. Anterior glide of the scapula on the humerus.
4. Posterior glide of the humerus on the scapula.

Teaching Points

Correct Answer: 2
The convex humerus moves on the concave glenoid fossa. To improve abduction, the head of the humerus needs to be mobilized inferiorly or the opposite direction of the glide of the bone.

Incorrect Choice:
Superior glides of the glenohumeral joint often result in impingement and should be used judiciously. Anterior glides typically increase lateral (external) rotation while posterior glides assist with flexion and medial (internal) rotation of the glenohumeral joint.

Type of Reasoning: Deductive
This question requires the test taker to recall the proper procedures for joint mobilization techniques. This is a factual procedure that requires recall of facts and knowledge and necessitates deductive reasoning skill. For this case, when performing joint mobilization techniques of the glenohumeral joint, the assistant should perform an inferior glide of the humerus on the scapula. If answered incorrectly, review joint mobilization procedures of the upper extremity, especially of the glenohumeral joint.

C47

Nonsystem | Therapeutic Modalities

The physical therapist's plan of care for a patient with acute low back pain identifies the use of interferential current. Where should the physical therapist assistant place the electrodes?

Choices:
1. Immediately adjacent and parallel to the spinal column with one channel on each side.
2. Channel one perpendicular to the spinal column.
3. Diagonally so the channels cross near the area of most pain.
4. Channel one parallel to the spinal column crossing the mid-thoracic spine paravertebrals.

Teaching Points

Correct Answer: 3
The crisscrossed electrode configuration over the lower back allows current interference and focuses treatment on the muscles involved.

Incorrect Choice:
The incorrect options do not allow for the currents from both channels to interfere with each other and create the interferential current pattern.

Type of Reasoning: Inductive
The use of clinical judgment in determining the best electrode placement is paramount to arriving at a correct conclusion for this question. This requires inductive reasoning skill. For this case the patient with low back pain should have the electrode configuration placement diagonal to the spinal column so the channels cross near the area of most pain. Review electrode placement for interferential current with low back pain if answered incorrectly.

C48

Musculoskeletal | Data Collection

A patient who is substituting with the sartorius muscle during manual muscle testing of the iliopsoas muscle would demonstrate which of the following deviations?

Choices:
1. Lateral (external) rotation and abduction of the hip.
2. Medial (internal) rotation and abduction of the hip.
3. Flexion of the hip and extension of the knee.
4. Extension of the hip and knee.

Teaching Points

Correct Answer: 1

The iliopsoas is the prime flexor of the hip. Substitution of the sartorius muscle for a weak iliopsoas will result in lateral (external) rotation and abduction of hip.

Incorrect Choice:
The gluteus minimus muscle performs medial (internal) rotation and abduction of the hip. The rectus femoris would produce extension of the knee with flexion of the hip. Extension of the hip and knee would require simultaneous co-contraction of the anterior and posterior leg muscles.

Type of Reasoning: Inferential
This question requires one to infer or draw a reasonable conclusion about the likely substitution pattern for a weak iliopsoas muscle. Questions that require one to determine what may be true of a situation often require inferential reasoning. In this situation, a patient with a weak iliopsoas muscle will likely demonstrate lateral rotation and abduction of the hip. If answered incorrectly, review typical substitution patterns for weak muscles, especially of the lower extremity.

C49

Musculoskeletal | Diseases and Conditions Impacting Intervention

An infant with developmental dysplasia of the hip will likely require splinting in which of the following hip positions?

Choices:
1. Flexion and adduction.
2. Extension and adduction.
3. Extension and abduction.
4. Flexion and abduction.

Teaching Points

Correct Answer: 4
To allow the acetabulum and the head of the femur to form correctly, the hip must be placed in a position causing the least amount of stress on and most congruence of the joint. This position is hip flexion and abduction.

Incorrect Choice:
The position that often results in developmental dysplasia is hip extension and adduction. The incorrect answers do not have the appropriate combination of positioning: hip flexion and abduction.

Type of Reasoning: Inferential

One must infer or draw a reasonable conclusion about what is likely to be true for an infant with developmental dysplasia of the hip. This requires inferential reasoning skill. For this situation, the patient is likely to come to therapy in a hip flexion and abduction splint, also known as a Pavlik harness. If answered incorrectly, review signs and symptoms of developmental dysplasia of the hip and splinting procedures.

C50

Musculoskeletal | Data Collection

Manual muscle testing strength of the lower trapezius muscle (for scapular depression and adduction) with good (4/5) to normal (5/5) strength should be conducted with the patient prone and the shoulder in what position?

Choices:
1. 180° of abduction and fully externally rotated.
2. 145° of abduction, the forearm in neutral with the thumb pointing at the ceiling.
3. 90° of abduction, elbow flexed to 90°, and the forearm in neutral with the thumb pointing inward.
4. Neutral position at the side and the shoulder and forearm internally rotated with the thumb pointing inward.

Teaching Points

Correct Answer: 2
To get the full effects of gravity for the lower trapezius muscle, the patient is positioned prone with the shoulder in 145° of abduction to align the arm with the fiber direction of the lower trapezius muscle.

Incorrect Choice:
A position of 180° is inappropriate as muscles are rarely tested at the end range where the muscle is physiologically weaker. At 90° of abduction in the prone position with the elbow flexed, the examiner is testing the rhomboids. The lower trapezius muscle cannot be tested with the shoulder in the neutral position at the side.

Type of Reasoning: Deductive
This question requires the recall of the procedures for manual muscle testing of the lower trapezius muscle. This is factual recall of information, which is a deductive reasoning skill. For this case, the muscle should be tested with the shoulder positioned in 145° of abduction and the forearm neutral with the thumb pointing at the ceiling. If answered incorrectly, review manual muscle testing procedures, especially testing of the lower trapezius muscle.

C51

Musculoskeletal | Interventions

To relieve pressure on the patient's calcaneus while the patient is in supine position, where should the physical therapist assistant position a 2-inch towel roll?

Choices:
1. Under the posterior tibia/fibula just distal to the fossa of the knee.
2. Laterally at the proximal femur, running along the length of the femur.
3. Under the distal posterior tibia at the area of the Achilles tendon.
4. Medially at the medial condyle of the femur, running distally along the length of the tibia.

Teaching Points

Correct Answer: 3
A towel roll placed at the Achilles tendon and distal calf will relieve pressure on the posterior area of the calcaneus—a common area of breakdown in individuals confined to bed.

Incorrect Choice:
Something placed on the posterior surface and distal to the knee will have the potential to increase extension pressure on the knee joint itself. Towel rolls placed along the length of the femur are used to control medial (internal) and lateral (external) rotation of the hip and to protect the medial or lateral malleolus (as well as bony landmarks on the medial and lateral side of the lower extremities) but not the calcaneus.

Type of Reasoning: Inductive
This question requires one to utilize clinical judgment to determine the best place to place a towel roll to relieve pressure on the patient's calcaneus. This requires inductive reasoning skill. For this case the assistant should place the towel roll under the distal posterior tibia at the area of the Achilles tendon. If answered incorrectly, review pressure relief techniques, including use of towel rolls for pressure relief.

C52

System Interactions | Diseases and Conditions Impacting Intervention

A physical therapist assistant is working in the intensive care unit of the hospital with a patient who was admitted for a flare-up of inflammatory bowel disease and dehydration. The physical therapy plan of care includes ambulation activities for endurance and lower extremity strengthening exercise. Which of the following interventions is **MOST** important for the physical therapist assistant?

Choices:
1. Limit lower-extremity exercise to active exercise and avoid resisted exercises.
2. Frequently offer water throughout treatment.
3. Exercise in a semi-Fowler's (head elevated) position.
4. Closely monitor heart rate and blood pressure with upright activities.

Teaching Points

Correct Answer: 4
A patient with hypovolemia (dehydration) is subject to problems with blood pressure and heart rate management secondary to the condition. A patient with hypovolemia may also present with irritable muscles (muscle fatigue, twitching, and cramping), a lower tolerance for exercise, and a higher resting heart rate. Older patients' systems will be less able to compensate for hypovolemia by increasing the heart rate, especially if they are on a cardiac medication such as a beta blocker or digoxin.

Incorrect Choice:
There are no indications to lower extremity active or resistive exercise. A patient in intensive care for dehydration will likely be receiving IV fluids making it unnecessary to offer fluid throughout treatment. There is no indication to keep the head elevated during this treatment.

Type of Reasoning: Inferential
One must determine the most important activity to complete with a patient in an intensive care unit who has inflammatory bowel disease and dehydration. This requires knowledge of both intensive care unit guidelines and the diagnosis of the patient, plus determination of the best course of action, which is an inferential reasoning skill. For this case, the assistant should closely monitor heart rate and blood pressure with upright activities because of the patient's propensity for problems with blood pressure and heart rate management. Review activities for patients with inflammatory bowel disease and hypovolemia if answered incorrectly, especially activities for patients in intensive care.

C53

Musculoskeletal | Interventions

A physical therapist assistant is working with a patient who has a complete spinal cord injury at the level of C6. The plan of care includes instructing the family in exercises to maintain passive range of motion. What should the physical therapist assistant instruct the family to focus on?

Choices:
1. Providing range of motion to individual muscles according to specific functional needs.
2. Keeping all muscles fully ranged through normal range of motion.
3. Keeping muscles fully ranged, with hyperflexibility in the low back extensors and hamstrings.
4. Limiting range of motion in the shoulders to promote stability.

Teaching Points

Correct Answer: 1
Selective stretching techniques are indicated for the patient with spinal cord injury. A patient with a spinal cord injury at the C6 level will need flexible shoulders, and will also need some residual tension in the long finger flexors to achieve a tenodesis grasp.

Incorrect Choice:
Not all muscles are ranged through their full range of motion when an individual has a spinal cord injury. Overstretching the long finger flexors will result in loss of tenodesis grasp. Overstretching the back extensors will result in loss of sitting stability. The shoulders need increased flexibility to achieve function, not less range of motion.

Type of Reasoning: Inductive
This question requires one to utilize clinical judgment to determine a best course of action for a patient with cervical spinal cord injury. Questions that require knowledge of therapeutic techniques and approaches often necessitate inductive reasoning skill. For this case, the assistant should instruct the family to provide range-of-motion to individual muscles according to specific functional needs. If answered incorrectly, review family training guidelines for patients with spinal cord injury, especially range-of-motion techniques.

C54

Neuromuscular | Diseases and Conditions Impacting Intervention

Children with spastic diplegia often have a crouched gait pattern. What positions does the common crouched gait pattern associated with spastic diplegia include?

Choices:
1. Hip flexion, abduction, lateral (external) rotation, and knee flexion.
2. Hip flexion, adduction, medial (internal) rotation, and knee flexion.
3. Hip flexion, adduction, lateral (external) rotation, and knee extension.
4. Hip extension, abduction, medial (internal) rotation, and knee extension.

Teaching Points

Correct Answer: 2
Children with the spastic diplegia form of cerebral palsy characteristically present with spasticity in their hip adductors, internal rotators, medial hamstrings, and ankle plantar flexors and significant weakness in their hip extensors, abductors, knee extensors and ankle plantar flexors. They stabilize themselves by adducting and medially (internally) rotating their hips to compensate for their weakness.

Incorrect Choice:
Characteristic patterns of spastic muscles in spastic diplegia do not include hip abduction, hip extension, hip lateral rotation, or knee extension.

Type of Reasoning: Inferential
One must determine the likely gait pattern for a child with spastic diplegia to arrive at a correct conclusion. This requires knowledge of the diagnosis and mobility patterns, which is an inferential reasoning skill. For this situation, one should anticipate hip flexion, abduction, internal rotation and knee flexion. Review gait patterns for children with spastic diplegia if answered incorrectly.

C55

Nonsystem | Equipment and Devices

What is an appropriate modification to accommodate a plantar flexion contracture during gait training?

Choices:
1. Use of a heel lift.
2. The addition of a metatarsal pad.
3. Use of a dorsiflexion assist ankle–foot orthosis.
4. Electrical stimulation of the tibialis anterior.

Teaching Points

Correct Answer: 1
A heel lift will accommodate a plantar flexion contracture and attempt to approximate a heel strike on the side with the contracture.

Incorrect Choice:
A dorsiflexion assist ankle–foot orthosis is used to assist a patient with a weak tibialis anterior. Use of an ankle–foot orthosis with a muscle contracture may result in tissue breakdown. A metatarsal pad may assist in decreasing abnormal tone in a lower extremity. Electrical stimulation of the tibialis anterior is appropriate if the muscle is weak.

Type of Reasoning: Inductive
One must determine the most appropriate modification to accommodate a plantar flexion contracture to arrive at a correct conclusion. This requires clinical judgment, which is an inductive reasoning skill. For this scenario, the use of a heel lift is most appropriate as it will accommodate the contracture and approximate a heel strike on the side with the contracture. If answered incorrectly, review ankle contractures, especially plantar flexion contractures and appropriate orthotic devices.

C56

Cardiac | Data Collection

While reviewing a patient's medical record prior to treatment, the physical therapist assistant notes that the patient has a diagnosis of congestive heart failure with right ventricular involvement. Which of the following is the patient **MOST** likely to present with?

Choices:
1. Pulmonary edema.
2. Progressive dyspnea.
3. Dependent edema.
4. Renal changes with increasing blood volume.

Teaching Points

Correct Answer: 3
Right ventricular failure is failure of the ventricle to adequately pump blood into the lungs, which results in peripheral edema and venous congestion. The accumulation of fluids in the venous system results in peripheral edema, a back-up of fluids into both lungs. Jugular venous distention and accumulation of fluid in the liver can also develop.

Incorrect Choice:
Pulmonary edema, progressive dyspnea, and renal changes are most closely associated with left-sided ventricular failure. Renal changes resulting in increasing blood volumes are associated with failure on both sides of the heart; however, they are more evident with left-sided failure.

Type of Reasoning: Inferential
This question requires the test taker to infer the most likely symptoms for a patient with congestive heart failure with right ventricular involvement. This requires knowledge of the diagnosis to correctly determine symptoms, which is an inferential reasoning skill. For this case, one should expect the patient to have dependent edema. If answered incorrectly, review symptoms of congestive heart failure, especially right ventricular failure.

C57

Nonsystem | Equipment and Devices

An active child with left hemiplegia including mild knee hyperextension and foot drop has a prescription to obtain an orthosis to correct the lower extremity problems. Which of the following devices **BEST** addresses this patient's dysfunction?

Choices:
1. A knee–ankle–foot orthosis.
2. A posterior leaf spring orthosis.
3. An ankle–foot orthosis.
4. A hip–knee–ankle–foot orthosis.

Teaching Points

Correct Answer: 3
An ankle–foot orthosis, which is set in neutral ankle dorsiflexion or a few degrees of dorsiflexion, will prevent mild knee hyperextension, maintain neutral ankle position, and assist with heel strike (initial contact).

Incorrect Choice:
A knee–ankle–foot orthosis provides knee and ankle control but is bulky and is best for individuals who have decreased hip control and poor to absent knee and ankle control. A posterior leaf spring orthosis provides control for excessive knee flexion with weight bearing. A hip–knee–ankle–foot orthosis provides support at the hips, knees, and ankles and this provides too much support for a child with mild lower extremity weakness.

Type of Reasoning: Analytical
One must analyze the deficits of the child and then determine the most appropriate orthotic device to correct the lower extremity problems. This requires analytical reasoning skill. For this situation, the best device to correct the problems is an ankle–foot orthosis or AFO. If answered incorrectly, review lower-extremity orthotic devices, especially orthoses to correct knee hyperextension and foot drop.

C58

Nonsystem | Equipment and Devices

A physical therapist assistant is working with an active young child who is ready for a new orthosis. The patient has good ankle dorsiflexion and plantar flexion strength and excessive pronation. The patient will require an orthosis to maintain the foot in neutral alignment and provide medial/lateral stability at the ankle while allowing free ankle dorsiflexion and plantar flexion. Which of the following devices is the **MOST** therapeutic for this patient?

Choices:
1. Hip–knee–ankle–foot orthosis.
2. Hinged ankle–foot orthosis.
3. Knee–ankle–foot orthosis.
4. Supramalleolar orthosis.

Teaching Points

Correct Answer: 4

A supramalleolar orthosis provides positioning at the foot and medial/lateral support at the ankle but does not block ankle dorsiflexion or plantar flexion or offer knee support.

Incorrect Choice:
The hip–knee–ankle–foot orthosis, hinged ankle–foot orthosis, and knee–ankle–foot orthosis all offer too much support and limit both knee and ankle movement.

Type of Reasoning: Analytical
One must determine the most effective orthosis that will provide medial/lateral stability at the ankle and neutral alignment of the foot. This requires knowledge of orthotic devices and analysis of their features, which is an analytical reasoning skill. For this situation, the most effective device is a supramalleolar orthosis. If answered incorrectly, review lower-extremity orthotic devices, especially supramalleolar orthoses.

C59

Neuromuscular | Interventions

A patient who is comatose and has loss of ankle dorsiflexion range of motion due hypertonicity is MOST likely to benefit from which of the following interventions?

Choices:
1. Serial casting and positioning to maintain flexibility.
2. PNF to promote strengthening.
3. Therapeutic exercise for sitting balance and coordination.
4. Weight-bearing activities.

Teaching Points

Correct Answer: 1

Serial casting and positioning will assist with maintaining flexibility for this individual and do not require active participation of the patient.

Incorrect Choice:
Because the patient is in a coma he or she will most likely not be able to actively participate in strengthening, therapeutic exercise for balance and coordination or weight-bearing activities. The priority at this time is to maintain joint range of motion and muscle flexibility. Upright positioning in a safe device such as a wheelchair, adapted seat, or tilt table is likely indicated; however, while it may address hypertonicity, it will not address loss of range of motion.

Type of Reasoning: Inductive
This question requires one to utilize knowledge of therapy processes that will be most effective for a patient who has severe traumatic brain injury. This is an inductive reasoning skill. For this case, the most effective intervention for this patient to address the loss of range of motion is serial casting and positioning to maintain flexibility. If answered incorrectly, review approaches to improve range of motion in patients who are comatose.

C60

Nonsystem | Professional Responsibility

A patient's adult children would like to look at the patient's medical record. What is the **MOST** appropriate action for the physical therapist assistant?

Choices:
1. Give the children the chart as a family member has a right to view the information.
2. Deny access to the chart unless written permission is granted from the patient, and then refer the children to the physical therapist.
3. Do not let the children view the chart under any circumstances.
4. Let the children look at the chart, but only with the physical therapist present.

Teaching Points

Correct Answer: 2
After the family member has received written permission from the patient, the physical therapist can discuss and review the chart with the family member(s).

Incorrect Choice:
The issue is patient confidentiality. Family members do not have access to medical information unless they have consent either from the patient or from a health care proxy if the patient is deemed incompetent. In accordance with the American Physical Therapy Association's Guide for Professional Conduct Principle 1: Physical therapist assistants respect the rights and dignity of all individuals.

Type of Reasoning: Evaluative
This question requires one to use both knowledge of guidelines as well as ethical reasoning to determine a best course of action. Questions of this nature often require evaluative reasoning skill to weigh the merits of each approach and determine the one that best addresses the issue at hand. For this situation, the assistant should deny access to the chart unless written permission is granted from the patient and then refer the son or daughter to the physical therapist. Ultimately, the physician in charge is the only one qualified to comment on the medical record if permission has been granted.

C61

Pulmonary | Diseases and Conditions Impacting Intervention

Which of the following contraindications to joint mobilization is common for patients with chronic pulmonary disease?

Choices:
1. Reflex muscle guarding.
2. Long-term corticosteroid therapy.
3. Concurrent inhalation therapy.
4. Functional chest wall immobility.

Teaching Points

Correct Answer: 2
Very often patients with chronic pulmonary disease have been managed with corticosteroid therapy. Long-term steroid use affects ligamentous integrity, which often produces joint hypermobility.

Incorrect Choice:
Reflex muscle guarding is a precaution or possible reaction to joint mobilization. Concurrent inhalation therapy is not a contraindication to joint mobilization. Chest wall immobility is a likely indication for joint mobilization.

Type of Reasoning: Deductive
This question requires one to recall the contraindications to joint mobilization to arrive at a correct conclusion. This is factual recall of information, which is a deductive reasoning skill. For this case, the typical contraindication to joint mobilization for patients with chronic pulmonary disease is long-term corticosteroid therapy. Review joint mobilization guidelines and contraindications, especially for patients with chronic pulmonary disease, if answered incorrectly.

C62

Musculoskeletal | Interventions

The supervising physical therapist completed an initial examination with the patient and recommended a treatment program addressing chronic lateral epicondylitis. What are the **MOST** appropriate intervention strategies for this patient?

Choices:
1. Cryotherapy, cross-friction massage followed by electrical stimulation, then flexibility.
2. Cryotherapy prior to activities, practice using power tools with review of proper ergonomic positioning and body mechanics, and heat therapy after activities.
3. Heat therapy prior to activities, practice using power tools with review of proper ergonomic positioning and body mechanics, and cryotherapy after activities.
4. Heat therapy, then ultrasound followed by strengthening activities.

Teaching Points

Correct Answer: 3
Heat therapy will assist with relaxing muscles and will warm tissues, followed by protected activity, and cryotherapy will assist with controlling pain after activities. Reviewing proper ergonomic technique and body mechanics is essential to prevent further injury and irritation to the affected area.

Incorrect Choice:
Massage, electrical stimulation, and ultrasound may be correct passive interventions; however, because it has been several months, a more active approach needs to be taken to return to normal function.

Type of Reasoning: Inductive
Knowledge of treatment guidelines for chronic lateral epicondylitis is paramount for arriving at a correct conclusion. Utilizing knowledge of treatment approaches and processes often requires inductive reasoning skill. For this situation, the most appropriate intervention strategies should include heat prior to activities, ergonomic training while using power tools, and cryotherapy after activities. Review guidelines for treatment of chronic lateral epicondylitis if answered incorrectly.

C63

Neuromuscular | Diseases and Conditions Impacting Interventions

What should typical physical therapy management for a child with myelomeningocele (spina bifida) at the T4–5 level focus on?

Choices:
1. Gait training with a knee–ankle–foot orthosis and crutches.
2. Strengthening of the hip extensors and quadriceps muscles.
3. Standing balance activities with a hip–knee–ankle–foot orthosis.
4. Wheelchair mobility training.

Teaching Points

Correct Answer: 4
Wheelchair mobility training is the most appropriate and functional intervention for this level. Children with a high thoracic lesion will have innervation to the neck, upper extremity, and some trunk muscles.

Incorrect Choice:
Because there is no innervation distal to T5, the patient will not be able to gain strength in his or her hip extensors or quadriceps muscles. Standing may be included for some children for physiological benefits; however, to do so, a parapodium or standing frame should be used. The child will need extensive wheelchair training as this will be the child's primary mode of mobility.

Type of Reasoning: Inductive
One must utilize knowledge of therapeutic processes for children with thoracic spina bifida to arrive at a correct conclusion, which is an inductive reasoning skill. For this case, children with thoracic spina bifida should receive wheelchair mobility training as this will be the child's primary mode of mobility. If answered incorrectly, review therapeutic activities for children with spina bifida, especially thoracic-level involvement.

C64

Pulmonary | Interventions

A patient who is recovering from surgery is receiving postural drainage as part of the physical therapy plan of care. When should the physical therapist assistant discuss decreasing the frequency of sessions per day with the physical therapist?

Choices:
1. If consistency of the sputum changes.
2. If the patient becomes febrile.
3. When the amount of productive secretions decreases.
4. When the patient experiences decreased postoperative pain.

Teaching Points

Correct Answer: 3
The purpose of postural drainage is to help remove secretions. If the amount of drainage diminishes, the treatment is likely successful and the frequency can be decreased.

Incorrect Choice:
Development of increased postoperative pain, a fever, or a change in the consistency of the sputum does not indicate readiness to decrease frequency of postural drainage.

Type of Reasoning: Inferential
One must determine the situation that would warrant decreasing the frequency of treatment sessions for a patient receiving postural drainage. This requires one to infer or draw a reasonable conclusion about what is likely to be true. For this situation, the frequency of sessions should be decreased if the patient demonstrates a decreased amount of productive secretions. If answered incorrectly, review treatment guidelines for patients requiring postural drainage techniques and frequency of treatment sessions.

C65

Musculoskeletal | Interventions

A patient sustained a left rectus femoris strain while playing volleyball 2 weeks ago. The plan of care indicates to begin a stretching program to promote a functional gain in range of motion. The patient has complained of pain and discomfort with knee flexion greater than 80°. Which is the **MOST** appropriate intervention following 20 minutes of moist heat?

Choices:
1. Immediate static stretching at end range with a 10- to 20-second stretch.
2. Immediate static, progressive stretching just beyond tissue resistance with a 30- to 60-second stretch.
3. Immediate ballistic stretching with 10 passive stretches to end range; repeat two sets.
4. Three repetitions of hold-relax with a 30-second hold and 10-second relax with stretch at end range.

Teaching Points

Correct Answer: 2
Static stretching at end range with a 30- to 60-second hold just beyond tissue resistance has been reported to increase the length of soft tissues (joint capsule, muscle, and tendon). Moist heat applied prior to the stretching helps improve elasticity of the tissues.

Incorrect Choice:
Ballistic stretching is not appropriate when pain, discomfort, or muscle strain are present. Static stretching with a 10- to 20-second hold has not been shown to be as effective as a 30- to 60-second hold. Hold-relax techniques can increase tissue length; however, up to a 10-second hold followed by a 30- to 60-second static progressive hold is effective, whereas a 30-second hold and 10-second stretch is not.

Type of Reasoning: Inductive

This question requires knowledge of treatment guidelines for a patient with rectus femoris strain to arrive at a correct conclusion. Knowledge of treatment guidelines often necessitates inductive reasoning skill. For this case, the most appropriate treatment program for this patient should include moist heat followed by immediate static, progressive stretching just beyond tissue resistance. If answered incorrectly, review treatment activities for muscle strain, especially rectus femoris strain.

C66

Neuromuscular | Interventions

Which of the following interventions is **MOST** effective in decreasing tone in a patient with hypertonia?

Choices:
1. A warm whirlpool to relax muscles and increase range of motion.
2. Use of a weighted vest or belts to increase proprioceptive feedback.
3. Passive range-of-motion activities and avoiding strength training.
4. Active weight bearing with aligned limbs and trunk.

Teaching Points

Correct Answer: 4

Persons with hypertonia generally have poor motor control and poor muscle strength. Using the principles of biomechanics, positioning limbs and trunk with muscles in a mid-position, not over-lengthened or in a shortened position, helps to facilitate active control. Even though the patient has hypertonia, strengthening can be emphasized. Concerns of increasing spasticity are not warranted as it has been proven that strengthening a muscle with increased tone does not increase that tone or spasticity.

Incorrect Choice:

Although passive range of motion will be an important part of treatment, it should be incorporated with active interventions. Whirlpools may assist with relaxing the muscles temporarily, but there is no lasting effect and it would be difficult to work on stretching and strengthening in a whirlpool. Weighted vests may be helpful for children with sensory dysfunction or movement disorder such as ataxia.

Type of Reasoning: Inductive

One must have knowledge of the therapeutic approaches that are most effective in decreasing hypertonia to arrive at a correct conclusion. Clinical judgment is utilized in this situation, which is an inductive reasoning skill. For this case, the most effective way to reduce hypertonia is to have the patient perform active weight bearing with aligned limbs and trunk. Review therapeutic approaches for decreasing hypertonia if answered incorrectly.

C67

Nonsystem | Equipment and Devices

A physical therapist assistant has observed a child with cerebral palsy to present with severe extensor posturing of the lower extremities. Which wheelchair modification is **MOST** appropriate for this individual?

Choices:
1. Seat position to create flexion less than 90° at the hip and knees.
2. Seat position to create flexion greater than 90° at the hip and knees.
3. Seat positioned in the anterior tilt direction.
4. Hip adductor wedge included in the seat.

Teaching Points

Correct Answer: 2
Hip and knee flexion greater than 90° facilitates flexion and would assist in inhibiting tone by assisting to keep the lower extremities in a flexed posture.

Incorrect Choice:
Hip flexion less than 90° will facilitate hip extension, which would cause the child's pelvis to slide forward and out of the wheelchair. The same will occur if the chair seat is in an anterior tilt. If the chair seat is tilted, it should be in a posterior direction to assist in keeping the pelvis back in the chair. Extensor posturing is often accompanied by adductor spasticity. A wheelchair seat should minimize adduction by including an abductor wedge.

Type of Reasoning: Inferential
Knowledge of wheelchair positioning for children with cerebral palsy is paramount to arriving at a correct conclusion for this question. For this scenario, the wheelchair seat should position the hip and knee to create flexion greater than 90° in a child with severe extensor posturing of the lower extremities. If answered incorrectly, review wheelchair positioning guidelines, especially for children with cerebral palsy.

C68

Musculoskeletal | Interventions

A patient presents with a grade 2 lateral ankle sprain incurred during a volleyball game the previous night. Today, the patient ambulates into the clinic non–weight-bearing using bilateral axillary crutches, has a compression wrap on the involved ankle and rates the pain a 5/10. What is an appropriate intervention during this early phase of rehabilitation?

Choices:
1. Encourage full-range-of-motion exercises.
2. Incorporate muscle-setting exercises.
3. Perform isotonic exercise at 60% maximum strength.
4. Train in partial weight-bearing gait pattern.

Teaching Points

Correct Answer: 2
An early goal is to protect the joint from further injury. Thus, muscle setting without motion is appropriate.

Incorrect Choice:
This injury occurred yesterday, and tissues are still healing. During the maximum protection phase of rehabilitation, full range of motion, resisted (isotonic) exercise, and partial weight bearing all place too much stress on the healing tissues.

Type of Reasoning: Inductive
This question requires the test taker to determine the most appropriate treatment intervention for a patient with grade 2 lateral ankle sprain. This requires clinical judgment, which is an inductive reasoning skill. For this case, the assistant should incorporate muscle-setting exercises during the early maximum protection phase. Review exercises for ankle sprains, especially during the early phase of rehabilitation.

C69

Nonsystem | Equipment and Devices

A young child with cerebral palsy presents with severe spastic quadriplegia, poor head and trunk control, no functional use of upper extremities, and musculoskeletal weakness. What equipment will **BEST** assist with standing activities?

Choices:
1. Mobile stander.
2. Upright stander.
3. Supine stander.
4. Prone stander.

Teaching Points

Correct Answer: 3

A supine stander provides posterior support for head and neck control in addition to support for musculoskeletal weakness.

Incorrect Choice:

A mobile stander is best suited to a child who has more strength and mobility. An upright stander is more appropriate for a child with mild to moderate physical impairments. A prone stander requires active upper body strength.

Type of Reasoning: Inductive

One must determine the most appropriate piece of equipment for a child with cerebral palsy and severe spastic quadriplegia. This requires the test taker to understand the effects of cerebral palsy and then assess which equipment piece will provide the most benefit. This requires inductive reasoning skill. For this case, a supine stander will provide the most benefit for the child's diagnosis and symptoms. Review therapeutic equipment for children with cerebral palsy if answered incorrectly.

C70

Neuromuscular | Interventions

Which represents the **BEST** strategy to get a 4-year-old child with pervasive developmental disorder (PDD) to participate in strengthening activities?

Choices:
1. Progressive resistive exercises using cuff weights and resistive band.
2. Daily activities such as climbing stairs, running on the playground, and ball activities.
3. Imaginative games and role playing of the patient's favorite characters.
4. PNF patterns using timing for emphasis at the end range of motion.

Teaching Points

Correct Answer: 2

Using familiar activities and functional activities is most appropriate for this child. Children with PDD do best with familiar and routine activities.

Incorrect Choice:

Children with PDD often have impaired receptive and expressive language skills and have difficulty with lots of verbal instructions, making it difficult to instruct them in an exercise program or PNF techniques. Children with PDD also often have impairments in imagination, thereby making it difficult for the child to participate in imaginative games.

Type of Reasoning: Inductive

This question requires one to utilize clinical judgment to determine a best course of action for a child with PDD. This is an inductive reasoning skill. For this scenario, children with PDD often respond positively to strengthening activities such as climbing stairs, running on the playground, and ball activities, as these are familiar activities. If answered incorrectly, review therapeutic activities for children with PDD, especially strengthening activities.

C71

Neuromuscular | Interventions

A patient recovering from traumatic brain injury is unable to bring the right foot up on the stair during stair-climbing training. What is the **MOST** functional method to develop this skill?

Choices:
1. Have the patient practice marching in place.
2. Passively place the foot on the next step.
3. Practice stair climbing inside the parallel bars using a 3-inch step.
4. Strengthen the patient's hip flexors by using an isokinetic training device before attempting stair climbing.

Teaching Points

Correct Answer: 3

The most appropriate functional activity to promote the skill of stair climbing is practice by using a 3-inch step in the parallel bars.

Incorrect Choice:

Passive movements do not promote active learning. Marching in place and isokinetic training may improve the strength of the hip flexors but do not promote the same synergistic patterns of muscle activity as the desired skill.

Type of Reasoning: Inductive

One must utilize clinical judgment and reasoning to determine the most functional method to develop stair-climbing skill. Questions of this nature, where determining the most therapeutic course of action is paramount to arriving at a correct conclusion, require inductive reasoning skill. For this scenario, the most functional method to develop this skill is to practice stair climbing inside the parallel bars by using a 3-inch step. Review stair-climbing training guidelines if answered incorrectly.

C72

Pulmonary | Diseases and Conditions Impacting Intervention

Which intervention is the primary focus for a child with cystic fibrosis?

Choices:
1. Postural drainage.
2. Pursed-lip breathing.
3. Assisted cough.
4. Diaphragmatic breathing.

Teaching Points

Correct Answer: 1
Chest physical therapy, including percussion, vibration, and postural drainage, is a primary physical therapy intervention for children with cystic fibrosis to maintain clear airways because of the excessive mucus production caused by cystic fibrosis. To clear these secretions and allow for good aeration, aggressive techniques must be used.

Incorrect Choice:
Pursed-lip breathing is used with patients with chronic obstructive pulmonary disease for them to exhale fully. Diaphragmatic breathing and assisted cough are techniques used with patients with spinal cord injuries to assist weak muscles.

Type of Reasoning: Inferential
One must infer the symptoms and therapeutic processes for children with cystic fibrosis to arrive at a correct conclusion. This requires inferential reasoning skill. For this situation, young children with cystic fibrosis primarily require postural drainage techniques to maintain clear airways because of excessive mucus production. If answered incorrectly, review the symptoms of cystic fibrosis and treatment interventions for this diagnosis.

C73

Musculoskeletal | Data Collection

A patient is being seen in physical therapy following a tibial fracture and has developed a compression injury of the peroneal nerve. The physical therapist assistant should expect to see altered motor and sensory responses in what dermatome?

Choices:
1. L5.
2. L4.
3. L3.
4. S1.

Teaching Points

Correct Answer: 1
The L5 dermatome covers the anterolateral lower extremity, medial dorsal foot and plantar aspect of the great toe; to think of the L5 dermatome covering the toes (one has five toes) may be a helpful study tool.

Incorrect Choice:
The L3 dermatome covers the distal anteromedial thigh and knee. L4 covers the anteromedial lower extremity. S1 covers the lateral dorsal foot and most of the plantar foot.

Type of Reasoning: Inferential
This question requires the test taker to infer the symptoms of a patient with a status of post-tibial plateau fracture with compression injury to the peroneal nerve. One must infer the likely dermatome that is affected with this type of injury, which requires inferential reasoning skill. In this case, the L5 dermatome is likely to be damaged. If answered incorrectly, review compression injury to the peroneal nerve and dermatome involvement for the L5 distribution.

C74

Neuromuscular | Interventions

A physical therapist assistant is working with a patient who has Stage 5: moderately severe decline Alzheimer's disease and a recent total hip arthroplasty. The patient is having difficulty following directions for ambulation activities with a walker. What should the PTA do to **BEST** facilitate ambulation with the walker?

Choices:
1. Use single-step verbal directions.
2. Physically assist the patient to perform the activities.
3. Perform ambulation activities on the treadmill.
4. First demonstrate the activity and then provide physical guidance.

Teaching Points

Correct Answer: 4
A person with middle-stage Alzheimer's disease will likely be able to "repeat" activities that have been demonstrated to him or her. Patients will likely do better if they receive some visual and tactile cueing to accomplish activities.

Incorrect Choice:
In earlier stages of Alzheimer's disease, patients may be able to follow single-step verbal direction; however, as the disease progresses, this approach is no longer effective. Manually performing the tasks with the patient may result in involuntary muscle resistance to movement. A patient with middle-stage Alzheimer's disease and a recent total hip arthroplasty will likely be unable to handle the speed of a treadmill and this may present a risk for the recent surgery.

Type of Reasoning: Inductive
One must determine the best therapeutic approach to assist a patient with Alzheimer's disease to use a walker for ambulation activities. This requires clinical judgment, which is an inductive reasoning skill. For this scenario, the assistant should first demonstrate the activity and then provide physical guidance, as patients with this condition in the middle stages respond positively to visual and tactile cueing. If answered incorrectly, review therapeutic approaches for patients with Alzheimer's disease, especially ambulation activities.

C75

Neuromuscular | Diseases and Conditions Impacting Intervention

Vertebral instability at the atlantoaxial joint is most often associated with which of the following conditions?

Choices:
1. Cerebral palsy.
2. Down syndrome.
3. Spina bifida.
4. Duchenne's muscular dystrophy.

Teaching Points

Correct Answer: 2
Children with Down syndrome have an increased incidence of atlantoaxial instability. This is an important consideration when one is implementing treatment with this patient population; care must be used to avoid extremes of range of motion in the cervical spine.

Incorrect Choice:

Instability at the atlantoaxial joint is not a hallmark in the diagnosis of cerebral palsy, spina bifida, or Duchenne's muscular dystrophy.

Type of Reasoning: Deductive

This question requires factual recall of information about Down syndrome and common deficits, which is a deductive reasoning skill. For this case, children with Down syndrome commonly have issues with vertebral instability at the atlantoaxial joint. If answered incorrectly, review signs and symptoms of Down syndrome, especially atlantoaxial instability.

C76

Neuromuscular | Diseases and Conditions Impacting Intervention

Which of the following postural deviations is commonly seen in individuals with Duchenne's muscular dystrophy?

Choices:
1. Forward flexion at the hips.
2. Internal rotation of the hips.
3. Hyperextension of the knees.
4. Supination of the forefoot.

Teaching Points

Correct Answer: 3

An individual with Duchenne's muscular dystrophy has lower extremity weakness and hypotonicity. Due to this weakness, individuals then tend to "lock their knees" and hyperextend their knees in standing.

Incorrect Choice:

Due to weak abdominals and back exetensors, as well as hypotonicity while standing, individuals will hang on their Y ligament of their hip and stand in slight hip extension (not flexion). In order to increase their base of support and increase their stability in standing, individuals will stand with external rotation of the hips, not internal rotation of the hips. Due to weakness pronation will be seen, not supination. The postural deviations of internal rotation of the hips, forward flexion of the hips and supination of the feet tend to be seen in individuals with spasticity or hypertonicity such as cerebral palsy.

Type of Reasoning: Inferential

One must infer or draw a reasonable conclusion about the common deviation observed with boys with Duchenne's muscular dystrophy when standing from the floor. This requires inferential reasoning skill. For this scenario, the common deviation is the use of the upper extremities to push on his knees and walk his hands up the legs because of insufficient lower-extremity strength to stand from the floor. If answered incorrectly, review functional abilities of boys with Duchenne's muscular dystrophy, especially mobility patterns.

C77

Musculoskeletal | Diseases and Conditions Impacting Intervention

A patient is receiving physical therapy following a Colles' fracture and the subsequent diagnosis of osteoporosis. The fracture is now well healed and the plan of care includes the development of a home exercise program. At a minimum, what should the exercise program include?

Choices:
1. Wall push-ups and upper-extremity resistive band exercises.
2. Aerobic activity and exercises that use eccentric muscle contractions.
3. Active upper-extremity diagonals and core stability exercises.
4. Submaximal upper-extremity active exercise and bike riding.

Teaching Points

Correct Answer: 1
For exercises to promote an increase in bone density they must be performed in a weight-bearing or loading capacity; wall push-ups and resistance exercises will meet those criteria.

Incorrect Choice:
Exercising muscles eccentrically, aerobic activities, sub-max or active upper extremity will not stimulate bone growth. Bike riding will likely increase upper-extremity weight bearing; however, submaximal exercises will not be beneficial for this patient.

Type of Reasoning: Inductive
One must utilize clinical judgment to determine the best exercise program for a patient with a healed Colles' fracture. Questions that require one to determine the best therapeutic approach often require inductive reasoning skill. For this scenario, the exercise program should include wall push-ups and upper-extremity resistive band exercises. Review exercise guidelines for patients with Colles' fracture if answered incorrectly.

C78

Musculoskeletal | Data Collection

Following a hip fracture that is now healed, a patient presents with weak hip flexors with a muscle grade of poor (2/5). All other muscles are within functional limits. What gait deviation is this patient **MOST** likely to present with?

Choices:
1. Forward trunk lean.
2. Circumducted gait.
3. Excessive hip flexion.
4. Backward trunk lean.

Teaching Points

Correct Answer: 2
Circumduction is a compensation for weak hip flexors or an inability to shorten the lower extremity (weak knee flexors and ankle dorsiflexors). Hip hiking can also compensate for an abnormally long lower extremity (lack of knee flexion and dorsiflexion).

Incorrect Choice:
Excessive hip flexion is a compensation for foot drop. Forward trunk lean and backward trunk lean are stance phase deviations that compensate for quadriceps weakness and gluteus maximus weakness, respectively.

Type of Reasoning: Inferential
This question requires one to infer or draw a reasonable conclusion about what is likely to be true for a patient with weak hip flexors. This requires inferential reasoning skill. For this case, one should expect that the patient will walk with a circumducted gait. If answered incorrectly, review gait patterns for patients with lower-extremity weakness, especially weak hip flexors.

C79

Musculoskeletal | Interventions

The physical therapist assistant is working with a 2-month-old child who sustained an avulsion injury to the brachial plexus during the delivery and is now 2 weeks postsurgical repair of the avulsion. Which of the following interventions should be initiated?

Choices:
1. Gentle range-of-motion exercises.
2. Developmental activities such as prone on elbows.
3. Introduction of assistive devices to promote functional skills.
4. Active strengthening exercises.

Teaching Points

Correct Answer: 1

Following surgical repair of an avulsion injury, the infant's arm is usually positioned across the chest in adduction and medial (internal) rotation for approximately 1–2 weeks to promote healing. Gentle range-of-motion exercises to prevent contractures is recommended for the next few weeks followed by more aggressive exercises including weight-bearing and reaching activities.

Incorrect Choice:

Because the child is only 2 months old, developmental activities such as prone on elbows are too developmentally advanced. It is also too early at this stage for use of assistive devices or strengthening exercises.

Type of Reasoning: Inductive

One must utilize clinical judgment to determine the best intervention for an infant with brachial plexus injury. Inductive reasoning skills are utilized whenever one must determine a best therapeutic process. For this situation, intervention should include gentle range-of-motion exercises. If answered incorrectly, review intervention approaches for brachial plexus injuries in infants.

C80

System Interactions | Diseases and Conditions Impacting Intervention

A physical therapist assistant is treating a patient who has Paget's disease. The medical management for this patient includes a medication to improve bone strength. What is a possible side effect of medications for building bone strength?

Choices:
1. Impaired blood-clotting times.
2. Hypotension.
3. Dizziness and lightheadedness.
4. Swelling of the feet or abdomen.

Teaching Points

Correct Answer: 1

One medication used to treat disorders of the bone is raloxifene (Evista); this medication can impair blood-clotting times. Physical therapist assistants working with patients who are taking this medication should be sure to observe the patient for bruising and encourage the patient to get regular blood tests of blood-clotting times.

Incorrect Choice:

A patient taking ACE inhibitors may be at risk for swelling of the feet or abdomen. Multiple different medications can cause hypotension (e.g., calcium channel blockers, fish oil). Diuretics can cause symptoms of lightheadedness or dizziness.

Type of Reasoning: Deductive

One must recall the side effects of medications that build bone strength to arrive at a correct conclusion. This is factual information, which is a deductive reasoning skill. In this situation, the possible side effect of such medications is impaired blood-clotting times. If answered incorrectly, review side effects of medications for patients with Paget's disease, especially bone-building medication.

C81

Integumentary | Diseases and Conditions Impacting Intervention

A physical therapist assistant is discussing the benefits of wheelchair cushions with a patient who has paraplegia. What should the physical therapist explain is the primary cause of pressure ulcers?

Choices:
1. Friction.
2. Excess moisture.
3. Soap cleansers.
4. Excess pressure.

Teaching Points

Correct Answer: 4

A pressure ulcer is formed from the pressure of prolonged sitting.

Incorrect Choice:

Friction requires the rubbing of two surfaces, and this is most likely to occur during a transfer or during bed mobility activities. Moisture softens the skin and soap cleansers may contain toxic chemicals, contributing to skin breakdown.

Type of Reasoning: Deductive

One must recall the causes of pressure ulcers to arrive at a correct conclusion. This is factual recall of information, which is a deductive reasoning skill. In this case, the primary cause of pressure ulcers is excess pressure, most commonly attributable to prolonged sitting. If answered incorrectly, review pressure ulcer guidelines, especially causes of pressure ulcers.

C82

System Interactions | Diseases and Conditions Impacting Intervention

A patient who has had diabetes since childhood is now receiving hemodialysis. Which of the following is an indication that the hemodialysis is not optimally effective?

Choices:
1. Persistent cough.
2. Increased peripheral edema.
3. Jaundiced coloring.
4. Hyperreflexia.

Teaching Points

Correct Answer: 2

Patients with type 1 diabetes suffer kidney failure; therefore, they need hemodialysis to replace the kidney's function. The kidney's function is to clear waste products, toxins, and excess fluid from the blood. If this is not done satisfactorily there will be an excessive peripheral edema caused by the increased fluid and toxins in the blood and tissues. This manifests itself as edema in the periphery.

Incorrect Choice:

Persistent cough, jaundiced coloring, or hyperreflexia are not caused by increased fluid in the peripheral tissues, and they are not indications of inadequate hemodialysis.

Type of Reasoning: Inferential

One must infer the symptom that would indicate that hemodialysis is not optimally effective. Questions that require the test taker to determine what may be true of a situation often require inferential reasoning skill. In this case, a person with increased peripheral edema demonstrates that hemodialysis is not optimally effective. If answered incorrectly, review hemodialysis guidelines and symptoms indicating ineffective dialysis.

C83

Musculoskeletal | Interventions

A basketball player is undergoing rehabilitation status post-left knee anterior cruciate ligament reconstruction. The orthopedic surgeon utilized a bone-patellar tendon-bone graft and has ordered an accelerated rehabilitation protocol. Which **BEST** describes the positive impact of utilizing closed-chain kinetic exercises as part of an accelerated rehabilitation protocol?

Choices:
1. Facilitates long axis distraction of the joint.
2. Enhances functional movement in the transverse plane.
3. Promotes the functional recruitment of motor units.
4. Creates shear forces at the articular level.

Teaching Points

Correct Answer: 3

Closed-chain exercises encourage functional recruitment of motor units, specifically co-contraction of the flexor and extensor groups.

Incorrect Choice:

Closed joint compression versus joint distraction occurs as a part of closed-chain exercise. The primary motion of the knee occurs in the sagittal plane, with flexion and extension; the screw home mechanism occurs in the transverse plane; however, it is an accessory movement, thus one that is not selectively exercised. Closed-chain exercises actually reduce shear forces, not promote forces at a joint.

Type of Reasoning: Inductive

This question requires one to determine the positive impact of utilizing closed-chain kinetic exercises as part of an accelerated rehabilitation protocol. This necessitates clinical judgment, which is an inductive reasoning skill. For this case, closed-chain kinetic exercises promote the functional recruitment of motor units. If answered incorrectly, review the benefits of closed-chain kinetic exercises, especially after athletic injuries and anterior cruciate ligament reconstruction.

C84

Cardiovascular | Diseases and Conditions Impacting Impairment

A physical therapist assistant is instructed to begin treating a distance runner who has been referred to physical therapy for ankle pain. Prior to beginning treatment the patient's blood pressure is 100/60 mm Hg and the resting heart rate is 48 bpm. Which is the **BEST** conclusion based on this information?

Choices:
1. The patient is poorly hydrated, provide water prior to treatment.
2. The patient is hypotensive; monitor vitals throughout treatment.
3. The patient is aerobically fit; exercise as pain tolerates.
4. The patient's endurance training has resulted in a lower heart rate, the patient will tolerate exercise.

Teaching Points

Correct Answer: 4
A benefit of endurance training is that it can result in a decreased resting heart rate and lower resting blood pressure with improved functional capacity. The blood pressure is within normal ranges and should not lead the physical therapist assistant to become concerned.

Incorrect Choice:
There are no signs and symptoms observed that would lead the physical therapist assistant to suspect dehydration, hypotension, or low blood sugar level.

Type of Reasoning: Inductive
One must utilize clinical judgment to determine the meaning of a patient with a resting heart rate of 48 bpm and a blood pressure of 100/60 mm Hg. Given that the patient is a distance runner, one should conclude that endurance training has resulted in a lower heart rate and that the patient will tolerate exercise. The patient's blood pressure is unremarkable. If answered incorrectly, review vital sign guidelines in athletes, especially distance runners.

C85

Neuromuscular | Diseases and Conditions Impacting Intervention

Persons with Duchenne's muscular dystrophy often progressively lose the ability to ambulate. At what age does wheelchair mobility typically become necessary?

Choices:
1. 4–9 years of age.
2. 9–14 years of age.
3. 14–19 years of age.
4. 19–24 years of age.

Teaching Points

Correct Answer: 2
Patients with Duchenne's muscular dystrophy often lose their ambulation skills between the ages of 9 and 14 years.

Incorrect Choice:
Between 3 and 8 years of age, children show signs of weakness with gait deviations, decreased endurance, and tripping; however, they are still able to ambulate. Adolescents between 15 and 17 years of age often use powered mobility and may need ventilator assistance because of respiratory complications. Individuals aged 18 years and older demonstrate increased dependence and respiratory compromise.

Type of Reasoning: Deductive

One must recall the typical age range that a child with Duchenne's muscular dystrophy will progressively lose the ability to ambulate to the point of needing a wheelchair for mobility. This is factual information, which is a deductive reasoning skill. For this situation, a boy with Duchenne's muscular dystrophy will typically decline in strength and need to use a wheelchair for mobility between 9 and 14 years of age. If answered incorrectly, review symptoms of Duchenne's muscular dystrophy and mobility patterns as the disease progresses.

C86

Neuromuscular | Safety and Protection

What should a physical therapist assistant working with a patient who is exhibiting signs and symptoms of autonomic dysreflexia do?

Choices:
1. Lay the patient down and monitor blood pressure and pulse rate.
2. Administer chest compressions.
3. Allow the patient to rest then resume exercise activities at a lighter pace.
4. Activate emergency protocols and check for and eliminate irritants to the patient's system.

Teaching Points

Correct Answer: 4

Autonomic dysreflexia is an emergency situation encountered by patients with spinal cord lesions, generally at the T7 and above level. It is a dangerous condition in which hypertension will persist if it is not treated immediately. It is generally triggered by noxious stimuli, which initiate an autonomic response that the autonomic system cannot control and correct normally. The most common irritant to the system is bladder distension; other irritants can include rectal distension, pressure sores, bladder infections, and noxious cutaneous stimuli (e.g., tight clothing).

Incorrect Choice:

While it may be appropriate to monitor vital signs, this action does not address the immediate need to eliminate the irritant to the patient's autonomic system. Simply resting and then resuming activities does not eliminate the irritant to the patient's autonomic system. Administering chest compressions is only appropriate if the patient's heart has stopped beating.

Type of Reasoning: Deductive

This question requires the test taker to recall factual guidelines regarding how to intervene when a patient exhibits signs and symptoms of autonomic dysreflexia. Using factual information to determine a correct course of action often necessitates deductive reasoning skill. For this situation, the assistant should activate emergency protocols and check for and eliminate irritants to the patient's system. If answered incorrectly, review guidelines for intervening during episodes of autonomic dysreflexia.

C87

Neuromuscular | Interventions

A physical therapist assistant is instructing a nurse to properly position a patient who is status post a cerebrovascular accident with resulting upper extremity posturing into a flexion synergy. What position should the patient be positioned in order to BEST facilitate a decrease in the upper extremity synergy pattern?

Choices:
1. Flexion, pronation, and radial deviation with extension, respectively.
2. Extension, pronation, and ulnar deviation with extension, respectively.
3. Extension, supination, and radial deviation with flexion, respectively.
4. Flexion, supination, and ulnar deviation with flexion, respectively.

Teaching Points

Correct Answer: 2

To decrease spasticity, the extremity is positioned out of the synergy pattern. The upper-extremity flexor synergy pattern consists of elbow flexion with forearm supination, and wrist and finger flexion. Positioning the elbow into extension, forearm in pronation, and the wrist and fingers into extension will inhibit the flexor tone.

Incorrect Choice:

The other positions listed are positions that will inhibit flexor synergy tone.

Type of Reasoning: Deductive

One must recall the out-of-synergy pattern for a patient with a status of post–cerebrovascular accident to arrive at a correct conclusion. This is factual information, which is a deductive reasoning skill. For this situation, the out-of-synergy pattern consists of elbow, forearm, and wrist extension, pronation, and ulnar deviation with extension. If answered incorrectly, review synergy patterns with cerebrovascular accidents, especially out-of-synergy patterns.

C88

Musculoskeletal | Interventions

A patient presents for outpatient physical therapy services with the diagnosis of hypermobility of the shoulder. The physical therapist directs the physical therapist assistant to provide therapeutic exercise to address the hypermobility. What is the **MOST** appropriate therapeutic exercise?

Choices:
1. Taping and stabilization exercises.
2. Grade 2 and 3 manual peripheral joint mobilization.
3. Rotator cuff stretching exercises.
4. Overhead strengthening exercises.

Teaching Points

Correct Answer: 1

For a hypermobile joint, the proper intervention is to stabilize the joint functionally through corrective exercises or taping.

Incorrect Choice:

If a joint is hypermobile, no joint mobilization is warranted. Because the joint has such hypermobility, the assistant should not do strengthening exercises at the end range in the overhead position; instead, strengthening should be done in the beginning to midrange. Stretching exercises are not indicated for a hypermobile joint.

Type of Reasoning: Inductive

One must utilize clinical judgment to determine the most appropriate therapeutic exercise for shoulder hypermobility. Questions that require one to determine an appropriate therapeutic approach often necessitate inductive reasoning skill. For this situation, the most appropriate therapeutic exercise is taping and stabilization exercises. If answered incorrectly, review therapeutic exercises for joint hypermobility, especially shoulder hypermobility.

C89

Nonsystem | Safety and Protection

While walking through the parking lot to work, a physical therapist assistant comes upon an individual who is calling for help. The individual is on the ground and reports that he or she fell on the ice. Upon visual inspection the assistant notes a swollen ankle that is resting at an extreme range of inversion. The appropriate first aid intervention is to call for help and/or call the emergency response system. What should the PTA do next?

Choices:
1. Encourage the patient, with verbal cueing only, to come into a sitting position and assess the individual's heart rate.
2. Cover the patient for warmth and discourage active movement or weight bearing until help arrives.
3. Straighten the ankle and fabricate and apply a splint from available material.
4. Attempt to transfer the patient from the ground into an available vehicle and apply ice to the ankle until help arrives.

Teaching Points

Correct Answer: 2
The safest intervention for this patient is to initiate steps to get emergency response and comfort the patient until help arrives. Because the ankle is disfigured and swollen, there is a potential for fracture and/or sprain.

Incorrect Choice:
Attempting to move a patient in this situation could result in further injury to the ankle or lower extremity, including further damage to bone, nerve or other soft tissue. Attempting to transfer the patient into a car could result in further injury to the patient or cause injury to the rescuer. Keeping the patient warm with a jacket or blanket will prevent him or her from going into shock.

Type of Reasoning: Deductive
This question requires one to recall first aid guidelines to arrive at a correct conclusion. The recall of factual guidelines necessitates deductive reasoning skill. For this scenario, the assistant should cover the patient for warmth and discourage active weight bearing or movement until help arrives. If answered incorrectly, review first aid guidelines and care for injured joints. Additional information on first aid guidelines is located in the Management, Safety and Professional Roles chapter.

C90

Musculoskeletal | Interventions

Following a compound fracture of the tibia at mid-shaft, a patient's tibia is immobilized with an external fixation device. While the external fixator is in place, what should a rehabilitation program for the affected limb include?

Choices:
1. Isometric exercises of the distal limb and resisted exercise of the hip and knee musculature.
2. Increasing cardiovascular fitness through aerobic exercises.
3. Maintaining or increasing muscle strength of the affected limb by using cuff weights at the ankle.
4. Increasing muscle strength by using closed-chain activities.

Teaching Points

Correct Answer: 1
It is a goal to prevent or minimize muscle atrophy of the entire limb, yet care needs to be taken not to disturb the integrity of the healing site. This is best accomplished by isometric exercises of the distal limb, and resisted exercise of hip and knee (resistance can be as little as gravity itself); active movement is likely not contraindicated at the hip and knee.

Incorrect Choice:
Increasing cardiovascular fitness will not be contraindicated; however, this will not address the goal of maintaining or increasing strength of the affected limb. Increasing strength through closed-chain activities should be a goal of treatment once the fixator is removed. Cuff weights placed at the ankle should be distal to the fracture and create increased stress at the fracture site; at the same time a cuff weight applied proximal to the fracture will not be contraindicated.

Type of Reasoning: Inductive
Knowledge of rehabilitation guidelines after lower-extremity fractures is paramount to arriving at a correct conclusion for this question. This requires clinical judgment, which is an inductive reasoning skill. For this case, the patient's fracture of the tibia at mid-shaft warrants isometric exercises of the distal limb and resisted exercise of the hip and knee musculature. If answered incorrectly, review exercises for the lower extremity after fracture, especially tibial fractures.

C91

Gastrointestinal | Interventions

A patient is recovering from a mild stroke and demonstrates trunk extensor weakness and postural instability. The patient also suffers from severe heartburn and says that previous physical therapy treatments have made it worse. Prior exercises have included holding in side-lying, bridging, and prone on elbows. What is the **BEST** choice to maximize recovery while minimizing side effects?

Choices:
1. Perform trunk stabilization exercises with the patient in a semi-Fowler's position.
2. Reduce the number of repetitions of bridging and focus on dynamic reversals, not holding.
3. Perform rhythmic stabilization with the patient sitting.
4. Assure the patient that the heartburn is not aggravated by exercise and suggest taking antacids before physical therapy.

Teaching Points

Correct Answer: 3
Heartburn is a common symptom of gastrointestinal disorders and can be aggravated by supine and prone positioning. Modifying the patient's position to upright can alleviate the symptoms and demonstrate to the patient the assistant's concern.

Incorrect Choice:
Recommending medications is outside the scope of the physical therapist assistant. Trunk stabilization exercises in a semi-Fowler's position may address heartburn but will not effectively work to develop trunk stabilization. Reducing the number of repetitions and focusing on dynamic reversals does not address the problematic position of lying supine.

Type of Reasoning: Inductive
One must utilize clinical judgment to determine the best exercise to perform with a patient who experiences severe heartburn during exercise. Questions that require one to determine a best therapeutic approach often necessitate inductive reasoning skill. For this situation, exercise in an upright position is best; therefore, performing rhythmic stabilization with the patient sitting is best. If answered incorrectly, review exercise approaches for patients with heartburn.

C92

Musculoskeletal | Diseases and Conditions Impacting Intervention

A patient has been admitted to a skilled nursing facility following an open reduction internal fixation to the right hip for a femoral neck fracture. The physical therapy plan of care includes strengthening the lower extremities, gait training, transfer training, and patient education. Which of the following complications is **LEAST** likely to be an issue with this patient?

Choices:
1. Avascular necrosis.
2. Deep vein thrombosis.
3. Dislocation of the hip joint.
4. Respiratory compromise.

Teaching Points

Correct Answer: 3
Hip dislocation is more often associated with a total hip arthroplasty than with an open reduction internal fixation.

Incorrect Choice:
Avascular necrosis, deep vein thrombosis, and respiratory compromise are all possible complications of surgery. Avascular necrosis is possible because the blood supply to the head of the femur is often compromised after a femoral neck fracture. The patient will initially have mobility problems. A decrease in mobility can cause a compromise in the peripheral circulation, which can then lead to a deep vein thrombosis. Respiratory compromise is also possible because of decreased mobility as well as a potential side effect from anesthesia during the surgery.

Type of Reasoning: Inferential
One must draw a reasonable conclusion about the least likely complications for a patient with a status of post-open reduction internal fixation of the hip. This requires the test taker to determine what may be true of a patient, which requires inferential reasoning skill. For this scenario, dislocation of the hip joint is the least likely complication after open reduction internal fixation as this is more characteristic of a total hip replacement. If answered incorrectly, review complications after hip open reduction internal fixation.

C93

Musculoskeletal | Diseases and Conditions Impacting Intervetion

The supervising physical therapist is concerned that a patient may have a pars interarticularis defect (spondylolisthesis) that is responsible for lower back pain symptoms. Until a patient's condition can be verified through radiographic imaging, what exercises should be avoided?

Choices:
1. Isometric strengthening of the abdominals.
2. Stretching of the hamstrings.
3. Isometric strengthening of the back extensors.
4. Isotonic strengthening of the back extensors.

Teaching Points

Correct Answer: 4
Spondylolisthesis is the definition of a defect with forward slippage of one vertebra on the one below it. Excessive motion especially with extension of the spine can exacerbate symptoms or potentially cause more damage. Activities that include extension of the spine in the area of the spondylolisthesis should be avoided. When one is performing isotonic strengthening exercises, there is movement about the joint that needs to be avoided.

Incorrect Choice:
Isometric strengthening is permissible because there is not movement about the joint. Often there is hamstring tightness associated with spondylolisthesis and to decrease the stress on the spinal segments the hamstrings should be at their optimal length; therefore, hamstring stretching should be encouraged.

Type of Reasoning: Inductive
One must utilize clinical judgment to determine a best course of action for this question. Questions that require knowledge of therapeutic approaches often require inductive reasoning skill. For this situation, a patient with suspected spondylolisthesis should avoid performing isotonic strengthening exercises of the back extensors. Review signs and symptoms of spondylolisthesis and contraindications for exercises if answered incorrectly.

C94

Integumentary | Data Collection

The physical therapist assistant is completing gait training with a patient who is using a prosthesis for a transtibial amputation. During therapy, the physical therapist assistant notes that the patient has developed a small nonblanchable red area on the distal-lateral aspect of the residual limb. What should the physical therapist assistant do?

Choices:
1. Discontinue use of the prosthesis and contact the physical therapist immediately.
2. Continue using the prosthesis and make arrangements for the prosthetist to be present at the next treatment session.
3. Discontinue use of the prosthesis and make arrangements for the prosthetist to be present at the next treatment session.
4. Continue using the prosthesis and tell the physical therapist about the reddened area at the next treatment session.

Teaching Points

Correct Answer: 1
With an ulcer already forming, the patient must stop using the prosthesis immediately to prevent further skin breakdown. Because there is a change of patient status (presentation of a skin ulcer), the physical therapist must complete a reexamination of the patient.

Incorrect Choice:
There will need to be a change in the plan of care because of the patient's status change, and that change in the plan of care needs to be determined by the physical therapist. A visit to the prosthetist may be indicated; however, before this occurs, the therapist needs to determine whether there are other factors affecting the patient's change in status.

Type of Reasoning: Evaluative
This question requires the test taker to weigh the merits of the potential courses of action and determine the one that best resolves the patient's issue. This requires evaluative reasoning skill. For this scenario, it would be best to instruct the patient to discontinue use of the prosthesis and contact the physical therapist immediately.

C95

Musculoskeletal | Data Collection

The clinician in the photograph is testing the strength of which muscle?

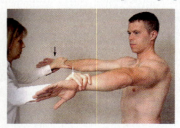

Magee D (2002). *Orthopedic Physical Assessment,* 4th ed. Philadelphia, W. B. Saunders, Figure 5-94, page 278, with permission.

Choices:
1. Supraspinatus.
2. Anterior deltoid.
3. Middle deltoid.
4. Upper trapezius.

Teaching Points

Correct Answer: 1

The muscle being tested is the supraspinatus. The empty-can position puts the supraspinatus muscle in its most effective position for contraction. Weakness may be the result of inflammation, neuropathy of the suprascapular nerve or a tendon tear.

Incorrect Choice:

The test position for the anterior deltoid is 90° of forward flexion of the shoulder, slight elbow flexion and forearm pronation. The test position for the middle deltoid is 90° of shoulder abduction, slight elbow flexion and forearm pronated. The test position for upper trapezius is sitting with arms resting at the sides.

Type of Reasoning: Analytical

This question requires one to evaluate the information presented in the photo to determine which muscle is being tested. Information that is evaluated through pictures and graphs often requires analytical reasoning skill. For this situation, the photo depicts strength testing of the supraspinatus. If answered incorrectly, review muscle testing of the shoulder, especially photos of muscle-testing procedures.

C96

Musculoskeletal | Interventions

A patient with rheumatoid arthritis is being treated in physical therapy during an acute flare-up. The patient presents with bilateral ulnar drift and swan neck deformities that affect the patient's ability to button shirts, comb hair, and brush teeth. During this acute flare-up what intervention **BEST** focuses on preventing further deformity and loss of function?

Choices:
1. Paraffin baths.
2. Stretching the intrinsic hand muscles and long finger flexors.
3. Fabrication of custom resting splints.
4. Strengthening the intrinsic hand muscles and long finger flexors.

Teaching Points

Correct Answer: 3
Splints to help limit the effects of the deformity are appropriate first steps in preventing further loss of function and deformity. The patient is in an acute flare-up; therefore, any intervention needs to be carefully administered.

Incorrect Choice:
Paraffin baths are a heating agent and are generally contraindicated for a patient who is in an acute flare-up; avoid any modality that could potentially increase the swelling of the joint. Strengthening and stretching the intrinsic hand muscles and finger flexors is appropriate but not during active flare-ups of rheumatoid arthritis. It is best to prevent further deformity and attempt to relieve some of the discomfort by fabrication and donning of splints.

Type of Reasoning: Inductive
One must determine the best course of action for a patient with an acute rheumatoid arthritis flare-up. This necessitates clinical judgment, which is an inductive reasoning skill. For this patient, intervention should focus on the fabrication of custom resting splints to address the ulnar drift and swan neck deformity of both hands. If answered incorrectly, review therapeutic approaches for rheumatoid arthritis, especially splinting of the hands.

C97

Musculoskeletal | Interventions

The patient has a diagnosis of shoulder impingement syndrome and the physical therapist plan of care includes thermal modalities and shoulder joint mobilization grades 1 and 2. What purpose do the joint mobilization techniques serve in this plan of care?

Choices:
1. Increase joint nutrition and diminish pain.
2. Maintain joint mobility and increase strength.
3. Increase joint mobility and reeducate the neuromuscular proprioceptors.
4. Increase capsular mobility and decrease pain.

Teaching Points

Correct Answer: 1
The effects of grade 1 and 2 joint mobilization are to maintain joint nutrition and decrease pain responses.

Incorrect Choice:
Only grades 3 and 4 maintain or increase capsular mobility. Joint mobilization techniques do not directly affect strength; however, they may improve biomechanics within a joint and indirectly improve strength or function of a joint. Joint mobilization does not reeducate joint proprioceptors.

Type of Reasoning: Inferential
One must determine the purpose of joint mobilization for a patient with shoulder impingement syndrome. This requires the test taker to determine what may be true of a therapeutic approach, which is an inferential reasoning skill. For this case, the purpose of joint mobilization for this patient is to increase joint nutrition and diminish pain. If answered incorrectly, review purposes and categories of joint mobilization and use of joint mobilization for shoulder impingement syndrome.

C98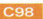

Cardiac, Pulmonary | Diseases and Conditions Impacting Intervention

A patient has developed congestive heart failure after a myocardial infarction. What pulmonary signs and symptoms may be present?

Choices:
1. Inspiratory wheezing and shortness of breath.
2. Crackles and cough.
3. Cough productive of thick yellow secretions.
4. Crackles and barrel chest.

Teaching Points

Correct Answer: 2

Patients who present with a myocardial infarction and congestive heart failure have changes to their pulmonary exam, the most common being crackles and dry cough.

Incorrect Choice:

Inspiratory wheezing occurs with extreme airway narrowing, which is a hallmark of an obstructive disease process and not of congestive heart failure. The cough associated with congestive heart failure is most likely nonproductive. Crackles or adventitious sounds as well as a barrel-shaped chest are all symptoms of emphysema.

Type of Reasoning: Inferential

This question requires the test taker to infer or draw a reasonable conclusion about the likely pulmonary signs and symptoms of a patient with congestive heart failure. This requires inferential reasoning skill as one must determine what may be true of a diagnosis. For this situation, one should anticipate pulmonary signs of crackles and cough. If answered incorrectly, review signs and symptoms of congestive heart failure, especially pulmonary signs and symptoms.

C99

Nonsystem | Professional Responsibility

A patient fell out of a wheelchair while in physical therapy. What should the incident report of this event include?

Choices:
1. The cause of the incident, the name of the injured, and the date of the incident.
2. The cause of the incident, the corrective actions taken, and names of those involved.
3. The names of those involved, witnesses, what occurred, and where it occurred—only in the event of an injury.
4. The name of those involved, witnesses, what occurred, time of incident, and where it occurred.

Teaching Points

Correct Answer: 4

An incident report should avoid interpretive information such as cause of the occurrence or corrective actions that were taken. The typical information included on an incident report includes the name of those involved inclusive of witnesses, what occurred, when it occurred, and where it occurred.

Incorrect Choices
The cause of the incident as well as the corrective action are determined upon review of the incident/occurrence. There is no presumption that someone was injured. It is sometimes called an "occurrence" report.

Type of Reasoning: Deductive
One must recall the factual guidelines for the completion of an incident report. Deductive reasoning skills are often utilized when one is recalling factual guidelines and procedures. For this scenario, an incident report should include the names of those involved, witnesses, what occurred, time of incident, and where it occurred. If answered incorrectly, look over incident report guidelines and procedures.

C100

Nonsystem | Safety and Protection

What should the physical therapist assistant do when working with a patient who is coughing and exhibiting signs and symptoms of influenza?

Choices:
1. Wear a moisture barrier gown while providing care.
2. Ensure that the patient wears gloves prior to touching equipment that is being used by other patients.
3. Provide the patient with a trash can to dispose of used tissues.
4. Ensure that the patient wears a mask while exercising in the common gym area.

Teaching Points

Correct Answer: 4
Standard precautions are based on the principle that all blood and body fluids, secretions and excretions, except sweat, are infections and may contain transmissible infectious agents. By ensuring that the patient wears a mask when out of his or her room, the assistant ensures that the public and other patients will be shielded from any potential pathogens.

Incorrect Choice:
This situation does appear to present a threat to the physical therapist assistant that requires the use of a gown. In addition to the assistant providing a container to dispose of the used tissues, the patient should be offered alcohol-based hand rub or the ability to wash his or her hands after coughing, sneezing, or blowing his or her nose. Any equipment used by the patient should be disinfected according to procedure.

Type of Reasoning: Evaluative
This question requires the test taker to weigh the benefits and merits of each of the potential courses of action and then determine the action that best resolves the issue at hand. Questions of this nature often require evaluative reasoning skill. For this situation, a patient who is coughing and demonstrates symptoms of influenza should wear a mask while exercising in the common gym area. If answered incorrectly, go over standard precautions for patients with viral illness, including influenza.

C101

System Interactions | Data Collection

A physical therapist assistant is reading a plan of care for a patient with the diagnosis of long-standing rheumatoid arthritis. Which of the following clinical presentations is consistent with this diagnosis?

Choices:
1. Morning stiffness, Herberden's nodules, joints of the hand, knee, and hip involved.
2. Morning stiffness, nodules over bony prominences, joints of the cervical spine, hand, and elbow involved.
3. Pain with weight bearing, ulnar drift, and subluxation of the wrist joint, joints of the wrist, hand, elbow, and cervical spine involved.
4. Stiffness following periods of rest, deformities of interphalangeal joints, joints of the lumbar spine, hips, and knees involved.

Teaching Points

Correct Answer: 2

Rheumatoid arthritis is an autoimmune-type disorder in which the synovial joints become affected, typically the smaller joints of the body. The associated signs and symptoms include morning stiffness and bilateral involvement of smaller joints such as the joints of the hand, wrists, elbow, shoulders, and the cervical spine. Inflammatory signs within the joint are common. Common joint deviations associated with rheumatoid arthritis include ulnar drift, swan neck deformity, boutonniere deformity, hallux valgus, splayfoot, and hammer toes.

Incorrect Choice:

Osteoarthritis is a pathological condition in which the articular cartilage of the joints is destroyed and bony overgrowth occurs within the joint. The larger, weight-bearing joints of the body are more typically affected. Osteoarthritis tends to affect individual joints, unlike the bilateral involvement in rheumatoid arthritis. Joints typically involved include, but are not limited to the lumbar spine, hip, knee, and first metatarsal phalangeal joint; the upper-extremity joints can include the carpal metacarpals, distal interphalangeals, and proximal interphalangeals.

Type of Reasoning: Inferential

This question requires one to infer or draw a reasonable conclusion about the likely symptoms for a patient with rheumatoid arthritis. This requires inferential reasoning skill. For this case, the most likely symptoms include morning stiffness, nodules over bony prominences and involvement of the cervical spine, hand, and elbow joints. If answered incorrectly, review signs and symptoms of rheumatoid arthritis.

C102

System Interactions | Diseases and Conditions Impacting Intervention

A patient with congestive heart failure is on a regimen of diuretics and calcium channel blockers. What potential side effects should the physical therapist assistant be mindful of?

Choices:
1. Orthostatic hypotension and dizziness.
2. Reflex tachycardia and unstable blood pressure.
3. Gastrointestinal upset and extreme fatigue.
4. Decreased electrolytes and electrical instability evidenced by increased arrhythmias.

Teaching Points

Correct Answer: 1

The adverse side effects that diuretics or calcium channel blockers have in common are orthostatic hypotension and dizziness. These represent a safety risk during functional training and gait.

Incorrect Choice:

Other symptoms listed are potential side effects of other medication and conditions.

Type of Reasoning: Deductive

One must recall the potential side effects of both diuretics and calcium channel blockers. This is factual recall of information, which is a deductive reasoning skill. For this case, the likely side effects are orthostatic hypotension and dizziness. If answered incorrectly, review side effects of congestive heart failure medication, especially diuretics and calcium channel blockers.

C103

Nonsystem | Therapeutic Modalities

What are the therapeutic guidelines for using intermittent traction to alleviate symptoms of a lumbar herniated disc protrusion?

Choices:
1. Utilize 75% of the patient's actual body weight.
2. Utilize the highest force tolerable by the patient to alleviate symptoms.
3. Utilize the lowest force possible to alleviate symptoms.
4. Utilize a fixed force, between 80 and 180 pounds.

Teaching Points

Correct Answer: 3

The correct answer is to use the lowest force that alleviates the symptoms of pain and discomfort associated with disc herniation and protrusion.

Incorrect Choice:

A fixed percentage of the patient's actual body weight, one-quarter to one-half of the patient's body weight, is typically utilized as a starting point for the amount of force to use, not 75%. When one is utilizing a traction table that is not friction free, one half of the patient's body weight is needed just to overcome the effects of gravity. Utilizing the highest force possible to alleviate symptoms can increase joint hypermobility and possibly cause collateral damage.

Type of Reasoning: Deductive

This question requires the recall of therapeutic guidelines for use of intermittent traction to treat lumbar herniated disc protrusion. This requires the recall of factual guidelines, which is a deductive reasoning skill. For this situation the guidelines for intermittent traction are to utilize the lowest force possible to alleviate symptoms. If answered incorrectly, review intermittent traction guidelines and use of traction for lumbar herniated discs.

C104

Nonsystem | Safety and Protection

A physical therapist assistant is preparing to perform cardiopulmonary resuscitation (CPR) on a 14-year-old who has just collapsed in the therapy gym. Where should the physical therapist assistant place the heel of their hand to perform CPR on this patient?

Choices:
1. On the distal one-third and parallel to the length of the sternum, with the heel of the other hand directly over it.
2. On the patient's forehead to stabilize the neck; the other hand is placed with the second and third fingertips over the sternum just below the nipple line.
3. On the middle portion of and parallel to the length of the sternum; the heel of the other hand is placed directly over the top of it.
4. Two finger widths proximal to the xiphoid process on the length of the sternum; the other hand is placed just proximal to that hand on the length of the sternum.

Teaching Points

Correct Answer: 1

The correct hand placement is on the distal one-third of the sternum, parallel to it and two finger widths proximal to the xiphoid process.

Incorrect Choice:

The heels of both hands on the sternum or hands placed in the middle portion of the sternum would not deliver effective compression forces to the heart and may put the patient at greater risk for fracture of the ribs or puncture of organs lying below the ribs. One hand placed on the forehead and fingertips placed on the sternum to deliver compressions is correct for performing CPR on an infant; a 14-year-old is considered an adult and the physical therapist assistant should use the same placement as that for an adult.

Type of Reasoning: Deductive

One must recall the guidelines for performing CPR to arrive at a correct conclusion. This is factual information, which is a deductive reasoning skill. For this scenario, the assistant should place the heel of one hand on the distal one-third and parallel to the length of the sternum with the heel of the other hand directly over it. If answered incorrectly, review CPR guidelines, especially adult CPR guidelines.

C105

Integumentary | Interventions

A patient is being seen as an outpatient in the wound care center at the local hospital. The patient presents with a wound that is draining copious amounts of serous fluid. The physical therapist plan of care calls for cleaning and a dressing change. Which represents the **MOST** appropriate dressing for this wound?

Choices:
1. A transparent dressing.
2. An autolytic debrider covered with a gauze wrap.
3. An alginate covered with a cushioned dressing.
4. An absorbent dressing.

Teaching Points

Correct Answer: 4

An absorbent dressing is best to absorb serous drainage from this wound.

Incorrect Choice:

A transparent dressing would cover the wound but would likely not be able to contain the amount of drainage from this wound; copious means a large amount of drainage. Autolytic agents or alginates are most often used to debride eschar and slough, respectively.

Type of Reasoning: Inductive

This question requires clinical judgment to determine the most appropriate course of action. Questions of this nature, which require knowledge of therapeutic processes, often require inductive reasoning skill. For this case, the most appropriate dressing for the wound is an absorbent dressing. Review wound care guidelines, especially use of absorbent dressings for wound drainage, if answered incorrectly.

C106

Musculoskeletal | Interventions

A patient presented with reports of persistent wrist pain after painting a house 3 weeks ago. The physical therapist plan of care includes soft tissue management for de Quervain's tenosynovitis. What structures should be included in soft tissue work?

Choices:
1. Abductor pollicis longus and extensor pollicis brevis muscle and tendons.
2. Transverse ligament at the distal radial and ulna.
3. Flexor pollicis longus and opponens pollicis muscle and tendons.
4. Adductor pollicis muscle and tendon.

Teaching Points

Correct Answer: 1

De Quervain's tenosynovitis is an inflammation of the abductor pollicis longus and extensor pollicis brevis tendons. Soft tissue work on the muscles and tendons can help decrease pain and soft tissue restrictions.

Incorrect Choice:

Soft tissue massage over the transverse ligament does not address affected tissues. The adductor pollicis, flexor pollicis longus, or opponens pollicis tendons are not associated with de Quervain's tenosynovitis.

Type of Reasoning: Inductive

This question requires knowledge of treatment procedures for de Quervain's tenosynovitis to arrive at a correct conclusion. Knowledge of therapeutic processes often requires inductive reasoning skill. For this situation, the assistant should perform soft tissue massage on the abductor pollicis longus and extensor pollicis brevis tendons. If answered incorrectly, review treatment techniques for de Quervain's tenosynovitis, especially soft tissue massage techniques.

C107

Musculoskeletal | Interventions

A physical therapist assistant is seeing a patient in the outpatient setting 4 weeks after an open repair of the rotator cuff of the right shoulder. The short-term goals include maintenance of range of motion and pain and inflammation control. The physical therapist has directed the assistant to provide therapeutic exercise and modalities to address the goals. Which represents the **BEST** choice of interventions at this time?

Choices:
1. Passive range-of-motion activity.
2. Active range-of-motion activity within pain-free range.
3. Isometric exercise in the midrange position at 50% effort.
4. Cold pack and interferential current.

Teaching Points

Correct Answer: 1
Passive range-of-motion activity will be the most effective method to prevent loss of motion and at the same time protect the musculoskeletal repairs at 4 weeks post-op.

Incorrect Choice:
Active range-of-motion activity will help prevent a loss of motion but may also disrupt the healing process. Isometric muscle contractions, especially at 50% effort, would clearly cause potential harm to the surgically repaired tissue; isometrics do not protect against loss of motion. Cold pack and interferential current do address the short-term goal of pain and inflammation control; however, they do not address maintenance of range of motion.

Type of Reasoning: Inductive
One must determine the best choice for intervention for a patient with open repair of the rotator cuff. This requires clinical judgment, which is an inductive reasoning skill. For this case, the best choice of intervention for a patient who is 4 weeks post-op is passive range-of-motion activity. If answered incorrectly, review intervention activities for patients with acute rotator cuff repair, including range-of-motion activities.

C108

Neuromuscular | Interventions

After demonstration of a functional activity being completed correctly, which of the following interventions will **BEST** reinforce the concepts of motor learning for the patient?

Choices:
1. Ask the patient to verbally repeat the functional activity just observed.
2. Allow the patient to perform the functional activity in whatever manner is needed to accomplish it, even with errors.
3. Assist the patient to perform the functional activity.
4. Request the patient perform the functional activity if it can be accomplished without error.

Teaching Points

Correct Answer: 3
The principles of motor learning emphasize the patient observing and performing functional activities and tasks to improve performance. Early in the learning the patient learns by observation and guided practice; there is allowance for some trial-and-error learning to occur.

Incorrect Choice:
Having the patient verbally repeat what has been done will not involve the motor system and will limit learning through movement. Guidance is provided to allow the patient to accomplish a task relatively well, versus learning and reinforcing poor movement patterns.

Type of Reasoning: Inductive
One must utilize clinical judgment to determine the best functional activity for a patient with a cerebrovascular accident. This requires knowledge of motor learning principles, which is an inductive reasoning skill. For this scenario, the assistant should demonstrate the functional activity and then assist the patient to perform the task, which coincides with the principles of motor learning theory. If answered incorrectly, review motor learning principles and engagement in functional activity.

C109

System Interactions | Data Collection

A patient with a 10-year history of diabetes reports cramping, pain, and fatigue of the right buttock after walking 400 feet or climbing stairs. When the patient stops exercising, the pain goes away immediately. The skin of the involved lower extremity is cool and pale. The physical therapist assistant checks the record and finds no mention of this problem. What are these observations an indication of?

Choices:
1. Radiating pain.
2. Muscle cramps.
3. Intermittent claudication.
4. Delayed onset of muscle soreness.

Teaching Points

Correct Answer: 3
Intermittent claudication, often the earliest indication of peripheral arterial disease, is manifested by cramping, pain or fatigue in the muscles during exercise that is typically relieved by rest. Peripheral arterial disease is a common result of long-standing diabetes. The calf muscle is most commonly affected, but discomfort may also occur in the thigh, hip, or buttock. Cessation of pain immediately upon stopping the exercise is characteristic of intermittent claudication, not other spinal problems. With severe disease, however, pain may be present even at rest.

Incorrect Choice:
The findings/observations cannot explain the Incorrect Choices identified.

Type of Reasoning: Analytical
This question requires the test taker to analyze the symptoms presented and then determine the most likely diagnosis. This requires analytical reasoning skill. For this situation, the symptoms are most consistent with intermittent claudication. If answered incorrectly, review signs and symptoms of peripheral arterial disease, including intermittent claudication.

C110

System Interactions | Interventions

A patient in chronic renal failure is being seen in physical therapy for deconditioning and decreased gait endurance. The assistant needs to schedule the patient's sessions around dialysis, which is received three mornings a week. The patient is also hypertensive and requires careful monitoring. What is the **BEST** approach to monitor blood pressure?

Choices:
1. Before and after activities, using the non-shunted arm.
2. In the seated position, when activity has ceased.
3. In the supine position, using the shunted arm.
4. Every 10 minutes during activity, using the shunted arm.

Teaching Points

Correct Answer: 1
Use the non-shunted arm. Pre- and postexercise measurements are appropriate; taking blood pressure during walking can result in inaccurate measurements.

Incorrect Choice:
A dialysis shunt interferes with taking blood pressure and should not be used. A blood pressure reading obtained in the seated or supine position may not accurately reflect the workload of the heart.

Type of Reasoning: Inductive
This question requires clinical judgment to determine a best course of action for a patient with chronic renal failure requiring blood pressure monitoring. This necessitates inductive reasoning skill. For this case, blood pressure should be taken before and after activities, using the non-shunted arm. If answered incorrectly, look over blood pressure techniques, including taking blood pressure for patients on dialysis with shunt access on the upper extremity.

C111

Nonsystem | Therapeutic Modalities

A patient presents with partial and full-thickness burns on the chest and neck region. The assistant plans to apply transcutaneous electrical nerve stimulation (TENS) prior to debridement to modulate pain. Which TENS mode should provide the **BEST** relief?

Choices:
1. Conventional (high-rate) TENS.
2. Acupuncture-like (low-rate) TENS.
3. Modulated TENS.
4. Brief intense TENS.

Teaching Points

Correct Answer: 4
Brief intense TENS is used to provide rapid-onset but short-term relief during painful procedures. The pulse rate and pulse duration are similar to that with conventional TENS; however, the current intensity is increased high enough to reach the limits of the patient's tolerance.

Incorrect Choice:
Conventional TENS and modulated TENS provide pain relief while the modality is on; however, they provide very little carryover to assist with tolerating a painful procedure. Acupuncture-like TENS better addresses pain tolerance over several hours after the modality has been applied.

Type of Reasoning: Inductive
One must determine the appropriate TENS mode that will best provide pain relief for a patient with partial- and full-thickness burns. This requires knowledge of therapeutic processes, which is an inductive reasoning skill. For this case, brief intense TENS is best to provide rapid-onset, short-term relief during painful procedures such as debridement. If answered incorrectly, review TENS guidelines, including use of TENS for debridement.

C112

Musculoskeletal | Diseases and Conditions Impacting Intervention

A patient who had a transtibial amputation 3 months ago is receiving physical therapy services. During the therapy session today the patient reports a knifelike pain and electrical shocks in the missing limb. How should this be documented in the medical record?

Choices:
1. Local pain.
2. Phantom pain.
3. Phantom sensation.
4. Referred pain.

Teaching Points

Correct Answer: 2

Following amputation, it is common for the majority of individuals to experience a phantom limb sensation. For most patients these feelings usually recede. Phantom sensation is usually not painful and is the sensation the patient feels that part or the entire limb is present. Some may experience painful sensations called phantom pain. Phantom pain may be local or diffuse, and may be continuous or intermittent.

Incorrect Choice:

Local pain refers to pain that is specific to an injured area such as a bruise, cut nerve endings at that specific spot, or pressure from a prosthesis. Referred pain is usually involved in problems related to areas where pain is referred from the original nerve root down its pathway. One example is in the back where pain can be referred down the lower extremity because of compression of a nerve root as it exits the spine.

Type of Reasoning: Analytical

One must analyze the symptoms presented and then determine the likely cause of the pain to enter into the medical record. Questions that require the test taker to analyze information to draw conclusions often require analytical reasoning skill. For this situation, the symptoms are indicative of phantom pain. If answered incorrectly, review phantom sensations and pain after amputation.

Nonsystem | Therapeutic Modalities

The initial evaluation identifies that a patient has weakness of the knee muscles, grade poor (2/5) resulting from an anterior cruciate ligament injury, moderate pain (5/10) and excessive translation of the tibia during active knee extension. The plan of care includes functional electrical stimulation (FES) to improve knee stability during gait. How should the FES be applied to the affected limb?

Choices:
1. Stimulate the quadriceps at toe off.
2. Stimulate the hamstrings immediately followed by the quadriceps at foot flat.
3. Stimulate the hamstrings at midstance.
4. Stimulate the quadriceps immediately followed by the hamstrings at mid-swing.

Teaching Points

Correct Answer: 2

Stimulating the hamstrings just prior to stimulating the quadriceps at foot flat will assist to stabilize the knee and prevent anterior tibial translation during knee extension and stance.

Incorrect Choice:

Stimulating the quadriceps at toe off will place torque on the knee by activating knee extension in a non–weight-bearing position. Stimulating the hamstrings at mid-stance without simultaneous quadriceps stimulation will create a knee flexion response creating a more unstable knee. Stimulating the quadriceps immediately followed by the hamstrings at mid-swing will not assist with knee stability during gait.

Type of Reasoning: Deductive

One must recall the guidelines for use of FES with patients demonstrating lower-extremity weakness to arrive at a correct conclusion. The recall of factual information is a deductive reasoning skill. For this case, FES should consist of stimulation of the hamstrings immediately before the quadriceps to produce co-contraction. Review applications of FES for lower-extremity weakness if answered incorrectly.

C114

Musculoskeletal | Data Collection

A patient with diabetes who had a transtibial amputation 3 months ago has recently been fitted with a prosthesis. During ambulation the patient reports pain in the distal and posterior portion of the residual limb. Upon inspection, the physical therapist assistant notes a reddened area developing on the distal tibia. Which of the following should be the physical therapist assistant's response?

Choices:
1. Initiate strengthening exercises for the quadriceps muscles.
2. Instruct the patient to avoid excessive lateral thrust of the residual limb during mid-stance.
3. Adjust the sock layers and continue with gait training, closely monitoring the patient's response.
4. Contact the prosthetist to make modifications to the prosthesis.

Teaching Points

Correct Answer: 3

Patients with new amputations fluctuate in volume and use various layers of socks within their temporary prosthesis to maintain proper fit. If a patient uses too few layers of socks it will allow them to "bottom out" in the prosthesis, or fit too far down into it and bear weight on the distal end of the residual limb versus the weight-bearing areas of the socket.

Incorrect Choice:

Weak quadriceps strength can lead to a gait deviation of excessive knee flexion in the early stance phase. Excessive lateral thrust is likely because of the prosthetic foot being inset too far. If this caused tissue irritation it would likely be on the lateral tibia. Insufficient plantar flexion built into the prosthesis will likely lead to a gait deviation of early knee flexion during stance phase, but would not likely lead to the development of reddened areas in this pattern.

Type of Reasoning: Evaluative

One must assess the benefits of the courses of action presented and then determine a course of action that effectively resolves the patient's issue. Weighing information to determine its merits often requires evaluative reasoning skill. For this situation, the assistant should respond by adjusting the sock layers and continue with gait training, closely monitoring the patient's response. If answered incorrectly, review prosthetic training guidelines and appropriate responses for reddened areas on the residual limb after ambulation.

C115

Neuromuscular | Diseases and Conditions Impacting Intervention

A physical therapist assistant is providing physical therapy interventions for a 9-year-old with myelomeningocele (spina bifida) lesion at L4–5. The plan of care indicates continuation of mobility training. What level of function **BEST** represents typical function for a patient with this diagnosis?

Choices:
1. Community mobility with a power wheelchair.
2. Household ambulation with crutches and knee–ankle–foot orthosis.
3. Household ambulation with reciprocating gait orthosis and walker, and wheelchair for community mobility.
4. Community ambulation with crutches and ankle–foot orthosis.

Teaching Points

Correct Answer: 4

Children with L4–5 lesions generally have good strength in their hip flexors, adductors, knee flexors and extensors, and ankle dorsiflexors. They also have some muscle control in their hip extensors and abductors and ankle plantar flexors. Therefore, they usually can ambulate community distances with ankle–foot orthoses and crutches.

Incorrect Choice:

Children with this diagnosis typically do not need reciprocating gait orthoses, knee–ankle–foot orthoses, or power wheelchairs because they have functional hip and knee strength.

Type of Reasoning: Inferential

One must infer or draw a reasonable conclusion about the likely mobility status of a child with spina bifida at L4–5. This requires knowledge of the diagnosis and typical mobility patterns, which is an inferential reasoning skill. For this case, one should expect the patient's mobility status to include community ambulation with crutches and use of ankle–foot orthoses. If answered incorrectly, review mobility patterns for children with spina bifida affecting the lumbar region.

C116

Nonsystem | Safety and Protection

How should the physical therapist assistant instruct a patient caregiver to assist the patient while performing a sliding board transfer?

Choices:
1. By using a wide base of support and bending at the hips and knees.
2. By using a narrow base of support and bending at the hips.
3. By maintaining an upright posture in the back.
4. By flexing at the hips and extending at the knees.

Teaching Points

Correct Answer: 1

A wide base of support increases balance as well as lowers the center of gravity. Bending at the hips and knees helps the caregiver to utilize the stronger muscles of the hips and lower extremities to assist with the transfer.

Incorrect Choice:

In contrast to a wide base of support, a narrow base of support decreases balance and raises the center of gravity, which will decrease the biomechanical advantage of the caregiver. Maintaining the back in an upright posture is correct body mechanics; however, it does nothing to affect the base of support. Correct body mechanics call for flexing both the hips and knees; this also lowers the center of gravity.

Type of Reasoning: Deductive

One must recall the guidelines for how to achieve a lower center of gravity during sliding board transfers. This is factual information, which is a deductive reasoning skill. For this scenario, using a wide base of support will achieve a lower center of gravity. If answered incorrectly, review biomechanical guidelines for transfer techniques, including sliding board transfers.

C117

Neuromuscular | Diseases and Conditions Impacting Intervention

A physical therapist assistant is treating a 2-year-old child with Down syndrome who frequently uses a "W" sitting position. Why is this sitting position discouraged?

Choices:
1. It has the potential to promote abnormally low tone because of reflex activity.
2. There is the potential to develop femoral torsion and create medial knee stress.
3. It promoted a developmental delay of normal sitting.
4. It promotes hip subluxation and causes lateral knee stress.

Teaching Points

Correct Answer: 2
"W" sitting is a stable and functional position but may cause later orthopedic problems of femoral torsion and knee stress.

Incorrect Choice:
Children with Down syndrome typically exhibit low tone and hyper extensibility. "W" sitting is not likely to affect low tone or reflex activity. Hip subluxation is unlikely.

Type of Reasoning: Inductive
This question requires the test taker to utilize clinical judgment to determine the main reason to discourage "W" sitting for a child with Down syndrome. This requires inductive reasoning skill. For this situation, the main reason to discourage "W" sitting is that it may cause femoral torsion and medial knee stress. If answered incorrectly, review sitting posture in children with Down syndrome, including "W" sitting.

C118

Nonsystem | Equipment and Devices

The supervising physical therapist has instructed a physical therapist assistant to order a wheelchair for an elderly patient whose status is post–total hip arthroplasty surgery. What is the **MOST** important adaptation to this wheelchair?

Choices:
1. Anti-tip attachments.
2. Elevating adjustable leg rests.
3. Adjustable arm rests.
4. A solid seat.

Teaching Points

Correct Answer: 4
The solid seat helps maintain the hips in a neutral position and avoid hip internal rotation that occurs with a sling seat.

Incorrect Choice:
The sling seat promotes the medially (internally) rotated hip position, which is contraindicated following hip arthroplasty surgery. The elevating leg rests might be nice to have and could potentially help with any edema but are not critical. Adjustable arm rests and anti-tip attachments again are nice options but do not seem to be indicated for this individual.

Type of Reasoning: Inductive

One must determine the most appropriate wheelchair feature for a patient whose status is post–hip arthroplasty. This requires clinical judgment, which is an inductive reasoning skill. For this situation, the assistant should order a wheelchair with a solid seat to maintain the hips in a neutral position. If answered incorrectly, review wheelchair prescription guidelines, especially for patients with a status of post–total hip arthroplasty.

C119

Integumentary | Diseases and Conditions Impacting Intervention

An elderly and frail resident of a nursing home has developed a stage III pressure ulcer. The wound is open with necrosis of the subcutaneous tissue down to the fascia. How might this elderly patient, when compared with a younger patient with the same type of ulcer, differ?

Choices:
1. Decreased vascular and immune responses.
2. Increased scarring with healing.
3. Increased elasticity and eccrine sweating.
4. Increased vascular responses with significant erythema.

Teaching Points

Correct Answer: 1
Age-associated changes in the integumentary system include decreased vascular and immune responses that result in impaired healing. Rate of healing is considerably slower.

Incorrect Choice:
In the elderly, scarring is typically less than in a younger individual. Both elasticity and eccrine sweating are decreased in the elderly. Vascular responses are typically diminished when compared to a younger individual.

Type of Reasoning: Inferential
One must determine the likely characteristics of wound healing for an elderly patient versus a younger patient. This requires one to determine what may be true of the situation, which is an inferential reasoning skill. For this case, the elderly patient can be expected to demonstrate decreased vascular and immune responses resulting in impaired healing compared with a younger patient with the same type of ulcer. If answered incorrectly, review wound healing guidelines, especially in the elderly.

C120

Cardiac | Interventions

A physical therapist assistant is following the plan of care for treatment of a patient on the coronary care unit 2 days after a coronary artery bypass surgery. What will an appropriate exercise regimen at this stage of the patient's recovery include?

Choices:
1. Ankle pumps and heel slides to increase the heart rate 15 beats over the resting level.
2. Shoulder flexion and abduction, and elbow flexion with a 3-pound weight at an intensity to increase the heart rate 15–25 beats per minute.
3. Exercises that increase the heart rate 30 beats over the resting level, such as upper-extremity exercises using a 1-pound weight, or marching in place while seated.
4. Ankle pumps and marching in place while seated, at an intensity to increase the heart rate 10–15 beats over the resting level.

Teaching Points

Correct Answer: 4

For a patient in phase I of a cardiac program, it is important to increase circulation in the lower extremities to decrease the chances of a deep vein thrombosis.

Incorrect Choice:

For a patient in phase I of a cardiac program, it is important to increase circulation in the lower extremities to decrease the chances of a deep vein thrombosis. Exercises should be in the 1–3 MET range and the heart rate should not exceed 20 bpm above the resting heart rate. Exercising that increases the heart rate only 1–5 beats over the resting level is not enough to build up endurance. Upper-extremity exercises will increase the heart rate more quickly than lower-extremity exercises; in addition, they do not achieve the added benefit of promoting blood flow in the lower extremities.

Type of Reasoning: Inductive

One must determine the best therapeutic approach for a patient on the coronary care unit after coronary artery bypass surgery. This requires clinical judgment, which is an inductive reasoning skill. For this situation, a patient who has had a recent coronary artery bypass graft should perform ankle pumps and marching in place, while seated, at an intensity to increase the heart rate 10–15 beats over the resting level. If answered incorrectly, review cardiac rehabilitation guidelines, especially for patients in the initial phases of rehabilitation.

C121

Neuromuscular | Diseases and Conditions Impacting Intervention

An outpatient client had an open-reduction internal fixation repair of a lower cervical fracture 21 days ago. What type of stabilization device should the physical therapist assistant anticipate the patient will have at this stage of recovery?

Choices:
1. A halo with vest attachment.
2. A soft cervical collar.
3. A hard cervical collar.
4. A body jacket.

Teaching Points

Correct Answer: 3

Following surgical fixation of a lower cervical spine fracture, a patient will most likely present with a hard cervical collar to limit cervical range of motion and protect the surgical repair.

Incorrect Choice:

A halo with vest attachment is more typically used for stabilizing upper cervical spine injuries and repairs. A soft cervical collar will not provide sufficient support following open-reduction surgical repair of the cervical spine. A body jacket will protect the thoracic or lumbar spine; however, it will offer no protection for the cervical spine.

Type of Reasoning: Inferential

This question requires the test taker to infer the likely stabilization device that will be utilized with a patient who has sustained a cervical fracture. This requires inferential reasoning skill. For this case, one should anticipate that the patient will wear a halo with vest attachment. If answered incorrectly, review stabilization devices for spinal cord injury, including cervical injuries.

C122

Nonsystem | Equipment and Devices

Where should a physical therapist assistant stand to appropriately guard a patient who is descending stairs for the first time using crutches and who is non–weight-bearing on the right side?

Choices:
1. Behind and slightly to the right side.
2. In front and slightly to the right side.
3. In front and slightly to the left side.
4. Behind and slightly to the right side.

Teaching Points

Correct Answer: 2

The correct guarding position is to stand in front and slightly to the involved side of the patient (the right side in this case). During ascent, the therapist should stand behind and slightly to the involved side.

Incorrect Choice:

The other guarding positions described are incorrect.

Type of Reasoning: Inductive

One must utilize clinical judgment to determine the best guarding position for a client who is descending stairs using crutches and who is non–weight-bearing on the right side. Questions of this nature often require inductive reasoning skill as knowledge of therapeutic guidelines is paramount to arriving at a correct conclusion. For this situation, the assistant should stand in front and slightly to the right side. If answered incorrectly, review stair negotiation guidelines including use of crutches while negotiating stairs.

C123

Musculoskeletal | Interventions

What is the therapeutic disadvantage of ballistic stretching?

Choices:
1. Is likely to elicit a stretch reflex, which will prohibit a full stretch.
2. Will promote plastic elongation of the muscle and tendons.
3. Will not facilitate safer shortening of the muscle and tendons.
4. Is likely to inhibit the stretch reflex that will allow for a full stretch.

Teaching Points

Correct Answer: 1
Quick or ballistic stretching activates the stretch reflex and triggers shortening of the muscle by stimulating the muscle and musculotendinous proprioceptors, not elongation of the muscle. Eliciting the stretch reflex makes stretching the muscle more difficult.

Incorrect Choice:
Quick stretches do not promote plastic elongation of muscle or tendon fibers and do not facilitate safer shortening of the muscle and tendons. Ballistic or quick stretching is likely to elicit a stretch reflex.

Type of Reasoning: Inductive
One must determine the therapeutic disadvantage of ballistic stretching to arrive at a correct conclusion. This requires clinical judgment, which is an inductive reasoning skill. For this case, the therapeutic disadvantage of ballistic stretching is that it is likely to elicit a stretch reflex, which will trigger shortening of the muscle and prohibit a full stretch. If answered incorrectly, review stretching technique guidelines, especially ballistic stretching techniques.

C124

Neuromuscular | Diseases and Conditions Impacting Intervention

How is a child with autism who encounters a change in his or her routine at school likely to respond?

Choices:
1. By demonstrating increased excitement and the inability to sit still, disturbing classmates by talking and distracting them.
2. By eliciting others to participate in the new routine to make coping easier.
3. By refusing to participate, disagreeing verbally with direction or withdrawing by going to sleep.
4. By having a temper tantrum, screaming, displaying stereotypical behaviors such as hand flapping, or social withdrawal.

Teaching Points

Correct Answer: 4
Autism is a neurobehavioral disability that includes differences in behavior, speech, socialization, and interaction with the environment. Stereotypical behaviors such as hand flapping, as well as difficulty with changes in routine leading to temper tantrums, characterize autism.

Incorrect Choice:
Poor social skills and poor expressive language skills are also characteristic and would likely make it difficult to elicit participation from others. Because changes in routine are difficult for children with autism to handle, it is unlikely that this child would demonstrate excitement, verbal interactions, or appropriate social skills such as directing his peers.

Type of Reasoning: Deductive
One must recall the common behaviors of children with autism to arrive at a correct conclusion. This necessitates the recall of factual information, which is a deductive reasoning skill. For this scenario one should anticipate the child reacting by having a temper tantrum, screaming, displaying stereotypical behaviors such as hand flapping, or social withdrawal. If answered incorrectly, review signs and symptoms of autism and autistic behaviors.

C125

Neuromuscular | Data Collection

The physical therapist has finished an evaluation on a patient who suffered a traumatic brain injury in a motor vehicle accident 2 weeks ago. The patient is able to respond to simple commands and requires a structured environment. The patient's memory is severely impaired; however, past memory is better than recent memory. Communication is difficult, as the patient tends to confabulate. Which of the following indicate an improvement in the patient's cognitive functioning?

Choices:
1. The patient follows simple commands in an inconsistent or delayed manner; reacts inconsistently to stimuli.
2. The patient shows carry-over for relearned tasks and little carry-over for new tasks, and demonstrates goal-oriented behavior with instruction.
3. The patient appears in a deep sleep, completely unresponsive to any stimuli.
4. The patient shows heightened activity levels with bizarre and nonpurposeful behavior that is not relative to the immediate environment.

Teaching Points

Correct Answer: 2
The patient in the question is functioning at Rancho Level V, confused–inappropriate. By demonstrating goal-oriented behavior and carry-over of relearned tasks the patient is functioning at a Rancho Level VI, which is an improvement in cognitive functioning.

Incorrect Choice:
A patient who is unresponsive to stimuli and appears to be in a deep sleep is functioning at Level 1 and is not showing an indication of improvement. A patient who is functioning at Level IV will demonstrate heightened activity levels and demonstrate bizarre and nonpurposeful behaviors that are unrelated to the immediate environment.

Type of Reasoning: Analytical
This question requires the test taker to analyze the patient's current status and deficits to determine the symptoms that indicate an improvement in cognitive functioning. This requires analytical reasoning skill. For this case, the patient is showing carry-over for relearned tasks and little carry-over for new tasks with goal-oriented behavior, which would indicate an improvement in cognitive functioning. If answered incorrectly, review traumatic brain injury signs and symptoms, including the Rancho Levels of Cognitive Functioning Scale.

C126

Neuromuscular | Interventions

A physical therapist assistant is working with a patient who has Parkinson's disease. The patient demonstrates a pattern of slow movements, resting tremors, and decreased postural reflexes. What intervention will **MOST** likely help meet the identified goal of improved ambulation activities?

Choices:
1. Sitting "pelvic clock" exercises on a physio-ball.
2. Assisted segmental rolling activities.
3. Standing marching and foot-placing activities.
4. Frenkel's lower-extremity coordination exercises.

Teaching Points

Correct Answer: 3

Standing marching and foot-placing activities will help improve a patient's ability to weight shift and advance the foot for ambulation.

Incorrect Choice:

Physio-ball activities and segmental rolling will assist with trunk mobility. Frenkel's exercises will help with lower-extremity control but may not transfer into improved gait activities.

Type of Reasoning: Inductive

This question requires one to use clinical judgment to determine the best intervention activities for a patient with Parkinson's disease. This requires inductive reasoning skill. For this case, the best intervention activities should include standing marching and foot-placing activities. If answered incorrectly, review intervention activities for patients with Parkinson's disease, including ambulation activities.

C127

Nonsystem | Professional Responsibilities

What federal law mandates that individualized educational services be provided free of charge, and in the restrictive environment, to qualifying children (from birth to 21 years of age) with disabilities?

Choices:
1. Section 504 of the Rehabilitation Act.
2. Individuals with Disabilities Education Act (IDEA).
3. Americans with Disabilities Act.
4. Technology Assistance Act.

Teaching Points

Correct Answer: 2

Both Section 504 of the Rehabilitation Act and the Americans with Disabilities Act are civil rights legislation. These acts legislate access for children to go to school but do not mandate their education.

Incorrect Choice:

The Technology Assistance Act provides for technology information and supports for individuals with disabilities but does not mandate educational services for young children. IDEA mandates educational and related services for children with disabilities.

Type of Reasoning: Deductive

This question requires one to recall factual information about federal laws, which is a deductive reasoning skill. For this situation, the federal mandate described is that of the Individuals with Disabilities Education Act or IDEA. Review information regarding federal mandates for individuals with disabilities, especially IDEA.

C128

Neuromuscular | Data Collection

A physical therapist assistant is treating a patient with Duchenne's muscular dystrophy. Which of the following **BEST** describes characteristics of this disorder?

Choices:
1. Progressive muscular weakness from proximal to distal musculature.
2. Hypersensitivity in the tissues of the lower extremity, typically associated with an insult to the central nervous system or a systemic disease process.
3. General weakness of the facial nerves of one side of the face, affecting expression and eyelid control.
4. Bilateral lower extremities affected; gait pattern is dominated by a scissoring gait.

Teaching Points

Correct Answer: 1

Duchenne's muscular dystrophy is a genetic disorder characterized by progressive weakness in the proximal musculature, progressing to the distal musculature. The child progressively loses mobility and self-care skills by the preteen years, and survives until the late teens or twenties and then most commonly succumbs to respiratory or cardiac problems.

Incorrect Choice:

Reflex sympathetic dystrophy is a sympathetically mediated response, often following some type of central nervous system lesion or systemic disease process, and leads to severe hypersensitivity of the affected extremity or trunk portion. Bell's palsy affects the facial nerve and leads to weakness or paralysis of the facial muscles. A patient with spastic cerebral palsy will often demonstrate a scissoring gait pattern.

Type of Reasoning: Inferential

This question provides a diagnosis, and the test taker is to determine the likely symptoms associated with this disorder. This requires inferring the symptoms, which is an inferential reasoning skill. For this situation, the expected characteristics of the disorder include progressive muscular weakness from proximal to distal musculature. If answered incorrectly, review signs and symptoms of Duchenne's muscular dystrophy.

C129

Nonsystem | Equipment and Devices

A physical therapist assistant is working with a patient who has just received a new plastic, solid ankle–foot orthosis. As a part of the adjustment and breaking-in period, what areas should be closely monitored for proper relief or tissue breakdown?

Choices:
1. Calf band, fibular head, popliteal fossa, malleoli, and styloid process of the 5th metatarsal.
2. Tibial condyles, tibial tuberosity, anterodistal tibia, and metatarsal heads.
3. Pelvic band, quadriceps tendon, popliteal space, tibial tuberosity, and navicular.
4. Popliteal space, posterior calf musculature, malleoli, Achilles tendon, and base of the metatarsals.

Teaching Points

Correct Answer: 1

When a patient receives a new ankle–foot orthosis it is important to implement patient education regarding wearing and tissue breakdown areas. Physical therapists and physical therapist assistants should carefully monitor the tissues of the limb to avoid skin breakdown caused by improper fit, as well as teach these to the patient and family members. Common areas for tissue breakdown are over bony prominences. Common bony prominences in the lower extremity that would be involved include, but are not limited to, calf band, fibular head, popliteal fossa, malleoli, and styloid process of the 5th metatarsal.

Incorrect Choice:

The tibial condyles and tibial tuberosity are often areas of potential breakdown with a transtibial prosthesis. An ankle–foot orthosis does not come into contact with the pelvis or thigh so it is unnecessary to inspect this area on this patient.

Type of Reasoning: Inferential

One must infer or draw a reasonable conclusion about the likely areas to be closely monitored for tissue breakdown in a patient with a new ankle–foot orthosis. This requires inferential reasoning skill. For this case, the likely areas that will be monitored include the calf band, fibular head, popliteal fossa, malleoli, and styloid process of the 5th metatarsal. If answered incorrectly, review prosthetic fitting guidelines, including monitoring for proper fit.

C130

Neuromuscular | Data Collection

A physical therapist assistant is preparing to treat a patient with an injury to the posterior knee that crushed the tibial nerve. The physical therapy evaluation identifies both motor and sensory involvement. What deficits should the physical therapist assistant expect the patient to present with?

Choices:
1. Decreased muscle tone of the knee flexors, as well as paresthesia of the posterior thigh and knee.
2. Increased muscle tone and spasticity of the knee flexors, as well as absent sensation over the posterior thigh area.
3. Decreased muscle tone of the plantar flexors and invertors of the ankle, as well as paresthesia of the posterior calf and plantar surface of the foot.
4. Increased muscle tone and spasticity of the plantar flexors and invertors of the ankle, as well as absent sensation over the posterior calf and plantar surface of the foot.

Teaching Points

Correct Answer: 3

Lesions in the upper motor neuron area cause motor spasticity and hyperreflexive muscle responses. A lesion to the nerve at the posterior thigh involves a peripheral nerve, or lower motor neuron. This will result in decreased muscle tone and reflexes.

Incorrect Choice:

The sciatic nerve splits just proximal to the knee to form the tibial, and common and deep peroneal (fibular) nerves. The common peroneal nerve serves motor and sensory function to the antero-lateral distal limb. The tibial nerve supplies the posterior calf area. It innervates the gastrocnemius, soleus, plantaris, tibialis posterior, flexor digitorum longus, and flexor hallucis longus.

Type of Reasoning: Inferential

One must determine the likely symptoms for a patient who has a crushed tibial nerve. This requires the test taker to infer the symptoms, which is an inferential reasoning skill. For this case, one should expect the patient to present with decreased muscle tone of the plantar flexors and inverters of the ankle, with paresthesia of the posterior calf and plantar surface of the foot. If answered incorrectly, review signs and symptoms of lower-extremity nerve injury, especially tibial nerve damage.

C131

Cardiac | Data Collection

A phase 2 outpatient cardiac rehabilitation program uses circuit training with different exercise stations for the 50-minute program. One station uses upper-extremity ergometry. What principles hold true when comparing upper-extremity exercise to lower-extremity exercise, at a given workload?

Choices:
1. Higher systolic and diastolic BP.
2. Exercise capacity is reduced owing to higher stroke volumes.
3. Heart rate (HR), systolic, and diastolic blood pressure (BP) will all be higher.
4. HR will be higher while systolic BP will be lower.

Teaching Points

Correct Answer: 3

Upper-extremity ergometry uses a smaller muscle mass than leg ergometry, resulting in a lower maximal oxygen uptake. In upper-extremity exercise, both HR and BP will be higher than for the same level of work in the lower extremities.

Incorrect Choice:
Choice one only accounts for a raise in BP and not HR. Exercise capacity is not reduced secondary to higher stroke volumes with upper-extremity exercise. It is not expected that the systolic BP decreases with upper-extremity exercise.

Type of Reasoning: Analytical
One must analyze the different types of exercises presented to determine their effects on HR and BP. This requires analytical reasoning skill. For this case, one should expect both HR and systolic and diastolic BP to be higher when comparing upper-extremity exercise to lower-extremity exercise. If answered incorrectly, review cardiac rehabilitation guidelines, especially effects of exercise on HR and BP.

C132

Nonsystem | Professional Responsibilities

What source should be referenced to find out if a physical therapist assistant is legally permitted to supervise a physical therapy aide in a specific state?

Choices:
1. Jurisdiction (state) practice act.
2. Departmental policy and procedure manual.
3. American Physical Therapy Association's Guide for Conduct of the Physical Therapist Assistant.
4. American Physical Therapy Association's Standards of Practice.

Teaching Points

Correct Answer: 1
Each state will set its own supervision requirements for personnel. These can typically be referenced in the state's practice act or in the state's rules and regulations for practice.

Incorrect Choice:
The American Physical Therapy Association sets acceptable standards for physical therapy and physical therapy personnel; individual states can choose to use those or other requirements. A department's policy and procedure manual is not a reference for legal supervisory requirements.

Type of Reasoning: Deductive
This question requires the test taker to determine the appropriate resource to refer to in order to find whether an assistant is able to supervise a physical therapy aide. This is factual information, which requires deductive reasoning skill. For this situation, the best resource to refer to is the appropriate practice act for the state in which the physical therapist assistant resides. If answered incorrectly, review supervision of personnel guidelines.

C133

Neuromuscular, Nervous | Interventions

A physical therapist assistant is working with a patient who has right hemiparesis and is demonstrating good recovery. Both involved limbs demonstrate some ability to move in patterns that are out of synergy. The patient is ambulatory with a small-base quad cane. What activity is **MOST** appropriate for a patient at this stage of recovery?

Choices:
1. Supine, bending the hip and knee up to the chest, and slowly lowering the foot back to the mat.
2. Standing with the hip extended while flexing the knee and slowly lowering the foot back to the floor.
3. Sitting, marching in place, and incorporating elbow flexion with the marching pattern.
4. Supine, performing active assistive diagonal flexion patterns with the lower extremities.

Teaching Points

Correct Answer: 2
This stage of recovery is characterized by some movement combinations that do not follow the paths of either flexion or extension synergies. Knee flexion in standing is a movement that is an out-of-synergy movement pattern.

Incorrect Choice:
All other choices identified represent synergistic movements.

Type of Reasoning: Inductive
This question requires clinical judgment about an appropriate therapeutic activity for a patient with a cerebrovascular accident. Questions of this nature where one must determine a most appropriate therapeutic activity often require inductive reasoning skill. For this case, a most appropriate activity is standing with the hip extended while flexing the knee and slowly lowering the foot back to the floor. If answered incorrectly, review therapeutic exercises for patients with cerebrovascular accident, especially stages of recovery.

C134

Musculoskeletal | Diseases and Conditions Impacting Intervention

A physical therapist assistant is helping to plan a scoliosis screening for a local school. The assistant should plan it for girls who are between what years of age?

Choices:
1. 6 and 8.
2. 9 and 11.
3. 12 and 14.
4. 15 and 17.

Teaching Points

Correct Answer: 2

The most effective age to screen girls for scoliosis is just before the pubescent growth spurt, between ages 9 and 11 years, when the scoliotic curve can increase dramatically.

Incorrect Choice:

Other choices are not representative of the age group most susceptible to developing scoliosis. Boys should be screened between 11 and 13 years of age because of differences in the age of puberty onset between girls and boys.

Type of Reasoning: Deductive

One must recall the guidelines for the assessment of scoliosis in young females to arrive at a correct conclusion. This is factual information, which necessitates deductive reasoning skill. For this situation, the assistant should plan to assess girls between the ages of 9 and 11 years. If answered incorrectly, review scoliosis screening guidelines, especially in females.

C135

Neuromuscular | Diseases and Conditions Impacting Intervention

A physical therapist assistant is working with a patient who is recovering from a complete spinal cord injury at the C6 neurological level. The physical therapist has directed the physical therapist assistant to strengthen the available musculature. Which of the following muscles would the physical therapist assistant focus on?

Choices:
1. Shoulder flexion, extension, and all elbow motions.
2. Scapular elevation and respiration.
3. Shoulder lateral (external) rotation and abduction.
4. All shoulder motions as well as all elbow motions.

Teaching Points

Correct Answer: 1

A patient with an intact spinal cord to the C6 level will have intact shoulder flexion, extension, and medial (internal) rotation; elbow flexion and extension; pronation; and wrist extension.

Incorrect Choice:

A patient with an intact spinal cord to the C5 level will have intact shoulder lateral (external) rotation and abduction, elbow flexion, and supination. A patient with an intact spinal cord to the C7 level will have intact all shoulder motions, elbow flexion and extension, wrist flexion and extension, and finger extension. A patient with an intact spinal cord to the C4 level will have intact scapular elevation and respiration.

Type of Reasoning: Inferential

This question requires one to draw a reasonable conclusion about the likely muscles that will be focused on for a patient with C6 spinal cord injury. Questions that require one to determine what may be true of a situation often necessitate inferential reasoning skill. For this case, the assistant is likely to focus on shoulder flexion and extension, and all elbow motions. Review intact musculature for cervical spinal cord injury, including C6 injury, if answered incorrectly.

C136

Neuromuscular | Data Collection

A physical therapist assistant is working on dynamic sitting balance with an infant with Down syndrome. What type of tone would this child most likely present with?

Choices:
1. Hypertonia.
2. Hypotonia.
3. Fluctuating tone patterns.
4. Absent tone.

Teaching Points

Correct Answer: 2
Most individuals with Down syndrome present with low or hypotonic muscle tone.

Incorrect Choice:
Hypertonia is rarely, if ever, present in an individual with Down syndrome. Fluctuating tone is common in a child with athetoid cerebral palsy. Absent tone is associated with a lesion of the peripheral nervous system.

Type of Reasoning: Inferential
This question requires one to infer the likely tone that is present for a child with Down syndrome. Determining what may be true of a situation often necessitates inferential reasoning skill. For this case, one should expect the infant's tone to be hypotonic. If answered incorrectly, review signs and symptoms of Down syndrome.

C137

Musculoskeletal | Data Collection

What angle should the shoulder be abducted to in order to correctly perform a manual muscle test for grade good (4/5) muscle strength of the sternal head of the pectoralis major muscle?

Choices:
1. 120°.
2. 90°.
3. 60°.
4. 160°.

Teaching Points

Correct Answer: 1
To test the sternal head of the pectoralis major the shoulder needs to be abducted to 120° for best alignment of the muscle fibers.

Incorrect Choice:
The whole muscle is tested in 90° of abduction, the sternal head requires 120° of abduction and the clavicular head is tested in 60° of abduction. Grade poor (2/5) or lower is tested with the upper extremity supported or with the patient sitting with the upper extremity supported on a horizontal surface at the level of the axilla.

Type of Reasoning: Deductive
This question requires the test taker to recall the procedure for manual muscle testing of the sternal head of the pectoralis major. This is factual information, which is a deductive reasoning skill. For this scenario, the correct testing position is with the patient supine and the shoulder in 120° of abduction. If answered incorrectly, review manual muscle testing procedures, including testing the pectoralis major.

C138

Cardiac | Interventions

A patient recovering from surgery for triple coronary artery bypass grafts is scheduled to begin a phase III cardiac rehabilitation program. During the resistance portion of the circuit training program, why should the patient be instructed to **AVOID** the Valsalva maneuver?

Choices:
1. To avoid elevating the heart rate and blood pressure.
2. To avoid accumulation of peripheral fluid and resulting edema.
3. Because it may produce slowing of pulse and increased venous pressure.
4. Because a cholinergic or vagal response may occur.

Teaching Points

Correct Answer: 3
The Valsalva maneuver results from forcible exhalation with the glottis, nose, and mouth closed. It increases intrathoracic pressure and causes slowing of the pulse, decreased return of blood to the heart, and increased venous pressure.

Incorrect Choice:
A cholinergic or vagal response is the result of parasympathetic nervous system stimulation. The Valsalva maneuver does not result in peripheral edema or elevated heart rate or blood pressure.

Type of Reasoning: Inductive
One must determine the reasons to avoid the Valsalva maneuver with a patient who has a status of post-coronary artery bypass grafting. This requires clinical judgment, which is an inductive reasoning skill. For this situation, the reasons to avoid the Valsalva maneuver are the possibility of slowing of the pulse and increased venous pressure. If answered incorrectly, be aware of precautions and contraindications for patients in cardiac rehabilitation.

C139

Nonsystem | Interventions

A patient is having difficulty learning how to transfer from mat to wheelchair. The patient cannot coordinate the movement even after numerous attempts. During early motor learning, what is the **MOST** effective feedback method?

Choices:
1. Include increased verbal feedback as the patient fatigues.
2. Use verbal feedback for the correct technique and proprioceptive feedback for incorrect technique.
3. Incorporate tactile and visual feedback for correct technique.
4. Focus on visual feedback rather than other forms of feedback.

Teaching Points

Correct Answer: 3
During the early stage of motor learning, learners benefit from seeing the whole task performed correctly as dependence on visual input is high. Tactile feedback for correct technique also provides appropriate feedback into the system. Developing a reference of correctness and success (knowledge of results) is critical to ensure early skill acquisition.

Incorrect Choice:
Increased verbal feedback as the patient fatigues is unlikely to achieve positive results. Proprioceptive feedback for incorrect techniques is inappropriate. A focus on visual feedback rather than incorporating other forms of feedback is unlikely to enhance motor learning.

Type of Reasoning: Inductive
This question requires the test taker to determine the most effective feedback approach to facilitate motor learning during transfer training. This requires knowledge of therapeutic approaches for transfer training, which necessitates inductive reasoning skill. For this case, one should incorporate tactile and visual feedback for correct technique. Review transfer training guidelines using motor learning approaches if answered incorrectly.

C140

Pulmonary | Interventions

What is the appropriate action with a patient who reports feeling lightheaded during use of an incentive spirometer?

Choices:
1. Take a rest period and only use the device 10 times per hour.
2. Take a deeper breath on the following attempt.
3. Lie down while using the spirometer.
4. Try to use the spirometer more frequently to get used to it.

Teaching Points

Correct Answer: 1
If a patient feels lightheaded with an incentive spirometer, it may be because of blowing off too much CO_2 by hyperventilating.

Incorrect Choice:
An incentive spirometer should always be used in the most upright position possible to attain the highest values possible. Lying down may not change the feeling of lightheadedness. Taking a deeper breath during inhalation will create further lightheadedness and may lead to the patient losing consciousness. More frequent use of the device with poor results is not an effective solution.

Type of Reasoning: Evaluative

One must weigh the benefits of the courses of action presented to determine the approach that will most effectively resolve the patient's issue. This requires evaluative reasoning skill. For this situation, the assistant should instruct the patient who is using an incentive spirometer to take a rest period and only use the device 10 times per hour. If answered incorrectly, review guidelines for use of incentive spirometers.

C141

Neuromuscular | Interventions

What can isokinetic traning be useful for during later stages of recovery from a cerebrovascular accident?

Choices:
1. Building strength of synergistic muscle groups.
2. Assisting with initiation of movements.
3. Creating better control of isolated muscles at slower speeds.
4. Developing control of movements at faster speeds.

Teaching Points

Correct Answer: 4

Patients during later stages of recovery from stroke frequently exhibit problems with control of faster movements. They are able to move at slow speeds, but as speed of movement increases, control decreases. An isokinetic device can be an effective training modality to remediate this problem.

Incorrect Choice:

The use of isokinetic equipment is not likely to build strength of synergistic muscle groups nor is it likely to assist with initiation of movements. Isokinetic equipment works with muscle groups not isolated muscles.

Type of Reasoning: Inductive

One must utilize clinical judgment to determine the benefits of using isokinetic training for patients with CVA. This requires inductive reasoning skill. For this case, the benefits of isokinetic training include improving control of movements at faster speeds. If answered incorrectly, review isokinetic training guidelines, especially for patients with a status of post-CVA.

C142

Neuromuscular | Interventions

A patient with a traumatic brain injury is inconsistently oriented to time and place. The patient is unable to remember recent events and shows little or no carry-over for new learning. What is the primary focus of rehabilitation at this stage of recovery?

Choices:
1. Develop an environment and daily structure in which the patient is best able to process stimuli cognitively.
2. Promote independence in problem-solving skills and provide as little verbal or tactile input as possible.
3. Increase functional independence in bed mobility and transfers.
4. Promote increased arousal and attention through the use of sensory stimulation techniques.

Teaching Points

Correct Answer: 1

This patient demonstrates recovery consistent with a confused state (Rancho Los Amigos Levels V/VI). The main focus of treatment should be on providing environmental and daily structure to reduce distractions and help the patient process stimuli.

Incorrect Choice:

Independence in problem solving or functional independence in bed mobility are inappropriate focus areas at this stage of recovery and are too advanced for this individual. This patient is already functioning higher than requiring sensory stimulation.

Type of Reasoning: Inductive

This question requires the test taker to determine the primary focus for rehabilitation of a patient with traumatic brain injury. This requires clinical judgment, which is an inductive reasoning skill. For this situation, a patient at this stage of recovery would benefit from developing an environment and daily structure where the patient is best able to process stimuli cognitively. If answered incorrectly, review the Rancho Los Amigos Levels of recovery and therapeutic approaches for patients with traumatic brain injury, especially patients at Levels V and VI of recovery.

C143

Musculoskeletal | Data Collection

A patient is walking with a transtibial prosthesis and demonstrates terminal swing impact. Which gait deviation should be expected?

Choices:
1. Hip external (lateral) rotation at midswing.
2. Decreased hip flexion at heel strike.
3. Knee hyperextension at heel strike.
4. Hip abduction at swing.

Teaching Points

Correct Answer: 3

Terminal swing impact refers to the sudden stopping of the prosthesis as the knee extends during late swing. Possible causes can include insufficient knee friction or too much tension in the extension aid; the assistant should note knee hyperextension at heel strike. Additionally, if the patient with an amputation fears the knee will buckle at heel strike (initial contact), the patient can use forceful hip flexion to extend the knee.

Incorrect Choice:

Hip external rotation at mid-swing, decreased hip flexion at heel strike, and hip abduction at swing are not described with this terminology.

Type of Reasoning: Inferential

One must infer or draw a reasonable conclusion about the likely gait pattern of a patient who is using a below-knee prosthesis. Questions that ask one to determine what may be true of a patient often necessitate inferential reasoning skill. For this case, the patient with a terminal swing impact is likely to perform the hyperextension at heel strike. If answered incorrectly, review gait patterns for patients who are using lower-extremity prostheses, especially terminal swing impact.

C144

Neuromuscular | Interventions

The physical therapist has just finished the evaluation of a patient with the diagnosis of L4–5 paraplegia. The physical therapist has met with the orthotist and discussed the most appropriate orthotic device to use in the continued care of this patient. This patient is able to perform all transfers independently, perform independent skin inspections, can stand and ambulate with forearm crutches, and is independent in all activities of daily living. What orthosis is **MOST** appropriate to facilitate improved gait for this individual?

Choices:
1. Bilateral solid ankle–foot orthosis.
2. Bilateral knee–ankle–foot orthosis.
3. A hip–knee–ankle–foot orthosis.
4. A thoracic–lumbar–sacral orthosis.

Teaching Points

Correct Answer: 2
A Craig-Scott knee–ankle–foot orthosis is the most common orthosis used for persons with a spinal cord injury at the L4–5 level. It has a shoe attachment and ankle and knee joints with controls and shells for the thigh and calf.

Incorrect Choice:
A patient at an L4–5 spinal injury level does not have enough support with an ankle–foot orthosis because of poor knee stability. A thoracic–lumbar–sacral orthosis could limit mobility too much and would not provide the support needed at the hips and knees for standing. A hip–knee–ankle–foot orthosis is very bulky and would likely limit the patient's ability to efficiently perform activities of daily living.

Type of Reasoning: Inductive
This question requires one to determine the most appropriate orthosis for a patient with an L4–5 spinal cord injury. This requires knowledge of the diagnosis and orthotic devices to arrive at a correct conclusion, which is an inductive reasoning skill. For this case, the most appropriate orthotic device is a bilateral knee-ankle-foot orthosis. If answered incorrectly, review lower-extremity orthotics for patients with spinal cord injury.

C145

System Interactions | Diseases and Conditions Impacting Intervention

A woman who is 12 weeks pregnant asks a physical therapist assistant if it is safe to continue with her aerobic exercise. Currently she jogs 3 miles three times a week and has done so for the past 10 years and wants to continue throughout her pregnancy. After discussion with the therapist, what is the **BEST** reply to this client?

Choices:
1. Jogging is safe as long as the target heart rate does not exceed 140 beats per minute.
2. Jogging is safe at mild to moderate intensities whereas vigorous exercise is contraindicated.
3. Continue jogging only until the fifth month of pregnancy.
4. Swimming is preferred over walking or jogging for all phases of pregnancy.

Teaching Points

Correct Answer: 2
According to the American College of Sports Medicine, women can continue to exercise regularly (three times a week) at mild to moderate intensities throughout pregnancy if no additional risk factors are present. After the first trimester, women should avoid exercise in the supine position because this position is associated with decreased cardiac output.

Incorrect Choice:
Typically heart rate limitations are made based on the age of the mother; no age is given to determine the best range for this client. There is no protocol that identifies a pregnant client can only jog until the fifth month of pregnancy. Non–weight-bearing exercise (swimming) is an appropriate alternative to walking or jogging, depending on the patient's skill and interests; however, it is not applicable in all phases of pregnancy.

Type of Reasoning: Evaluative
This question requires one to determine a best course of action and to evaluate the benefits of such an action with a patient who is pregnant and who wishes to continue aerobic exercise. This requires evaluative reasoning skill. For this situation, the best reply to the patient is that jogging is safe at mild to moderate intensities, whereas vigorous exercise is contraindicated. If answered incorrectly, review exercise guidelines for patients who are pregnant.

C146

Nonsystem | Therapeutic Modalities

Evaluation findings for a 10-year-old include pain and limited range of motion following a surgical repair of the medial collateral ligament and the anterior cruciate ligament. The plan of care includes use of physical agents for pain control and tissue healing. What modality should be avoided?

Choices:
1. Pulsed shortwave diathermy.
2. Pulsed ultrasound.
3. Transcutaneous electrical stimulation.
4. Interferential current.

Teaching Points

Correct Answer: 2
Ultrasound is contraindicated for patients whose epiphyseal areas are still active. The epiphyseal plates close at the end of puberty.

Incorrect Choice:
All the other physical agents can be used without adverse physiological effects and would contribute to pain control.

Type of Reasoning: Deductive
One must recall the contraindications for use of specific physical agent modalities to arrive at a correct conclusion. This is recall of factual guidelines, which is a deductive reasoning skill. For this situation, the assistant should avoid use of pulsed ultrasound, as the patient's epiphyseal areas are still active. If answered incorrectly, review contraindications for use of physical agent modalities, especially ultrasound, in children.

C147

Integumentary | Interventions

Which dressing is **MOST** appropriate when treating an infected and draining stage IV pressure ulcer?

Choices:
1. Transparent film.
2. Hydrogel covered with a lightly absorbent wrap.
3. Hydrocolloid dressing.
4. Alginate covered with absorbent dressings.

Teaching Points

Correct Answer: 4

A stage IV pressure ulcer will include disruption of the deep tissues such as fascia, muscle, and joint structures. It will likely present with necrotic tissue and have exudate. This type of wound needs intervention to clean up the necrotic tissue, such as an alginate to rid the wound of necrotic tissue and dressings to absorb the drainage or exudate.

Incorrect Choice:

Clean stage I and stage II wounds can be better managed with the transparent film or hydrocolloid; these are designed to provide protection to the wound. A hydrogel dressing is **BEST** used on stage II and III wounds to maintain a moist wound bed.

Type of Reasoning: Inferential

One must infer the likely treatment approach for an infected and draining stage IV pressure ulcer. Ultimately, such ulcers are managed surgically after infection clears. This requires one to determine what may be true, which is an inferential reasoning skill. For this case, one would most likely include the application of an alginate covered with absorbent dressings. If answered incorrectly, review treatment guidelines for pressure ulcers, especially stage IV.

C148

System Interactions | Diseases and Conditions Impacting Intervention

A physical therapist assistant is providing treatment in a long-term care center for a patient who has decreased core strength with an additional diagnosis of gastroesophageal reflux disease. The patient reports being unable to tolerate lying on his back to perform exercises. Which is the **BEST** choice for modification?

Choices:
1. Performing exercise with the patient prior to eating.
2. Modify exercise to include light jogging and avoid lying down.
3. Modify the supine position to right side-lying.
4. Encouraging the patient to eat a heavy snack prior to exercise.

Teaching Points

Correct Answer: 1

Performing exercise prior to eating is the best solution for persons who have gastroesophageal reflux. The stomach acids are less likely to be active during this time.

Incorrect Choice:
Patients with gastroesophageal reflux disease may have difficulty tolerating exercise that can increase stomach churning (e.g., jogging, running). Fatty foods or high-calorie foods prior to exercise can trigger the reflux response. Reflux symptoms may be decreased in the left side-lying position.

Type of Reasoning: Inductive
This question requires one to determine a best course of action for a patient with gastroesophageal reflux disease. This requires knowledge of the diagnosis and therapeutic courses of action to arrive at a correct conclusion, which is an inductive reasoning skill. For this situation, the assistant should modify the intervention approach by performing exercise with the patient prior to the patient eating to reduce the likelihood of symptoms. If answered incorrectly, review signs and symptoms of gastroesophageal reflux disease and guidelines for exercise.

C149

Neuromuscular | Data Collection

As a result of a drug overdose, a patient suffered permanent damage to the basal ganglia. Which of the following conditions will **MOST** likely be present?

Choices:
1. Hypotonia.
2. Ataxia.
3. Poor motor planning.
4. Dysdiadochokinesia.

Teaching Points

Correct Answer: 3
The basal ganglia functions to convert general motor activity into specific, goal-oriented action plans. Dysfunction results in problems with motor planning and scaling of movements and postures.

Incorrect Choice:
Dysdiadochokinesia is the inability to quickly substitute antagonistic motor impulses to produce antagonistic muscular movements. Hypotonia is decreased muscle tone. Parkinson's disease is an example of a disorder that also affects the basal ganglia; however, the patient presents with difficulty initiating movements.

Type of Reasoning: Inferential
One must infer the likely symptoms of a patient who has damage to the basal ganglia. This requires the test taker to determine what may be true of this patient, which is an inferential reasoning skill. For this case, the patient would most likely demonstrate poor motor planning with damage to the basal ganglia. If answered incorrectly, review signs and symptoms of patients with basal ganglia damage.

C150

Pulmonary | Interventions

Which of the following methods will **BEST** to teach a patient segmental breathing?

Choices:
1. Place a hand over the area of hypoventilation, apply firm pressure just prior to inspiration then ask the patient to breathe in against the resistance of the hand.
2. Place both hands gently over the lower ribs, apply gentle pressure throughout exhalation, and increase pressure at the end of exhalation by asking the patient to inhale against the resistance.
3. Place a hand over the lower abdomen and apply pressure at or near the end of exhalation.
4. Place the incentive spirometer in the patient's mouth and encourage the patient to breathe in as deeply as possible.

Teaching Points

Correct Answer: 1
To assist with segmental breathing the clinician places a hand over the area of hypoventilation and applies firm pressure just prior to inspiration and asks the patient to breathe in against the resistance of the hand.

Incorrect Choice:
In diaphragmatic breathing, the clinician places both hands gently over the lower ribs, applies gentle pressure throughout exhalation, increases pressure at the end of exhalation, and asks the patient to inhale against the resistance. During pursed-lip breathing, the exhalation phase can be prolonged by the clinician gently applying pressure through the abdomen near the end of expiration. An incentive spirometer assists with overall inhalation, not inhalation of a specific segment.

Type of Reasoning: Inductive
For this question, the test taker must utilize knowledge of segmental breathing techniques to arrive at a correct conclusion. This requires inductive reasoning skill. For this case, the assistant should teach the patient segmental breathing by placing a hand over the area of hypoventilation and applying firm pressure just prior to inspiration followed by asking the patient to breathe in against the resistance of the hand. If answered incorrectly, review segmental breathing techniques.

References

References comprehensive of PT practice. References particularly useful for the physical therapist assistant candidate appear in bold print.

Adler S, Beckers D, Buck M (2013). *PNF in Practice*, 4th ed. New York, Springer.

American College of Sports Medicine (2017). *ACSM's Guidelines for Exercise Testing and Prescription*, 10th ed. Philadelphia, Lippincott Williams & Wilkins.

American Physical Therapy Association (2014). *Guide to Physical Therapist Practice, Version 3.0*. Alexandria, VA, APTA.

American Physical Therapy Association. *Occupational Health Physical Therapy Guidelines: Prevention of Work-Related Injury/Illness*. Initial BOD11-99-25-71, APTA;

The Role of the Physical Therapist in Occupational Health. BOD 03-97-27-71, APTA.

Physical Therapist Management of the Acutely Injured Worker. BOD 03-01-17-56, APTA.

Evaluation Functional Capacity. BOD11-01-07-11, APTA.

Work Conditioning and Work Hardening Programs. BOD 03-01-17-58, APTA.

Armstrong A, Hubbard M (2015). *Essentials of Musculoskeletal Care*, 5th ed. Rosemont, IL, American Academy of Orthopedic Surgeons.

Avers D, Brown M (2018). *Daniels and Worthingham's Muscle Testing: Techniques of Manual Examination and Performance Testing*, 10th ed. St. Louis, Elsevier.

Baranoski S, Ayello E (2015). *Wound Care Essentials: Practice & Principles*, 4th ed. Philadelphia, Lippincott Williams & Wilkins.

Barrett C (2017). *Physical Therapist Practice for Physical Therapist Assistant*, 3rd ed. Burlington, MA, Jones & Bartlett Learning.

Bear M, Connors B, Paradiso M (2015). *Neuroscience—Exploring the Brain*, 4th ed. Philadelphia, Lippincott Williams & Wilkins.

Belanger AY (2014). *Therapeutic Electrophysical Agents*. 3rd ed. Philadelphia, Lippincott Williams & Wilkins.

Bellew J, Michlovitz, S et al. (2016). *Michlovitz's Modalities for Therapeutic Intervention*, 6th ed. Philadelphia, FA Davis.

Bickley L (2016). *Bates' Guide to Physical Examination and History Taking*, 12th ed. Philadelphia, Lippincott Williams & Wilkins.

Biel A (2013). *Trail Guide to the Body: A Hands-on Guide to Locating Muscles, Bones, and More*, 5th ed. Books of Discovery.

Bircher W (2018). *Documentation for Physical Therapist Assistants*, 5th ed. Philadelphia, FA Davis.

Boissonnault W (2011). *Primary Care for the Physical Therapist—Examination and Triage*, 2nd ed. St Louis, Elsevier.

Cameron M (2018). *Physical Agents in Rehabilitation*, 5th ed. St. Louis, Elsevier.

Campbell S (2016). *Physical Therapy for Children*, 5th ed. St Louis, Elsevier.

Carter R, Lubinski J, Domholdt E (2015). *Rehabilitation Research*, 5th ed. St. Louis, Elsevier.

Ciccone C (2015). *Davis Drug Guide for Rehabilitation Professionals*, 5th ed. Philadelphia, FA Davis.

Clarkson H (2013). *Musculoskeletal Assessment*, 3rd ed. Philadelphia, Lippincott Williams & Wilkins.

Cleland J, Koppenhaver S, Su J. (2016). *Netter's Orthopaedic Clinical Examination: An Evidence-based Approach*, 3rd ed. St Louis, Elsevier.

Clynch H (2017). *The Role of the Physical Therapist Assistant*, 2nd ed. Philadelphia, FA Davis.

Cook C, Hegedus E (2012). *Orthopedic Physical Examination Tests: An Evidence-Based Approach*, 2nd ed. Upper Saddle River, NJ, Prentice Hall.

Davis C and Musolino G. (2016). *Patient Practitioner Interaction: An Experiential Manual for Developing the Art of Health Care.* Thorofare NJ, Slack Inc.

Denegar C, Saliba E (2015). *Therapeutic Modalities for Musculoskeletal Injuries*, 4th ed. Champaign, IL, Human Kinetics.

DeTurk W, Cahalin L (2010). *Cardiovascular and Pulmonary Physical Therapy*, 2nd ed. New York, McGraw-Hill.

DiFabio R (2013). *Essentials of Rehabilitation Research: A Statistical Guide to Clinical Practice.* Philadelphia, FA Davis.

Doherty R, Purtilo R (2015). *Ethical Dimensions in the Health Professions*, 6th ed. St Louis, Elsevier.

Donatelli R, Wooden M (2010). *Orthopedic Physical Therapy*, 4th ed. New York, Churchill Livingstone.

Drake R, Vogl A, Mitchell A (2010). *Gray's Anatomy for Students*, 2nd ed. Maryland Heights, MO, Elsevier.

Drench M, Noonan A, Sharby N, Ventura S (2012). *Psychosocial Aspects of Health Care*, 3rd ed. Upper Saddle River, NJ, Prentice Hall.

Durstine J, et al (2016). *ACSM's Exercise Management for Persons with Chronic Diseases and Disabilities*, 4th ed. Champaign, IL, Human Kinetics.

Dutton M (2016). *Orthopaedic Examination, Evaluation, and Intervention*, 4th ed. New York, McGraw-Hill.

Dutton M (2019). *Orthopaedics for the Physical Therapist Assistant*, 2nd ed. Burlington, Jones & Bartlett.

Edelstein J, Moroz A (2010). *Lower-Limb Prosthetics and Orthotics: Clinical Concepts.* Thorofare NJ, Slack Inc.

Effgen S (2012). *Meeting the Physical Therapy Needs of Children*, 2nd ed. Philadelphia, FA Davis.

Equal Employment Opportunity Commission, https://www.eeoc.gov/laws/practices/, 2018.

Erickson M, Utzman R, McKnight G (2014). *Physical Therapy Documentation: From Examination to Outcome*, 2nd ed. Thorofare, NJ, Slack.

Fairchild S, Kuchler O'Shea R, Washington R (2018). *Principles and Techniques of Patient Care*, 6th ed. St. Louis, MO, Elsevier.

Field-Fote E (2009). *Spinal Cord Injury Rehabilitation*. Philadelphia, FA Davis.

Frownfelter D, Dean E (2012). *Cardiovascular and Pulmonary Physical Therapy: Evidence and Practice*, 5th ed. St Louis, Elsevier Mosby.

Goodman C, Fuller K (2015). *Pathology: Implications for the Physical Therapist*, 4th ed. St Louis, Elsevier.

Goodman C, Marshall C (2015). *Recognizing & Reporting Red Flags for the Physical Therapist Assistant*. St. Louis, Elsevier.

Goodman C, Snyder T (2017). *Differential Diagnosis in Physical Therapy: Screening for Referral*, 6th ed. St Louis, Elsevier.

Grossman S, Porth C (2013). *Porth's Pathophysiology: Concepts of Altered Health Status*, 9th ed. Philadelphia, Lippincott Williams & Wilkins.

Guccione A, Wong R, Avers D (2012). *Geriatric Physical Therapy*, 3rd ed. St Louis, Elsevier.

Gulic D (2018). *Ortho Notes: Clinical Examination Pocket Guide*, 4th ed. Philadelphia, FA Davis.

Guyton A, Hall J (2015). *Textbook of Medical Physiology*, 13th ed. St Louis, Elsevier.

Hack L, Gwyer J (2013). *Evidence into Practice: Integrating Judgment, Values, and Research*. Philidelphia, FA Davis.

Hall C, Brody L (2017). *Therapeutic Exercise—Moving Toward Function*, 4th ed. Philadelphia, Lippincott Williams & Wilkins.

Hengeveld E, Banks K (2014). *Maitland's Peripheral Manipulation: Management of Neuromusculoskeletal Disorders, Vol 2*, 5th ed. Philadelphia, Elsevier.

Hengeveld E, Banks K (2014). *Maitland's Peripheral Manipulation*. 5th ed. Philadelphia: Elsevier.

Hengeveld E, Banks K (2014). *Maitland's Vertebral Manipulation: Management of Neuromuscular Disorders, Vol 1*, 8th ed. Philadelphia, Elsevier.

Hillegass E (2016). *Essentials of Cardiopulmonary Physical Therapy*, 4th ed. St Louis, Elsevier.

Hoppenfeld S (1982). *Physical Evaluation of the Spine and Extremities*. New York, Appleton-Century-Crofts.

Irion J, Irion G (2010). *Women's Health in Physical Therapy*. Baltimore, Lippincott Williams & Wilkins.

Jenkins D (2009). *Hollinshead's Functional Anatomy of the Limbs and Back*, 9th ed. Maryland Heights, MO, Elsevier.

Jewell D (2015). *Guide to Evidence-Based Physical Therapy Practice*, 3rd ed. Sudbury, MA, Jones & Bartlett.

Johansson C, Chinworth S (2012). *Mobility in Context: Principles of Patient Care Skills*. Philadelphia, FA Davis.

Kaltenborn F (2012). *Manual Mobilization of the Joints, Vol 2 The Spine*, 6th ed. The Spine, 4th ed. Oslo, Norway, Olaf Norlis Bokhandel.

Kaltenborn F (2014). *Manual Mobilization of the Joints. Vol 1. The Extremities*, 8th ed. Oslo, Norway, Olaf Norlis Bokhandel.

Kandel E, Schwartz J, Jessell T, et al (2012). *Principles of Neural Science*, 5th ed. New York, McGraw-Hill.

Kauffman T, Scott R (2014). *A Comprehensive Guide to Geriatric Rehabilitation*, 3rd ed. St Louis, Churchill Livingstone Elsevier.

Kendall F, McCreary E, Provance P, et al (2005). *Muscle Testing and Function*, 5th ed. Philadelphia, Lippincott Williams & Wilkins.

Kenney W, Wilmore J (2015). *Physiology of Sport and Exercise*, 6th ed. Champaign, IL, Human Kinetics.

Kisner C, Colby L (2017). *Therapeutic Exercise Foundations and Techniques*, 7th ed. Philadelphia, FA Davis.

Law M, MacDermid J (2013). *Evidence-Based Rehabilitation: A Guide to Practice*, 3rd ed. Thorofare, NJ, Slack.

Lescher P (2011). *Pathology for the Physical Therapist Assistant*, Philadelphia, FA Davis.

Levangie P, Norkin C (2011). *Joint Structure and Function: A Comprehensive Analysis*, 5th ed. Philadelphia, FA Davis.

LeVeau B (2010). *Biomechanics of Human Motion: Basics and Beyond for the Health Professions*. Thorofare NY, Slack Inc.

Levine, D, Richards, J (2012). *Whittle's Gait Analysis*, 5th ed. St Louis, Churchill Livingstone Elsevier.

Lewis C, Bottomley J (2007). *Geriatric Rehabilitation—A Clinical Approach*, 3rd ed. Upper Saddle River, NJ, Pearson Education.

Lippert L (2011). *Clinical Kinesiology and Anatomy*, 5th ed. Philadelphia, FA Davis.

Lundy-Ekman L (2013). *Neuroscience*, 4th ed. St Louis, Elsevier.

Lusardi M, Jorge M, Nielsen C (2012). *Orthotics and Prosthetics in Rehabilitation*, 3rd ed St Louis, Elsevier Saunders.

Lusardi M, Jorge M, Nielsen C (eds) (2013). *Orthotics and Prosthetics in Rehabilitation*, 3rd ed. St Louis, Elsevier Butterworth-Heinemann.

Magee D (2014). *Orthopedic Physical Assessment*, 6th ed. St Louis, Elsevier.

Magee D, Zachazewski J (2015). *Pathology and Intervention in Musculoskeletal Rehabilitation*. 2nd ed. St Louis, Elsevier.

Malone T, Hazle C, Grey M et al (2016). *Imaging for the Health Care Practitioner*. New York, McGraw-Hill.

Mansfield P, Neumann D (2014). *Essentials of Kinesiology for the Physical Therapist Assistant*, 2nd ed. St. Louis, MO, Elsevier.

Manske R (2015). *Fundamental Orthopedic Management for the Physical Therapist Assistant*, 4th ed. St. Louis, Elsevier.

Martin, S and Kessler, M (2015). *Neurologic Interventions for Physical Therapy*, 3rd ed. St Louis, Elsevier Saunders.

McArdle W, Katch F, Katch V (2014). *Exercise Physiology: Energy, Nutrition and Human Performance*, 8th ed. Philadelphia, Lippincott Williams & Wilkins.

McCulloch J, Kloth L (2010). *Wound Healing: Evidence-Based Management* (Contemporary Perspectives in Rehabilitation, 4th ed. Philadelphia, FA Davis.

McKinnis L, Mulligan M (2014). *Musculoskeletal Imaging Handbook: A Guide for Primary Practitioners*. 4th ed. Philadelphia, FA Davis.

Michlovitz S, Bellew J (2016). *Modalities for Therapeutic Intervention*, 6th ed. Philadelphia, FA Davis.

Minor SM, Minor MS (2013). *Patient Care Skills*, 7th ed. Upper Saddle River, NJ, Prentice Hall Health.

Moore K, Agur A, Dalley A (2014). *Essential Clinical Anatomy*, 5th ed. Baltimore, Lippincott Williams & Wilkins.

Myers B (2012). *Wound Management: Principles and Practice*, 3rd ed. Upper Saddle River, NJ, Prentice Hall.

Netter FH (2014). *Atlas of Human Anatomy*, 6th ed. St Louis, Elsevier.

Neumann DA (2016). *Kinesiology of the Musculoskeletal System: Foundations for Physical Rehabilitation*, 3rd ed. St Louis, Elsevier.

Norkin C, White J (2016). *Measurement of Joint Motion: A Guide to Goniometry*, 5th ed. Philadelphia, FA Davis.

Nosse L, Friberg D (2013). *Managerial and Supervisory Principles for Physical Therapists*, 3rd ed. Philadelphia, Lippincott Willliams & Wilkins.

Oatis C (2016). *Kinesiology: The Mechanics & Pathomechanics of Human Movement*. 3rd ed. Philadelphia, Lippincott Williams & Wilkins.

OConnell D, OConnell J, Hinman M (2011). *Special Tests of Cardiopulmonary, Vascular and Gastrointestinal Systems*. Thorofare NJ, Slack Inc.

Olson KA (2015). *Manual Physical Therapy of the Spine*. 2nd ed. St Louis, Elsevier.

O'Sullivan S, Schmitz T (2016). *Improving Functional Outcomes in Physical Rehabilitation*, 2nd ed. Philadelphia, FA Davis.

O'Sullivan S, Schmitz T, Fulk GD (2019). *Physical Rehabilitation*, 7th ed. Philadelphia, FA Davis.

Paz J, West M (2013). *Acute Care Handbook for Physical Therapists*, 4th ed. St Louis, Elsevier.

Perry J, Burnfield J (2010). *Gait Analysis—Normal and Pathological Function*, 2nd ed. Thorofare NJ, Slack Inc.

Portney L, Watkins M (2015). *Foundations of Clinical Research*, 3rd ed. Philadelphia, FA Davis Co.

Purtilo R, Haddad A (2013). *Health Professional and Patient Interaction*, 3rd ed. St Louis, Elsevier.

Quinn L, Gordon J (2015). *Documentation for Rehabilitation: A Guide for Clinical Decision-Making,* 3rd ed. St Louis, Elsevier.

Reese N (2011). *Muscle and Sensory Testing,* 3rd ed. St Louis, Elsevier.

Reese NB, Bandy WD (2016). *Joint Range of Motion and Muscle Length,* 3rd ed. St Louis, Elsevier.

Robinson A, Snyder-Mackler L (2008). *Clinical Electrophysiology—Electrotherapy and Electrophysiologic Testing,* 3rd ed. Philadelphia, Lippincott Williams & Wilkins.

Roy S, Wolf S, Scalzitti D (2012). *The Rehabilitation Specialist's Handbook,* 4th ed. Philadelphia, FA Davis.

Rubin M, Safdieh J (2016). *Netter's Concise Neuroanatomy.* St Louis, Elsevier.

Sahrmann S (2011). *Movement System Impairment Syndromes of the Extremities, Cervical and Thoracic Spines.* St Louis, Elsevier. Mosby.

Schmidt R, Lee T (2018). *Motor Control and Learning,* 6th ed. Champaign, IL, Human Kinetics.

Scifers J (2008). *Special Tests for Neurologic Examination.* Thorofare, NJ, Slack.

Scott R (2009). *Promoting Legal and Ethical Awareness: A Primer for Health Professionals and Patients.* St Louis, Elsevier.

Scott R, Petrosinol L (2008). *Physical Therapy Management.* St Louis, Elsevier.

Shumway-Cook A, Woollacott M (2016). *Motor Control—Theory and Practical Applications,* 5th ed. Philadelphia, Lippincott Williams & Wilkins.

Snell R (2009). *Clinical Neuroanatomy,* 7th ed. Philadelphia, Lippincott Williams & Wilkins.

Somers M (2009). *Spinal Cord Injury Rehabilitation,* 3rd ed. Upper Saddle River, NJ, Prentice Hall.

Starkey C, Ryan J (2015). *Evaluation of Orthopedic and Athletic Injuries,* 4th ed. Philadelphia, FA Davis.

Starkey C (2013). *Therapeutic Modalities,* 4th ed. Philadelphia, FA Davis.

Straus S, Sackett, D, et al (2011). *Evidence-Based Medicine,* 4th ed. Philadelphia, Churchill Livingstone.

Swain J, Bush K, Brosing J (2009). *Diagnostic Imaging for Physical Therapists.* St Louis, Elsevier.

Tecklin J (2014). *Pediatric Physical Therapy,* 5th ed. Philadelphia, Lippincott Williams & Wilkins.

Umphred D (ed) (2013). *Neurological Rehabilitation,* 6th ed. St Louis, Elsevier Mosby.

Watchie J (2009). *Cardiovascular and Pulmonary Physical Therapy: A Clinical Manual,* 2nd ed. St Louis, MO, Elsevier.

Watson T (ed) (2008). *Electrotherapy: Evidenced-Based Practice,* 12th ed. St Louis, Elsevier.

Waxman S (2016). *Clinical Neuroanatomy,* 28th ed. New York, McGraw-Hill.

White N, Delitto A, Manal, T, et al (2015). *The American Physical Therapy Association's Top Five Choosing Wisely Recommendations.* Phys Ther 95:9-24.

Wise, C. (2015). *Orthopaedic Manual Physical Therapy.* Philadelphia, FA Davis.

Young P, Young P, Tolbert D (2015). *Basic Clinical Neuroscience.* 3rd ed. Philadelphia, Lippincott Williams & Wilkins.

Quick Facts Index

CONTENT	QUICK FACTS BOX NUMBER	PAGE
Active vs. Passive Learner Comparison	Quick Facts 12-1	436
American Spinal Injury Association (ASIA) Levels	Quick Facts 3-6	127
Angina Scale	Quick Facts 4-6	150
Bone Loss – Diseases and Mediations Affecting	Quick Facts 8-3	311
Borg Rate of Perceived Exertion Scale	Quick Facts 4-13	160
Claudication Pain Rating Scale	Quick Facts 4-18	176
Common Gait Deviations: Stance Phase	Quick Facts 11-1	400
Common Gait Deviations: Swing Phase	Quick Facts 11-2	401
Conditions Observed	Quick Facts 4-9	152
Contraindications for Contrast Bath	Quick Facts 10-12	373
Contraindications for Iontophoresis	Quick Facts 10-26	388
Contraindications for Massage	Quick Facts 10-24	382
Contraindications for Paraffin	Quick Facts 10-4	369
Contraindications for Use of SWD	Quick Facts 10-18	377
Depression – Symptoms of	Quick Facts 8-5	326
Determine Maximum Heart Rate	Quick Facts 4-15	170
Distribution of Motor Involvement with CP	Quick Facts 9-8	354
Dyspnea Scale	Quick Facts 5-2	195
Early Ambulation Characteristics	Quick Facts 9-4	343
Effects of Ion Concentration Changes	Quick Facts 4-4	145
Exercise Precautions for Individuals Who Are Overweight or Obese	Quick Facts 6-2	264
FIM Scale	Quick Facts 3-2	104
First Year Milestones	Quick Facts 9-2	338
FITT Equation	Quick Facts 1-2	7
Gait Achievements	Quick Facts 9-3	343
Gait Deviations – Following CNS Insult	Quick Facts 3-1	100
Goals and Indications for Aquatic Therapy	Quick Facts 10-7	371
Goals and Indications for Cryotherapy	Quick Facts 10-9	373
Goals and Indications for Paraffin Use	Quick Facts 10-3	369
Goals and Indications for Pneumatic Compression	Quick Facts 10-21	380
Goals and Indications for Superficial Thermotherapy	Quick Facts 10-1	367
Goals and Indications for Tilt Table	Quick Facts 10-23	382

CONTENT	QUICK FACTS BOX NUMBER	PAGE
Goals and Indications for Use of Intermittent Traction	Quick Facts 10-19	378
Goals and Indications for Use of Non-Thermal Ultrasound	Quick Facts 10-14	375
Goals and Indications for Use of Phonophoresis	Quick Facts 10-16	377
Goals and Indications for Use of SWD	Quick Facts 10-17	377
Goals and Indications for Use of Thermal Ultrasound	Quick Facts 10-13	375
Heart Chambers and Conduction	Quick Facts 4-1	142
Hepatitis Review	Quick Facts 6-1	233
Herpes Infections	Quick Facts 7-1	277
Indications for Contrast Bath	Quick Facts 10-11	373
Indications for Hydrotherapy	Quick Facts 10-5	370
Indications for Percussion and Shaking Techniques	Quick Facts 5-4	206
Injury Reduction Techniques	Quick Facts 7-7	295
Learning Strategies Early-to-Progression	Quick Facts 3-4	112
Learning Theories	Quick Facts 12-2	437
Levels of Amputation	Quick Facts 11-3	415
Maturing Gait Pattern	Quick Facts 9-5	343
Meaning of Ankle Brachial Index Measures	Quick Facts 7-5	290
Measuring the Pulse	Quick Facts 4-5	147
Mobilization Techniques	Quick Facts 2-3	32
Muscle Fiber Types	Quick Facts 1-1	2
Muscles of Respiration	Quick Facts 5-1	192
NDT to PNF Comparison	Quick Facts 3-3	106
One-Way vs. Two-Way Communication	Quick Facts 12-3	443
Parasitic and Fungal Infections	Quick Facts 7-2	278
Parkinson's Stages (Hoehn and Yahr Classification)	Quick Facts 8-4	323
Pathological Vision Problems in the Geriatric Population	Quick Facts 8-1	305
Patient Education for Lymphedema Management	Quick Facts 4-19	182
Physical Therapy Interventions for Immune Disorders of the Skin	Quick Facts 7-3	279
Positioning to Prevent Contracture Development	Quick Facts 7-4	287
Possible Effects of Physical Training/Cardiac Rehabilitation	Quick Facts 4-16	173
Postural Reactions	Quick Facts 9-1	338
Precautions and Contraindications for Aquatic Therapy	Quick Facts 10-8	371
Precautions and Contraindications for Cryotherapy	Quick Facts 10-10	373
Precautions and Contraindications for ES	Quick Facts 10-25	386
Precautions and Contraindications for Immersion Hydrotherapy	Quick Facts 10-6	370
Precautions and Contraindications for Intermittent Traction	Quick Facts 10-20	380
Precautions and Contraindications for Pneumatic Compression	Quick Facts 10-22	381
Precautions and Contraindications for Superficial Thermotherapy	Quick Facts 10-2	367
Precautions and Contraindications for Ultrasound	Quick Facts 10-15	376
Progression of Duchenne Muscular Dystrophy	Quick Facts 9-10	359
Progression of Preambulation Activities	Quick Facts 3-5	115
Pulse Grading Scale	Quick Facts 4-10	152
Pulse Locations	Quick Facts 4-7	151
Receptor Control Mechanisms	Quick Facts 4-3	145
Right- and Left-Sided Heart Failure	Quick Facts 4-12	159
Scar Tissue Formation – Phases of	Quick Facts 2-1	27

CONTENT	QUICK FACTS BOX NUMBER	PAGE
Signs of Decompensation	Quick Facts 4-17	175
Skin Color Changes	Quick Facts 4-8	152
Spinal Cord Injury – Changes Associated with Recovery	Quick Facts 3-7	129
Subjective Pain Ratings with Intermittent Claudication	Quick Facts 4-11	153
Tendinitis vs. Tendinosis	Quick Facts 2-4	45
Tissue Immobilization – Effects of	Quick Facts 2-2	28
Types of Down Syndrome	Quick Facts 9-9	358
Types of Foot Orthosis	Quick Facts 11-4	415
Types of Osteogenesis Imperfecta (OI)	Quick Facts 9-7	351
Types of Pneumonia	Quick Facts 5-3	200
Types of Thoracolumbosacral Orthoses	Quick Facts 9-6	347
Typical Home Discharge Instructions	Quick Facts 4-14	169
Vascular System Structures	Quick Facts 4-2	144
Visual and Auditory Loss Compensatory Adaptations	Quick Facts 8-2	305
Wound Cleansing Agents and Delivery Systems	Quick Facts 7-6	291

Index

Note: Page numbers with *f* indicate figures, those with *t* indicate tables, and those with *b* indicate boxes.

A

A1C Test, 260
ABCDEs of malignant melanoma, 280*t*
Abdominal aortic aneurysm (AAA), 68
Abdominal musculature, patients who lack, 192
Abdominal pain in GI conditions, 245, 245*t*
Abdominal strengthening, 211
Abducens nerve (CN VI), 90*t*, 95*t*
Abnormal synergy patterns associated with cerebral stroke, 121
Above elbow (AE) prosthesis, 417
Abrasion, 280
Absence or petit mal seizures, 133
Absent pulse, 152*b*
Abstract reasoning, 93
Abuse and neglect, 458
Acapella device, 210
Acceleration injuries of the cervical spine (whiplash), 66–67
Acceptance stage, 271
Accessory joint movement, grading of, 31
Accessory muscles of ventilation, 192, 192*b*
Acclimatization, 9
ACE Inhibitors, 160, 163*t*, 314*t*
Acetyl cholinesterase inhibitors, 315*t*
Achalasia, 244
Achilles' tendinitis/tendonosis, 61
Acid-base balance, 254–55
  abnormal, 197, 198*t*
Acquired immunodeficiency syndrome (AIDS), 223–24
  AIDS awareness training, I-6
Acromioclavicular joint, 29*t*, 30*t*, 35*t*, 50
Actinic keratosis, 279
Activated partial thromboplastin time (APTT), 236
Active compression (O'Brien) test, 35*t*
Active cycle of breathing technique (ACBT), 209
Active inhibition techniques, 11
Active ROM (AROM), 4, 16, 46, 100
Active stretching, 10
Active *vs.* passive learning, 436

Active weight shifts, 15
Activities of daily living (ADL), 104
Activity, defined, 449*b*
Activity limitations, defined, 449*b*
Activity pacing, 16
Acute bacterial prostatitis, 252
Acute coronary syndrome (ACS), 157–59
  angina pectoris, 157–58
  characteristics, 157
  heart failure (HF), 158–59, 159*t*
  myocardial infarction (MI), 158, 158*f*
  surgical interventions for, 162*t*
Acute musculoskeletal conditions, 73–74
  acute (inflammatory) phase/maximal protection, 73
  functional restoration/minimal protection phase, 74
  subacute phase/moderate protection, 73–74
Acute (inflammatory) phase/maximal protection, 73
Acute pulmonary diseases, 199–201
  Pneumocystis carinii pneumonia (PCP), 200
  pneumonia, 199, 200*b*
  severe acute respiratory syndrome (SARS), 200
  standard precautions, 225–28*b*
  tuberculosis (TB), 199
Adapting mechanism, 269
Addison's Disease (primary adrenal insufficiency), 265
Adenosine triphosphate (ATP), 8
Adherence-enhancing behavioral strategies, 114
Adhesions, 11
  early flexibility for preventing, 60
  early PROM for preventing, 51, 61
  mobilization of patella for preventing, 72
  scar tissue formation, 27, 27*b*
  soft tissue/massage techniques for preventing, 73
  tissue mobilization, 28*b*
Adhesive capsulitis (frozen shoulder), 51
Adhesive taping, 413–14
Adrenal androgens (dehydroepiandrosterone [DHEA]), 257

Adrenal cortex, 257
Adrenal disorders, 265
Adrenal medulla, 258
Adrenocorticotropic hormone (ACTH), 43, 257
Adson's test, 35*t*, 37*f*
Adult-onset diabetes, 259
Adult respiratory distress syndrome (ARDS), 204
Adult respiratory rate, 149
Adventitious (unusual) sounds, 149
Aerobic capacity and endurance, 93–94
Aerobic exercise
  to modify effects of aging, 28
  for obesity, 264
Aerobic training, 8
Agility activities test, 102*t*
Aging, definitions and theories of, 299
Aging patients, 297–331
  chapter review questions and answers, 331, 508–9
  cognitive disorders affecting, 323–27
  definitions and theories of aging, 299
  demographics, mortality, and morbidity, 299–300
  musculoskeletal system conditions associated with, 27–28, 310–19
  neurological disorders and diseases affecting, 320–23
  patient care concepts, 300–302
  physiological changes and adaptations associated with, 302–10
    body fat composition, 303
    cardiovascular system, 308
    cellular changes, 302
    cognitive changes, 307–8
    endocrine system, 310
    gastrointestinal system, 309–10
    hepatic, renal, and genitourinary systems, 310
    integumentary system, 309
    neurological system, 303–4
    pulmonary system, 308–9
    sensory systems, 304–7
    skeletal system, 303
    soft tissue changes, 302–3

809

Aging patients (*Cont.*)
  problem areas for, 327–30
  socioeconomic costs, 299–300
Agnosia, 96
Agranulocytes (monocytes), 235
AIDS awareness training, I-6
Air plethysmography (APG), 153
Airway
  chronic obstructive diseases, 202
  clearance techniques, 208–9
  lower, 191
  maintaining in burns, 285
  upper, 191
Akathisia (motor restlessness), 330
Akinesia, 88*b*, 100*b*, 100*t*, 118
Alarm system, 455
Alcohol-related dementia, 325
Aldosterone (mineral corticosteroids), 257
Alendronate, 312*t*
All-or-none principle, 86
Alpha blockers for cardiovascular disease, 163*t*
Altered basic life functions (body temp, thirst, hunger, sleep/wake cycles), 88*b*
Altered consciousness, 88*b*, 133
Altered relay of sensory information, 88*b*
Altered respiratory patterns, 88*b*
Alternate heel to knee; heel to toe test, 101*t*
Alternate nose to finger test, 101*t*
Alveolar ventilation, 194
Alzheimer's disease, 133, 244, 256, 303, 315*t*, 324*t*, 325
Ambulation independence, promoting, 114–16
  preambulation mat activities, with progression, 114–15, 115*b*
  preambulation parallel activities, 115
Ambulatory aids, 402–5
  bariatric equipment, 403
  canes, 402–3
  crutches, 403
  gait devices, additions to, 403
  gait patterns, use of assistive devices, 404–5
  guarding, 405
  locomotor training, 405
  walkers, 403
Ambulatory monitoring (telemetry), 168
American Physical Therapy Association (APTA), 469–81
  direction and supervision of PTAs, 474–75
  Guide for Conduct of the Physical Therapist Assistant (Guide), 476–81
  guidelines for documentation of patient/client management, 469–70
  Standards of Practice, 471–73
American Spinal Injury Association (ASIA) Impairment Scale, 126, 127*b*
Americans with Disabilities Act (ADA), 457
Amnesia, 123
Amperage, 384*t*
Amputation, levels of, 414, 415*b*
Amyotrophic lateral sclerosis (ALS), 117
Analysis in critical reasoning, I-13
Anaphylactic shock, 459
Anatomy and physiology
  cardiovascular system, 142–45
  female reproductive system, 248, 249*f*
  gastrointestinal system, 243, 244*f*
  immune system, 222
  lymphatic system, 143–44, 178*f*
  male reproductive system, 251–52, 251*f*
  musculoskeletal system, 23–28
  neuromuscular system, 85–91
  pulmonary system, 191–94, 191*f*
Anemia, 237
Anger stage, 271
Angina pectoris, 150, 157–58
Angina scale, 150*b*
Angiotension II receptor blockers (ARBs) for cardiovascular disease, 160
Angle of Louis (sternal angle), 191
Ankle. *See* Foot and ankle
Ankle-Brachial Index (ABI), 181
Ankle-foot orthosis (AFO), 347
Ankylosing spondylitis (Marie-Strümpell, Bechterew's, rheumatoid spondylitis), 42, 43
Anorexia, 244
Anosognosia, 88*b*, 96
Anterior border of bony thorax, 191
Anterior cerebral artery syndrome, 119, 120*t*
Anterior compartment syndrome (ACS), 60
Anterior cord syndrome, 127, 128*t*
Anterior cruciate ligament (ACL), 58, 60, 71, 72, 72*t*
Anterior drawer test, 36*t*
Anterior instability tests, 35*t*
Anterior pituitary gland, 88*b*
Anterior rolling walker, 347
Anterior tibial periostitis (shin splints), 60
Anterior/ventral regions, 90
Anthropometric characteristics, in physical therapy examination, 34
Anti-adrenergics for cardiovascular disease, 163*t*
Antiarrhythmics for cardiovascular disease, 161, 161*t*
Antibiotics, 78*t*, 79*t*, 213, 238, 315*t*
Antibodies, 222
Anticholinergics, 213, 244, 315*t*
Anticipatory timing activities, 15
Anti-citrullinated protein antibody (ACPA), 44
Anticoagulation therapy, 78*t*, 79*t*, 121, 164, 314–15*t*
Antidiuretic hormone (ADH), 253, 257
Antiepileptic medications, 133
Antigen, 222
Antihypertensives, 160, 161*t*
Anti-inflammatory agents, 213
Antiretroviral therapies (ARTs), 224
Antisocial behaviors, 88*b*
Anxiety, 269
Anxiety disorders (anxiety neurosis), 269
Aortic arch, 89
Aortic valve, 147
Ape hand deformity, 56, 56*f*
Aphasia
  Broca's, 88*b*, 120, 120*t*
  fluent, 121
  global, 120*t*, 121
  nonfluent, 120
  treatment considerations with, 445
  Wernicke's, 88*b*, 120*t*, 121
Apical pulse, 151*b*
Apley's test, 58
Appendicitis, 247
Apprehension test, 35*t*
Apraxia, 96–97, 120*t*
  constructional, 88*b*
  ideational, 97
  ideomotor, 97
  verbal, 120
Aquatic exercise, 17–18
  contraindications, 18
  exercise applications, 17–18
  goals and outcomes, 17
  physics related to, 17
  precautions, 18
  special equipment, 17
  strategies, 17
  thermodynamics, 17
Aquatic therapy, 371, 371*b*
Arachnoid layer, 89
Archimedes' principle, 17
Arm ergometry (dynamic arm exercise), 169
Arousal, 93
Arrhythmias (dysrhythmias), 148
  medications used for, 314*t*
Arterial blood gases (ABGs), 155*t*, 197, 198*t*
Arterial disease, 164, 176–77
Arterial lines, 215
Arterial oxygenation, 193
Arterial ulcer, 288
Arteries, 142, 143*f*, 144*b*
Arteriosclerosis obliterans (atherosclerosis), 157, 164
Arthritic conditions
  aging patients, 317–19
  degenerative joint disease (DJD), 36*t*, 42, 42*t*, 47
  osteoarthritis (OA), 42, 42*t*
  psoriatic arthritis, 43
  rheumatoid arthritis (RA), 44, 47, 75–76, 318–19
Arthrography, 41
Arthrogryposis multiplex congenita, 44, 351–52
Arthrokinematics, 28, 29
Articulatory techniques, 75–76
  joint mobilization, 75–76
  joint oscillation, 75
  manipulation, 76
  traction, 76
Asepsis and wound care, 285
Ashworth's scale for spasticity, 97, 97*t*
Aspirational pneumonia, 200*b*
Aspirin, 161, 161*t*, 312*t*, 313*t*
Assessment. *See also* Pain assessment and relief
  cough, 149
  motor function, 97
  Neonatal Behavioral Assessment Scale (NBAS), 344
  osteoporosis, 311
  outcome and assessment information set (OASIS), 104
  pediatric patients, 344
  performance/learning, 442–43
  sensory testing, 94–95
  tissue, 280–81
  wound, 289–90
Assessment scales
  Neonatal Behavioral Assessment Scale (NBAS), 344
  in stress management/lifestyle adaptation techniques, 16

Assisted cough, 209
Assisted transfers, 425
　devices for, 426–27
Assistive and adaptive devices, 104
Associated stage characteristics in motor learning, 111t
Asthma, 201, 202
Ataxia, 99t, 121, 123, 168, 169b, 354, 355t
Atelectasis, 205, 205t
Atherosclerosis (arteriosclerosis obliterans), 157, 164
Athetosis, 88b, 100t
Athlete's foot (tinea pedis), 277
Atraumatic instability, 48
Atrial filling pressure, 143
Atrioventricular (AV) nodes and valves, 142, 142b
Attention, 93
Attention deficits, 88b, 112
Auditory loss, 305–6, 305b
Augmented feedback, 110, 112, 112b
Auscultation, 147, 147t, 149
　landmarks, 147
　with stethoscope, 196
Authorization-to-test letter, I-6
Autogenic drainage, 209–10
Autogenic facilitation, 91
Autoimmune diseases, 222–23
Automatic implantable cardioverter defibrillators (AICDs), 175–76
Autonomic dysreflexia (autonomic hyperreflexia, hyperreflexia), 129b, 130
Autonomic nervous system (ANS), 88b
Autonomous stage characteristics in motor learning, 112t
Avascular necrosis (AVN, osteonecrosis), 56–57
Axillary or forearm support crutches, 347
Axonal degeneration, 134
Axonotmesis, 134

B

Babinski reflex, 98, 98t
Bacterial infections, 276
Bacterial pneumonia, 200b
Bacteroides, 248
Balance, 100, 101, 102–4
　in aging patients, 306
　assessing, 100, 102
　　dynamic/functional balance, 102, 104t
　　maximum sway, 102
　　static balance, 102, 104t
　control, 101
　　base of support (BOS), 101, 102
　　center of mass (COM), 101
　　limits of stability (LOS), 101
　deficits, 88b, 95t
　interventions to improve, 15–16
　　disturbed balance activities, 15
　　exercises to improve ROM, strength, and synergistic responses, 15
　　functional training activities, 15
　　safety education/fall prevention, 16
　　sensory training, 15–16
　systems contributing to, 101, 102
　　musculoskeletal system, 102
　　somatosensory system, 102
　　vestibular system, 102
　　visual system, 101
　testing, 102
　　functional balance grades, 104t
　　functional balance tests, 103t
　training (*See* Coordination and balance training)
Balance Efficacy Scale (BES), 103t
Ballistic stretching, 10
Bankart lesion, 49
Barbiturates, 123
Bargaining stage, 271
Bariatric equipment, 403, 426–27
　assisted devices for transfer, 426–27
　equipment, 426
　facility modifications, 427
　lift devices, 427
Bariatric surgery, 263, 263t
Barognosis, 94t, 96
Baroreceptors (pressoreceptors), 145b
Basal ganglia, 87, 88b, 90b, 99, 100b, 100t
Base of support (BOS), 12, 14, 15, 101, 102
Basic activities of daily living (BADL), 14
Basic life support and CPR, 460–61b
Basophils, 235
Bechterew's disease, 42, 43
Behavioral changes in TBI, 123
Behavioral inhibition, lack of, 93
Behavioral shaping techniques, 113
Bell's palsy (facial paralysis), 95t, 134
Below elbow (BE) prosthesis, 417
Bending fracture, 352
Benign nevus (common mole), 279
Benign paroxysmal positional vertigo (BPPV), 266b, 306
Benign tumors, skin, 279
Berg Balance Scale, 103t
Beta-2 agonists for pulmonary disease, 213
Beta-blockers, 145, 160, 161, 161t, 163t, 313t, 314t
Bicarbonate ions within the arterial blood (HCO_3^-), 194
Biceps load II test, 35t
Biceps rupture "Popeye" sign, 35t
Bicipital tendinitis, 51
Bilateral edema, 152
Bilateral symmetrical involvement of peripheral nerves, 134
Bilateral transfer, 110
Biofeedback, 12, 15, 16
　electrodes, 391–92
Biological response modifiers (BRMs), 43
Biomechanical alignment, 14, 17
Biomechanics, 28–31
　capsular positions, 29–31
　　close-packed position, 29, 30t
　　end-feels, 29
　　grading of accessory joint movement, 31
　　resting or loose-packed position, 29, 30t
　　selected capsular patterns, 29, 30t
　kinematics, 28–29
　　arthrokinematics, 28
　　convex-concave rule, 29, 29t
　　motions describing movement of one joint surface on another, 28–29
　　osteokinematics, 29
　levers, 28
　muscle substitutions, 31
Biotherapy, 240, 241t
Bipolar disorder (manic-depressive illness), 270
Bisphosphonates, 79t
Biventricular heart failure, 158, 159t
Bleeding (hypocoagulopathy), 236–37
Blocked practice, 110, 112
Blood-brain barrier, 89
Blood clotting, medications used to inhibit, 314–15t
Blood composition, 235
Blood glucose testing, 260
Blood pressure (BP), 148–49
　ACC/AHA guidelines, 149t
　measurement, 148–49
　monitoring during exercise, 168, 170
　monitoring in intensive care unit, 215
　pediatric blood pressure by age, 149t
Blood screening tests, 235
Blood sugar levels, 260, 260t
Blood supply, 89
　anterior system, 89
　Circle of Willis, 89
　posterior system, 89
Blood urea nitrogen (BUN), 253
Blood values, 197
Bloom's Taxonomy, I-10
Blumberg's sign (rebound tenderness), 247
Body fat composition, in aging patients, 303
Body functions, defined, 449b
Body image disorders, 96
Body mass index (BMI), 34, 262
Body mechanics, 463–64
　inpatient care, 464
　instructions for patient/client, 464
　other injury prevention information, 464
　principles, 463–64
Body of bony thorax, 191
Body position, effects on ventilation, 194
Body scheme disorder (somatognosia), 96
Body structure, defined, 449b
Body weight support (BWS), 16
Bone disorders, medications used for, 312t
Bone fracture
　in aging patients, 317
　bending fracture, 352
　buckle fracture, 352
　clinical implications, 317
　complete fracture, 27
　distal humeral fracture, 52
　epiphyseal fracture, 352
　foot and ankle fractures, 61
　greenstick fracture, 27, 352
　hip fracture, 317
　incomplete fracture, 27
　knee fracture, 60
　open fracture, 27
　open reduction internal fixation (ORIF), 27, 71
　in pediatric patients, 352
　proximal humeral fractures, 51
　rib fracture, 204
　risks, 317
　spinal fracture, 352
　stabilization, in spinal cord injury, 131
　stress fracture, 27, 61, 317
　vertebral compression fractures, 317

Bone loss, diseases and mediations affecting, 311b
Bone marrow (stem cell) transplant, 240, 241t
Bone mineral density and treatment recommendations, 311t
Bone remodeling, 24, 25t, 27
Bone scan (osteoscintigraphy), 41
Bone tissue
  function of, 24
    healing times, 25t
    stress and, 27
Bone tumors, 68
Bony thorax, 191
Borg Modified Dyspnea Scale, 149t
Borg Rate of Perceived Exertion (RPE) scale, 160, 160b, 168, 170
Boston orthosis, 347b
Botox or baclofen for spasticity, 123
Bounding pulse, 152b
Boutonnière deformity, 55, 55f, 319
Bowel and bladder dysfunction in spinal cord injury, 130
Boxer's fracture, 56
Brachial plexus, 91
Brachial plexus injury, 353
Brachial pulse, 151b
Bradykinesia, 88b, 100t, 118
Braiding (preambulation parallel activity), 115
Brain, 87–90
  abscess, 116
  arachnoid layer, 89
  basal ganglia, 87, 88b, 90b, 100b
  blood-brain barrier, 89
  blood supply, 89
  brainstem, 87, 88b, 90b, 95t, 97t, 98t, 117, 123
  caudate, 87
  central sulcus, 87
  cerebellum, 88b, 89, 90b
  cerebrospinal fluid, 89
  cerebrum, 87
  cranial nerves, 89, 90t, 95t
  diencephalon, 87
  dura matter, 89
  dysfunction patterns of brain based on area of damage, 88b
  frontal lobe, 87
  functional areas of, 87f
  function of key structures, 90b
  globus pallidus, 87
  gray matter, 87
  gyri, 87
  hemispheres, 87, 89b, 119, 120, 120t
  hypothalamus, 87, 88b, 90b, 95t
  impairment, gait deviations following CNS insult, 100b
  lateral central fissure, 87
  limbic system, 87
  lobes, 87, 88b, 89t
  longitudinal cerebral fissure, 87
  medulla oblongata, 87, 90b
  meninges, 89
  midbrain, 87
  organic brain syndromes, 324t
  parietal lobe, 87
  pia mater, 89
  pons, 87
  putamen, 87
  skull, 89
  sulci, 87
  support structures, 89
  temporal lobe, 87
  thalamus, 87, 88b
  unmyelinated axons, 87
  white matter, 87
Brainstem, 87, 88b, 90b, 95t, 97t, 98t, 117, 123
Brandt-Daroff habituation exercise, 267, 268, 268b
Breathing exercises, 210–11
  abdominal strengthening, 211
  diaphragmatic breathing, 210
  to promote relaxation, 16
  pursed lip breathing, 211
  segmental breathing, 210–11
  sustained maximal inspiration (SMI), 211
Breathing mechanisms, 193
Bridging (preambulation mat activity), 114
Brief, repetitive isometric exercise, 6
Broca's aphasia, 88b, 120, 120t
Broca's area, 89t, 120
Bronchial drainage, 206, 207f, 208t
Bronchiectasis, 202
Bronchogenic carcinoma, 203–4
Bronchopulmonary dysplasia, 202
Bronchoscopy, 197
Broviac catheter, 214
Brown-Séquard syndrome, 127, 128t
Bruit, 147t
Buckle fracture, 352
Buerger's disease (thromboangiitis obliterans), 164
Buoyancy, 15, 17–18, 369, 371
Buoyant dumbbells (swimmers), 17
Burns, 284–87
  burn healing, 285
  burn injury, complications of, 284, 285
  burn management, 285
  burn wound classification, 284t
  medical management, 285–86
  pathophysiology, 284
  physical therapy goals, outcomes, and interventions, 286–87
  positioning to prevent contracture development, 287b
Bursitis, 46
  pes anserine (knee), 59
  subacromial/subdeltoid (shoulder), 50
  trochanteric (hip), 57

C

Calcitonin, 312t
Calcium, 254
Calcium channel blockers, 161, 161t, 163t, 313t
Caloric testing, 266
Cancer, 239–43
  bronchogenic carcinoma, 203–4
  cancer treatments, side effects/clinical considerations, 241t
  characteristics, 239–40
  fatigue, 241
  grades, 240
  hospice care, 241
  medical interventions, 240
  metastasis, 241, 242
  overview of, 239–41
  pain, 241, 242
  pathophysiology, 240
  physical therapy goals, outcomes, and interventions, 241–43
  skin, 279–80
  staging, 240
Cancer pain syndrome, 241
Canes, 402–3
Capacity, defined, 449b
Capillaries, 144b
Capsular positions, 29–31, 30t
  close-packed position, 29, 30t
  end-feels, 29
  grading of accessory joint movement, 31
  resting or loose-packed position, 29, 30t
  selected capsular patterns, 29, 30t
Carcinoma, 240
Cardiac catheterization (coronary angiogram, or cath), 154t
Cardiac cycle, 142, 142b, 143f, 148, 148f
Cardiac output (CO), 143
Cardiac rehabilitation program, guidelines for, 172t
Cardiac syncope, 156t, 157
Cardiac transplant, 175
Cardiogenic pulmonary edema, 204
Cardiogenic shock, 459
Cardiopulmonary disorders in aging patients, 327
Cardiopulmonary resuscitation (CPR), 460–61b
Cardiorespiratory endurance activities, 169
Cardiovascular compromise, 156, 156t
Cardiovascular disease. See also Congestive heart failure (CHF)
  activity restriction, 161–62
  arrhythmias, medications used for, 314t
  congestive conditions, medications used for, 314t
  diagnostic tests, 153, 154t
  evaluation, diagnosis, and prognosis, 157–63
    acute coronary syndrome (ACS) (coronary artery disease), 157–59
    atherosclerosis, 157
    hypertension, 159–60
  intervention strategies for patients with, 166–76
    cardiac rehabilitation program, guidelines for, 172t
    exercise prescription, 166–71, 167b, 175–76
    exercise tolerance test (ETT), 166
    phase 1: inpatient cardiac rehabilitation, 171–73, 172t
    phase 2: outpatient cardiac rehabilitation, 172t, 173–74
    phase 3: community exercise programs, 174
    resistance exercise training, 174
  ischemic conditions, medications used for, 313t
  laboratory tests and values, 154–56, 155t
  lipid panel ranges, 154b
  medical management, 160, 161, 161t, 163t
  risk factors for, 146t

signs and symptoms of, 156–57, 156t
   cardiac syncope, 156t, 157
   cardiovascular compromise, 156, 156t
   chest pain or discomfort, 156, 156t
   claudication, 156t, 157
   cyanosis, 156t, 157
   diaphoresis, 156, 156t
   dyspnea, 156t, 157
   fatigue, 156t, 157
   nausea or vomiting, 156, 156t
   pallor, 156, 156t
   palpitations, 156–57, 156t
   peripheral edema, 156t, 157
spine and, 68
surgical interventions, 162, 162t
Cardiovascular endurance strategies, 6, 7
Cardiovascular system, 146–56. See also Cardiovascular disease; Peripheral vascular disease
  aging patients, 308
  anatomy and physiology, 142–45
    heart and circulation, 142–43
    neurohumoral influences, 144, 145
    vascular system, 143–44, 144b
  physical therapy examination and data collection, 146–56
    blood pressure (BP), 148–49
    cardiovascular diagnostic tests, 153, 154t
    electronic measurement of heart rhythm, 148
    heart rate (HR)/pulse measurement, 146, 147
    heart sounds, 147
    laboratory tests and values, 154–56, 155t
    oxygen saturation, 149–50
    pain assessment, 150
    peripheral arterial circulation, tests of, 153
    peripheral venous circulation, tests of, 152–53
    physical examination: peripheral vascular system, 150–52
    PTA's role and responsibilities, 146
    respiration, 149
  sample exercise programs per MET level, 185–86
Caregiver definition and roles, 465–68
Carotid pulse, 151b
Carpal tunnel syndrome (repetitive stress syndrome), 54
Case-control study, 489
Case report study, 489
Catatonia, 270
Cauda equina, 90, 127, 128t
Caudate, 87
CD molecules, 222
Cellular changes, in aging patients, 302
Center of gravity (COG), 92t, 102t
Center of mass (COM), 12, 14, 15, 101
Centers for Disease Control and Prevention (CDC) standard precautions, 225–28b, 234–35
  infection precautions, 234
  physical therapy-related infection control, 234–35
Central control centers, 194
Central cord syndrome, 127, 128t

Central line, 215
Central nervous system (CNS), 14, 85, 85f
Central posterior bulge/herniation, 66
Central sulcus, 87
Central venous access devices (CVAD), 214–15
Cerebellum, 88b, 89, 90b, 99, 99t
Cerebral angiography, 92
Cerebral anoxia, 119
Cerebral edema, 119
Cerebral infarction, 119
Cerebral palsy (CP), 353–56
Cerebral vascular accident (CVA, stroke), 119–22
  in aging patient, 320, 321–22t
  anticoagulation therapy for prevention, 121
  cerebral anoxia, 119
  cerebral edema, 119
  cerebral infarction, 119
  constraint-induced movement therapy, 122
  dysphagia, 121
  embolus, 119
  gait deficits, 121, 121t
  hemisphere lesions, 119–20, 120t, 321–22t
  hemorrhage, 119
  medical management, 121
  motor impairments, 121
  pathophysiology, 119
  perceptual dysfunction, 121
  physical therapy management, 122
  sensory impairments, 121
  speech and communication impairments, 120–21
  surgical intervention: carotid endarterectomy, 121
  syndromes, 119, 120t
  thrombus, 119
  tissue plasminogen activator (TPA), 121
Cerebrospinal fluid, 89
Cerebrum, 87
Certified lymphedema therapist (CLT), 183
Cervical nerves, 90
Cervical traction, 379
Cervicothoracolumbosacral orthosis (CTLSO), 347b
Cesarean childbirth, 251
Change-of-support strategies, 15
Chapter review questions and answers, 493–517
  cardiac, vascular, and lymphatic physical therapy, 187, 500–501
  functional training, equipment, and devices, 433, 514
  geriatric physical therapy, 331, 508–9
  integumentary physical therapy, 296, 506–7
  management, safety, and professional roles, 482, 516
  musculoskeletal physical therapy, 81, 496–97
  neuromuscular physical therapy, 138, 498–99
  other systems, 272, 504–5
  pediatric physical therapy, 363, 510–11
  pulmonary physical therapy, 217, 502–3

  research and evidence-based practice, 491, 517
  teaching and learning, 446, 515
  therapeutic exercise foundations, 19, 494–95
  therapeutic modalities, 393, 512–13
Charcot-Marie-Tooth disease, 63
Chemoreceptors, 145b
Chemotherapy, 240, 241t
Chest pain or discomfort
  cardiovascular disease, 156, 156t
  lung disease, 205t
Chest tubes, 214
Chest wall excursion, 195–96
Chest x-ray for cardiovascular disorders, 154t
Childbirth education classes, 249
Cholesteatoma, 266b
Cholesterol, 154b
Cholesterol-lowering medications, 313t
Chorea, 88b, 100t
Christmas disease, 238
Chronic fatigue syndrome (CFS), 224–25, 229
Chronic musculoskeletal conditions, 74
  determine possible causative factors, 74
  reduce stresses to tissues, 74
  regain structural integrity, 74
  resume optimal patient function and prevention of reoccurrence, 74
Chronic obstructive diseases, 201–2
  airway, 202
  asthma, 201, 202
  bronchiectasis, 202
  bronchopulmonary dysplasia, 202
  chronic obstructive pulmonary disease (COPD), 201
  classification of, 197, 198t
  common findings in, 201t
  cystic fibrosis (CF), 202
  exercise, 202
  medical management, general, 202
  medications, 202
  physical therapy management, 202
  prevention, 202
  respiratory distress syndrome (RDS), 202
Chronic obstructive pulmonary disease (COPD), 201
Chronic postthrombotic syndrome, 165
Chronic prostatitis, 252
Chronic renal failure, 256
Chronic restrictive diseases, 203, 203t
Chronic Traumatic Encephalopathy (CTE), 126
Chronic venous insufficiency (CVI), 177
Chronic venous stasis/incompetence, 165
Circle of Willis, 89
Circuit training, 3, 6, 8
Circulation
  coronary, 142–43, 143f, 144f
  integumentary, 275
  lymph, 179
  peripheral venous tests, 152–53
Circumferential measurements for edema, 152t
Circumflex artery (Circ), 142
Classic concussion, 123
Claudication, 156t, 157
Clinical prediction rule (CPR), 484, 485

813

Clonus, 97
Closed-chain exercise, 6
Closed head injury, 122
Close-packed position, 29, 30t
Clostridium difficile (C. difficile), 232t
Clotting factor IX deficiency (hemophilia B or Christmas disease), 238
Clotting factor VIII deficiency (hemophilia A), 238
Clubbing, 152b, 201t, 205t
Clubfoot (talipes equinovarus), 62
Coccygeal segments, 90
Cognition, 93
Cognitive changes, in aging patients, 307–8
Cognitive disorders affecting aging patients, 323–27
　cardiopulmonary disorders and diseases, 327
　delirium, 323, 324t
　dementia, 324–25
　depression, 326–27
　integumentary disorders and diseases, 327
　medications used for, 314–15t
　metabolic pathologies, 327
Cognitive stage characteristics in motor learning, 111t
Cognitive strategies
　in coordination and balance training, 15
　in relaxation training, 16
Cogwheel rigidity, 97t
Cohesion, 17, 18, 369, 371
Cohort study, 489
Coil/cable of application, 378
Cold application, 372, 372t
Cold packs, 372–73
Collaboration, principles of, 465
Collagen, 11, 23
Colles' fracture, 54
Color of skin, changes in, 282t
Combined (cortical) sensations, 94t, 96
Common law, 462–63
Communication, 443–45
　aphasia, treatment considerations with, 445
　nonverbal, 443
　speech/language disorders, 444–45
　strategies, effective, 444
　verbal, 443
Community activities, 15
Community and work (job/school/play) integration/reintegration, 105
Community exercise programs (phase 3), 174
Compensated heart failure, 159
Compensatory strategies, 14, 106
Compensatory training approach, 108, 109
Complete blood count (CBC), 155t, 235, 236t
Complete cord syndrome, 128t
Complete decongestive therapy (CDT), 183, 184
Complete fracture, 27
Complete spinal cord injury, 126, 127b
Complex partial seizure, 133
Complex regional pain syndrome (CRPS), 47, 136–37
　abnormal response of peripheral nerve, 136
　clinical picture, 136–37

clinical stages, 136–37, 137t
　etiology, 136
　medical management, 137
　physical therapy management, 137
　variations, 136
Compound action potentials (CAP), 391
Compression bandaging/garments, 183
Computed tomography (CT scan), 36, 40, 92
Computerized dynamic posturography (CPD), 266
COMT inhibitors, 315t
Concentric exercise, 5, 5t
Concurrent validity, 487
Concussion, 122–23, 125–26
Conductive hearing loss, 305
Congestive heart failure (CHF), 158, 160b
　clinical manifestations of, 159t
　compensated, 167b
　compression therapy and, 177
　edema associated with, 152, 154t
　gallop rhythm, 147t
　medications used for, 314t
　pulse location, 151b
　resistance exercise training and, 174
　types of, 163t
　uncompensated, 167b
Connective tissue, 23
Connective tissue mobilization
　for lengthening, 31–32
　　duration, 31–32
　　frequency, 32
　　intensity, 32
　　mode of stretch, 32
　　speed, 31
　for tissue tension, 31
　　fascia techniques, 31
　　muscle techniques, 31
　　transverse friction techniques, 31
　　transverse muscle techniques, 31
Constipation, 244
Constraint-induced (CI) movement therapy, 114, 122
Constructional apraxia, 88b
Construct validity, 487
Content Outline for the PTA Exam, I-1, I-8
Content validity, 487
Contextual factors, defined, 449b
Continuing education, I-7, 454
Continuous electrocardiogram (ECG), 215
Continuous exercise tolerance test (ETT), 166
Continuous passive motion (CPM), 58, 71, 381–82
Continuous quality improvement (CQI), 452–53
Contractile tissue, 10–11
Contract-relax, 107t
Contract-relax-active contraction (CRAC), 11
Contracture, 11, 51
Contralateral hemiparesis, 88b
Contralateral sensory motor loss, 120t
Contralateral weakness, 88b
Contrast baths, 373–74, 373b
Controlled mobility, 12
Contusion, 280
Conversion disorder (hysterical paralysis), 270
Convex-concave rule, 29, 29t
Cool-down period, 8, 9

Coordination and balance training, 14–16
　aerobic capacity and muscular endurance, interventions to improve, 16
　balance, interventions to improve, 15–16
　coordination, interventions to improve, 15
　disturbed balance activities, 15
　exercises to improve ROM, strength, and synergistic responses, 15
　functional training activities, 15
　goals and outcomes, 14
　safety education/fall prevention, 16
　sensory training, 15–16
　training strategies, 14
Coping mechanism, 269
Coping skills, in stress management, 16
Core temperature, 9, 17
Coronary artery bypass graft (CABG), 162, 162t, 171
Coronary artery disease. See Acute coronary syndrome (ACS)
Coronary artery occlusion, 158
Coronary circulation, 142–43
　arteries, 142, 143f, 144b
　capillaries, 144b
　veins, 143, 144b, 144f
Cortical blindness, 88b, 120t
Corticosteroids, 42, 43, 44, 57, 78t, 312t
Corticotropin-releasing hormone (CRH), 257
Cortisol (glucocorticoids), 42, 78t, 257
Cough, 149, 208
Coup-contrecoup injury, 122
COX-2 inhibitors, 78t, 80, 312t
Coxa vara and coxa valga, 57
Crackles (rales), 149, 159t, 201t, 205t
Cranial nerve palsy, 88b
Cranial nerves, 89, 90t
　abducens nerve (CN VI), 90t, 95t
　facial nerve (CN VII), 90t, 95t
　glossopharyngeal nerve (CN IX), 90t
　hypoglossal nerve (CNXII), 90t
　neural screens performed by PTA, 94t
　oculomotor nerve (CN III), 90t, 95t
　olfactory nerve (CN I), 90t
　optic nerve (CN II), 90t
　spinal accessory nerve (CN XI), 90t, 95t
　trigeminal nerve (CN V), 90t, 95t
　trochlear nerve (CN IV), 90t, 95t
　vagus nerve (CN X), 90t, 95t
　vestibulocochlear nerve (CN VIII), 90t, 95t
Credentials evaluation, I-6
Crescendo angina (unstable angina), 158
Crisis drugs for pulmonary disease, 213
Critical reasoning
　in licensure exam performance, role of, I-12
　resources and references, I-15
　self-assessment questions, I-14t
　skills, I-14–I-15
　skills, improving, I-14–I-15
　subtypes of, I-12–I-3
　　analysis, I-13
　　deductive reasoning, I-13
　　evaluation, I-13
　　inductive reasoning, I-12–I-13
　　inference, I-13
Crohn's disease, 247
Cromolyn sodium, 213

Cross-linking, 26, 28b
Cross-section, 90, 90f
Crutches, 347, 403
Cryo-cuff, 374
Cryotherapy, 45, 46, 52, 77t, 371–74
Culture and sensitivity, 197
Cushing's syndrome, 265
Cyanosis, 152b, 156t, 157, 201t, 205t
Cystic fibrosis (CF), 202
Cytokines, 222
Cytology, 197
Cytotoxic drugs, 43

D

Data collection
  cardiovascular system, 146–56
  hypertension, 160
  integumentary system, 280–82
  lymphatic system, 153
  musculoskeletal system, 34–41
  neuromuscular system, 91–105
  pediatric patients, 344–45
  pulmonary system, 195–99
  roles and responsibilities of PTA in, 34–36
Data types, 486, 486t
Dead space, 194
Death and dying, 271
Deceleration injuries of the cervical spine (whiplash), 66–67
Decerebrate rigidity, 97t, 123
Decompensation, 175, 175b
Decorticate rigidity, 97t, 123
Deductive reasoning, I-13
Deep inspiration, 192t
Deep partial thickness burn, 284t
Deep tendon reflexes (DTRs), 97, 97t
Deep thermotherapy, 374–78
  electromagnetic energy: diathermy, 377–78
  ultrasound, biophysics related to, 374–77
Deep vein thrombosis (DVT), 129b, 130, 164, 165t
Degenerative arthritis/osteoarthritis (OA), 317–18
Degenerative diseases of CNS, 117–19
  amyotrophic lateral sclerosis (ALS), 117
  multiple sclerosis (MS), 117–18
  Parkinson's disease (PD), 118–19
Degenerative joint disease (DJD), 42, 42t
  in temporomandibular joint (TMJ) conditions, 47
  tests for, 36t
Dehydration, 253
Dehydroepiandrosterone (DHEA), 257
Delayed-onset muscle soreness (DOMS), 4, 5t
Delayed or poor initiation, 88b
Delirium, 323, 324t
Dementia, 324–25, 324t
Demographics, of aging patients, 299–300
Denial stage, 271
Dense connective tissue, regular and irregular, 23
Density, of water, 17
Dependent transfers, 425
Depolarization, 86
Depression, 269
  aging patients, 326–27

Depression stage, 271
Depth/distance perception disorder, 96
de Quervain's tenosynovitis, 35t, 54
Dermal healing, 285
Dermatitis, 276
Dermatome distribution, 90, 91f
Dermis, 275t
Desipramine, 315t
Development, 335–43
  developmental milestones by age and domain, 336, 338b, 339–42t
  human development and learning/development theories, 335
  motor control and motor learning, 335
  neonatal development, 335–36
  posture and gait, 338, 342–43
  tests commonly used by therapists, 344
Developmental delay, in pediatric patients, 360
Developmental disability, in pediatric patients, 360
Developmental dysplasia of the hip (DDH), 348
Devices in physical therapy examination, 36
Diabetes mellitus (DM), 258–62
  blood sugar levels, 260t
  characteristics, 258
  complications, 259–60
  diagnostic criteria, 260
  exercise precautions, 262b
  exercise prescription, 176
  medical goals and interventions, 260
  medications and associated precautions, 261t
  physical therapy goals, outcomes, and interventions, 260, 261, 262
  signs and symptoms, 259, 261–62b
  types, 258–59
Diabetic angiopathy, 164
Diabetic autonomic neuropathy (DAN), 259–60
Diabetic polyneuropathy, 259
Diabetic ulcer, 288, 288f
Diagnostic ultrasound, 41
Dialysis, 256
Dialysis dementia, 256
Dialysis disequilibrium, 256
Diaphoresis, 156, 156t
Diaphragmatic breathing, 210
Diarrhea, 244, 245t
Diastasis rectus abdominis, 250
Diastole, 142
Diastolic failure, 163t
Diastolic filling time, 143
Diathermy, 377–78
Dicyclomine, 245t
Diencephalon, 87
Diffuse axonal injury, 122
Digitalis compounds, 161, 161t, 314t
Diminished pulse, 152b
Disability
  in aging patients, 327–28
  PTA Exam candidates with documented, I-6
Discal with nerve root compromise, 42t
Discharge plan, 450
Discharge summary, 450
Discography, 40

Disease-modifying antirheumatic drugs (DMARDs), 43, 44, 312t
Disinfection, 234–35
Dislocations, elbow, 53
Distal humeral fracture, 52
Distal interphalangeal (DIP) joint, 55, 319
Distraction techniques, 33
Distributed practice, 110, 112
Disturbed balance activities, 15
Disuse atrophy, 3
Diuretics, 161, 163t, 314t
Diverticular disease, 247
Diverticulitis, 247
Diverticulosis, 247
Divided attention, 93
Dix-Hallpike maneuver, 267, 268b
Dizziness in cardiovascular disease, 57, 149, 150, 155t, 163t, 168, 169b, 175b
Documentation. *See* Medical records management
Doppler Ultrasound, 153, 181
Dorsal (posterior) rami, 91
Dorsal roots, 90
Dorsiflexion sign (Homan's sign), 130, 165
Dosing, systems of
  Kaltenborn, 32b, 33, 33f
  Maitland, 32–33, 32b
Double-blind study, 487
Down Syndrome (trisomy 21), 65, 66, 67, 75, 76, 358, 358b
Drawing a circle test, 101t
Drop arm test, 35t
Drug-induced movement disorders, 330
Drug toxicity, 329–30
Drum method of application, 378
Dual task training, 15
Duchenne muscular dystrophy (pseudohypertrophic muscular dystrophy), 358–59
Dupuytren's contracture, 55, 55f
Dura matter, 89
Dynamic arm exercise (arm ergometry), 169
Dynamic flexibility, 9
Dynamic/functional balance, 102, 104t
Dynamic Gait Index (DGI), 103t
Dynamic reversals (slow reversals), 107t
Dynamic stabilization, 12
Dynamic standing test, 102t
Dynamic stretching, 10
Dysarthria, 99t, 121
Dysdiadochokinesia, 88b, 99t, 117
Dysfunction and mobility restriction tests, 36t
Dyskinesias, 330
Dyslipidemia, 259
Dysmetria, 88b, 99t, 117
Dysphagia, 121, 244
Dyspnea
  cardiovascular disease, 149, 150, 156t, 157, 159t
  lung disease, 201t, 205t
  scale, 195b
Dyspnea on exertion (DOE), 149, 157
Dysrhythmias (arrhythmias), 148

E

Eccentric exercise, 5, 5t
Ecchymosis, 280

Echocardiogram (echo), 154t
E. coli, 248
Edema
  bilateral, 152
  cancer, 241–42
  cerebral, 119
  circumferential measurements for, 152t
  congestive heart failure (CHF), 152, 152t
  peripheral, in cardiovascular disease, 152, 152t, 156t, 157
  pitting, 152
  pulmonary, 204, 205t
  skin, 281t
  traumatic brain injury (TBI), 122
  urinary regulation of fluids and electrolytes, 253–54
Educational theories, 436–37
  active vs. passive learning, 436
  educational concepts, 437
  learning styles, 436
  learning theories, 436–37
Effect size, 487
Egocentricity, 93
Eichhoff's test, 35t, 37f, 38f
Ejection fraction (EF), 143
Elasticity, 2, 11, 24
Elastin fibers, 23
Elbow
  abnormal synergies, 99t
  capsular patterns, 30t
  conditions of, 51–53
    distal humeral fracture, 52
    elbow contractures, 51
    elbow dislocations, 53
    lateral epicondylitis ("tennis elbow"), 52
    medial epicondylitis ("golfer's elbow"), 52
    nerve entrapments, 53
    osteochondrosis of humeral capitellum, 52
    ulnar collateral ligament injuries, 53
  in convex-concave rule, 29t
  flexion test, 35t
  joint positions, 30t
  patterns of spasticity in upper motor neuron syndrome, 92t
  tests for, 35t
Electrical current, 384t
Electrical safety considerations in hydrotherapy, 371
Electrical stimulation (ES), 383–87
  applying, guidelines for, 385–87
  basic concepts of electricity, 384t
  treatments, 387–92
    electromyographic (EMG) biofeedback, 391–92
    high-voltage pulsed galvanic stimulation, 389–90
    interferential current (IFC), 390–91
    iontophoresis, 387
    neuromuscular electrical stimulation (NMES), 391
    transcutaneous electrical nerve stimulation (TENS), 387–89
Electrocardiogram (ECG)
  for cardiovascular disorders, 154t
  for heart rhythm, 148
  for monitoring during exercise, 168
  pulmonary examination, 197

Electroconvulsive therapy (ECT), 326
Electrodiagnostic testing, 41
  electroneuromyography (ENMG), 41
  in musculoskeletal physical therapy, 41
  nerve conduction velocity (NCV), 41
Electroencephalography (EEG), 92
Electromagnetic energy (diathermy), 377–78
Electromyographic (EMG) biofeedback, 391–92
Electroneuromyography (ENMG), 41
Electronic measurement of heart rhythm, 148
Electronystagmography (ENG), 266
Electrotherapeutic agents, in musculoskeletal physical therapy, 77
Electrotherapy, 77, 77t
Elevation activities, 15
Ely's test, 39f
Embolus, 119
Emergency plans, 455
Emergency preparedness, 455
Emotional responses/behaviors, 93
Employee training in emergency preparedness, 455
Encephalitis, 116
End-feels, 29
Endocardium, 142
Endocrine and metabolic systems, 257–65
  adrenal disorders, 265
  diabetes mellitus (DM), 258–62
  endocrine system, overview of, 257–58, 258t
  glucose control, 258
  hormonal regulation, 257–58
  Islets of Langerhans, hormones released by, 258
  metabolic system, overview of, 258
  obesity, 262–65
  thyroid disorders, 265
Endometriosis, 251
Endorsement, I-7
Endoscope, 197
Endotracheal suctioning, 209
Endurance training, 6–9
  aerobic training, 8
  cardiovascular endurance strategies, 6, 7
  FITT equation, 7, 7b
  individual differences principle, 7
  muscular endurance strategies, 6
  overload principle, 6
  pulmonary endurance strategies, 7, 8
  reversibility principle, 7
  specificity principle, 6
  training errors to avoid, 9
Energy conservation, 16, 212
English language proficiency, tests of, I-6
Enlarged heart, 155t
Entrapment syndrome, 134
Environmental factors, defined, 449b
Environment and equipment considerations, 104–5, 427–28
  assistive and adaptive devices, 104
  community and work (job/school/play) integration/reintegration, 105
  environment, home, and work (job/school/play) barriers, 104
  functional considerations for intervention, 105b
  in motor learning, 112, 112b

  orthotic, protective, and supportive devices, 104
  self-care and home-management (including ADL), 104
Environments of care, for pediatric patients, 361
Eosinophils (granulocytes), 235
Epicardium, 142
Epidermal healing, 285
Epidermis, 275t
Epilepsy, 131, 133
  characteristics, 131, 133
  classifications of seizures, 133
  common causes of seizures, 133
  exam/determine, 133
  medical management, 133
  signs and symptoms, 133
Epinephrine, 258
Epiphyseal fracture, 352
Equilibrium boards, 15
Equilibrium tests of coordination, 100, 102t
Equinus, 62, 121
Equipment, use of, 456
Erectile dysfunction (ED) (impotence), 252
Ergometers, 16
Ergonomics, 429–32
Erythrocytes (red blood count), 235, 236t
Erythrocyte sedimentation rate (ESR), 155t, 235
Esophagus, 245–46
Essential tremor, 330
Estrogen, 248
Evaluation in critical reasoning, I-13
Evidence, evaluating, 489–90, 490t
  definitions, 489
  levels of evidence and grades of recommendation, 489, 490t
Evidence-based practice (EBP), 484. See also Research and evidence-based practice
Examination
  cardiovascular system, 146–56
  diagnostic
    arthrography, 41
    bone scan (osteoscintigraphy), 41
    computed tomography (CT scan), 36, 40
    diagnostic ultrasound, 41
    discography, 40
    magnetic resonance imaging (MRI), 40, 41
    in musculoskeletal physical therapy, 36–41
    myelography, 41
    plain film radiography (x-ray), 36
  flexibility, 34
  functional mobility, 36
  integumentary system, 280–82
  lymphatic system, 153, 179–82
  medical record review, 34
  motor function, 34
  musculoskeletal system, 34–41
  neuromuscular system, 91–105
  patient history, 34
  pediatric patients, 344–45
  peripheral vascular system, 150–52
  posture, 34
  pulmonary system, 197–99
  range of motion (ROM), 34

roles and responsibilities of PTA in, 34–36
spinal cord injury (SCI), 127
vestibular system, 267, 268b
Exercise. *See* Therapeutic exercise
Exercise-induced asthma (EIA), 8
Exercise prescription
cardiovascular disease, 166–71, 167b, 175–76
activity levels: METs (metabolic equivalents), 168, 172t
adverse responses to inpatient care, 169b, 171
ambulatory monitoring (telemetry), 168
cardiac transplant, 175
considerations following surgical procedures, 168–69
diabetes, 176
duration, 170
entry into programs, 166, 167b
exercise prescription for post-CABG, 171
exercise prescription for post-PTCA, 171
exercise type, 169–70
frequency, 170
guidelines for exercise prescription, 169–71
heart failure (HF), 175, 175t
home discharge instructions, 169b
intensity, 170
maximum heart rate, determining, 170b
monitoring during exercise and recovery, 168
pacemakers and AICDs, 175–76
patients requiring special considerations, 175–76
possible effects of physical training/ cardiac rehabilitation, 171, 173b
progression, 171
resistance exercise training, 174
transtelephonic ECG monitoring, 168
diabetes mellitus, 260, 261
obesity, 264, 265
Exercise tolerance test (ETT), 9, 154t, 166, 197
Expiratory muscles of ventilation, 192, 192t
Expiratory reserve volume (ERV), 193
Expressive dysfunction, 120–21
Extension synergy, 99t
Extensor carpi radialis brevis (ECRB) tendon, 52
External validity, 487
Exteroceptive stimulation techniques, 109t
Extra-ocular muscle movement, impaired, 88b
Extremity coordination, lack of, 88b
Eye movement test, 266

F

FABER (Patrick's) test, 36t, 38f
Facet joint conditions/dysfunction, 42t, 66
Face validity, 487
Facial nerve (CN VII), 90t, 95t
Facilitated stretching, 10–11
active inhibition techniques, indications for, 11
contract-relax-active contraction (CRAC), 11
hold-relax (HR), 10–11
hold-relax-active contraction (HRAC), 11
Facilitation techniques, 109t
Facility department management, 449–55
emergency preparedness, 455
human resource responsibilities, 453–55
medical records management, 449–51
policy and procedures, 452
quality assurance/continuous quality improvement, 452–53
risk management, 451–52
Facility modifications, 427
Falls
in aging patients, 328–29
balance testing, 456
in obese patients, 263
risk and prevention, 16, 455–56
Fascia techniques, 31
Fast-twitch (ST) fibers, 2, 2b
Fatigue
cancer-related, 241
in cardiovascular disease, 156t, 157, 159t
Federation of State Boards of Physical Therapy (FSBPT). *See also* National Physical Therapist Assistant Exam (PTA)
authorization-to-test letter, I-6
candidates with documented disabilities, I-6
contact information, I-8
Content Outline for the PTA Exam, I-1, I-8
list of texts used in PTA programs, I-2
overview of, I-2
passing criterion or standard established by, I-5
Performance Feedback Request Form, I-6–I-7
sanctioning of scores by, due to fraud, I-17
scheduling, I-16
Score Transfer Service/Score Transfer Request Form, I-6–I-7
scoring and reporting results of exam, I-6
Security Agreement, I-2
state information, I-9
Feedback
in coordination and balance, 14, 15
in motor control, 110
in progression, 18t
in relaxation of muscles, 12
Feedforward in motor control, 110
Fees, licensure, I-6
Feldenkrais movement, 75
Female reproductive system, 248–51
anatomy and physiology, 248, 249f
breasts, 248
disorders of, 251
pregnancy: normal, 248–50
pregnancy-related pathologies, 250–51
sexual reproduction functions, 248
Femoral anteversion and antetorsion, 57
Femoral fracture, open reduction internal fixation (ORIF) for, 27, 71
Femoral pulse, 151b
Fibrocartilage, 23–24
Fibromyalgia syndrome (FMS), 229–30
Fibrosis, 27b, 28b
Figure-ground discrimination disorder, 96
Finger opposition test, 101t
Finger to assistant's finger test, 101t
Finger to finger test, 101t
Finger to nose test, 101t
Finkelstein's test, 35t
First aid, 458–59
basic life support and CPR, 460–61b
bleeding
external, 458–59
internal, 459
shock (hypoperfusion), 459
First-class lever, 28
Fish oil, 313t
Fistula, 266b
FITT equation, 7, 7b
Fixation or position holding test, 101t
Flaccidity, 97t, 121
Flail chest, 204
Flat foot (pes planus), 62
Flex-foot orthosis, 415b
Flexibility, 9, 34
Flexion synergy, 99t
Flexor hallucis tendonopathy, 62
Floor-to-standing rises, 15
Flow rates, 193
Flu, 231t
Fluent aphasia, 121
Fluid imbalances, 253–54
Fluid replacement therapy
burns, 286
core temperature, 9
FLUTTER device, 210
Focal lesion, 122
Focused attention, 93
Follicle-stimulating hormone (FSH), 257
Foot and ankle
abnormal synergies, 99t
ankle-foot orthosis (AFO), 347
conditions of, 61–64
Achilles' tendinitis/tendinosis, 61
Charcot-Marie-Tooth disease, 63
equinus, 62
flexor hallucis tendonopathy, 62
forefoot/rearfoot deformities, 63–64
fractures, 61
hallux valgus, 62
ligament sprains, 61
metatarsalgia, 62–63
metatarsus adductus, 63
pes cavus (hollow foot), 62
pes planus (flat foot), 62
plantar fasciitis, 63
talipes equinovarus (clubfoot), 62
tarsal tunnel syndrome, 61
in convex-concave rule, 29t
deformities, in pediatric patients, 352–53
foot deformities, 319
foot orthosis, 414, 415b
gait deficits, 121t
joint positions, 30t
patterns of spasticity in upper motor neuron syndrome, 92t
Forced expiration, 192t, 193
Forced inspiration, 192t
Forefoot/rearfoot deformities, 63–64
Form constancy disorder, 96
Fraction of oxygen in the inspired air (FiO_2), 193
Fracture. *See* Bone fracture

Freezing of Gait Questionnaire, 118
Frontal lobe, 87, 88b, 89t
Frozen shoulder (adhesive capsulitis), 51
Full-arc exercise, 5
Full-thickness burn, 284t
Functional balance grades, 104t
Functional balance tests, 103t
Functional incontinence, 256
Functional Independence Measure (FIM), 104, 104b
Functional massage, 74–75
Functional mobility, 36
Functional rating scales, 104
Functional Reach (FR), 103t
Functional residual capacity (ERV + RV), 193
Functional restoration/minimal protection phase, 74
Functional training, equipment, and devices, 15, 395–433
   adhesive taping, 413–14
   ambulatory aids, 402–5
   bariatric equipment, 426–27
   chapter review questions and answers, 433, 514
   environmental considerations, 427–28
   ergonomics, 429–32
   gait, 397–402
   orthotics, 406–13
   prosthetics, 414–21
   transfer training, 425
   wheelchairs, 421–24
Functional training activities, 15
Furniture and equipment, 464
Fusobacterium, 248

G

Gait, 397–402
   activities, 15
   cycle, phases of, 397–400
   deficits, 121, 121t
   deviations, 400–402
   devices, additions to, 403
   in human development, 338, 342–43
   locomotion and, 100, 100b
   patterns, use of assistive devices, 404–5
   prosthetic gait deviations, 419–21, 420t
   trainers, 347
Gallop rhythm, 147t
Gamekeeper's thumb, 56
Gastric bypass, 263t
Gastritis, 246
Gastroesophageal reflux disease (GERD), 245, 245t, 246
Gastrointestinal (GI) bleeding, 245
Gastrointestinal (GI) conditions, affecting spine, 68
Gastrointestinal (GI) system, 243–48
   aging patients, 309–10
   anatomy and physiology, 243, 244f
   disorders, 244–45
   esophagus, 245–46
   intestines, 246–48
   medical management, 245, 245t
   overview of, 243–45
   rectum, 248
   stomach, 246

Gastrointestinal (GI) tract, 243, 244f
General adaptation syndrome (GAS), 269
Generalizability, 487
Generalized manipulation, 76
Generalized seizures, 133
Genetic disorders, 353–61
   cerebral palsy (CP), 353–56
   Down Syndrome (trisomy 21), 358
   Duchenne muscular dystrophy (pseudohypertrophic muscular dystrophy), 358–59
   intellectual disability/developmental disability/developmental delay, 360
   pervasive developmental disorder (PDD), 359–60
   sickle cell anemia, 360–61
   spina bifida, 356–58
   traumatic brain Injury (TBI), 356
Genital/reproductive system, 248–52
   female reproductive system, 248–51
   male reproductive system, 251–52
Gentle rocking techniques, 13, 16
Genu varum and valgum, 59–60
Geriatric rehabilitation, principles of, 300–301
Gestational diabetes mellitus (GDM), 259
Glasgow Coma Scale (GCS), 93, 93t, 123, 123t
Glenohumeral joint, 29t, 30t, 35t
Glenohumeral rhythm, 68
Glenohumeral subluxation and dislocation, 48
Glide movement, 28–29
Gliding techniques, 33
Global aphasia, 120t, 121
Global Initiative for Obstructive Lung Disease (GOLD), 197, 198t, 201
Globus pallidus, 87
Glossopharyngeal nerve (CN IX), 90t
Glucagons, 258
Glucocorticoids (cortisol), 42, 78t, 257
Glucose control, 258
Glucose-polymer drinks, 9
Gold therapy compounds, 312t
Golfer's elbow (medial epicondylitis), 52
Golgi tendon organ (GTO), 10–11
Gout, 43
Graded compression stockings (GCS), 164
Graded exercise test, 154t, 166, 197, 199t
Grades, cancer, 240
Grades of recommendation, 489, 490t
Grading of accessory joint movement, 31
Grading scale for muscle reflexes, 98, 98t
Gram-negative/positive bacteria, 200b
Gram stain, 197
Granulation/fibroblastic phase of scar tissue formation (phase 2), 27b
Granulocytes (eosinophils), 235
Graphesthesia, 94t, 96
Gravity-dependent/independent area of the lung, 194
Gray matter, 87, 90
Greenstick fracture, 27, 352
Grief process, 270
Grind (scouring) test, 38f
Growth hormone (GH), 257
Growth hormone–releasing hormone (GHRH), 257
Guarding, 405

Guided imagery, 16
Guide for Conduct of the Physical Therapist Assistant (Guide), 476–81
Guillain-Barré Syndrome (GBS), 95t, 134–35
Gynecological conditions affecting spine, 68
Gyri, 87

H

Hair, changes in, 282t
Half-kneeling (preambulation mat activity), 115
Hallux valgus, 62
Hamstrings, 57, 59, 72, 72t
Hand. *See* Wrist and hand
Handheld dynamometry, 99
Hassles Scale, 16
Hawkins-Kennedy test, 35t
Health Insurance Portability and Accountability Act (HIPAA), 457
Hearing
   in aging patients, 304, 305–6, 305b
   impairments (dominant), 88b
   loss, 305–6, 305b
Heart and circulation, 142–43
   anatomy of heart, illustrated, 143f
   cardiac cycle, 142, 142b, 143f
   coronary circulation, 142–43, 143f, 144f
   heart chambers and conduction, 142b
   heart tissue, 142
   hemodynamics, 143
   myocardial fibers, 143
Heartburn, 245
Heart chambers and conduction, 142b
Heart failure (HF), 175, 175t
Heart rate (HR)/pulse measurement, 146, 147, 148, 168, 170, 170b
Heart rate reserve (HRR), 7b
Heart rhythm, electronic measurement of, 148
Heart sounds, 147
Heart tissue, 142
Heart valves, 142b
Heat
   application, 367b, 368t
   relaxation of muscles and, 11–12
   for soft tissue conditions, 27b, 77, 77t
   transmission, 367
Heel on shin test, 101t
Helicobacter pylori, 246
Helper T cells, 223
Hematocrit (Hct), 155t, 197, 236t
Hematological system, 235–39
   anemia, 237
   blood composition, 235
   blood screening tests, 235
   hematopoiesis, 235
   hemophilia, 238–39
   hemostasis, 235, 236
   hypercoaguability disorders, 236
   hypocoagulopathy (bleeding), 236–37
   overview of, 235–37
   shock, 237
   sickle cell disease, 237–38
Hematopoiesis, 235
Hemiplegia, 88b, 107, 108, 119, 120t
Hemispherectomy, 133

Hemisphere lesions, 119–20, 120t, 321–22t
Hemispheres, 87, 89b, 119, 120, 120t
Hemodynamics, 143
Hemoglobin (Hgb), 155t, 197, 236t
Hemophilia, 238–39
Hemoptysis, 205t
Hemorrhage, 119
Hemorrhagic shock, 459
Hemorrhoids (piles), 248
Hemostasis (clotting/bleeding times), 155t, 235, 236
Hemothorax, 204
Heparin, 315t
Heparin-induced thrombocytopenia (HIT), 164
Hepatitis, 231t, 232, 233b
Herpes infections, 223, 224, 231t, 277b
Herpes zoster (shingles), 276, 277, 277b
Heterogeneity, 489
Heterotopic bone formation (ectopic bone), 129b, 130
Heterotopic ossification, 130, 130b
Hiatal hernia, 246
Hickman catheter, 214
Hidrosis, 282t
High altitudes, exercising at, 9
High-density lipoproteins (HDL), 154b
Higher-level cognitive abilities, 93
High-pressure positive expiratory pressure (PEP) mask, 210
High-voltage pulsed galvanic stimulation, 389–90
Hip
  abnormal synergies, 99t
  capsular patterns, 30t
  conditions of, 56–58
    avascular necrosis (AVN, osteonecrosis), 56–57
    coxa vara and coxa valga, 57
    femoral anteversion and antetorsion, 57
    hip scour test, 36t
    ITB tightness/friction disorder, 57
    Legg-Calvé-Perthe's disease (osteochondrosis), 58
    piriformis syndrome, 57–58
    slipped capital femoral epiphysis, 58
    total hip replacement (THR)/arthroplasty, 70, 70t
    trochanteric bursitis, 57
  in convex-concave rule, 29t
  gait deficits, 121t
  insufficient pelvic rotation during swing, 121
  joint positions, 30t
  patterns of spasticity in upper motor neuron syndrome, 92t
  PNF diagonal patterns, 108t
  tests for, 36t
Hip disarticulation prosthesis, 417
Hip hiking (preambulation parallel activity), 115
Hip-knee-ankle-foot orthosis (HKAFO), 347
Hip scour test, 36t
Hoehn & Yahr Disease Stage I, II, III, IV, 118, 322, 323b
Hold-relax (HR), 10–11, 107t
Hold-relax-active contraction (HRAC), 11
Hollow foot (pes cavus), 62

Holmes-Rahe Social Readjustment Scale, 16
Homan's sign (dorsiflexion sign), 130, 165
Home exercise program (HEP), 173
Homeostasis, 253
Homogeneity, 489
Homonymous hemianopsia, 88b, 96, 120t
Homonymous visual deficits, 88b
Hook-lying (preambulation mat activity), 114
Horizontal adduction test, 35t
Hormonal regulation, 257–58
Hormonal therapy, 240
Hospice care, 241
Hot packs, 368
Hot weather conditions, exercising in, 9
Hubbard tank, 17, 370
Huffing, 209
Human development and learning/development theories, 335
Human immunodeficiency virus (HIV), medical interventions, 224
Human resource responsibilities, 453–55
  continuing education, 454
  interview, 453
  job descriptions, 454
  OSHA, 454
  performance review/appraisal, 454
  sexual harassment, 454–55
Humeroradial joint, 29t, 30t
Humeroulnar joint, 29t, 30t
Hyaluronic acid (HA), 42
Hydration to modify effects of aging, 28
Hydrostatic pressure, 17
Hydrotherapy, 369–71
  aquatic therapy, 371, 371b
  electrical safety considerations, 371
  Hubbard tank, 370
  indications for, 370b
  precautions and contraindications, 370b
  principles of, 369
  temperature for, 370b
  whirlpool, 369–70
Hyperactive reflexes, 97
Hypercalcemia, 145b, 254
Hypercapnea, 201t
Hypercoaguability disorders, 236
Hyperglycemia, 262b
Hyperkalemia, 145b, 254
Hypermagnesemia, 254
Hypermobile spinal segments, 67
Hypernatremia, 145b, 254
Hyperpnea, 149
Hypertension, 159–60
Hyperthyroidism, 265
Hypertonia, 97, 97t
Hypertrophy, 2
Hyperventilation, 9
Hypoactive reflexes, 97
Hypocalcemia, 145b, 254
Hypocapnea, 201t, 202, 205t
Hypochondria, 270
Hypocoagulopathy (bleeding), 236–37
Hypoglossal nerve (CNXII), 90t
Hypoglycemia, 176, 261, 261b
Hypokalemia, 145b, 254
Hypolipidemic agents for cardiovascular disease, 161, 161t
Hypomagnesemia, 254
Hyponatremia, 145b, 254

Hypoperfusion (shock), 237, 459
Hypotension, 148, 149, 159t
Hypothalamus, 87, 88b, 90b, 95t, 257, 258f
Hypothesis, 486
Hypothyroidism, 265, 306
Hypotonia, 97, 97t, 99t, 121, 123, 134
Hypoxemia, 150, 201t, 205t
Hypoxia, 9, 150, 159t
Hypoxic-ischemic injury, 122
Hysterical paralysis (conversion disorder), 270

I

Ibuprofen, 312t
Ice massage, 373
Ice packs, 373
Ideational/ideomotor apraxia, 97
Idiopathic scoliosis, 47
Iliotibial band (ITB), 31, 57
Illegal practice and malpractice, 462–63
  common law, 462–63
  nondiscrimination laws, 462
  statutory laws impacting physical therapy, 462
Imaging in musculoskeletal physical therapy, 36–41
Immediate recall, 93
Immobility, in aging patients, 327–28
Immobilization, tissue, 28, 28b
Immune cells, 222
Immune disorders of skin, 278–79
Immune response, 222
Immune system, 222–30
  acquired immunodeficiency syndrome (AIDS), 223–24
  anatomy and physiology, 222
  autoimmune diseases, 222–23
  chronic fatigue syndrome (CFS), 224–25, 229
  fibromyalgia syndrome (FMS), 229–30
  human immunodeficiency virus (HIV), 224
  immune response, 222
  immunodeficiency diseases, 222
Immunodeficiency diseases, 222
Impaired glucose tolerance (IGT), 259
Impairments, defined, 449b
Impingement syndrome, 50
Impotence (erectile dysfunction) (ED), 252
Impulsivity, 93
Incident reporting, 451
Incomplete fracture, 27
Incomplete spinal cord injury, 126, 127b
Independent secretion removal techniques, 209–10
  active cycle of breathing technique (ACBT), 209
  autogenic drainage, 209–10
  FLUTTER or acapella device, 210
  high-pressure positive expiratory pressure (PEP) mask, 210
  low-pressure positive expiratory pressure (PEP) mask, 210
Individual differences principle, 7
Individuals with Disabilities Education Act (IDEA), 457–58

Inductive reasoning, I-12–I-13
Infection control, physical therapy-related, 234–35
Infection precautions, 225–28b, 234
   standard precautions, 225–28b, 234
   universal precautions, 234
Infections
   bacterial, 276
   parasitic, 278
   viral, 276–77
Infectious diseases, 230–34
   healthcare-associated infections, 231–32t
   hepatitis, 231t, 232, 233b
   modes of transmission and protective measures, 231t
   staphylococcal infections, 230
   streptococcal infections, 230, 232
   tuberculosis (TB), 233–34
Infectious disorders, neuromuscular, 116
   brain abscess, 116
   encephalitis, 116
   meningitis, 116
   physical therapy management, 116
Inference in critical reasoning, I-13
Inferior instability tests, 35t
Inflammatory bowel disease (IBD), 247
Inflammatory disorders, medications used for, 312t
Inflammatory/proliferative phase of scar tissue formation (phase 1), 27b
Informed consent, 487
Inhibitory techniques, 109t
Initial transient flaccidity with subsequent long-lasting spasticity, 123
Injury prevention, 463–64
Inpatient cardiac rehabilitation (phase 1), 171–73, 172t
   exercise/activity goals and outcomes, 171, 173
   exercise/activity guidelines, 173
   home exercise program (HEP), 173
   patient and family education goals, 173
Inpatient care, 464
Insight Assessment, Inc., I-15
Inspiratory capacity (IRV + TV), 193
Inspiratory muscles of ventilation, 191, 192b, 192t
Inspiratory muscle trainer (IMT), 212
Inspiratory reserve volume (IRV), 193
Instability
   in aging patients, 328–29
   shoulder, 48–49
   traumatic/atraumatic, 48
Instruction, 437–40
   implementation of instruction, 439–40
   instructional activities, 438
   instructional modes, 438–39
   instructional process, 437–38
Instrumental activities of daily living (IADL), 14
Instrumentation, 487
Insulin, 258
Insulin-dependent diabetes, 258–59
Insulin glucose homeostasis, 260
Insulin resistance, 259
Insulin resistance syndrome, 259
Integumentary system, 273–96
   aging patients, 309, 327
   burns, 284–87

burn healing, 285
burn management, 285
complications of burn injury, 284, 285
medical management, 285–86
pathophysiology, 284
physical therapy goals, outcomes, and interventions, 286–87
chapter review questions and answers, 296, 506–7
circulation, 275
conditions/pathology/diseases with intervention, 276–80
   bacterial infections, 276
   dermatitis, 276
   immune disorders of skin, 278–79
   other infections, 277–78
   parasitic infections, 278
   skin cancer, 279–80
   skin trauma, 280
   viral infections, 276–77
physical therapy examination and data collection, 280–82
   other symptoms, 281
   PTA's role in, 280
   skin conditions and descriptions, 281–82t
   tissue assessment, 280–81
preferred practice patterns, 283t
skin conditions and descriptions, 281–82t
skin or integument, 275
   immune disorders of, 279b
   integrity, in physical therapy examination, 36
   layers of, 275t
   physical therapy intervention for impaired, 283
skin ulcers, 287–95
   arterial ulcer, 288
   diabetic ulcer, 288, 288f
   pressure injury (decubitus ulcer or bed sore), 288–89
   venous ulcers (stasis ulcers), 287–88
   wound assessment, 289–90
   wound care, 290–95
Intellectual disability, in pediatric patients, 360
Intensive care unit, physical therapy in, 214–16
   arterial lines, pulmonary artery catheter (Swan-Ganz catheter), central line, 215
   central venous access devices (CVAD), 214–15
   chest tubes, 214
   intravenous lines (IVs), 214
   mechanical ventilation, 214
   monitors/oscilloscopes, 215
   peripherally inserted central catheters (PICC Line), 215
   supplemental oxygen, 215–16
Intention tremors, 88b, 99t, 117, 118, 120t
Interferential current (IFC), 390–91
Intermittent claudication, 153, 153b
Intermittent pneumatic compression, 380–81
Intermittent traction. See Mechanical spinal traction
Internal carotid artery syndrome, 119, 120t

Internal derangement of joint, 48
Internal disc disruption, 65
Internal (posterior) impingement, 50–51
Internal validity, 487
International Classification of Functioning, Disability, and Health Resources (ICF) model, 449
Interphalangeal (IP), 30t
Interval scale, 486, 486t
Interval training, 8
Intervertebral stenosis, 65
Interview, in human resources, 453
Intestines, 246–48
Intracerebral pressure, monitoring, 123
Intrapleural space, 191
Intravascular stents for cardiovascular disease, 162, 162t
Intravenous lines (IVs), 214
Intrinsic feedback, 110, 112
Involuntary movement, 98t, 119, 120t
Ion concentration changes, 145, 145b
Iontophoresis, 387
Irreversible contracture, 11
Irritable bowel syndrome (IBS), 247
Ischemic cardiac pain, 150
Ischemic conditions of the heart, medications used for, 313t
Islets of Langerhans, hormones released by, 258
Isokinetic dynamometry, 99
Isokinetic exercise, 5, 5t
Isometric exercise, 4, 5t
Isotonic exercise, 4, 5, 5t
Isotonics (agonist reversals), 107t
ITB tightness/friction disorder, 57

Jacobson's progressive relaxation technique, 16
Jendrassik's maneuver, 98
Jerk test, 35t
Job descriptions, 454
Joint Commission of Accreditation of Healthcare Organizations (JCAHO), 452, 456
Joint deformities, 319
Joint mobilization, 32–33
   application considerations, 33
   articulatory techniques, 75–76
   contraindications, 32t, 76
   force and direction of movements, 33
   grades, 32b
   indications, 32t, 76
   pain assessment, 33
   techniques, 32–33, 32b
      Kaltenborn, 32b, 33, 33f
      Maitland, 32–33, 32b
Joint oscillation, 75
Joint positions, 29–31, 30t
   close-packed position, 29, 30t
   end-feels, 29
   grading of accessory joint movement, 31
   resting or loose-packed position, 29, 30t
   selected capsular patterns, 29, 30t
Jumper's knee (Osgood-Schlatter), 59
Juvenile-onset diabetes, 258–59
Juvenile rheumatoid arthritis (JRA), 44, 350

K

Kaltenborn joint mobilization, 32b, 33, 33f
Karvonen's formula, 7b
Katz's index of ADL, 104
Kidney
   1,25-dihydroxyvitamin D released by, 258
   anatomy, 252
   functions, 253
Kidney stones (renal calculi), 255, 256
Kinematics/kinesiology, 28–29, 33
   arthrokinematics, 28
   convex-concave rule, 29, 29t
   motions describing movement of one joint surface on another, 28–29
      combinations of, 29
      glide, 28–29
      roll, 28
      spin, 29
   osteokinematics, 29
Kinesthesia, 94t, 96, 128t
Kinesthetic awareness, 12, 17
Kitchen sink exercises, 15
Knee
   abnormal synergies, 99t
   capsular patterns, 30t
   conditions of, 58–60
      fractures, 60
      genu varum and valgum, 59–60
      ligamentous repairs of (ACL/PCL reconstructive surgery), 71, 72, 72t
      ligament sprains, 58
      meniscal injuries, 58–59
      Osgood-Schlatter (jumper's knee), 59
      patellofemoral conditions, 59
      pes anserine bursitis, 59
      total knee replacement (TKR)/ arthroplasty, 71, 71t
   in convex-concave rule, 29t
   gait deficits, 121t
   joint positions, 30t
   ligamentous repairs of, 71, 72, 72t
   patterns of spasticity in upper motor neuron syndrome, 92t
   tests for, 36t
Knee-ankle-foot orthosis (KAFO), 347
Knee disarticulation prosthesis, 417
Kneeling (preambulation mat activity), 114–15
Knowledge of performance (KP), 14, 110, 112
Knowledge of results (KR), 14, 110, 112
Kübler-Ross stages of death and dying, 271

L

Laboratory tests
   cardiovascular, 154–56, 155t
   musculoskeletal, 41
   pulmonary, 197
Labral tears, 49
Labyrinthitis, 266b
Laceration, 280
Lachman stress test, 36t, 40f
Language comprehension, impaired, 88b
Lap band procedure, 263t
Lateral border of bony thorax, 191
Lateral central fissure, 87
Lateral collateral ligament (LCL), 58
Lateral epicondylitis (tennis elbow), 52
Lateral patellar tracking, 59
Lateral retinacular release, 72
LDL/HDL ratio, 154b
Leadpipe rigidity, 97t
Leaf-spring shank, 415b
Learning deficits, 88b
Learning/development theories, 335, 436–37
Learning styles, 436
Learning to Think Things Through: A Guide to Critical Thinking in the Curriculum (Nosich), I-15
Left anterior descending artery (LAD), 142
Left atrium (LA), 142b
Left coronary artery (LCA), 142
Left-sided heart failure. *See* Congestive heart failure (CHF)
Left ventricle, 142b
Left ventricular end-diastolic pressure (LVEDP), 143
Leg, conditions of lower, 60–61
   anterior compartment syndrome (ACS), 60
   anterior tibial periostitis (shin splints), 60
   media tibial stress syndrome, 60
   stress fractures, 61
Legg-Calvé-Perthes disease (LCPD), 58, 348–49
Lengthening, connective tissue mobilization for, 31–32
Length tension relationship, 2
Lesions
   Bankart, 49
   in bowel and bladder dysfunction, 130
   focal, in TBI, 122
   hemisphere, in CVA, 119–20, 120t
   level of, in spinal cord injury, 126, 130
   skip, 247
   SLAP, 35t, 48, 49
Leukemias, 240
Leukocytes (white blood count), 155t, 197, 236t, 325
Leukotriene receptor antagonists for pulmonary disease, 213
Level of cognitive functioning (LOCF), Rancho Los Amigos, 123, 124t
   management with decreased response levels (LOCF I–III), 124–25
   management with high-level recovery (LOCF VII–VIII), 125
   management with mid-level recovery (LOCF IV–VI), 125
Levels of evidence, 489, 490t
Levers, 28
Lice (pediculosis), 278
License, procedure for obtaining and retaining, I-6–I-7
   AIDS awareness training, I-6
   candidates with documented disabilities, I-6
   continuing education, I-7
   credentials evaluation, I-6
   endorsement, I-7
   English language proficiency, tests of, I-6
   fees, I-6
   fingerprinting, FBI check, vaccination, malpractice insurance, I-6
   FSBPT's role in, I-6
   jurisprudence examination, I-6
   license/regulation renewal, I-7
   retaking PTA Exam, I-7
   temporary license, I-6
   transfers of scores to other jurisdictions, I-6–I-7
Life Events Scale, 16
Lifestyle modification, 16
Life support and CPR, 460–61b
Lift devices, 427
Ligamentous instability tests, 35t
Ligamentous repairs of the knee, 71, 72, 72t
Ligaments
   healing times, 24–25t
   in tissue, 23
Ligament sprains
   foot and ankle, 61
   knee, 58
Lightheadedness in cardiovascular disease, 149, 155t, 157, 175b
Light touch, 94t, 96, 109t, 127, 128t
Limbic system, 87
Limits of stability (LOS), 15, 101
Lipedema, 179, 180f
Lipid panel ranges, 154b
Lipodermatosclerosis, 181
Lobectomy, 212
Lobes, brain, 87, 88b, 89t
   frontal, 88b, 89t
   occipital, 88b, 89t
   parietal, 88b, 89t
   temporal, 88b, 89t
Lobes, lung, 191
Local brain damage, 122
Locked-in syndrome, 120t
Locomotor training, 405
Long-acting beta-2 agonists for pulmonary disease, 213
Longitudinal cerebral fissure, 87
Long-term recall, 93
Loose, irregular connective tissue, 23
Loose-packed position, 29, 30t
Loperamide, 245t
Low back pain, pregnancy-related, 250
Low-density lipoproteins (LDL), 154b
Lower airways, 191
Lower extremities (LEs)
   abnormal synergies, 99t
   amputations, 415b
   in aquatic exercise, 17, 18
   conditions of
      foot and ankle, 61–64
      hip, 56–58
      knee, 58–60
      leg, 60–61
   in coordination and balance training, 15, 16
   orthopedic surgical repairs, 70–73
   patterns of spasticity in upper motor neuron syndrome, 92t
   in postural stability training, 13
   in relaxation training, 16
   tests for, 36t
   venous pooling in, 8
Lower-limb orthoses, components/terminology, 406–10

Lower-limb prosthetics (LLPs), 414–17
  hip disarticulation prosthesis, 417
  immediate postoperative prosthesis (rigid dressing), 417
  knee disarticulation prosthesis, 417
  partial-foot prosthesis, 414
  transfemoral (above-knee) prosthesis, 416–17
  transtibial (below knee) prosthesis, 414, 415–16, 415b
Lower motor neuron (LMN) syndrome, 98, 98t
Low-molecular-weight heparin (LMWH), 164
Low-pressure positive expiratory pressure (PEP) mask, 210
Lumbar nerves, 90
Lumbar traction, 379–80
Lumbosacral plexus, 91
Lung capacities, 193, 193f
Lung contusion, 204
Lung structures, 191
Lung volume reduction surgery (LVRS), 212
Lung volumes, 193, 193f
Lupus erythematosus, 278, 279
Luteinizing hormone (LH), 257
Lymphadenopathy, 179
Lymphangiectasia, 181
Lymphangiography, 153
Lymphangitis, 179
Lymphatic system, 143–44, 178–84
  anatomy and physiology, 143–44, 178f
  examination, 153, 179–82
    diagnostic tests, 181–82
    history, 179–80
    in physical therapy examination and data collection, 153
    quality of life issues, 181
  intervention/rehabilitation guidelines for lymphedema, 182–84
  lymph circulation, 179
  lymph vessel contraction, 179
  lymph vessels and nodes, 143–44, 178, 178f
  pathophysiology/common pathologies, 179
Lymph circulation, 179
Lymphedema
  intervention for asymptomatic patients at risk for, 182–83
  lipedema differentiated from, 179, 180f
  outcome measures/self-report instruments, 184
  pathophysiology, 179
  patient education for managing, 182b
  phase II management, 183–84
  phase I management: edema secondary to lymphatic dysfunction, 183
  summary, 182t
Lymph nodes, 143–44, 178, 178f, 222
  palpation, 153, 181
  transplantation, 184
Lymphocytes, 222, 235
Lymphoma, 240
Lymphorrhea, 181
Lymphoscintigraphy, 181
Lymph system, 222
Lymph vessel contraction, 179
Lymph vessels, 143–44, 178, 178f

M

Macrophages, 222
Macrovascular disease, 259
Magnesium, 254
Magnetic resonance imaging (MRI), 40, 41, 92
Maintenance drugs for pulmonary disease, 213
Maitland joint mobilization, 32–33, 32b
Major histocompatibility complex (MHC), 222
Malabsorption syndrome, 246–47
Male reproductive system, 251–52
  anatomy and physiology, 251–52, 251f
  disorders of, 252
Malignant tumor, 240, 279–80
Malingering (symptom magnification syndrome), 80
Mallet finger, 56, 56f
Management and professional roles, 447–82
  American Physical Therapy Association (APTA), 469–81
  chapter review questions and answers, 482, 516
  facility department management, 449–55
  illegal practice and malpractice, 462–63
  roles and responsibilities, 464–68
Manic-depressive illness (bipolar disorder), 270
Manipulation, 76
Manual lymphatic drainage (MLD), 183, 184
Manual muscle testing, 99
Manual resistance, 3
Manual secretion removal techniques, 206–8
  conditions that do not respond to, 206
  indications for, 206
  percussion, 206, 206b, 208t
  postural/bronchial drainage, 206, 207f, 208t
  shaking (vibration), 206, 206b, 208, 208t
Manual static, passive stretching, 10
Manual therapy approaches in rehabilitation, 77
Manubrium, 191
Marie-Strümpell disease, 42, 43
Massage, 382–83
  functional, 74–75
  ice, 373
  for relaxation of muscles, 12
  transverse friction, 75
Massed practice, 110, 112
Mass grasp test, 101t
Maturation phase of scar tissue formation (phase 3), 27b
Maximal ETT, 166
Maximum sway, 102
McBurney's point, 247
McConnell (patellofemoral) taping, 59
McGill pain questionnaire, 34
McMurray's test, 36t, 41f, 58
Measurement, levels of, 486
Mechanical agents, 378–82
  continuous passive motion (CPM), 381–82
  intermittent pneumatic compression, 380–81
  mechanical spinal traction (intermittent traction), 378–80
  tilt table, 382
Mechanical resistance, 3
Mechanical spinal traction, 378–80, 378b
  application methods, 379–80
    cervical traction, 379
    lumbar traction, 379–80
  effects of, 378–79
  goals and indications for, 378b
  precautions and contraindications, 380b
Mechanical ventilation, 214
Mechanoreceptors, 6
Medial collateral ligament (MCL), 58
Medial epicondylitis (golfer's elbow), 52
Media tibial stress syndrome, 60
Medical diagnostic exams and imaging
  arthrography, 41
  bone scan (osteoscintigraphy), 41
  computed tomography (CT scan), 36, 40
  diagnostic ultrasound, 41
  discography, 40
  magnetic resonance imaging (MRI), 40, 41
  in musculoskeletal physical therapy, 36–41
  myelography, 41
  plain film radiography (x-ray), 36
Medical management. See also Medications
  burns, 285–86
  cardiovascular disease, 160, 161, 161t, 163t
  cerebral vascular accident (CVA, stroke), 121
  chronic obstructive disease, 202
  complex regional pain syndrome (CRPS), 137
  epilepsy, 133
  gastrointestinal system, 245, 245t
  hypertension, 159, 160
  neoplasms, CNS, 117
  osteoporosis, 311, 312–15t
  rheumatoid arthritis (RA), 319
  spinal cord injury (SCI), 130–31
  traumatic brain injury (TBI), 123
Medical record review, 34, 91–93
Medical records management, 449–51
  basic principles of documentation, 450
  discharge plan, 450
  discharge summary, 450
  documentation format, 449
  documentation methods, 449
  guidelines for documentation, 450, 469–70
    documentation authority for physical therapy services, 469
    general guidelines, 469–70
    visit encounter, 470
  ICF model, 449
  payment denials, 451
  problem oriented medical record (POMR), 449
  progress notes, 450
  reasons for documenting, 449–50
  reevaluation/reassessment, 450
  successful documentation practices, 451
  terminology, 449b

Medication errors, in aging patients, 329–30
Medications. *See also* Medical management
   antiepileptic, 133
   arrhythmias, 314*t*
   blood clotting, 314–15*t*
   bone disorders, 312*t*
   cholesterol-lowering, 313*t*
   chronic obstructive diseases, 202
   cognitive disorders, 314–15*t*
   congestive conditions, 314*t*
   diabetes mellitus (DM), 261*t*
   errors, in aging patients, 329–30
   inflammatory disorders, 312*t*
   ischemic conditions, 313*t*
   musculoskeletal conditions, 77–80
   renal and urological disorders, 255*t*
   spinal cord injury (SCI), 130
   symptom modifying, 315*t*
Medulla oblongata, 87, 90*b*
Medullary lesion, 322*t*
Memory, 88*b*, 93
Meninges, 89, 90
Meningitis, 116
Meniscal arthroscopy, 72
Meniscal injuries, 58–59
Meniscus tear tests, 36*t*
Mental practice, 110, 112
Mentation, 93
Metabolic acidosis, 254
Metabolic alkalosis, 254
Metabolic effects of strength training, 3
Metabolic equivalents (METs), 168, 170, 171*t*
   activity chart, 171*t*
   levels, 186*t*
   sample exercise program, 185–86*b*
Metabolic pathologies in aging patients, 327
Metabolic shock, 459
Metabolic syndrome, 259
Metabolic system. *See* Endocrine and metabolic systems
Metacarpophalangeal (MCP) joint, 30*t*, 55
Metastasis, 240, 241, 242
Metatarsalgia, 62–63
Metatarsophalangeal (MTP) joint, 63
Metatarsus adductus, 63
Methicillin-resistant *Staphylococcus aureus* (MRSA), 230, 232*t*
Methods, research, 485
Methylprednisolone, 312*t*
Methylxanthines for pulmonary disease, 213
Microvascular disease, 259
Midbrain, 87
Midbrain lesion, 321*t*
Middle cerebral artery syndrome, 119, 120*t*
Midrange manipulation, 76
Midsternotomy, 213
Mild concussion, 123
Mild TBI, 123*t*
Milwaukee orthosis, 347*b*
Mineral corticosteroids (aldosterone), 257
Mini-Mental Status Examination (MMSE), 93
Mitral valve, 147
Mobilization
   connective tissue
      for lengthening, 31–32
      for tissue tension, 31
   joint, 32–33

Mobility and flexibility training, 9–12
   common errors in, 12
   flexibility, 9
   relaxation of muscles, 11–12
      biofeedback and, 12
      heat and, 11–12
      local relaxation techniques, 11
      massage and, 12
   stretching, 10–11
Modalities in musculoskeletal physical therapy, 77
Moderate TBI, 123*t*
Modified Ashworth's scale for spasticity, 97, 97*t*
Modified Functional Reach Test (MFRT), 103*t*
Modified Ober test, 39*f*
Modified plantigrade (preambulation mat activity), 115
Mole, common, 279
Monitors/oscilloscopes, 215
Monoclonal antibodies, 240
Monocytes (agranulocytes), 235
Mononeuropathy, 134
Monosynaptic stretch reflex, 91, 97, 97*t*
Morbidity/mortality, in aging patients, 299–300
Mosaic Down Syndrome, 358*b*
Motions describing movement of one joint surface on another, 28–29
   combinations of, 29
   glide, 28–29
   roll, 28
   spin, 29
Motor control, 109–10
   feedback, 110
   feedforward, 110
   motor learning and, 335
   motor plan, 109–10
   motor program, 109
   motor skill acquisition, 110
   stages of, 110
Motor fiber type, 2, 2*b*
Motor function, 97–100
   assessment, 97
   muscle performance, 98–99, 98*t*
   muscle tone, 97, 97*t*
   in physical therapy examination, 34
   reflex integrity, 97–98, 97*t*
   voluntary movement patterns, 99–100
Motor impairments in TBI
   Brunnstrom's Stages of Motor Recovery, 121
   muscle performance impairments, 121
   muscle tone, 121, 123
   voluntary movement patterns, 121
Motor learning, 110–12, 440–43
   description, 440
   effective, strategies for, 110, 112, 112*b*
   environment, 112, 112*b*
   feedback, 110, 112, 112*b*
   frequency, 110, 112*b*
   general concepts, 110
   intervention or instruction, implications for, 442
   measures of, 110
   motor control and, 335
   performance/learning, assessment of, 442–43

   phases of, 440–42
   practice, 110, 112
   stages of, 110, 111–12*t*
   strategies, 14
   transfer, 110
Motor plan, 109–10
Motor program, 109
Motor restlessness (akathisia), 330
Motor skill acquisition, 110
Motor unit action potentials (MUAP), 391
Motor unit potentials (MUP), 391
Movement adaptation syndrome (MAS), 16
Movement decomposition, 99*t*
Multidirectional Reach Test (MDRT), 103*t*
Multi-infarct dementias (MIDs), 324*t*, 325
Multilevel vertebral fusion, 73
Multi-lumen catheters, 215
Multiple choice questions on PTA Exam, strategies for answering, I-10–I-12
   clues, I-11
   crucial for survival, I-12
   key words, I-10, I-11
   negative words or phrases, I-12
   opposites, I-11
   overanalyze, I-12
   overlapping facts, I-12
   similar choices, I-11
Multiple sclerosis (MS), 117–18
Murmurs, 147*t*, 159*t*
Muscle
   adaptations of strength training, 2–3
   endurance strategies, 6
   energy techniques, 75
   function and strength, concepts of, 2
   length/strength involvement tests, 36*t*
   performance, 98–99, 98*t*
   relaxants, 80
   strain, 46
      degree of, 26*t*
      spinal, 64
   substitutions, 31
   techniques, 31
   tissue, 24, 25*t*
   tone, 97, 97*t*
   of ventilation, 191–92, 192*t*, 194
Musculoskeletal system, 21–81
   aging patients, 310–19
      degenerative arthritis/osteoarthritis (OA), 317–18
      fractures, 317
      osteoporosis, 310–16
      Paget's disease (osteitis deformans), 316
      rheumatoid arthritis (RA), 318–19
   anatomy and physiology, 23–28
      aging, effects on structure and function, 27–28
      immobilization, effects of, 28
      stress, response to, 24, 26–27
      tissue structure and function, 23–24
   balance and, 102
   biomechanics, 28–31
   chapter review questions and answers, 81, 496–97
   conditions/pathology/diseases with intervention, 42–73, 73–80
      acute conditions, 73–74
      acute (inflammatory) phase/maximal protection, 73

Musculoskeletal system (Cont.)
  arthritic conditions, 42
  articulatory techniques, 75–76
  chronic conditions, 74
  functional restoration/minimal protection phase, 74
  lower extremity conditions—foot and ankle, 61–64
  lower extremity conditions—hip, 56–58
  lower extremity conditions—knee, 58–60
  lower extremity conditions—leg, 60–61
  manual therapy approaches in rehabilitation, 77
  modalities and electrotherapeutic agents, 77, 77t
  neural tissue mobilization, 76
  neurodynamic exercises, 76
  orthopedic surgical repairs—lower extremity, 70–73
  orthopedic surgical repairs—upper extremity, 68–70
  pharmacology, relevant, 77–80, 78–79t
  psychosocial considerations, 80
  rheumatoid conditions, 42–44
  skeletal conditions, 44
  soft tissue, 45–48, 74–77
  soft tissue/myofascial techniques, 74–75
  spinal conditions, 64–68
  subacute phase/moderate protection, 73–74
  therapeutic exercise for musculoskeletal conditions, 76–77
  upper extremity conditions—elbow, 51–53
  upper extremity conditions—shoulder, 48–51
  upper extremity conditions—wrist and hand, 54–56
  dysfunction, intervention strategies for patients with, 31–33
  connective tissue mobilization for lengthening, 31–32
  connective tissue mobilization for tissue tension, 31
  joint mobilization, 32–33
  examination and data collection, 34–41
  electrodiagnostic testing, 41
  laboratory tests, 41
  medical diagnostic exams and imaging, 36–41
  PTA's role and responsibilities, 34–36
  kinematics/kinesiology, 28–29, 33
Myasthenia gravis, 95t, 135
Mycobacterium tuberculosis, 199, 233
Myelography, 41
Myelomas, 240
Myelomeningocele, 62, 356, 357t
Myocardial fibers, 143
Myocardial infarction (MI), 150, 158, 158f
Myocardial oxygen demand (MVO_2), 143
Myocardial perfusion imaging, 154t
Myocardium, 142
Myoelectric system, 417

Myofascial pain syndrome, 45
Myositis ossificans, 46–47
Myositis ossificans, 130, 130b
Myostatic contracture, 11

N

Nails, changes in, 282t
Naproxen, 312t
Narcotic analgesics, 78t, 80
National Physical Therapist Assistant Exam (PTA), I-1–I-17. *See also* Federation of State Boards of Physical Therapy (FSBPT)
  areas covered in, I-2
  breaks and timing during exam, I-9
  content for PTA, I-2–I-5
    category A (physical therapy data collection), I-3
    category B (diseases and conditions impacting intervention), I-4
    category C (intervention), I-4
    category D (equipment, devices, technologies, and therapeutic modalities), I-4
    category E (safety, protection, professional responsibilities, research and evidence-based practice), I-5
    number of questions by body system, I-3t
  critical reasoning skills, I-14–I-15
  development of, I-2
  examination items/questions, successfully managing, I-10–I-13
    critical reasoning, I-12–I-15
    exam item difficulty, taxonomy of, I-10
    levels of exam questions, I-10, I-11t
    multiple choice questions, strategies for answering, I-10–I-12
    strategies to avoid, I-12
    test item strategies, I-10
  format, I-9
  grading, I-5
  number of questions on, I-9
  purpose of, I-8–I-9
    protection of public, I-8
    PTA Exam is not a jurisprudence examination, I-8–I-9
  question format, I-9
  retaking, I-7
  review, organizing, I-15–I-16
    practice exam(s), when to take, I-16
    study sessions, structuring, I-15–I-16
    study time, I-15, I-15t
  score reporting, I-5
  success, planning for, I-8, I-16–I-17
    attitude, I-17
    break, I-17
    communication, I-17
    during exam, I-16–I-17
    length of exam, I-16
    morning of exam, I-16
    personal items, I-16
    required identification, I-16
    scheduling, I-16
    skipping questions, I-17
    time management, I-17
    travel, I-16
    tutorial, I-17
    what will be provided, I-16–I-17
  web links and e-mail addresses, I-8
Nausea and vomiting, 156, 156t, 244
Needle electrodes/sensors, 391
Neer's test, 35t, 37f
Neglect, 458
Neonatal Behavioral Assessment Scale (NBAS), 344
Neonatal development, 335–36
Neoplasm, cancer, 240
Neoplasm, CNS, 116–17
  clinical picture: dependent upon location of lesion, 116
  medical management, 117
  physical therapy management, 117
  primary CNS neoplasms, 116
  secondary CNS neoplasms, 116
Neoplastic disease, 42t
Nerve conduction velocity (NCV), 41
Nerve entrapments, 53
Nervous system, organization of, 85
  central nervous system (CNS), 85, 85f
  parasympathetic division, 85, 86f
  peripheral nervous system (PNS), 85
  sympathetic division, 85, 85f
Neural screens performed by PTA, 94t
Neural tissue
  grouping of, 86
  mobilization, 76
Neurapraxia, 134
Neurodevelopmental treatment (NDT), 106, 106b
Neurodynamic exercises, 76
Neurogenic bladder management, 130
Neurogenic shock, 459
Neuroglia, 86
Neurohumoral influences on cardiovascular system, 144, 145
  additional control mechanisms, 145, 145b
  ion concentration changes, 145, 145b
  parasympathetic stimulation, 145
  sympathetic and parasympathetic systems, 144
  sympathetic stimulation (adrenergic), 144, 145
Neurological conditions, painful, 136–37
Neurological disorders
  in aging patients, 320–23
    cerebrovascular accident (stroke, CVA), 320–22
    neurological rehabilitation, intervention considerations for, 320
    Parkinson's disease, 322–23
  genetic, 353–61
    cerebral palsy (CP), 353–56
    Down Syndrome (trisomy 21), 358
    Duchenne muscular dystrophy (pseudohypertrophic muscular dystrophy), 358–59
    intellectual disability/developmental disability/developmental delay, 360
    pervasive developmental disorder (PDD), 359–60
    sickle cell anemia, 360–61
    spina bifida, 356–58
    traumatic brain Injury (TBI), 356

Neurological dysfunction, intervention strategies for patients with, 105–16
  ambulation independence, promoting, 114–16
    preambulation mat activities, with progression, 114–15, 115b
    preambulation parallel activities, 115
  intervention approaches, 106–9
    compensatory training approach, 108, 109
    hemiplegia, movement therapy in, 107, 108
    neurodevelopmental treatment (NDT), 106, 106b
    proprioceptive neuromuscular facilitation (PNF), 106–7, 106b
    proprioceptive techniques, 109t
    sensory stimulation techniques, 108
  motor control, 109–10
    feedback, 110
    feedforward, 110
    motor plan, 109–10
    motor program, 109
    motor skill acquisition, 110
    stages of, 110
  motor learning, 110–12
    effective, strategies for, 110, 112, 112b
    environment, 112, 112b
    feedback, 110, 112, 112b
    frequency, 110, 112b
    general concepts, 110
    measures of, 110
    practice, 110, 112
    stages of, 110, 111–12t
    transfer, 110
  PTA's role and responsibilities, 105–6
    exercise/activity difficulty, 106, 106t
    general intervention considerations, 105–6
    implementing treatment, 105
  task-specific training strategies, 113–14
    adherence-enhancing behavioral strategies, 114
    behavioral shaping techniques, 113
    constraint-induced (CI) movement therapy, 114
    general concepts, 113, 113b
    locomotor training, 114
    task selection, 114
    tests, 35t
Neurological system in aging patients, 303–4
Neuroma, 266b
Neuromodulators, 86
Neuromuscular electrical stimulation (NMES), 391
Neuromuscular system, 83–138
  anatomy and physiology, 85–91
    brain, 87–90
    nervous system, organization of, 85
    physiology, 86–87
    spinal cord, 90–91
    structural components, 85–86
  chapter review questions and answers, 138, 498–99
  complex regional pain syndrome (CRPS), 136–37
    abnormal response of peripheral nerve, 136
    clinical picture, 136–37
    clinical stages, 136–37, 137t
    etiology, 136
    medical management, 137
    physical therapy management, 137
    variations, 136
  conditions/pathology/diseases with intervention, 116–36
    cerebral vascular accident (CVA, stroke), 119–22
    concussion, 125–26
    degenerative diseases of CNS, 117–19
    epilepsy, 131, 133
    infectious disorders, 116
    neoplasms, CNS, 116–17
    peripheral nervous system (PNS) disorders, 133–36, 135
    spinal cord injury (SCI), 126–31
    traumatic brain injury (TBI), 122–25
  neurological conditions, painful, 136–37
  neurological dysfunction, intervention strategies for patients with, 105–16
    ambulation independence, promoting, 114–16
    intervention approaches, 106–9
    motor control, 109–10
    motor learning, 110–12
    PTA's role and responsibilities, 105–6
    task-specific training strategies, 113–14
  physical therapy examination and data collection, 91–105
    aerobic capacity and endurance, 93–94
    arousal, mentation, and cognition, 93
    balance, 100, 101, 102–4
    environment and equipment considerations, 104–5
    gait and locomotion, 100, 100b
    motor function, 97–100
    patient history and medical record review, 91–93
    perceptual dysfunction, 96–97
    PTA's role and responsibilities, 91
    sensory testing, 94–96, 94t
Neuron, 85
Neuropathies (peripheral neuropathy), 134
  entrapment syndrome, 134
  mononeuropathy, 134
  polyneuropathy, 134
  radiculopathy, 134
  traumatic nerve injury, 134
Neurotmesis, 134
Neurotransmitters, 86
Neutrophils, 235
Newborn respiratory rate, 149
Nitrates (vasodilators), 160, 161t, 163t, 313t
Nitroglycerine, 160, 161t, 163t, 313t
Nodes of Ranvier, 86
Nominal scale, 486, 486t
Nonbacterial inflammatory prostatitis, 252
Non-cardiogenic pulmonary edema, 204
Noncontinuous ETT, 166
Noncontractile tissue, 6, 10, 11
Nondiscrimination laws, 462
Nondisjunction Down Syndrome, 358b
Nonequilibrium tests of coordination, 100, 101t
Nonfluent aphasia, 120
Nonimmersion irrigation, 371
Non-insulin dependent diabetes, 259
Noninvasive blood pressure cuff (NIBP), 215
Nonnarcotic analgesics, 80
Nonsteroidal anti-inflammatory drugs (NSAIDS), 312t
  for gastrointestinal disorders, 246
  for musculoskeletal conditions, 77, 78t, 79t, 80
    acute, 73
    arthritic, 42, 43, 44
    elbow, 51, 52, 53
    foot and ankle, 61, 62, 63
    hip, 57, 58
    knee, 58, 59, 60
    lower leg, 60, 61
    shoulder, 48, 49, 50, 51
    soft tissue conditions, 45, 46, 47, 48
    spine, 64, 65, 66, 67
    wrist and hand, 54, 55, 56
  side effects, monitoring for, 246
Nontransmural infarction, 158
Nonverbal communication, 443
Norepinephrine, 258
Normal physiological end-feel, 29
Normal pulse, 152b
Norovirus, 231t
Nortriptyline, 315t
Nosich, G. M., I-15
Numeric pain scale (NPS), 34
Nutrition
  deficiencies, in aging patients, 330
  for modifying aging effects on musculoskeletal system, 28

Ober's test, 36t, 39f
Obesity, 262–65
  body mass index (BMI), 262
  exercise evaluation (ACSM guidelines, 2017), 264, 264b
  exercise precautions, 264b
  exercise prescription (ACSM guidelines, 2017), 264, 265
  exercising in heat and, 9
  medical problems associated with, 262
  physical problems associated with, 263
  physical therapy interventions and considerations with, 264
  prevention and management, 263
  surgical intervention, 263, 263t
Objectivity in research, 488
O'Brien (active compression) test, 35t
Obsessive-compulsive behavior, 269
Obstipation, 244
Obstructive disorders, 255, 256
Occipital lobe, 88b, 89t
Occupational Safety and Health Administration (OSHA), 454
Occurrence/incident report, 451
Oculomotor nerve (CN III), 90t, 95t
Oculomotor nerve palsy, 120t
Ohm's Law, 384t
Olfactory nerve (CN I), 90t
Omeprazole, 245t

Index

1-plane anterior instability tests, 36t
1-plane medial-lateral instability tests, 36t
1-plane posterior instability tests, 36t
1,25-dihydroxyvitamin D released by, 258
Open-chain exercise, 6
Open fracture, 27
Open head injury, 122
Open reduction internal fixation (ORIF), 27, 52, 71
Opioid dependency, 80
Optic nerve (CN II), 90t
Optimal respiration, 194
Ordinal scale, 486, 486t
Organic brain syndromes, 324t
Orthopedic disorders, 348–53
   arthrogryposis multiplex congenita, 351–52
   brachial plexus injury, 353
   developmental dysplasia of the hip (DDH), 348
   foot and ankle deformities, 352–53
   juvenile rheumatoid arthritis (JRA), 350
   Legg-Calvé-Perthes disease (LCPD), 348–49
   osteogenesis imperfecta (OI), 351
   pediatric fractures, 352
   slipped capital femoral epiphysis (SCFE), 349, 350
Orthopedic surgical repairs
   lower extremity, 70–73
      lateral retinacular release, 72
      ligamentous repairs of the knee, 71, 72, 72t
      meniscal arthroscopy, 72
      multilevel vertebral fusion, 73
      open reduction internal fixation (ORIF) after femoral fracture, 71
      physical therapy goals, outcomes, and interventions following surgery, 73
      surgical repairs of spine, 72–73
      total hip replacement (THR)/arthroplasty, 70, 70t
      total knee replacement (TKR)/arthroplasty, 71, 71t
   upper extremity, 68–70
      rotator cuff tear, 68
      tendon injuries and repairs of the hand, 69–70
Orthopnea, 149, 159t
Orthostatic hypotension, 149
Orthotics, 104, 406–13
   general concepts, 406
   lower-limb orthoses, components/terminology, 406–10
   physical therapy intervention, 412–13
   spinal (trunk) orthoses, components/terminology, 410–11
   upper-limb orthoses or splints, components/terminology, 411–12
Oscilloscopes, 215
Osgood-Schlatter (jumper's knee), 59
Osteitis deformans (Paget's disease), 47, 306, 316
Osteoarthritis (OA), 42, 42t
Osteochondritis dissecans, 44
Osteochondrosis of humeral capitellum, 52
Osteogenesis imperfecta (OI), 44, 351
Osteokinematics, 29
Osteomalacia, 44
Osteomyelitis, 44
Osteonecrosis, 56–57
Osteoporosis, 44, 310–16
   assessment, 311
   bone loss, diseases and mediations affecting, 311b
   bone mineral density and treatment recommendations, 311t
   characteristics, 311
   diagnostic criteria, 310
   disease process, 310
   etiological factors, 310, 311
   intervention, implications, and compensatory strategies, 316
   medical management, 311, 312–15t
   resistance exercises and, 4
Osteoscintigraphy (bone scan), 41
Otosclerosis, 306
Outcome and assessment information set (OASIS), 104
Outpatient cardiac rehabilitation (phase 2), 172t, 173–74
   eligible patients, 173
   exercise/activity goals and outcomes, 173–74
   exercise/activity guidelines, 174
Ovaries, 248
Overflow incontinence, 256
Overground training (TT) with least restrictive device (LRD), 114
Overload principle, 3, 6
Overstretching, 11
Oxybutynin, 255t
Oxygen saturation, 149–50, 168
Oxygen transport, 8, 9
Oxytocin, 257

P

Pacemakers, 175–76
Paget's disease (osteitis deformans), 47, 306, 316
Pain assessment and relief, 34
   burns, 285
   cancer, 241, 242
   in cardiovascular disease, 150
   claudication pain rating scale, 176b
   gastrointestinal, 245
   in joint mobilization, 33
   pregnancy, 250
   subjective, in intermittent claudication, 153b
Palliative intervention, 240
Pallor, 152b, 153, 156, 156t
Palpitations, 156–57, 156t
Pancreatic islet cells, 258
Panic attacks, 269
Papillomatosis, 181
Paraffin, 369, 369b
Paranoia, 270
Paraplegia, 126
Parapodium, 347
Parasitic infections, 278
Parasympathetic division, 85, 86f
Parasympathetic stimulation, 145
Parasympathetic system, 144
Parathyroid glands, 258
Paresthesias, 153
Parietal lobe, 87, 88b, 89t
Parietal pleura, 191
Parieto-occipital cortex, damage to, 120
Parkinsonism, 330
Parkinson's disease (PD), 118–19, 322–23, 325
Parkinson's Disease Questionnaire (PDQ-39), 118
Parkinson's Fatigue Scale, 118
Paroxysmal nocturnal dyspnea (PND), 149, 159t
Partial-foot prosthesis, 414
Partial or focal seizures, 133
Partial pressure of carbon dioxide within the arterial blood ($PaCO_2$), 194
Partial pressure of oxygen in the atmosphere (PaO_2), 193
Partial thromboplastin time (PTT), 155t, 235, 236
Partial weight-bearing (PWB), 18, 70t
Participation, defined, 449b
Participation restrictions, defined, 449b
Part-whole transfer, 110, 112
Pascal's law, 17
Passive finger flexion, 31
Passive flexibility, 9
Passive ROM (PROM), 46
Patella alta, 59
Patella baja, 59
Patellar tendinitis, 59
Patellofemoral conditions, 59
Patellofemoral pain syndrome (PFPS), 59
Patellofemoral (McConnell) taping, 59
Pathological end-feel, 29
Patient/client rights, 457–58
   abuse and neglect, 458
   ADA, 457
   HIPAA, 457
   IDEA, 457–58
   sexual harassment, 458
Patient history, 34, 91–93
Patient safety and protection, 455–61
   equipment, use of, 456
   fall risk and prevention, 455–56
   first aid, 458–59
   life support and CPR, 460–61b
   patient/client rights, 457–58
   restraints, use of, 456–57
Patrick's (FABER) test, 36t, 38f
Payment denials, 451
Pedal pulse, 152b
Pediatric patients, 333–63
   chapter review questions and answers, 363, 510–11
   development, 335–43
   intervention, 345–48
      adaptive equipment, 346–48
      approaches, 345
      overview of, 345
      physical therapy tools for working with children, 345–46
   neurological and genetic disorders, 353–61
   orthopedic disorders, 348–53
   physical therapy examination and data collection, 344–45

special considerations when working with, 361–62
Pediculosis (lice), 278
Pelvic floor disorders/exercises, 250
Pelvic inflammatory disease (PID), 251
Pelvic pain, pregnancy-related, 250
Peptic ulcer disease, 246
Perceptual dysfunction, 96–97, 121
   agnosia, 96
   anosognosia, 96
   apraxia, 96–97
   body image disorders, 96
   body scheme disorder (somatognosia), 96
   homonymous hemianopsia, 96
   right/left discrimination disorder, 96
   spatial relations disorders, 96
   use as guide, 96
   visual spatial neglect (unilateral neglect), 96
Percussion, 206, 206b, 208t
Percussion test, 152
Percutaneous transluminal coronary angioplasty (PTCA), 162, 162t, 171
Performance, defined, 449b
Performance Feedback Request Form, I-6–I-7
Performance/learning, assessment of, 442–43
Performance-Oriented Mobility Assessment (POMA, Tinetti), 103t
Performance review/appraisal, 454
Performance scales measuring function and outcomes of therapy, 344–45
Perfusion (blood flow, or Q), 194
Pericardium, 142
Peripheral arterial circulation, tests of, 153
Peripheral arterial disease (PAD)
   in diabetes mellitus (DM), 258
   exercise training for patients with, 176–77
   intermittent claudication (IC), 150
   lower extremity exercise, 177
   outpatient cardiac rehabilitation, 173
Peripheral edema, 152, 152t, 156t, 157
Peripherally inserted central catheters (PICC Line), 215
Peripheral nervous system (PNS), 85
Peripheral nervous system (PNS) disorders, 133–36
   axonal degeneration, 134
   Bell's palsy (facial paralysis), 134
   clinical picture, 134
   Guillain-Barré Syndrome (GBS), 134–35
   medical management, 136
   myasthenia gravis, 135
   neuropathies (peripheral neuropathy), 134
   pathology, 133–34
   postpolio syndrome, 135
   segmental demyelination, 134
   symptoms, 134
   trigeminal neuralgia (tic douloureux), 135–36
   Wallerian degeneration, 133
Peripheral vascular disease
   arterial disease, 164, 176–77
   differential diagnosis, 165–66t

evaluation, diagnosis, and prognosis, 164–66
intervention, 176–77
venous disease, 164–66, 177
Peripheral vascular system, physical examination of, 150–52
   edema, 152, 152t
   extremities, 150
      conditions observed, 152b
      pulse grading scale, 152b
      pulse locations, 151–52b
      skin color changes, 152b
   intermittent claudication, 150
   PTA's responsibilities in, 150
Peripheral venous circulation tests, 152–53
   air plethysmography (APG), 153
   Doppler ultrasound, 153
   percussion test, 152
   Trendelenburg's test, 153
Peritoneum, 248
Peritonitis, 248
Perseveration, 270
Personal factors, defined, 449b
Personality changes, 88b, 125
Pervasive developmental disorder (PDD), 359–60
Pes anserine bursitis, 59
Pes cavus (hollow foot), 62
Pes planus (flat foot), 62
Petechiae, 280
Petit mal seizures, 133
Phalen's test, 35t, 38f
Pharmacology. See Medications
Phenazopyridine, 255t
Phobias, 269
Phonophoresis, 376–77, 377b
Physical agents, 367–74
   cryotherapy, 371–74
   hydrotherapy, 369–71
   nonimmersion irrigation, 371
   superficial heat agents, methods of application, 368–69
   superficial thermotherapy, 367–68
Physical therapist assistants (PTA), I-5
   direction and supervision of, 474–75
   license, procedure for obtaining and retaining, I-6–I-7
      AIDS awareness training, I-6
      candidates with documented disabilities, I-6
      continuing education, I-7
      credentials evaluation, I-6
      endorsement, I-7
      fees, I-6
      fingerprinting, FBI check, vaccination, malpractice insurance, I-6
      FSBPT's role in, I-6
      jurisprudence examination, I-6
      license/regulation renewal, I-7
      retaking PTA Exam, I-7
      temporary license, I-6
      tests of English language proficiency, I-6
      transfers of scores to other jurisdictions, I-6–I-7
   PT/PTA team, roles and responsibilities, 464–65
   web links and e-mail addresses, I-8

Physical therapist assistants (PTA), roles and responsibilities
   cardiovascular disease, 146
   examination and data collection, 34–36
      anthropometric characteristics, 34
      electrodiagnostic testing, 41
      functional mobility and use of devices, 36
      integumentary integrity, 36
      laboratory tests, 41
      medical diagnostic exams and imaging, 36–41
         arthrography, 41
         bone scan (osteoscintigraphy), 41
         computed tomography (CT scan), 36, 40
         diagnostic ultrasound, 41
         discography, 40
         magnetic resonance imaging (MRI), 40, 41
         myelography, 41
         plain film radiography (x-ray), 36
   motor function, 34
   neurological dysfunction, 105–6
      exercise/activity difficulty, 106, 106t
      general intervention considerations, 105–6
      implementing treatment, 105
   neuromuscular physical therapy, 91
   pain, 34
   patient history and medical record review, 34
   in peripheral vascular system exam, 150–52
   posture, 34
   prior to and throughout patient care, 34
   range of motion/flexibility, 34
   special tests, 34, 35–36t
      active compression, 35t
      Adson's test, 35t, 37f
      anterior drawer test, 36t
      apprehension test, 35t
      biceps load II test, 35t
      biceps rupture "Popeye" sign, 35t
      drop arm test, 35t
      Eichhoff's test, 35t, 37f, 38f
      elbow flexion test, 35t
      Ely's test; negative, 39f
      Ely's test; positive, 39f
      Finkelstein's test, 35t
      grind (scouring) test, 38f
      Hawkins-Kennedy test, 35t
      hip scour test, 36t
      horizontal adduction test, 35t
      jerk test, 35t
      Lachman stress test, 36t, 40f
      for lower extremities, 36t
      McMurray's test, 41f
      McMurray test, 36t, 41f
      modified Ober test, 39f
      musculoskeletal, 34
      Neer's test, 35t, 37f
      Ober's test, 36t, 39f
      Patrick's (FABER) test, 36t, 38f
      Phalen's test, 35t, 38f
      posterior drawer test, 36t
      posterior sag sign, 36t
      PTA's role regarding, 34
      Roos elevated arm test, 35t

Physical therapist assistants (PTA), roles and responsibilities (*Cont.*)
    sulcus sign, 35*t*
    supraspinatus (empty can test), 35*t*, 37*f*
    Thomas test, 36*t*, 38*f*
    Tinel's sign, 35*t*
    Trendelenburg sign, 36*t*, 40*f*
    two-point discrimination test, 35*t*
    for upper extremities, 35*t*
    varus/valgus stress tests, 35*t*, 36*t*
    Yergason test, 35*t*
Physical therapy examination and data collection. *See* Data collection; Examination
Physical therapy management, 122
Physiology. *See* Anatomy and physiology
Pia mater, 89
Pigmentation of skin, changes in, 282*t*
Piles (hemorrhoids), 248
Piriformis syndrome, 57–58
Pitting edema, 152
Pituitary gland, 257
Pituitary tumors, 265
Plain film radiography (x-ray). *See* X-ray (plain film radiography)
Plantar fasciitis, 63
Plasma, 235
Plasticity of soft tissue, 24
Platelets (PLTs), 155*t*, 235, 236*t*
Pleura, 191
Pleural effusion, 205
Pleural injury, 204
Plexuses, 91
Plyometric training, 6
Pneumatic compression pumps, 184
Pneumococcal pneumonia, 200*b*
Pneumocystis carinii pneumonia (PCP), 200
Pneumonectomy, 212
Pneumonia, 199, 200*b*
Pneumothorax, 204
PNF hold-relax-contract technique, 75
Pointing and past pointing test, 101*t*
Point of maximal impulse (PMI), 151*b*
Policy and procedures, 452
Polymyositis (PM), 279
Polyneuropathy, 134
Polysynaptic or inverse stretch reflex, 91
Pons, 87
Pontine lesion, 321*t*
Popliteal pulse, 151*b*
Position in space deficit, 96
Positive expiratory pressure (PEP) masks, 210
Postconcussion syndrome, 126
Posterior border of bony thorax, 191
Posterior cerebral artery syndrome, 119, 120*t*
Posterior cord syndrome, 127, 128*t*
Posterior cruciate ligament (PCL), 58, 71, 72
Posterior/dorsal regions, 90
Posterior drawer test, 36*t*
Posterior instability tests, 35*t*
Posterior rolling walker, 347
Posterior sag sign, 36*t*
Posterior tibial pulse, 151*b*
Posterolateral bulge/herniation, 65–66
Postpolio syndrome, 135
Postthrombotic syndrome (PTS), 164
Posttraumatic ischemia, 130
Posttraumatic stress disorder (PTSD), 269–70

Postural awareness training, 15
Postural/bronchial drainage, 206, 207*f*, 208*t*
Postural control, 12, 14, 17
Postural stability training, 12–14
    common errors in, 13
    dynamic stabilization, controlled mobility, 12
    dynamic stabilization, static-dynamic control, 12
    guidelines to develop postural stability, 12–13
    stability (static postural control), 12
    stability ball training, 13–14
Postural stress syndrome (PSS), 16
Postural sway (weight shifts), 15
Postural tremor, 99*t*
Posture
    in human development, 338, 342–43
    in physical therapy examination, 34
Potassium, 254
Preambulation mat activities, with progression, 114–15, 115*b*
Preambulation parallel activities, 115
Prediabetes, 258
Predictive validity, 487
Prednisone, 312*t*
Preeclampsia, 250–51
Pregnancy, normal, 248–50
Pregnancy-related pathologies, 250–51
Preinfarction (unstable angina), 158
Presbycusis, 306
Presenile dementia Alzheimer's type (PDAT), 324*t*
Pressoreceptors (baroreceptors), 145*b*
Pressure injury (decubitus ulcer or bed sore), 288–89
Primary adrenal insufficiency (Addison's Disease), 265
Primary brain damage, 122
Primary CNS neoplasms, 116
Primary degenerative dementia, 325
Prinzmetal's angina (variant angina), 158
Problem oriented medical record (POMR), 449
Profile of Function and Impairment Level Experience with Parkinson's Disease (PROFILE PD), 118
Program evaluation, 453
Progression, general principles of, 18, 18*t*
Progressive resistive exercise (PRE), 6
Progress notes, 450
Prolonged mechanical stretching, 10
Pronation/supination test, 101*t*
Prone on elbows/hands (preambulation mat activities), 114
Prone stander, 347
Proprioception, 89*t*, 94*t*, 102, 127, 128*t*
Proprioceptive neuromuscular facilitation (PNF), 106–7, 106*b*
    in coordination and balance training, 15, 16
    diagonal patterns, 108*t*
    feedback, 112
    in mobility and flexibility training, 10
    NDT differentiated from, 106*b*
    in postural stability training, 13
    in strength training, 3
    techniques for, 75, 107*t*, 109*t*
Prospective review, 453

Prostatitis, 252
Prosthetics, 414–21
    amputation, levels of, 414, 415*b*
    general concepts, 414
    lower-limb prosthetics (LLPs), 414–17
    physical therapy intervention, 417–21
    preprosthetic management, 418–19
    prosthetic gait deviations, 419–21, 420*t*
    prosthetic management, 419
    upper-limb prosthetics (ULPs), 417
Prothrombin time (PT), 155*t*, 235, 236
Provision of services for pediatric patients, legislation guiding, 361–62
Proximal humeral fractures, 51
Proximal interphalangeal (PIP) joint, 30*t*, 55, 319
Pruritus, 281*t*
Pseudohypertrophic muscular dystrophy (Duchenne muscular dystrophy), 358–59
Pseudomonas aeruginosa, 202
Psoriasis, 278
Psoriatic arthritis, 43
Psychiatric conditions, 269–71
    death and dying, 271
    grief process, 270
    interventions, 271
    pathologies, 269–70
    psychiatric states/mechanisms, 269
Psychogenic shock, 459
Psychosocial considerations, in musculoskeletal physical therapy, 80
Psychosomatic disorders (somatoform disorders), 270
Pulmonary artery catheter (Swan-Ganz catheter), 215
Pulmonary edema, 204, 205*t*
Pulmonary embolism (PE), 164, 165, 204, 205, 205*t*
Pulmonary endurance strategies, 7, 8
Pulmonary function tests (PFTs), 197
Pulmonary system
    aging patients, 308–9
    anatomy and physiology, 191–94, 191*f*
        bony thorax, 191
        breathing mechanisms, 193
        control of ventilation, 194
        internal structures, 191
        muscles of ventilation, 191–92, 192*b*, 192*t*
        perfusion (blood flow, or Q), 194
        respiration, 193–94
        ventilation, 193, 194
    chapter review questions and answers, 217, 502–3
    intensive care unit management, 214–16
    medical tests and examinations, 197–99
        abnormal acid-base balance, 197, 198*t*
        arterial blood gases (ABGs), 197, 198*t*
        bronchoscopy, 197
        classification of obstructive lung disease, 197, 198*t*
        exercise tolerance test (ETT), 197
        graded exercise test termination criteria, 199*t*
        laboratory tests, 197
        lung volumes, 199*f*
        radiographic examination, 197, 197*f*

physical dysfunction/impairments, 199–205
  acute diseases, 199–201
  bronchogenic carcinoma, 203–4
  chronic obstructive diseases, 201–2
  chronic restrictive diseases, 203
  other pulmonary conditions, 204–5
  trauma, 204
physical therapy examination and data collection, 195–99
  auscultation with stethoscope, 196
  chest wall excursion, 195–96
  data collection, 195–96
  medical tests and examinations, 197–99
  observation, 195–96
  patient interview, 195
  vital signs, 195
physical therapy intervention, 206–13
  airway clearance techniques, 208–9
  breathing exercises, 210–11
  functional abilities, activities for increasing, 211–12
  independent secretion removal techniques, 209–10
  in intensive care unit, 214–16
  manual secretion removal techniques, 206–8
  medical management, 213
  postsurgical care, 211
  surgical management, 212–13
spine and, 68
Pulmonic valve, 147
Pulsed lavage, 371
Pulsed short-wave diathermy (PSWD), 377–78
Pulse grading scale, 152b
Pulse measurement, 146, 147
Pulse oximetry, 216
Pursed lip breathing, 211
Pusher syndrome, 120t
Putamen, 87

Q

Q angle, 59
Quadruped (preambulation mat activity), 114
Quality assurance (QA), 452–53
Quality-of-life questionnaire, 118
Questions on PTA Exam
  critical reasoning
    in licensure exam performance, role of, I-12
    resources and references, I-15
    self-assessment questions, I-14t
    skills, improving, I-14–I-15
    subtypes of, I-12–I-3
  exam item difficulty, taxonomy of, I-10
  format, I-9
  levels of exam questions, I-10, I-11t
  multiple choice questions, strategies for answering, I-10–I-12
    clues, I-11
    crucial for survival, I-12
    key words, I-10, I-11
    negative words or phrases, I-12
    opposites, I-11
    overanalyze, I-12
    overlapping facts, I-12
    similar choices, I-11
  number of, I-9
  strategies to avoid, I-12
    change answer, I-12
    patterns, I-12
  successfully managing, I-10–I-13
  test item difficulty, I-10
  test item strategies, I-10

R

Radial pulse, 151b
Radiation therapy, 240, 241t
Radiculopathy, 134
Radiographic examination, pulmonary system, 197, 197f
Rales (crackles), 149, 159t, 201t, 205t
Raloxifene, 312t
Randomized controlled trial (RCT), 489
Random practice, 110, 112
Random sample, 486
Range of motion (ROM)
  active ROM (AROM), 4, 16
  aquatic exercise and, 17
  balance and, 15
  coordination and, 15
  exercise, 3, 4, 5–6, 5t
  flexibility and, 9, 12
  length tension relationship and, 2
  in physical therapy examination, 34
  relaxation and, 16
  resistance exercise and, 3, 5–6
  spinal, 12
  stretching and, 10–11
Rash, 281t
Rate of Perceived Exertion (RPE) scale, 160, 160b, 168, 170
Rate pressure product (RPP), 168
Rating of perceived exertion (RPE), 7b, 168
Ratio scale, 486, 486t
Raynaud's disease or phenomenon, 164
Rebound tenderness (Blumberg's sign), 247
Rebound test, 101t
Receptive dysfunction, 121
Receptors, 194
Reciprocal inhibition, 91
Reciprocating gait orthosis (RGO), 347
Rectal fissure, 248
Rectum, 248
Red blood cells (RBCs, erythrocytes), 155t, 236t
Referred pain, 150
Reflex arc, 91
Reflex bowel management programs, 130
Reflex integrity, 97–98, 97t
  Babinski reflex, 98
  deep tendon reflexes commonly tested, 97t
  grading scale for muscle reflexes, 98, 98t
Reflex sympathetic dystrophy (RSD), 136
Refractory periods, 86
Relative refractory period, 86
Relaxation training, 16–17, 170
  common errors in, 16–17
  relaxation, 16
  strategies to promote relaxation, 16
Reliability of research, 488
Remedial strategies, 14
Remodeling, 2
  bone, 24, 27
  phase of scar tissue formation, 27b
Renal and urological systems, 252–57
  aging patients, 310
  anatomy, 252–53, 253f
  disorders, 255–57
    medications and precautions, 255t
    obstructive disorders, 255, 256
    renal cystic disease, 255
    renal failure, 256
    urinary incontinence, 256–57
    urinary tract infections (UTIs), 255
  kidney functions, 253
  urinary regulation of fluids and electrolytes, 253–55
  urine, normal values of, 253
Renal calculi (kidney stones), 255, 256
Renal cystic disease, 255
Renal failure, 256
Repeated stretch (repeated contractions), 107t
Repetition maximum (RM), 6
Repetitive/cumulative trauma to the back, 68
Repetitive stress syndrome (carpal tunnel syndrome), 54
Repolarization, 86
Rescue drugs for pulmonary disease, 213
Research and evidence-based practice, 483–91
  chapter review questions and answers, 491, 517
  clinical prediction rule (CPR), 484, 485
  evidence, evaluating, 489–90, 490t
  evidence-based practice (EBP), PTs and PTAs use of, 484
  research design, 485–88
  roles and responsibilities, 484
Research design, 485–88
  hypothesis, 486
  informed consent, 487
  instrumentation, 487
  measurement, levels of, 486
  methods, 485
  objectivity, 488
  reliability, 488
  research quality, determining, 487–88
  responsiveness, 488
  sampling, 486, 487
  sensitivity and specificity, 488
  subjectivity, 488
  validity, 487–88
  variables, 485–86
Research quality, determining, 487–88
Residual volume (RV), 193
Resistance, electrical, 384t
Resistance exercise, 4–6. *See also* Strength training
  for cardiovascular disease, 174
  contraindications, 4
  errors associated with, 3
  exercise regimes, 6
    brief, repetitive isometric exercise, 6
    circuit weight training, 6
    plyometric training, 6
    progressive resistive exercise (PRE), 6

Index

Resistance exercise (Cont.)
  goals and indications for, 4
  manual, 3
  mechanical, 4
  precautions, 4
  resistance training specificity chart, 6t
  types, 4–6, 5t
    closed-chain exercise, 6
    concentric exercise, 5, 5t
    eccentric exercise, 5, 5t
    isokinetic exercise, 5, 5t
    isometric exercise, 4, 5t
    isotonic exercise, 4, 5, 5t
    open-chain exercise, 6
    range of motion exercise, 3, 4, 5–6, 5t
Resistance training specificity chart, 6t
Respiration, 149, 193–94
Respiratory acidosis, 254
Respiratory alkalosis, 255
Respiratory distress syndrome (RDS), 202
Respiratory rate (RR), 149
Respiratory shock, 459
Responsiveness in research, 488
Resting expiration, 192t
Resting heart rate (RHR), 7b
Resting inspiration, 192t
Resting or loose-packed position, 29, 30t
Resting posture, 91
Resting potential, 86
Resting tremors, 88b, 100t, 118
Restraints, use of, 456–57
Retaking PTA Exam, I-7
Reverse scapulothoracic rhythm, 31
Reversibility, 3
Reversibility principle, 7
Reversible dementia, 324–25
Rheumatoid arthritis (RA), 44, 318–19
  articulatory techniques and, 75, 76
  characteristics, 318
  description, 318
  intervention, 319
  joint protection principles, 319t
  joints deformities, 319
  joints impacted, 318–19
  juvenile rheumatoid arthritis (JRA), 44
  medical management, 319
  other tissues, 319
  in temporomandibular joint (TMJ), 47
Rheumatoid conditions, 42–44. See also Rheumatoid arthritis (RA)
  ankylosing spondylitis (Marie-Strümpell, Bechterew's, rheumatoid spondylitis), 42, 43
  gout, 43
  psoriatic arthritis, 43
  rheumatoid spondylitis, 42, 43
Rheumatoid factor (RF), 44
Rheumatoid spondylitis, 42, 43
Rhythmic initiation, 107t
Rhythmic rotation (RRo), 16, 107t
Rhythmic stabilization (RS), 13, 107t
Rib cage, 191, 193
Rib fracture, 204
Right atrium (RA), 142b
Right coronary artery (RCA), 142
Right/left discrimination disorder, 96
Rights, patient/client, 457–58
Right-sided heart failure, 158, 159t, 160b, 163t
Rigidity, 88b, 97t, 100t, 118, 123
Ringworm (tinea corporis), 277
Risk management, 451–52
Roles and responsibilities, 464–68, 484. See also Physical therapist assistants (PTA), roles and responsibilities
  caregiver definition and roles, 465–68
  clinical prediction rule (CPR), 484, 485
  collaboration, principles of, 465
  evidence-based practice (EBP), 484
  PT/PTA team, 464–65
Rolling (preambulation mat activity), 114
Rolling walker, 347
Roll movement, 28
Romberg's test, 102
Roos elevated arm test, 35t
Rotary-chair testing, 266
Rotator cuff
  pathology tests, 35t
  tear, 68
  tendinitis, 50
Rotavirus, 231t
Rubor, 152b, 153

S

S1 sound ("lub"), 147t
S2 sound ("dub"), 147t
Sacral nerves, 90
Sacral sparing, 127
Sacroiliac joint (SIJ) conditions, 67–68, 250
Safety
  body mechanics, 463–64
  fall prevention, 16, 455–56
  illegal practice and malpractice, 462–63
  injury prevention, 463
  patient safety and protection, 455–61
Saltatory conduction, 86
Sampling, 486, 487
Sarcoma, 240
Scabies (mites), 278
Scaphoid fracture, 54
Scapular stabilizers, 31
Scar mobilization, 169
Scar tissue adhesions, 11
Scar tissue formation, 26, 27, 27b
  phases of, 26, 27, 27b
  tissue healing times, 24–25t
Schedule
  feedback, 110
  practice, 112
Scheduling PTA Exam, I-16
Schizophrenia, 270
Scissoring, 121
Scleroderma, 279
Scores, PTA Exam
  reporting, I-5, I-6
  sanctioning of, due to fraud, I-17
  Score Transfer Service/Score Transfer Request Form, I-6–I-7
  transfers of, to other jurisdictions, I-6–I-7
Score Transfer Service/Score Transfer Request Form, I-6–I-7
Screening tests, for pediatric patients, 344
Seborrheic keratosis, 279
Secondarily generalized seizures, 133
Secondary adrenal insufficiency, 265
Secondary brain damage, 122
Secondary CNS neoplasms, 116
Secondary diabetes, 259
Secondary gain for staying ill, 80, 270, 271
Second-class lever, 28
Second-impact syndrome, 126
Secretion removal techniques
  airway clearance techniques, 208–9
  independent, 209–10
  manual, 206–8
Security Agreement, I-2
Segmental breathing, 210–11
Segmental demyelination, 134
Seizures, classifications of
  absence or petit mal seizures, 133
  complex partial seizure, 133
  generalized seizures, 133
  partial or focal seizures, 133
  secondarily generalized seizures, 133
  status epilepticus, 133
  temporal lobe seizure, 133
Selective serotonin reuptake inhibitors (SSRIs), 315t
Self-care and home-management (including ADL), 104
Semilunar valves, 142b
Senile dementia Alzheimer's type (SDAT), 324t, 325
Sensitivity and specificity in research, 488
Sensorineural hearing loss, 306
Sensory axons, 86–87
Sensory conflict situations, 16
Sensory control, 14, 17
Sensory impairments, 121
Sensory stimulation techniques, 108
Sensory systems
  in aging patients, 304–7
    hearing, 304, 305–6, 305b
    somatosensory, 306–7
    taste and smell, 307
    vestibular/balance control, 306
    vision, 304, 305b
  in aquatic exercise, 17
  in coordination and balance, 14
Sensory testing, 94–96, 94t
  assessment completed, 94–95
  combined (cortical) sensations, 94t, 96
  exteroceptive (superficial) sensations, 94t, 96
  neural screens commonly performed, 95t
  proprioceptive (deep) sensations, 94t, 96
  sensory testing commonly performed, 94t
  testing considerations, 96
Sensory training, 15–16
Sentinel event, 451–52
Septic shock, 459
Serial practice, 110, 112
Serotonin and norepinephrine reuptake inhibitors (SNRIs), 315t
Serum lipids panel, 156
Severe acute respiratory syndrome (SARS), 200
Severe concussion, 123
Severe TBI, 123t
Sex hormones, 248
Sexual dysfunction in spinal cord injury, 130
Sexual harassment, 454–55, 458
Shaking (vibration) techniques, 206, 206b, 208, 208t

Sharp/dull discrimination, 94t, 96
Sharpened or tandem Romberg, 102
Shingles (herpes zoster), 276, 277, 277b
Shin splints (anterior tibial periostitis), 60
Shock (hypoperfusion), 237, 459
Short-acting beta-2 agonists for pulmonary disease, 213
Short-arc exercise, 5
Short Physical Performance Battery (SPPB), 103t
Short-term recall, 93
Short-wave diathermy (SWD), 377–78, 377b
Shoulder
 abnormal synergies, 99t
 capsular patterns, 30t
 conditions of, 48–51
  acromioclavicular and sternoclavicular joint disorders, 50
  adhesive capsulitis (frozen shoulder), 51
  bicipital tendinitis, 51
  glenohumeral subluxation and dislocation, 48
  impingement syndrome, 50
  instability, 48–49
  internal (posterior) impingement, 50–51
  labral tears, 49
  proximal humeral fractures, 51
  rotator cuff tendinitis, 50
  subacromial/subdeltoid bursitis, 50
  thoracic outlet syndrome (TOS), 49–50
 in convex-concave rule, 29t, 30t
 patterns of spasticity in upper motor neuron syndrome, 92t
 PNF diagonal patterns, 108t
 tests for, 35t
 traction injuries to flaccid, avoiding, 105
Shoulder girdle, 191
Shunt, 194
Sickle cell anemia, 360–61
Sickle cell crisis, 238
Sickle cell disease, 237–38
Sinemet, 119, 322
Single axis foot orthosis, 415b
Sinoatrial (SA) node, 142
Sit-down (SIT) activity, 15
Sitting (preambulation mat activity), 114
Sitting tests, 102
Sit-to-stand (STS) activity, 15
Skeletal system. *See also* Musculoskeletal system
 in aging patients, 303
 conditions, 44
Skin cancer, 279–80
Skin or integument, 275
 conditions and descriptions, 281–82t
 skin cancer, 279–80
 skin trauma, 280
Skin ulcers, 287–95
 arterial ulcer, 288
 diabetic ulcer, 288, 288f
 pressure injury (decubitus ulcer or bed sore), 288–89
 venous ulcers (stasis ulcers), 287–88
 wound assessment, 289–90
 wound care, 290–95

Skip lesions, 247
Skull, 89
SLAP lesion (superior labrum anterior to posterior), 35t, 48, 49
Slipped capital femoral epiphysis (SCFE), 58, 349, 350
Slow-twitch (ST) fibers (Type I), 2b
Smell in aging patients, 307
Smith's fracture, 54
Socioeconomic costs, of aging patients, 299–300
Sodium, 254
Soft tissue
 in aging patients, 302–3
 conditions, 45–48
  bursitis, 46
  complex regional pain syndrome (CRPS), 47
  idiopathic scoliosis, 47
  muscle strains, 46
  myofascial pain syndrome, 45
  myositis ossificans, 46–47
  Paget's disease (osteitis deformans), 47
  temporomandibular joint (TMJ) conditions, 47–48
  tendinitis, 45, 45b
  tendinosis, 45b, 46
  torticollis, 47
 degree of strain or sprain, 26, 26t
 elasticity, 24
 grades of movement, 26f
 healing/scar tissue formation in, 26, 27, 27b
 plasticity, 24
 response to stress, 24, 26
 specific interventions, 74–77
  articulatory techniques, 75–76
  neural tissue mobilization, 76
  neurodynamic exercises, 76
  soft tissue/myofascial techniques, 74–75
  therapeutic exercise for musculoskeletal conditions, 76–77
Soft tissue/myofascial techniques, 74–75
Solid ankle cushion heel (SACH) foot orthosis, 415b
Solid ankle flexible endoskeleton (SAFE) foot orthosis, 415b
Somatoform disorders (psychosomatic disorders), 270
Somatognosia (body scheme disorder), 96
Somatosensory system, 14, 15, 17
 in aging patients, 306–7
 balance and, 102
Somatostatin, 258
Space occupying lesion, 266b
Spasticity, 97t, 121, 127, 129b
 modified Ashworth's scale for, 97, 97t
 typical patterns of, 92, 92t
Spatial relations deficit/disorders, 96
Specificity principle, 6
Specific manipulation, 76
Speech and communication impairments, 120–21
 damage to parieto-occipital cortex, 120
 dysarthria, 121
 expressive dysfunction, 120–21
 fluent aphasia, 121
 global aphasia, 121

nonfluent aphasia, 120
 receptive dysfunction, 121
 verbal apraxia, 120
Speech/language disorders, 444–45
Spina bifida, 356–58
Spinal accessory nerve (CN XI), 90t, 95t
Spinal conditions, 64–68. *See also* Spinal cord injury (SCI)
 acceleration/deceleration injuries (whiplash), 66–67
 bone tumors, 68
 cardiovascular and pulmonary conditions, 68
 central posterior bulge/herniation, 66
 disc, 65–66
 facet joint conditions, 66
 fracture, 352
 gastrointestinal conditions, 68
 hypermobile spinal segments, 67
 multilevel vertebral fusion for, 73
 muscle strain, 64
 repetitive/cumulative trauma to the back, 68
 sacroiliac joint (SIJ) conditions, 67–68
 spina bifida, 356–58
 spinal disc conditions, 65–66
 spinal or intervertebral stenosis, 65
 spinal shock, 129b
 spinal stenosis, 42, 42t, 43t
 spondylolysis/spondylolisthesis, 64
 surgical repairs of, 72–73
 Urological and gynecological conditions, 68
 visceral tumors, 68, 69f
Spinal cord anatomy, 90–91
 anterior/ventral regions, 90
 cross-section, 90, 90f
 gray matter, 90
 meninges, 90
 posterior/dorsal regions, 90
 purpose and structure, 90
Spinal cord dysesthesia, 130
Spinal cord injury (SCI), 126–31
 abdominal musculature, patients who lack, 192
 autonomic dysreflexia (autonomic hyperreflexia, hyperreflexia), 129b, 130
 basic information, 126
 bowel and bladder dysfunction, 130
 changes associated with recovery, 127, 129b
  autonomic dysreflexia (autonomic hyperreflexia, hyperreflexia), 129b
  deep venous thrombosis (DVT), 129b
  heterotopic bone formation (ectopic bone), 129b
  spasticity/spasms, 127, 129b
  spinal shock, 129b
 classification, 126
 clinical picture, 126–27
 clinical syndromes, 127, 128t
  anterior cord syndrome, 127, 128t
  Brown-Séquard syndrome, 127, 128t
  cauda equina, 127, 128t
  central cord syndrome, 127, 128t
  complete cord syndrome, 128t
  posterior cord syndrome, 127, 128t
  sacral sparing, 127

831

Spinal cord injury (SCI) (Cont.)
  deep venous thrombosis (DVT), 129b, 130
  degree of injury, 126
    American Spinal Injury Association (ASIA) Impairment Scale, 126, 127b
    complete, 126, 127b
    incomplete, 126, 127b
  examination, 127
  functional table, 132t
  heterotopic bone formation (ectopic bone), 129b, 130
  level of injury: UMN injury, 126
    lesion level, 126
    paraplegia, 126
    tetraplegia (quadriplegia), 126
  medical management, 130–31
    fracture stabilization, 131
    medication to limit posttraumatic ischemia and address secondary complications, 130
  other clinical considerations, 129–30
    autonomic dysreflexia (autonomic hyperreflexia, hyperreflexia), 129b, 130
    bowel and bladder dysfunction, 130
    deep venous thrombosis (DVT), 129b, 130
    heterotopic bone formation (ectopic bone), 129b, 130
    sexual dysfunction, 130
    spinal cord dysesthesia, 130
  physical therapy goals, outcomes, and interventions, 127, 129
  physical therapy management, 131
  sexual dysfunction, 130
  spinal cord dysesthesia, 130
Spinal nerves, 90–91
  brachial plexus, 91
  cauda equina, 90
  cervical, 90
  coccygeal segments, 90
  dermatome distribution, 90, 91f
  dorsal (posterior) rami, 91
  dorsal roots, 90
  lumbar, 90
  lumbosacral plexus, 91
  plexuses, 91
  sacral, 90
  thoracic, 90
  ventral (anterior) rami, 91
  ventral roots, 90
Spinal (trunk) orthoses, components/terminology, 410–11
Spinal range of motion (ROM), 12
Spinal reflexes, 91
Spinal shock, 129b
Spinal stenosis, 42, 42t, 43t, 65
Spin movement, 29
Spleen, 222
Spondylolysis/spondylolisthesis, 64
Sprains, foot and ankle, 61
Sputum studies, 197
Stability ball training, 13–14, 15
Stabilizing reversals (alternating isometrics), 107t
Stable angina, 158
Staff management, 464
Stages, death and dying (Kübler-Ross), 271

Staging, cancer, 240
Stance phase, 397, 399
Standard precautions, 225–28b, 234
Standards of Practice, 471–73
Standing (preambulation mat activity), 115
Standing tests, 102, 102t
Staphylococcal infections, 202, 230
Staphylococcus aureus (SA), 202, 230
Static balance, 102, 104t
Static-dynamic control, 12
Static standing test, 102t
Status epilepticus, 133
Statutory laws impacting physical therapy, 462
Stem cell (bone marrow) transplant, 240, 241t
Stemmer's sign, 181
Stepping/step test, 102t, 166
Stepping strategies, 15
Stereognosis, 94t, 96, 128t
Sterilization, 234
Sternal angle (angle of Louis), 191
Sternoclavicular joint, 29t, 30t, 50
Sternocleidomastoid (SCM) muscle, 47
Sternum, 191
Steroids, 312t
Stocking/glove distribution, 134
Stomach, 246
Stratified sample, 487
Strength training, 2–4. *See also* Resistance exercise
  common errors associated with, 3
  exercises to improve strength and range, 3–4
  guidelines to develop strength, 3
  to improve aerobic capacity and muscular endurance, 16
  metabolic effects of, 3
  to modify effects of aging, 28
  motor fiber type, 2, 2b
  muscle function and strength, concepts of, 2
  muscular adaptations of, 2–3
  overload principle, 3
  positive changes in response to, 3
  reversibility, 3
  specificity of training, 3
  strength, defined, 2
Streptococcal infections, 230, 232
Stress
  management, in relaxation training, 16, 17
  musculoskeletal system affected by, 24, 26–27
Stress fracture, 27, 61
Stress incontinence, 256
Stretching, 10–11
  contractile tissue in, 11
  contracture, 11
  effective, 10
  to improve aerobic capacity and muscular endurance, 16
  noncontractile tissue in, 11
  overstretching, 11
  purpose of, 10
  types of, 10–11
    active stretching, 10
    ballistic stretching, 10
    determining, 10
    dynamic stretching, 10

    facilitated stretching, 10–11
    manual static, passive stretching, 10
    prolonged mechanical stretching, 10
Stretch-protection reflex, 91
Stretch reflex, 97, 97t
Stretch-shortening activity, 6
Stretch weakness, 11
Stroke. *See* Cerebral vascular accident (CVA, stroke)
Stroke volume (SV), 143
Subacromial impingement tests, 35t
Subacromial/subdeltoid bursitis, 50
Subacute phase/moderate protection, 73–74
Subarachnoid hemorrhage, 119
Subcutaneous tissues, 275t
Subdermal burn, 284t
Subdural hemorrhage, 119
Submalleolar orthosis (SMO), 347
Submalleolar shoe insert, 347
Submaximal ETT, 166
Sulci, 87
Sulcus sign, 35t
Sulfamethoxazole/trimethoprim, 255t
Sunrise view, 59
Superficial burn, 284t
Superficial heat agents, methods of application, 368–69
Superficial partial thickness burn, 284t
Superficial thermotherapy, 367–68, 367b
Superior labrum anterior to posterior (SLAP lesion), 35t, 48, 49
Supine stander, 347
Supplemental oxygen, 215–16
Supportive feedback, 112
Supraspinatus (empty can test), 35t, 37f
Surface electrodes/sensors, 391
Surgical intervention. *See also* Transplantation
  acute coronary syndrome (ACS), 162t
  cardiovascular disease, 162, 162t
  carotid endarterectomy, 121
  lung volume reduction surgery (LVRS), 212
  obesity, 263, 263t
  orthopedic
    lateral retinacular release, 72
    ligamentous repairs of the knee, 71, 72, 72t
    lower extremity, 70–73
    meniscal arthroscopy, 72
    multilevel vertebral fusion, 73
    open reduction internal fixation (ORIF) after femoral fracture, 71
    physical therapy goals, outcomes, and interventions following surgery, 73
    rotator cuff tear, 68
    surgical repairs of spine, 72–73
    tendon injuries and repairs of the hand, 69–70
    total hip replacement (THR)/arthroplasty, 70, 70t
    total knee replacement (TKR)/arthroplasty, 71, 71t
    upper extremity, 68–70
  pulmonary system, 212–13
  spinal conditions, 72–73
Sustained attention, 93
Sustained maximal inspiration (SMI), 211
Swan-Ganz catheter, 215

Swan neck deformity, 55–56, 55f, 319
Sweating with immersion, 17
Swimmers (buoyant dumbbells), 17
Swing phase, 399–400
Swiss ball, 13
Symmetrical weight distribution, 14, 17
Sympathetic division, 85, 85f
Sympathetic stimulation (adrenergic), 144, 145
Sympathetic system, 144
Symptom modifying medications, 315t
Synapse, 86
Syndrome X, 259
Systemic review (SR), 489
Systemic sample, 487
Systole, 142
Systolic heart failure, 163t

T1/T2 imaging, 40–41
Tachycardia, 147, 155t, 159t, 163t, 168, 175, 201t, 205t
Tachypnea, 149, 201t, 205t
Tactile localization, 94t, 96
Talipes equinovarus (clubfoot), 62
Talocrural joint, 63
Tapping test, 101t
Tarsal tunnel syndrome, 61
Task selection, 114
Task-specific training strategies, 113–14
  adherence-enhancing behavioral strategies, 114
  behavioral shaping techniques, 113
  constraint-induced (CI) movement therapy, 114
  general concepts, 113, 113b
  locomotor training, 114
  task selection, 114
Taste in aging patients, 307
Teaching and learning, 435–46
  chapter review questions and answers, 446, 515
  communication, 443–45
  educational theories, 436–37
  instruction, 437–40
  motor learning, 440–43
Telemetry (ambulatory monitoring), 168
Temperature of skin, changes in, 282t
Temperature sensation, 94t, 96
Temporal lobe, 87, 88b, 89t
Temporal lobe seizure, 133
Temporary license, I-6
Temporomandibular joint (TMJ)
  acceleration/deceleration injuries (whiplash), 66
  capsular patterns, 30t
  conditions, 47–48
  in convex-concave rule, 29t
  dysfunctions (TMD), 47–48
  positions, 30t
Tendinitis, 45, 45b
  Achilles', 61
  bicipital, 51
  patellar, 59
  rotator cuff, 50
Tendon injuries and repairs of the hand, 69–70

Tendonosis, 45b, 46, 61
Tennis elbow (lateral epicondylitis), 52
Tensor fascia latae (TFL), 31
Tetraplegia (quadriplegia), 126
Texts used in PTA programs, I-2
Texture recognition, 94t, 96
Thalamic pain syndrome, 88b, 120t
Thalamus, 87, 88b
Therapeutic exercise, 2–18
  aquatic exercise, 17–18
    contraindications, 18
    exercise applications, 17–18
    goals and outcomes, 17
    physics related to, 17
    precautions, 18
    special equipment, 17
    strategies, 17
    thermodynamics, 17
  chapter review questions and answers, 19, 494–95
  coordination and balance training, 14–16
    goals and outcomes, 14
    interventions to improve aerobic capacity and muscular endurance, 16
    interventions to improve balance, 15–16
    interventions to improve coordination, 15
    training strategies, 14
  endurance training, 6–9
    aerobic training, 8
    cardiovascular endurance strategies, 6, 7
    FITT equation, 7, 7b
    individual differences principle, 7
    muscular endurance strategies, 6
    overload principle, 6
    pulmonary endurance strategies, 7, 8
    reversibility principle, 7
    specificity principle, 6
    training errors to avoid, 9
  mobility and flexibility training, 9–12
    common errors in, 12
    flexibility, 9
    relaxation of muscles, 11–12
    stretching, 10–11
  musculoskeletal conditions, 76–77
  postural stability training, 12–14
    common errors in, 13
    dynamic stabilization, controlled mobility, 12
    dynamic stabilization, static-dynamic control, 12
    guidelines to develop postural stability, 12–13
    stability (static postural control), 12
    stability ball training, 13–14
  progression, general principles of, 18, 18t
  relaxation training, 16–17
    common errors in, 16–17
    relaxation, 16
    strategies to promote relaxation, 16
  resistance exercise, 4–6 (See also Strength training)
    contraindications, 4
    errors associated with, 3
    exercise regimes, 6
    goals and indications for, 4

    manual, 3
    mechanical, 4
    precautions, 4
    resistance training specificity chart, 6t
    types of, 4–6, 5t
  strength training, 2–4
    common errors associated with, 3
    exercises to improve strength and range, 3–4
    guidelines to develop strength, 3
    to improve aerobic capacity and muscular endurance, 16
    metabolic effects of, 3
    motor fiber type, 2, 2b
    muscle function and strength, concepts of, 2
    muscular adaptations of, 2–3
    overload principle, 3
    positive changes in response to, 3
    reversibility, 3
    specificity of training, 3
    strength, defined, 2
  weather conditions, 9
Therapeutic modalities, 365–93
  chapter review questions and answers, 393, 512–13
  deep thermotherapy, 374–78
  electrical stimulation (ES), 383–87
  massage, 382–83
  mechanical agents, 378–82
  physical agents, 367–74
Thermodynamics, 17
Third-class lever, 28
Thomas test, 36t, 38f
Thoracic nerves, 90
Thoracic outlet syndrome (TOS), 35t, 49–50
Thoracolumbosacral orthosis (TLSO), 347, 347b
Thoracotomy, 213
Thrill, 147t
Thromboangiitis obliterans (Buerger's disease), 164
Thrombolytic therapy for cardiovascular disease, 161t
Thrombus, 119
Thumb deformities, 319
Thymus gland, 222
Thyroid C cells, 258
Thyroid disorders, 265
Thyroid gland, 258
Thyrotropin-releasing hormone (TRH), 257
Thyroxine, 258
Tidal volume (TV), 193
Tightness/friction disorder, 57
Tilt table, 382
Timed tests for power and endurance, 99
Timed Up and Go (TUG), 103t
Tinea corporis (ringworm), 277
Tinea pedis (athlete's foot), 277
Tinel's sign, 35t
Tissue
  assessment, integumentary system, 280–81
  healing times, 24–25t, 26
  immobilization, 28, 28b
  response to stress, 24–27
  soft tissue, 24, 26
  structure and function, 23–24

Tissue (Cont.)
    articular cartilage, 23
    bone, 24, 25t, 27
    collagen types I and II, 23, 25t
    dense, irregular connective tissue, 23
    dense, regular connective tissue, 23
    elastin fibers, 23
    fibrocartilage, 23–24
    loose, irregular connective tissue, 23
    muscle, 24, 25t
  tension, connective tissue mobilization for, 31
    fascia techniques, 31
    muscle techniques, 31
    transverse friction techniques, 31
    transverse muscle techniques, 31
Tissue plasminogen activator (TPA), 121
T-lymphocytes, 223
Toe to examiner's finger test, 101t
Topographical disorientation, 96
Torticollis, 47
Total hip replacement (THR)/arthroplasty, 70, 70t, 115
Total knee replacement (TKR)/arthroplasty, 71, 71t
Total lung capacity (IRV + TV + ERV + RV), 193
Touch-down weight bearing (TDWB), 70t, 71t
Tracheal stimulation, 209
Traction, 76
Training level or target (THR), 7b
Training programs. *See* Therapeutic exercise
Training strategies, 14
Tranquilizers for cardiovascular disease, 161, 161t
Transcutaneous electrical nerve stimulation (TENS), 45, 239, 242, 251, 387–89
Transfemoral (above-knee) prosthesis, 416–17
Transfer, assisted devices for, 426–27
Transfer, in motor learning, 110
Transfer training, 425
Transitional stabilization, 13
Translocation Down Syndrome, 358b
Transmural infarction, 158
Transplantation
  cardiac, 162, 162t
  lung, 203
  lymph node, 184
  renal, 238, 255, 256
  stem cell (bone marrow), 240, 241t
Transtibial (below knee) prosthesis, 414, 415–16, 415b
Transverse friction massage, 75
Transverse friction techniques, 31
Transverse muscle techniques, 31
Trauma. *See also* Traumatic brain injury (TBI)
  nerve injury, 134
  pulmonary system, 204
  repetitive/cumulative, to the back, 68
  skin, 280
Traumatic brain injury (TBI), 122–25
  amnesia, 123
  behavioral changes, 123
  clinical picture, 123
  focal lesion, 122
  Glasgow Coma Scale (GCS), 123
  level of cognitive functioning (LOCF), Rancho Los Amigos, 123, 124t
  levels of brain injury, 123, 123t
  mechanism of injury, 122
  medical management, 123
  motor impairments and muscle tone, 123
  pathophysiology, 122–23
    concussion, 122–23
    primary brain damage, 122
    secondary brain damage, 122
  in pediatric patients, 356
  physical therapy management, 123–25
    issues to be addressed, 123, 124
    management with decreased response levels (LOCF I–III), 124–25
    management with high-level recovery (LOCF VII–VIII), 125
    management with mid-level recovery (LOCF IV–VI), 125
  types of head injury, 122
Traumatic instability, 48
Traumatic nerve injury, 134
Treadmill training (TT), 16, 114, 166
Trendelenburg sign, 36t, 40f, 121, 153
Triceps surae, 60, 61, 62, 63, 72
Tricuspid valve, 147
Tricyclics, 314t
Trigeminal nerve (CN V), 90t, 95t
Trigeminal neuralgia (tic douloureux), 95t, 117, 135–36
Trigger point injections, 48, 64, 65, 66, 67
Trigger points, 45
Triglycerides, 154b
Triiodothyronine, 258
Trisomy 21 (Down Syndrome), 65, 66, 67, 75, 76, 358, 358b
Trochanteric bursitis, 57
Trochlear nerve (CN IV), 90t, 95t
Trunk coordination, lack of, 88b
Trunk movements, 15
Tuberculosis (TB), 199, 233–34
Tumor necrosis factor (TNF) inhibitors, 43
Tumors
  bone, 68
  brain, 353
  malignant, 240, 279–80
  medical interventions, 240, 241t
  pituitary, 265
  skin, 279
  visceral, 68, 69f
Tunneled CVAD, 214
Turbulence, 17, 18, 371
Two-point discrimination, 35t, 94t, 96, 128t
Type 1 diabetes mellitus (T1DM), 258–59
Type 2 diabetes mellitus (T2DM), 259

U

Ulcerative colitis (UC), 247
Ulnar collateral ligament injuries, 53
Ultrasound, 374–77
  application, methods of, 376–77
    direct contact, 376
    indirect contact, 376
    phonophoresis, 376–77, 377b
  applicator, 374
  biophysics related to, 374–77
  conversion, 374
  goals and indications for use of non-thermal, 375b
  physiological effects of, 375
  precautions and contraindications, 376b
  spatial characteristics of, 374
  temporal characteristics of, 374–75
  transducer size, 374
Unfractionated heparin (UFH), 164
Unhappy triad, 58
Unified Rating Scale for Parkinsonism (MDSUPDRS), 118
Unilateral edema, 152
Unilateral neglect (visual spatial neglect), 96
Universal precautions, 234
University of California Biomechanics Laboratory (UCBL) shoe insert, 347
Unmyelinated axons, 87
Unstable angina (preinfarction, crescendo angina), 158
Upper airways, 191
Upper extremities (UEs)
  abnormal synergies, 99t
  amputations, 415b
  conditions of
    elbow, 51–53
    shoulder, 48–51
    wrist and hand, 54–56
  in coordination and balance training, 15, 16
  orthopedic surgical repairs, 68–70
  patterns of spasticity in upper motor neuron syndrome, 92t
  in postural stability training, 12
  tests for, 35t
  upper-limb orthoses or splints, 411–12
  upper-limb prosthetics (ULPs), 417
Upper-limb orthoses or splints, 411–12
Upper-limb prosthetics (ULPs), 417
Upper motor neuron (UMN) syndrome, 92t, 98, 98t
Uremia, 256
Urge incontinence, 256
Urinalysis findings, 253
Urinary incontinence, 256–57
Urinary regulation of fluids and electrolytes, 253–55
  acid-base balance, 254–55
  calcium, 254
  fluid imbalances, 253–54
  homeostasis, 253
  magnesium, 254
  potassium, 254
  sodium, 254
Urinary tract infections (UTIs), 130, 252, 255
Urine, normal values of, 253
Urological conditions affecting spine, 68
Urticaria, 281t
Utilization review (UR), 452–53

V

Vaccinations for pulmonary disease, 213
Vagus nerve (CN X), 90t, 95t
Validity, research, 487–88
  threats to, 487–88
  types, 487

Valsalva's maneuver, 3, 4, 5t, 170, 246
Vancomycin-resistant enterococci (VRE), 232t
Vancomycin-resistant *Staphylococcus aureus* (MRSA), 230
Variable practice, 110
Variables, research, 485–86
Variant angina (Prinzmetal's angina), 158
Varicose veins, 164, 250
Varus foot, 121
Varus/valgus stress tests, 35t, 36t
Vascular claudication, 42t
Vascular system, 143–44, 144b
Vastus medialis oblique (VMO) muscle, 59
Veins, 143, 144b, 144f
Venous disease
  evaluation, diagnosis and prognosis, 164–66
  rehabilitation guidelines, 177
Venous filling time, 153
Venous thromboembolism (VTE), 164, 177
Venous ulcers (stasis ulcers), 287–88
Venous valvular insufficiency, 165
Ventilation, 193, 194
  control of, 194
  defined, 7
  muscles of, 191–92, 192t, 194
Ventilation perfusion gravity dependent, 194
Ventilation perfusion ratio (V/Q ratio), 194
Ventral (anterior) rami, 91
Ventral roots, 90
Ventricular assist device (VAD) for cardiovascular disease, 162, 162t
Ventricular function, impaired, 158, 162, 162t
Verbal apraxia, 120
Verbal communication, 443
Vermiform appendix, 247
Vertebral canal, 90
Vertebrobasilar artery syndrome, 119, 120t
Vertical disorientation, 96
Vertical sleeve gastrectomy, 263t
Vertigo, 266, 266b
Vestibular control in aging patients, 306
Vestibular evoked myogenic potential (VEMP) test, 266
Vestibular pathology, dizziness or nausea associated with, 14
Vestibular stimulation, 16, 109t
Vestibular system, 266–68
  balance and, 102
  etiology, 266–68
  examination, 267, 268b
  medical evaluation and testing, 266–67
  overview of, 266
  physical therapy evaluation, 267
  physical therapy goals, outcomes, and interventions, 267, 268
  vertigo, 266, 266b

Vestibulocochlear nerve (CN VIII), 90t, 95t
Vibration, 94t, 96, 127, 128t, 131
Videostagmography (VNG), 266
Viral gastroenteritis, 231t
Viral infections, 276–77
Viral pneumonia, 200b
Visceral pleura, 191
Visceral tumors, 68, 69f
Vision
  in aging patients, 304, 305b
  changes, 15
  compensation strategies, 15
  deficit, 88b
  sensory control, 17
Visit encounter, 470
Visual agnosia, 88b, 120t
Visual analog scale (VAS), 34
Visual feedback, 112
Visual signals, 12
Visual spatial neglect (unilateral neglect), 96
Visual system, balance and, 101
Vital capacity (IRV + TV + ERV), 193
Vital signs
  burns, 285
  cancer treatment, 241
  immune system examination, 229
  internal bleeding, 382
  neuromuscular examination, 122, 127, 135, 195
  pulmonary examination, 195
  renal failure, 256
  tilt table, 382
Voltage, 384t
Voluntary movement patterns, 99–100
  abnormal synergies, 99, 99t
  basal ganglia dysfunction signs and tests, 99, 100t
  cerebellar dysfunction signs and tests, 99, 99t
  testing guidelines, 100
  tests, 100
Voluntary movement patterns in TBI, 123
Vomiting, 156, 156t, 244

Walkers, 403
Walking test, 102t
Wallenberg's Syndrome, 120t
Wallerian degeneration, 133
Warfarin, 315t
Warm-up period, 8, 9
Weak pulse, 152b
Weather conditions, exercising in, 9
Wedge resection, 212
Weight bearing at tolerated (WBAT), 25t, 70t, 71t

Weight shifts (postural sway), 15
Wells Criteria Score for DVT, 164, 165t
Wernicke's aphasia, 88b, 120t, 121
Wernicke's area, 87f, 89t, 121
Wheelchairs, 421–24
  components, 421–23
  wheelchair measurements, 423–24
  wheelchair training, 424
Wheezing, 149, 159t, 201t
Whirlpool, 369–70
White blood cells (WBC, leukocytes), 155t, 197, 236t, 325
White matter, 87, 90
Wobble board, 15
Wolf's law, 25t, 27
Wound assessment, 289–90
Wound care, 290–95
Wrist and hand
  capsular patterns, 30t
  conditions of, 54–56
    ape hand deformity, 56, 56f
    Boutonnière deformity, 55, 55f
    Boxer's fracture, 56
    carpal tunnel syndrome (repetitive stress syndrome), 54
    Colles' fracture, 54
    de Quervain's tenosynovitis, 54
    Dupuytren's contracture, 55, 55f
    gamekeeper's thumb, 56
    mallet finger, 56, 56f
    scaphoid fracture, 54
    Smith's fracture, 54
    swan neck deformity, 55–56, 55f
    tendon injuries and repairs of the hand, 69–70
  in convex-concave rule, 29t
  joint positions, 30t
  patterns of spasticity in upper motor neuron syndrome, 92t
  tests for, 35t

Xeroderma, 281t
Xiphoid process, 191
X-ray (plain film radiography), 36, 154t

Yergason test, 35t

Zone of infarction, 158
Zone of injury, 158
Zone of ischemia, 158